PATHO PHYSIOLOGY

Adaptations and Alterations in Function

Karla Wise
Class of '87
FJC

PATHO

PHYSIOLOGY

Adaptations and Alterations in Function

Barbara L. Bullock, R.N., M.S.N.
Assistant Professor,
Ida V. Moffett School of Nursing,
Samford University,
Birmingham, Alabama

Pearl Philbrook Rosendahl, R.N., Ed.D.
Associate Professor,
Boston University School of Nursing;
University Hospital,
Boston

Little, Brown and Company
Boston/Toronto

To our husbands and children without whom it never could have materialized

To Pete, Sheila, Brian, and Doug, with my love and appreciation B. L. B.

To Winston, Sonya, Rana, Jinja, and my mother P. P. R.

First Edition

Library of Congress Catalog Card No. 83-81577

ISBN 0-316-11479-0

Printed in the United States of America

DON

CONTENTS

CONTRIBUTING AUTHORS

Gaylene Altman, R.N., M.S.
Assistant Professor,
University of Washington School of Nursing,
Seattle

Gloria Anderson, R.N., M.S.N.
Associate Professor of Nursing,
University of Alabama School of Nursing-Huntsville,
Huntsville

Joseph L. Andrews, Jr., M.D.
Clinical Assistant Professor,
Harvard Medical School, Boston;
Senior Staff, Respiratory Section,
Lahey Clinic Medical Center,
Burlington, Massachusetts

Pamela Appleton, R.N., M.N.
Assistant Professor of Nursing,
University of Alabama School of Nursing-Huntsville,
Huntsville

Sue H. Baldwin, Ed.D.
Associate Professor of Nursing,
University of North Alabama School of Nursing,
Florence

Anne Roome Bavier, M.N.
Associate Professor,
Medical-Surgical Nursing Program,
Yale University School of Nursing,
New Haven

Joan P. Bufalino, R.N., M.S.N.
Clinical Nurse Specialist,
Department of Surgery,
Loyola University Medical Center,
Maywood, Illinois

Barbara L. Bullock, R.N., M.S.N.
Assistant Professor,
Ida V. Moffett School of Nursing,
Samford University,
Birmingham, Alabama

Concepcion Y. Castro, R.N., M.S.
Associate Professor, College of Nursing,
University of Rhode Island;
Project Director,
Primary Health Care–Family Nurse Practitioner Program,
College of Nursing,
University of Rhode Island,
Kingston

Jules Constant, M.D.
Clinical Associate Professor of Medicine,
Department of Medicine,
State University of New York at Buffalo School of Medicine;
Attending Physician,
Buffalo General Hospital,
Buffalo

Virginia Earles, D.S.N.
Professor of Nursing,
Russell Sage College,
Troy, New York

Ann Estes Edgil, R.N., D.S.N.
Associate Professor,
University of Alabama School of Nursing,
Birmingham

Thomas Mark Fender, B.S.N.
Orthopedic Specialist,
Orthopedic Associates,
Huntsville, Alabama

Shirley Freeburn, R.N., G.N.P., M.S.
Assistant Professor, School of Nursing,
The University of Colorado Health Sciences Center,
Denver

Janet L. Gelein, R.N., M.S.N., G.N.P.
Doctoral Candidate,
University of Rochester School of Nursing,
Rochester, New York

Doris J. Heaman, M.S.N.
Assistant Professor,
University of Alabama School of Nursing-Huntsville,
Huntsville

Reet Henze, R.N., M.S.N.
Associate Professor,
University of Alabama School of Nursing-Huntsville,
Huntsville

Joan T. Hurlock, R.N.C., F.N.P., Ed.D.
Associate Professor of Nursing,
University of Northern Colorado,
Greeley

Karen E. Jones, R.N., M.N.
Adjunct Assistant Professor,
University of Alabama School of Nursing-Huntsville;
Director of Nursing,
Ambulatory Care Center of the
School of Primary Medical Care,
University of Alabama School of Nursing-Huntsville,
Huntsville

June H. Larrabee, R.N., M.S.
Assistant Professor of Nursing,
University of Central Florida,
Orlando

Carla A. Bouska Lee, R.N., Ed.S., F.A.A.N.
Assistant Professor and Chairperson,
Nurse Clinician Department,
College of Health Related Professions,
Wichita State University,
Wichita, Kansas

John A. R. Marino, M.D.
Chief, Division of Diabetes,
Niagara Falls Memorial Medical Center,
Niagara Falls, New York

Gretchen S. McDaniel, R.N., M.S.N.
Assistant Professor,
Ida V. Moffett School of Nursing,
Samford University,
Birmingham, Alabama

M. S. Megahed, M.D., F.R.C.P.
Associate Clinical Professor,
School of Nursing,
State University of New York,
Buffalo

Frances Donovan Monahan, R.N., Ph.D.
Chair, Department of Nursing,
Rockland Community College,
Suffern, New York

Jennie L. Moore, R.N., M.P.H.
Formerly, Instructor in Nursing,
University of Alabama School of Nursing-Huntsville,
Huntsville

Emilie Musci, R.N., M.S.N.
Assistant Professor,
Department of Nursing,
San Jose State University,
San Jose

Betty Norris, R.N., M.S.N.
Cardiovascular Nurse Specialist,
University of Alabama,
Baptist Medical Center,
Birmingham

Leah F. Oakley, R.N., M.S.N.
Clinical Nurse Specialist in Adult Health,
Internal Medicine,
Decatur, Alabama

Donna Rogers Packa, R.N., M.S.N.
Assistant Professor,
School of Nursing,
University of Alabama,
Birmingham

Marilyn Nelsen Pase, R.N., M.S.N.
Assistant Professor,
University of Alabama School of Nursing-Huntsville,
Huntsville

Helen F. Ptak, R.N., Ph.D.
Associate Dean and Professor, School of Nursing,
University of Texas Medical Branch;
Director, Nursing Research and Evaluation,
University of Texas Medical Branch Hospitals,
Galveston

Cammie M. Quinn, R.N., M.S.N.
Department of Neurosurgery,
University of Alabama Hospitals,
Birmingham

Pearl Philbrook Rosendahl, R.N., Ed.D.
Associate Professor,
Boston University School of Nursing;
University Hospital,
Boston

Sharon P. Schlosser, R.N., M.S.N.
Assistant Professor, Parent Child Health Nursing,
Ida V. Moffett School of Nursing,
Samford University;
Staff Nurse, Department of Obstetrics and Gynecology,
Baptist Medical Center, Birmingham,
Alabama

Therese B. Shipps, R.N., M.S.
Adjunct Assistant Professor,
Boston University, Boston;
Nursing Studies Coordinator,
Mount Auburn Hospital,
Cambridge, Massachusetts

Eileen Ledden Sjoberg, R.N., M.S.
Assistant Professor,
Fitchburg State College,
Fitchburg, Massachusetts

Carol A. Stephenson, R.N., Ed.D.
Assistant Professor,
Harris College of Nursing,
Texas Christian University,
Fort Worth

Camille P. Stern, R.N., M.S.N.
Instructor, Ida V. Moffett School of Nursing,
Samford University,
Birmingham, Alabama

Metta Fay Street, M.S.
Assistant Professor and Community Health Coordinator,
Ida V. Moffett School of Nursing,
Samford University;
Consultant, Bureau of Nursing,
Jefferson County Department of Public Health,
Birmingham, Alabama

Joan M. Vitello, R.N., M.S.N., C.C.R.N.
Graduate Student, University of Alabama,
Birmingham

Linda Hudson Williams, M.S.
Assistant Professor,
University of Alabama School of Nursing-Huntsville,
Huntsville

Joan W. Williamson, R.N., M.S.N.
Associate Professor,
University of Alabama School of Nursing-Huntsville,
Huntsville

PREFACE

Pathophysiology can be defined as the study of the physiologic changes that result from different pathologic processes. The study of pathophysiology can expand a previously learned base of knowledge in the sciences, especially anatomy, physiology, and chemistry. This study helps the student understand how alterations in structure and function can disrupt the human body as a whole. Inherent in the study is an increased understanding of the adaptive powers utilized by the human body to maintain the steady state.

All alterations cause a disruption of normal basic cellular processes that ultimately lead to tissue or organ alterations. Alterations placed on the human body are adjusted and changed by the adaptive and compensatory mechanisms also at the cellular level. For this reason, cellular processes are discussed in depth and alterations to these processes are described throughout the book. The concept of feedback and information sharing within the body is detailed. This concept is related to the open systems theory discussed in Chapter 3. In health, the body functions in a negative feedback pattern that allows the return of the normal or steady state. In some pathologic processes a positive feedback pattern is established, which, if unchecked, will result in death.

This book was written to help the baccalaureate level student in any health care discipline. Higher level students may also find the book useful due to the extensive coverage of pathologic processes and complex concepts. Some emphasis on physical and laboratory findings is found in appropriate sections; treatment aspects for diseases are not included for the most part unless it is supportive to understanding of the process.

The book is organized into 3 sections, 17 units, and 53 chapters. The first section provides a basis for subsequent chapters — covering cellular dynamics, stress effects, and fluid and electrolyte balance. Section II covers bodily defense mechanisms and effects of alterations to defense mechanisms. Section III describes organ and system function and dysfunction and relates the alterations described in other chapters to the aging population.

Learning objectives placed at the beginning of each chapter provide a framework for study. The student is encouraged to use these objectives as a study guide. Each chapter is referenced for the assistance of those wishing to pursue specific topics in greater depth; a bibliography is provided at the end of each unit.

The authors acknowledge with enduring appreciation the support and guidance provided by many talented persons at Little, Brown, specifically,

Ann West, Nursing Developmental Editor, for sticking with us from start to finish, offering many helpful suggestions, and doing much of the footwork in putting the manuscript finally together.

Susan Pioli, Medical Book Editor, for excellent assistance and guidance throughout the publication process.

Julie Stillman, former Nursing Editor, for helping us to get started and for handling so much of the detail work.

The outstanding art program in this book is the work of the Boston University Educational Media Support Center at Boston University. We would like to thank especially JoEllen Murphy, Biomedical Illustrator, and Marcia Williams and Mark Lefkowitz, Medical Illustrators.

We are indebted to our contributors, whose commitment to this project shows, we believe, in every chapter of the book.

We are also grateful to Penny Shook who typed and retyped manuscript and helped us to meet deadlines. She endured so cheerfully our changes and revisions from start to final completion of the manuscript. Becky Vaughan and Eloise Rasberry also assisted with manuscript typing, and their help is appreciated.

Our reviewers, through their critical analyses, helped us to clarify and complete this manuscript. Through their careful scrutiny, logical decisions were made about what aspects should be included to make this book appropriate for the intended level. They provided an invaluable service. We thank the following: Gloria Grissett of The University of Alabama-Huntsville; Harry Peery, Tompkins Cortland Community College, Dryden, New York; Richard Pflanzer, Indiana University/Purdue University, Indianapolis; and Cleo Richards, Northern Illinois University, De Kalb.

The book would not have been possible without the understanding of the deans at our schools of nursing. Special appreciation goes to Dean Martha Hearn of the Ida V. Moffett School of Nursing, Samford University, and to Dean Carmen Westwick and Associate Deans Julia A. Sullivan and Margery Chisholm of Boston University.

Special thanks go to a colleague who supported the efforts and stress involved in the project: Janice Thomas, Assistant Professor, Ida V. Moffett School of Nursing, Samford University. We want to add a special note of appreciation to Helen King who worked diligently on the initial drafts of the manuscript.

B. L. B.
P. P. R.

SECTION I

INTRODUCTION TO PATHOPHYSIOLOGY

Adaptations and Alterations in Cellular Function

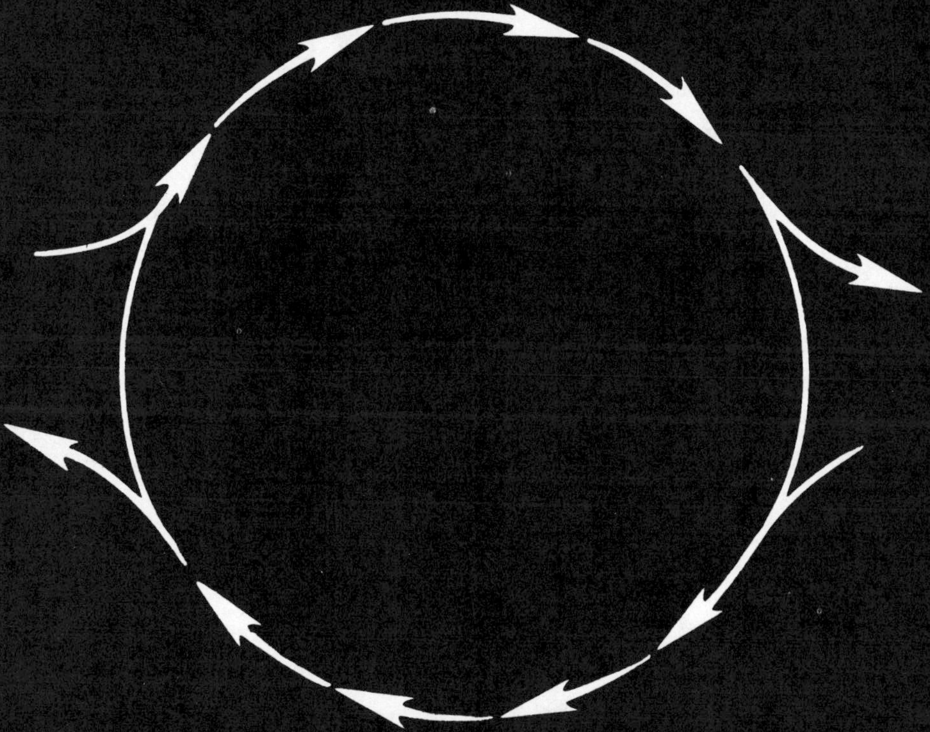

UNIT 1
CELLULAR DYNAMICS

Barbara L. Bullock

Since the cell is the basis of life, it is appropriate to begin the study of pathophysiology with a review of the normal cellular processes. Understanding of these processes is necessary for the understanding of concepts in every other unit of the text. The material presented can be found in many anatomy and physiology textbooks but is presented here as a convenient, available reference. Sources for the more detailed aspects of cellular function can be found in the bibliography at the end of Unit 1.

Chapter 1 describes normal cellular function with special emphasis on the cellular organelles and on movement of materials across the cell membrane. Chapter 2 of this unit details the alterations in cells when they are exposed to a changing, hostile environment. Cellular adaptation, injury, and death are explored in terms of their effect on body function. Mechanisms by which the steady state can be maintained even at the expense of altered intracellular metabolism are explored. Altered cellular function ending finally in lethal change is described.

The reader is encouraged to utilize the learning objectives at the beginning of each chapter as a study guide outline for essential concepts. The bibliography at the end of the unit provides general and specific resources for further study.

CHAPTER 1
NORMAL CELLULAR PROCESSES

LEARNING OBJECTIVES

1. Describe the differences in cell structure between the four major types of cells in the human body.
2. Define the purposes of the three types of epithelial cells.
3. Differentiate between skeletal, cardiac, and smooth muscle on the basis of histologic appearance.
4. Briefly describe the components of the neuron.
5. List the major types of connective tissue cells.
6. Identify the structure and function of each type of connective tissue.
7. Explain briefly the negative feedback pattern seen with the reproduction of cells of the body.
8. Classify cells according to their ability to regenerate.
9. Briefly describe the process of mitosis.
10. Define *organelle.*
11. Differentiate between intracellular and extracellular electrolyte composition.
12. Describe, in detail, the structure and function of the following organelles: cell membrane, mitochondria, ribosomes, endoplasmic reticulum, Golgi apparatus, lysosomes, microtubules, centrioles, nucleus, and nucleolus.
13. Explain the major ways by which adenosine triphosphate (ATP) is formed.
14. Describe the process of protein synthesis from DNA-RNA transcription to manufacture of proteins.
15. Compare the function of the smooth endoplasmic reticulum with the rough endoplasmic reticulum.
16. Explain the mechanisms of transport across the cell membrane.
17. Identify the process of facilitated passive transport including the mechanism and what facilitates it.
18. Clearly explain the purpose of the sodium pump.
19. Differentiate between pinocytosis and phagocytosis.
20. Describe the purpose of exocytosis.
21. Draw a cell exhibiting ameboid motion.
22. Describe the process of muscle contraction.
23. Compare smooth, cardiac, and skeletal muscle contraction.
24. Briefly explain the electrical properties of cells including depolarization and repolarization.
25. Define the *absolute refractory* and *relative refractory periods*.

An understanding of the structure and function of the cell is essential to the study of pathophysiology. This chapter reviews the important and relevant aspects of cellular function to assist the student in understanding alterations of cellular processes.

Cells are the units of tissues, organs, and finally, systems of the human body (Fig. 1-1). The human body contains over 75 trillion cells, each of which performs specific functions that are determined by genetic differentiation and are controlled by a highly specific information system that directs the activity of cellular organelles and inclusions.

Some cells have the major function of carrying out the activities of the organ and as such are called *parenchymal cells.* This means that the parenchyma of an organ actually does its function. Some examples of parenchymal cells include hepatocytes, neurons, gastric parietal cells, osteocytes, and myocardial cells. Other cells make it possible for the parenchymal cells to effect their function by providing the supporting structure or the architectural framework to hold the organ in place. Examples include neuroglia, gastric capillary endothelial cells, and cardiac connective tissue cells.

Although cells have different functions, they are alike in many ways. The similarities include how nutrients are used, what type of nutrients are needed, how oxygen is utilized, and the disposition of excretory products.

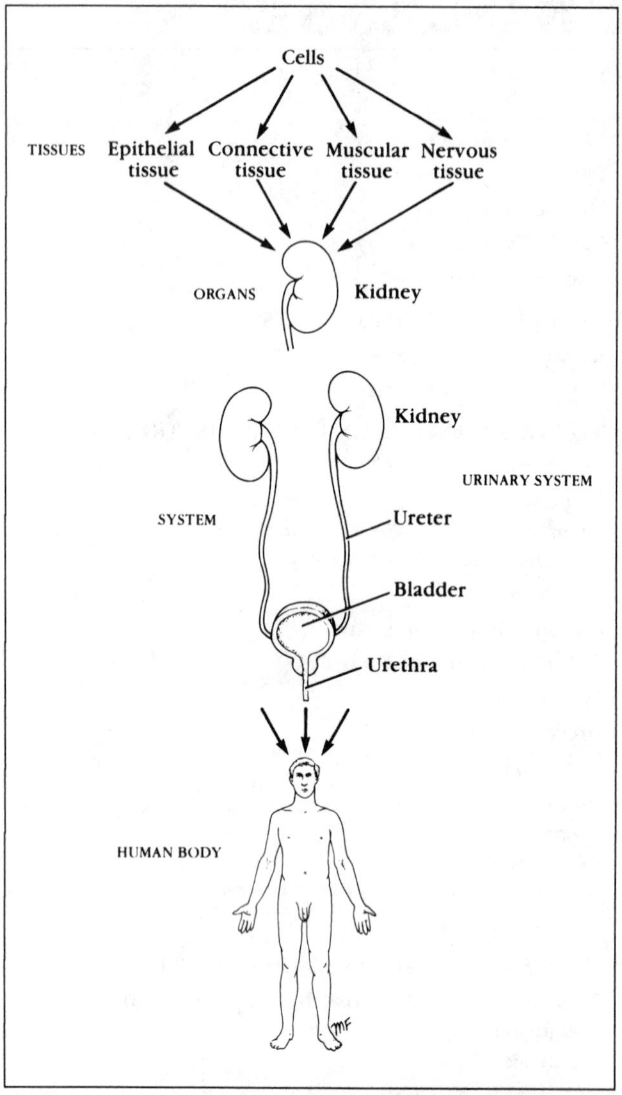

FIGURE 1-1. Structural subunits of the body: cells, tissues, organs, and systems. (From R. S. Snell, *Clinical Histology for Medical Students.* Boston: Little, Brown, 1984.)

TYPES OF TISSUES

Basically, the human body is composed of four types of tissues: epithelial, muscle, nerve, and connective. Each type is subdivided into subgroups of different types of cells. The broad subgroups are discussed in this section. The reader is referred to the bibliography for further information.

Epithelial Tissues

Epithelial tissues occur as coverings of most of the internal and external surfaces of the body. In this way, they may function as protective barriers or they may be involved with absorption of materials, excretion of waste products, and secretion of specialized products into the cavities.

Epithelial tissue is classified according to its thickness in number of layers. *Simple squamous epithelium* exists as single layers of flattened, pancakelike cells. *Simple cuboidal epithelial cells* assume the appearance of cubes. *Simple columnar epithelial cells* have the appearance of columns (Fig. 1-2).

Squamous epithelial cells may be found in single or multiple layers. Single layers allow for diffusion of material across the cell wall while multiple layers provide for continuous replenishment or regeneration of cells. Simple squamous cells line the heart and blood vessels, form the alveoli, and exist in many other areas.

Cuboidal epithelial cells are usually found in single layers and frequently function in forming secretions. These cells line the ducts and are the parenchymal cells of many glands.

The *columnar epithelial cells,* in various forms, line the walls of the gastrointestinal and respiratory systems and are involved with the secretion of mucus. They may exist as goblet cells or with projections, called microvilli or cilia, present on their surfaces (Fig. 1-3).

Stratified squamous epithelium exists in multiple layers functioning to replenish superficial layers as they are sloughed off. The skin is an excellent example of stratified squamous epithelium, but this tissue is also found lining the mouth, esophagus, vagina, and pharynx.

Transitional epithelial cells are usually considered to be cuboidal except that the appearance of the cells varies depending on the stretch of the organ. These cells, then, at different times, appear to be flattened, or spherical. They are best exemplified by the epithelial cells in the bladder.

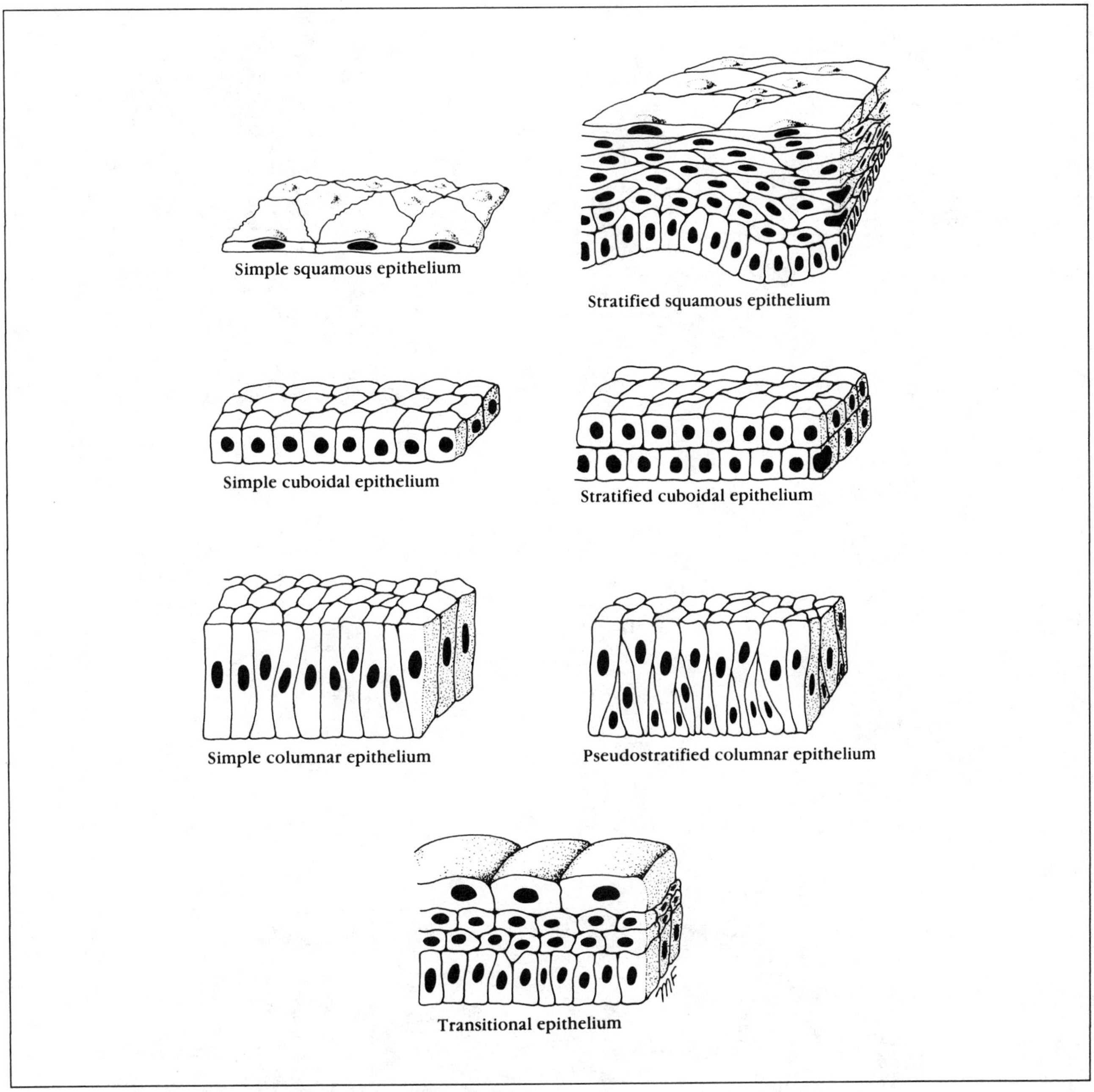

FIGURE 1-2. Different types of epithelium. (From R. S. Snell, *Clinical Histology for Medical Students.* Boston: Little, Brown, 1984.)

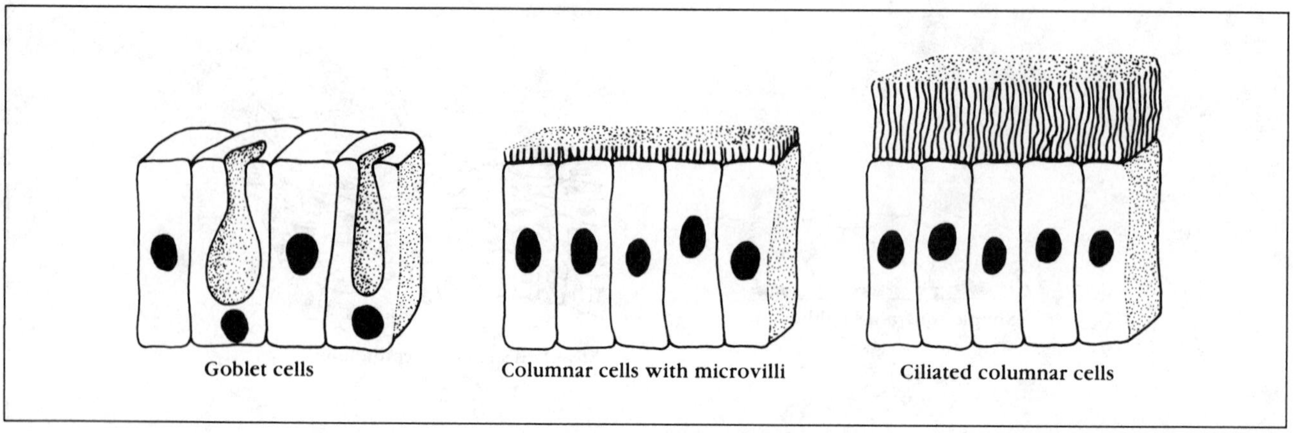

FIGURE 1-3. Specialized columnar cells. (From R. S. Snell, *Clinical Histology for Medical Students.* Boston: Little, Brown, 1984.)

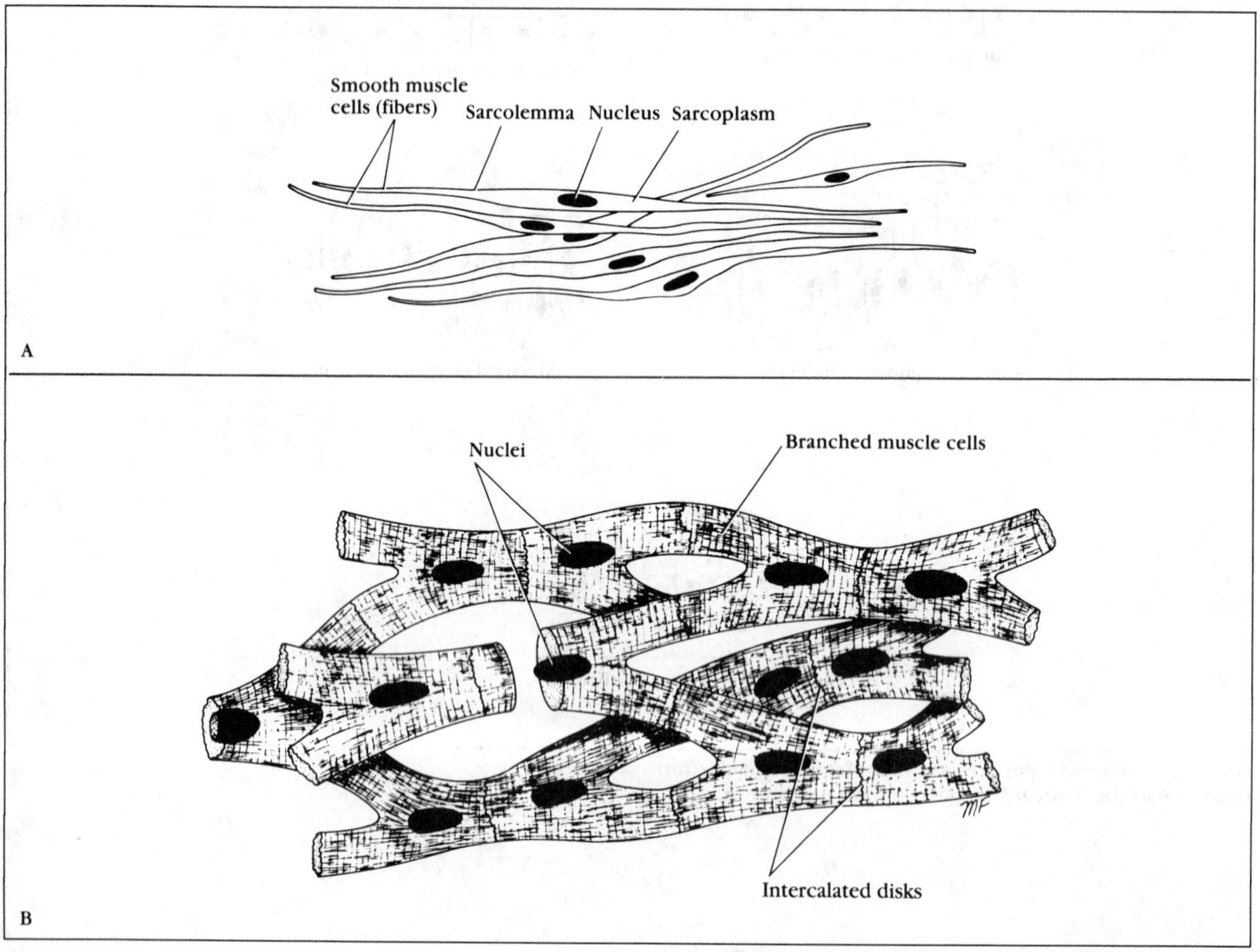

FIGURE 1-4. A. Group of smooth muscle cells (fibers). B. Group of branched cardiac muscle cells (fibers). (From R. S. Snell, *Clinical Histology for Medical Students.* Boston: Little, Brown, 1984.)

Muscle Tissues

The microstructure and functions of the muscle cells that make up muscle tissues are discussed in depth in Unit 13. In general, muscles are classified as *skeletal, cardiac,* and *visceral* muscles according to their appearance and function (Fig. 1-4).

Striated skeletal muscle provides for voluntary movement of the body. The characteristic striated appearance results from an ordered sequence of contractile proteins. These proteins form or constitute numerous *myofibrils,* the contractile units of the muscle cell. Skeletal muscle cells are multinucleate with the nuclei located at the periphery of the cell under the cell membrane.

Cardiac muscle forms the walls of the heart, which are the working, or contractile, portions of this organ. Its appearance is similar to that of striated skeletal muscle except that a nucleus is centrally located and the myocardial cells lie very closely approximated one with another. The importance of myocardial construction in relation to cardiac contraction is detailed in Unit 8.

Visceral, or *smooth, muscle* does not exhibit the characteristic striations of skeletal or cardiac muscle, but smooth muscle cells have many fibrils that extend the length of the cell. A single nucleus lies near the center of each cell. Smooth muscle cells are located in the viscera, the blood vessels, the uterus, and many other areas.

Nerve Tissues

Nerve tissue is made up of nerve cells called neurons (Fig. 1-5). The typical nerve cell has a large central nucleus, multiple dendrites, and a single axon. Detailed function of the neuron is described in Chapter 42.

Connective Tissues

Connective tissue is generally that tissue that forms the framework for other cells and helps to bind various tissues and organs together. Many types of cells are included in the classification of tissue (Fig. 1-6). The major groups are described in the following section. Blood cells, described in detail in Unit 7, are classified as *specialized connective tissue cells.*

Loose connective tissue (areolar tissue) contains numerous cells, especially fibroblasts and macrophages. It also functions to attach the skin to the body and help to hold the organs and blood vessels in place. Spaces between cells allow for fluid storage and discharge of cellular products, which are then returned to the bloodstream.

Dense irregular connective tissue is compact and forms the reticular layer of the dermis of the skin. Sheets of this tissue comprise sheaths of many types and can withstand stretching in the direction in which their fibers run [4]. The layers of the dermis are composed of cells with fibers and ground substance that constantly undergo synthesis and degradation. Collagen fibers interlace with each other to provide strength to the dermis. Elastic fibers lie randomly dispersed throughout this layer, which allows for flexibility.

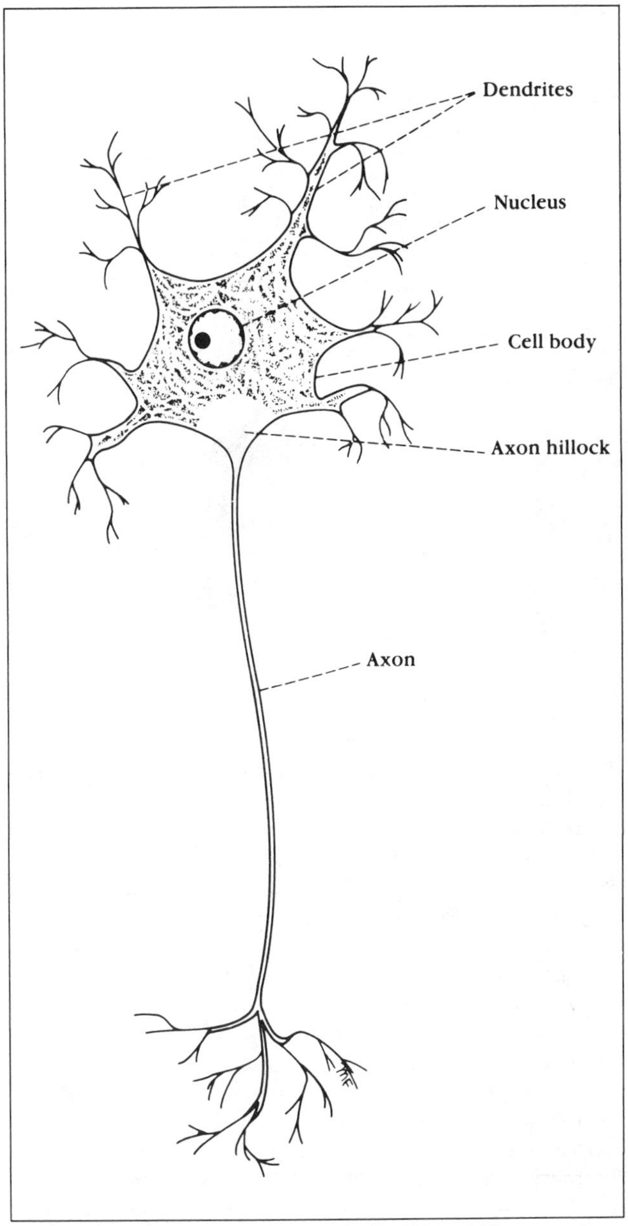

FIGURE 1-5. A neuron. (From R. S. Snell, *Clinical Neuroanatomy for Medical Students.* Boston: Little, Brown, 1980.)

Dense regular connective tissue is composed of white fibrous material. The cells are mainly fibrocytes, located in a regular or ordered plane [4]. Rows of fibrocytes with large amounts of intracellular substance, especially collagen, form the *tendons* that attach muscle to bone. *Ligaments* that attach bone to bone and *fascia* that provide the coverings for muscles are included in this category of connective tissue. The *aponeuroses,* which are similar to tendons with a wider base, function to attach muscles to other structures.

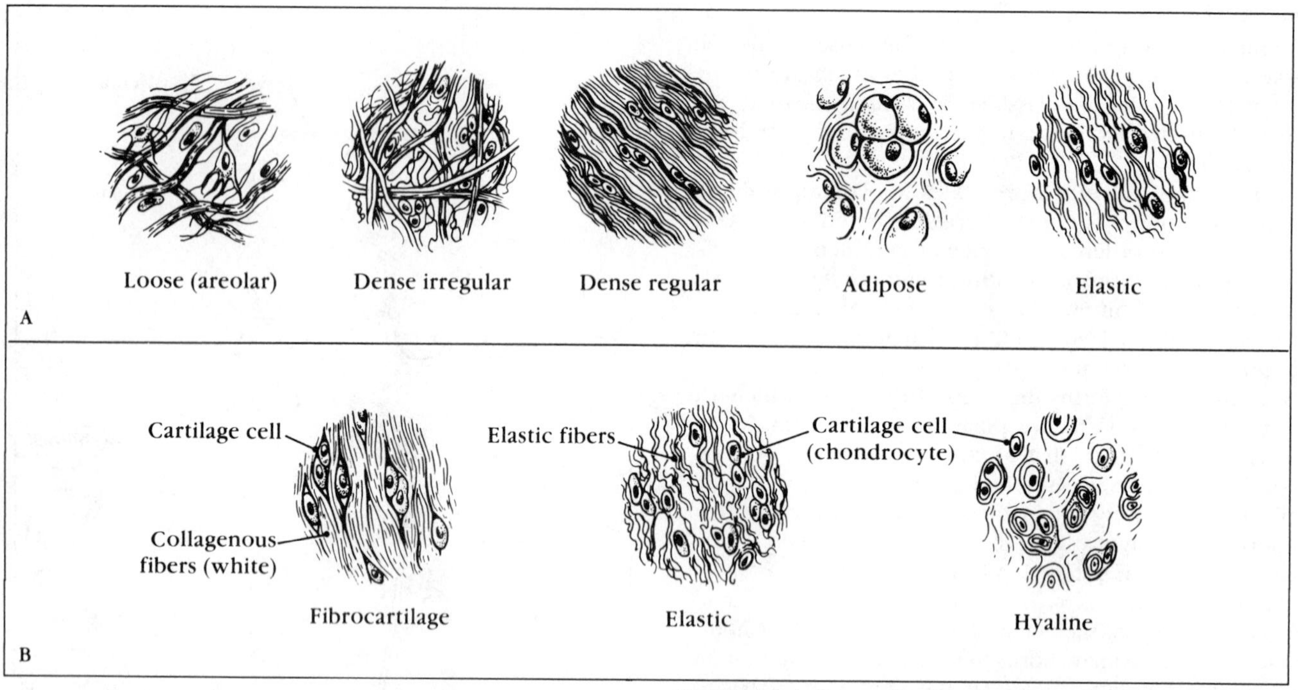

FIGURE 1-6. A. Types of connective tissues. B. Types of cartilage.

Adipose tissue cells are those whose cytoplasm is filled with lipid or fatty material. This storage area for lipids serves as a protective and insulating layer in the body. Layers of adipose are normally found around the kidney and intestine. In many areas of the body, substances not metabolized within the cell are converted to fat. This process is greatly influenced by insulin, a pancreatic hormone (see Chap. 33).

Elastic connective tissue allows for the properties of elasticity and extensibility, especially in the arteries and vocal cords. This is further discussed in Units 8 and 9.

Cartilage, a connective tissue that is made up of cells called *chondrocytes,* is of differing types, depending on the number of collagenous fibers associated with it. It functions to provide structural strength with some degree of flexibility. It is found in the costal cartilage, trachea, intervertebral disks, external ear, and other areas. In children the long bones have two ends, a diaphysis and an epiphysis, separated by epiphyseal cartilage, which allows for increasing bone length. Growth in length occurs as cartilage cells grow away from the shaft and are replaced by bone, resulting in an increased length of the shaft [1]. When maturity is reached this cartilage is replaced by bone, called *closure of the epiphysis.*

Bone, the hardest of the connective tissue, functions to provide the structural framework of the body as well as a plentiful reservoir for the minerals calcium and phosphorus. It is composed of cells, fibers, and extracellular components, which are calcified and hard. This material encloses the hematopoietic marrow, which functions to supply most of the blood cells of the body. Periosteum covers most bones and is lacking only in special areas. Bone tissue is organized in two ways, as *compact* or as *cancellous (spongy) bone* (Fig. 1-7). Compact bone forms a solid mass and has few spaces in its continuity. Cancellous bone forms a network of intercommunicating projections called *trabeculae* [1]. Compact bone generally is located on the outer shell while spongy bone usually assists in the internal framework. The principal cells of adult bone are called *osteocytes,* which with the other bone cells—osteoblasts, osteoclasts, and osteoprogenitor cells—form and repair the bone tissue. All of these distinct cells may be different functional states of the same cell type [1]. Bone cells adjust their number in proportion to the amount of physical stress placed on them. For example, increased deposition of collagen fibers and inorganic salts occurs in response to prolonged increase in workloads. Conversely, salts are pulled from bone when stress or weight bearing is decreased (see Chap. 39).

REPRODUCTIVE ABILITY OF CELLS

Most cells have the ability to reproduce themselves. This involves the complex process of *mitosis.* In the normal adult, the new cells take the place of old cells in a rigidly defined order that maintains cellular numbers but allows only for the replacement of the needed cells. The turnover rate is billions of cells per day in the normal individual, but rigid controls inherently limit the number of cells to be reproduced.

Specific controls on the reproductive process of cells function to produce precisely the correct quantity of cells. For example, if the red blood cell count decreases, erythropoietic stimulating factors cause the bone marrow to increase production of erythrocytes, leading ultimately

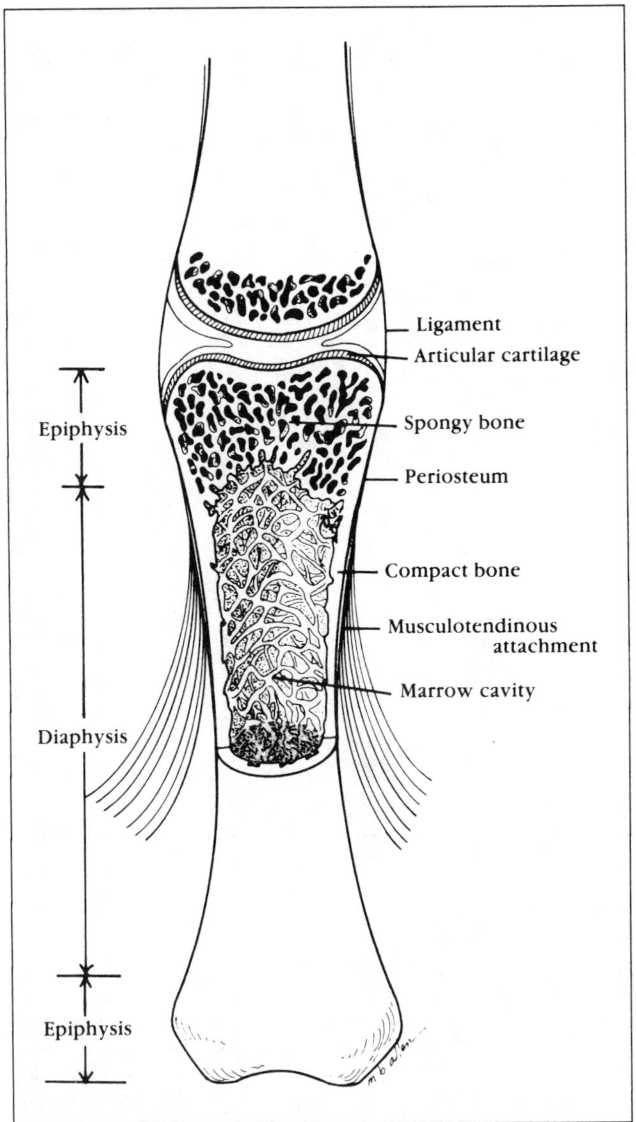

FIGURE 1-7. Vertical section through the proximal part of the femur showing the arrangement of the compact and spongy (cancellous) bone. (From M. Borysenko, et al., *Functional Histology* [2nd ed.]. Boston: Little, Brown, 1984.)

to increased numbers of circulating red blood cells (see Chap. 14). Another stage in the process of erythropoiesis occurs when the appropriate level of red blood cells is reached. Some factor, either diminished stimulation or an inhibitor, suppresses further production of red cells.

Regeneration of Cells

As stated earlier, almost all cells have the ability to reproduce themselves. This ability is called the *regenerative capacity* of cells. Cells that regenerate frequently and have a very short life span are called *labile cells* with a usual life span measured in hours or days. Some examples of labile cells include white blood cells and epithelial cells. Other cells retain the ability to regenerate or reproduce, but do so only under special circumstances. These are called the *stable cells* and their life span is measured in years or, sometimes through the entire life span of an organism. Some examples of stable cells are the osteocytes of the bone, the parenchymal cells of the liver, and the cells of the glands of the body. In the normal liver cell, for example, mitotic figures are rare, but following injury mitoses are abundant because the liver has a remarkable ability for self-repair. The third type of cells, the *permanent cells,* live for the entire life of the organism. This type includes the nerve cell bodies and probably most of the muscle cells. The neuron does not divide after birth but has the ability in certain circumstances, to regenerate its axon and dendrites (see Chap. 42). Myocardial muscle does not regenerate; when it dies it is repaired by the formation of scar tissue.

Reproduction of Cells

Reproduction, or the process of *mitosis,* begins in the nucleus and involves duplication or replication of all of the deoxyribonucleic acid (DNA) in the cell (Fig. 1-8). The stages of the cell cycle include *mitosis,* the actual growth stages, and *interphase,* the "resting" stages between mitotic division. Interphase consists of three separate phases, G1, which follows mitosis, S, and G2 (Fig. 1-9). Mitosis itself consists of four stages, *prophase, metaphase, anaphase,* and *telophase* (Fig. 1-10). The activities that occur during these phases are summarized in Table 1-1. The cytokinesis, (cytoplasmic separation) and karyokinesis (nuclear separation), result in the formation of two identical daughter cells that contain the complete complement of genetic information. In other words, all of the genetic information has been duplicated by the DNA and the new cell is a perfect image of its parent cell. The process progresses in a highly specialized manner, apparently initiated by certain specific stimulating factors. Vital aspects of mitosis are discussed in more detail in Chapter 12. The reader is also referred to the bibliography for further information.

CELLULAR ORGANELLES AND THEIR FUNCTION

The cell is composed of many different structures, which carry out its complex functions. Within the cell are highly organized physical structures called *organelles.* These structures are suspended in the fluid medium called *protoplasm.* This substance includes the *cytoplasm,* which is outside the nucleus of a cell, and the *nucleoplasm,* which is within the nucleus. The general structures of the cell are schematically diagrammed in Figure 1-11.

Protoplasm is composed mostly of water, but it also contains specific amounts of electrolytes, proteins, lipids, and carbohydrates. The intracellular electrolyte balance is closely regulated and differs from that of the extracellular fluid (Table 1-2). Proteins compose about 10 to 20 percent of the content of the protoplasm and function to help the cellular inclusions maintain structural strength and form.

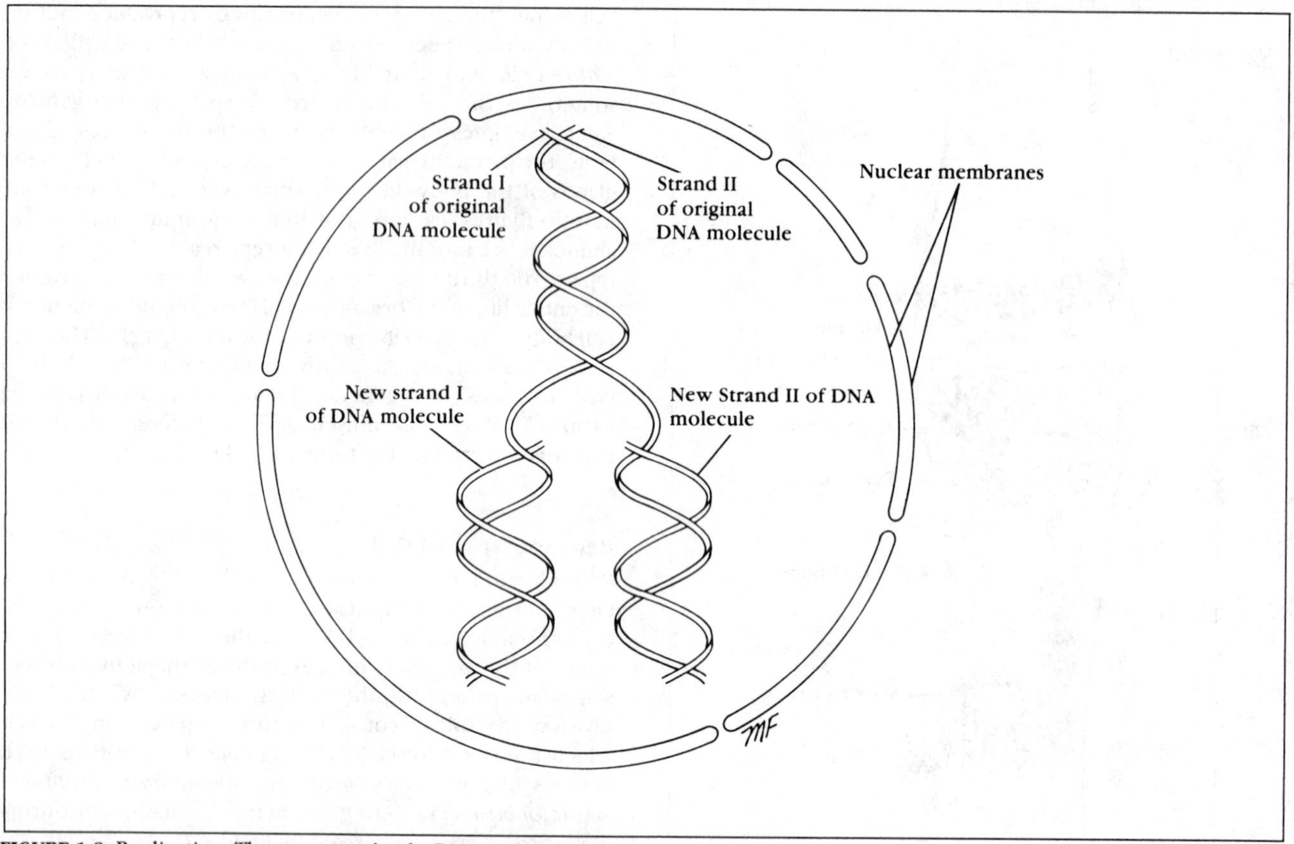

FIGURE 1-8. Replication. The two strands of a DNA molecule first separate and a new strand is synthesized alongside each of the separate strands. The result is that each newly-formed double-stranded molecule is identical to the original molecule whose strands became separated. (From R. S. Snell, *Clinical Histology for Medical Students.* Boston: Little, Brown, 1984.)

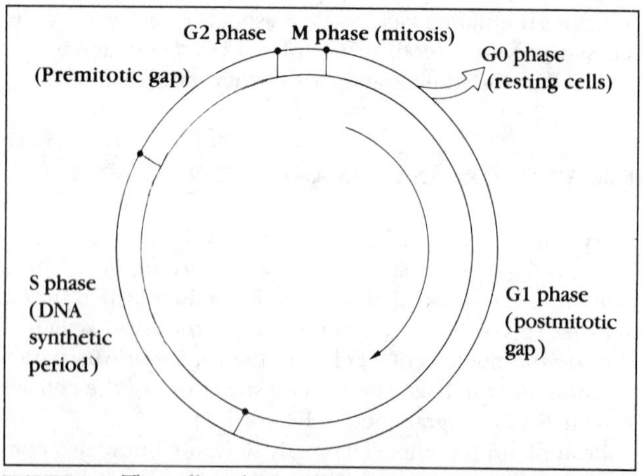

FIGURE 1-9. The cell cycle. A cell that has just completed mitosis enters the G1 phase. It may either stop cycling and enter the G0 phase or proceed to replicate its DNA in the S phase. After the entire genomic DNA has been replicated the cell is tetraploid and proceeds through the G2 phase to mitosis in the M phase. (From J. Stein [ed.], *Internal Medicine.* Boston: Little, Brown, 1983.)

TABLE 1-1. The process of cell division

Stage	Processes
Prophase	Chromosomes that doubled during the S phase become distinct. Each is composed of two strands called *chromatids.* Nucleoli disappear; centrioles duplicate and migrate to opposite poles of the nucleus. The nuclear membrane disappears.
Metaphase	The mitotic spindle is formed and chromosomes line up in preparation for migration to opposite poles of the dividing cell. The spindle is responsible for later precise separation of chromosome halves.
Anaphase	The chromosomes split with movement of chromatids to opposite poles of the spindle. The spindle elongates itself, which may be due to the contractile filaments, actin, and myosin (which are associated).
Telophase	The separated chromatids, now daughter chromosomes, uncoil; segments of the nuclear envelope reform; and karyokinesis (nuclear separation) becomes complete. The nucleoli also reform. Constriction of the cytoplasm, called a cleavage furrow occurs, bridged briefly at the midpoint by dense material, which gives way with contraction to pull the daughter cells apart. The process of cytoplasmic separation is called *cytokinesis.*

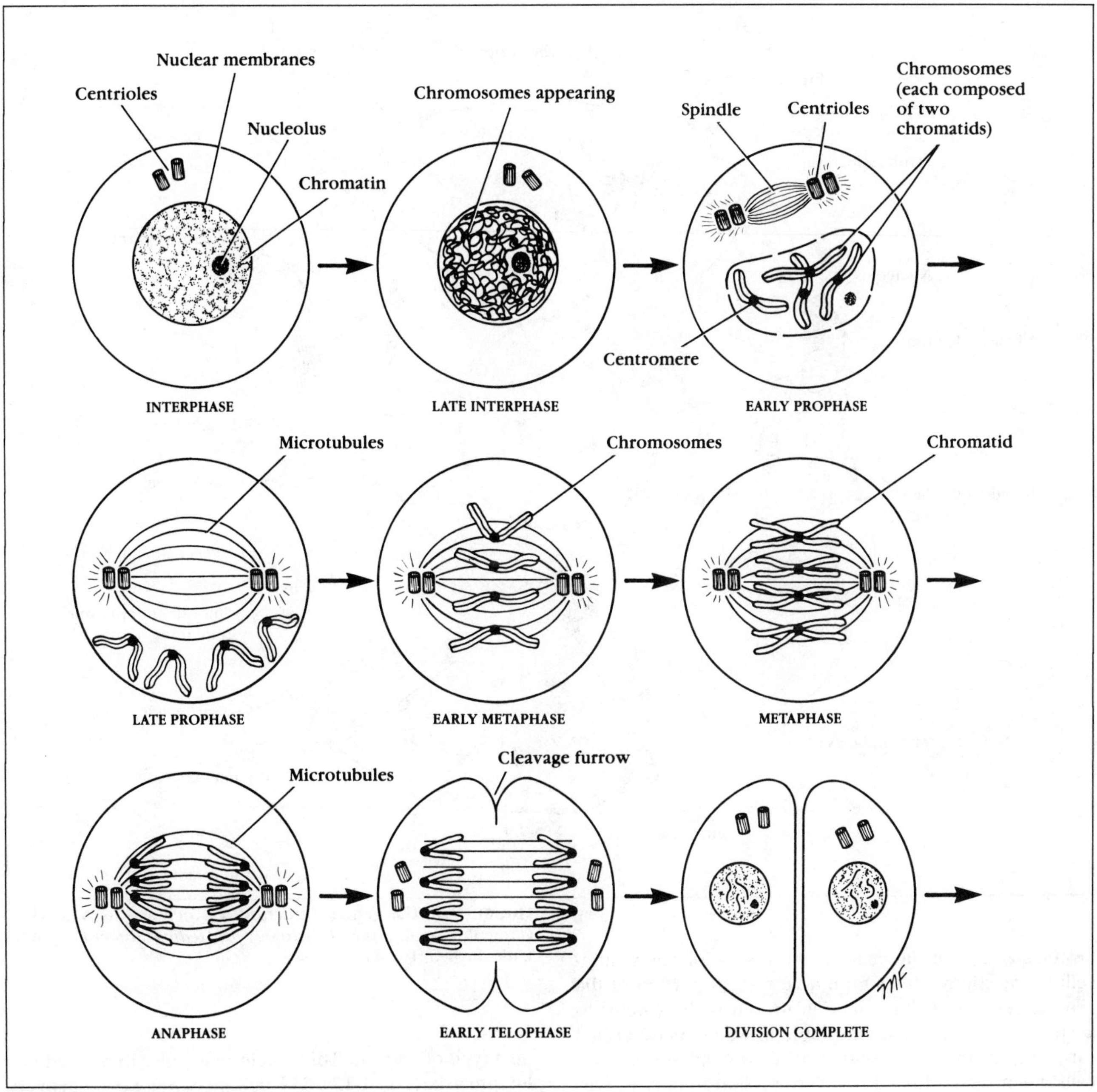

FIGURE 1-10. The main nuclear changes in mitotic division. (From R. S. Snell, *Clinical Histology for Medical Students.* Boston: Little, Brown, 1984.)

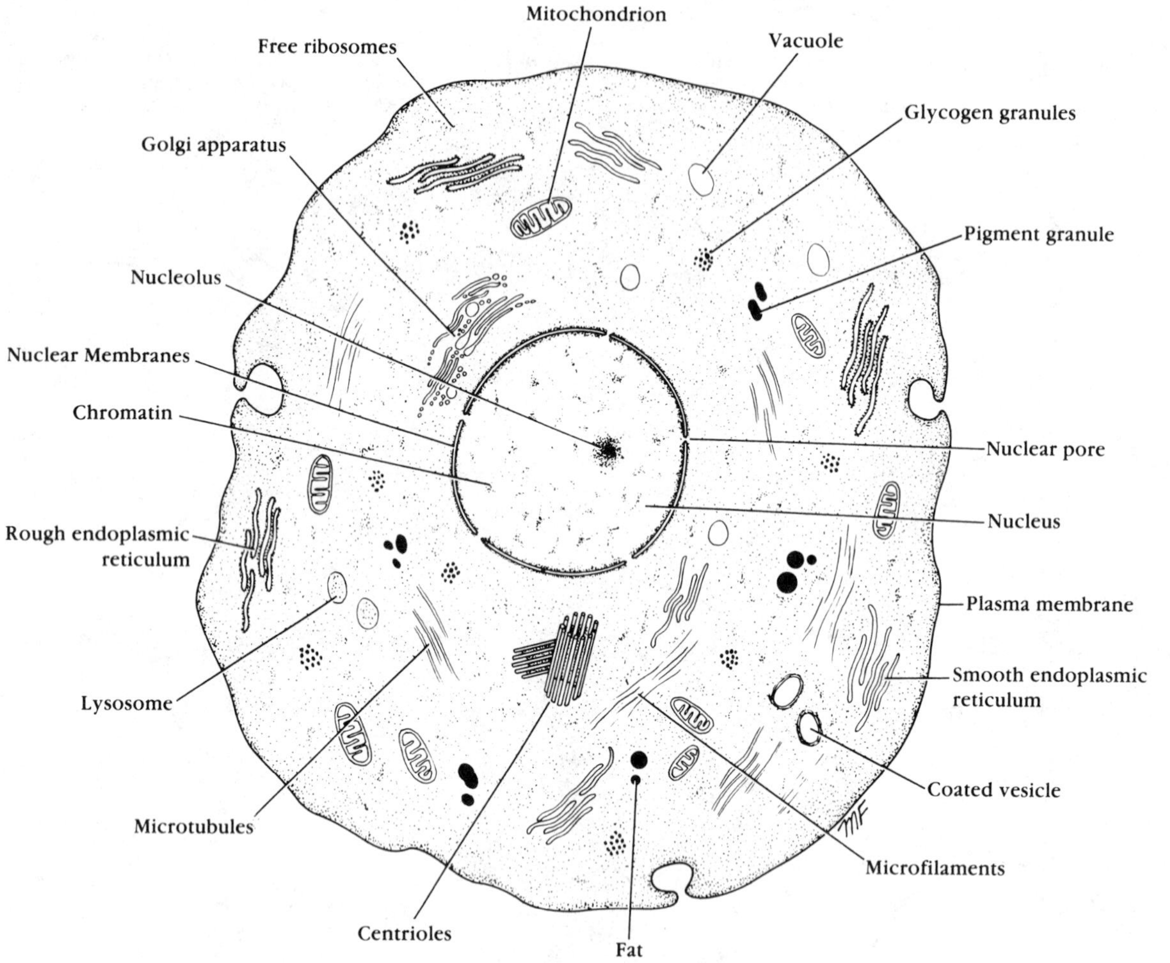

FIGURE 1-11. The general structure of a cell and its organelles. (From R. S. Snell, *Clinical Histology for Medical Students.* Boston: Little, Brown, 1984.)

Proteins also form the enzymes necessary for many intracellular reactions. Lipids form a very small portion of the general cell and mainly function to join with proteins to keep the cell membranes insoluble in water. As described earlier, lipids may be deposited in the cytoplasm of some cells when it is not needed for conversion to energy. Carbohydrates compose a very small amount of the cytoplasm and are utilized mainly in forming ATP for energy.

Cell Membrane

All cells are surrounded by a limiting membrane called the outer cell membrane. All the other organelles within the cell, with the exception of the nucleolus, are bounded by a membrane similar to the outer cell membrane. These limiting membranes, whether outer cell or organelle, consist of phospholipids, glycolipids, and neutral lipids, which are variably bound to proteins in the form of glycoproteins or lipoproteins. There are also structural proteins that make up a type of *"mosaic"* of protein molecules imbedded in a lipid matrix (Fig. 1-12). The cell membrane contains very small pores that allow for the passage of very small molecules across it.

The proteins and glycoproteins act as structural elements. Protein enzymes act as reactors in the transport system of molecules. Other proteins act as *"pumps"* for active transport of materials and as *receptor sites* for hormones and other substances.

The structure of the cell membrane allows for the selective movement of substances into and out of the cell. A normal and intact cell membrane is essential in the usual process of active transport, which establishes the proper electrochemical environment intracellularly and, ultimately, extracellularly. This process is further described

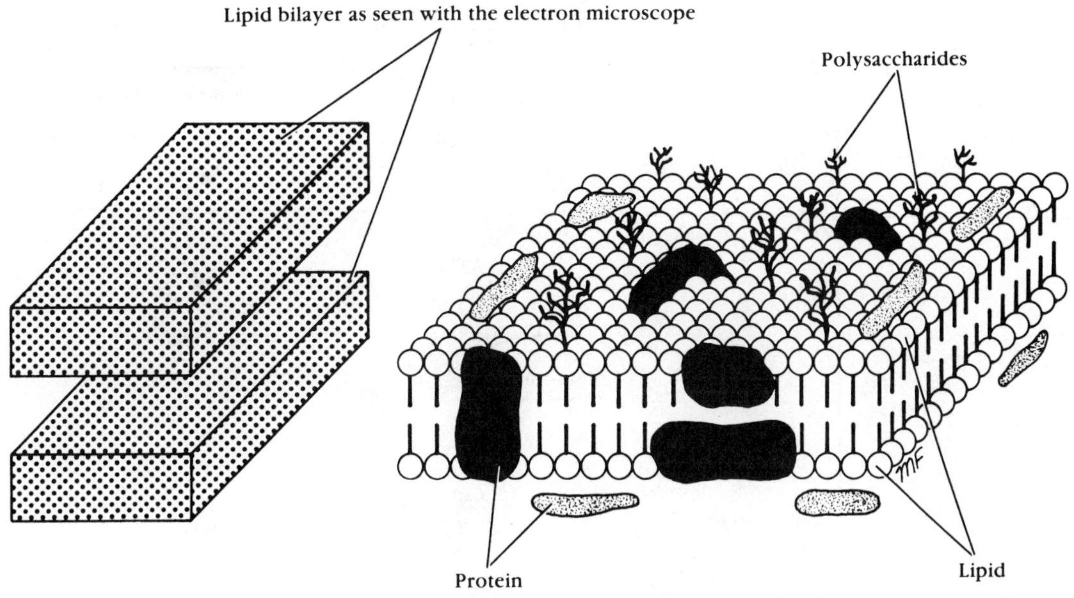

FIGURE 1-12. The probable structure of a cell membrane. (From R. S. Snell, *Clinical Histology for Medical Students.* Boston: Little, Brown, 1984.)

in the section on movement across the cell membrane (pp. 22–27).

Mitochondria

These organelles are the powerhouse, or workhorses, of the cell (Fig. 1-13). Most of the adenosine triphosphate (ATP) needed for energy to carry out cellular processes is manufactured here. The number of mitochondria within a cell varies from 0 to 1500 according to the metabolic activity of the cells [6].

Mitochondria are able to regenerate themselves under conditions of increased energy need. They contain a special type of DNA that resembles bacterial DNA rather than cellular DNA [2].

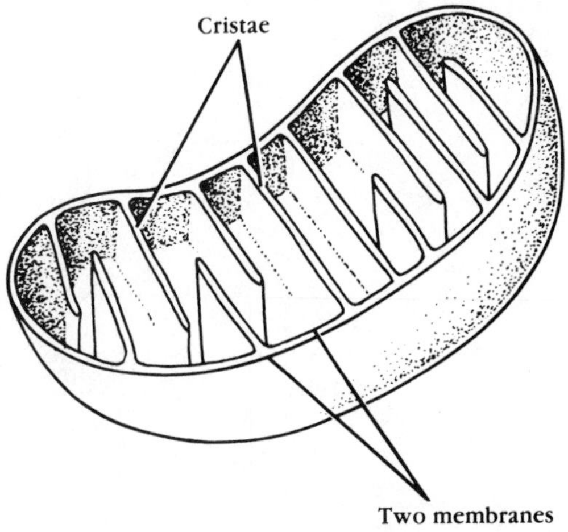

FIGURE 1-13. Schematic representation of a mitochondrion. (From R. S. Snell, *Clinical Histology for Medical Students.* Boston: Little, Brown, 1984.)

Formation of ATP with Oxygen

The process used by the mitochondria to form ATP is called *oxidative phosphorylation.* It requires simple forms of carbohydrates, proteins, and fats. These substances enter the mitochondria and utilizing oxidative enzymes, form ATP through the citric acid or Krebs cycle (Fig. 1-14). High-energy phosphate radicals are formed that later release their energy when the ATP is catabolized or reduced to adenosine diphosphate (ADP). The ADP can, through reentering the mitochondria, receive another phosphate radical and form ATP anew. The process of catabolizing ATP to ADP results in energy release. Adding the phosphate radical to the ADP is called *rephosphorylation.*

The *major* source of acetyl coenzyme A, the common intermediary in carbohydrate, protein, and fat metabolism, is

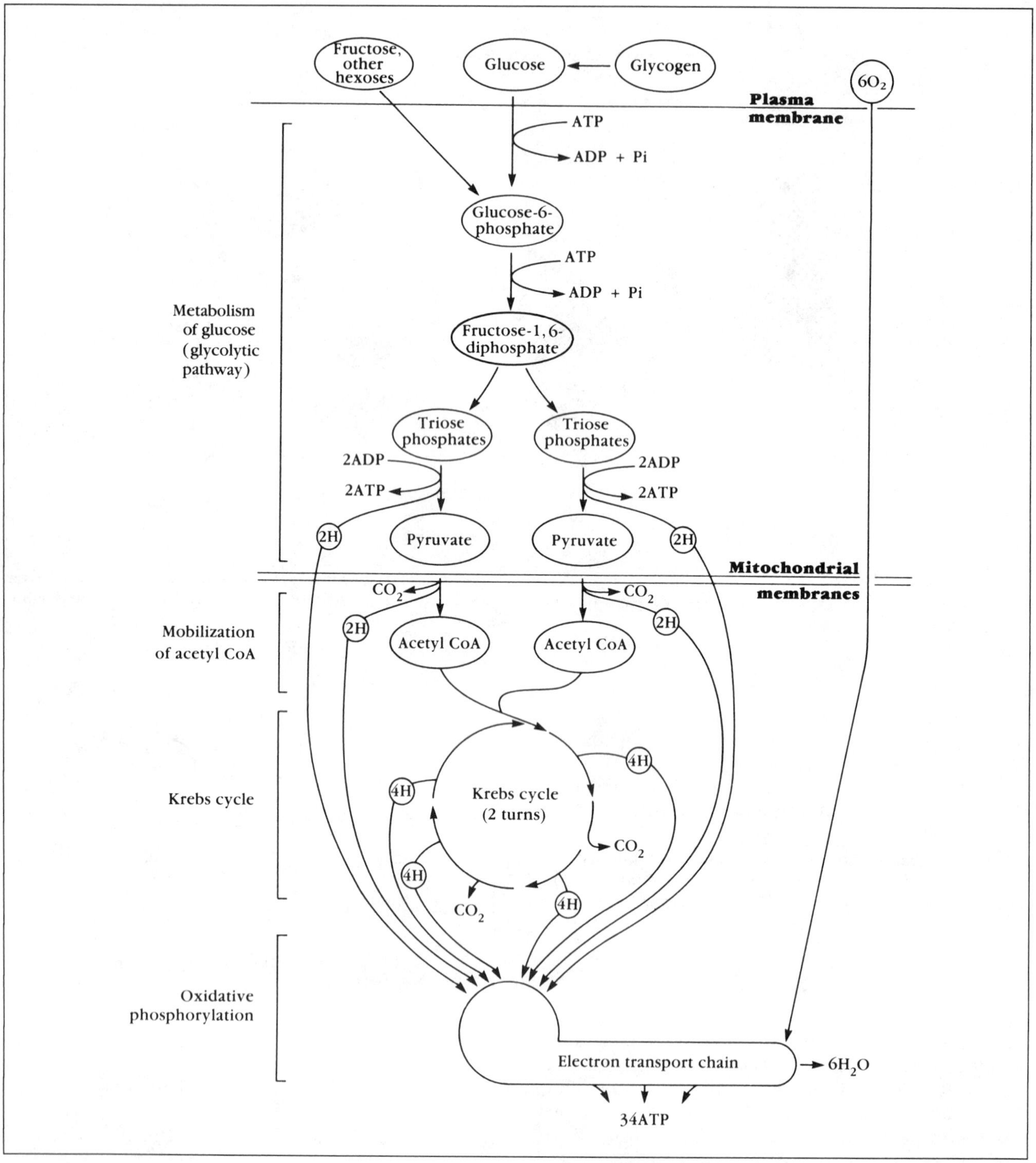

FIGURE 1-14. Metabolism of glucose in the formation of ATP. (From C. P. Hickman, Jr., L. S. Roberts, and F. M. Hickman, *Integrated Principles of Zoology* [7th ed.]. St. Louis: Mosby, 1984.)

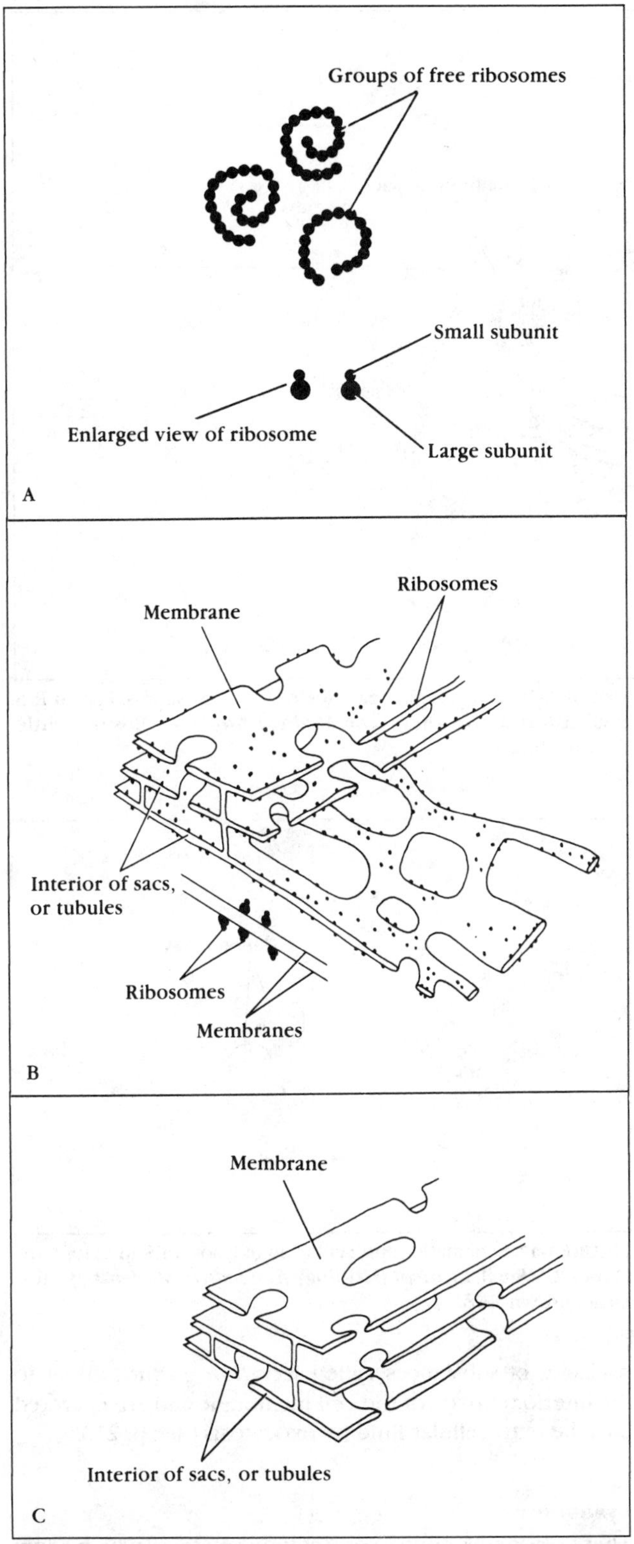

FIGURE 1-15. Electron microscopic appearance of structures of A. Ribosomes. B. Rough endoplasmic reticulum. C. Smooth endoplasmic reticulum. (From R. S. Snell, *Clinical Histology for Medical Students.* Boston: Little, Brown, 1984.)

glucose. Fats and proteins can be metabolized to intermediates that can be fed into Krebs cycle.

Approximately 95 percent of ATP is formed in the mitochondria through a sequence of chemical reactions requiring oxidative enzymes. The process involves glycolysis and then oxidation of the end product to form ATP. Many successive steps in the process allow for the release of 38 moles of ATP for each mole of glucose. Actually, 40 moles of ATP are produced with 2 moles being spent to initiate the process and 4 moles being produced outside the mitochondria. The efficiency in energy formation is about 44 percent with the remaining 56 percent being given off as heat and not utilized by the cells in specific cellular functions [3].

Formation of ATP Without Oxygen

A small amount of ATP can also be formed by glycolysis in the absence of oxygen. Figure 1-14 shows that glycolysis (Embden-Meyerhof pathway) itself is an anaerobic process. Glycolysis proceeds to produce pyruvic acid (pyruvate). Important in the process is a coenzyme called NAD (nicotinamide adenine dinucleotide), which functions to accept hydrogen ions. Normally, NAD picks up hydrogen and passes it to another acceptor in order to pick up more hydrogen. In the oxidative cycle this acceptor is oxygen, resulting in the formation of water. Without available oxygen, hydrogen ions accumulate in the form of lactic acid. The system is inefficient but it can keep certain cells viable for short periods of time. In the normal, unstressed cell, anaerobic metabolism provides less than 5 percent of the ATP requirements of the cell. The resulting lactic acid diffuses out of the cell into the tissues and plasma. This glycolytic process occurs during periods of intense muscular exertion in which oxygen consumption exceeds oxygen supply; subsequently, the accumulation of lactic acid in the muscle causes pain. The process produces an *oxygen debt* of the muscle that requires deep breathing following exercise to restore the balance of ATP. The lactic acid remaining within the muscle cell can be reconverted to glucose or pyruvic acid in the presence of oxygen. The lactic acid that leaves the cell during exercise is carried to the liver where it becomes converted to glycogen and carbon dioxide. The heart has been shown to be particularly capable of converting lactic acid to pyruvic acid until extreme hypoxia occurs when it produces more lactic acid than it can metabolize.

Ribosomes

These cytoplasmic organelles are necessary for the synthesis of protein. They are found free in the cytoplasm or attached to the endoplasmic reticulum (Fig. 1-15).

The free ribosomes are the sites where intracellular proteins are synthesized. These proteins are utilized to produce cellular structures and enzymes. Ribosomes on the endoplasmic reticulum synthesize the proteins, which are secreted by the cell through the process of exocytosis.

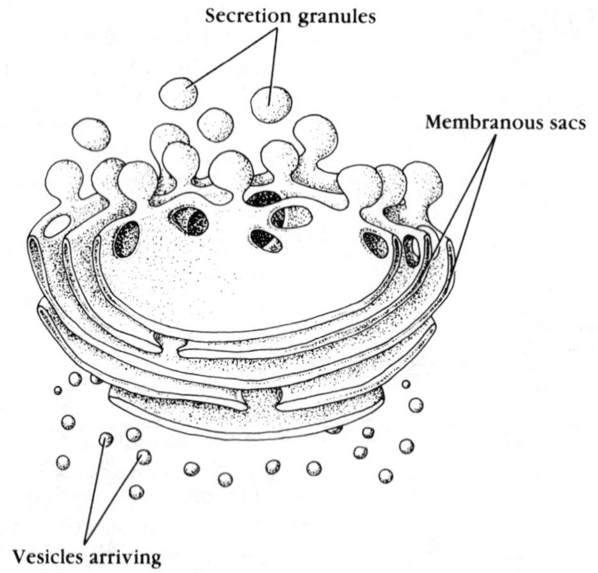

FIGURE 1-16. Probable appearance of Golgi apparatus. (From R. S. Snell, *Clinical Histology for Medical Students.* Boston: Little, Brown, 1984.)

They also function in the synthesis of lysosomal enzymes, which are packaged by the Golgi apparatus.

The ribosomes synthesize their specific proteins after reading a specific code from the ribonucleic acid (RNA). Messenger RNA (mRNA) contains the genetic code for specific ordering of amino acids. The code is transcribed on the mRNA from the DNA, ending finally in the manufacture of special proteins to carry out the various functions of the cell (see p. 20).

Endoplasmic Reticulum

This organelle is an intricate network of tubules, which may or may not have ribosomes on its surface. Endoplasmic reticulum (ER) with ribosomes on its surface, is called *granular* or *rough endoplasmic* reticulum (see Fig. 1-15B). ER without these ribosomes is called *agranular,* or *smooth, endoplasmic reticulum.*

Granular ER functions to synthesize proteins and these combine with fats or carbohydrates. Agranular ER functions in fat metabolism, in biotransformation of substances, in calcium storage in some cells, and it probably provides an intracellular transport system. The liver and pancreatic cells are examples of cells that contain a large amount of endoplasmic reticulum within their cytoplasm.

Golgi Apparatus or Complex

This organelle has a characteristic bowllike appearance, which has been demonstrated with the aid of the electron microscope (Fig. 1-16). It contains important enzyme systems that apparently package or encase manufactured substances and make important chemical additions. The packages of substances called *secretion granules* float to the interior surface of the cell membrane and are excreted into the extracellular fluid by exocytosis (see p. 27).

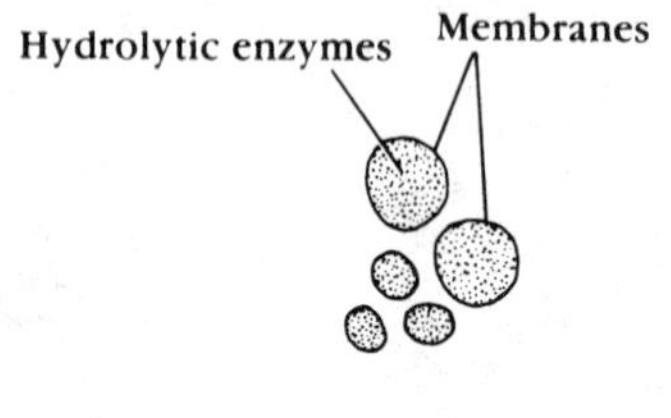

FIGURE 1-17. Schematic representation of lysosomes in cytoplasm. (From R. S. Snell, *Clinical Histology for Medical Students.* Boston: Little, Brown, 1984.)

Lysosomes

These organelles contain proteolytic enzymes, which allow for intracellular digestive activities within the cytoplasm (Fig. 1-17). The enzymes are hydrolases, which are capable of degrading complex compounds to simpler ones. In processes termed *pinocytosis* and *phagocytosis,* lysosomes attach to the complex material or to the foreign protein and fuse to the membrane of the material. A common vesicle or vacuole is formed, which allows the hydrolytic enzymes to diffuse into the area. Lysosomes are a very important part of the phagocytic cells in the destruction of foreign proteins (see Chap. 8).

Microtubules

These organelles are located in all nucleated cells at some time during the life of the cell, and when found close together they add structural strength to the cell (Fig. 1-18). These structures are also probably a part of the flagellum of sperm and the filaments of ciliated cells (Fig. 1-19). They have been observed to have many functions in different cells, including the following: a role in cellular division; transport along nerve axons; secretion of hormones; maintaining cell shape; transport of substances through their tubules; and cell movement.

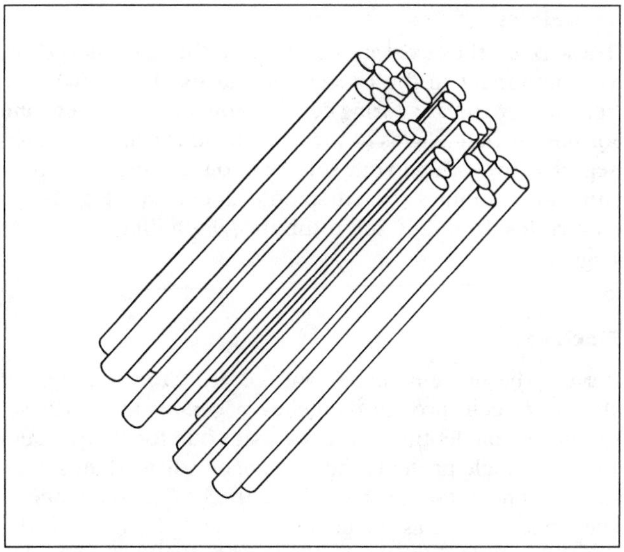

FIGURE 1-18. Microtubules. (From R. S. Snell, *Clinical Histology for Medical Students.* Boston: Little, Brown, 1984.)

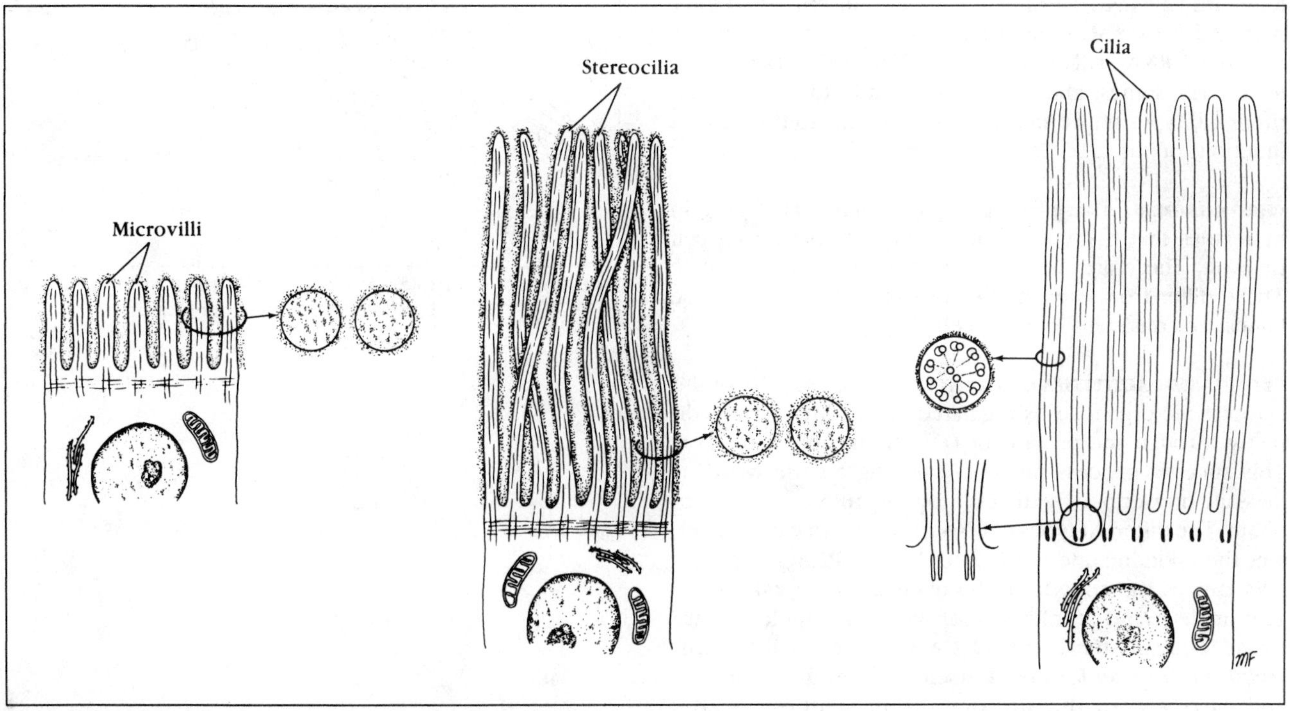

FIGURE 1-19. Examples of cells that have microtubules. (From R. S. Snell, *Clinical Histology for Medical Students.* Boston: Little, Brown, 1984.)

Centrioles

These organelles exist in pairs outside the nucleus and are very important in the process of mitosis (Fig. 1-20). The centrioles replicate during cell division with each new one forming at right angles to the old. The four centrioles then separate, two going to one side, two to the other. Here they form microtubules, called spindle fibers (see Fig. 1-19). Centrioles form all microtubules, including cilia and flagella.

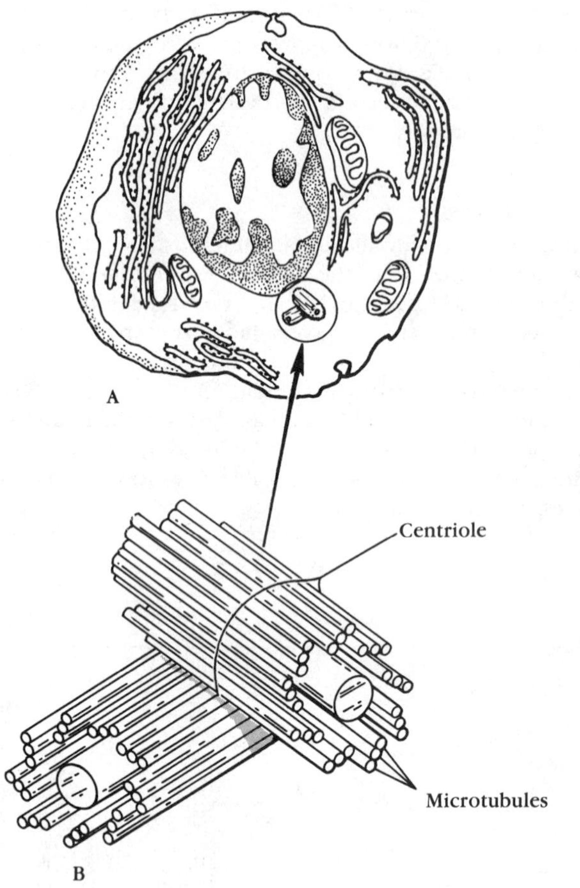

FIGURE 1-20. Centrioles. A. Placement in relationship to the nucleus. B. Appearance and composition of centriole.

Nucleus

GENES. The nucleus directs and controls the activities of the entire cell through the genes. A *gene* is the linear sequence of nucleotides on DNA that code for the production of a single protein. The sequence is divided into units of three nucleotides, each called a triplet. The sequence of the nucleotide bases (guanine, thymine, cytosine, and adenine) determines the unique code and ultimately codes for a single amino acid. The genes transcribe the specific code on the RNA. The gene is actually located on one of the two DNA strands called the master strand, which serves as the template for messenger RNA (mRNA) transcription. Other parts of DNA serve as templates for transfer RNA (tRNA) or ribosomal RNA (rRNA) formation. The code, transmitted to the ribosomes, allows for the manufacture of several thousand types of proteins that are essential to the various functions of human cells.

CHROMOSOMES. These are groups of genes and protein molecules that become visible as an X shape during cell division. There are 46 chromosomes in the human cell. These differ from one another in size and shape, but the bands are consistent in every cell (Fig. 1-21).

CYTOPLASMIC ACTIVITIES OF THE NUCLEUS. The activity of the cytoplasmic organelles is regulated either directly or indirectly through the process of DNA transcription of RNA. This specific process involves carrying a code word or message transcribed by the DNA on the mRNA to the cytoplasm. The different types of RNA necessary to carry and effect the code include mRNA, tRNA, and rRNA. *Messenger RNA* carries the code from the nucleus to the cytoplasm. The single strand of mRNA is formed as a complementary strand to the master strand of DNA in a process called *transcription. Transfer RNA* binds itself to a specific amino acid and carries it to the site of protein synthesis in the ribosome. It functions to sequence amino acids so that specified proteins are formed. The ribosomal RNA composes about 40 to 50 percent of the ribosome. Assembling of the coded amino acids occurs here and specific proteins are formed (Fig. 1-22).

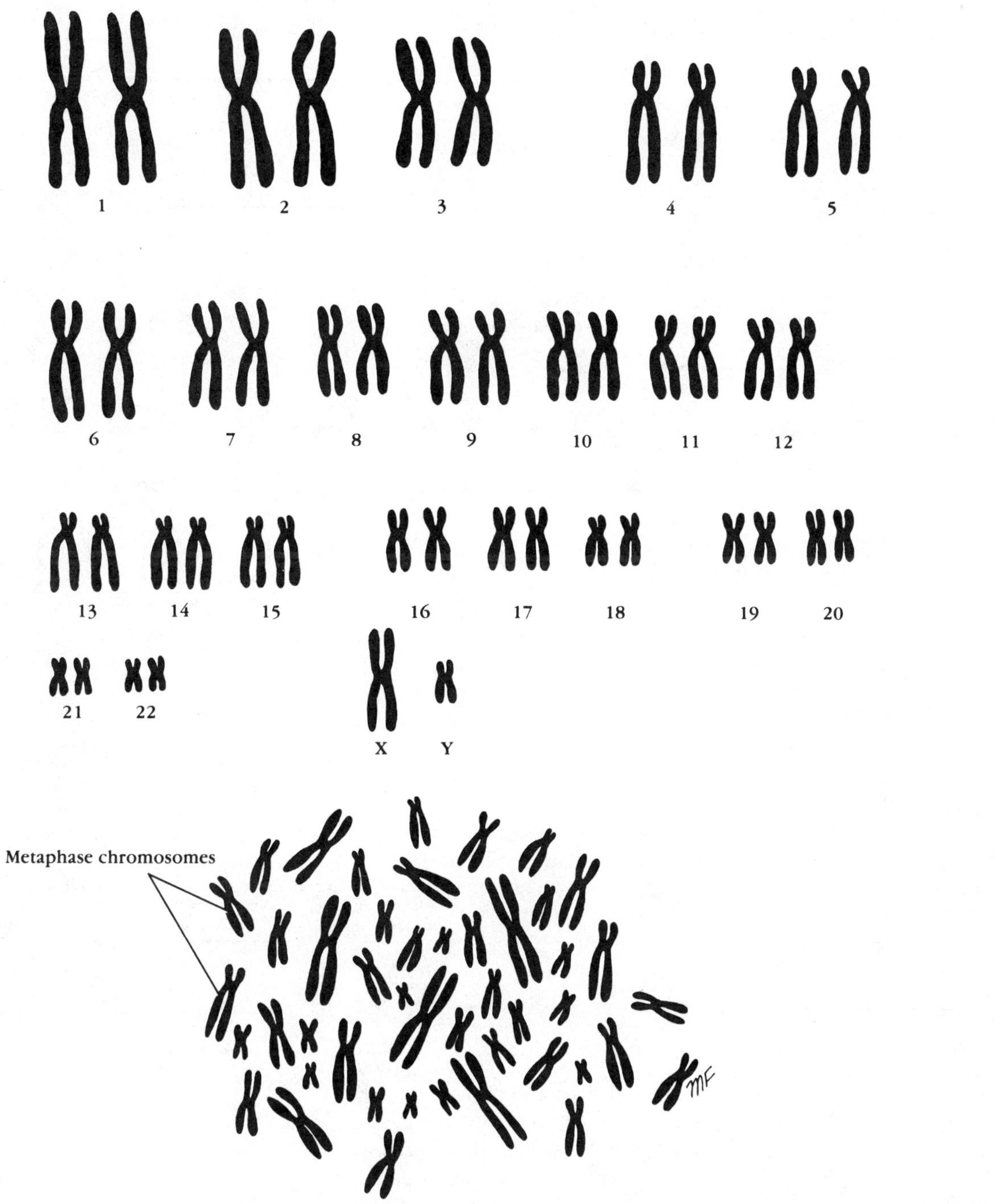

FIGURE 1-21. Structures of chromosomes showing a human male karyotype. Note the presence of X and Y sex chromosomes. (From R. S. Snell, *Clinical Histology for Medical Students.* Boston: Little, Brown, 1984.)

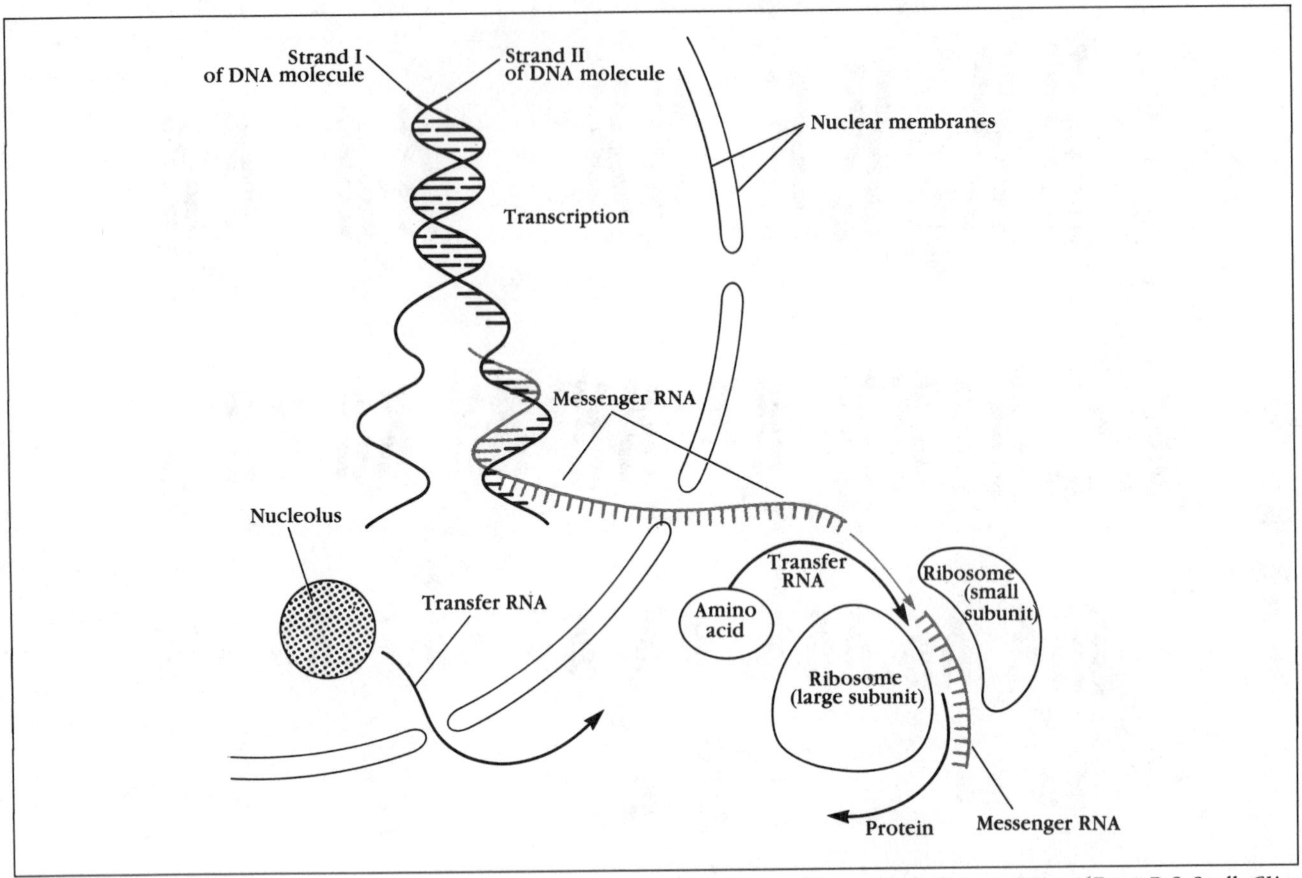

FIGURE 1-22. The process of transcription. (From R. S. Snell, *Clinical Histology for Medical Students.* Boston: Little, Brown, 1984.)

Nucleolus

This organelle is of various sizes and lies within the nucleus of the cell (see Fig. 1-9). It does not have a limiting membrane as do the other organelles and appears to be a region for RNA storage. It may supply the transfer RNA necessary for assembling amino acids.

MOVEMENT OF MATERIALS ACROSS THE CELL MEMBRANE

The intracellular fluid (ICF) is of a different electrolyte composition than the extracellular fluid (ECF). (Refer to Table 1-2.) This difference is maintained by a complex, well-regulated system of transport across the semipermeable cell membrane. Movement of particles across the cell membrane occurs through the following three mechanisms: (1) passive transport, including diffusion, facilitated diffusion, and osmosis; (2) active transport; and (3) endocytosis and exocytosis.

TABLE 1-2. Approximate chemical composition of extracellular and intracellular fluid

	Extracellular	Intracellular
Na^+	142 mEq/L	10 mEq/L
K^+	3.5–5.0 mEq/L	141 mEq/L
Ca^{2+}	5 mEq/L	1 mEq/L
Mg^{2+}	3 mEq/L	58 mEq/L
Cl^-	103 mEq/L	4 mEq/L
HCO_3^-	28 mEq/L	10 mEq/L
Phosphates	4 mEq/L	75 mEq/L
Glucose	90 dl	0–20 dl
pH	7.4	7.0

Source: A. C. Guyton, *Medical Physiology* (6th ed.). Philadelphia: Saunders, 1981. P. 41.

Passive Movement Across the Cell Membrane

DIFFUSION. This activity is commonly defined as the movement of a substance from a region of higher concentration to a region of lower concentration. The most important factor in this movement is the permeability of the cell membrane to the substance. Diffusion is *passive* because no energy (ATP) is expended in moving substances into or out of the cell. The structure of the cell membrane allows for the movement of oxygen, carbon dioxide, alcohol, fatty acids, and a few other substances that become dissolved in the lipid of the cell membrane and move across the membrane toward a lower concentration gradient. Because of this unrestricted diffusion, substances can move freely in either direction, depending on the concentration gradients on either side (Fig. 1-23).

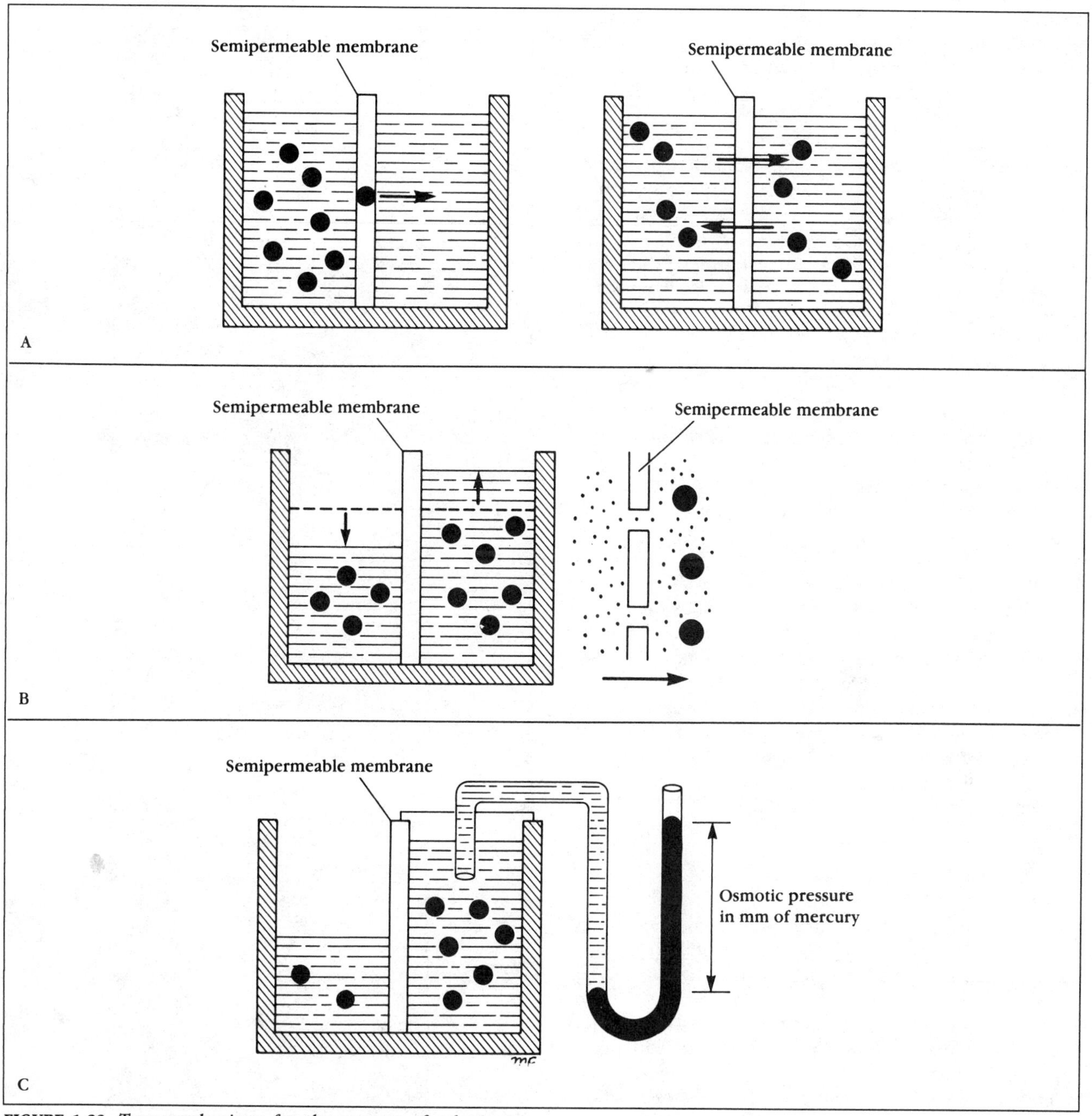

FIGURE 1-23. Two mechanisms for the passage of substances through a plasma membrane. A. Diffusion. B. Osmosis. C. A simple method of measuring osmotic pressure. (From R. S. Snell, *Clinical Histology for Medical Students.* Boston: Little, Brown, 1984.)

OSMOSIS. Water moves across the cell membrane through the membrane pores utilizing the principles of *osmosis*. Because of its small molecular size, water moves freely down its concentration gradient. Water moves through very small membrane pores, not through the cell membrane. The lipid and protein bilayer structure of the cell membrane keep the cell insoluble in water, but the membrane pores allow for free movement of water back and forth between ECF and ICF. When the ECF contains too many electrolytes it becomes *hypertonic* to the ICF, and water will attempt to equalize concentrations by moving toward the hypertonic fluid. The reverse is also true. When the ECF contains too few electrolytes, it becomes *hypotonic* to the ICF and water moves into the cell causing cellular swelling (Fig. 1-24).

FACILITATED DIFFUSION. This process of assisted diffusion is especially important in moving glucose from the ECF to the ICF. Normally, there is a very small reserve of glucose for energy metabolism within the cell, so the cell is very dependent on the transport of glucose from the ECF. Glucose is not soluble in the lipid of the cell membrane and is too large to pass through the membrane pores. The mechanism of facilitated passive transport involves the combination of glucose with specific carrier molecules that are in the cell membrane. After combining with the carrier molecule, the glucose is carried into the cell by simple diffusion (Fig. 1-25). This process requires no ATP but is assisted by the pancreatic hormone insulin, which has been shown to increase the rate of glucose transport seven- to tenfold [3]. Substances move only from an area of high concentration to low concentration, and the process seems to be enhanced when a greater differential exists between ICF and ECF.

Active Transport

Active transport is a process that involves moving of substances in and out of the cell against an electrochemical concentration gradient. This is the method by which sodium and potassium gradients are maintained. Other substances are also moved by active transport and include the following: calcium, some amino acids, glucose in special places of the body, and magnesium. The exact mechanism of active transport is unknown, but it is postulated that the substances are transported across the membrane on energy-driven (ATP) carriers. The process involves an enzymatic reaction that allows the substance to be released from the carrier when it reaches the intracellular fluid. Specificity of the carrier for its substance is an important aspect of active transport. It is thought that one carrier system transports excess intracellular sodium to the outside while bringing potassium to the inside [5] (Fig. 1-26). Other active systems bring in sugars, amino acids, and other ions.

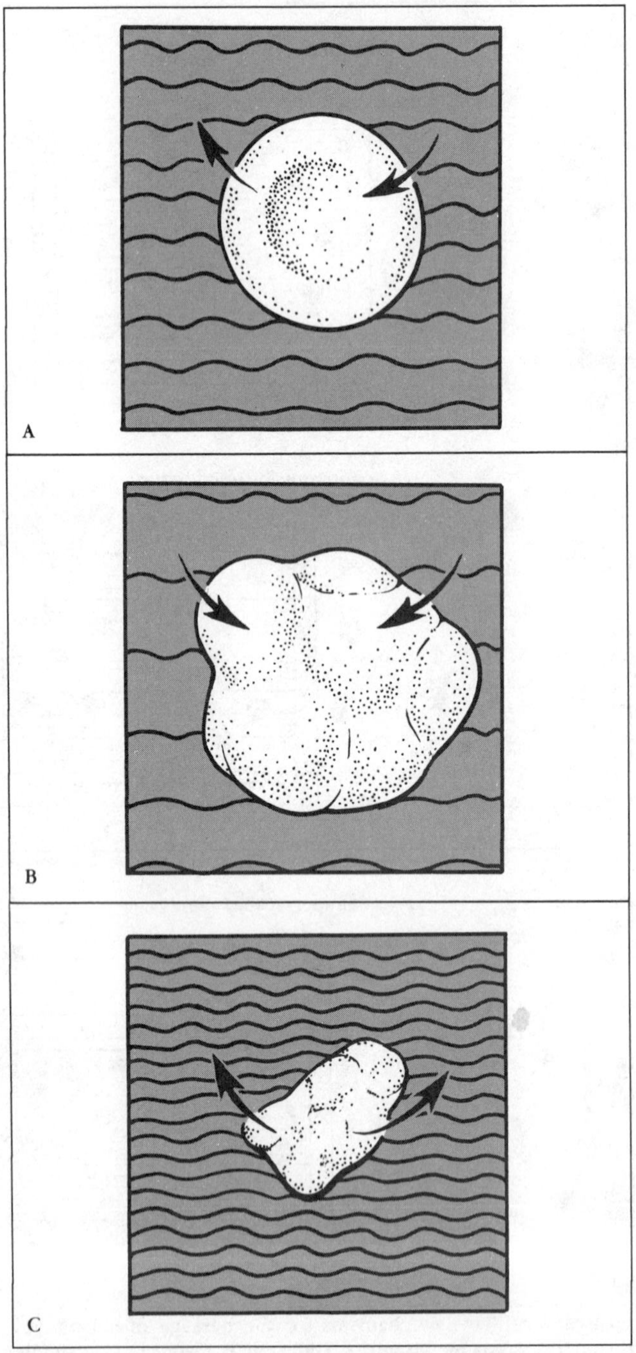

FIGURE 1-24. A. Appearance of a red blood cell placed in fluids with the same osmotic pressure as the ICF (isotonic). B. Appearance of a red blood cell placed in fluid with a lower osmotic pressure than the ICF (hypotonic). C. Appearance of a red blood cell placed in fluid with a higher osmotic pressure than the ICF (hypertonic).

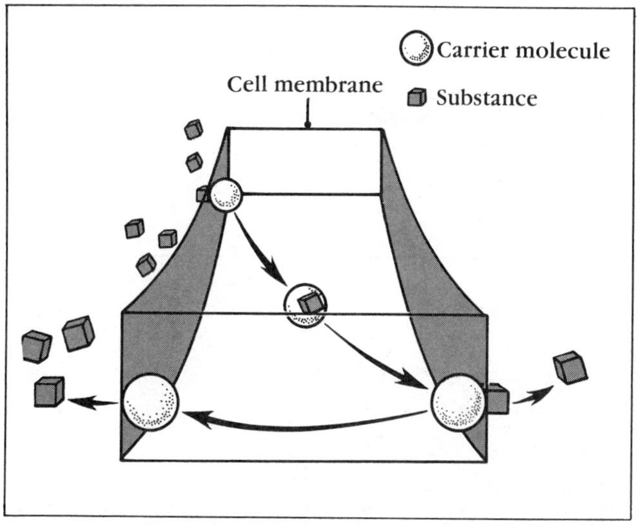

FIGURE 1-25. Example of facilitated transport with substance combining with carrier molecule and moving it to the inside of the cell, down its concentration gradient and without the expenditure of energy.

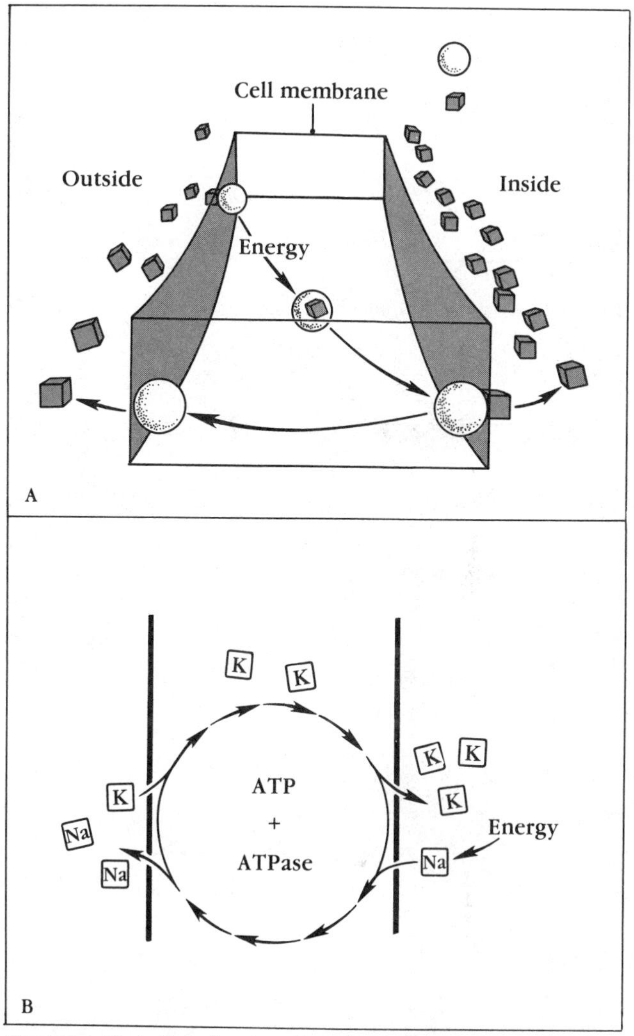

FIGURE 1-26. A. Postulated carrier system for moving substances across the cell membrane; like facilitated diffusion except movement is against a concentration gradient and requires energy. B. Postulated mechanism for moving sodium out of the cell and potassium to the interior of the cell.

SODIUM PUMP. Much attention has been directed to the *sodium pump,* which functions in all cells of the body. This pump prevents accumulation of sodium within the cell, thus preventing water influx into the cell and cellular swelling. Accumulation of sodium in ICF tends to cause osmosis of water toward the interior of the cell. The sodium pump, as a part of active transport, overcomes the continual tendency for water to enter the cell. Most important, when cellular metabolism ceases or decreases, adequate ATP is not available and cellular swelling begins immediately [3].

Active transport then functions to bring in essential substances to the interior of the cell and to actively excrete many others. The regulation of this transport system is dependent on certain hormones that may accelerate or inhibit the transport process. Examples of these hormones include insulin, somatotrophic hormone, glucocorticoids, and the sex hormones.

Endocytosis and Exocytosis

Endocytosis and *exocytosis* are methods for bringing particles into the cell and releasing secretions to the exterior of the cell. These processes are schematically illustrated in Figure 1-27. Both processes are essential in carrying out the functional capabilities of specific cells.

Endocytosis refers to the bringing in of proteins and other substances through invagination of the outer cell membrane. This process occurs in the following two ways:

1. *Pinocytosis* involves movement of complex proteins and some strong electrolyte solutions into the cell. The protein is seen to adhere to the outer cell membrane, which stimulates invagination of the membrane. The material is encased or enclosed in a vesicle and floats into the cytoplasm. Lysosomes attach to the vesicle surface, release hydrolytic enzymes into the vesicle, and break down the complex material for use within the cells. A residual body may be left within the lysosome or excreted through the cell membrane to the ECF.

2. *Phagocytosis* involves essentially the same process, but the material brought into the cell is in solid or particulate form and frequently is a microorganism (see Unit 4).

Exocytosis has been termed *reverse pinocytosis* and is an active release of soluble products to the ECF. Secretion granules are formed, as described earlier, by the Golgi complex and are secreted through the process of adherence to the inner cell membrane, outpouching of the membrane,

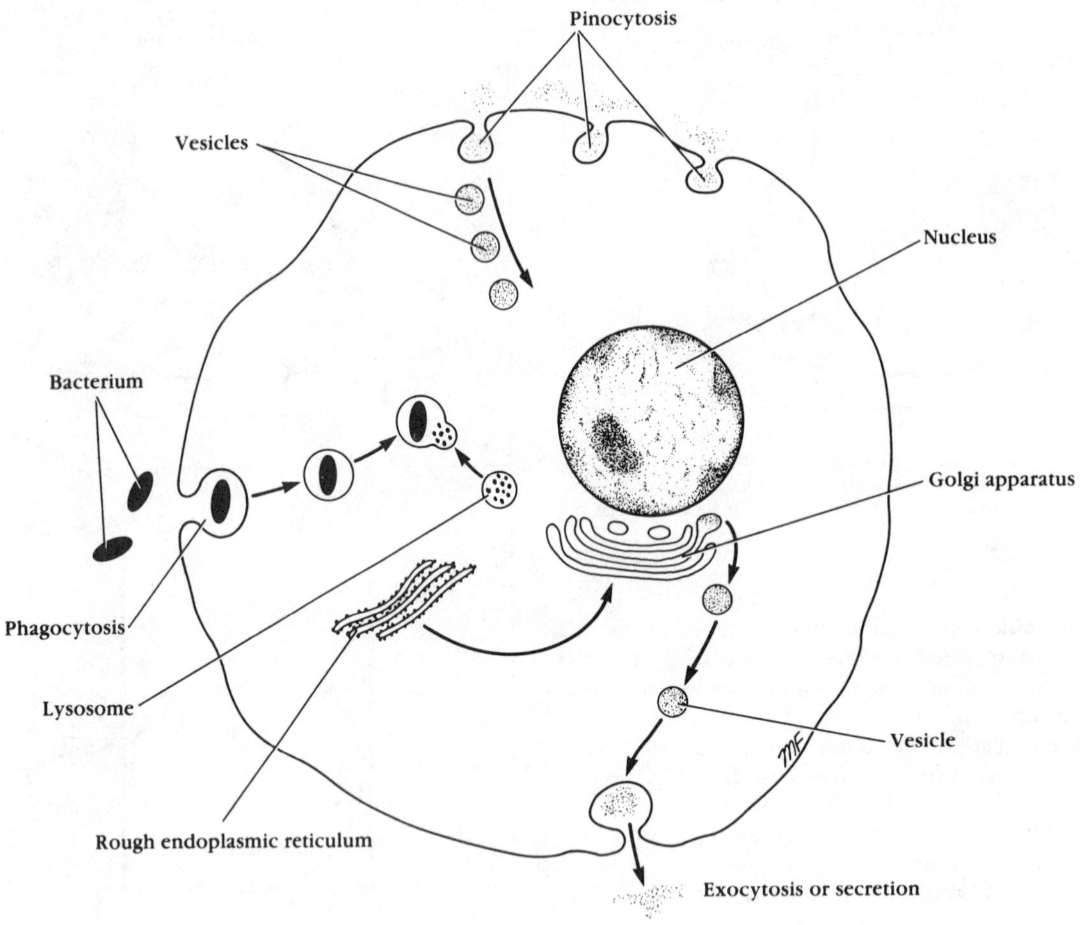

FIGURE 1-27. Schematic illustration of processes of endocytosis (pinocytosis and phagocytosis) and exocytosis. (From R. S. Snell, *Clinical Histology for Medical Students.* Boston: Little, Brown, 1984.)

and release of contents into the ECF. The secretory products are vital to maintenance of the steady state of the host and include secretions necessary for digestion, glandular secretion, neural transmission, etc.

Both endocytosis and exocytosis are processes that require energy and are affected by cellular ability to synthesize ATP. Both processes require enzymatic reactions to enhance the rate of reactions.

TYPES OF CELL MOVEMENT

Many cells exhibit the ability to move. Movement may involve locomotion from one place to another or it may involve movement of filaments within the cell. The three types of movement that are considered in this section are ameboid motion, myofilament motion resulting in muscular contraction, and movement of projections from the cells (cilia and flagella).

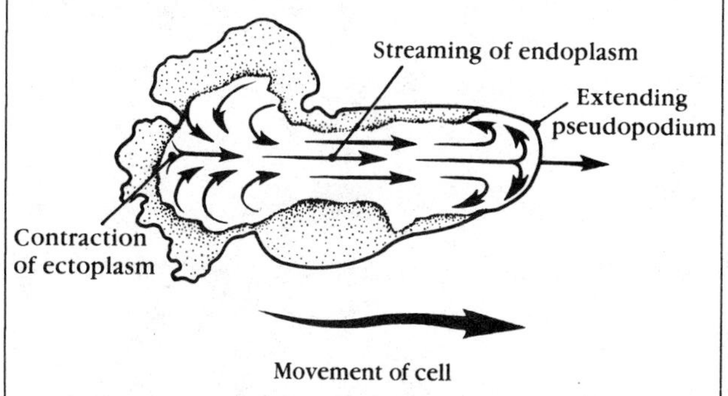

FIGURE 1-28. Method of ameboid motion of a cell, showing contraction of ectoplasm, extended pseudopodium, streaming of endoplasm toward the projected pseudopodium.

Ameboid Motion

Ameboid motion refers to the ability of a cell to move from one location to another. In the embryo, most of the cells exhibit ameboid motion in order to migrate to their appropriate location. This property of ameboid movement is retained by certain defensive cells of the body, especially the leukocytes, and allows these cells to move from the bloodstream to the tissue spaces to contact and destroy a foreign protein (see Chap. 8).

Utilizing energy (ATP) and calcium ions, the process is accomplished by the forward projection of a portion of the cell, called the *pseudopodium* (Fig. 1-28). It probably depends on contraction of microfilaments in the outer portion of the cytoplasm that push out or project the pseudopodium. The remainder of the cell follows the projected area by a streaming motion and allows for the rapid delivery of cells into an area.

Muscular Contraction

Approximately 50 percent of the body mass is skeletal, smooth, and cardiac muscle. The contraction of these muscles make possible both involuntary and voluntary movements. The details of muscular contraction are further described in Chapters 17, 34, and 38.

Both electrical and mechanical processes exist in muscle, and the initiation of most contractions is through electrical stimulation from the nerve terminals. The electrical events are followed immediately by the mechanical events in a sequential way. Electrical properties of cells are described in this chapter on pages 31–32. Electrical activation causes *depolarization*, which initiates the mechanical movement of contractile proteins on each other and causes a shortening of the muscle fiber. The muscle fiber is illustrated in Figure 1-29, which shows the subunits of the fiber finally terminating in two contractile proteins called actin and myosin.

Skeletal muscle has a striated appearance because of its regularly ordered proteins. These proteins make up the contractile portions of the muscle fiber. The process of skeletal muscle contraction basically follows this course: A nerve stimulation causes the release of acetylcholine at the myoneural junction (Fig. 1-30). *Acetylcholine,* a chemical neurotransmitter, causes a change in muscle cell permeability that is spread throughout the muscle cell membrane and to the t tubules that carry the stimulus to the interior of the cell. The transfer of stimulus by the t tubules to the sarcoplasmic reticulum (SR) causes the release of calcium from the SR. Calcium binds with the inhibitory protein, troponin causing troponin to interact with tropomyosin, resulting in the uncovering of the active sites on actin, which allows for free interaction with myosin. Actin (thin filament) then slides on myosin (thick filament), causing a shortening of the entire sarcomere unit (Fig. 1-31). Calcium is immediately taken back up into the SR and troponin-tropomyosin regain their normal inhibitory function. Large quantities of ATP are necessary to provide energy to pump the calcium back into the sarcoplasmic reticulum. During this process sodium also leaks into the cell, and an active sodium pump becomes necessary to prevent accumulation of water in the muscle cell.

Cardiac muscle is also striated and follows the same general pattern for contraction but exhibits basic differences. Cardiac muscle is rapidly depolarized and contracts immediately after stimulation, but repolarizes much more slowly than skeletal muscle. This slow repolarization apparently prevents cardiac muscle from tetany, a phenomenon that may be seen in skeletal muscle. Also, depolarizing impulses depolarize the entire muscle, either atrial or ventricular, rather than individual fiber depolarization as seen with skeletal muscle. This characteristic occurs because of the close proximity of one cardiac cell to the next (Fig. 1-32).

Smooth muscle cells are smaller than skeletal muscle cells and do not appear to have regularly ordered myofibrils. Contraction occurs generally in the same manner as with skeletal muscle except that it is relatively slow

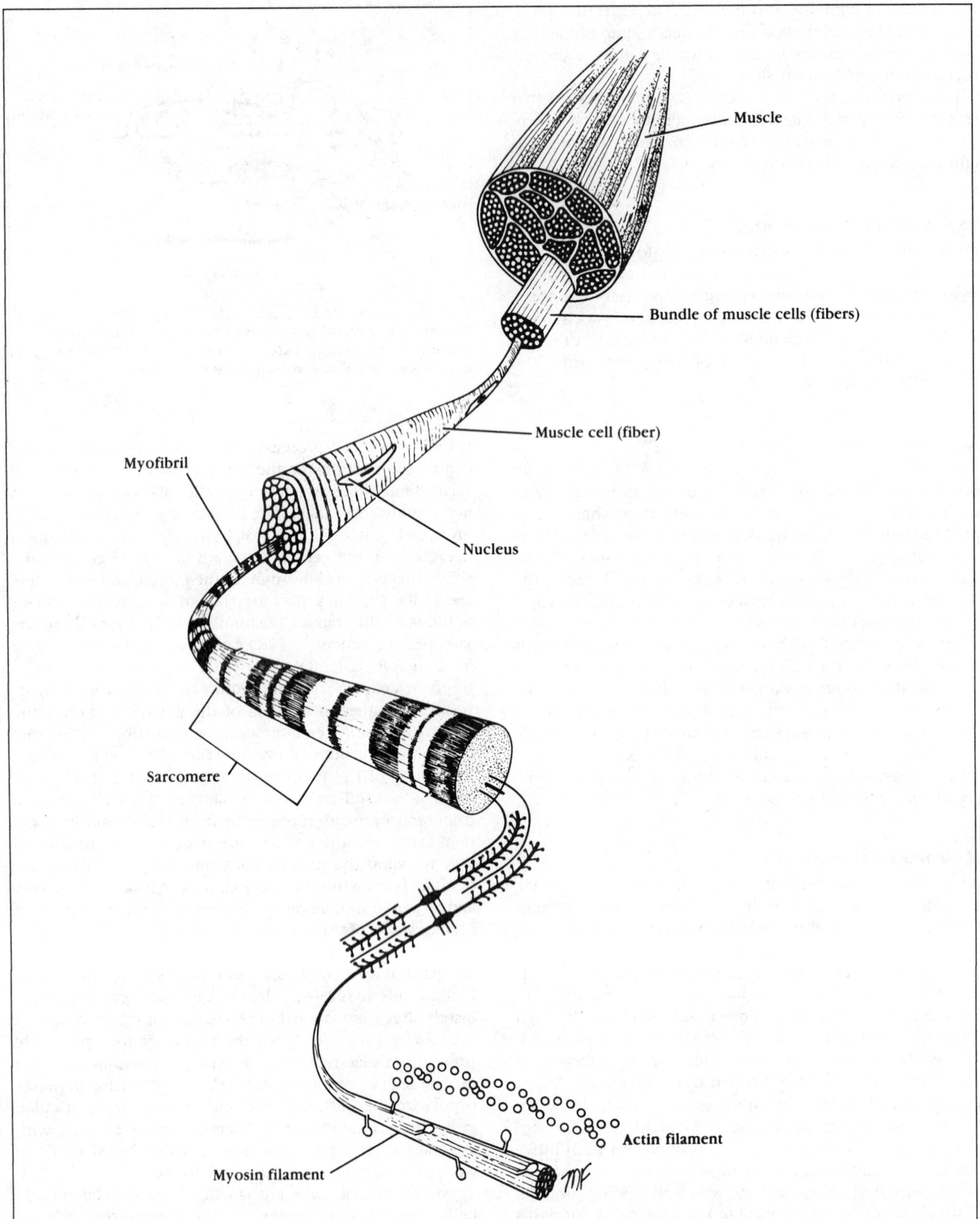

FIGURE 1-29. Illustration of gross to microscopic components of a muscle fiber. (From R. S. Snell, *Clinical Histology for Medical Students.* Boston: Little, Brown, 1984.)

Karla Wise
Class of '87 - FJC

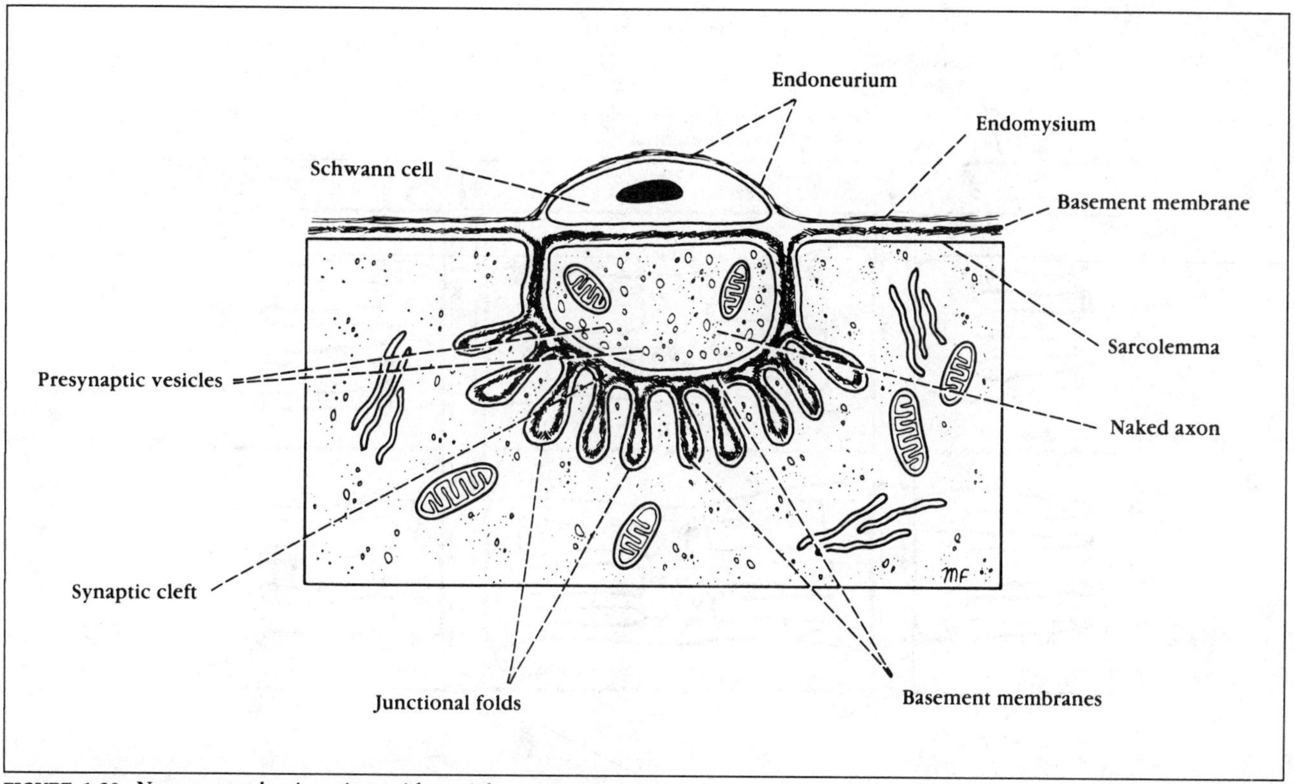

FIGURE 1-30. Neuromuscular junction with vesicles containing acetylcholine and synaptic cleft. (From R. S. Snell, *Clinical Histology for Medical Students.* Boston: Little, Brown, 1984.)

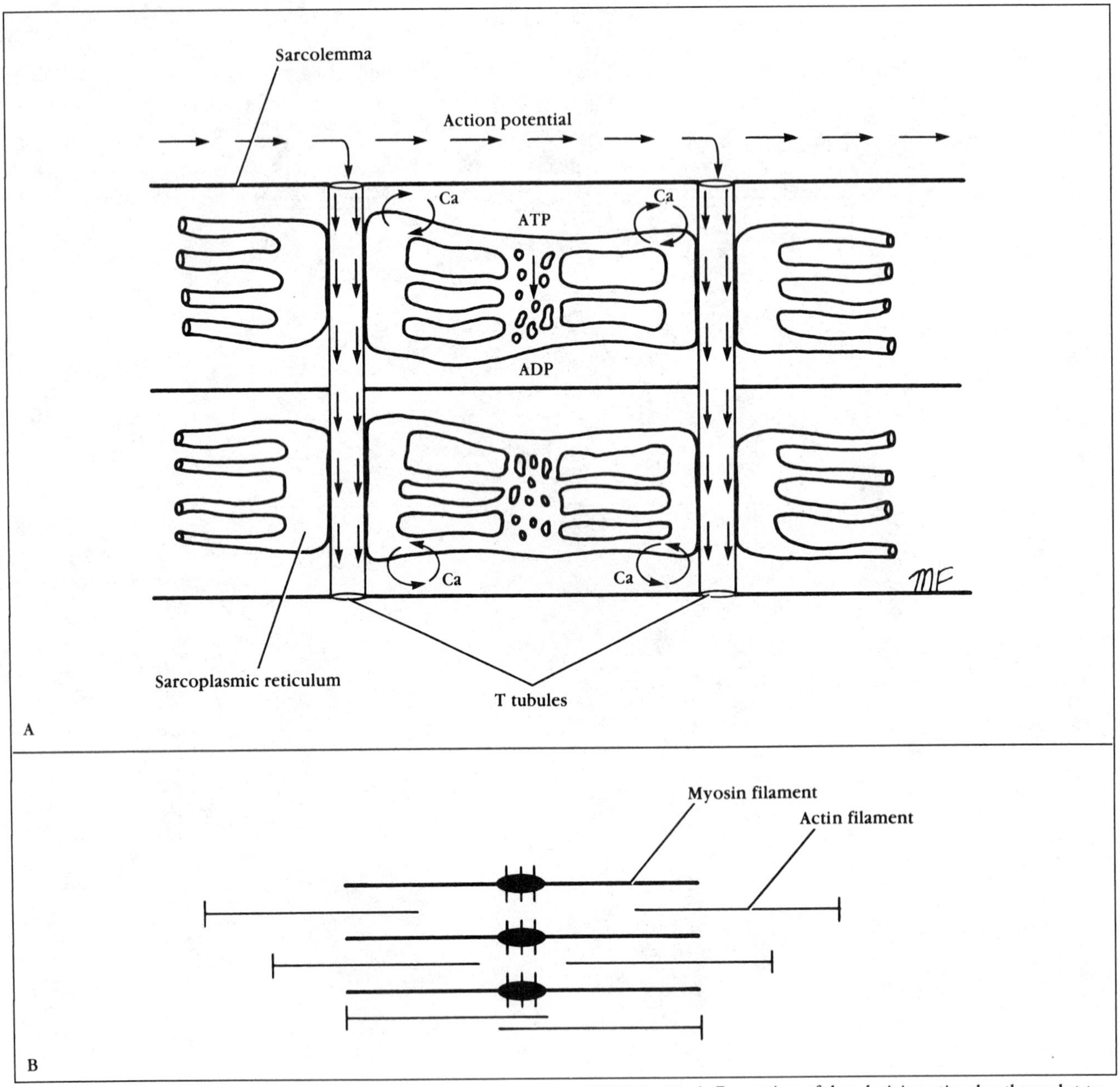

FIGURE 1-31. A. Reception of depolarizing stimulus through t tubules, release of calcium by sarcoplasmic reticulum, and degradation of ATP. B. Resting position of actin and myosin filaments. (From R. S. Snell, *Clinical Histology for Medical Students.* Boston: Little, Brown, 1984.)

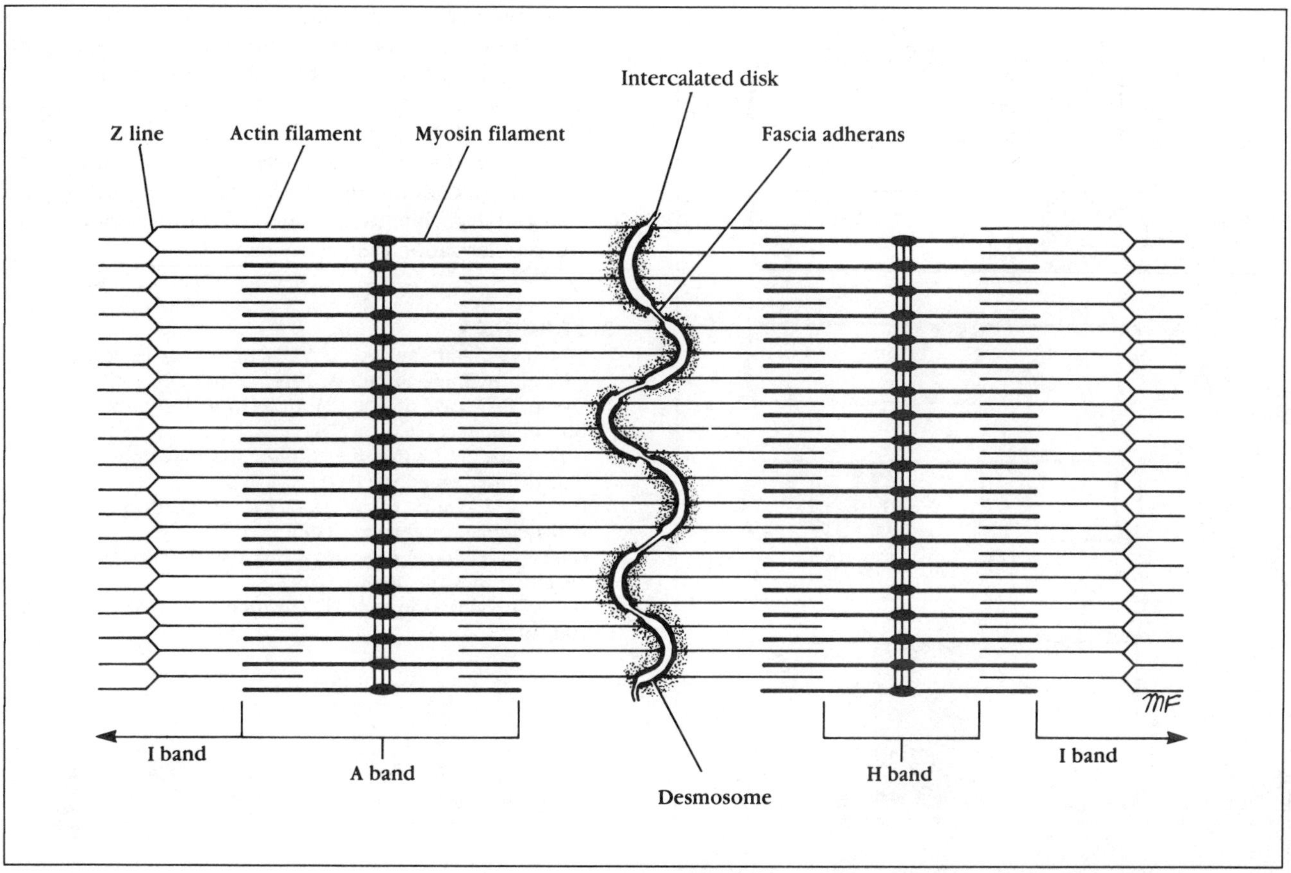

FIGURE 1-32. Schematic microscopic representation of myocardial muscle cell. (From R. S. Snell, *Clinical Histology for Medical Students.* Boston: Little, Brown, 1984.)

and contractions can be sustained for periods of time. Rhythmic contractions or waves of contractions result from the influence of nerve impulses as well as from many chemical agents.

Ciliary and Flagellar Movement

Many cells that lie on the surface of the respiratory tract and in the fallopian tubes have minute projections on their surfaces. These projections, cilia and flagella respectively, have a very important function in moving fluid forward. The structures of the cilia and flagella are alike. The cilia move with a swift forward movement and a slow backward stroke. This motion functions to propel fluid forward, which is an effective way to clear the respiratory tract and move an ovum along the fallopian tubes (see Fig. 1-16).

The movement of cilia is coordinated so that stimulation must be passed from one cilium to the next to allow for the movement. The motion of flagella and cilia is caused by contractile filaments, which contract rhythmically in a liquid medium. The spermatozoan is propelled by a single flagellum. This active process is dependent on ATP and a proper electrochemical balance. Cilia can be regenerated by the cell if they are destroyed.

ELECTRICAL PROPERTIES OF CELLS

Differences in electrical potential across the cell membrane are characteristic of all living cells. Some cells have the ability to respond to various types of stimuli, especially *electrochemical* stimuli. This response is called the cell's *excitability* and refers to the changing or altering of the electrical potential across the cell membrane. Two major types of cells, nerve and muscle, are considered to be excitable cells because they can change membrane potential, effect an action or response, and return to the resting state.

The excitable tissue or cell receives a *stimulus,* which rapidly changes its membrane potential. This *action potential* is followed by the action of the cell, which may be a contraction, transmitting the action potential to the next cell, or other actions. The cell then returns to the normal resting state, the *resting potential.*

Many changes occur in the cell membranes when an action potential is elicited. First, the stimulus causes release of a chemical transmitter, which causes increased permeability of the cell membrane to sodium. Sodium rushes into

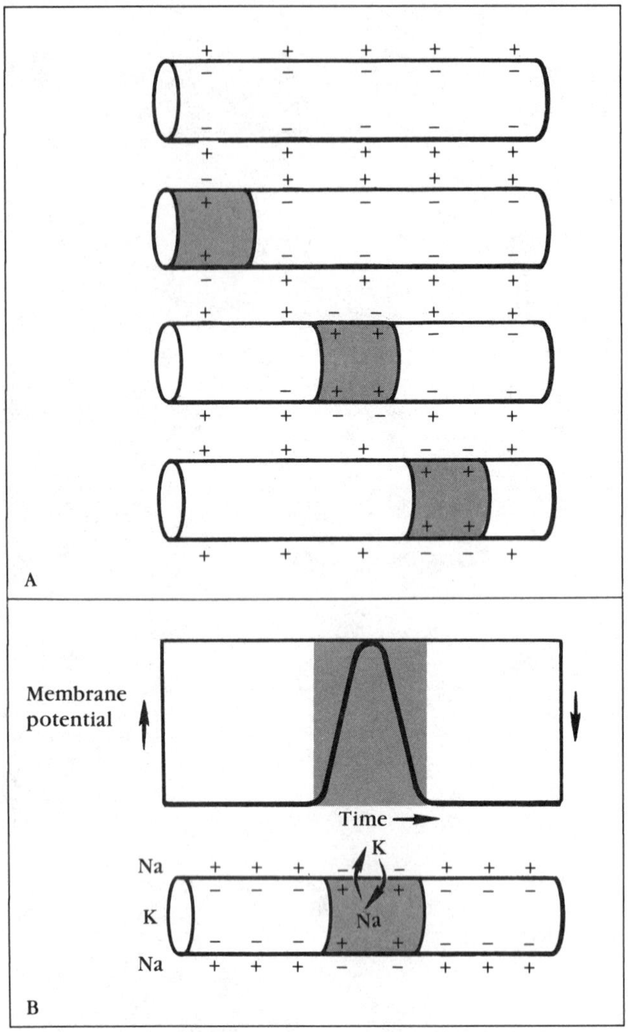

FIGURE 1-33. A. A resting nerve fiber, a depolarizing wave as the impulse passes rapidly down the nerve fiber. B. The membrane potential with depolarization occurring when the membrane is permeable to sodium causing more positive ions on the interior of the cell membrane. This requires an active sodium pump to rid the cell of excess sodium.

the cell and some potassium moves from the intracellular to the extracellular fluid, setting up appropriate conditions for the action of the cell. In the muscle cell, as previously mentioned, the stimulus causes the release of calcium, which effects the contraction of the muscle fiber. Following cellular action, the cell membrane decreases its permeability to sodium. Excess sodium trapped within the cell must be actively pumped out by the *sodium pump.* Some movement of potassium back into the cell also occurs, which requires a pumping system (Fig. 1-33).

The phases of the action potential have been divided into *refractory periods* depending on the receptiveness of the tissue to a new action potential. The *absolute refractory period* refers to that period of time when the cell is already stimulated or responding to its fullest and cannot respond no matter how strong the stimulus is. During the period of time when the cell is returning to the resting state, a strong stimulus may elicit a new action potential causing the cell to respond again. This period of time is called the *relative refractory period.* The absolute refractory period occurs during depolarization and subsequent cellular activity while the relative refractory period occurs during repolarization (see also Chaps. 38 and 42).

REFERENCES

1. Bloom, W., and Fawcett, D.W. *Textbook of Histology* (10th ed.). Philadelphia: Saunders, 1975.
2. Dyson, R.D. *Cell Biology: A Molecular Approach* (2nd ed.). Boston: Allyn & Bacon, 1978.
3. Guyton, A.C. *Textbook of Medical Physiology* (6th ed.). Philadelphia: Saunders, 1981.
4. Ham, A.W., and Cormack, D.H. *Histology* (8th ed.). Philadelphia: Lippincott, 1979.
5. Selkurt, E.E. *Basic Physiology for the Health Sciences* (2nd ed.). Boston: Little, Brown, 1982.
6. Weiss, L., and Greep, R.O. *Histology.* New York: McGraw-Hill, 1977.

CHAPTER 2
ALTERATIONS IN NORMAL CELLULAR PROCESSES RESULTING IN ADAPTIVE OR LETHAL CHANGE

STIMULI THAT CAN CAUSE CELLULAR INJURY OR ADAPTATION

INTRACELLULAR AND EXTRACELLULAR CHANGES RESULTING FROM CELLULAR ADAPTATION OR INJURY

- **Cellular Swelling**
- **Lipid Accumulation**
- **Glycogen Depositions**
- **Pigmentation**
- **Calcification**
- **Hyaline Infiltration**

CELLULAR CHANGES DUE TO INJURIOUS STIMULI

- **Atrophy**
- **Dysplasia**
- **Hypertrophy**
- **Hyperplasia**
- **Metaplasia**

INJURY AND DEATH OF CELLS DUE TO LACK OF OXYGEN

- **Ischemia**
- **Thrombosis**
- **Embolism**
- **Infarction**
- **Necrosis**
- **Somatic Death**

LEARNING OBJECTIVES

1. Define *adaptation.*
2. Describe alterations in cells that can occur because of stimuli.
3. List the six categories of stimuli that can cause cellular alterations.
4. Differentiate between endogenous and exogenous substances.
5. Describe the abnormal intracellular accumulations that result from noxious stimulation.
6. Define the common pigments that may accumulate in the cytoplasm.
7. Differentiate between the following pathologic cellular adaptations: atrophy, dysplasia, hypertrophy, hyperplasia, and metaplasia.
8. Define *autophagic vacuoles* and *residual bodies.*
9. Differentiate between ischemia and infarction.
10. Define and describe the factors producing thrombosis and embolism.
11. Describe the pathologic classification of infarcts.
12. Specify areas where bacterial supergrowth may be seen.
13. List and describe the three major types of necrosis.
14. Briefly explain the major changes that occur following somatic death.

The life cycle of a cell exists on a continuum that includes normal activities and adaptation, injury, or lethal changes. The pathologic changes exhibited may be obvious or very difficult to detect. The cell constantly makes adjustments to a changing, hostile environment in order to keep the organism functioning in a normal steady state. These adjustments are termed *adaptation* and are necessary to ensure the survival of the organism. *Adaptive changes* may be temporary or permanent. The separation between the adapted cell and the injured cell is the point at which the cell cannot functionally keep up with the stressful environment affecting it. Injured cells exhibit alterations that may affect body function and be manifested as disease.

Chapters 3 and 4 more explicitly define the concepts of stress and stressors to illustrate how the stress response can cause the manifestations of disease. Prevention of disease is dependent on the capacity of the affected cells to undergo self-repair and regeneration. This process of repair prevents cellular injury and death and may prevent the death of the host.

Specifically, adaptation is a return of the internal environment of the body to the steady state or normal balance following exposure to some alteration. The rigid electrolyte and water balance between the intracellular and extracellular fluid must be maintained. This process is described in Chapter 1 and in Unit 3. The steady state may be attained at the expense of altered intracellular metabolism and may continue for a certain period of time after which the cell, no longer able to adapt, may undergo injurious or lethal changes.

When cells are confronted with a stimulus that alters normal cellular metabolism, they may do any one or more of the following: (1) increase concentrations of normal cellular constituents; (2) accumulate abnormal substances; (3) change the cellular size or numbers; or (4) undergo a lethal change. These concepts are considered briefly in this chapter and further delineated in specific content areas. Categories of stimuli that can provoke changes and the types of changes that may occur are discussed in this chapter.

STIMULI THAT CAN CAUSE CELLULAR INJURY OR ADAPTATION

Because the cell is constantly making adjustments to a changing, hostile environment, many agents potentially can cause cellular injury or adaptation. Cellular injury may lead to further injury and death of the cell, or the cell may respond to the noxious stimulation by undergoing a change in itself in order to tolerate the invasion.

Stimuli that can alter the steady state can be grouped into the following categories: (1) physical agents, (2) chemical agents, (3) microorganisms, (4) hypoxia, (5) genetic defects, and (6) immunologic reactions (Table 2-1).

TABLE 2-1. Stimuli that can cause cellular injury

Physical agents	Trauma, thermal, electrical, atmospheric pressure changes, irradiation
Chemical agents	Drugs, poisons, foods, toxic, and irritating substances
Microorganisms	Viruses, bacteria, fungi, protozoa
Hypoxia	Shock, localized areas of inadequate blood supply, hypoxemia
Genetic	Inborn errors of metabolism, gross malformations
Immunologic	Hypersensitivity reactions to foreign protein

Physical agents include such factors as mechanical trauma, temperature gradients, electrical stimulation, atmospheric pressure gradients, and irradiation. Physical stimuli directly damage cells, cause rupture or damage of the cell walls, and disrupt cellular reproduction.

Chemical agents include a variety of chemicals that can cause cellular injury. These may include simple compounds such as glucose or complex agents such as poisons. Therapeutic drugs often chemically disrupt the normal cellular balance.

Microorganisms cause cellular injury in a variety of ways depending on the type of organism and the innate defense of the human body. Some bacteria secrete exotoxins, which are injurious to the host. Others liberate endotoxins when they are destroyed. Viruses interfere with the metabolism of the host cells and cause cellular injury by releasing viral proteins toxic to the cell (see Chap. 7).

Hypoxia is the most common cause of cellular injury and may be produced by inadequate oxygen in the blood or by decreased perfusion of blood to the tissues. The end result is a disturbance of cellular metabolism and local or generalized release of lactic acid (see Chap. 6).

Genetic defects can affect cellular metabolism through inborn errors of metabolism or gross malformations. The mechanisms for cellular disruption vary widely with the genetic defect but may result in intracellular accumulations of abnormal material.

Immunologic agents may cause cellular injury, especially when hypersensitivity reactions occur, causing the release of excess histamine and other substances. This response is discussed in more detail in Unit 5.

INTRACELLULAR AND EXTRACELLULAR CHANGES RESULTING FROM CELLULAR ADAPTATION OR INJURY

Abnormal intracellular accumulations often result from an environmental change or the inability of the cell to process materials. Normal or abnormal substances that cannot be metabolized may accumulate in the cytoplasm. These substances may be *endogenous* (produced within the body) or *exogenous* (produced in the environment) and stored by an originally normal cell. Abnormal exogenous substances include such things as carbon particles, silica, and metals that are deposited and accumulate because the cell cannot degrade them or transport them to other sites [5].

Cellular changes discussed in this section include: cellu-

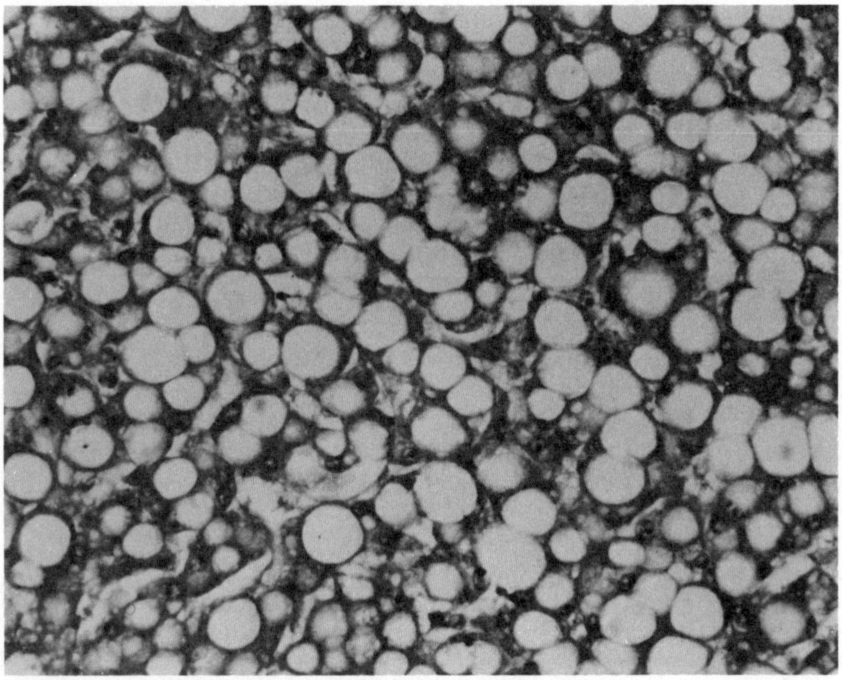

FIGURE 2-1. Fatty change of liver. (Magnification before reduction: x400) (From F. Miller, *Peery and Miller's Pathology* (3rd ed.). Boston: Little, Brown, 1978.)

lar swelling, lipid accumulation in organs, glycogen depositions, pigments, calcification, and hyaline infiltration. These are the most common changes in and around cells resulting from abnormal stimulation.

Cellular Swelling

Cellular swelling is a response of the cell to disruption of cellular metabolism, most frequently seen when the ability of the cell to synthesize adenosine triphosphate (ATP) is impaired. It results in increased cytoplasmic water and a cloudy intracellular swelling with enlargement of the cells. Ultimately, organs are affected. Cellular swelling is frequently reversible when sufficient oxygen is delivered to the cell and normal ATP synthesis resumes. *Hydropic degeneration* is a more severe form of cellular swelling in which much of the cytoplasm is occupied by small or large vacuoles of water [1].

Lipid Accumulation

This condition refers to a *fatty change process* that occurs within the cytoplasm of parenchymal cells of certain organs. Fat droplets accumulate as a result of improper metabolism and most commonly are seen in degenerative liver conditions. The heart and kidney also can undergo fatty change when placed under abnormal stimulation.

Large, fatty intracellular accumulations have been shown to stimulate progressive necrosis, fibrosis, and scarring of organs. This leads to functional impairment of the involved organ (Fig. 2-1).

Because fatty change of the liver is very common, this condition will be further described. Pathologically, the liver is enlarged, yellow, greasy in appearance, and infiltration may be seen to involve all or only a portion of the organ [1]. Microscopically, the cytoplasm may be filled with lipid, which pushes the nucleus and other cytoplasmic structures to one side. The predominant lipid involved in fatty change of the liver is triglyceride, which may be a result of increased synthesis of triglyceride or decreased secretion of this lipid from the cell. This fatty change is the initial change seen in the alcoholic liver because alcohol may interfere with the release of lipids from the hepatic cell and may increase the transport of fatty acids from subcutaneous fat to the liver. Other hepatotoxins may also cause this change. The fibrous scarring of cirrhosis, discussed in Chapter 37, appears to result from a reaction to the lipid infiltration in the cytoplasm of hepatocytes.

The heart and kidney also undergo fatty changes under abnormal stimulation. It most commonly occurs in the heart following chronic hypoxia and may be patchy or diffuse. If diffuse, severe infections or toxic states are usually the causative factors. The kidney shows increased fatty change around the proximal convoluted tubule of the nephron and this may be induced by exposure to certain nephrotoxins or poisons.

Associated with intracellular lipid accumulation is *interstitial fatty infiltration,* a condition that is associated with obesity. In this situation there is accumulation of fat cells between the parenchymal cells of an organ, and this probably results from the transformation of interstitial connective tissue cells to fat cells [1]. This condition rarely seems to affect the function of the organ and localizes most frequently in the heart and pancreas of the obese individual. Other effects of obesity involve fat cells laid down during gestation, during the first year of life, and immediately after puberty. The obese child develops an increased number of fat cells that remain for life but decrease in size after dieting [3]. Adult-onset obesity, for the most part, occurs when caloric intake exceeds energy requirements and the excess is converted to fat. Areas of subcutaneous fat distribution are related to hereditary characteristics much like body build or hair color.

Glycogen Depositions

Excess deposition of glycogen in organs and tissues is seen with genetic disorders called *glycogen storage diseases.* Most of these disorders result from specific enzyme deficiencies. Different forms of glycogen accumulate in skeletal and cardiac muscle as well as in the liver and kidneys.

Glycogen disturbances are also found in diabetes mellitus with a greater than normal storage of glycogen in the proximal convoluted tubule and in the liver [5]. This disturbance is related to a deficiency in the pancreatic hormone, insulin.

Pigmentation

Pigments are substances that have color and accumulate within the cells. Many types have been described in the literature but only the most common forms are discussed in this section.

Lipofuscin pigmenting of the skin is common in the aging person. The pigment responsible is *lipofuscin* or *lipochrome,* which is the "wear and tear" pigment and is predominant in cells that have atrophied or are chronically injured [2]. It may be seen in the brain, liver, heart, and ovary of the aged individual. The pigments gradually accumulate with the age of the person and apparently do not cause cellular dysfunction.

Melanin is a pigment that is formed by the melanocytes of the skin. It is one of the pigments that impart color to the skin. It also functions to absorb light and protects the skin from direct sun rays. Excessive deposition of melanin in the skin is common with Addison's disease (see Chap. 31), many skin conditions, and melanomas that arise from these cells. In the aged person, melanocytes are lost and the skin becomes paler.

Hemosiderin, a derivative of hemoglobin, is a pigment that is formed from excess accumulation of storage iron. It is often a hemoglobin-derived substance but also may be formed from excess intake of dietary iron or impaired utilization of iron. Excesses of hemosiderin are found with many pathologic states. One example is the common bruise, which is an accumulation of excess hemosiderin after the erythrocytes in the injured area are broken down by macrophages. The excess hemoglobin thus released becomes hemosiderin. The colors displayed occur as the hemoglobin is transformed first to biliverdin, a green color, then bilirubin, a yellow color, and the golden-yellow hemosiderin [5]. Deposits of hemosiderin in organs and tissues is called *hemosiderosis,* which may be seen with excess of absorbed dietary iron, impaired utilization of the iron, or with the hemolytic anemias [5]. For the most part, accumulation of hemosiderin does not interfere with organ function unless it is extreme. In extreme hemosiderosis, liver fibrosis may result.

Calcification

Pathologic calcification may occur in the skin, the soft tissues, blood vessels, heart, and kidneys. Normally, calcium is deposited only in the bones and teeth under the influence of various hormones. It may precipitate in areas of chronic inflammation or areas of dead or degenerating tissue. Calcium that precipitates into areas of unresolved healing is called *dystrophic calcification* (Fig. 2-2). *Metastatic calcification* results from calcium-phosphorus imbalances associated with excess circulating calcium. Calcium precipitates into many areas including kidneys, blood vessels, and connective tissue.

Hyaline Infiltration

Hyaline is a term used to indicate a characteristic alteration within cells or in the extracellular space that appears as a homogeneous, glassy, pink inclusion on stained histologic section [5]. Because it does not represent a specific pattern of accumulation, different mechanisms are responsible for its formation. Intracellular hyaline change may include excessive amounts of protein, aggregates of immunoglobulin, viral nucleoproteins, closely packed fibrils, or other substances [5]. Extracellular hyaline refers to the appearance of precipitated plasma proteins and other proteins across a membrane wall. This change is particularly well seen in and around the arterioles and the renal glomeruli. A variety of mechanisms causes the hyaline change and the implications of this deposition differ depending on the underlying process.

CELLULAR CHANGES DUE TO INJURIOUS STIMULI

In some cases, cells will undergo an actual change in order to adapt to an injurious agent. The changes often manifested are atrophy, dysplasia, hypertrophy, hyperplasia, and metaplasia. The cellular adaptations are ways in which the cells stay alive and adjust workload to demand.

Atrophy

Atrophy refers to a decrease in cell size resulting from a decreased workload, loss of nerve supply, decreased blood supply, inadequate nutrition, or loss of hormonal stimulation [5]. Atrophy implies previous normal development of

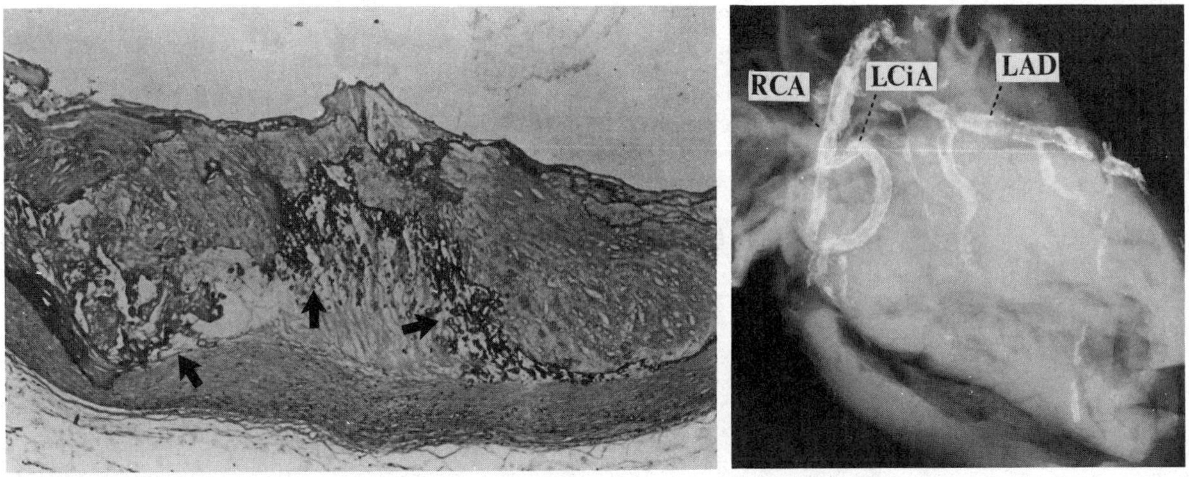

A B

FIGURE 2-2. Calcification. A. Photomicrograph of section of left anterior descending coronary artery. There is marked atheromatous thickening of the intima. Calcification of the wall (*arrows*) is prominent and is found microscopically at autopsy in the coronary arteries of a majority of patients over 60. B. X-ray film of postmortem heart. Dense calcification is visible in virtually all branches of the coronary arteries, including the left anterior descending, the left circumflex, and the right coronary arteries. Note that the lumen in the presence of calcification may be quite adequate, but that in this patient severe atherosclerosis has occluded the distal left anterior descending coronary artery and narrowed multiple branches. (From H. L. Abrams [ed.]. *Coronary Arteriography*. Boston: Little, Brown, 1983.)

the cell and that the cell has lost structural components and substance (Fig. 2-3). Physiologic atrophy occurs with aging in many areas and allows for survival of cells with a decreased function. The cells tend to reproduce less readily. Physiologic atrophy is seen in the thymus gland in adulthood and in the uterus after menopause. Many cells in other glands and muscles also undergo atrophy with aging. Cells may develop an increase in the number of autophagic vacuoles in the cytoplasm that isolate and destroy injured organelles. The triggering mechanism for autophagia is unknown, but it may result in incompletely digested material called *residual* bodies [5]. An example of this is the lipofuscin or brownish pigment seen in the aging cell. Atrophy may progress to cellular injury and death, and the cells may be replaced with connective and/or adipose tissue.

Disuse atrophy is a common occurrence following immobilization of an extremity in a cast. The decreased workload placed on the affected muscles results in a decreased size of the entire muscle. When the workload is again restored, the muscle often enlarges to its preinjury size.

Loss of nerve supply may also cause muscular atrophy. An example of this is the spinal cord injury that interrupts nervous stimulation to the muscles below the level of injury. Atrophy of muscles may also be seen with chronic ischemic disease of the lower extremities. The decreased blood supply impairs the metabolism within the cell and atrophy occurs to keep the tissue viable.

Dysplasia

Dysplasia refers to cells that have undergone some atypical changes in response to chronic irritation. It is not a true adaptive process in that it serves no specific function. Dysplasia is presumably a controlled reproduction of cells, but it is closely related to malignancy in that it may transform into uncontrolled, rapid reproduction. Epithelial cells are the most common types to exhibit dysplasia; cellular changes include alterations in the size and shape of the cells causing loss of normal architectural orientation of one cell with the next. Dysplastic changes most frequently occur in the bronchi of chronic smokers and in the cervix [5].

Hypertrophy

This cellular change refers to an increase in individual cell size, resulting in an increased tissue mass without an increase in the number of cells. It usually represents the response of a specific organ to an increased demand for work. Hypertrophied cells increase their number of organelles, especially the mitochondria. A good example of physiologic hypertrophy is the enlargement of muscles of athletes or weight lifters. The individual muscle cells enlarge but do not proliferate and this provides for increased strength. It is not understood what the limiting factors to hypertrophy are but it may have to do with limitation to the vascular supply or the energy production capabilities of the cells. Hypertrophy may also be pathologic and frequently affects the myocardium (Fig. 2-4).

Hyperplasia

This is a common condition seen in cells that are under an increased physiologic workload or stimulation. Hyperplasia is defined as increase of tissue mass due to an increase

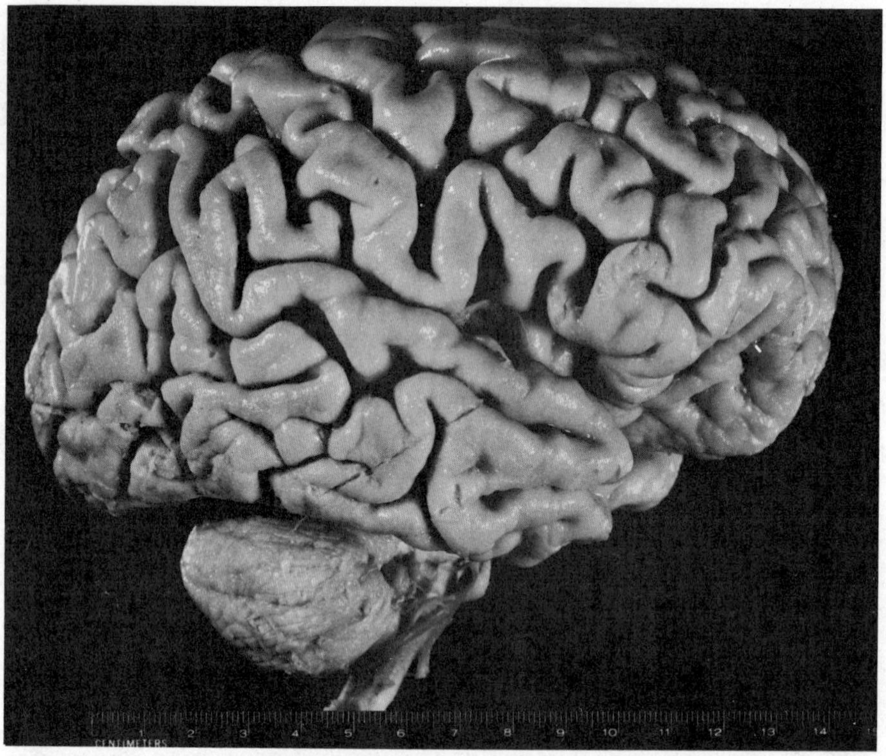

FIGURE 2-3. Atrophy of the cerebral cortex. There has been pronounced shrinking of the rounded folds that normally constitute the brain's outer surface. Severe, generalized shrinkage of this sort is uncommon, and the cause is unknown. So-called senile changes in the brains of most elderly persons are much less severe than the degree of shrinkage shown here. (From F.K. Widmann, *Pathobiology: How Disease Happens.* Boston: Little, Brown, 1978.)

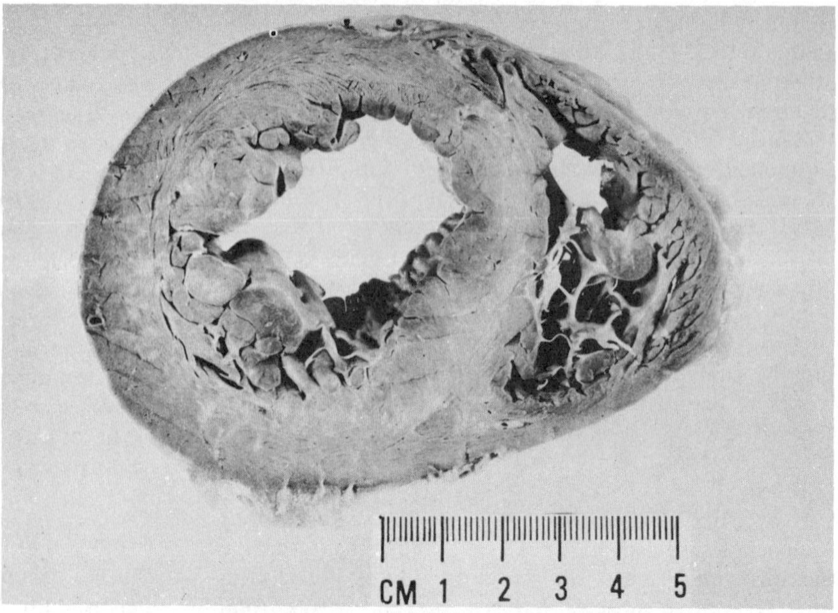

FIGURE 2-4. Hypertrophy of myocardium. (From F. Miller, *Peery and Miller's Pathology* (3rd ed.). Boston: Little, Brown, 1978.)

in the number of cells. Cells that undergo hyperplasia are those that are capable of cell division and thus of increasing their numbers. Whether hyperplasia, rather than hypertrophy, occurs depends on the regenerative capacity of the specific cell.

Physiologic hyperplasia is a normal outcome of puberty and pregnancy. *Compensatory hyperplasia* occurs in organs that are capable of regenerating lost substance. An example is regeneration of the liver when part of its substance is destroyed. *Pathologic hyperplasia* is seen in conditions of abnormal stimulation of organs with cells that are capable of regeneration. Examples of the latter situation are enlargement of the thyroid gland secondary to stimulation by the thyroid-stimulating hormone from the pituitary, and parathyroid hyperplasia due to renal failure (see Chaps. 29, 30, and 32).

Hyperplasia is induced by a known stimulus and almost always stops when the stimulus has been removed. This controlled reproduction is an important differentiating feature of hyperplasia from neoplasia. There is a close relationship between certain types of pathologic hyperplasia and malignancy.

Metaplasia

This condition is a reversible change in which one type of adult cell is replaced by another type. It is probably an adaptive substitution of one cell type, more suited to the hostile environment, by another [5]. Metaplasia is commonly seen in chronic bronchitis; the normal columnar, ciliated goblet cells are replaced by stratified squamous epithelial cells. The latter cells are better suited for survival in the face of chronic, irritating smoke inhalation or environmental pollution. The metaplasia increases the chances of cellular survival but decreases the protective aspect of mucus secretion. Certain types of metaplasia are closely related to malignancy, which probably means that the chronic irritation causes the initial change.

INJURY AND DEATH OF CELLS DUE TO LACK OF OXYGEN

As stated earlier in this chapter, lack of oxygen is the most common cause of cellular injury and death. The following conditions can produce this problem: ischemia, thrombosis, embolism, infarction, necrosis, and somatic death. In some instances the injury is reversible or it may progress to a permanent, lethal change.

Ischemia

Ischemia refers to a critical lack of blood supply to a localized area. It is reversible in that tissues will be restored to normal function when oxygen is again supplied to them. Ischemia may precede infarction or death of the tissue or it may occur sporadically when the oxygen need outstrips the oxygen supply. It is important to differentiate between ischemia, a clinical change, and infarction, a pathologic change.

Ischemia usually occurs in the presence of atherosclerosis in the major arteries. Atherosclerosis, more fully described in Unit 8, is a lipid-depositing process with fibrofatty accumulations, or plaques, on the intimal layers of the artery. The medial layer of the artery may also become involved, predisposing it to atherosclerotic aneurysm formation. Atherosclerosis often gives rise to the formation of clots or thrombi on the plaque. All of this compromises blood flow through the artery, which then impairs oxygen supply during increased need. In the later stages there is impairment to blood supply even at rest. The classic conditions resulting from ischemia are angina pectoris and intermittent claudication. The former refers to ischemia affecting the heart and the latter refers to ischemia of the lower extremities on exertion. Ischemia is often relieved by rest and the tissues return to normal function. Ischemia may progress to *ischemic infarction,* which involves cell death due to lack of blood supply or oxygen. Lack of oxygen supply to the brain, heart, and kidney can be tolerated for only a few minutes before irreversible damage occurs. The fibroblasts of connective tissue, however, have been shown to survive for up to 2 weeks without oxygen [4].

Ischemia also has been shown to occur following vasospasm of coronary arteries or other vessels that are unaffected by atherosclerosis. Vasospasm may be induced by nicotine, exposure to cold, and in some cases, stress.

Thrombosis

This term refers to the formation of a clot in the intimal lining of the blood vessels or the heart. It may decrease blood flow through the vessel or totally occlude it.

The most common factor in thrombosis is disruption of the endothelial lining of the blood vessels and heart. This endothelial layer is continuous from the heart to the arteries to the capillaries to the veins and back to the heart. When trauma, atherosclerosis, or other factors disrupt this layer, platelets may accumulate and the intrinsic clotting mechanism is initiated. The body spontaneously initiates its fibrinolytic system to dissolve the clot and reopen the vessel. This may or may not be successful in reestablishing the flow of blood. Stasis of blood and increased blood viscosity also enhance coagulability of blood (Fig. 2-5).

Thrombosis most frequently occurs in the deep veins of the legs but mural thrombosis may occur on the endocardial lining of the heart. If this thrombosis occurs in the left ventricle, the risk for arterial embolization is quite high (Fig. 2-6). Thrombosis in an artery can disrupt blood flow to the area supplied by the vessel causing ischemia or infarction. Thrombosis in the deep veins may embolize and lodge in the pulmonary circuit.

Embolism

A thrombus may break off and become a traveling mass in the blood, which is called *embolization.* The most common types of emboli are derived from thrombi, but other substances such as fat, vegetations from valves, or foreign

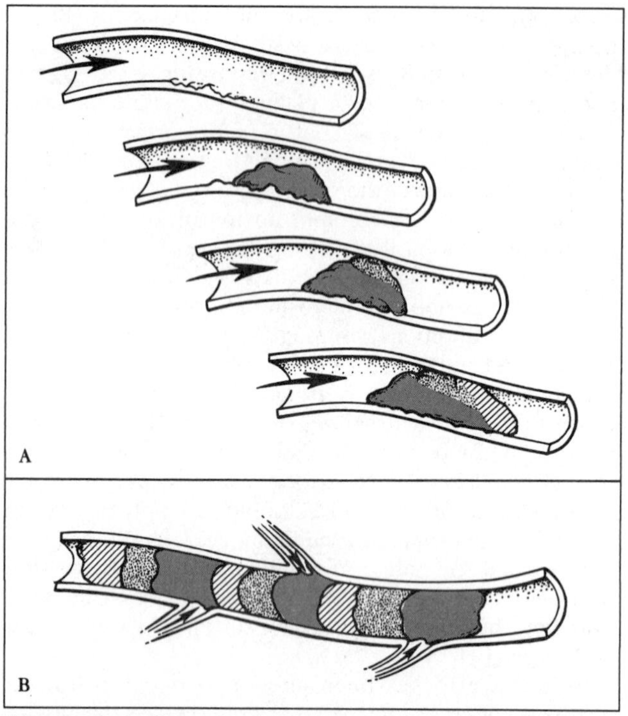

FIGURE 2-5. A. Stages in the development of phlebothrombosis: (1) intimal damage, sluggish circulation; (2) platelet aggregation; (3) occlusion of the lumen of the vein; (4) blood clot propagates. B. Clot propagates clot at each point of entry of the small veins.

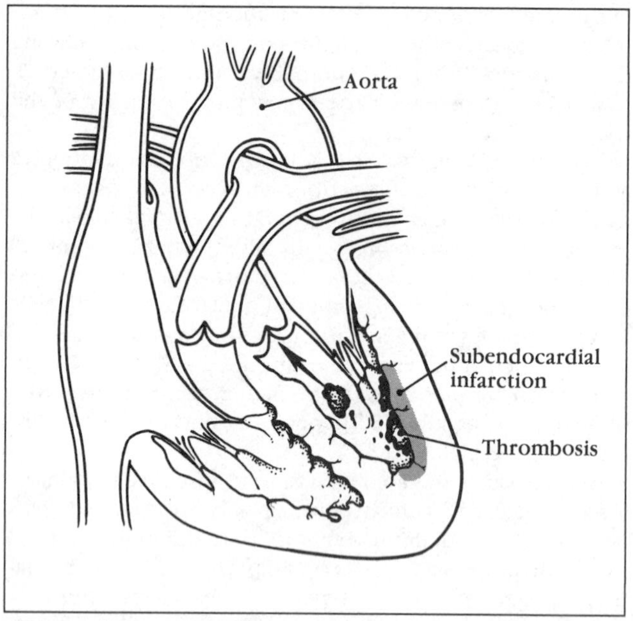

FIGURE 2-6. Disruption of the endocardial surface, such as that following a subendocardial infarction, may lead to a thrombosis that may become an arterial embolus.

particles may embolize. The obstruction caused by an embolus is termed *embolism*.

If the embolus arises in the venous circuit, it will be carried to and trapped in the vasculature of the pulmonary capillary bed. Depending on the size of the embolus, a varying clinical picture may be seen (see Chap. 25).

If the embolus arises in the left side of the heart, it may travel to any of the arteries branching off the aorta. Arterial embolism may also occur from a larger artery, such as one affected by atherosclerosis, to a smaller artery and it again compromises blood flow to the area.

Infarction

Occlusion of the blood supply of an artery causes *infarction*. This term refers to a localized area of tissue death due to lack of blood supply. It usually refers to ischemic necrosis and may occur in any organ or tissue.

Infarcts may cause different pathologic characteristics. They are frequently classified as *pale infarcts, hemorrhagic infarcts,* and *infarcts with bacterial supergrowth. Pale infarcts* are seen in solid tissue deprived of its arterial circulation as a result of ischemia. *Red* or *hemorrhagic infarcts* are seen more frequently with venous occlusion or with congested tissues. The infarcted tissue has a red appearance that may be poorly defined, causing difficulty in differentiating viable and nonviable tissue [5]. *Bacterial supergrowth* is common and may be present in the area or

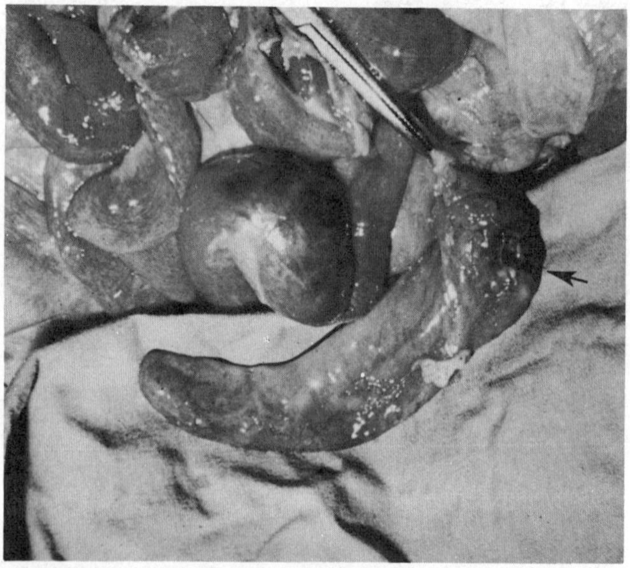

FIGURE 2-7. Acute gangrenous appendicitis with perforation. (From F. Miller, *Peery and Miller's Pathology* [3rd ed.]. Boston: Little, Brown, 1978.)

may be brought to the area. The lesion is converted to an abscess when it is septic and the inflammatory response is initiated. Gangrene is an example of infarction in which the ischemic cell death is followed by bacterial overgrowth leading to liquefaction of the tissues (Fig. 2-7). This term is frequently used to describe conditions of the extremities and the bowel.

Necrosis

The term *necrosis* refers to cell or tissue death causing characteristic cellular changes. As cells die, the mitochondria swell, functions become disrupted, membranes rupture, and the lysosomes may be released into the tissues [4]. The nucleus undergoes specific changes that may include shrinking, fragmenting, or gradual fading [1]. Necrosis is commonly described in terms of the following three patterns: coagulative, caseous, and liquefactive necrosis.

Coagulative necrosis results from lack of blood supply to an area. It is seen most frequently in organs such as the heart and kidney, or may result from chemical injury. In this type of necrosis, the architectural outline of the dead cell is preserved but the nucleus is lost. Eventually, the necrotic cell is removed by phagocytosis.

Caseous necrosis has long been described in relation to tuberculosis, but may be seen in a few other conditions. The central area of necrosis is soft and friable and this is surrounded by an area exhibiting a cheesy, crumbly appearance. The cellular architecture is destroyed. The area is walled off from the rest of the body and may become rimmed with calcium. Areas of caseous necrosis may localize in areas of tuberculous infestation.

Liquefactive necrosis is a pattern of necrosis most frequently seen in the brain tissue and results from fatal injury of the neuron. The breakdown of the neuron causes release of lysosomes and other constituents into the surrounding area. Lysosomes cause liquefaction of the cell and surrounding cells leaving pockets of liquid, debris, and cystlike structures. Liquefactive necrosis is most frequently described in brain infarction but also may be seen with bacterial lesions because of the release of bacterial and leukocytic enzymes [5].

Somatic Death

Death of the body occurs with the cessation of respiratory and cardiac function. The individual cells remain alive for differing periods of time, but irreversible changes occur and some of these make it difficult to determine exact premortem pathology. Postmortem changes include rigor mortis, livor mortis, algor mortis, intravascular clotting, autolysis, and putrefaction.

Rigor mortis develops because of depletion of ATP in the muscles, beginning in the involuntary muscles and in 2 to 4 hours affecting the voluntary muscles. The result is stiffening of the muscles and the onset and disappearance is variable with different individuals [1].

Livor mortis is the reddish-blue discoloration of the body that results from the gravitational pooling of blood [1].

Algor mortis is the term used for the cooling of the body that occurs after death. The rate of cooling depends on the premortem temperature and the postmortem environmental temperature [1].

Intravascular clotting results in a clot that is not adherent to the lining of the blood vessels and heart. These clots may be layered in appearance with streaks or layers of yellowish, fatty material [1].

Autolysis refers to the digestion of tissues from released substances such as enzymes and lysosomes. Organs may be swollen and spongy in appearance [1].

Putrefaction results from saprophytic organisms entering the dead body, usually from the intestines. This results in a greenish discoloration of the tissues and organs and the organisms may produce gases leading to foamy or spongy organs [1].

REFERENCES

1. Anderson, W. A. D., and Scotti, T. M. *Synopsis of Pathology* (10th ed.). St. Louis: Mosby, 1980.
2. Burnside, I. *Nursing and the Aged* (2nd ed.). New York: McGraw-Hill, 1981.
3. Luckmann, J., and Sorensen, K. *Medical-Surgical Nursing* (2nd ed.). Philadelphia: Saunders, 1980.
4. Purtillo, D. *A Survey of Human Disease.* Reading, Mass.: Addison-Wesley, 1978.
5. Robbins, S., and Cotran, R. *Pathologic Basis of Disease* (2nd ed.). Philadelphia: Saunders, 1979.

BIBLIOGRAPHY

Anderson, W. A. D., and Scotti, T. M. *Synopsis of Pathology* (10th ed.). St. Louis: Mosby, 1980.

Boyd, W., and Sheldon, H. *An Introduction to the Study of Disease* (7th ed.). Philadelphia: Lea & Febiger, 1977.

Brunner, L., and Suddarth, D. *Textbook of Medical Surgical Nursing* (4th ed.). Philadelphia: Lippincott, 1980.

Burnside, I. *Nursing and the Aged* (2nd ed.). New York: McGraw-Hill, 1981.

DeCoursey, R. *The Human Organism* (4th ed.). New York: McGraw-Hill, 1974.

Eccles, J. *The Understanding of the Brain.* New York: McGraw-Hill, 1973.

Frohlich, E. *Pathophysiology* (2nd ed.). Philadelphia: Lippincott, 1976.

Gilbert, E., and Huntington, R. W. *An Introduction to Pathology.* New York: Oxford University Press, 1978.

Gröer, M., and Shekleton, M. *Basic Pathophysiology: A Conceptual Approach.* St. Louis: Mosby, 1979.

Guyton, A. C. *Textbook of Medical Physiology* (6th ed.). Philadelphia: Saunders, 1981.

Isselbacher, K., et al. (eds.). *Harrison's Principles of Internal Medicine* (9th ed.). New York: McGraw-Hill, 1980.

Jensen, D. *The Principles of Physiology* (2nd ed.). New York: Appleton-Century-Crofts, 1980.

Lechtman, M., Roohk, B., and Egan, R. *The Games Cells Play.* Menlo Park, Calif.: Benjamin-Cummings, 1979.

Luckmann, J., and Sorensen, K. *Medical-Surgical Nursing* (2nd ed.). Philadelphia: Saunders, 1980.

Macleod, A. G. *Scope Monograph on Cytology.* Kalamazoo, Mich.: The Upjohn Co., 1972.

Muir, B. *Pathophysiology: An Introduction to the Mechanisms of Disease.* New York: Wiley, 1980.

Noback, C., and Demarest, R. *The Human Nervous System* (2nd ed.). New York: McGraw-Hill, 1975.

Price, S., and Wilson, L. *Pathophysiology: Clinical Concepts of Disease Processes* (2nd ed.). New York: McGraw-Hill, 1982.

Purtillo, D. *A Survey of Human Diseases.* Reading, Mass.: Addison-Wesley, 1978.

Robbins, S., and Cotran, R. *Pathologic Basis of Disease* (2nd ed.). Philadelphia: Saunders, 1979.

Selkurt, E. *Basic Physiology for the Health Sciences* (2nd ed.). Boston: Little, Brown, 1982.

Snell, R. S. *Clinical Anatomy for Medical Students* (2nd ed.). Boston: Little, Brown, 1981.

Snell, R. S. *Clinical Histology for Medical Students.* Boston: Little, Brown, 1984.

Snell, R. S. *Clinical Neuroanatomy for Medical Students.* Boston: Little, Brown, 1980.

Spence, A., and Mason, E. B. *Human Anatomy and Physiology.* Menlo Park, Calif.: Benjamin-Cummings, 1979.

Stephens, G. J. *Pathophysiology for Health Practitioners.* New York: Macmillan, 1980.

Tortora, G., Evans, R., and Anagnostakos, N. *Principles of Human Physiology.* Philadelphia: Harper & Row, 1982.

Walter, J. B. *An Introduction to the Principles of Disease* (2nd ed.). Philadelphia: Saunders, 1982.

UNIT 2
STRESS

Barbara L. Bullock
PHYSIOLOGIC EFFECTS OF STRESS
STRESS AND DISEASE

Janet B. Gelein
GENERAL SYSTEMS THEORY
GENERAL ADAPTATION SYNDROME

This unit contains two chapters that describe the physiologic response of the body to stress and how the stress response can cause disease. The general systems theory is utilized as the framework for understanding the physiologic effects of stress. Chapter 3 also describes adaptation that allows the body to withstand the stressors in response to tension-producing stimuli. This response occurs until a critical point is reached and exhaustion begins. The susceptibility of the individual to stress effects is related to the critical point at which these effects can cause actual disease development. Chapter 4 deals with some of the disease processes that are directly or indirectly related to stress effects. It is an introduction to the effects of stress in the production of disease; further information can be found in the unit bibliography. The reader is encouraged to be guided by learning objectives at the beginning of each chapter.

CHAPTER 3
PHYSIOLOGIC EFFECTS OF STRESS

LEARNING OBJECTIVES

1. Describe the general systems theory.
2. Compare and contrast open and closed systems.
3. Illustrate examples of negative and positive feedback.
4. Clearly define the terms *stress* and *stressors.*
5. Describe the general adaptation syndrome according to Hans Selye's studies.
6. Explain the chemical and hormonal mediators important in the stress response.
7. Differentiate between the general and local adaptation syndromes.
8. Define the terms *adaptation* and *compensation.*
9. Describe the three physiologic mechanisms that respond to the stress stimulation.

In considering factors that cause alterations to health, it is important to realize that other variables besides direct biologic phenomena frequently cause disease or dysfunction. Chapter 4 deals with some of the disease processes that are directly and indirectly related to stress. The physiologic factors concerning stress are considered in this chapter and the general systems theory is utilized as a framework to facilitate understanding.

GENERAL SYSTEMS THEORY

It is appropriate to review the systems theory in order to explain the physiologic reaction of the body to stress. Indeed, the open, physiologic organism utilizes relationships between its component parts to achieve a state of equilibrium or a steady state.

The general systems theory is a model for organizing and examining relationships between units. It describes *closed systems* as those that do not interact or exchange energy with their environments. The sciences of physics and physical chemistry are limited to the examination of closed systems. Conversely, *open systems* do exchange matter, energy, and information with their environments [5]. A dynamic equilibrium is achieved, which is called the *steady state,* a relative state of balance. It exists when the composition of the system is constant, despite continuous exchange of components. The three fundamental qualities of open systems are *structure, process,* and *function. Structure* refers to the arrangement of all defined elements at a given point in time. *Process* is the transformation of matter, energy, and information between the system and the environment. *Function* relates to the unique manner that each open system utilizes to achieve its required end [2].

A feedback scheme is used to describe the fundamental qualities of open systems. This means that if a factor becomes excessive or inadequate in the body, initiation of alterations in function will occur to decrease or increase that factor to bring it to normal range. The processes used in this scheme include input, throughput, output, and feedback.

Input is the energy, matter, or information absorbed by the system. *Throughput* is the transformation of this energy into useful information, matter, or energy that is utilized by the system. The excess information, matter, or energy is discharged to the environment in a process called *output.*

Feedback, an essential component, is the process of self-regulation by which open systems determine and control the amount of input and output in the system. The two types of feedback are called *negative* and *positive feedback. Negative feedback* refers to a process of returning to the steady state while *positive feedback* indicates movement away from the steady state [2]. In the human body, then, negative feedback indicates a return to the balanced steady state and positive feedback, unchecked, will lead to death. In the human organism, negative feedback can be easily illustrated by many functions (Fig. 3-1). Loss of hormonal controls, for example, cause disease states because the response of the body is detrimental to the organism.

Decreased circulating thyroid hormone
↓
Increased secretion of hypothalamic thyrotrophic hormone-releasing factor (TRF)
↓
Stimulation of anterior pituitary for increased synthesis of thyroid-stimulating hormone (TSH)
↓
Stimulation of thyroid gland to increase synthesis and secretion of thyroid hormone
↓
Increased levels of circulating thyroid hormone
↓
Decreased secretion of TRF
↓
Decreased secretion of TSH
↓
Decreased secretion of thyroid hormone (→ back to top)

FIGURE 3-1. Feedback system illustrating functions that keep the circulating thyroid hormone in balance.

In considering the open systems theory, one must enlarge the perspective beyond the physiologic and pathophysiologic basis. The individual, as a system, has physiologic, psychosocial, environmental, and other stresses, which are illustrated in Figure 3-2. These factors may join to produce a diseased or altered state or they may have the opposite effect, one of reinforcing adaptive behavior.

STRESS AND ADAPTATION IN THE HUMAN BODY

The study of the effects of stress on the human body was pioneered by Hans Selye. He studied the nonspecific response of the body to a demand and noted differences in individual abilities to withstand the same demands. He defined *stress* as a specific syndrome that is nonspecifically induced. He also defined *stressors* as tension-producing stimuli that potentially could cause disequilibrium. The perception of the significance of the stressor is important and varies among different persons. It is believed that psychologic stressors have as great an impact on disease states as physical stressors. Selye noted that laboratory animals reacted to different stressors, physiologically, by enlargement of the adrenal cortex, atrophy of the thymus gland, and development of gastric ulcers. Further study has revealed a pattern including fatigue, loss of appetite, joint pains, gastric upset, and other similar nonspecific complaints.

Selye noted a similarity in sickness patterns, which he called, at first, "the syndrome of just being sick" and later described as the *general adaptation syndrome (GAS)* [3].

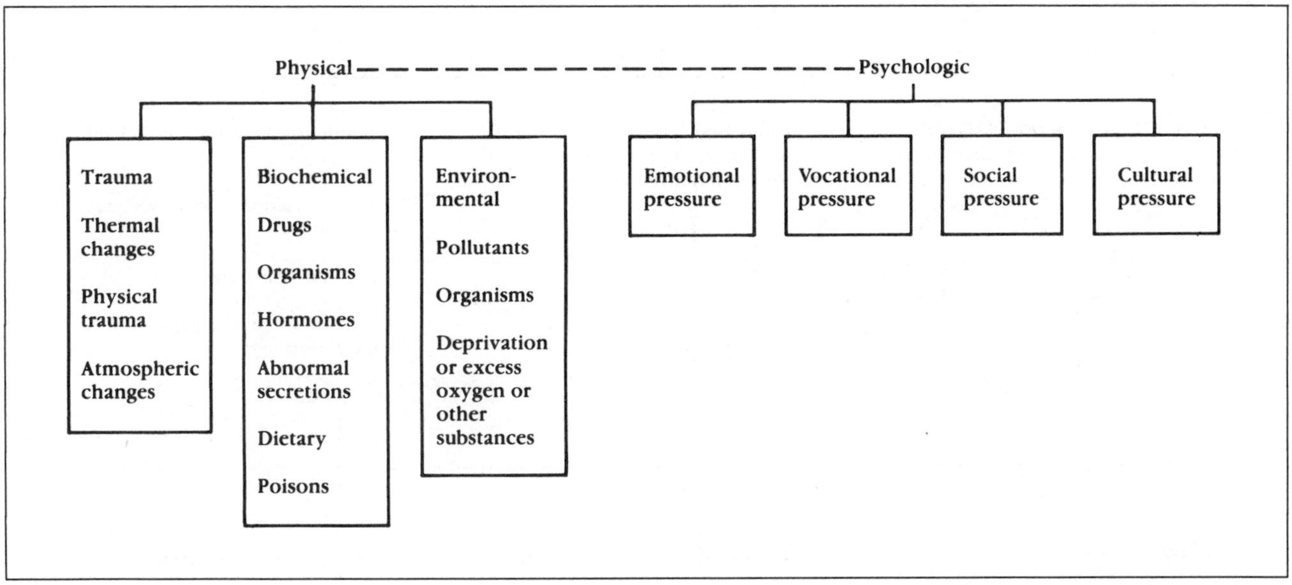

FIGURE 3-2. Stressors. This chart illustrates types of stimuli that can provoke the stress response.

The GAS may be elicited by a variety of stimuli or stressors and may be of a physiologic, psychogenic, sociocultural, or environmental nature, or it may be from any grouping of these categories. It is described in the following three stages: (1) alarm reaction, (2) stage of resistance, and (3) stage of exhaustion.

In the *alarm stage,* the defensive abilities of the body are mobilized. The "fight or flight" mechanism is activated, mainly through the sympathetic nervous system, which releases two catecholamines, norepinephrine and epinephrine. The physiologic action of these hormones causes vasoconstriction, increased blood pressure, and increased rate and force of cardiac contraction. All of these physiologic actions prepare the body for an assault.

In the *stage of resistance,* the corticosteroids, thyroid hormones, and aldosterone are increased. The adrenal cortex enlarges and becomes hyperactive. The result of this process increases blood sugar for available energy and stabilizes the inflammatory response. In this period, the immune system becomes depressed causing a suppression of T cells and atrophy of the thymus, which leads to a depression of primary antigen-antibody response, due either to a hypothalamus response or excess corticosteroids. The end result, immunologically, is suppression and atrophy of immune tissue (see Unit 5). If infection is present it will lead to delayed clearing of the organisms and delayed healing.

If stage 3, *exhaustion,* occurs, it will lead to a depletion of resistance to the stressor and ultimately to death, frequently caused by the lack of immunologic defense. This would be considered an immunodeficiency secondary to stress. Selye proposes that *exhaustion* is a correct term for aging, a wearing down of the human body from lifelong stress [3]. This theory is supported in some studies and contested in others. Figure 3-3 summarizes the three stages of the GAS.

Localized reaction to stressors is called the *local adaptation syndrome (LAS),* which is well illustrated by the process of inflammation. The LAS follows the same general pattern as the GAS with an acute phase followed by a resistance phase and exhaustion, which allows for spreading of the localized process and a generalized response.

ADAPTATION

Adaptation is defined as a person's positive response to a changing environment. It refers to adjustments that are made as a result of stimulation or change with the end result of modifying the original situation. Adaptive responses are a type of negative feedback that keep the organism in the steady state. Physiologic adaptation refers to the adjustments made by the organs and systems to stress or physiologic disruption. This response is often termed *compensation* for abnormal stimuli. Maladaptation is disruptive or tending toward positive feedback, a disordering of the physiologic response.

ORGAN AND SYSTEM FUNCTION IN MAINTAINING THE STEADY STATE

Three physiologic mechanisms respond to the stress stimuli and can be classified into the following: neurologic, endocrine, and immunologic. These mechanisms work together to react with the stressor or stressors.

Neurologic Mechanisms

Both the voluntary and autonomic divisions of the nervous system are reactive to stress. The voluntary system is mediated through the cerebral cortex, which is responsive

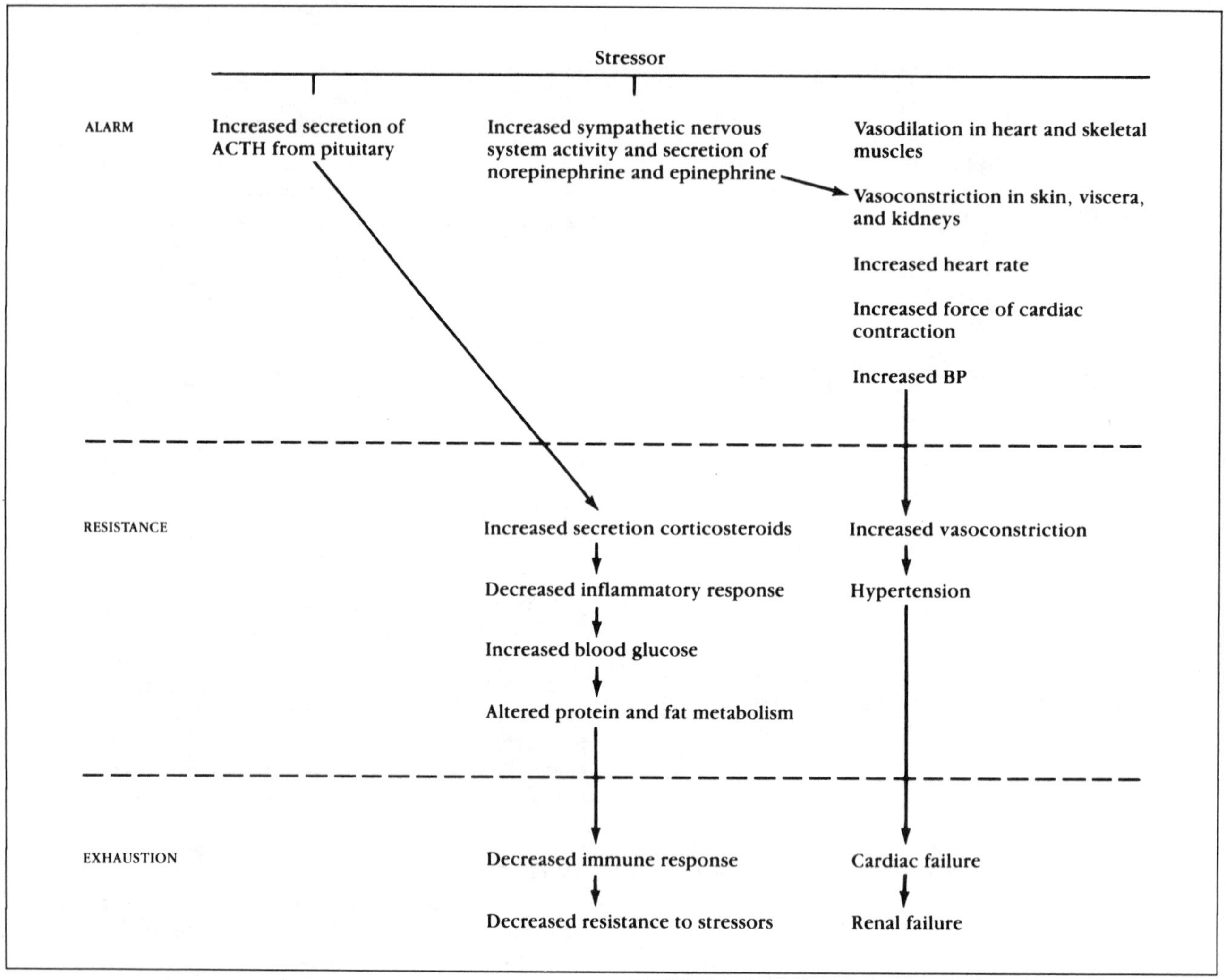

FIGURE 3-3. Stages in Selye's general adaptation syndrome.

to the stimulus. The cerebral cortex directs the muscles to move to avoid danger and effects the flight response. The autonomic nervous system (ANS) is involuntary and is regulated through the hypothalamus. In the stress response, stimulation of the sympathetic nervous system (SNS) occurs, which causes an increased heart rate, constriction of many arterioles, increased respiratory rate, bronchial dilatation, dilatation of the pupils, and inhibition of the gastrointestinal tract.

Two hormones, epinephrine and norepinephrine, are necessary components of the stress response. Epinephrine and norepinephrine are synthesized in the adrenal medulla and released when the sympathetic nervous system is activated. Norepinephrine is also synthesized and secreted at adrenergic (sympathetic) nerve terminals throughout the body and is directly released when the SNS is stimulated. These hormones are classified as *catecholamines*, and circulating levels can be measured in the urine and bloodstream (see Chap. 31). Epinephrine is excreted rapidly in the urine after being biotransformed in the liver. Norepinephrine, liberated at the axon ending, is actively taken up, restored, or biotransformed here.

Epinephrine has as its primary action an increased rate and force of cardiac contraction. It is secreted in the stress response from the SNS stimulation of the adrenal medulla [4]. It is interesting to note that epinephrine is a potent stimulus for glycogenolysis in the liver, which leads to an increased blood glucose level [1].

Norepinephrine is secreted in small quantities in the flight-or-fight response and in acute physical or mental stress. Studies have shown a constant increase in norepinephrine levels in individuals under chronic, unremitting stress. Individuals affected often feel a sense of loss of control over their lives [2]. Norepinephrine exerts its primary control over the arterioles leading to intense vasoconstriction and increased peripheral vascular resistance (PVR), causing an increased blood pressure and increased cardiac workload (Fig. 3-4).

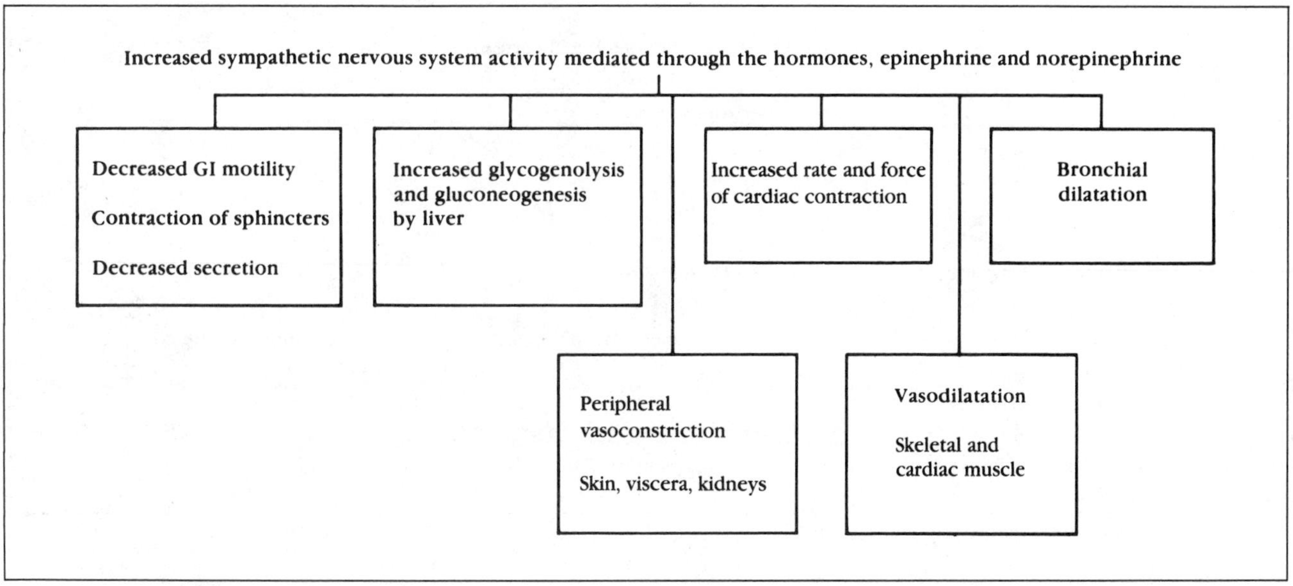

FIGURE 3-4. Sympathetic nervous system response to stress.

Endocrine Mechanisms

The hormones are increased in the stress response through hypothalamic stimulation of the pituitary leading to stimulation of target organ secretion. The relationship is illustrated in Figure 3-5. Stimulation of the pituitary can increase secretion of the adrenocorticotrophic hormone (ACTH), the antidiuretic hormone (ADH), the thyroid stimulating hormone (TSH), and others. Secretion of aldosterone is also increased from the adrenal cortex.

ACTH. The target organ of ACTH is the adrenal gland. Stimulation from this hormone causes an increased synthesis of the glucocorticoids, especially cortisol, cortisone, and small amounts of hydrocortisone. These substances function to increase serum glucose and to metabolize carbohydrates, fat, and protein. The glucocorticoids are normally thought to be synchronized by light. During sleep, the blood and urine concentration decreases and rises to its highest levels in the early morning. This pattern of glucocorticoid secretion follows a particular rhythm called the *circadian rhythm* or *pattern.* The early morning rise drops about 10 A.M., increases again about 2 P.M., and gradually declines until 10 P.M. Changes in circadian rhythms may relate to illness in that phase relationships seem to be consistent in particular maladies. One example is that of persons with peptic ulcer disease who frequently have increased gastric acid secretion causing pain in the late night or early morning hours. Low blood levels of glucocorticoids increase the sensitivity to sounds, tastes, and smells.

TSH. The stress response increases the secretion of TSH from the anterior pituitary, which leads to an increased synthesis and secretion of the thyroid hormones and an increased basal metabolism rate (BMR). The thyroid

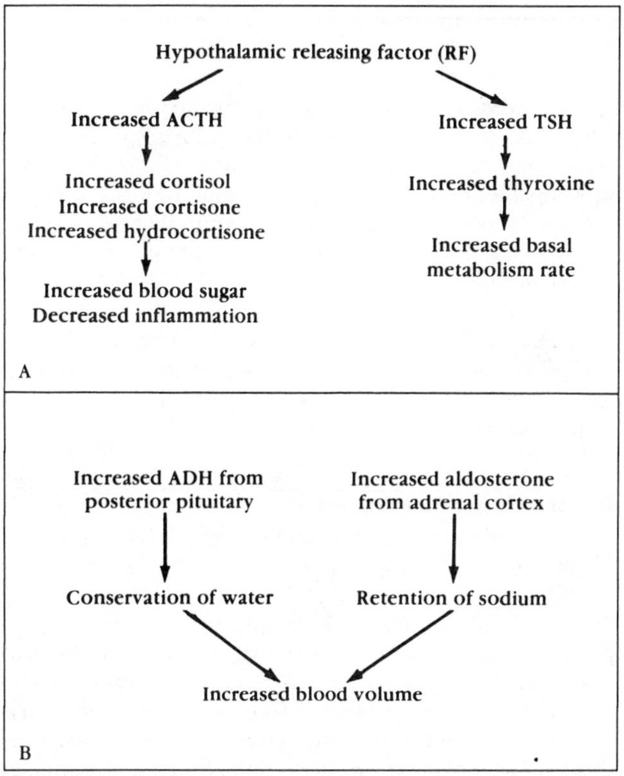

FIGURE 3-5. A. Effects of stress on hypothalamic-pituitary-target organ axis. B. Related hormonal effects of stress, possibly due to sympathetic stimulation.

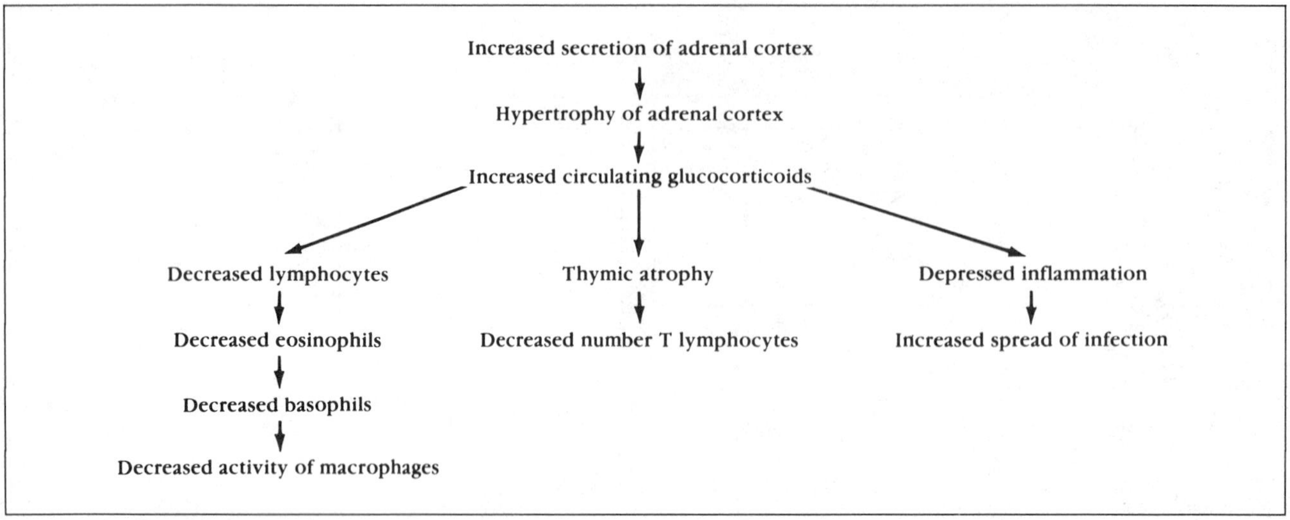

FIGURE 3-6. Effects of stress on the immune system.

hormone, thyroxine, apparently makes the body more responsive to the effects of epinephrine. It is believed that epinephrine is the more efficient responder in short-term stress while thyroxine works when stress is prolonged.

ALDOSTERONE. This is the major mineralocorticoid of the adrenal cortex. It is increased in the stress response, possibly as a result of increased renin secretion or as a response to sympathetic stimulation. Aldosterone increases the retention of sodium and water and thus increases blood volume. See Chapter 31 for further discussion of this important hormone.

ADH. The antidiuretic hormone is released from the posterior pituitary following the stress stimulus. ADH then acts on the renal tubules to conserve water, which leads, in turn, to an increased blood volume.

Immunologic Mechanisms

The effect of stress on the immune system has been the target of much study in recent years. The reader is referred to the bibliography at the end of this unit for a detailed listing of related material for further study. In general, stress apparently lowers the body's defense and this may be partially due to increased corticosteroid production. There have been studies on the relationship of the central nervous system and the immune system that tend to support the connection between the hypothalamus and immunosuppression. Immunosuppression occurs as a result of the increased corticosteroid secretion.

The end result of the stress response is acceleration of the normal atrophy of the thymus gland in the adult. The T cells, normally processed and matured in the thymus gland, are decreased so the body cannot recognize and process antigen as effectively as it can during the prestress period (Fig. 3-6).

REFERENCES

1. Guyton, A. C. *Textbook of Medical Physiology* (6th ed.). Philadelphia: Saunders, 1981. Chap. 57.
2. Miller, J. Living Systems: Basic Concepts. In W. Gray, et al., *General Systems Theory and Psychiatry.* Boston: Little, Brown, 1969. Pp. 51–133.
3. Selye, H. *The Stress of Life.* New York: McGraw-Hill, 1956.
4. Usdin, E., Kvetnansky, R., and Kopin, I. *Catecholamines and Stress: Recent Advances.* New York: Elsevier, 1980.
5. von Bertalanffy, L. *General Systems Theory.* New York: Brazille, 1968.

CHAPTER 4
STRESS AND DISEASE

LEARNING OBJECTIVES

1. Identify factors that increase the risk of disease.
2. Define *genetic susceptibility*.
3. Briefly explain the weak organ theory.
4. Identify examples of unhealthful behaviors.
5. Describe and give examples of how personalities and attitudes can contribute to development of disease.
6. Relate diet and stressful living conditions to coronary artery disease.
7. Briefly explain catecholamine effect on lipids.
8. State Pelletier's theory on the relationship of stress and blood pressure.
9. Define the *type A personality*.
10. Describe the effect of stress on the immune system.
11. Relate stress to activation of malignancy.
12. Relate stress to the development of stress, duodenal, and gastric ulcers.

Many studies have been conducted to relate stress effects with actual disease development. Psychologic and physical stressors have been studied correlating personality traits, genetic predisposition, environmental, emotional, occupational, and social factors with specific diseases.

Some similarities in disease development have been noted around such concepts as the weak or target organ theory; driving or submissive personality traits; chronic, excessive, unrelenting stress factors; and/or environmental alterations. With the caution that these areas are under study, this chapter describes some of the relationships between physical and/or psychologic stress and specific disease phenomena. Several of the prominent stress-related diseases are presented.

FACTORS RELATED TO DEVELOPMENT OF DISEASE

A maladaptive response of the body to stressors increases the risk of disease development. Factors that increase the risk of disease include one or a combination of the following: (1) biologic predisposition, (2) weak organ theory, (3) unhealthful behaviors, and (4) personalities and attitudes toward life. Each of these areas can be influenced by the amount of physical and/or emotional stress placed on the individual at one time.

Biologic Predisposition

Stressors of sufficient strength or intensity can cause an alteration in normal functioning of the body. If one has a genetic or hereditary susceptibility to the stressors, the alteration may be manifested as disease.

Genetic susceptibility refers to a myriad of conditions that "run in the family" and seem to make the individual react in a particular way to certain stressors. A common example is an exaggerated allergic response that predisposes members of families to specific pollens. When the pollen count is seasonally high, these persons will suffer different types of allergic responses. In this example, the stressor is the pollen count but the response is heightened by a hyperactive, hereditary immune reaction (see Chap. 11).

Many other diseases seem to be familial in nature, and development of actual disease may or may not require additional stressors to trigger the process. Coronary artery disease may develop in an individual with or without the associated risk factors of obesity, type A personality, hypertension, or others.

Weak Organ Theory

The weak organ theory is associated with hereditary factors. In different individuals, not all organs seem to be equally resistant to stressors. Some individuals under equal stress conditions will develop cardiovascular disorders, while others will develop peptic ulcers. Still others may suffer migraine headaches or other maladies. Why some persons have the heart as the target organ, while others target the stomach or other organs, is not known. It is known that a variety of ailments is induced, or at least aggravated, by stressful living conditions. In some cases, the major cause of the disease is not stress, but stress precipitates complications and intensity of the disease.

Unhealthful Behaviors

Some examples of unhealthful behaviors as stressors include the following: overeating, excessive alcohol intake, smoking, drug abuse, and lack of exercise. The unhealthful behavior is a destructive force that serves as the stressor and development of disease is correlated with the behavior. Disease does not always occur and individuals with high stressor levels due to destructive behavior may have no residual health problems. More frequently, when a person actually develops the related disease, a pattern of behavior emerges that includes a combination of other risk factors. An example of this is coronary artery disease with the combination of family history, obesity, high blood pressure, and smoking as major risk factors.

Personalities and Attitudes Toward Life

Of great interest in recent studies is the relationship between attitude and health. Social isolation, such as is often seen in the aged person, correlates with an increase in chronic disease. Children who are not loved and fondled after birth fail to thrive. The opposite effect may be seen when persons with a high number of risk factors have strong support groups and develop disease significantly less often than the general population with the same risk factors [11].

Faith and hope, as personality factors, have been studied in relation to cancer prognosis. A dramatic example cited by Bruno Klopfer illustrated that a person with far advanced malignancy, who believed that the injections he received would significantly alleviate his cancer, showed much improvement both in tumor size and clinical condition. This individual had hope that the tumor treatment would cure him, and actual improvement occurred even though the treatment consisted of injections of sterile water [4].

In a study of cervical dysplasia, the personality trait of hopelessness was studied in order to predict which of the women would actually have cancer. The predictions made on the basis of personality testing alone were 73 percent accurate [9].

The type A personality has been extensively studied in relation to the development of coronary artery disease. The type A person is described as one constantly driven to participate in a multitude of events in an ever-decreasing amount of time [12]. This so-called hurry sickness leads, in some cases, to an increased incidence of hypertension, along with increased serum lipoprotein levels [1]. While some studies have attempted to refute the relationship between personality factors and myocardial infarction, the weight of the evidence seems to support the relationship.

TABLE 4-1. Selye's classification of stress-induced diseases

1.	Hypertension
2.	Heart and blood vessel disease
3.	Kidney disease
4.	Eclampsia
5.	Arthritis
6.	Skin and eye inflammation
7.	Infections
8.	Allergic and hypersensitivity diseases
9.	Nervous and mental diseases
10.	Sexual derangements
11.	Digestive diseases
12.	Metabolic diseases
13.	Cancer
14.	Diseases of resistance

Further support is the evidence that norepinephrine levels are increased when there is chronic, unrelenting stress, especially when the person feels a sense of loss of control over his or her life situation. Epinephrine, the other catecholamine, is seen to increase in fear and acute arousal states [12].

It is important to consider all of the previous information in order to understand that while stress seems to be a significant factor in development of different diseases, and while biochemical phenomena have been described, the conclusions do not support direct relationships. Disease conditions must be considered individually in respect to their relationship to stress. It must also be remembered that while some studies support the stress/disease concepts, other, equally valid studies, may cast some doubt on the relationship.

STRESS AND DISEASE

Wolff describes stress in terms of adaptive reaction patterns and systematically relates life stress to bodily manifestations [13]. Selye refers to the production of disease as maladaptation and categorizes stress-induced diseases as indicated in Table 4-1 [10]. In the subsequent material, the following diseases are discussed in relation to their stress connection: (1) cardiovascular diseases, (2) immune deficiency diseases, and (3) digestive diseases.

Cardiovascular Disease

For many years it has been recognized that stress is important in the etiology of coronary artery disease. This stress can be in the form of emotional, occupational, societal, cultural, hereditary, and physical stressors. The importance of occupational origin of coronary artery disease has received great attention in recent years.

Several theories of the pathogenesis of coronary artery disease have resulted from studies of the relationship between high-fat diet, stressful living situations, and development of disease. Individuals who develop hypercholesteremia have a greater risk of developing atherosclerotic heart disease than those with normal levels. The mechanism for the production of hypercholesteremia is unclear. In contrast, however, studies have supported the protective nature of certain serum lipoproteins called ***high-density lipoproteins (HDLs),*** which may delay or prevent the development of atherosclerosis. HDL is seen in greater serum concentrations in women than in men, which is consistent with studies showing that estrogen functions to increase HDL while androgens tend to decrease the HDL levels [6]. During stressful periods, the serum cholesterol has been shown to rise leading to the conclusion that lipid-regulating mechanisms are responsive to stress. Studies have been conducted showing that catecholamine release leads to an increased rate of lipolysis, increased serum-free fatty acids, and a subsequent rise in serum cholesterol [13]. Correlate studies also link serum lipid levels and personality patterns.

Pelletier theorizes that a relationship exists between chronic stress and blood pressure. The stress leads to increased blood pressure, which, in turn, leads to a weakening and tearing of the linings of the blood vessels, thus providing a focal point for the deposition of cholesterol plaques on the vessel lining. The end result is narrowing of the lumen of vessels, leading to an increased peripheral vascular resistance and further increase in blood pressure levels. To compensate for the elevated blood pressure, the left ventricle undergoes hypertrophy and requires greater blood and oxygen supply. A relationship between high blood pressure and coronary artery disease has not been found consistently, but the correlation is significant enough to consider hypertension as a major risk factor [7].

The increase in incidence of coronary artery disease has prompted investigations into many facets of the current life-style in the United States. One area of study is the commonly observed personality pattern in which the person feels a loss of control over his or her occupational or social environment. Friedman and Rosenman also identified a behavior pattern consistent with hypertension and heart attack. It includes competitiveness in work, fast work pace, time pressure, and inability to relax at work or play. Other risk factors also were studied, but the personality pattern apparently offered the greatest risk [2].

Stress-Induced Immune Deficiency

The decreased immune response following stressful situations appears to be due to an increased secretion of the glucocorticoids from the adrenal cortex. The major effect is on the T lymphocytes, which in turn reduces the cell-mediated immune response. Both T and B lymphocytes are shown to be affected by the glucocorticoid release, but the lymphopenia (decreased numbers of lymphocytes) is due to a redistribution rather than loss of T cells [3]. Physiologically or psychologically stressful events precipitate a decrease in lymphocytes and other leukocytes.

The administration of the glucocorticoids in conditions of hypersensitivity or exaggerated response has long been shown to be beneficial. This is especially true in such conditions as rheumatoid arthritis, acute asthmatic attacks, and specific types of malignancy, especially leukemia.

Conversely, the stress-induced response of decreased immunity can be very detrimental in conditions such as cancer. It is often seen that an individual who was declared "cured" of cancer may undergo relapse following an acute stressful situation, such as the death of a loved one. The stress-induced depression of the immune system may allow for an increased rate of malignant growth (see Unit 6).

Digestive Diseases

The relationship of stress and peptic ulcers has been studied for many years. Three types of stress-induced ulcer disease are described in this section and in further detail in Chapter 35.

Overwhelming stress frequently leads to the development of *stress ulcers.* These may be related to gastric mucosal ischemia and gastric acid secretion. The mechanism for the related gastric acid secretion is not entirely understood, but may be due to cerebral stimulation of the dorsal motor nucleus of the vagus nerve [5]. Hypersecretion has only been clearly demonstrated in the development of Cushing's ulcers, which are associated with brain lesions [6].

The occurrence of an increased rate of gastric secretion between meals has been demonstrated in patients having *duodenal ulcers* while patients with *gastric ulcers* often have a normal or decreased secretion of hydrochloric acid. It would appear that the duodenal ulcers result from a chronic increase in gastric acid secretion and affect the duodenum before the alkalinizing secretions can buffer the acid. Gastric ulcers seem to be related to gastritis and to a decreased mucosal resistance in the gastric mucosa [5, 8].

Stress has been indicated in many other digestive conditions including such diverse conditions as constipation, diarrhea, ulcerative colitis, and Crohn's disease. Personality and stress factors with ulcerative colitis and regional enteritis have been extensively studied, adding much knowledge concerning the very complex pathogenesis of these conditions.

One can see that the response of the body to stressors is individual and depends on a number of factors. Most of the diseases of humans have stress as one element. Stress enters into the pathogenesis of the disease or results from the abnormalities inflicted from the process. A few examples of stress-induced diseases have been mentioned in this chapter. Others are described throughout the text. Further study of the stress response will clarify relationships between personalities, life stressors, and genetic predisposition to disease.

REFERENCES

1. Carruthers, M., and Taggart, P. Behavior Patterns and Emotional Stress in the Etiology of Coronary Heart Disease: Cardiological and Biochemical Correlates. In D. Wheatley, *Stress and the Heart.* New York: Raven Press, 1977.
2. Friedman, R., and Dahl, L. L. Psychic and Genetic Factors in the Etiology of Hypertension. In D. Wheatley, *Stress and the Heart.* New York: Raven Press, 1977.
3. Fudenberg, H. H., et al. *Basic and Clinical Immunology* (3rd ed.). Los Altos, Calif.: Lange, 1980.
4. Garfield, C. *Stress and Survival.* St. Louis: Mosby, 1979.
5. Guyton, A. C. *Textbook of Medical Physiology.* Philadelphia: Saunders, 1981.
6. Isselbacher, K. J., et al. (eds.). *Harrison's Principles of Internal Medicine* (10th ed.). New York: McGraw-Hill, 1983.
7. Pelletier, K. *Mind as Healer, Mind as Slayer.* New York: Dell, 1977.
8. Robbins, S., and Cotran, R. *Pathologic Basis of Disease* (2nd ed.). Philadelphia: Saunders, 1979.
9. Schmale, A. H., and Iker, H. Hopelessness as a Predictor of Cervical Cancer. In P. J. McEwan (ed.), *Social Science and Medicine* (vol. 5). Elmsford, N. Y.: Pergamon, 1971.
10. Selye, H. *The Stress of Life.* New York: McGraw-Hill, 1956.
11. Stout, C., et al. Unusually low incidence of death from myocardial infarction. *J. A. M. A.* 188:382, 1964.
12. Wheatley, D. *Stress and the Heart.* New York: Raven Press, 1977.
13. Wolff, H. G. *Stress and Disease* (2nd ed.). Springfield, Ill.: Thomas, 1968.

BIBLIOGRAPHY

Ashton, K. The many faces of stress. *Nurs. Times* 75:1297, 1979.

Bahlmann, J., and Liebau, H. *Stress and Hypertension.* New York: Karger, 1982.

Bogolin, L., and Harris, J. Meeting the immunological challenge: Rush-Presbyterian, St. Lukes Medical Center Symposium. *Heart Lung* 9:643, 1980.

Brockway, B.J. Situational stress and temporal changes in self respondents and vocal measurements. *Nursing Res.* 28:20, 1979.

Bruhn, J. G., and Wolf, S. *The Roseto Story: An Anatomy of Health.* Norman, Okla.: The University of Oklahoma, 1979.

Burnside, I. *Nursing and the Aged* (2nd ed.). New York: McGraw-Hill, 1981.

Cassem, H.H., et al. Reactions of coronary patients to the CCU nurse. *Am. J. Nurs.* 70:3194, 1970.

Claus, K., and Bailey, J. *Living with Stress and Promoting Well-Being: A Handbook for Nurses.* St. Louis: Mosby, 1980.

Cox, T. *Stress.* Baltimore: University Park Press, 1980.

Critical care nursing stress: The findings revisited. *Nursing Res.* 30:182, 1981.

Cromwell, R.L., et al. *Acute Myocardial Infarction.* St. Louis: Mosby, 1977.

DePue, R. *The Psychobiology of the Depressive Disorders.* New York: Academic, 1979.

Dowdall, S. Breathing techniques that help reduce hypertension. *RN* 40:73, 1977.

Ebersole, P., and Hess, P. *Toward Healthy Aging.* St. Louis: Mosby, 1981.

Fauci, A.S., Dale, D.C., and Balow, J.E. Glucocorticosteroid therapy: Mechanism of action and clinical considerations. *Ann. Intern. Med.* 8:304, 1976.

Folinsbee, L.J. *Environmental Stress: Individual Human Adaptations.* New York: Academic, 1978.

Fromm, D. Stress ulcer. *Hosp. Med.* 14:5, 1978.

Garfield, C. *Stress and Survival: The Emotional Realities of Life Threatening Illness.* St. Louis: Mosby, 1979.

Gelein, J.L. Introduction to the Systems Approach. In W.J. Phipps (ed.), *Medical-Surgical Nursing: Concepts and Clinical Practice* (2nd ed.). St. Louis: Mosby, 1983.

Gersten, H., et al. The subjective aspects of coronary care. *Nursing Res.* 25:211, 1976.

Getty, C., and Humphreys, W. *Understanding the Family.* New York: Appleton-Century-Crofts, 1981.
Glass, D. *Behavior Patterns, Stress and Coronary Disease.* Hillsdale, N.Y.: Lawrence Erlbaum, 1977.
Gunderson, E., and Rahe, R. *Life Stress and Illness.* Springfield, Ill.: Thomas, 1974.
Guyton, A. *Textbook of Medical Physiology* (6th ed.). Philadelphia: Saunders, 1981.
Hall, J., and Weaver, B. *A Systems Approach to Community Health.* New York: Lippincott, 1977.
Hemenway, J. A. Sleep and the cardiac patient. *Heart Lung* 9:453, 1980.
Henry, J. P., and Stephens, P. H. *Stress, Health and the Social Environment.* New York: Springer-Verlag, 1977.
Jalowiec, A. Stress and coping in hypertensive and emergency room patients. *Nurs. Res.* 30:10, 1981.
Jasmin, S., Hill, L., and Smith, N. The art of managing stress. *Nurs. 81* 11:52, 1981.
Jensen, D. *The Principles of Physiology* (2nd ed.). New York: Appleton-Century-Crofts, 1980.
Luckmann, J., and Sorensen, K. *Medical-Surgical Nursing* (2nd ed.). Philadelphia: Saunders, 1980.
Maher, A. A systems approach to nursing the patient with multiple systems failure. *Heart Lung* 10:866, 1981.
Marcinek, M. Stress in the surgical patient. *Am. J. Nurs.* 77:1809, 1977.
Meissner, J. Measuring patient stress with the hospital stress rating scale. *Nurs. 80* 10:70, 1980.
Miller, C., et al. Personality and emotional stress measurement on hypertensive patients with essential and secondary hypertension. *Inter. J. Nurs. Stud.* 16:85, 1979.
Miller, J. *Living Systems.* New York: McGraw-Hill, 1978.
Miller, J. Living Systems: Basic Concepts. In W. Gray, et al. (eds.), *General Systems Theory and Psychiatry.* Boston: Little, Brown, 1969.
Motta, G. J. Stress and the elderly: Coping with a change in body image. *J. Enteros. Ther.* 8:21, 1981.
Murray, R., and Zentner, J. *Nursing Concepts for Health Promotion* (2nd ed.). Englewood Cliffs, N.J.: Prentice-Hall, 1979.
Neurnberger, P. Freedom from stress: A holistic approach. *Nurs. Life* 1:61, 1981.
Northouse, L. L. Living with cancer. *Am. J. Nurs.* 81:960, 1981.
Raab, W. Emotional and sensory stress factors in myocardial pathology. *Am. Heart J.* 72:538, 1966.
Roberts, S. *Behavioral Concepts and Nursing Throughout the Life Span.* Englewood Cliffs, N.J.: Prentice-Hall, 1978.
Roundtable. When stress tips the clinical balance. *Patient Care* 15:7, 1981.
Schlesinger, Z., and Barzilay, J. Prolonged rehabilitation of patients after acute myocardial infarction and its effects on a complex of physiological variables. *Heart Lung* 9:1038, 1980.
Schmale, A. H., and Iker, H. Hopelessness as a predictor of cervical cancer. *Social Science and Medicine* 5:95, 1971.
Scully, R. Stress in the nurse. *Am. J. Nurs.* 80:911, 1980.
Selkurt, E. *Basic Physiology for the Health Sciences* (2nd ed.). Boston: Little, Brown, 1982.
Selye, H. *The Physiology and Pathology of Exposure to Stress.* Montreal: Acta, 1950.
Selye, H. *The Stress of Life.* New York: McGraw-Hill, 1956.
Selye, H. *Stress Without Distress.* Philadelphia: Lippincott, 1974.
Siegrist, J., and Halhuber, M. J. *Myocardial Infarctions and Psychosocial Risks.* New York: Springer-Verlag, 1981.
Sivarajan, E., and Halpenny, C. J. Exercise testing. *Am. J. Nurs.* 79:2162, 1979.
Stephenson, C. A. Stress in critically ill patients. *Am. J. Nurs.* 79:1606, 1977.
Stout, C., et al. Unusually low incidence of death from myocardial infarction. *J.A.M.A.* 188:845, 1964.
Sutterley, D., and Donnelly, G. *Perspectives in Human Development.* Philadelphia: Lippincott, 1973.
Taché, J., Selye, H., and Day, S. *Cancer, Stress and Death.* New York: Plenum, 1979.
Tierney, M. J., and Strom, S. Type A behavior in the nurse. *Am. J. Nurs.* 80:915, 1980.
Usdin, E., Kvetnansky, R., and Kopin, I. *Catecholamines and Stress: Proceedings of the International Symposium* (2nd ed.). New York: Elsevier North-Holland, 1980.
Vansom, S. R. Stress effects on patients in critical care units from procedures performed on others. *Heart Lung* 9:494, 1980.
von Bertalanffy, L. *General Systems Theory: Foundations, Development and Applications.* New York: Braziller, 1968.
Wheatley, D. *Stress and the Heart.* New York: Raven Press, 1977.

UNIT 3
FLUID, ELECTROLYTE, AND ACID-BASE BALANCE

Barbara L. Bullock
NORMAL AND ALTERED FLUID, ELECTROLYTE, AND ACID-BASE BALANCE

Helen Ptak
FLUID AND ELECTROLYTE BALANCE

The maintenance of the steady state of fluid, electrolyte, and acid-base balance is achieved through the complex cooperation of various systems of the body. Continual movement and exchange of water results in a regulated balance between plasma and interstitial and intracellular fluid. Because the subject encompasses many other systems, the intent of this unit is to provide the basis for further exploration in the specific systems of the body.

Chapter 5 summarizes water and electrolyte balance and explores the major alterations that can occur with disease states. Edema and shock are presented in this chapter because they represent alterations in or a shift of fluid volume between compartments. Specific reference to electrolyte and water regulation is found in many other areas of the text. Chapter 6 deals with the basic concepts of the regulation of acid-base balance and how alterations in the balance can result. Respiratory alterations are described in greater detail in Unit 9 and the metabolic alterations are specifically explored in Unit 10. Other systems that function in the regulation of hydrogen ion concentration are noted in Units 7, 11, 12, and 15.

The reader is encouraged to utilize the learning objectives as a study guide outline; the bibliography listed at the end of the unit can aid in further investigation of the topic.

CHAPTER 5

NORMAL AND ALTERED FLUID AND ELECTROLYTE BALANCE

REGULATION OF FLUID AND ELECTROLYTE BALANCE

Regulation of Water Balance

Thirst

ADH

Aldosterone

Prostaglandins

Glucocorticoids

Fluid Balance in Body Compartments

Movement of Fluids at the Capillary Line

Sodium, Water, and Volume Deficits and Excess

Sodium

Hyponatremia

Hypernatremia

Potassium

Hypokalemia

Hyperkalemia

Calcium

Relationship of Calcium to Phosphate

Hypocalcemia

Hypercalcemia

Chloride

Magnesium

Hypomagnesemia

Hypermagnesemia

EDEMA

Decreased Colloid Osmotic Pressure

Increased Capillary Hydrostatic Pressure

Increased Capillary Permeability

Obstruction of the Lymphatics

Sodium and Body Water Excess

Types of Edema

Distribution of Edema

SHOCK

Compensatory Mechanisms in Shock

Sympathetic Nervous System (SNS) Stimulation

Anaerobic Production of ATP

Fluid Shifts and Renal Conservation

Stages of Shock

Cardiogenic Shock

Pump Failure

Decreased Venous Inflow

Blood Volume Decrease (Hypovolemic Shock)

Hemorrhagic Shock

Burn Shock

Dehydration Shock

Changes in Peripheral Resistance

Neurogenic Shock

Septic or Toxic Shock

Anaphylactic or Allergic Shock

LEARNING OBJECTIVES

1. Describe the mechanisms by which water balance is normally regulated.
2. List the normal serum concentrations of the major electrolytes and plasma proteins.
3. Show the relationship of fluid and electrolyte composition between the intracellular and extracellular compartments.
4. Describe in detail the normal fluid dynamics at the capillary line.
5. Define the terms *hydrostatic pressure*, *oncotic pressure*, *colloid osmotic pressure*, and *outward and inward forces* as they relate to capillary fluid dynamics.
6. Briefly describe the role of the lymphatic system in controlling extravascular fluid volume.
7. Describe the role of sodium in controlling osmotic pressure in the extracellular fluid.
8. Differentiate between the clinical effects of hypernatremia and hyponatremia.
9. Define *dilutional hyponatremia*.
10. Discuss how SIADH can cause hyponatremia.
11. Describe the function of potassium in the body.
12. Differentiate between the pathophysiologic changes resulting from hypokalemia and hyperkalemia.
13. Discuss the multiple functions of calcium in the body.
14. List several causes of hypocalcemia.
15. Describe the physiologic effects of hypocalcemia and hypercalcemia.
16. Explain how hypochloremia is related to metabolic alkalosis.
17. Describe the effects of magnesium on the body.
18. Discuss the five pathologic mechanisms that can produce edema and their relation to each other.
19. Diagram the positive feedback mechanism associated with decreased colloid osmotic pressure.
20. Differentiate between pitting and nonpitting edema.
21. Describe in detail the three physiologic mechanisms in the production of shock.
22. Explain the compensatory mechanisms used by the body in response to hypotension.
23. Explain the significance of the stages of shock.
24. List at least three factors that can cause hypovolemic shock.
25. Describe the major pathologic processes that can cause decreased peripheral resistance in shock.

In order to maintain body function an equilibrium between intake and output of water and solutes must be maintained. Continual movement and exchange of water and electrolytes occur with intake being equal to the output. The protein composition of the plasma is also important in the regulation of fluid movement at the capillary line. This chapter presents a brief review of water and electrolyte balance and those alterations that can occur with stress and disease.

REGULATION OF FLUID AND ELECTROLYTE BALANCE

Water balance refers to an equilibrium maintained between water intake and output. Intake of water comes from liquids ingested, from water in foods, and from water produced by oxidation of foodstuffs. Water is utilized in the many metabolic processes of the body and is necessary to carry waste products for excretion through the urine, skin, lungs, and feces.

The composition of the body fluids is further regulated by the kidneys and lungs with input from the heart and the glands of the body. Hormones, especially aldosterone and antidiuretic hormone (ADH), function to regulate the composition of the plasma and the other fluid compartments.

Water accounts for approximately 60 percent of body weight in the adult. This amount normally decreases with age and is affected by body weight. The lean individual has a greater percentage of body water than an obese individual because fat cells contain less water than muscle cells. The amount of water necessary to maintain life in the adult is about 1500 ml/day. Usually, water intake is higher with a total of 2000 ml/day being average. It is directly conserved by the antidiuretic hormone and indirectly conserved by aldosterone.

Intake of water must be balanced by output. Obligatory urinary output to eliminate waste and maintain minimal renal function is 300 to 500 ml per 24 hours. The kidneys function to rid the body of excess water. Excretion volume can be increased tremendously in order to maintain the composition of the body fluids. Water is also lost through the lungs, skin, and feces. This loss is termed *insensible water loss*.

Water functions to cushion, protect, and provide for structure or appearance in the skin of the human body. Skin turgor is reflected by the resiliency of the skin and normally provides a soft, smooth appearance.

Volume disturbances can involve both water depletion and water excess. Depletion is called dehydration and may be associated with sodium depletion (hypotonic dehydration) or with sodium excess (hypertonic dehydration). Body water loss is enhanced by elevated body temperature, diarrhea, vomiting, and other excessive volume losses such as occur through the kidney, skin, lungs, and the gastrointestinal tract. Water excess often occurs in association with sodium retention, but it also may occur with excess ADH secretion or with excessive ingestion of water.

Regulation of Water Balance

THIRST. When the extracellular fluid becomes depleted or hypertonic, rapid stimulation of the osmoreceptors in the hypothalamus occurs. The two results of this stimulation are the release of ADH and thirst. The sensation of thirst causes the person to take in fluid. The release of ADH causes an increase in the permeability of the collecting tubule. Water is resorbed, thus decreasing the osmolarity of the extracellular fluid. With resorption of water, there is a decrease in urinary output.

Loss of 10 percent of plasma volume leads to secretion of ADH and thirst stimulation. Any condition that decreases the circulating blood volume leads to this compensatory reaction. The ADH-thirst mechanism is also a major feedback for control of the sodium concentration in the extracellular fluid because anything that increases the osmolarity of the plasma leads to thirst and an increased secretion of ADH. Conversely, when the osmolarity is decreased, the thirst stimulus subsides and the ADH is suppressed, which results in increased urinary output.

ADH. ADH is secreted from the neurohypophysis after its formation in the hypothalamus. It functions to increase resorption of water at the collecting ducts, leading to a decrease in the urinary output. This returns the osmolarity to normal. The major stimulus for ADH secretion is an increase in the osmolarity of the extracellular fluid. ADH is also called *vasopressin* and has a minor vasoconstrictive effect on the arterioles, which can increase the blood pressure. A significant decrease in ADH secretion causes diabetes insipidus, which leads to a massive increase in the urinary output and can cause rapid depletion of the water balance. An increased secretion of ADH may be stimulated by extrapituitary tumors or from pituitary hypersecretion, evidenced by a marked decrease in the serum osmolarity, an increase in blood volume, and a decrease in the urinary output. This is known as the syndrome for inappropriate secretion of ADH (SIADH).

ALDOSTERONE. This hormone, secreted by the adrenal gland, acts on the renal tubules to increase the sodium uptake (see Chap. 31). The increased sodium retention causes an increase in the retention of water. Aldosterone release is stimulated by changes in potassium concentration, by serum sodium concentrations, and by the renin-angiotensin system (see Chap. 26). Normally, the rate or amount of aldosterone secretion is closely regulated by the potassium concentration and is very effective in controlling hyperkalemia.

PROSTAGLANDINS. The prostaglandins are naturally occurring fatty acids that are present in many of the tissues of the body, and function in the inflammatory response, in blood pressure control, in uterine contractions, and in gastrointestinal motility. In the kidney, the renal prostaglandins may play a role in the regulation of renal circulation, in the renal effect on ADH, and in sodium resorption [11]. Renal constriction due to any mechanism stimulates prostaglandin release, which promotes renal vasodilatation and prevents renal ischemia. ADH may stimulate prostaglandin release or synthesis and prostaglandins may decrease the ADH effect. Prostaglandins in small amounts may promote sodium excretion but this is probably not a major physiologic factor [11].

GLUCOCORTICOIDS. The glucocorticoids also exert a weak mineralocorticoid activity and promote the resorption of sodium and water, thus promoting increased blood volume and sodium retention. Alterations in the glucocorticoids cause alterations in the blood volume balance.

Fluid Balance in Body Compartments

Fluids are maintained in strict volume and concentration in each of the three compartments: (1) extracellular, intravascular (plasma); (2) extracellular, extravascular (interstitial fluid); and (3) intracellular fluid. Figure 5-1 shows the relationship of fluid balance and composition of these three compartments. Body fluid is normally distributed with about 70 percent being intracellular and the rest being extracellular in the form of interstitial, plasma, and secretion/excretion fluids. The relationship of cations, anions, and volumes must be maintained rigidly to preserve life. Interstitial fluid and plasma basically contain the same electrolyte composition but plasma contains a large amount of protein. Intracellular electrolyte composition is quite different from the extracellular composition but the numbers of charges (cations and anions) are basically equal between the two compartments. In order to maintain life, fluid containing oxygen and nutrients from the blood is filtered into the interstitial spaces and carried to the intracellular fluid, while excess carbon dioxide and other cellular waste products are returned to the bloodstream to be circulated and excreted by the lungs and kidneys (see Chap. 1). The process requires the constant movement and exchange of fluids and gases.

Movement of Fluids at the Capillary Line

The capillaries are formed of endothelium, which is permeable to all of the solutes and water of the plasma. It is impermeable to the large molecules and cells in the plasma. Substances move through the gaps or spaces in the endothelial cells and some substances—CO_2, O_2, small solutes—move through the endothelial membrane as well. The process occurs by diffusion so that a near equilibrium exists at the capillary line. The amount of fluid leaving the capillary nearly equals the amount resorbed. This equilibrium occurs mostly through a balance achieved between the hydrostatic pressure of the blood and the colloid osmotic pressure within the capillaries.

Blood that enters the capillary comes in at a *hydrostatic pressure* that is generated by the heart. This hydrostatic pressure is variable in the different systemic arterioles but is always higher at the arteriolar end of the capillary than at the venular end (Fig. 5-2). As fluid filters out of the capillary into the tissue spaces, the hydrostatic pressure decreases. The high pressure exerted at the arteriolar end of the capillary has been called a simple *outward force*, which moves fluid from the vessel to the interstitial spaces [3]. The average hydrostatic pressure at the arteriolar end is 32 mm Hg, which drops to 15 mm Hg at the venous end [11]. This hydrostatic pressure provides the main outward force, but it is enhanced by a negative interstitial pressure and the interstitial fluid colloid osmotic pressure (ISCOP) as shown in Figure 5-2. The ISCOP results from plasma proteins that are leaked into the interstitial spaces and exert a colloid, or water-pulling, effect. The pressure exerted by the plasma proteins, the *colloid osmotic (COP)* or *oncotic pressure*, is an osmotic pulling or *inward force*, which draws water toward it. Because the plasma proteins cannot move into the interstitial area they exert their colloidal effect by drawing water back into the vessel. The average COP is 25 mm Hg, a pressure that remains constant across the capillary. Referring to Figure 5-2, note that at the arteriolar end of a schematic capillary the hydrostatic pressure exceeds the colloid osmotic pressure by about 7 mm Hg, causing fluid movement to the interstitial area. At the venous end, the hydrostatic pressure has dropped to 15 mm Hg so that the hydrostatic pressure is now less than the colloid osmotic pressure, which causes the movement of fluid into the capillary. The colloid osmotic pressure in the capillaries is mainly generated by albumin because it is the most abundant of the plasma proteins. Table 5-1 lists the relative concentrations of plasma proteins.

TABLE 5-1. Concentration of major plasma proteins

Total serum proteins	6.0–8.0 gm/dl
Albumin	3.5–5.5 gm/dl
Globulin	1.5–3.0 gm/dl
Fibrinogen	200–400 mg/dl
Electrophoresis	
Albumin	45–55% of total
Globulin	
$Alpha_1$	5–8% of total
$Alpha_2$	8–13% of total
Beta	11–17% of total
Gamma	15–25% of total

Source: J. Wallach, *Interpretation of Diagnostic Tests* (3rd ed.). Boston: Little, Brown, 1978.

It has been noted that while fluid filtered out of the vessel nearly equals fluid resorbed, a smaller excess is filtered into the tissue spaces than is resorbed. Also, small amounts of protein escape into the tissue spaces during the process of fluid movement and cannot be resorbed by the blood vessels. This excess fluid and protein are absorbed by the *lymphatic system* and returned via lymphatic channels to the blood. The lymphatic system provides the only means to return plasma proteins in the tissues to the bloodstream [3].

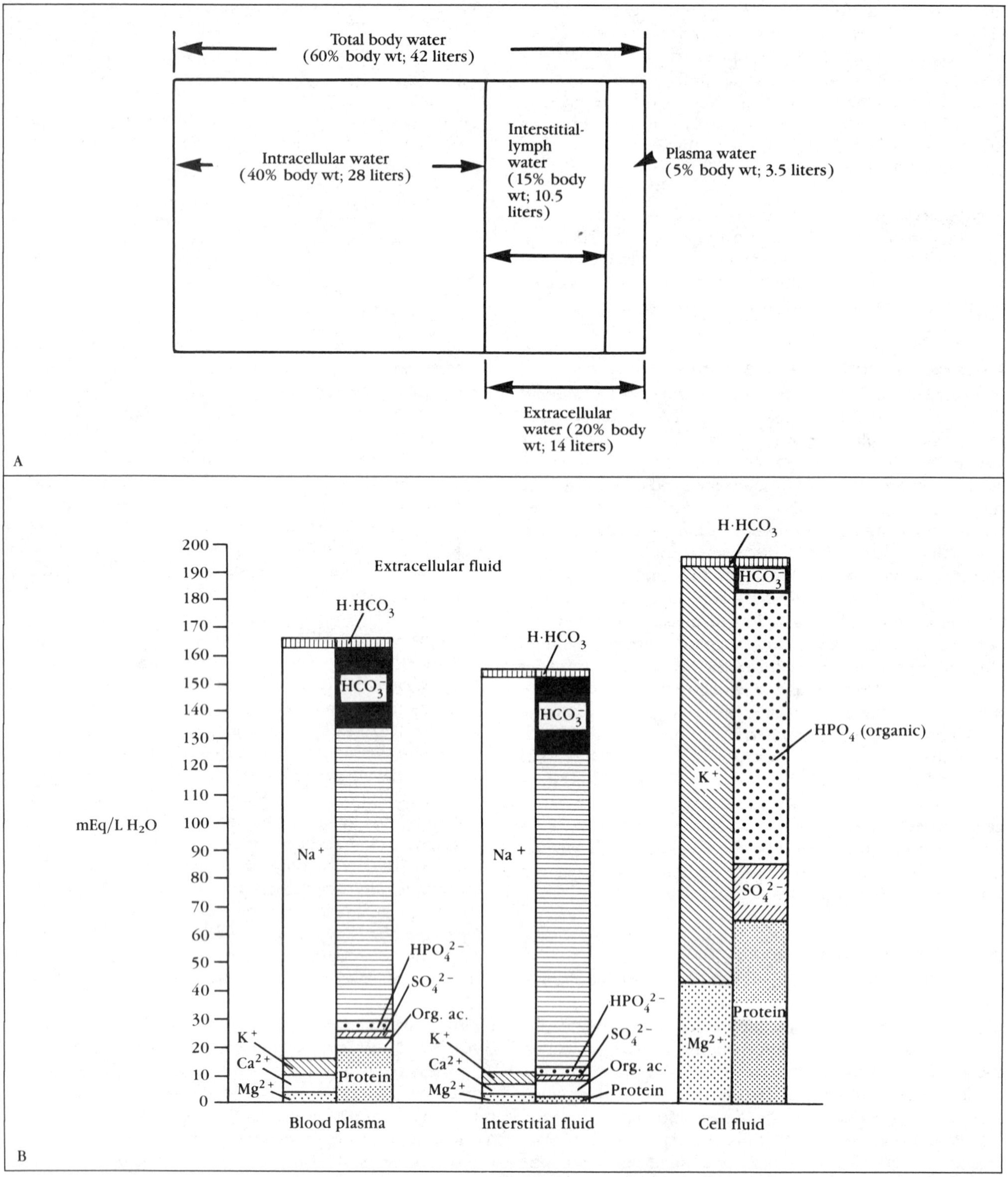

FIGURE 5-1. Fluid balance and composition. A. Distribution of water in the body. Percentages and volumes are for an idealized 70-kg young adult male. (From E. Selkurt, *Basic Physiology for the Health Sciences* [2nd ed.]. Boston: Little, Brown, 1982.) B. Electrolyte composition of the body fluid compartments.

Edema does not normally occur until there is a 10 to 15 mm Hg increase in the gradient favoring filtration, or the outward force [11]. This is because the lymph channels can increase the amount of fluid carried and thus can compensate for increased fluid escaping into the tissue spaces. Edema does result when there is significant alteration in either the inward (ISCOP) or outward (hydrostatic) forces.

Sodium, Water, and Volume Deficits and Excess

SODIUM. Sodium is the major cation of the ECF (Table 5-2). It regulates the osmotic pressure of the ECF and markedly affects the osmotic pressure of the ICF. Water balance is so closely associated with sodium that the alterations in sodium balance are considered with water balance changes in this chapter. Sodium intake comes from the diet with a requirement for body needs of approximately 500 mg/day [7]. The average daily intake in the United States is 6 to 15 gm [9]. Sodium is also an essential component in neuromuscular excitability and is responsible for depolarization of the cell membranes of excitable cells. It participates in acid-base balance by combining with the bicarbonate radical. Sodium exists in combination with various anions, especially chloride and bicarbonate. Sodium concentration is directly regulated by aldosterone as previously described.

HYPONATREMIA. Deficits of sodium in the serum can be caused by excessive loss of sodium and water through the skin, gastrointestinal tract, or urinary system. Inadequate intake of sodium can also lead to this condition. Diuresis may be initiated by many types of drugs, by hyperglycemia, and by decreased amounts of circulating ADH. In volume loss, serum sodium levels may or may not be decreased depending on the composition of the fluid lost. If water is lost in excess of sodium, hypernatremia may actually result.

The signs of water deficit include loss of body weight, excessive thirst, and decreased urinary output. The skin turgor becomes less resilient, and the eyeballs feel soft to the touch. Plasma loss is reflected in an increased compensatory heart rate and postural hypotension.

Serum sodium depletion may be the result of sodium loss without water loss or of water gains in excess of sodium (called *dilutional hyponatremia*). SIADH causes excessive conservation of water and may produce this syndrome (see p. 60). The effect of hyponatremia is the production of a hypotonic ECF, which leads to intracellular swelling, and affects the brain and other systems of the body.

Symptoms of hyponatremia include weakness, confusion, and muscle cramps; it may terminate in convulsions and vasomotor collapse. The specific gravity of the urine in hyponatremia is usually very low, in the range of 1.001 to 1.003, which reflects the conservation of sodium. In SIADH, however, this level is usually much higher, reflecting ADH retention of water and secretion of concentrated urine containing large amounts of sodium.

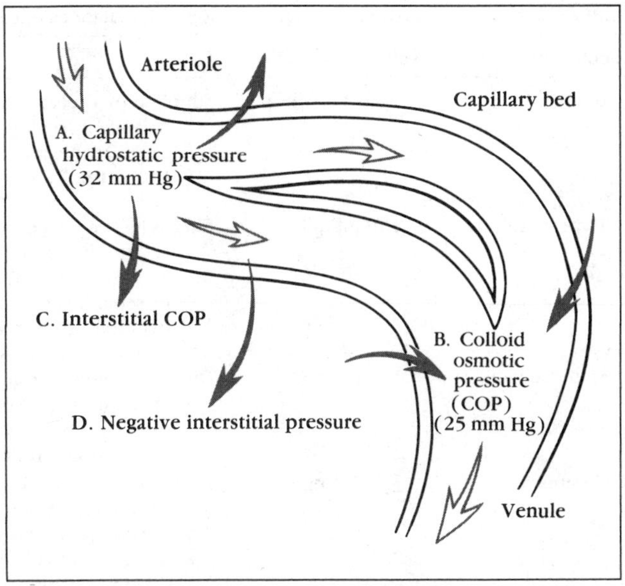

FIGURE 5-2. Fluid dynamics at the capillary line. A. Capillary hydrostatic pressure is higher at the arteriolar end and tends to push fluid out. B. Colloid osmotic pressure generated by the plasma proteins maintains a constant inward pull or force. C. Interstitial COP is an outward force. D. Negative interstitial pressure is an outward force.

HYPERNATREMIA. Retention of sodium is usually associated with retention of water. The conditions most frequently associated with this are heart failure, cirrhosis of the liver, and kidney failure. The increased volume leads to an increased circulating blood volume, increased blood pressure, weight gain, and edema, usually beginning peripherally and later affecting the face and torso (anasarca).

Serum sodium elevation may occur when there is increased intake of sodium or a decreased output. It occurs in those conditions in which more water is lost than sodium: ADH insufficiency, salt-water near-drowning, or some cases of diarrhea. If the thirst mechanism is inactivated for any reason the increased osmolarity may not be a stimulus for increased water intake. Hypernatremia causes an increased tonicity of the ECF and intracellular shrinkage. As water is pulled out of the cells, cellular dysfunction occurs, especially in the central nervous system. The kidneys respond by excreting large quantities of sodium. Clinical manifestations include excessive thirst; dry, sticky mucous membranes; decreased vascular volume; and decreased blood pressure. Severe hypernatremia may terminate in coma, convulsions, and death.

Potassium

Potassium is concentrated in the intracellular fluid. It directly affects the excitability of nerves and muscles, and contributes to the intracellular osmotic pressure (see Table 5-2). Secretions and excretions contain large amounts of potassium. The source of potassium is the diet and the nor-

TABLE 5-2. Normal electrolyte concentrations and imbalances of each

Electrolyte	Values*	Cause	Effects
Sodium	136–145 mEq/L	Supplied by diet; excreted by kidney; balance normally regulated by aldosterone and ADH; dominant ECF cation	Regulates fluid volume by maintaining osmotic pressure between compartments; functions in acid-base balance; functions in neuromuscular and muscular excitability
Hypernatremia	>150 mEq/L	Excess loss of water over sodium through GI system, lungs, or skin; excess administration of sodium through diet or renal insufficiency; essential hypernatremia may be due to hypothalamic lesions	Causes cellular shrinking due to hypertonic ECF, leads to CNS irritability, tachycardia, dry, flushed skin, hypotension; thirst excessive
Hyponatremia	<130 mEq/L	Dilutional hyponatremia from CHF, cirrhosis, nephrosis; sodium depletion, loss of body fluids, without replacement; diuretic therapy	Causes cellular swelling, may lead to cerebral edema, headache, stupor progressing to coma; peripheral edema, polyuria, absence of thirst
Potassium	3.5–5.0 mEq/L	Balance maintained by dietary intake, excess excreted by kidneys; increased potassium in plasma excreted under influence of aldosterone by kidneys; dominant cation in ICF	Regulates osmolarity of ICF, functions in neuromuscular and muscular excitability; competition with H^+ and Na^+ in renal tubule helps maintain acid-base balance
Hyperkalemia	>5 mEq/L	Renal failure or renal insufficiency — acute or chronic; hemolysis of RBC; acute increase in potassium intake*	Main effect is depression of conductivity in heart, peaked T waves, widened QRS on ECG; muscle cramping, paresthesias, nausea, diarrhea, associated with metabolic acidosis
Hypokalemia	<3.5 mEq/L	Lack of dietary intake; vomiting, gastric suction, potassium-depleting diuretics, aldosteronism, salt-wasting kidney diseases; major GI surgery without replacement	Cardiac effect-increased irritability, onset of U wave on ECG, arrhythmias, vomiting, paralytic ileus; thirst; associated with metabolic alkalosis; affect renal tubular function causing inability to concentrate urine
Calcium	4–5 mEq/L 8.5–10.5 mg/dl	Regulated by PTH and thyrocalcitonin; supplied by diet, absorbed under influence of activated vitamin D; 99% stored in bones and teeth; excreted by kidney and GI tract	Blocks sodium at cell membrane, decreases membrane excitability; enhances coagulation process; essential in complement cascade; makes up much of crystalline matrix of bone; reciprocal relationship with phosphate
Hypercalcemia	> 5.5 mEq/L >10.5 mg/dl	Excessive vitamin D, immobility, renal insufficiency; hyperparathyroidism, malignancies of bone or blood	Decreased neuromuscular excitability, muscle weakness, CNS depression, stupor to coma; ECG shows shortened Q–T interval; if due to increased absorption from bones, increased risk of fracture; vomiting, constipation, kidney stones
Hypocalcemia	<4.0 mEq/L <8.5 mg/dl	Hypoparathyroidism, surgical or idiopathic; malabsorption of calcium; insufficient or inactivated vitamin D; dietary lack of calcium or vitamin D; hypoalbuminemia	Increased neuromuscular excitability; Trousseau's and Chvostek's signs positive; skeletal muscle cramps, tetany, laryngospasm, asphyxiation, death
Chloride	100–106 mEq/L	Major anion of ECF; supplied by diet, excreted by kidney, GI tract	Functions in acid-base balance; essential in gastric acid; follows sodium in loss and gain
Hypochloremia	<95 mEq/L	Diuretic therapy, hyponatremia, metabolic alkalosis due to chloride loss, bicarbonate gain	Signs of hyponatremia and metabolic alkalosis
Magnesium	1.5–2.5 mEq/L 1.8–3.0 mg/dl	Major cation in ICF and bones; supplied in diet, excreted by kidneys; competes at renal tubule for reabsorption; PTH increases excretion	Promotes many intracellular enzyme reactions; depresses neuromuscular excitability, peripheral vasodilation
Hypomagnesemia	<1.5 mEq/L	Malabsorption related to GI disease; excess loss of GI fluids; acute alcoholism and cirrhosis of the liver; diuretic drug therapy; pancreatitis; sometimes hyper- or hypoparathyroidism	May cause hypocalcemia, and hypokalemia; neuromuscular irritability increased, positive Chvostek's and Trousseau's signs, tetany, convulsions; tachycardia, hypertension

*Source for values: J. Wallach, *Interpretation of Diagnostic Tests* (3rd ed.). Boston: Little, Brown, 1978.

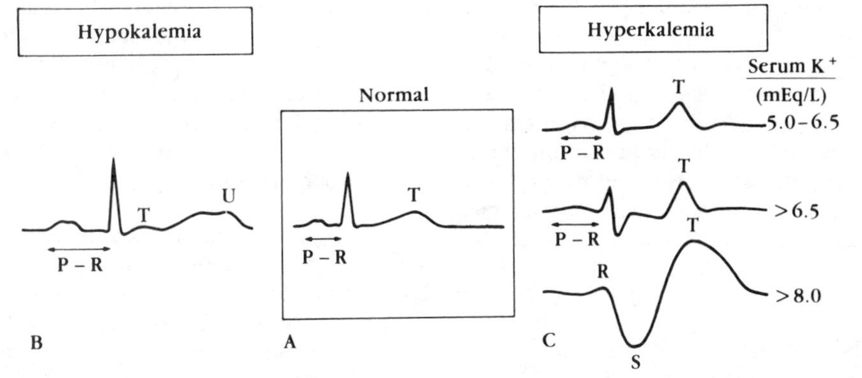

FIGURE 5-3. Altered cardiac conduction in hypokalemia and hyperkalemia. A. Normal ECG in the adult. B. In hypokalemia the T wave is flattened and the U wave is prominent. C. In hyperkalemia, the ECG changes do not always correspond to the serum potassium values given, but the progression from minor to severe changes correlates to some degree with the potassium level. With potassium concentration less than 6.5 mEq/L, the early ECG abnormality is peaking or tenting of the T waves. The next change, shown with a level of potassium concentration greater than 6.5, includes flattening of the P wave, prolongation of the P–R interval, and widening of the QRS complex, with development of a deep S wave. With severe hyperkalemia (8.0 mEq/L), ventricular fibrillation or cardiac arrest is imminent. (From R. Schrier, *Manual of Nephrology.* Boston: Little, Brown, 1981.)

mal diet provides much more potassium than is needed by the human body. Urine potassium concentrations vary, providing an efficient mechanism for the excretion of excess potassium in order to maintain the narrow normal serum concentrations.

Potassium moves into the cell during the formation of new tissues, the anabolic phase. During tissue breakdown, the catabolic phase, potassium leaves the cell. Potassium will not move into cells if there is a lack of oxygen, glucose, or insulin.

The human body very effectively excretes potassium but has little mechanism for renal conservation. Potassium deficit will occur in 2 to 3 days if there is no intake. This deficit is enhanced when there are conditions such as surgery that increase anabolic needs. Anything that increases the excretion of potassium, such as diuretics, may cause potassium depletion.

The major route for the loss of potassium is the kidneys but some of the loss can be through gastrointestinal secretions or the skin. In the kidney the final excretion of potassium is under the control of aldosterone at the distal tubule. At this point, hydrogen, potassium, and sodium tend to compete with each other for excretion. Sodium is usually preferred for absorption in the presence of aldosterone. If the plasma hydrogen ion concentration is high, the tubules tend to preferentially excrete hydrogen and conserve potassium, which leads to the hyperkalemia often seen in association with acidosis. The reverse is true in alkalosis when the hydrogen concentration is low, the potassium is preferentially excreted, and hydrogen is conserved, thus causing the problem of hypokalemia associated with alkalosis.

HYPOKALEMIA. A serum deficit of potassium may be caused by any of the following: (1) lack of intake, (2) diuretics (potassium-depleting), (3) major gastrointestinal surgical procedures especially with nasogastric suctioning and incomplete replacement, (4) excessive gastrointestinal secretions, (5) hyperaldosteronism, (6) malnutrition, and (7) posttrauma or burns.

Hypokalemia affects every system. In the gastrointestinal system anorexia, nausea, vomiting, and paralytic ileus may be seen. In the muscles, flaccidity and weakness may be exhibited, and finally may lead to respiratory muscle weakness and arrest. Cardiac arrhythmias are common and the electrocardiogram may show the presence of a U wave when it was not previously present (Fig. 5-3). Ventricular tachycardia and cardiac arrest may occur when the levels are very low. Central nervous system depression and decreased deep tendon reflexes also may be noted. Hypokalemia causes a decreased renal tubular ability to concentrate waste leading to increased water loss.

Hypokalemia causes an increased sensitivity to digitalis and may precipitate the effects of digitalis toxicity in persons taking one of these preparations. It enhances automaticity and may precipitate ventricular fibrillation.

HYPERKALEMIA. Excess potassium is usually secondary to temporary or permanent kidney dysfunction. It is frequently seen in association with renal failure. It also may be seen transiently (with normal renal function) following major tissue trauma or following the rapid transfusion of stored bank blood. As blood is stored, the red blood cells begin to break down and release their potassium into the surrounding fluid. One unit of blood, 1 day old, has approximately 7 mEq/L of potassium while that which is 21 days old has 23 mEq/L.

Hyperkalemia mainly affects the cardiovascular system.

A decreased membrane potential causes a decrease in the intensity of the action potential, resulting in a dilated, flaccid heart. Varying kinds of conduction defects may be noted along with ectopic arrhythmias. The electrocardiogram shows tall peaked T waves, a short Q–T interval, and widening of the QRS (Fig. 5-3C). In the gastrointestinal system nausea, vomiting, and diarrhea are common. Initial irritability of the skeletal muscles gives way to weakness and flaccid paralysis. Digital numbness and tingling may be described.

Calcium

Calcium is found in the body in the form of calcium salts, as ionized and as protein-bound calcium (see Table 5-2). Ninety-nine percent of the calcium is in the bones and teeth in the crystalline form, which gives hardness to these structures. Of the 1 percent that is circulating, approximately 40 percent is bound to the plasma proteins, especially the albumin. The ionized form of calcium is the active portion and functions in membrane integrity, coagulation, muscle contraction, and in the electrophysiology of the excitable cells.

Calcium can be released from its bound form especially in the presence of a decreased serum pH. The reaction simply stated is a reversible equation:

$$Ca^{2-} \text{ (protein bound)} + H^{+} \rightleftharpoons Ca^{2+} \text{ (ionized)} + H^{+} \text{ (protein complex)}$$

The reaction is driven toward the right in acidosis causing an increase in ionized serum calcium. In alkalosis the reaction is driven more toward the left, which can cause hypocalcemia. This is the method utilized by the body plasma proteins to buffer hydrogen ion [2] (see Chap. 6).

Calcium concentration in the blood is under the influence of the *parathyroid hormone* (PTH) and *thyrocalcitonin*. PTH is released by the parathyroid glands from the bone crystals and functions to increase serum calcium levels (see Chap. 32). Thyrocalcitonin enhances the deposition (uptake) of calcium into the bone when increased calcium levels are present and it inhibits bone resorption. Thyrocalcitonin is produced by the thyroid gland and functions to reduce serum calcium and phosphate.

Calcium functions to stabilize the cell membrane and block sodium transport into the cell. Because of this, decreased calcium levels increase the excitability of cells while increased calcium levels decrease excitability.

Vitamin D is produced in the skin through the action of ultraviolet light and is found also in most American diets. Vitamin D is changed by the liver to 25-hydroxycholecalciferol by hydroxylation and is further metabolized by the kidney with the aid of PTH to form the most active type 1,25-dihydroxycholecalciferol, which is important in enhancing calcium uptake from the gastrointestinal tract and to function with PTH in bone resorption [3, 11].

RELATIONSHIP OF CALCIUM TO PHOSPHATE. Phosphate is an anion that is also regulated by PTH and activated vitamin D. Normally, there is a constant total concentration of calcium and phosphate. If the calcium level increases, the phosphate level decreases. Calcium joins with phosphate to form calcium phosphate ($CaHPO_4$). When an excessive amount of $CaHPO_4$ is formed it is not ionizable and hypocalcemia results.

HYPOCALCEMIA. When calcium levels decrease, the blocking effect of calcium on sodium also decreases. As a result, depolarization of excitable cells occurs more readily as sodium moves in. Therefore, when the calcium levels are low increased central nervous system excitability and muscle spasms occur. Convulsions and tetany may be the end result.

Hypocalcemia may be seen with decreased activation of vitamin D, which is often associated with renal or liver disease. Pancreatitis may cause decreased serum calcium due to the release of pancreatic lipase, which combines with fatty acids and calcium. Blood transfusions may cause hypocalcemia as calcium binds with the citrate utilized in blood preparation, thus removing the ionizable calcium from the blood. Hyperphosphatemia, hypoalbuminemia, parathyroid disease, drug therapy such as ACTH or glucagon, surgical removal of the parathyroid glands, gastrointestinal tract disease, or neoplastic conditions may all be associated with hypocalcemia.

The results of hypocalcemia are osteoporosis, spasms and tetany, increased gastrointestinal motility, and cardiovascular problems. Muscle tetany is both common and dangerous especially when it involves laryngeal spasm. Trousseau's sign of hypocalcemia is elicited when a blood pressure cuff is inflated on an extremity for 1 to 3 minutes and a contraction of the fingers occurs. Chvostek's sign is elicited when the facial nerve at the temple is tapped, which causes a twitch on that side of the face (see Fig. 5-4). Cardiac problems include delayed depolarization and repolarization. Sometimes decreased cardiac contractility, and symptoms of heart failure result. A prolonged Q–T interval is seen in the presence of this electrolyte imbalance (Fig. 5-5).

HYPERCALCEMIA. Excessive levels of calcium increase the blocking effect on sodium in the skeletal muscles. This leads to decreased excitability of both muscles and nerves, eventually contributing to flaccidity. Hypercalcemia is associated with decreased phosphate levels. The major cause of hypercalcemia is hyperparathyroidism, which leads to increased PTH, which increases calcium uptake from the bones into the circulating blood. Some malignant tumors secrete PTH-like substances that function like the normal PTH. Excessive ingestion of vitamin D may cause the condition and occasionally it is seen with prolonged immobilization.

Hypercalcemia causes skeletal muscle weakness, anorexia, nausea and vomiting, constipation, weight loss, and increased excretion of calcium in the urine. The increased

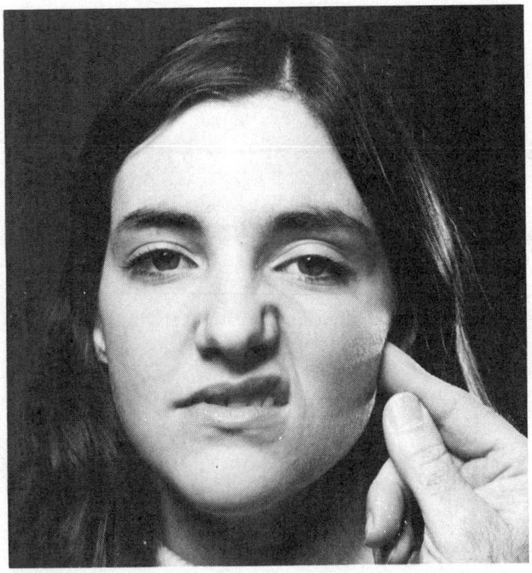

FIGURE 5-4. Facial muscle contraction in Chvostek's sign. (From M. Beyers and S. Dudas [eds.], *The Clinical Practice of Medical-Surgical Nursing* [2nd ed.]. Boston: Little, Brown, 1984.)

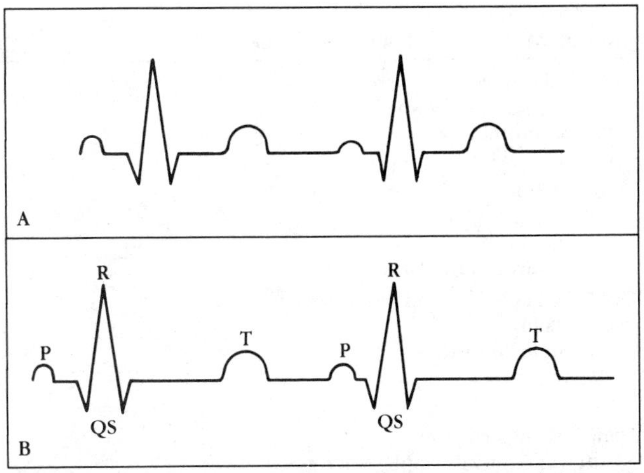

FIGURE 5-5. A. Normal ECG. B. ECG changes seen with hypocalcemia; prolongation of the Q–T interval is characteristic.

circulating calcium may be deposited anywhere but the kidneys are the most vulnerable and calcium deposition may result in kidney stones. Increased deposition in the arteries and cardiac valves also may be seen.

Chloride

The chloride ion is the major anion of the ECF (Table 5-2). The amount of chloride in the fluids closely parallels the sodium content. Chloride functions as a component of hydrochloric acid in the stomach. It also serves an essential role in the transport of carbon dioxide by the red blood cell (see Chap. 14). Chloride moves into the cell by passive transport.

Chloride depletion (hypochloremia) especially results from loss of gastrointestinal secretions, such as that which occurs from vomiting, excessive diarrhea, and nasogastric suctioning. Diuretic therapy commonly causes hypochloremia along with hyponatremia, but urinary loss of chloride may be greater than loss of sodium. Metabolic alkalosis results as bicarbonate is conserved to maintain cation-anion balance. The clinical manifestations of hypochloremia are usually related to the associated metabolic alkalosis (see Chap. 6).

Magnesium

This cation is found mostly within the cells and in the bones (see Table 5-2). It functions to activate a number of intracellular enzyme systems and is required for protein and nucleic acid synthesis. Magnesium is particularly essential in promoting neuromuscular integrity [8].

HYPOMAGNESEMIA. The most common cause of decreased serum magnesium is excessive ingestion of alcohol. Other causes include malnutrition, diabetes mellitus, liver failure, and poor intestinal absorption. The clinical manifestations include increased neuromuscular irritability, paresthesias, tetany, and convulsions.

HYPERMAGNESEMIA. This condition is rare but may be seen in individuals with renal failure, especially if they ingest magnesium-containing antacids [8]. Clinical manifestations include lethargy, coma, cardiac arrhythmias, respiratory failure, and death. Because dialysis in persons with chronic renal failure does not remove magnesium well these individuals should be restricted from ingesting magnesium-containing medications.

EDEMA

The term *edema* refers to an expansion or accumulation of interstitial fluid volume. It may be localized or generalized, pitting or nonpitting, depending on the etiologic basis for the condition. Edema is usually thought of as accumulation of excess fluid in the skin; however, the mechanism causing skin edema also can cause fluid shifts in other vulnerable areas of the body. These fluid shifts are sometimes termed *third-space* shifts and include ascites, pleural or pericardial effusions, and pulmonary edema [1]. Table 5-3 summarizes the etiologic mechanisms that may lead to the formation of edema and fluid shifts. Five interrelated mechanisms are commonly described [10].

1. Decreased colloid osmotic pressure
2. Increased capillary hydrostatic pressure
3. Increased capillary permeability
4. Lymphatic obstruction
5. Sodium and body water excess

Some forms of edema result from more than one mechanism.

TABLE 5-3. Examples of etiologic mechanisms for the formation of edema

- Increased capillary pressure
  - Congestive heart failure
  - Phlebothrombosis
  - Cirrhosis of liver with portal hypertension
- Vasodilatation
  - Inflammation
  - Allergic reactions
  - Burns (direct vascular injury)
- Decreased colloid osmotic pressure
  - Liver failure
  - Protein malnutrition
  - Nephrosis
  - Burns
- Lymphatic obstruction
  - Surgical removal lymph structures
  - Inflammation or malignant involvement of lymph nodes and vessels
  - Filariasis
- Sodium/body water excess
  - Congestive heart failure
  - Renal failure
  - Aldosteronism
  - Excess sodium intake

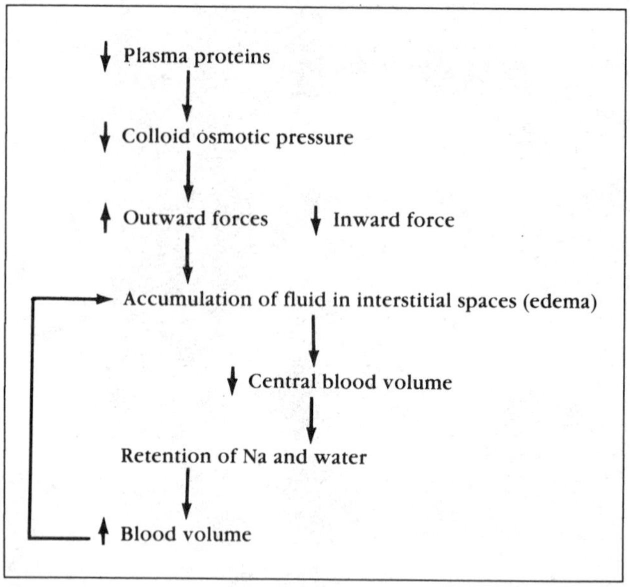

FIGURE 5-6. Positive feedback of compensatory mechanisms for decreased colloid osmotic pressure.

Decreased Colloid Osmotic Pressure

When the plasma proteins are depleted in the blood, the inward forces are decreased allowing the filtration effect to favor movement into the tissues (see p. 61). This leads to accumulation of fluid in the tissues with a decreased central volume of plasma. The kidneys respond to the decreased circulating volume by activation of the renin-angiotensin system, resulting in further resorption of sodium and water.

Hypoproteinemia causes decreased colloid osmotic pressure (COP) and may result from malnutrition, neoplastic wasting, liver failure, or protein loss from burns, kidneys, or the gastrointestinal tract. Albumin is the primary protein affected because it is the most abundant and also because it is rather small and can pass through damaged capillary endothelium or glomeruli. Loss of protein into the tissues causes a decreased resorption of tissue fluids and edema. The situation becomes a positive feedback response because as the central blood volume becomes depleted, the kidney conserves more sodium and water, and further edema is formed (Fig. 5-6). This response can be terminated by restoration of intravascular protein levels, which increases the intravascular colloid osmotic pressure and subsequently its volume.

The accumulation of ascitic fluid in cirrhosis of the liver is partly related to the hypoproteinemia from decreased hepatic production of albumin and partly due to increased hydrostatic pressure created by portal hypertension (see Chap. 37).

Increased Capillary Hydrostatic Pressure

The most common cause of increased capillary pressure is congestive heart failure (right heart failure) in which there is a combination of increased systemic venous pressure and increased blood volume. Left heart failure may also lead to an increase in the pulmonary capillary pressure (PCP). When the pressure exceeds 30 mm Hg pulmonary edema occurs. Other causes of increased hydrostatic pressure include renal failure with increased total blood volume, increased gravitational forces from standing for long periods of time, impaired venous circulation, and hepatic obstruction. Venous obstruction produces localized rather than generalized edema because only one vein or group of veins is usually affected.

Increased Capillary Permeability

Direct damage to blood vessels, such as with trauma and burns, may cause increased permeability of the endothelial junctions. Localized edema may occur in response to an allergen, such as a bee sting, and in certain individuals this allergen may precipitate an anaphylactic response with widespread edema initiated by the histamine or slow-reactive substance of anaphylaxis (SRS-A) type of reaction (see Chap. 11).

Inflammation causes hyperemia and vasodilation, which leads to accumulation of fluids, proteins, and cells in an affected area. This results in edematous swelling (exudation) of the affected localized area (see Chap. 8).

Obstruction of the Lymphatics

The most common cause of lymphatic obstruction is the surgical removal of a group of lymph nodes and vessels to prevent the spread of a malignancy. Radiation therapy, trauma, malignant metastasis, and inflammation may also lead to localized lymphatic obstruction. *Filariasis*, a rare

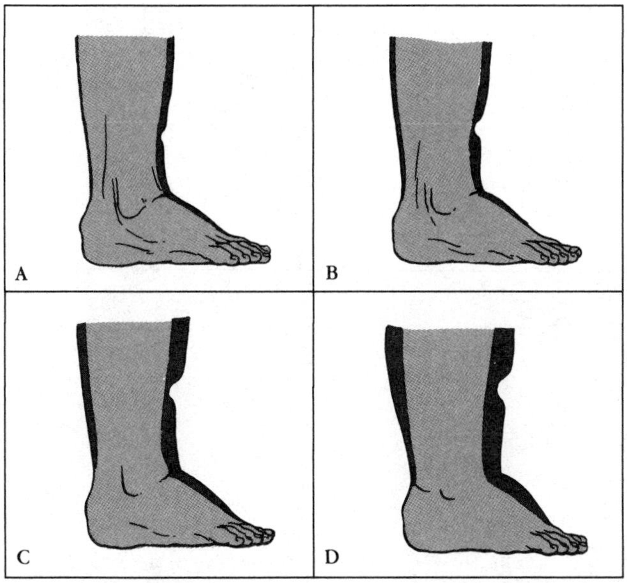

FIGURE 5-7. Grading of edema. A. 1+: slight pit, normal contours. B. 2+: deeper pit, fairly normal contours. C. 3+: deep pit, puffy appearance. D. 4+: deep pit, frankly swollen. (From R. Judge, G. Zuidema, and F. Fitzgerald, *Clinical Diagnosis* [4th ed.]. Boston: Little, Brown, 1982.)

parasitic infection of the lymph vessels, can cause widespread obstruction of the vessels.

Lymphatic obstruction leads to retention of excess fluid and plasma proteins in the interstitial fluid. As proteins accumulate in the interstitial (IS) spaces more water moves into the area. The edema is usually localized in nature.

Sodium and Body Water Excess

With congestive heart failure (and other conditions), cardiac output is decreased as the force of contraction decreases. To compensate, aldosterone causes the retention of sodium and water. Plasma volume increases as does venous intravascular capillary pressure. The failing heart is unable to handle this increased venous return, and fluid is forced into the interstitial space.

Types of Edema

Pitting edema refers to the displacement of interstitial water by finger pressure on the skin leaving a pitted depression. This is graded 1 to 4 according to the depth of pitting noted (Fig. 5-7). After the pressure is removed it often takes several minutes for the depression to be resolved. Pitting edema often appears in dependent positions such as the sacrum of a bedridden individual. Similarly, gravitational hydrostatic pressure increases the accumulation of fluid in the legs and feet of an upright individual.

Nonpitting edema may be seen in areas of loose skin folds such as the periorbital spaces of the face. Nonpitting edema may follow venous thrombosis especially of the superficial veins. Persistent edema leads to trophic changes

TABLE 5-4. Clinical picture exhibited by patient in shock

	Pump failure	Volume decrease	Change in resistance
Urinary output	↓	↓	Normal to ↓
Blood pressure	↓	↓	↓
Cardiac output	↓	↓	Normal to ↓ (early ↑)
Central venous pressure	↑	↓	Normal to ↓
Temperature	Normal	↓	↑ or ↓
Peripheral vascular resistance	↑	↑	↓

Source: C. V. Kenner, C. E. Guzzetta, and B. M. Dossey, *Critical Care Nursing*. Boston: Little, Brown, 1982. Used with permission.

in the skin. These changes may progress to stasis dermatitis and ulcers that heal very slowly (see Chap. 21). Nonpitting, brawny edema is also associated with thick, hardened skin and color changes. Serum proteins that have become trapped and coagulated in the tissue spaces are the cause of this type of edema.

Distribution of Edema

The distribution of edema can give clues as to its cause. If the edema is localized in one extremity it is probably due to venous or lymphatic obstruction. Edema resulting from hypoproteinemia is generalized but is especially pronounced in the eyelids and face in the morning, due to the recumbent position assumed at night and the aid of gravitational forces. Edema of heart failure is usually greatest in the legs of an ambulatory individual and it tends to accumulate throughout the day [4].

SHOCK

Shock refers to a syndrome that results in inadequate tissue perfusion. It is usually recognized by the classic symptoms of decreased blood pressure, rapid, thready pulse, increased respiration, cold, clammy skin, oliguria, and alterations in consciousness [12]. The most common classification utilizes the following mechanisms [5]:

I. Cardiogenic shock
   A. Pump failure
   B. Decreased venous inflow
II. Decreased blood volume
   A. Hemorrhage
   B. Burn shock
   C. Dehydration
III. Change in peripheral resistance
   A. Neurogenic shock
   B. Septic shock
   C. Allergic shock

Table 5-4 shows the differences in the clinical pictures that may be exhibited with the three mechanisms.

TABLE 5-5. Clinical picture exhibited by patient according to degree of shock

	Early	Middle	Late
Sensorium	Oriented to time, place, person	Remains oriented; words slurred	Disoriented
Pulse	Rate, 110–120 Quality, full to decreased	Rate, 120–150 Quality, decreased and variable	Rate, greater than 150 Quality, weak
Blood pressure	Normal to low (10–20% decrease but may be slightly increased as compensatory mechanism)	Decreased 40–50 mm Hg below normal (20–40% decrease)	Systolic less than 80 Diastolic may not be heard
Urinary output	35–50 ml/hr	20–35 ml/hr	Less than 20 ml/hr
Color	Pale	Pale	Mottled
Capillary refill	Circulation return slightly slowed	Circulation return slowed	Circulation return very slow; skin pale both before and after Large differences between rectal and big toe temperature

Source: C. V. Kenner, C. E. Guzzetta, and B. M. Dossey, *Critical Care Nursing*. Boston: Little, Brown, 1982. Used with permission.

Compensatory Mechanisms in Shock

SYMPATHETIC NERVOUS SYSTEM (SNS) STIMULATION. Whenever the blood pressure drops for any reason a reflex stimulation of the SNS occurs. The result of this stimulation is arteriolar vasoconstriction, tachycardia, and increased myocardial contractility.

ANAEROBIC PRODUCTION OF ATP. In order to maintain viability of the cell, ATP must be continually formed. In the absence of oxygen, ATP can be formed for a period of time without oxygen. This anaerobic metabolism is inefficient in production of ATP but does allow for cell survival for varying periods depending on the type of cell. The brain cells are very vulnerable to lack of oxygen and can survive only minutes without it. As anaerobic metabolism continues, its by-product, lactic acid, accumulates. The buildup of lactic acid causes intracellular acidity, leading finally to cellular membrane rupture and death. Lactic acidosis progresses to metabolic acidosis and leads to the irreversible stage of shock.

FLUID SHIFTS AND RENAL CONSERVATION. As the blood pressure falls the intravascular volume may be depleted. The intracellular and interstitial fluid is moved into the intravascular system in an attempt to restore central blood volume. The kidneys respond by decreasing urinary output and conserving sodium through the influence of the renin-angiotensin-aldosterone (RAA) system. Blood is shunted away from many organs by the process of vasoconstriction, and organ function is depressed in order to conserve oxygen.

Stages of Shock

The hemodynamic changes of shock have been classified as early, middle, or late (Table 5-5). The early stage is characterized by increased cardiac and sympathetic compensation. In the middle stage, the *classic* shock picture is usually expressed. The late stage is called the irreversible stage when compensatory mechanisms are failing and the prognosis is poor.

Cardiogenic Shock

PUMP FAILURE. In pump failure the heart is unable to adequately discharge its contents to the circulatory system because of intrinsic myocardial disease. The most common cause of pump failure is left ventricular failure resulting from myocardial infarction. Pump failure shock also may be seen with right heart failure (see Chap. 18). The cardiac output is decreased but the end-diastolic volume and pressure are increased. The result is a decrease in the systemic blood pressure and a concomitant increase in venous pressure. In response to the decreased blood pressure the kidneys secrete renin, which leads to vasoconstriction and volume retention. As the blood volume and peripheral vascular resistance increase, the load on an overtaxed heart is increased causing further decompensation. The sympathetic nervous system also is stimulated causing an increased heart rate and contractility. As the tissues suffer from oxygen deprivation the cells utilize anaerobic metabolism to sustain life. The entire process is a positive feedback mechanism that will progress irreversibly to death if treatment is not initiated.

DECREASED VENOUS INFLOW. Conditions such as cardiac tamponade (due to acute hemopericardium), mediastinal shift, or acute pericardial effusion decrease the blood inflow to the heart and subsequently decrease the cardiac output (Fig. 5-8). The source of the problem is not the heart muscle but external compression on the heart. The venous system becomes engorged with blood causing an increased central venous pressure, distended neck veins, tachycardia, orthopnea, hepatomegaly, and hypotension. The amount of fluid required to produce the tamponade effect can be as little as 250 ml in a rapid bleed or as much as 1000 ml in a slowly accumulating effusion. As the fluid accumulates, distant heart sounds and decreased QRS voltage on the ECG may be noted.

Blood Volume Decrease (Hypovolemic Shock)

HEMORRHAGIC SHOCK. Hemorrhagic or hematogenic shock

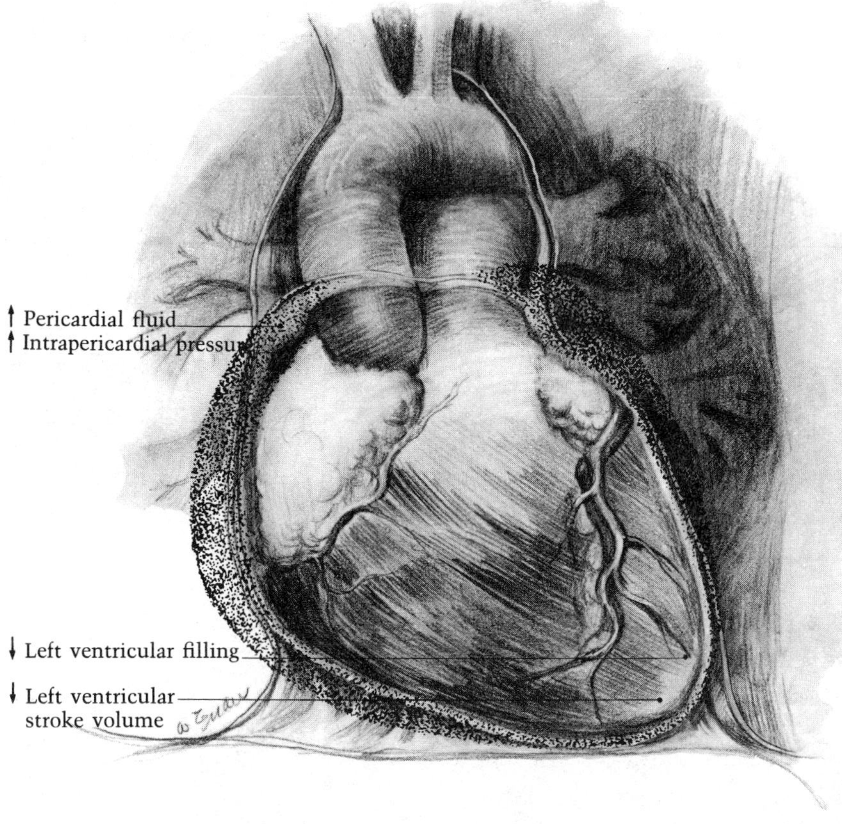

FIGURE 5-8. Pericardial effusion and cardiac tamponade. The following hemodynamic effects may result following pericardial effusion: (1) accumulation of pericardial fluid resulting in intrapericardial pressure; (2) elevation of right atrial pressure; (3) elevation of left ventricular end-diastolic pressure; (4) reduction in left ventricular end-diastolic volume and cardiac output; (5) elevated venous pressure. (From C. V. Kenner, C. E. Guzzetta, and B. M. Dossey, *Critical Care Nursing*. Boston: Little, Brown, 1982.)

results from loss of whole blood, including both plasma and cells. An actual decrease in blood volume occurs, which usually must be greater than 500 ml in the adult to cause symptoms. Acute blood loss of greater than 1 liter leads to a drop in cardiac output causing hypotension, tachycardia, vasoconstriction, oliguria, diaphoresis, and anxiety. If up to 50 percent of the blood volume is lost the anxiety gives way to stupor and coma, anuria, blood pressure below 60 mm Hg, and extreme tachycardia [9]. Hemorrhagic shock may result from external or internal blood loss, for example trauma or gastrointestinal bleeding.

The compensatory mechanisms initiated include SNS stimulation, RAA activation, vasoconstriction of the peripheral vessels, tachycardia, increased oxygen uptake, and anaerobic metabolism, all of which initially tend to promote a return to the steady state, or a negative feedback mechanism.

BURN SHOCK. Shock resulting from third-degree burns results from loss of plasma proteins and water into the interstitial areas. The resulting decreased colloid osmotic pressure leads to a decreased central volume and blood pressure. The central venous pressure decreases, the heart rate increases, and all compensatory mechanisms are initiated. The restoration of central volume and pressure often requires the replacement of plasma proteins.

DEHYDRATION SHOCK. Critical amounts of fluid volume can be lost through excessive gastrointestinal, skin, and urinary volume loss. Total body fluids are lost leading to decreased circulating plasma. Such diverse conditions as diarrhea, heat prostration, and lack of ADH can precipitate dehydration shock. As the blood volume decreases to a critical level, the blood pressure begins to fall and all of the compensatory mechanisms are activated to preserve life.

Changes in Peripheral Resistance

NEUROGENIC SHOCK. Neurogenic shock results from the loss of SNS control of the arterioles, which leads to sudden onset of vasodilation and peripheral pooling. Many conditions can precipitate this reaction including drug reactions, spinal cord injury, overwhelming stress reactions, and brain injuries. Even fainting is considered to be a transient form of neurogenic shock. The hemodynamic result of SNS interruption leads to decreased peripheral vascular resistance, peripheral pooling, decreased systemic blood pressure, and decreased central venous pressure. This condition is often transient, and restoration of SNS tone without intervention may occur.

SEPTIC OR TOXIC SHOCK. This condition has many names and is being recognized with increasing frequency in acute care settings. Toxic shock can produce a hyperdynamic or hypodynamic clinical picture or one state may progress to the next [6].

The *hyperdynamic* picture is also called *warm* or *pink shock*. The person affected often presents with high temperature, chills, mental confusion, severe tachycardia, and tachypnea. The blood pressure may be normal in the initial bacteremic stages but becomes decreased as the vasodilation becomes widespread. The hyperdynamic picture is often the initial reaction in bacteremia in the person who has an immunocompetent defense system. As vasodilation becomes severe, fluid shifts to the capillary bed and stagnant anoxia occur. Cell metabolism becomes impaired because of the poor circulation.

Cool shock is also called *normodynamic* shock. As the endotoxins are released decreased venous return and capillary leakage result. The blood pressure decreases, the body begins to compensate with vasoconstriction, and cool skin results. Tachycardia, oliguria, thirst, and blood pressure decrease are characteristic at this point.

Progression of the shock state leads to *hypodynamic* shock, which gives the external appearance of hemorrhagic shock. The hypodynamic picture is usually equivalent to the late or irreversible stage of shock and the prognosis for recovery is poor. The clinical manifestations include cold, clammy skin; severe hypotension; metabolic acidosis; anuria; and tachycardia. Disseminated intravascular coagulation (DIC) is a common complication that may result from toxin activation of the coagulation system. Circulatory collapse and severe metabolic acidosis may lead to death.

Blood cultures identify the organism responsible for the bacteremia. *Escherichia coli* is a common cause of this type of shock, especially in elderly or debilitated persons. Other laboratory studies reveal the effects of shock on the system and include blood gas abnormalities, blood urea nitrogen and creatinine elevations, and sometimes clotting disturbances.

ANAPHYLACTIC, OR ALLERGIC, SHOCK. This dangerous type of shock develops because of a hypersensitivity reaction to a specific allergen. The result is mediated by IgE antibody in which allergen and mast cell interactions cause a release of histamine, SRS-A, and other vasoactive substances. Widespread vasodilation and increased capillary permeability lead to hypotension, decreased venous pressure, and compensatory tachycardia. The clinical manifestations include any or all of the following: anxiety, hypotension, tachycardia, wheezing, coughing, hives, periorbital edema, and laryngospasm. This reaction can be rapidly fatal if the person is not treated immediately (see Chap. 11).

REFERENCES

1. Braunwald, E. Edema. In K. J. Isselbacher, et al. (eds.), *Harrison's Principles of Internal Medicine* (10th ed.). New York: McGraw-Hill, 1983.
2. Gröer, M. W. *Physiology and Pathophysiology of the Body Fluids*. St. Louis: Mosby, 1981.
3. Guyton, A. C. *Textbook of Medical Physiology* (6th ed.). Philadelphia: Saunders, 1981.
4. Isselbacher, K. J. et al. *Harrison's Principles of Internal Medicine* (10th ed.). New York: McGraw-Hill, 1983.
5. Kenner, C. V., Guzzetta, C. E., and Dossey, B. M. *Critical Care Nursing*. Boston: Little, Brown, 1982.
6. Lamb, L. S. Think you know septic shock? *Nurs. '82* 12:34, 1982.
7. Luckmann, J., and Sorensen, K. C. *Medical-Surgical Nursing: A Psychophysiologic Approach* (2nd ed.). Philadelphia: Saunders, 1980.
8. Metheny, N. M., and Snively, W. D. *Nurse's Handbook of Fluid Balance* (3rd ed.). Philadelphia: Lippincott, 1979.
9. Porth, C. *Pathophysiology Concepts of Altered Health States*. Philadelphia: Lippincott, 1982.
10. Robbins, S., and Cotran, R. *Pathologic Basis of Disease* (2nd ed.). Philadelphia: Saunders, 1979.
11. Rose, B. D. *Clinical Physiology of Acid-Base and Electrolyte Disorders*. New York: McGraw-Hill, 1977.
12. Shedden, H. E. Shock: Mechanisms at the cellular level. *Focus* 2:27, 1979.

CHAPTER 6
NORMAL AND ALTERED ACID-BASE BALANCE

LEARNING OBJECTIVES

1. Define the meaning of the symbol *pH*.
2. List the normal values of the blood gases and pH of the different body fluids.
3. Differentiate between volatile and nonvolatile acids.
4. Diagram the dissociation of carbonic acid.
5. Describe the three major buffer systems.
6. Describe specifically how the carbonic acid-bicarbonate system is affected by the respiratory and renal systems.
7. Explain how the ratio of H_2CO_3 with HCO_3^- is maintained.
8. Explain how the kidney excretes hydrogen ion without decreasing the pH of the urine below physiologic limits.
9. Describe the activity of hemoglobin as a protein buffer.
10. Differentiate between acidosis and alkalosis on the basis of physiologic disruption.
11. Describe the pathophysiology that underlies respiratory acidosis.
12. Compare respiratory acidosis and metabolic acidosis in terms of pathophysiology and compensatory mechanisms.
13. Define the term *anion gap* and relate it to an acid-base abnormality.
14. Differentiate the etiology of metabolic and respiratory alkalosis.
15. Describe the clinical manifestations of metabolic and respiratory alkalosis.

Many disease processes can alter the precise acid-base balance of the body, and the effect of the resulting acidosis or alkalosis may be more devastating than the disease itself. This chapter reviews the basic concepts of acid-base balance and discusses the major alterations in this balance. Detailed information concerning the calculation of the pH, other related chemical equations, and advanced application of the concepts is found in the bibliography at the end of the unit.

pH AND HYDROGEN ION

The pH is simply a negative logarithm of hydrogen ions (H^+) in a solution. One liter of water contains 0.0000001 gm of hydrogen ions. This figure is equal to $1/10^7$ or the following equation:

$$0.0000001 = 1/10{,}000{,}000 = 1/10 \times 10 \times 10 \times 10 \times 10 \times 10 \times 10 = 1/10^7 = 10^{-7}$$

This simplified formula denotes the negative notation of a pH of 7 for neutral water [4]. Therefore, if water is neutral at a pH of 7 and hydrogen ions are added to it, the solution becomes more acidic. The greater the hydrogen ion concentration the more acidic the solution and the pH number falls. Acidic solutions are scaled between 0 and 7. Alkalotic or basic solutions, on the other hand, have less hydrogen ion concentration and are scaled between 7 and 14. The smaller the hydrogen ion concentration the more alkaline is the solution. Table 6-1 shows the Sorensen pH scale as it relates to the approximate pH compositions of body fluids. Note that the relationship between the pH and the hydrogen ion figures is logarithmic rather than linear. This means that an increase or decrease of one pH unit represents a tenfold change in hydrogen ion concentration.

In the fluids of the human body the acceptable pH range is 7.35 to 7.45. Normal blood gas values are indicated in Table 6-2. Levels below 7.35 indicate a state of acidosis while levels above 7.45 indicate alkalosis. When the hydrogen ion concentration is in the normal range of 40 nEq/L, the pH is 7.40. A nEq, or nanoequivalent, is the same as a millimicroequivalent and represents a very small measurement [1]. Table 6-3 shows the relationship between the pH of the arterial blood and the H^+ concentration. The pH levels that are compatible with life are approximately 6.8 to 7.8.

Alterations in H^+ concentration alter the functioning of many enzyme and hormone systems, e.g., acidosis depresses the function of epinephrine. H^+ concentration also affects neurologic functioning and distribution of other ions.

In the processes of cellular metabolism acid is continually being formed. Fifty to 100 mEq of excess hydrogen is produced daily, which must be eliminated from the body to maintain the steady state. The acids formed are of two types: (1) *volatile* acids that are excretable by the lungs; and (2) *nonvolatile* acids that are excreted by the kidney.

The volatile acid is in the form of carbonic acid (H_2CO_3), a weak acid, which can be dissociated into carbon dioxide gas (CO_2) and water (H_2O). Because H_2CO_3 is a weak acid the following reversible equation results:

$$H_2CO_3 \underset{\text{(CARBONIC ANHYDRASE)}}{\rightleftharpoons} CO_2 + H_2O$$

The reaction proceeds more readily when the enzyme carbonic anhydrase is present.

The carbon dioxide gas diffuses readily across the alveolocapillary membrane and is removed in the process of ventilation (see Chap. 22).

Nonvolatile acids, such as sulfuric and phosphoric acid, are produced in the metabolism of proteins, carbohydrates, and fats. These acids are dependent on renal tubular function for their excretion.

BUFFER SYSTEMS

A buffer system refers to a weak acid and its salt, which function to pick up or donate sufficient hydrogen ions to keep the pH within a normal range. The major buffer systems for regulating acid-base balance are: (1) the carbonic acid–bicarbonate system, (2) the protein buffer, and (3) the phosphate buffer. These systems function together in an interrelated fashion with changes in one system influencing the others.

Carbonic Acid–Bicarbonate System

This system is the most important extracellular buffer because it can be regulated by both the lungs and the kidneys. Normally the carbonic acid (H_2CO_3)–bicarbonate (HCO_3^-) ratio is maintained at approximately 1:20. This ratio keeps the pH at approximately 7.40. The actual content required to maintain this balance is 1.2 mmol/liter of H_2CO_3 to 24 mEq/liter of HCO_3^-. As long as the ratio of 1:20 is maintained the pH will also be stabilized. If, for example, a retention of carbon dioxide and a reciprocal compensatory retention of bicarbonate occurs, the amounts might be 2.0 mmol/liter of H_2CO_3 and 40 mEq/L of HCO_3^-, which would still maintain the ratio (2:40 instead of 1:20) and the pH would remain at 7.40. The respiratory system works very rapidly in the excretion or retention of CO_2 while the renal system functions much more slowly to retain or excrete HCO_3^-.

RESPIRATORY REGULATION. As excess carbon dioxide is formed from cellular processes most of it is picked up by the red blood cells and carried to the lungs. The CO_2 combines with H_2O in a reversible equation that forms H_2CO_3 and $H^+ + HCO_3^-$. Therefore, increased amounts of carbon dioxide are the same as increased hydrogen ion and function to lower the blood pH.

Hypoventilation increases the carbon dioxide and thus the acid content of the blood, while hyperventilation decreases the CO_2 and makes the blood more alkalotic. An increase in alveolar ventilation of 2 times normal can in-

TABLE 6-1. pH scale showing the concentration of hydrogen ions from pH 1 to pH 14

H^+ concentration (gm/liter)	Scientific notation	pH units	Examples
0.1	10^{-1}	$-\log 10^{-1} = 1$	Gastric juice
0.01	10^{-2}	$-\log 10^{-2} = 2$	Gastric juice
0.001	10^{-3}	$-\log 10^{-3} = 3$	Gastric juice
0.0001	10^{-4}	$-\log 10^{-4} = 4$	
0.00001	10^{-5}	$-\log 10^{-5} = 5$	Urine
0.000001	10^{-6}	$-\log 10^{-6} = 6$	Urine
0.0000001	10^{-7}	$-\log 10^{-7} = 7$	Arterial blood
0.00000001	10^{-8}	$-\log 10^{-8} = 8$	Pancreatic juice
0.000000001	10^{-9}	$-\log 10^{-9} = 9$	
0.0000000001	10^{-10}	$-\log 10^{-10} = 10$	
0.00000000001	10^{-11}	$-\log 10^{-11} = 11$	
0.000000000001	10^{-12}	$-\log 10^{-12} = 12$	
0.0000000000001	10^{-13}	$-\log 10^{-13} = 13$	
0.00000000000001	10^{-14}	$-\log 10^{-14} = 14$	

Note: The approximate pH of some of the body fluids is indicated.
Source: Adapted from M. W. Groër, *Physiology and Pathophysiology of the Body Fluids.* St. Louis: Mosby, 1981.

TABLE 6-2. Normal blood gas values including anion gap

Plasma HCO_3^-	Adults: 23–25 mEq/L arterial
Plasma pH, arterial	7.38–7.42
Plasma HPO_4^-	1.7–2.6 mEq/L
Plasma PCO_2	38–42 mm Hg (arterial or arterialized blood)
Plasma PO_2	95–100 mm Hg (arterial or arterialized blood)
Anion gap = Na^+ (mEq/L) − (Cl^-[mEq/L] + HCO_3^- [mEq/L])	13 or below = normal or if acidosis caused by inorganic acids; above 13 = acidosis due to organic acids

Source: N. M. Metheny and W. D. Snively, *Nurses' Handbook of Fluid Balance* (3rd ed.). Philadelphia: Lippincott, 1979.

TABLE 6-3. Relationship between the pH and the H^+ concentration in the physiologic range

pH ↓	$[H^+]$ (nmol/L)
7.80	16
7.70	20
7.60	26
7.50	32
7.40	40
7.30	50
7.20	63
7.10	80
7.00	100
6.90	125
6.80	160

Source: B. D. Rose, *Clinical Physiology of Acid-Base and Electrolyte Disorders.* New York: McGraw-Hill, 1977. P. 169.

crease the pH of blood 0.23 pH units and depressing ventilation to one-fourth of normal decreases the pH by 0.4 pH units [2].

In normal respiratory control minute changes in H^+ (CO_2) affect the respiratory center in the medulla oblongata. The respirations are increased or decreased accordingly so that the pH remains in normal range (see Chap. 22).

RENAL REGULATION. The kidneys function to return the pH to normal range by increasing or decreasing the amount of bicarbonate ions in the extracellular fluid (ECF). This mechanism functions more slowly than the respiratory mechanism but it continues its action until the pH is returned to normal. The kidneys compensate by altering the rate of hydrogen ion resorption (which alters sodium and potassium exchange) and the bicarbonate formation and resorption. The mechanism involves: (1) the excretion of 50 to 100 mEq of H^+ produced daily, and (2) the resorption of filtered HCO_3^- [3].

The conservation of bicarbonate in the plasma depends on active secretion of H^+ from the capillaries into the renal tubules. Bicarbonate is filtered through the glomerulus and most of it is resorbed in the proximal tubule. In the proximal tubule the HCO_3^- receives secreted H^+ and H_2CO_3 is formed. This H_2CO_3 is split into $CO_2 + H_2O$ with the aid of carbonic anhydrase, an enzyme found on the brush border of proximal tubular cells. The reaction is as follows:

$$H^+ + HCO_3^- \longrightarrow H_2CO_3 \xrightarrow{\text{(CARBONIC ANHYDRASE)}} CO_2 + H_2O$$

The CO_2 and H_2O are resorbed, and in the capillary they again join to become H_2CO_3, which splits into H^+ and HCO_3^-. Active secretion of H^+ continues through the distal tubule and collecting ducts but the reconversion of CO_2 and H_2O does not occur as readily due to the lack of carbonic anhydrase in these areas. The tubular pH then falls indicating a hydrogen ion loss into the urine, or urinary acidification. A urine pH of 4.5 represents a H^+ concentration of almost 1000 times that of plasma [3].

Several weak acids that are filtered at the glomerulus and poorly resorbed also aid in buffering. These include the phosphate buffer and, to a lesser extent, uric acid and creatinine. The phosphate buffer is weak in the ECF of the blood but is much more powerful in the urine. It consists

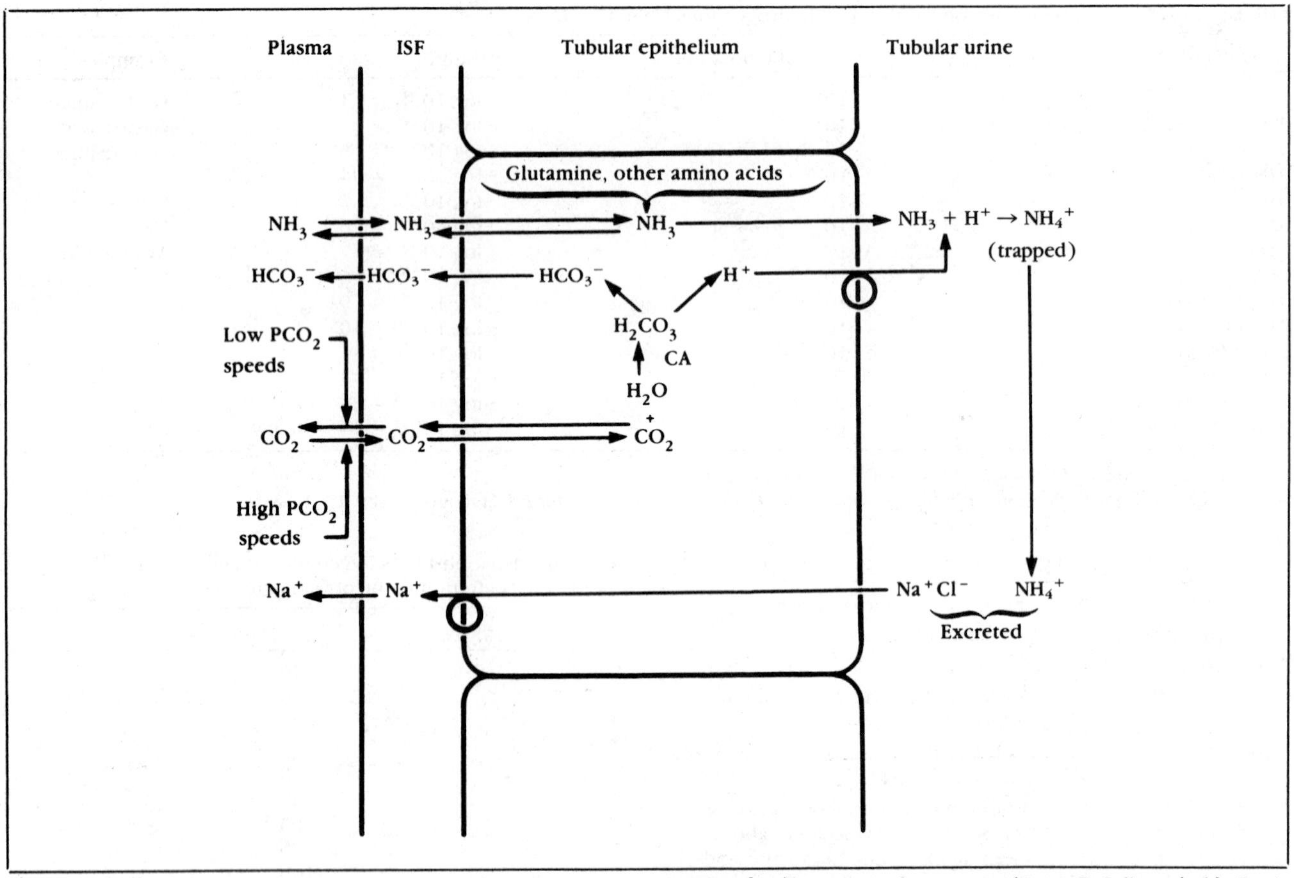

FIGURE 6-1. Excretion of ammonia. (From E. Selkurt (ed.), *Basic Physiology for the Health Sciences* [2nd ed.]. Boston: Little, Brown, 1982.)

of HPO_4^-, which picks up excess H^+ to become H_2PO_4. A sodium ion is resorbed for the hydrogen that is excreted. The end result is increased sodium bicarbonate ($NaHCO_3$) in the ECF [2]. This mechanism can increase its rate of activity when there is a decreased blood pH.

The ammonia-ammonium mechanism also assumes importance in renal adjustments of pH. The renal tubules synthesize *ammonia* (NH_3) from certain amino acids. The NH_3 diffuses into the renal tubules where it can add a hydrogen ion and become NH_4^+, or *ammonium*. This NH_4^+ radical joins with an anion such as chloride. Again, this reaction often serves to release a sodium ion, which is resorbed and adds another $NaHCO_3$ complex to the blood [2]. The actual tubular synthesis of NH_3 is controlled by the concentration or amount of H^+ ion to be secreted. The mechanism assumes great importance when a large number of hydrogen ions must be excreted from the body (Fig. 6-1). Physiologically, the pH of the urine cannot drop below 4.5 because the secretion of H^+ ion ceases. The ammonia-ammonium mechanism is only weakly acidic and affects the pH of the urine only slightly (see also Chap. 26). This mechanism allows a way to eliminate excess H^+ ion from the blood and is often seen with chronic acidotic conditions, such as chronic respiratory acidosis.

Protein Buffer

The most abundant buffer in the body is the protein buffer, which can involve both the cells and the plasma. This intracellular buffer affects the extracellular fluid because of the diffusion of hydrogen, carbon dioxide, and bicarbonate into the cell.

Hemoglobin is an effective protein buffer, which functions to attach carbon dioxide directly or indirectly (Fig. 6-2). The buffering results when carbon dioxide diffuses into the red blood cell forms H_2CO_3, which then dissociates into H^+ and HCO_3^-. The H^+ attaches to the hemoglobin molecule (see Chap. 22). The end result of the process is to make HCO_3^- available for buffering in the plasma. Most of the CO_2 is carried on the hemoglobin in the form of hydrogen hemoglobin (HHb), which is a weak acid.

Phosphate Buffer

The function of the phosphate buffer in the kidney tubule was described on p. 75. Phosphate is also an extremely important intracellular buffer due to its high concentration in ICF. In general, the ICF has a lower pH than the ECF,

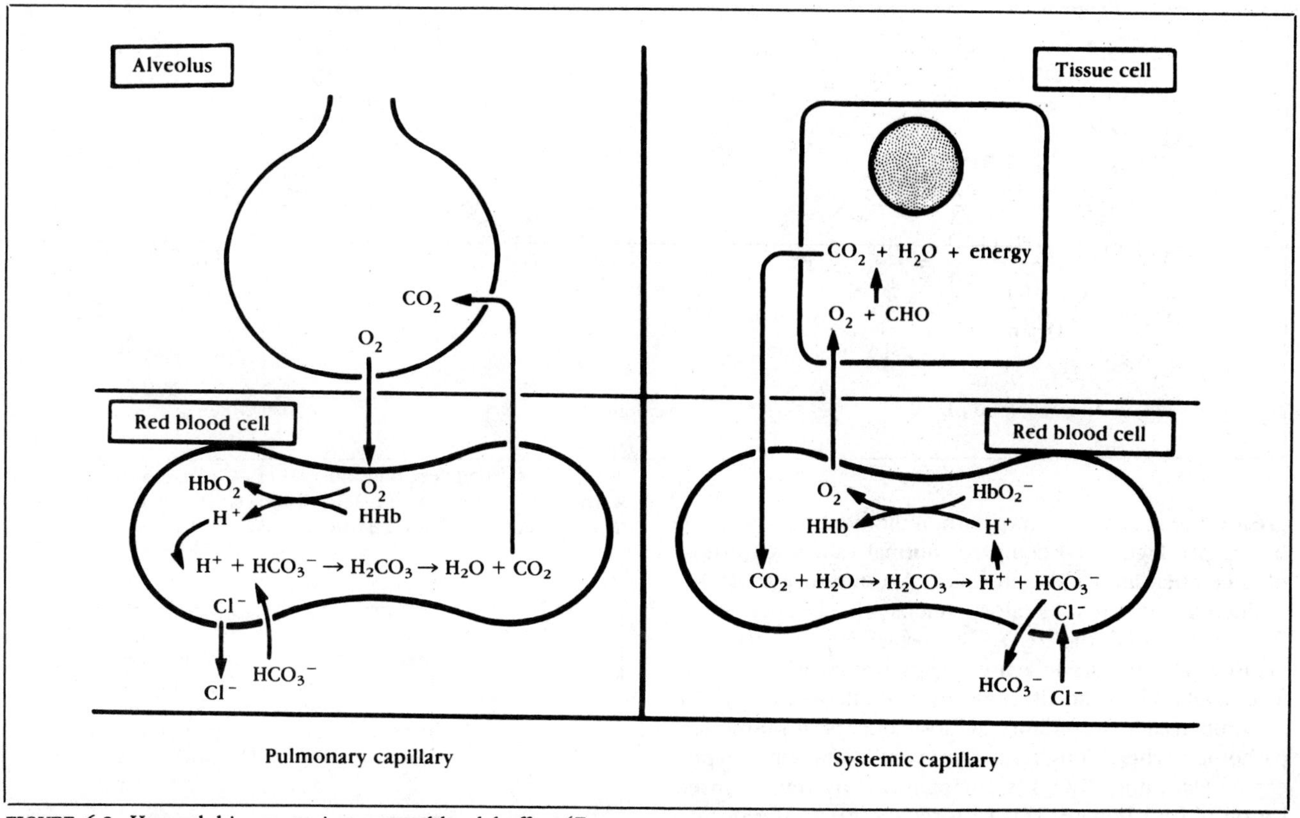

FIGURE 6-2. Hemoglobin as an important blood buffer. (From E. Selkurt [ed.], *Basic Physiology for the Health Sciences* [2nd ed.]. Boston: Little, Brown, 1982.)

and indirect methods estimate that the pH within the cell varies [3].

All of the buffer systems work together to buffer each other. Under normal conditions the venous H^+ and CO_2 will be higher than the arterial and the rate of their excretion will equal the rate of production.

ACIDOSIS-ALKALOSIS

Acidosis in the body fluids refers to an elevation of the H^+ concentration above normal or a decrease in the HCO_3^- below normal. The result of this alteration is a decrease in the pH of the body fluids below 7.35. The source of the excess hydrogen ion or altered H_2CO_3/HCO_3^- ratio can be respiratory (volatile) or metabolic (nonrespiratory or nonvolatile).

Alkalosis refers to a decrease in the H^+ concentration of the body fluids or an excess of the HCO_3^-. The pH of the body fluids increases above 7.45. The source of the depletion of hydrogen ion is either elimination of CO_2 (hyperventilation), or a primary base bicarbonate excess (metabolic). Table 6-4 summarizes some factors that tend to cause acidosis and alkalosis. Figure 6-3 shows the effect of altering the ratio of bicarbonate and carbonic acid on the blood pH. Other acids can similarly affect the blood pH.

TABLE 6-4. Some factors that tend to cause alkalosis and acidosis

Alkalosis	Acidosis
METABOLIC	METABOLIC
Steroid therapy	Uremia
Potassium deficiency	Diarrhea
HCO_3^- therapy	Abnormal organic acid
Nasogastric tube drainage or vomiting	Ketoacids (diabetes)
Thiazide diuretic therapy	Lactic acid (hypoperfusion)
RESPIRATORY	RESPIRATORY
Sepsis	COPD
Brain injury	Drug overdose
Asthma and many other lung diseases	Brain injury
Hyperventilation	Chest wall injury or paralysis
	Pneumothorax and hydrothorax

Source: H. A. Braun, F. W. Cheney, and C. P. Loehnen, *Introduction to Respiratory Physiology* (2nd ed.). Boston: Little, Brown, 1980.

Respiratory Acidosis

Respiratory acidosis may result from anything that depresses alveolar ventilation. Conditions such as pulmonary disease; depression of the central nervous system by drugs, disease, or injury; or restrictions of thoracic movement may lead to respiratory acidosis. Hypoventilation causes the accumulation of carbon dioxide, an increase in carbonic acid, and a shifting of the pH to the acidic side. The

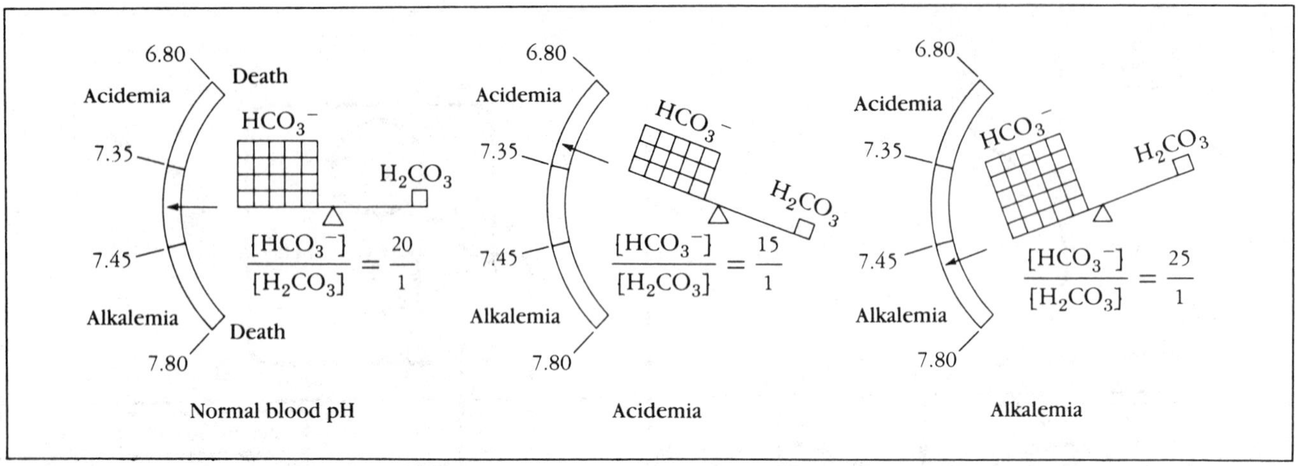

FIGURE 6-3. The effect on blood pH of a change in the ratio of bicarbonate ion to carbonic acid. (From G. H. Schmid, *The Chemical Basis of Life*. Boston: Little, Brown, 1982.)

greater the accumulation of carbon dioxide the lower will be the pH. Figure 6-4 compares normal values with those of uncompensated and compensated respiratory acidosis.

Uncompensated respiratory acidosis is seen when the PCO_2 is elevated, the HCO_3^- is normal, and the pH is decreased. This occurs in acute respiratory insufficiency before renal buffers can alter the pH (see Chaps. 24 and 25).

Compensated respiratory acidosis occurs in pulmonary pathology where long-term hypoventilation with hypercapnia (elevated PCO_2) is compensated by renal conservation of bicarbonate. This restores the pH to the normal range.

Clinical manifestations include the symptoms of the underlying problem. Carbon dioxide retention may lead to disorientation and coma. The urinary pH decreases, the serum bicarbonate increases after the renal buffers begin to function, and oxygen levels are often decreased.

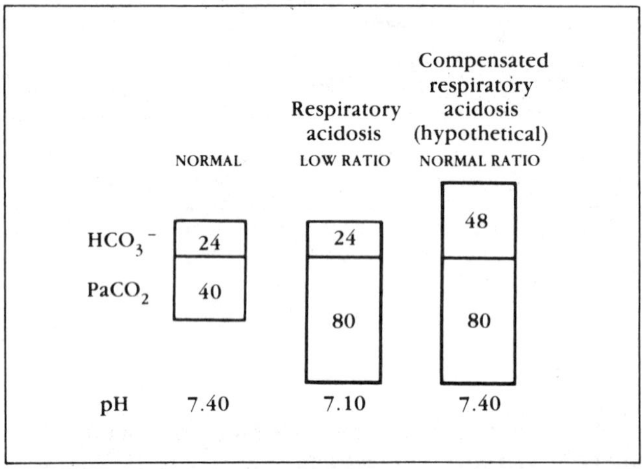

FIGURE 6-4. Changes of pH resulting from increased $PaCO_2$. (From H. A. Braun, F. W. Cheney, and C. P. Loehnen, *Introduction to Respiratory Physiology* [2nd ed.]. Boston: Little, Brown, 1980.)

Metabolic Acidosis

This condition results when there is a decrease in the bicarbonate levels or an increase in the retention of hydrogen ion. It results when an excess of organic or inorganic acids cannot be cleared by the kidneys. It may be associated with shock, diabetic ketoacidosis, uremia, starvation, drugs, hyperkalemia, or other conditions. Metabolic acidosis itself may cause a transient hyperkalemia when the kidney is secreting excess H^+ instead of K^+ in order to bring the pH into a normal range.

In metabolic acidosis the bicarbonate, pH, and PCO_2 levels are decreased. All of the buffers work together to buffer the excess H^+ that has accumulated in the body. Hyperventilation occurs within minutes and functions to cause a rapid decrease in the PCO_2 levels. This compensation may help to bring the pH into a more normal range. If the amount of metabolic acid is increasing rapidly, it overwhelms any respiratory compensation and the acidosis becomes more severe.

The existence of an *anion gap* may be helpful in determining the basis of acidosis. Anion gap refers to the difference between the sodium content and the sum of the bicarbonate and chloride levels [1]. Normally, there is about a 10- to 12-mEq difference, which increases to above 14 mEq with metabolic acidosis. It usually increases to greater than 25 mEq when the metabolic acidosis is due to organic acids, such as lactic acids. A normal anion gap in metabolic acidosis is seen in such conditions as diarrhea, ammonium chloride ingestion, and renal dysfunction, while a high anion gap may be seen with accumulation of organic acids such as ketoacids and lactic acids as well as certain drugs and poisons (Table 6-5). A normal gap is maintained by an increase in chloride ions so that the sum of the HCO_3^- and Cl^- remains constant. This situation is often called *hyperchloremic acidosis* [3]. A high anion gap occurs when there is a decrease in the sum of HCO_3^- and Cl^- due to the accumulation of other acids.

TABLE 6-5. Anion gap that may be seen in metabolic acidosis

Normal anion gap
Diarrhea, causing loss of HCO_3^-
Renal HCO_3^- loss in renal insufficiency
Drugs and parenteral fluids, e.g., ammonium chloride, hyperalimentation
Hypoaldosteronism
High anion gap
Ketoacidosis
Lactic acidosis
Loss of sulfates and phosphates in renal insufficiency
Salicylate intoxication
Other drugs or poisons, e.g., ethylene glycol, methanol, paraldehyde

Source: B. D. Rose, *Clinical Physiology of Acid-Base and Electrolyte Disorders*. New York: McGraw-Hill, 1977.

Clinical manifestations of metabolic acidosis include deep, rapid respirations (Kussmaul breathing), weakness, vasodilatation, nausea and vomiting and a decreased level of consciousness, which progresses to coma. Laboratory findings include an arterial blood pH below 7.35, a low urinary pH, and depressed serum bicarbonate levels.

Respiratory Alkalosis

The usual cause of respiratory alkalosis is alveolar hyperventilation. This condition may result from over-breathing, mechanical ventilation, fever, encephalitis, salicylate intoxication and a few other conditions.

Clinical signs may include light-headedness, convulsions, and coma. Laboratory findings include a pH above 7.45, a normal bicarbonate in the early stages that decreases if the condition progresses, and a gradual increase in the pH of the urine.

Metabolic Alkalosis

This condition may occur due to an elevation of the HCO_3^- level or a loss of H^+ concentration. It may be caused by chloride loss, hyperaldosteronism, excessive vomiting, gastrointestinal suction, diuretic therapy, hypokalemia, or excessive ingestion of a base such as bicarbonate of soda. Hyperaldosteronism leads to excessive sodium resorption, which increases the blood base content and encourages H^+ loss. When the chloride level is depleted, alkalosis occurs because bicarbonate is resorbed to balance the cations. This is often called *hypochloremic alkalosis*.

Inhibition of the respiratory center causes a decrease in the rate and depth of respiration and results in compensatory carbon dioxide retention. However, this does not markedly alter serum pH. Hyperactive reflexes, confusion, and convulsions may be seen as late manifestations. Laboratory findings usually include an alkaline urine, a plasma pH over 7.45, and a potassium of less than 4 mEq/L.

REFERENCES

1. Braun, H. A., Cheney, F. W. and Loehnen, C. P. *Introduction to Respiratory Physiology* (2nd ed.). Boston: Little, Brown, 1980.
2. Guyton, A. C. *Textbook of Medical Physiology* (6th ed.). Philadelphia: Saunders, 1981.
3. Rose, B. D. *Clinical Physiology of Acid-Base and Electrolyte Disorders*. New York: McGraw-Hill, 1977.
4. Toporek, M. *Basic Chemistry of Life*. St. Louis: Mosby, 1981.

BIBLIOGRAPHY

Aspinall, J. J. A simplified guide to managing patients with hyponatremia. *Nurs. 78* 8:32, 1978.

Burkhart, C. Upper GI hemorrhage: The clinical picture. *Am. J. Nurs.* 81:1817, 1981.

Cawson, R. A., McCracken, A. W., and Marcus, P. B. *Pathological Mechanisms and Human Disease.* St. Louis: Mosby, 1982.

Chan, J. Clinical disorders of sodium, potassium, chloride, and sulfur metabolism: Diagnostic approaches to children. *Urology* 12:504, 1978.

Corbett, J. V. *Laboratory Tests in Nursing Practice.* Norwalk, Conn.: Appleton-Century-Crofts, 1982.

Crumlish, C. M. Cardiogenic shock: Catch it early. *Nurs. 81* 11:34, 1981.

Felver, L. Understanding the electrolyte maze. *Am. J. Nurs.* 80:1591, 1980.

Groër, M. W. *Physiology and Pathophysiology of the Body Fluids.* St. Louis: Mosby, 1981.

Guyton, A. *Textbook of Medical Physiology* (6th ed.). Philadelphia: Saunders, 1981.

Isselbacher, K., et al. (eds.). *Harrison's Principles of Internal Medicine* (9th ed.). New York: McGraw-Hill, 1980.

Jensen, D. *The Principles of Physiology* (2nd ed.). New York: Appleton-Century-Crofts, 1980.

Keithley, J. K., and Faulini, K. E. What's behind that IV line? *Nurs. 82* 17:32, 1982.

Kubo, W. M. The syndrome of inappropriate secretion of antidiuretic hormone. *Heart Lung* 7:469, 1975.

Lamb, L. S. Think you know septic shock? Read this. *Nurs. 82* 12:34, 1982.

Lamphier, T. A., and Lamphier, R. A. Upper GI hemorrhage: Emergency evaluation and management. *Am. J. Nurs.* 81:1814, 1981.

Luckmann, J. and Sorensen, K. *Medical Surgical Nursing: A Psychophysiological Approach* (2nd ed.). Philadelphia: Saunders, 1980.

Manzi, C. Edema: How to tell if it's a danger signal. *Nurs. 77* 7:66, 1977.

Maxwell, M. H., and Kleeman, C. R. *Clinical Disorders of Fluid and Electrolyte Metabolism.* New York: McGraw-Hill, 1972.

Metheney, N. A. Perioperative fluids and electrolytes. *Am. J. Nurs.* 78:840, 1978.

Metheney, N. A., and Snively, W. D. *Nurses' Handbook of Fluid Balance* (3rd ed.). Philadelphia: Lippincott, 1979.

Miller, M., and Sherman, R. Metabolic acid-base disorders: Parts I, II, and III. *Am. J. Nurs.* 77, 78, 1977, 1978.

O'Dorisio, T. M. Hypercalcemia crisis. *Heart Lung* 7:425, 1978.

Phipps, W., Ling, B., and Woods, N. *Medical Surgical Nursing: Concepts and Clinical Practice.* St. Louis: Mosby, 1979.

Robbins, S. L., and Cotran, R. *Pathological Basis of Disease* (2nd ed.). Philadelphia: Saunders, 1979.

Roberts, S. L. Renal assessment: A nursing point of view. *Heart Lung* 8:105, 1979.

Rose, B. D. *Clinical Physiology of Acid-Base and Electrolyte Disorders.* New York: McGraw-Hill, 1977.

Shedden, H. E. Shock: Mechanisms at the cellular level. *FOCUS* 1979.

Shrabe, K. The ABC's of ABG's: Or how to interpret a blood gas value. *Nurs. 79* 9:26, 1979.

Stark, J. BUN/creatinine: Your keys to kidney function. *Nurs. 80* 10:33, 1980.

Stroot, V., Lee, C., and Schaper, A. *Fluids and Electrolytes: A Practical Approach* (2nd ed.). Philadelphia: Davis, 1977.

Sumner, S. M., and Grau, P. A. To defeat hypovolemic shock. *Nurs. 81* 11:47, 1981.

Tripp, A. Hyper and Hypocalcemia. *Am. J. Nurs.* 76:1142, 1976.

Twombly, M. The shift into third space. *Nurs. 78* 8:38, 1978.

White, S. IV fluids and electrolytes: How to head off the risks. *RN* 42:60, 1979.

Wilson, R. F. The diagnosis and management of severe sepsis and septic shock. Reprint from Department of Surgery, Wayne State University, 1979.

SECTION II
BODILY DEFENSE MECHANISMS
Adaptations and Alterations

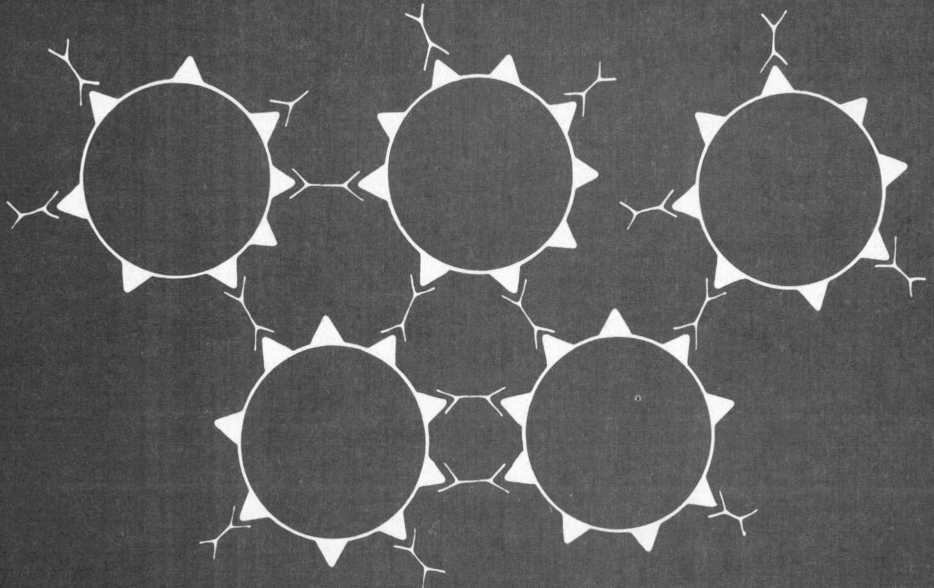

UNIT 4
INFLAMMATION AND REPAIR

Barbara L. Bullock
INFECTIOUS AGENTS
INFLAMMATION AND REPAIR

Marilyn Pase
INFECTIOUS AGENTS

Emilie Musci
WOUND HEALING

The inflammatory response is the reaction of the body to tissue injury. It is usually initiated by an injurious substance and results in the removal of the foreign material. It is a beneficial response that must be present for the maintenance of life. The most common causes of inflammation are the infectious agents. Chapter 7 presents a condensed review of the classifications of organisms that can cause inflammation. It also describes the normal mechanisms used by the body to prevent or inhibit organism entrance. The student may wish to expand the study of microbiology as it relates to pathophysiology; reference material is listed in the unit bibliography. Chapter 8 details acute and chronic inflammation as well as the resolution of the inflammatory process. Normal and aberrant resolutions are presented. Effects of the inflammatory process as they affect specific organs and systems are studied in other sections of the textbook.

The reader is encouraged to study Units 4 and 5 together to maximize the understanding of the entire process. Utilization of the learning objectives will facilitate understanding by providing an organized approach to the topic. The bibliographies at the end of the units provide further sources for investigative study.

CHAPTER 7
INFECTIOUS AGENTS

LEARNING OBJECTIVES

1. List the major characteristics of each type of infectious agent.
2. Explain how the various infectious agents are classified.
3. Describe the mode of viral infection and how they multiply.
4. List the events occurring as a cell is infected by a virus.
5. Describe at least six viral infections, differentiating DNA and RNA viruses, incubation periods, mode of transmission, and clinical effects.
6. Describe the pathologic effects of the rickettsial organism in spotted and typhus fevers.
7. Discuss the role of the toxins produced by the bacterial organisms.
8. Describe at least six gram-positive and gram-negative bacterial infections in terms of pathogenesis and clinical effects.
9. List three major classifications of fungi that are infectious to humans and describe the relationships between them.
10. List the protozoa that may be pathologic to humans.
11. Explain how protozoa move and reproduce.
12. Briefly describe three infections that may result from protozoa.
13. Categorize the types of helminths and describe how each can cause pathology in the body.

Infectious diseases are produced by living organisms: viruses, rickettsia, bacteria, fungi, protozoa, and nematodes. These diseases have been present in enormous numbers and have caused epidemics by their contagiousness in past decades. Developments in nutrition, insect control, immunization, sanitation, and drug therapy have decreased the mortality and morbidity of infectious diseases [4]. Still, the control of microbial infections has not eliminated this prevalent cause of disease. Microbes have developed mutant strains that are resistant to once effective antimicrobial therapy.

Infectious diseases still occur in great numbers and often are fatal to the very young or the debilitated victim. In 1976 there were approximately 50 million cases of acute infectious and parasitic diseases in the United States. The incidence of disease is greater in underdeveloped countries [4].

The occurrence of infectious diseases depends on many factors, including virulence of the organism, number of invading organisms, defense mechanisms of the body, and pathogenesis of the infection. *Virulence* is the ability of the infecting organism to cause disease, requiring a receptive host in which it can settle and multiply. A *number* of invading organisms sufficient to overwhelm the host's defenses must be present.

The defense mechanisms of the human body are found on the external and internal surfaces and include physical, chemical, and immune defense barriers. Whether or not the organism can cause disease depends largely on the success or failure of these defense mechanisms and barriers. The main physical, external barrier to infection is the skin, an intact epidermis being almost impervious to infection. The mucous membranes lining the various organs also function in the removal of organisms through the secretion of mucus that provides a washing effect and prevents membrane adherence by the organism. Chemical secretions, such as hydrochloric acid in the stomach and the usually acid pH of urine, contribute to the sterile environment within the bodily organs. The immune system targets pathogens or organisms for destruction. When organisms gain access to the body the lymphocytes recognize and destroy them, often without producing disease manifestations. The immune system also plays a major role in the outcome of infectious disease (see Chap. 9).

The defense mechanisms can be grouped into physical or chemical characteristics, immune factors, and nature of the host. These mechanisms are summarized in Table 7-1.

Pathogenesis of infection depends on the capability of the specific organism and its ability to bypass or inactivate the defense mechanisms of the body. Each microorganism is distinct and has its own means of invasion and reproduction. Once actual infection is established it often causes nonspecific signs and symptoms, which characteristically include fever, chills, muscle pain, lymph node enlargement, and variable elevations in the white cell count. The major classifications of living organisms are described in this chapter. The effects of the resultant diseases are also described in the chapters relating to specific organs and systems.

TABLE 7-1. Defense mechanisms of the body

Mechanism	Characteristics of defense
Physical	Intact epidermis Mucus-secreting membranes Mucus blanket movement in respiratory tract Connective tissue
Chemical	Hydrochloric acid in stomach Acid pH of urine Lysozyme enzyme present in many secretions Resident flora in mouth, on skin, in large intestine
Immune mechanisms	Specific ATG-ATB reactions IgA Inflammatory response
Host factors	Age Sex Genetic susceptibilities Nutritional balance Stress—physiologic or emotional Presence of other diseases

VIRUSES

Viruses are the smallest infectious agents known. They are not complete cells in themselves and exist essentially as parasites of living cells. These organisms use the biochemical products of other living cells in order to replicate.

Structure, Reproduction, and Pathogenesis of Viruses

Viruses vary in size, appearance, and behavior. They are classified as either DNA or RNA viruses according to their genetic material. Many viruses contain nucleic acid, which is protected by a closed protein shell called the *capsid*. Some viruses have a surrounding lipid envelope.

Mature virus particles are called *virions* (Fig. 7-1) [3]. Viruses appear to be species and organ specific and apparently can replicate only in permissive or receptive cells. Some viruses enter a receptive cell by pinocytosis after which the process of multiplication can begin.

While there is no one typical virus, the replication and transmission of this organism has been studied extensively by usage of the bacteriophage (virus that attacks bacteria). The genetic material of the bacteriophage is enclosed in an angular head or protein-containing capsid. This hollow head contains the viral genetic material and connects with a hollow cylinder of protein surrounded by protein contractile fibers. The contractile fibers coil around the cylinder like a spring. At the end of the tail, the fibers and an enzyme are important in attaching the virion to the host cell (Fig. 7-2).

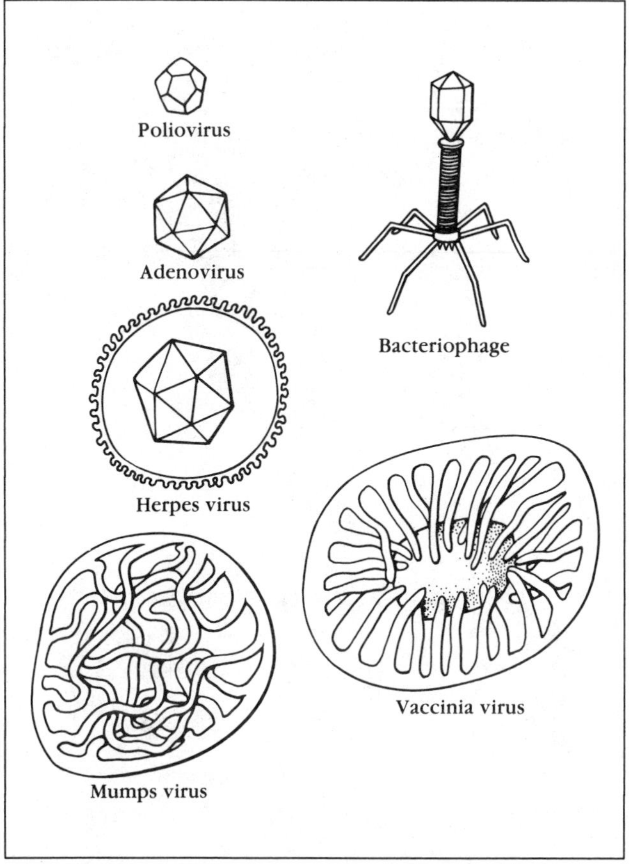

FIGURE 7-1. Various forms of viruses.

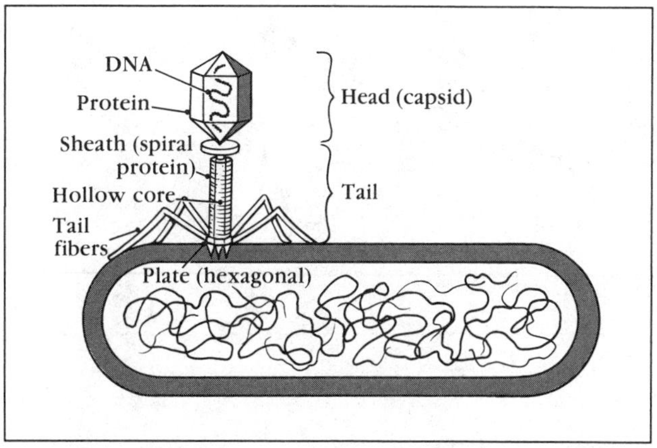

FIGURE 7-2. A bacteriophage.

Some viruses have amino acids that are similar to the actively transported substances in the cell membrane of the host. The virus can fool the cell, attach itself to receptor sites on the host cell, and block the movement of normally transported materials.

Viral multiplication usually occurs in several steps that result in lysis of the host cell. The first step is recognition and attachment of the virus to the host cell. The tail of the virus adsorbs to specific receptor sites on the host cell. It then digests a part of the host cell wall through lysosomal-like enzymes. The hole produced by the virus allows the injection of nucleic acid into the recipient cell. The tube portion of the virus enters the host cell through a hypodermiclike process. The viral shell (capsid and tail) remains attached to the host cell (as a "ghost" on the outside of the cell wall) after injection of the genetic material. Within the host cell, the viral particles may alter protein synthesis, cause chromosomal changes, or alter the genes of the host [6]. Synthesis of new viral DNA, proteins, and shells occurs, and new DNA is assembled into the hollow protein shells, a process that continues until the host cell ruptures and releases swarms of new infective viruses (Fig. 7-3). For example, in a few hours, the poliovirus can produce 100,000 poliovirus particles [1]. The formed particles can survive outside the host cell for variable periods of time, often until a new susceptible host cell can be found. Following attachment, an *eclipse* stage may be entered, during which the viral DNA becomes part of the host chromosome and remains latent. The greater the capability of a virus to initiate the rapid reproductive cycle, the more virulent the virus.

Activation or induction causes the latent viruses to become active. The process reprograms the cell for viral reproduction. It has been suggested that activation may be initiated by cold temperatures, carcinogens, or materials in food, air, or water. Each virus responds to a specific induction mechanism. Sometimes a few cells with viruses within them escape induction so that not all affected cells are lysed. In this way, the host cell carries viral DNA as part of its own DNA, and the virus can remain latent in the host tissues throughout the life span of the cell.

The structure of the virus has been studied with the electron microscope and is described according to its appearance. The complete infective particle is called a *virion*. The *capsid* is the protein coat, which is made up of protein subunits called *capsomeres*. Complex virions may contain additional layers, or envelopes.

The protein covering of the virus is type specific. The surface structure is responsible for attachment to particular cell receptors. Infection depends on the compatibility of the viral surface with the host cell receptors and the ability of the viral nucleic acid to use the host cell for manufacture of viral products. All viruses are similar in their method of attachment to the specific receptors on the host cell membrane, the so-called lock and key attachment.

Viruses affect and infect specific cells. Some B lymphocytes, for example, carry receptors for the Epstein-Barr virus while cells in the tracheal lining have receptors for the influenza virus. Viruses produce specific diseases involving specific tissues, but the mode of transmission and variety of diseases produced are numerous. Cells respond to viral infection in different ways. There may be no apparent cellular change because the viral DNA may adopt a symbiotic relationship with the host cell. Cellular pathologic effects, such as cell death or virus-induced hyperpla-

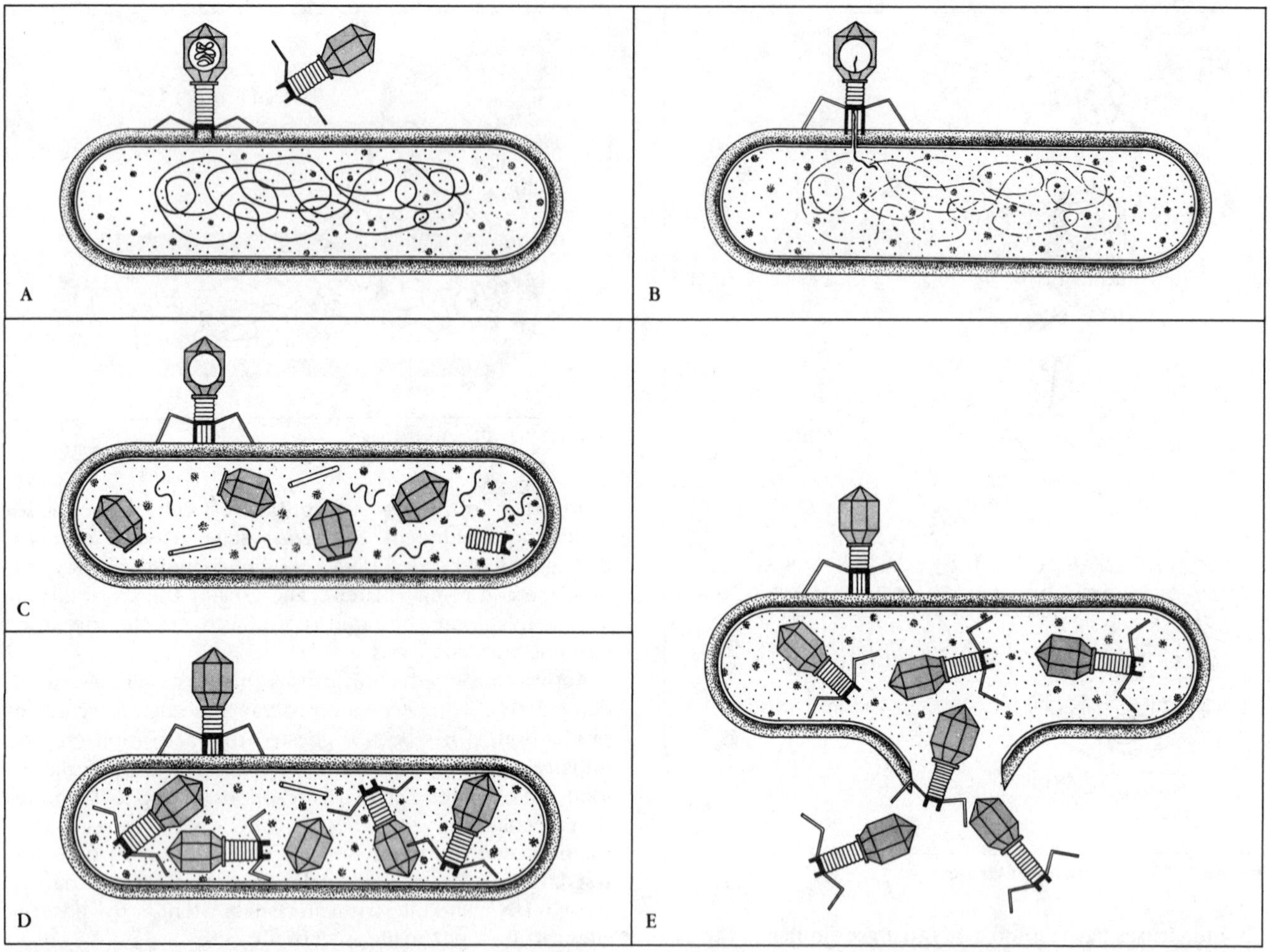

FIGURE 7-3. Development of a virulent phage in a susceptible bacterium. A. The polyhedral head of the phage is seen attached to the outer surface of the bacterium by its tail and tail fibers. B. Within a few seconds or minutes the bacterial cell wall and membrane have been perforated by lytic enzymes in the tail, and the DNA of the phage has entered the bacillus through the phage tail. Note the retraction of the tail sheath. The opening through the cell wall is resealed. The inert protein coat of the phage remains on the outside of the cell. Disintegration of the cell DNA begins at once. The phage, as such, is no longer demonstrable. C. During the next 12 minutes phage protein heads, tails, and phage DNA replicons are being synthesized. D. About 12 minutes later, following a brief period of maturation during which some of the heads, tails, and DNA molecules have been assembled, infective phage virions are first demonstrable by artificial rupture of the cell. E. About 12 minutes later, the assembly of parts into phage virions is complete and the now "eviscerated" cell, an inert sac, ruptures by enzymic lysis of the cell wall, liberating many new phage particles. Their number is characteristic of the burst size of the particular phage involved; in this case, six. The whole process, A–E, occupies about 30 to 40 minutes in this particular virus-cell system. In this diagram the phage virions have been drawn about 3 times as large proportionately in order to show more clearly certain structural details. (From M. Frobisher, et al., *Fundamentals of Microbiology* [9th ed.]. Philadelphia: Saunders, 1974.)

sia may occur. Cytopathic effects are common and include aggregation of host cells into clusters with shrinkage, lysis, and fusion of the cells. The effects differ and are affected by the effects of the virus on cellular synthesis of macromolecules, alteration in cellular organelles such as the lysosomes, and changes in the host cell membrane.

Viral infections stimulate the immune system with its antibody production. The initial response to viral infestation is usually by the mononuclear cells such as monocytes and lymphocytes. At the site of entry of viruses into the body, the immunocompetent (antigen-specific) cells accumulate and initiate the process of inflammation. Macrophages often attach to the virus and enhance the T and B cell interaction (see Chap. 9). Exposure to viral agents initially causes the synthesis of specific IgM antibodies, which is followed after about 10 days by IgG antibodies. When the virion is sufficiently coated with antibody it is rendered noninfectious. The specific T lymphocytes provide for long-term immunity. Viruses and other substances stimulate the production of *interferon,* an antiviral protein that inhibits viral spread from cell to cell [3].

Viral infections produce many varied diseases including hepatitis, meningoencephalitis, pneumonia, rhinitis, skin diseases, and many other disorders affecting almost every system of the body. Although there are multitudes of different types of viruses, most of them can be classified into DNA or RNA structural viruses. Table 7-2 presents this classification, listing the common disease-producing groups, their modes of transmission, and the resulting symptomology.

RICKETTSIA

Rickettsia, once thought to be related to viruses because of their small size, are small obligate parasitic organisms. They possess all of the features of bacteria except that they can multiply only within certain cells of susceptible hosts [5]. Their normal reservoir is most often the arthropods, especially ticks, mites, lice, and fleas in which they multiply without causing disease. Most rickettsial diseases are transmitted to humans through the bite or feces of the infected arthropod. An exception to this is Q fever, which is probably spread person-to-person by respiratory droplet. The classification of the rickettsia is based on the clinical features and epidemiologic aspects of the diseases they cause. The organisms are often organized into the (1) spotted fever group, (2) typhus group, and (3) others, including Q fever.

All rickettsial diseases cause fever, and most cause a skin rash that is the result of rickettsial multiplication in the endothelial cells of the small blood vessels. The cells become swollen and necrotic, leading to the vascular lesions noted on or through the skin. Aggregations of lymphocytes, granulocytes, and macrophages accumulate in the small vessels of the brain, heart, and other bodily organs.

Laboratory tests demonstrate the presence of rickettsial antigens and antibodies. Broad-spectrum antibiotics, such as tetracycline, suppress the growth of rickettsia but full recovery requires an intact immune system that can develop antibodies against the rickettsial organism.

The most common diseases resulting from rickettsial infection include Rocky Mountain spotted fever and the typhus fevers. These are summarized in Table 7-3.

BACTERIA

Unlike viruses, bacteria do not require living cells for growth. They are free living organisms that utilize the nutrients of the body as a food source and a favorable environment for growth. Bacteria can attach to epithelial tissue and, like viruses, prefer to infect specific sites. Pathogenic effects of bacterial infection usually result from substances such as enzymes or toxins produced by the bacteria, or injury from the inflammatory response of the body to the bacteria.

Bacteria are classified in many ways. They may be gram-positive or gram-negative depending on the chemical composition of their cell walls and absorption of staining dye. Gram-positive bacteria stain purple because their cell walls resist decolorization by acetone-alcohol. Gram-negative bacteria are decolorized and then stained with a red dye to make them stand out. Bacteria are also classified by their morphologic appearance. The spherical bacteria are cocci, the rod-shaped are bacilli, and the spiral are spirochetes. They can be pyogenic (pus producing), granulomatous, aerobic, or anaerobic. Organisms such as *mycobacterium tuberculosis* elicit a granulomatous inflammatory response that involves a chronic inflammatory process with a nodule of granulation tissue and actively growing fibroblasts and capillary buds (see Chap. 23).

Pathogenesis of Bacteria

All bacteria have the capability to localize in specific organs and often produce acute inflammatory reactions. The degree of tissue damage depends on the number of bacteria present, the virulence of the organism, the site of infestation, and the resistance of the host to the organism [4]. Table 7-4 presents a classification of some of the more common bacteria that affect humans. The list is necessarily incomplete because there are thousands of bacterial organisms.

The virulence of bacteria is enhanced by the elaboration of endotoxins and exotoxins. *Endotoxins* are produced by many gram-negative organisms that, when released, are pyrogenic and confer antigenic specificity to the toxin [5]. These enhance chemotaxis and some activate complement by the alternate pathway (see Chap. 8). *Exotoxins* are usually produced by gram-positive bacteria. These toxins have specific effects on target organs; for example, elaboration of diphtherial toxin causes the formation of a thick membrane on the respiratory structures and toxic effects on the heart and nervous system. Coagulase, a protein produced by many staphylococcal organisms, can initiate the coagulation sequence and produce coagulation in various areas.

TABLE 7-2. Common viruses that cause pathologic effects in humans

Type	Nucleic acid present	Incubation period	Mode of transmission	Clinical manifestations
Herpesviruses				
Varicella (chickenpox)	DNA	10–21 days	Highly contagious through respiratory droplets	Fever, disseminated vesicular eruption, profuse on trunk and on oral mucosa
Zoster (shingles)	DNA	Variable		Follows chickenpox, may occur years after a primary attack, spreads down peripheral nerves of skin, active ganglionitis causes burning or dull pain, vesicles follow nerve fibers
Herpes simplex				
Type 1	DNA	2–12 days	Skin contact (oral)	Fever, vesicular eruption of mucous membranes, conjunctivitis, oral lesions (fever blisters); encephalitis occasionally results when virus ascends to central nervous system
Type 2	DNA	2–5 days	Skin contact (genital) attack rate with sexual contact 1:3	Genital vesicles, fever, burning, urinary urgency in male, dysuria, vulvar burning, dyspareuria in female
Epstein-Barr	DNA	30–50 days	Respiratory droplet, transfusion	Called "kissing disease" of young persons; sore throat, lymphadenopathy, splenomegaly, supraorbital edema; virus has been isolated from Burkitt's lymphoma
Cytomegalovirus (CMV)	DNA	?20–50 days	Saliva, urine, feces, semen, transplacental, transfusion	Vary with age of onset: *Congenital:* failure to thrive, jaundice, respiratory distress, may be fatal *Postnatal:* infection may cause anemia, hepatomegaly, lymphocytosis *Adult form:* fever, lymphocytosis, Guillain-Barré syndrome *Immunosuppressed individuals:* interstitial pneumonia, increased incidence of rejection in transplant cases
Pox viruses				
Variola (smallpox)	DNA	7–17 days	Respiratory droplets	High fever, vesicles on mucous membranes, papules on face and trunk, bone marrow depression
Vaccinia	DNA	Approximately 2 weeks after vaccination	Innoculation for smallpox	Vaccinia virus probably a hybrid of variola or cowpox viruses; may cause widespread eczematous reaction or encephalomyelitis that causes death in 30–40% of individuals
Adenovirus (many strains identified)	DNA	5–10 days	High frequency in children and military recruits; respiratory aerosol or droplet	Febrile pharyngitis; headache, regional lymphadenopathy, nasal obstruction and discharge, conjunctivitis, *pneumonia*
Papovavirus (warts)	DNA	1–20 months	Skin contact, contact with contaminated secretions	Solid, rounded tumors with horny projections 1–2 cm in size; often asymptomatic unless located on area of irritation; often found on hands, neck, shins, and forearms
Picornavirus				
Coxsackieviruses A & B (many strains)	RNA	2–5 days	Fecal-oral contact, insects may be passive vectors	Depend on type; acute myocarditis, fever, muscle, pleuritic pain, vesicular lesions on soft palate, tonsils, pharyngitis, associated with many systemic problems

Rhinovirus (many strains)	RNA	1–2 days	Respiratory droplet	Common respiratory illness; fever, cough, croup, and pneumonia may develop in children; sore throat, nasal congestion, and nasal discharge without fever are common in the adult
Poliovirus	RNA	2–5 days	Fecal-oral contact	Undifferentiated febrile illness that may spread to involve anterior horn cells of spinal cord and motor nuclei of cranial nerves; causes various muscle paralyses, hemiplegia, paraplegia, bladder, and respiratory muscle dysfunction; poliovaccines can prevent the disease
Myxovirus				
Influenza A, B, and C	RNA	18–36 hours, up to 7 days	Epidemic, new strains evolve frequently; transmitted by infected respiratory secretions	Respiratory symptoms, cough, headache, muscle pain, fever, chills, sneezing, nasal discharge, prostration are common; symptoms between strains similar
Mumps	RNA	15–21 days	Very communicable in crowded conditions; transmitted by upper respiratory secretions	Painful enlargement of salivary glands; orchitis occurs in 20–35% postpubertal males; small percentage develop meningitis or may affect other glands
Arenavirus				
Rubella	RNA	14–21 days	Very communicable; confers immunity; naso-pharyngeal transmission	Rash begins on face, spreads to trunk and extremities; lasts 1–5 days; enlarged lymph nodes common, joint pains and encephalomyelitis are rare complications
Rhabdovirus				
Rabies	RNA	Variable average 2–6 weeks in humans	Animal bite of nonimmunized domestic dogs or cats or of wild animals such as skunks, foxes, raccoons, wolves, and bats	Virus introduced through mucous membranes or epidermis; replicates in striated muscle then spreads up peripheral nerve bundles to CNS; passes to all organs but major effects on CNS; acute encephalitis, brainstem dysfunction and death; rapidly fatal if not treated; hydrophobia (excessive salivation) characteristic
Arbovirus				
Four groups cause CNS disease	RNA	4–14 days	Mosquito bite transmits to man; can multiply in horses, birds, bats, snakes, and insects	Age-related; younger individuals often have high fever and convulsions; headache, fever, drowsiness, confusion, disorientation; some manifest mainly by lethargy, "sleeping sickness"; muscle weakness; residual effects range from none to convulsions; speech difficulties
Unclassified viruses				
Hepatitis A	RNA similar to picorna-viruses	15–45 days	Fecal-oral enhanced by poor hygiene, overcrowding, contaminated food, water; sexual, percutaneous transmission	Onset acute, more frequently seen in younger individuals; causes anorexia, malaise, and other symptoms followed by jaundice; dark urine, clay-colored stools; recovery usually complete
Hepatitis, non A, non B	RNA	15–160 days	Not known, possible fecal-oral or percutaneous	Clinical course variable; debilitation and liver dysfunction not infrequent
Hepatitis B	DNA-type	45–160 days	Percutaneous, sexual, fecal-oral transmission	Chronic active hepatitis may occur; jaundice, liver dysfunction may progress to liver failure; recovery slow

TABLE 7-3. Common rickettsia that cause pathologic effects in humans

Rickettsia	Morphology	Mode of transmission	Clinical effects
Spotted fevers *R. rickettsii* (Rocky Mountain spotted fever)	Small organism, stains purple; usually gram-negative cell wall antigenic; elaborates an endotoxinlike substance	Mutiply in nucleus and cytoplasm of infected cells of ticks and mammals; commonly occurs in Western Hemisphere; transmitted by bite of infected tick or through skin abrasions contacting tick feces or tissue juices; incubation period of 3–12 days	Swelling and degeneration of endothelial cells, vascular damage, myocarditis pneumonitis; peripheral vascular collapse may cause death; impairment of hepatic function and consumption coagualopathy may occur; severe headache, muscle pain, fever for 15–20 days; characteristic rash small discrete, nonfixed, pink lesions begin on wrists, ankles, forearms, etc.; becomes petechial; mortality approximately 7–10%
Typhus fevers *R. prowazekii* (epidemic typhus)	Small, gram-negative organism, always multiplies within the cytoplasm of cells	Inhalation of dried louse feces; louse feces often rubbed into broken skin as with scratching of the bite; incubation of approximately 1 week	Intense headache, continuous pyrexia for 2 weeks, a macular rash in axilla spreads to extremities; becomes petechial; peripheral vascular collapse as with Rocky Mountain spotted fever
R. mooseri (endemic typhus)	Similar to *R. prowazekii*	Transmitted by fleas, widespread in U.S. especially Southeastern and Gulf Coast states	Headache, fever, chills; fever up to 12 days; rash generalized, dull red macular, over thorax and abdomen; prognosis good with or without treatment
Q Fever *Coxiella burnetti*	Appearance similar to other rickettsiae	Inhalation of infected dust, of ticks on body and lice feces; sheep, goats, cows often affected; incubation period 2–4 weeks; found throughout the world	Fever, headache, weakness, interstitial pneumonitis; dry cough, chest pain; hepatitis and endocarditis may follow; rash is not characteristic

Coagulase may also cause the deposition of fibrin on the surface of staphylococci that may inhibit the ability of defensive phagocytes to destroy the bacteria. Laboratory tests often note whether a bacterium is coagulase-positive.

FUNGI

Fungus or mycotic diseases are disorders caused by yeasts and molds. These infections are often divided into three groups according to the part(s) of the body they infect. (1) The *systemic or deep mycoses* invade the internal organs or viscera. These pathogens can attack major systems and organs of the body and may result in death. (2) The *subcutaneous mycoses* infect the skin, subcutaneous tissue, fascia, and bone. Infection usually occurs from direct contamination with fungal spores or mycelial fragments into wounds or broken areas of the skin. (3) *Superficial mycoses* involve only the epidermis, hair, and nails. Their principal habitat is mammalian skin [2].

Unlike bacteria, most pathogenic fungi produce no extracellular toxic products. They usually stimulate a hypersensitivity to their antigenic components or metabolites that is thought to cause their pathogenicity. Of the many thousands of species of fungi, only about 50 cause pathology in man. The structure of these pathogenic fungi is similar to that of other fungi. Long, branching filaments called *hyphae* are produced, which may divide into a chain of cells by forming walls or septa. As these hyphae grow and branch, they form a mesh of growth called a *mycelium.* Fungi reproduce sexually by spores when there is fusion, or asexually by nuclei when there is no fusion [6].

Saprophytic fungi that grow in the soil usually cause a systemic type of mycosis. The infection is transmitted from the soil or the droppings of fowl to humans through the inhalation of spores. Most deep mycoses are caused by free-living organisms and are limited to certain geographic locations. The severity of the disease produced depends on the degree of hypersensitivity of the host. The usual pathologic lesion is a chronic inflammatory granuloma that can produce abscess and necrosis.

Saprophytic fungi in the soil or on vegetation can cause subcutaneous mycotic infection. This infection is opportunistic in that it occurs by direct implantation through a crack or sore on the skin. As with the systemic mycoses, necrotic, granulomatous lesions of any area may occur.

The superficial mycosis infections may represent allergic reactions to fungi. These mycoses do not invade deeper tissues or become disseminated.

TABLE 7-4. Bacteria that cause pathologic effects in humans

Bacteria	Gram's stain	Morphology	Mode of transmission	Clinical effects
Pseudomonas aeruginosa	Gram-negative	Motile rod; greenish-yellow pigment formed; saprophytic but can establish infection and invade when the host resistance is decreased	Commonly found on skin and mucous membranes; often attacks debilitated, immunosuppressed, burned, premature, or elderly individuals; transmitted by contact, especially to urinary tract, lungs, or damaged skin	Purulent drainage from wounds; characteristic greenish mucus from site of infection; bacteremia carries a 75% mortality; high fever, confusion, chills followed by circulatory collapse and sometimes leukopenia
Proteus	Gram-negative	Actively motile rod; hydrolyzes urea; actively decomposes protein	Commonly found in decaying matter, soil, water, and the human intestine; affects the skin, urinary tract, ears, and other areas secondarily in susceptible individuals	Causes localized purulent infections that may spread and cause bacteremia; causes symptoms of bacteremia; usually sensitive to penicillin therapy
Enterobacter-Klebsiella	Gram-negative	Short, plump, nonmotile rods; type-specific capsular antigens	Urinary tract and respiratory infections, especially pneumonia; often found in immunosuppressed, alcoholic, or individuals with diabetes mellitus	Symptoms of pneumonitis: productive cough, weakness, anemia; may resemble TB; responds well to aminoglycoside therapy
Shigella	Gram-negative	Nonmotile rods; aerobic or nearly anaerobic	GI tract resident; transmitted through fecal-oral route, or through contaminated food, water, swimming pools; common in countries where sanitation is poor; incubation is usually less than 48 hours	Fever, colicky abdominal pain, diarrhea; liquid greenish stools may contain various amounts of blood; dehydration may result
Escherichia coli	Gram-negative	Non-spore-forming rods; different strains characterized by their antigens	Normal inhabitant of colon; may spread to urinary tract directly or through hematogenous spread; opportunistic organism in debilitated individuals	Symptoms of UTI account for more than 75% of UTI; abscesses may form on any area; bacteremia characterized by fever, chills, dyspnea,may develop endotoxic shock
Salmonella *S. typhi* (typhoid fever)	Gram-negative	Motile; type identified by specific antigens	Ingestion of contaminated foods, water, or milk; transmitted through fecal contamination of foodstuffs; totally transmitted by human carriers; incubation period about 10 days	Rare in the U.S.; onset of fever, chills, abdominal pain, and distension; rash of small macules on upper abdomen and thorax; without treatment often causes intestinal bleeding and perforation
Other *Salmonella* organisms	Gram-negative		Food contamination; onset within hours of food ingestion	Enteritis, massive vomiting, and diarrhea, dehydration, fever; antibiotic treatment normally not helpful
Hemophilus *H. influenzae*	Gram-negative	Small, pleomorphic nonmotile, aerobic non-spore-forming	Respiratory transmission especially to very young and aged individuals	Nasopharyngitis may be epidemic especially in impoverished and rural populations; often outbreaks during winter months may develop into pneumonia, ear infections, rarely meningitis
H. pertussis (*Bordetella pertussis*)	Gram-negative	Small, aerobic slow growing	Respiratory droplets; very contagious; incubation period approximately 1 week	"Whooping cough"; characterized by a catarrhal stage followed by paroxysmal cough and laryngeal stridor; without immunization, epidemics are seen; immunization or disease does not provide lifelong immunity
Staphylococcus	Gram-positive	Spherical, grapelike clusters of organisms on solid media		
S. Aureus	Gram-positive	Coagulase positive; remains viable on surfaces of furniture or clothing	Commonly resides on skin and mucosal surfaces, invades skin through hair follicles, thence to bloodstream; occasionally through urinary or respiratory tract	Most common cause of ***skin infections,*** furuncles, boils, and carbuncles; may have localized lymphadenopathy; impetigo results from an exfoliative toxin from a form of *S. aureus.* ***Pneumonia*** more common in hospitalized individuals; causes fever, tachycardia with localized areas of pneumonia; also may cause empyema; ***bacteremia*** may produce fever, tachycardia with abscess throughout the body; often fatal, nearly 50% mortality; ***acute osteomyelitis*** commonly caused by this

TABLE 7-4. (continued)

Bacteria	Gram's stain	Morphology	Mode of transmission	Clinical effects
				organism; may result from skin or bloodborne infection or from open or closed trauma of the affected bone; causes high fever and bone pain; may cause much osseous destruction; usually responds well to antimicrobials; *urinary tract infections* most frequently result from contamination of an indwelling catheter, are ascending to kidneys from the bladder
Streptococci	Gram-negative	Spherical, anaerobe nonmotile, non-spore-forming		
Group A, *S. pyogenes* (at least 60 subtypes), B hemolytic	Gram-positive		Respiratory, droplet	Streptococcal *pharyngitis* very common in crowded living situations, greatest incidence between ages of 5 and 15; fever, extremely painful and inflamed pharynx, tonsils, uvula; *scarlet fever* may result when a specific strain of *Streptococcus* A produces a toxin causing rash, diffuse erythema, with petechiae on soft palate, scarlet "strawberry" tongue occurs in early stages; later, tongue becomes beefy in appearance called "raspberry" tongue; desquamation of the skin occurs up to 3–4 weeks postdisease; may occur prior to rheumatic fever; *rheumatic fever* may follow acute streptococcal infection and apparently is an immune reaction to the organism; *acute glomerulonephritis* also may follow a streptococcal infection; *erysipelas*, an acute infection of the skin and SQ tissue from *S. Pyogenes*, causes malaise, itching, erythema that spreads rapidly with edema and encrustation; localized skin lesions, cellulitis and pneumonia may also result from this organism
Group B, *S. pyogenes* B hemolytic	Gram-positive		Frequently colonize in the female genital tract, the throat, and rectum; may be transmitted to susceptible individual directly or by respiratory contact	Associated with UTI in both men and women; may be seen in the puerperium; often associated with diabetes mellitus; bacteremia may also result
S. Pneumoniae pneumococcus	Gram-positive	Diplococcal form, lancet-shaped	Transmitted by respiratory tract droplet; rapidly progressive once established	Preceded by "cold" or "sinus" complaints; fever, chills, pleuritic pain, cough productive of rusty sputum; hypoxia occurs with infiltration of lung tissue; progresses to atelectasis in one or more lobes; responds well to antibiotic therapy
Neisseria				
N. meningitides	Gram-negative	Single cocci, grows well in media with small amounts of oxygen	Resides in nasopharynx of carriers, spreads through respiratory droplets; transmitted by bloodstream to the meninges	*Meningococcemia* begins with cough, headache, sore throat followed by high fever and sometimes manifestations of endotoxic shock; *meningitis* is evidenced by evidence of the meningococcus in CSF and neurologic symptoms
N. gonorrhea (gonorrhea)	Gram-negative	Diplococcus	Humans are only natural hosts; transmitted almost solely through sexual intercourse; incubation period usually less than 1 week	Men develop dysuria urethral discharge; because of penicillin treatment complications are rare; women have dysuria, vaginal discharge, abnormal menstrual bleeding, Bartholin's gland may be involved; PID may result from the disease

Corynebacterium diphtheriae (diphtheria)	Gram-positive	Nonmotile red, club-shaped; elaborates exotoxin	Most frequently transmitted through respiratory tract but also may be transmitted by skin, genitalia; incubation period from 1 day to 1 week	Respiratory effect on pharynx, larynx, and trachea, formation of a thick, leathery membrane on these structures causing respiratory obstruction; exotoxin effects: heart, causing myocarditis; nervous system, causing peripheral neuritis, motor denervation; peripheral vascular collapse occurs in late stages; without antitoxin protection, mortality is about 35% with 90% of those having laryngeal involvement
Clostridium tetani (tetanus)	Gram-positive	Anaerobic, motile rod, spore-bearing; exotoxin production	Found in soil and in the intestinal tract of humans and some animals; puncture or laceration of skin usual mode of entry; incubation period variable, usually about 14 days	Exotoxin attacks the CNS causing muscle rigidity and spasms; pain and stiffness of jaw early symptoms; *lockjaw* refers to inability to open jaw; laryngospasm may lead to hypoxia; overall mortality: 40–60%
Mycobacterium M. tuberculosis (tuberculosis)		Aerobic, acid-fast: resists decolorization with acid or acid alcohol; curved, spindle-shaped	Respiratory droplet; reinfection or activation of dormant infection; incubation of 4–8 weeks if not walled off	*Primary TB:* usually lung involvement, macrophages wall viable organisms off; these may be seen on x-ray by rims of calcification; *clinical TB:* fever, pleurisy, night sweats, cough, weight loss; can spread to bone or cause liquefaction and cavitation of lung
M. lepromatous (leprosy)		Hansen's bacillus; acid-fast rod	Prolonged exposure, especially familial; skin or nasal mucosa may be portal of entrance; incubation period approximately 3–5 years; little immunity has been demonstrated; endemic regions: tropical countries and few states in U.S.	Destructive lesions of skin, peripheral nerves, upper respiratory passages, testes, and hands and feet; treatment may be curative
Treponema pallidum (syphilis)		Spiraled organism, with fibrils, 3 at each end, contractile elements for motility	Almost always transmitted by sexual contact; incubation period averages 3 weeks	The organism can penetrate any mucous membrane, enters blood and lymphatics; primary lesion at site of infection, heals; secondary effects are lymphadenopathy, skin rash, arterial inflammation; tertiary syphilis involves CNS changes, dementia, inflammatory changes of the aorta, etc.

TABLE 7-5. Common fungi that cause pathologic effects in humans

Fungus	Morphology	Mode of transmission	Clinical effects
Superficial Dermatophytoses: tinea pedis (athlete's foot), tinea capitus (scalp ringworm), tinea corporus (body ringworm)	Branching hyphae of fungus on microscopic examination; found on keratinized portion of skin, nail plate, and hair	Contact with fungus through skin; maceration or poor hygiene favor acquisition	Fissuring of toe webs, itching, irritation, areas of alopecia, and scaling; circumscribed lesion with round borders of inflammation lead to designation of *ringworm;* treatment is curative
Systemic Candidiasis *(C. albicans)*	Small, yeastlike cells; blastospores with budding; forms clusters of round growths on cornmeal agar	Contact with normal flora of mouth, stool, and vagina; may be superficial or systemic in susceptible immunosuppressed individuals	*Oral* lesions: white plaques on mouth and tongue, may cause fissures and open sores; *UTI* following broad-spectrum antibiotic therapy or individual with diabetes mellitus; *vaginal* discharge may be profuse and irritating, *Candida* in the serum may cause disseminated abscesses
Coccidioidomycoses *(C. immitis)*	Yeastlike cells, no budding is formed, divide into multiple small cells	Soil saprophyte in southern U.S., Mexico, South America; infection occurs with inhalation of arthrospores; symptoms begin 10–14 days after inhalation	*Primary form:* respiratory infection causes flulike symptoms, sometimes pneumonia; pleural effusion may occur; *progressive form:* dissemination to regional lymph nodes, skin, meninges, etc. may occur especially with immunosuppressed, other than Caucasian; fever, cough, chest pain, pulmonary coin lesion
Histoplasmosis *(H. capsulatum)*	Dimorphic fungus, forms a cottony white growth on glucose agar	Grows as a mold, prefers moist soil; airborne exposure by cleaning chicken coops, working with soil	Cough, fever, weight loss, hilar adenopathy; progressive fibrosis of mediastinal structures; difficult to diagnose; treatment with amphotericin B may or may not be helpful

Table 7-5 summarizes some of the common fungal infections in man. The reaction to these organisms often depends on host resistance and nutrition.

PROTOZOA

Protozoa are complex unicellular organisms that may be spherical, spindle-shaped, spiral, or cup-shaped [6]. Many protozoa absorb fluids through the cell membrane and all possess the ability to move from place to place. Pathogenesis caused by protozoa is often seen in the gastrointestinal tract, genitourinary tract, and the circulatory system.

The protozoa may be divided into four groups.

1. The *flagellates* (Mastigophora) have flagella or undulating membranes. They are considered to be some of the more primitive of protozoa. Members of this group include *Giardia, Trichomonas,* and *Enteromonas*, which infect the intestinal or genitourinary tracts. Other flagellates such as *Leishmania* or *Trypanosoma* are blood and tissue flagellates. *Trichomonas vaginalis*, a common protozoal infection in women, is discussed in Chapter 51.

2. Typical ameboid characteristics are seen in the group *Sarcodina.* Species such as *Entamoeba, Endolimax,* and *Iodamoeba* are representative of this group.

3. The *Sporozoa* group undergo a definite life cycle that usually involves two different hosts, one of which is often the arthropod and the other a vertebrate. *Plasmodium,* the malaria parasites, are representative of this group.

4. Along with the Sporozoa, the *Ciliates* are the most complex of the protozoa. These organisms have cilia distributed in rows or patches and two kinds of nuclei in each individual. *Balantidium coli* is the only representative pathogen in this group in humans. It is a rare cause of infection with only a few cases being recorded [2].

The motility of the protozoa is accomplished by pseudopod formation or by the action of flagella or cilia. *Pseudopod* movement is characteristic of many ameboid cells and

TABLE 7-6. Common protozoa that cause pathologic effects in humans

Protozoa	Morphology	Mode of transmission	Clinical effects
Amebiasis *Entamoeba histolytica*	Motile trophozoite usually seen in active disease; cyst form usual means of disease transmission; anaerobic	Cyst transmitted from human feces; contaminated food, poor personal hygiene	Chronic, mild diarrhea to fulminant dysentery; stools may contain mucus and blood, may persist for months or years; numerous trophozoites found in stools; fever, abdominal cramps, and hepatomegaly are common
Malaria *Plasmodium vivax* *Plasmodium ovale* *Plasmodium malariae* *Plasmodium falciparum*	Asexual phase passed in the human body; multiply in liver, called *exoerythrocytic* cycle; then enter RBC and multiply, *trophozoite* stage; as RBCs hemolyze, segments called *merozoites* are released into the blood	Transmitted by infected mosquito bite; only by female of *Anopheles* mosquito; incubation period varies with type of organism from 10 days to 7 weeks	Anemia due to loss of RBCs; hemolyzing process with release of parasites causes chills and fever; immunologic mechanisms cause normal as well as infected RBC hemolysis; debilitation is progressive; hepatic complications may cause permanent damage
Toxoplasmosis *Toxoplasma gondii*	Intracellular protozoa exists in trophozoite, cysts and oocysts form; trophozoites invade all cells; cyst form often that of transmission; *oocysts* transmitted through a cycle by the cat; form not seen in man	Transplacental transfusion or fecal-oral cysts route; may be in lamb or pork	Focal areas of necrosis, especially of eye but may cause CNS or disseminated effects; lymphadenopathy is common in immunosuppressed individuals, CNS involvement leads to high mortality; may infect the fetus of an affected mother

the projection is actively pressed foward, being rapidly followed by the rest of the organism. The movement is usually accomplished directionally, toward a specific focus. The *flagella* are whiplike projections that move the organism by their motions. These projections can cause very rapid movement of the organism from one place to the next. *Cilia* are shorter, more delicate, and are on the entire outer surface of the organism. The synchronous action of these structures provides for rapid motion by the organism.

Reproduction may be sexual or asexual depending on the species. The sexual cycle, when it occurs, occurs in the *definitive* host while the asexual cycle occurs in the intermediate host [6]. Those protozoa capable of sexual reproduction are called *gametes* while those of asexual reproduction are called *zygotes.* Protozoa also have the ability to form cysts, which means that they can surround themselves with a resistant membrane. This prevents destruction and allows them to live for a long period of time. Table 7-6 summarizes several common protozoal diseases of man.

HELMINTHS

The term *helminth* means worm and usually refers to the pathogenic worms, which are often parasitic. The common intestinal helminths are often divided into three general groups called the *nematodes* or the roundworms, the *trematodes* or flukes, and the *cestodes* or tapeworms. The helminths are very complex organisms in both their structure and life cycles. Many helminths spend part of their developmental periods in several locations and in various hosts such as fish, hogs, rats, snails, and humans. Often the eggs or larvae of the helminths are eliminated in the feces or urine of humans and may be found in the feces on microscopic examination. The mode of infection for intestinal helminths is often through fecal-oral transmission or through broken skin.

TABLE 7-7. Common helminths that cause pathologic effects in humans

Helminths	Morphology	Mode of transmission	Clinical effects
Trematodes (flukes) Schistosomiasis	Blood flukes grow and mature in the portal venous system, may attain 1–2 cm in length; life span of 4–30 years	Eggs of worm pair excreted in feces or urine of humans, hatch miracidia that penetrate a specific snail host and transform into infective larvae; these penetrate human skin and are carried to rest finally in the portal venous circulation; worldwide distribution	Usually asymptomatic; may cause dermatitis at focus of entry; cause mild fever and malaise; acute fever begins 1–2 months after exposure often associated with lymphadenopathy; eosinophilic levels elevate markedly; mucosa of bowel may become ulcerative and ova may be recovered from stool specimens
Cestodes (tapeworms) *Taenia saginata* (beef) *Taenia solium* (pork) *Hymenolepis nana* (dwarf) *Dipylidium caninum* (dog)	Segmented ribbon-shaped hermaphroditic worms; absorb food through their surface; attach to host intestinal mucosa by sucking cups; length varies with species from 1 cm–10 m	Transmitted when raw or poorly cooked beef or pork are eaten; other types may be transmitted by fecal-oral route, man to man or dog to man; usually matures in adult intestines	Weight loss, hunger, epigastric discomfort. In *T. solium,* encysted larvae may deposit in muscles, eye, and brain; leads to eosinophilia, weakness, muscular pain; anemia may result from tapeworm competition for nutrition
Nematodes	Elongated, cylindrical, unsegmented organisms from a few millimeters to a meter in length; life span 1–2 months up to 10 years		
Trichinosis *(T. spiralis)*		Encysted larvae of *T. spiralis* ingested in poorly cooked pork or bear meat; larvae are released in the intestinal mucosa, multiply, and new larvae migrate into vascular channels throughout the body; lodge in skeletal muscle, become encysted and grow for 5–10 years	Severe inflammation of muscles is found in major infestation of muscle; may begin with diarrhea and fever; muscle pain, conjunctivitis, and a rash may develop; eosinophilia is common
Enterobiasis (pinworm, threadworm)	Female of 10 mm, male of 3 mm live attached to mucosa of bowel; female deposits eggs on perianal skin at night, then dies	Fecal-oral transmission, transfer of eggs from anus to mouth; contamination of bed linens, remains viable 2–3 weeks; common infection in humans	Pruritis of the anal and genital region common, especially at night; bladder infection or other foci are relatively rare; simultaneous treatment of entire families and groups is essential
Hookworm *(Ancylostoma duodenale, necator americanus)*	Four prominent hooklike teeth attach worm to upper part of small intestine; adults about 1 cm in length	Affect about 700 million persons worldwide, greatest incidence in Africa, Asia, tropical Americas; transmitted by invasion of exposed skin by larvae, migrates through lungs and resides in GI tract; excretion of larvae in fecal material perpetuates cycle	Iron-deficiency anemia and hypoalbuminemia result from chronic intestinal blood loss; most infections are asymptomatic but may have GI distress or ulcerlike pain; eosinophilia is common

Table 7-7 summarizes some common diseases caused by helminth organisms. These conditions, while often not fatal, comprise an important source of disability worldwide.

REFERENCES

1. Braunstein, H. (ed.). *Outlines of Pathology.* St. Louis: Mosby, 1982.
2. Giese, A. C. *Cell Physiology.* Philadelphia: Saunders, 1979.
3. Lerner, A. M. Enteric Viruses. In K. Isselbacher, et al. (eds.), *Harrison's Principles of Internal Medicine* (9th ed.). New York: McGraw-Hill, 1980.
4. Purtilo, D. T. *A Survey of Human Diseases.* Reading, Mass. Addison-Wesley, 1978.
5. Robbins, S. L., and Cotran, R. *Pathological Basis of Disease* (2nd ed.). Philadelphia: Saunders, 1979.
6. Smith, A. L. *Principles of Microbiology* (8th ed.). St. Louis: Mosby, 1977.

CHAPTER 8
INFLAMMATION AND RESOLUTION OF INFLAMMATION

LEARNING OBJECTIVES

1. Define and describe different types of mechanical and physical wounds.
2. List factors that can cause inflammation.
3. Describe the vascular and cellular phases of acute inflammation.
4. Define *chemotaxis* and *chemotactic gradient*.
5. Utilize terminology of leukocyte response in inflammation.
6. Describe directional emigration.
7. Draw or describe the process of phagocytosis.
8. Briefly explain how organisms are actually killed.
9. Describe the functions of the major mediators of the inflammatory system.
10. Draw the classic and alternate pathways for complement activation.
11. Define the types of exudates and show familiarity with how they are named.
12. Differentiate chronic inflammation from acute inflammation.
13. Describe the reason for the systemic effects of inflammation including fever, leukocytosis, lymphadenopathy, lymphangitis, lymphadenitis, and neutropenia.
14. Briefly explain the process of simple resolution in inflammation.
15. Explain why regeneration occurs in some tissues and not in others.
16. Describe the process of repair by scar tissue.
17. Define *cicatrization*.
18. Differentiate between healing by first intention and healing by second intention.
19. Define *epithelialization* in wound healing.
20. Describe exuberant granuloma and keloid scar formation.
21. Define *contracture* as a normal and abnormal part of wound healing.
22. Define *stenosis*, *constriction*, *adhesion*, *dehiscence*, and *evisceration*.

In the process of living, injury to the body tissues and organs inevitably occurs. Healing and repair of these tissues and organs must proceed in order for life to be maintained. Wound healing and inflammation are a part of many disease processes. Many environmental and individual factors modify or alter the healing process. Healing is normally preceded by the process of inflammation, which sets the stage for a cellular environment conducive to healing.

A *wound* is a break or interruption of the continuity of a tissue caused by *mechanical* or *physical* means (Table 8-1). A mechanical wound is caused by some kind of trauma that damages the tissues. Physical wounds may result from organisms, chemical or thermal agents, or death of tissues or organs. Each type of wound results in *inflammation*, which is the reaction of the body to tissue injury. Many disease processes result in chemical changes that alter the process of healing and/or decrease resistance to infection. Examples of diseases that may result in alterations include atherosclerosis, diabetes mellitus, cirrhosis of the liver, and renal failure.

Inflammation is usually a beneficial response to invasion by microbial agents and/or a response to tissue injury. It normally proceeds on a continuum from the inflammatory phase to the healing phase. Inflammation can be defined as a tissue reaction to injury, which characteristically involves vascular and cellular responses working together in a coordinated manner to destroy substances recognized as being foreign to the body. The tissue is then restored to its previous state or repaired in such a way that the tissue or organ can retain viability. The process of inflammation is closely related to the process of immunity (see Chap. 9).

Healing ideally involves the return of tissue exactly to its previous state, but when this is not possible scar formation may result. Regeneration of tissue also participates in the healing process.

Inflammatory states may be classified as *acute* or *chronic* inflammation. The most common causes of inflammation include: (1) infection, from microorganisms in the tissues; (2) physical trauma, often causing blood in the tissues; (3) chemical, radiation, mechanical, or thermal injury, causing direct irritation to the tissues; and (4) immune reactions causing hypersensitivity responses in the tissues.

TABLE 8-1. Types of mechanical and physical wounds

Wound	Definition
Mechanical	
Incision	Caused by cutting instrument; wound edges are in close proximity, aligned
Contusion	Caused by blunt instrument, usually disrupting skin or organ surface; causes hemorrhage or ecchymosis of affected tissue
Abrasion	Caused by rubbing or scraping of epidermal layers of skin or mucous membranes
Laceration	Caused by tissue tearing, from blunt or irregular instrument; tissue is nonaligned with loose flaps of tissue
Puncture	Caused by piercing of tissue or organ with a pointed instrument, accidentally, such as with a nail, or intentionally, such as a venipuncture
Projectile or penetrating	Caused by foreign body entering the tissues at a high velocity; fragments of foreign missile may scatter to various tissues and organs
Avulsion	Caused by the tearing of a structure from its normal anatomic position; damage to vessels, nerves, and other structures may be associated
Physical	
Microbial agents	Living organisms may affect skin, mucous membranes, organs, and bloodstream; secrete exotoxins; or release endotoxins or affect other cells
Chemical agents	Agents that are toxic to specific cells of the body; these include pharmaceutic agents, agents released from cellular necrosis, acids, alcohols, metals, and others
Thermal agents	High or low temperatures can produce wounds of various thicknesses; these may lead in turn to cellular necrosis
Radiation	Ultraviolet light or radiation exposure affects epithelial and/or mucous membranes; large doses of whole body radiation causes changes in CNS, blood-forming system, and the GI system

ACUTE INFLAMMATION

Vascular Phase

When tissue injury occurs, large amounts of strong chemical substances are released in the tissue. These substances provide a "chemical wall" called a *chemotactic gradient*, which provides a source toward which fluids and cells begin to move. The initial reaction to injury is a neural reflex causing vasoconstriction, which serves to decrease the blood flow initially. It is rapidly followed by arteriolar and venular dilatation, which allows more fluids to cross from the capillaries into the tissue spaces. The increased permeability allows protein-rich fluid high in fibrinogen to move into the area of high concentration. This fluid may serve to dilute the injurious chemicals and bring complement, antibodies, and other chemotactic substances to the area. The plasma proteins leaked into the tissues provide an osmotic gradient, or pull, which brings more water in from the plasma (Fig. 8-1A).

Cellular Phase

The components of the fluid exudation cause a characteristic response by the leukocytes commonly described as margination and pavementing, directional emigration, aggregation, recognition, and phagocytosis (see also Chap. 15). The properties of the leukocytes allow for the

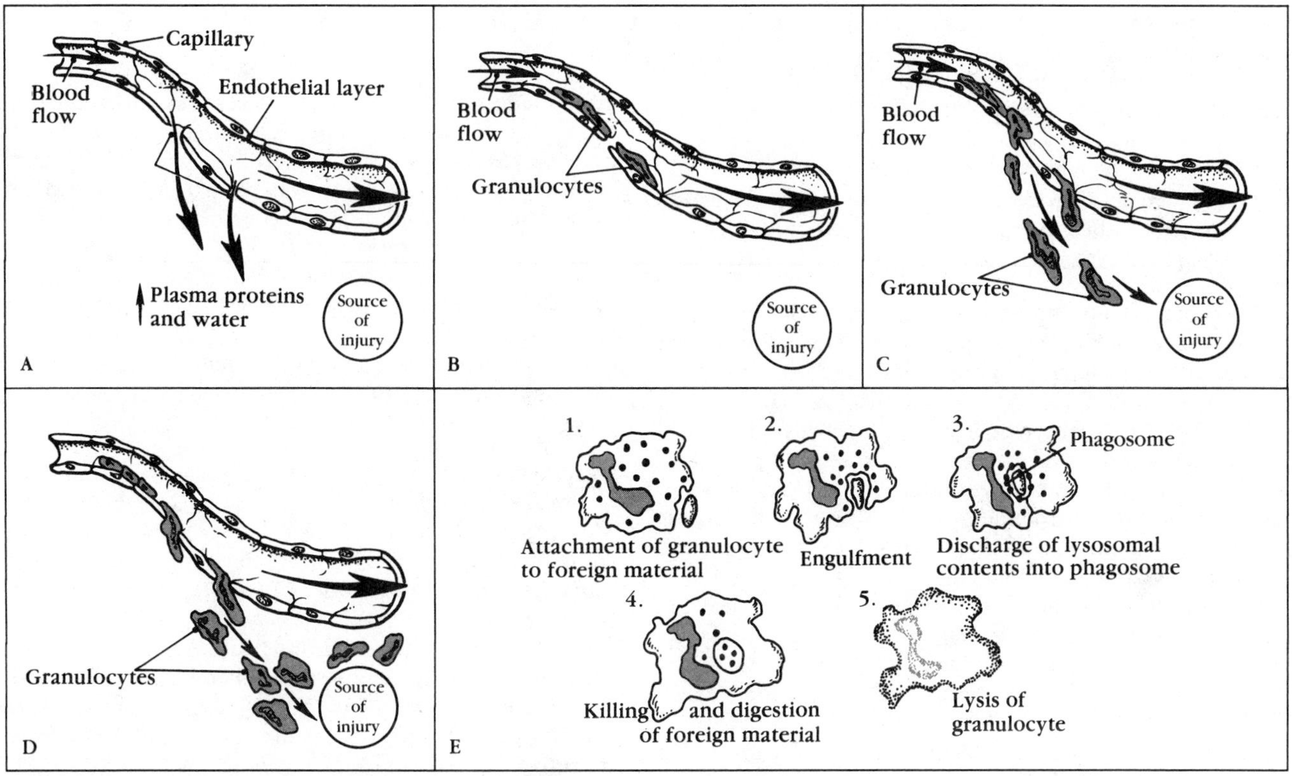

FIGURE 8-1. Acute inflammation. A. Vascular phase. Increased permeability of endothelial junctions allows the movement of plasma proteins into interstitial spaces, pulling water into the area and leading to edema. The stimulus for this increased permeability is induced by chemical mediators given off by the foreign agent or by body cells in reaction. It occurs immediately after the injury and primarily affects the venulae. B. Cellular phase. Granulocytes marginate to the wall of the blood vessel. This response is also probably a response to the chemical messengers. As groups stick to the endothelium, a pavementing pattern is seen. The leukocyte then begins to move by ameboid motion toward the endothelial junctions. C. Emigration. Granulocytes move by ameboid motion through the endothelial gaps and move toward the chemotactic source. D. Chemotaxis. Large numbers of granulocytes accumulate in the area of injury. E. Phagocytosis is utilized to engulf and destroy foreign material. In this process many granulocytes are also destroyed. These may release their lytic enzymes into surrounding tissues.

destruction of the foreign material and the removal of cellular debris. Properties of leukocytes are discussed in Chapter 15, which further describes the function of these cells in inflammation.

MARGINATION AND PAVEMENTING. Margination refers to the movement of granulocytes and monocytes toward the endothelial lining of the vessel. Because of the increased capillary permeability resulting from the initial injury, the blood movement is slowed. The polymorphonuclear leukocytes (PMNs) drop to the side of the venulae to form a layer closely approximated to the endothelial lining. This layer assumes a particular appearance called *pavementing* (Fig. 8-1B). The platelets and a few red blood cells may also join the PMNs on the endothelial lining [7]. Normally, the endothelial cells are charged so that blood cells are repelled but the changes occurring during inflammation appear to inhibit this endothelial property.

EMIGRATION. The movement of white blood cells to the area of injury is through the process of emigration. The neutrophils move by ameboid motion toward the chemotactic signal. Neutrophil movement is accomplished by the projection of a pseudopodium into the gap between two endothelial cells. This active process is followed by the streaming of the cytoplasm toward the projected extension (Fig. 8-1C) [7]. The entire leukocyte then arrives in the tissue spaces; the first ones arriving on the scene are neutrophils. Monocytes (macrophages) and lymphocytes arrive later. Red blood cells may also leak into the tissues passively following the PMNs or following hydrostatic pressure changes.

Directional orientation for the movement of the PMNs is through chemotaxis. *Chemotaxis* is the directional movement of ameboid cells along a concentration gradient composed of substances such as bacterial toxins, products of tissue breakdown, activated complement factors, and other factors. The gradient provides a directional force that draws phagocytic cells to the area (Fig. 8-1D).

RECOGNITION AND PHAGOCYTOSIS. Phagocytosis is a highly specific process that requires recognition of the foreign particle by the phagocyte before actual attack and engulfment takes place. The major phagocytes are the neutrophils and the macrophages (see Chap. 15). Neutrophils generally require the foreign material to be coated with a substance called *opsonin*. Opsonins include immunoglobulins, especially IgG and the opsonic fragment of C3 [7] (see pp. 114 and 118). Once the foreign particles are recognized, their receptors are attached by the leukocyte and phagocytosis occurs. Macrophages may respond to opsonized or other foreign material.

Phagocytosis involves the engulfment of foreign material. The cytoplasm of the phagocyte flows around the foreign particle, taking the particle into its cytoplasm. The cytoplasmic lysosomes attach to the ingested particle and release hydrolytic enzymes into it, which often kills the microorganisms or dissolves foreign proteins (Fig. 8-1E). In the process, the phagocyte often dies and releases its enzymes into the surrounding tissue. This activity causes injury to surrounding cells but also results in the digestion of the cell membrane of the phagocyte.

Accumulations of large numbers of phagocytes lead to pus accumulations and eventual destruction and removal of foreign material. The process of phagocytosis tends to localize or wall off foreign material preventing the spread of the process to other areas.

Phagocytosis is an energy-dependent process and stimulates the production of hydrogen peroxide within the lysosomes of the phagocyte. The pH of the lysosome drops to about 4.0, which enhances the action of the hydrolytic enzymes [7]. The quantities of hydrogen peroxide produced are apparently not sufficient to induce the bacteriocidal effect but they are increased in the presence of myeloperoxidase and a halide ion. Myeloperoxidase is found in the granules of the neutrophils [6]. Superoxide, formed during oxidative metabolism, has also been studied in bacterial killing during the process of phagocytosis [5].

Some organisms are virulent and quite resistant to destruction by the phagocytes. Others, such as the tubercle bacillus, are engulfed but not destroyed by a macrophage and live within the cell for years [7].

Complement and Other Mediators of the Inflammatory System

PROSTAGLANDINS. Prostaglandins are substances that can be synthesized by most connective tissue, blood, and parenchymal cells. During cell injury, phospholipids become available for conversion to prostaglandins. Other mediators of inflammation such as bradykinin also have been shown to stimulate prostaglandin synthesis. Prostaglandins function as vasodilators by enhancing vascular permeability. This leads to edema with increased concentrations of these substances in the fluids and exudates of inflammatory reactions. The mechanism by which prostaglandins increase fever is not known, but local production is thought to affect the hypothalamus, which then transmits the information to the vasomotor system resulting in sympathetic nervous system stimulation with vasoconstriction and fever.

KININS. Substances called *kinins* can cause vasodilation. *Bradykinin*, a small polypeptide, is activated by an enzyme called *kallikrein*. Kallikrein, present in the body fluids in an inactive form, can be activated by a decreased pH of body fluids, by changes in temperature, by contact with abnormal surfaces, and by activation of the Hageman factor (XII) of the clotting system. The Hageman factor may be activated by endotoxins, cartilage contact, and contact with basement membrane tissue. Bradykinin is a powerful vasodilator and kallikrein, which can be converted to bradykinin, has been shown to have chemotactic properties.

COMPLEMENT. The complement system has been identified as a major mediator of the inflammatory response. It contains at least 20 distinct proteins; their cleavage products are sequentially activated with each component serving to activate the next in the series (Fig. 8-2). The complement system functions to enhance chemotaxis, to increase vascular permeability, and in the final conversion, to cause cell lysis. Fixation or activation of complement at the C1 level is by antigen-antibody interaction. This *classic pathway* continues a reaction pattern until the C8 and C9 enzymes are activated (see p. 118).

The alternate pathway is initiated by cleavage or activation of the C3 portion by plasmin, trypsin, bacterial proteases, and other enzymes found in the tissues [7]. The C5 fragment also can be activated by many of these same substances. These may be important pathways for mediating the inflammatory process to clear agents that have little immunologic specificity such as some bacterial products and proteases found in normal tissue.

COAGULATION SYSTEM. This group of plasma proteins can be activated by factor XII, the Hageman factor, which initiates the formation of bradykinin and kallikrein (see above). Plasminogen may be activated to plasmin in the process that lyses fibrin clots but also activates the alternate pathway for complement. Several factors in this system lead to increased vascular permeability.

HISTAMINE AND SEROTONIN. In the immediate postinjury phase, histamine and serotonins are the major mediators of increased vascular permeability. Histamine is found mostly in mast cells, basophils, and platelets. The tissue release may result from such varied things as mast cell/IgE reaction, C3 and C5a fragments, trauma, heat, and lysosomes of neutrophils.

Some serotonin is found in the platelets but the major source of this amine is the enterochromatine and related cells of the gastrointestinal tract.

LYMPHOKINES. This group of vasoactive substances is released from the lymphocytes during immunologic reactions (see Chap. 9). They induce chemotaxis for PMNs and macrophages.

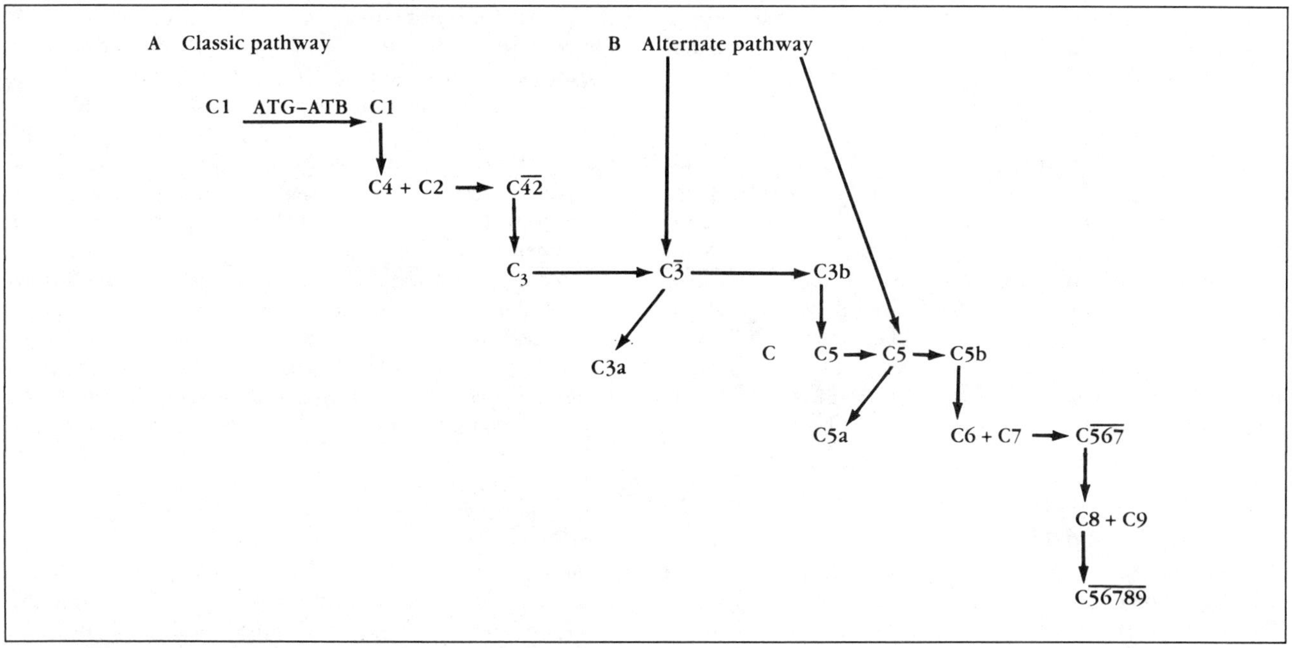

FIGURE 8-2. Complement activation. A. Classic pathway activated by ATG/ATB reaction. B. Alternate pathway at C3 activated by endotoxins, trypsin, plasmin, and tissue proteases. C. Alternate pathway at C5 activated by trypsin, bacterial proteases, and macrophages. *C3a* increases vascular permeability; anaphylatoxin causes liberation of histamine from mast cells and platelets; *C3b* is an opsonic factor; C5a increases chemotaxis and vascular permeability; $\overline{C567}$ complex is chemotactic, $\overline{C89}$ causes breakdown of cell membrane (cell lysis).

SRS-A. *The slow-reacting substance of anaphylaxis* is released from the mast cells during an anaphylactic reaction. It functions to increase vascular permeability, increase the histamine effect, and is the principal substance responsible for allergic bronchoconstriction in humans.

NEUTROPHILS. The lysosomes of neutrophils contain potent proteins and proteases, which can activate the alternate pathway for complement, release kininlike substance, and release cationic proteins, all of which increase vascular permeability [7]. As the neutrophils die and release their products into the surrounding tissue, chemotaxis and vasodilation are enhanced.

Exudates

In the process of inflammation, different types of exudates are formed, the analysis of which may offer clues as to the nature of the inflammatory process. The simplest exudate, the *serous* exudate, is the protein-rich fluid that escapes into the tissues in the early stages of inflammation. Because of its high protein content it draws more water and is responsible for the edema at the site of an inflammatory reaction. Depending on the source of the inflammation other types of exudation may be seen. These are described in Table 8-2, which shows that the nomenclature used for exudates depends on the constituents of the exudations.

TABLE 8-2. Types of exudates

Name	Description
Serous	Exudate fluid high in proteins; without cells
Fibrinous	Exudate has high content of fibrin; may lead to development of adhesions
Hemorrhagic	Usually suppurative exudation also containing red blood cells
Purulent	Refers to exudate that contains pus
Suppurative	Refers to exudate with pus and tissue damage from breakdown of neutrophils and macrophages; PMNs major cells in early suppurations; macrophages in old exudates
Abscess	Area of pus, usually located in an organ
Furuncle	Abscess of the skin
Carbuncle	Extensive abscess of skin that tends to spread
Cellulitis	Suppurative exudation with diffuse spread along tissue planes
Serofibrinous	Serous exudate with high fibrin content
Fibrinopurulent	Purulent exudate with high fibrin content

Summary of the Acute Inflammatory Response

Acute inflammation begins with the invasion of the body by an agent recognized as being foreign. The initial response is often vasoconstriction followed closely by vasodilatation. The vasodilatation or hyperemic response causes an increased vascular permeability, which leads to the exudation of serous protein-rich fluid into the area. This fluid, along with histamines and other substances, sets up a chemotactic gradient toward which leukocytes are attracted. These ameboid cells marginate and emigrate along the chemotactic gradient. The first cells to be delivered to the area are PMNs, which attack and phagocytose the foreign material once it is recognized as foreign. Recognition occurs through opsonization, which is the coating of the foreign material by antibody or through fragments of the complement factors. Complement, a major mediator of inflammation, is sequentially activated through the classic pathway with an antigen-antibody interaction. It may also be activated by tissue proteins and other substances at the C3 and C5 levels. Complement enhances hyperemia, chemotaxis, and opsonization, and causes cell lysis. When the foreign agent is destroyed, the cellular debris is removed by macrophages and neutrophils and resolution of the inflammation occurs.

CHRONIC INFLAMMATION

When an inflammatory process persists in the tissues and is not cleared by the body, certain patterns of response occur. The chronically inflamed area is usually infiltrated by mononuclear leukocytes, mostly macrophages and lymphocytes while the acute process mostly contains PMNs. Certain types of chronic inflammations, such as osteomyelitis, contain neutrophils for months while some types of acute inflammations have increased numbers of lymphocytes in the early phase. When macrophages are the predominant cell they divide and multiply and release chemotactic substances that attract more macrophages. The inflammatory process may begin as a low-grade, poorly cleared inflammation or it may begin as an acute inflammation that is not totally resolved by the body.

Chronic inflammation results in infiltration of the site with fibroblasts, increased amounts of collagen deposited, and varying amounts of scar tissue formation. The scar tissue and smoldering inflammation often cause organ dysfunction.

A distinctive pattern of chronic inflammation is the *granulomatous* inflammation, which is characterized by the accumulation of large *macrophages* or *histiocytes*. The offending foreign material is walled off from the rest of the body but not removed. In tuberculosis the resulting granuloma is called a *tubercle*, which is characterized by caseous necrosis and calcium infiltration at the rim of the granuloma [7].

SYSTEMIC EFFECTS OF INFLAMMATION

All types of inflammation have in common five cardinal signs, which were described many centuries ago: calor (heat), dolor (pain), rubor (redness), tumor (swelling), and loss of normal function. These result from vasodilatation, exudation, and irritation of nerve endings. If the inflammatory response is localized, the above effects will also be localized.

Inflammation also produces fever and leukocytosis. *Fever* is an almost universal phenomenon of illness, particularly of inflammation. It is thought to be caused by the release of *endogenous pyrogens* from macrophages and possibly eosinophils, which are activated by phagocytosis, endotoxins, immune complexes, and other products [2]. These pyrogens act to elevate the thermostat in the hypothalamus and allow for an increased setting, which elevates the body temperature [7]. Prostaglandins may interact with the pyrogen or with the hypothalamus to further increase the temperature.

Leukocytosis (Chap. 15) and an *elevated erythrocyte sedimentation rate* (ESR) are also components of the inflammatory response. An elevated ESR means that the red blood cells settle at a faster than normal rate in a test tube. This phenomenon probably occurs because of alterations in plasma components due to the inflammatory process.

Lymphadenopathy is a sign of a severe, localized infection. It results when the local lymph nodes and vessels drain the infected material, which becomes enmeshed in the follicular tissue of the lymph nodes.

Increased lymphatic flow is characteristic when there is localized inflammation. If an inflammation of the lymphatic vessel occurs it is termed *lymphangitis*. If it affects the lymph nodes it is termed *lymphadenitis*. The lymph system helps to keep infections localized and away from the bloodstream.

In advanced or overwhelming infection *neutropenia* may be seen. This denotes a depletion of neutrophils so that the individual is unable to mount an adequate defense.

RESOLUTION OF INFLAMMATION

For the body to maintain a steady state, foreign material must be removed or isolated to prevent its interaction with the defensive cells. This is accomplished through: (1) simple resolution, (2) regeneration, and/or (3) replacement by a connective tissue scar.

Simple Resolution

This type of resolution involves no destruction of normal tissue and probably goes on continuously in the human body. The offending agent is neutralized and destroyed. The vessels return to their normal permeability and excess fluid exudation is resorbed. Any defensive cells in the area are either resorbed or cleared by tissue macrophages.

Regeneration

The term *regeneration* refers to the process that occurs when lost or necrotic tissue is replaced by tissue of the same type. Intact healthy neighbor cells surrounding the dead cells undergo mitosis and proliferate to replace the cells lost in the tissue. This process generally occurs to a greater degree in epithelial tissue. Certain glands and organs can regenerate functional parenchymal cells if the intact architectural structure remains.

In the normal human body, how cell growth and reproduction occurs is still essentially unknown. Certain cells such as hematopoietic and epithelial cells reproduce continuously. Many other cells, such as bone and fibrous tissue, do not reproduce for years unless stimulated to do so. Other cells, such as the neuron, do not reproduce at all during the entire lifetime of an individual. If a person develops a deficiency of some cell types, these will reproduce rapidly until a precisely adequate number of cells are available. Other cells do not reproduce even when their numbers are depressed.

Very little is known about mechanisms and controls that keep adequate numbers of cells in the human body. Control substances are probably secreted by cells that act as a feedback mechanism to stop or slow growth when an adequate number of cells are produced [4]. Research has shown that cells removed from the body can be grown in a laboratory culture if the medium is suitable. These cells stop growing when small amounts of their own secretions are allowed to collect in the culture medium. The secretions are probably the control substances that limit cell growth and reproduction.

The classification of cells according to reproductive capability is discussed in Chapter 1. These cells react differently in the process of wound healing. All of the *labile* cells undergo complete regeneration by the proliferation of reserve cells. *Stable* cells regenerate if they are stimulated to do so. For example, bone injury causes fibroblasts to differentiate into osteoblasts and osteocytes. Muscle regeneration studies have shown that smooth muscle shows little regenerative ability while voluntary muscle may partially regenerate if conditions are optimal [1]. Synovial cells in the tendons may be reformed under optimal healing conditions. *Permanent* cells do not regenerate so that death of these cells requires replacement by scar tissue.

If tissue cells are to regenerate, the following two requirements are necessary: (1) preservation of a part of the original structure, and (2) preservation of the architectural framework of the injured tissue.

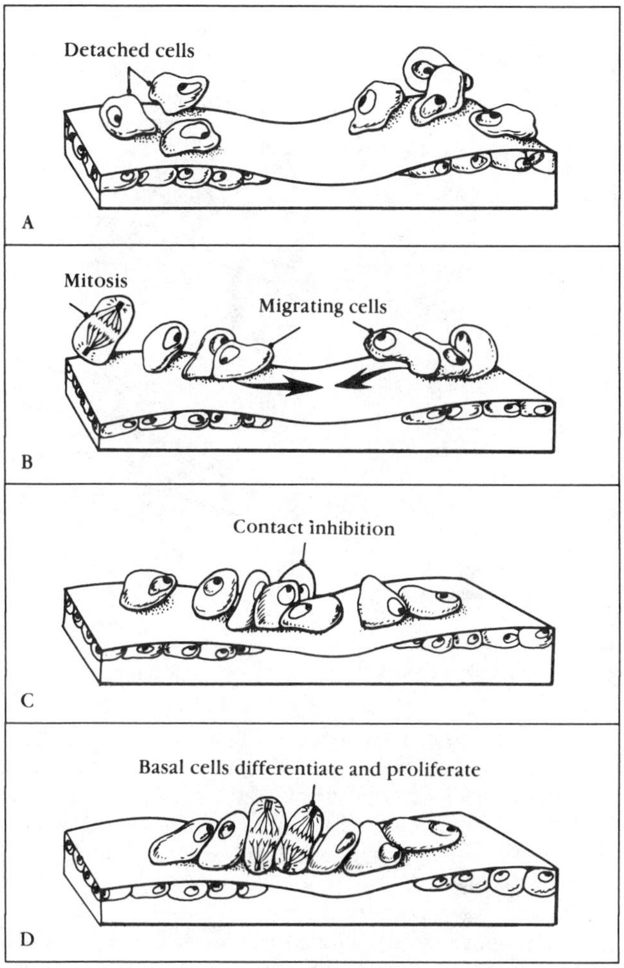

FIGURE 8-3. Epithelialization of a wound. A. With injury, epidermal cells detach from basement membrane and enlarge. B. Undifferentiated basal cells migrate toward center of wound defect. C. Contact inhibition occurs when migrating cells meet in the center and touch. D. Basal cells proliferate to restore epidermis.

Repair

The term *repair* refers to the process that occurs when dead tissue cells are replaced by viable cells that are different from the original cells. The new cells form granulation tissue, which later matures to fibrous scar tissue.

Wound healing begins with the process of inflammation. There is no distinct line between the two processes of healing and inflammation. The process for healing follows several typical steps or stages. The first stage requires a cleanup of cellular debris, organisms, or clot, which is carried out mostly by macrophages and a few neutrophils. When necrotic material, clot, or exudate is replaced by granulation tissue, the process is called *organization. Granulation tissue* is proliferative connective tissue that is highly vascularized. The gradual laying down of collagen by these connective tissue cells eventually causes a dense fibrous scar to form [1]. The scar begins as collagen, bridges the defect, and provides the initial strength to a wound. Epithelialization also occurs from the wound margins across the surface of the wound (Fig. 8-3).

As granulation tissue forms it is very vascular and bleeds readily. As the scar forms it tends to mold to the shape of the surrounding tissue and increases in tensile strength by compressing the collagen. In the early weeks the scar is red due to the many blood vessels infiltrating it. The color fades as vessels become smaller until the scar assumes a pale, white, fibrous appearance. Wound remodeling occurs throughout the process of healing. Wound contraction or shortening is effective in pulling the wound edges closer together in the early stages of scar formation.

Cicatrization is a term used to denote formation of mature scar tissue. It has been described as the erratic contracting of dense collagenous scar tissue. Extensive scarring may produce a large cicatrix, which causes deformity or immobilization in an area.

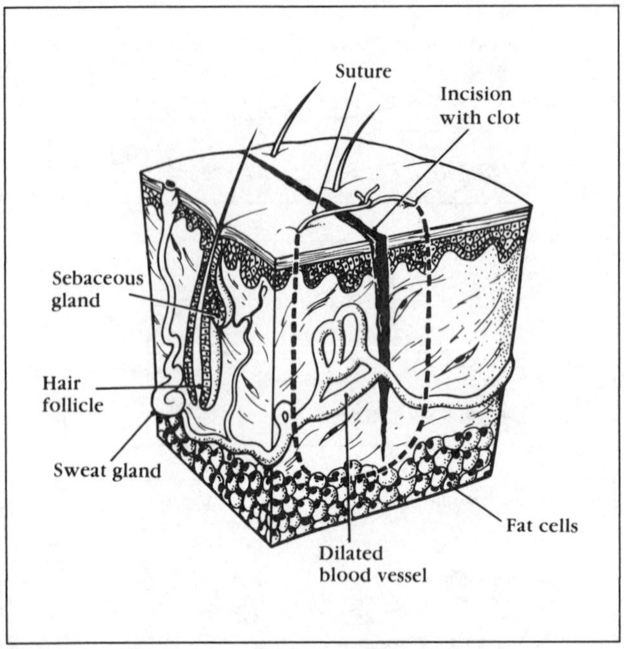

FIGURE 8-4. Initial stage of healing by first intention.

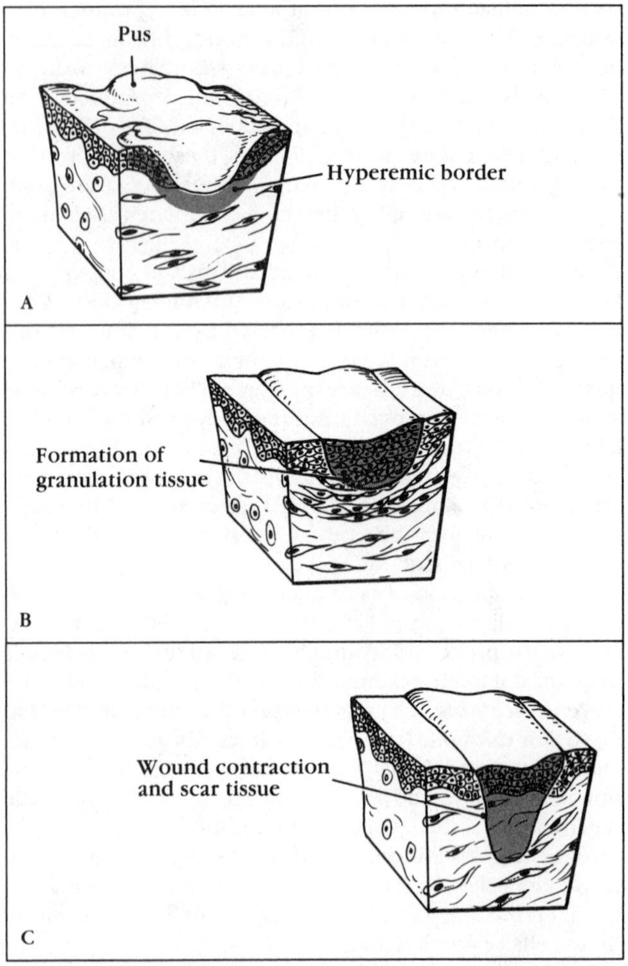

FIGURE 8-5. Healing by second intention. A. Hyperemic border around infected area. B. Formation of granulation tissue. C. Wound contraction and scar tissue.

HEALING BY FIRST INTENTION. First intention healing refers to scar tissue that is laid down across a clean wound whose edges are in close apposition. The edges are sealed together by a blood clot, which dries to protect and seal the wound. The best example is a clean surgical wound bound by sutures (Fig. 8-4).

An acute inflammatory reaction occurs within the first 24 hours with neutrophilic infiltration of the area. By the third day, macrophages have moved in to clear up cellular debris, and fibroblasts begin to synthesize collagen on the margins of the incision. By the fifth day the collagen fibrils begin to bridge the defect. The collagen continues to accumulate to form a firm, tough scar, progressively increasing in strength by the end of the first month. Epithelialization across the superficial layers restores a smooth contour. The scar is vascular initially and fades to a thin, white scar as vascularity decreases.

HEALING BY SECOND INTENTION. This type of healing parallels first intention healing except that it occurs in larger wounds in which large sections of tissue have been lost or in wounds complicated by infection. Much more time is necessary to remove the necrotic debris and infection from this type of wound.

Large amounts of granulation tissue must be formed. The wound must granulate from the margins and base with the collagen gradually filling the defect. As the wound is gradually filled, epithelialization across the scar occurs. Wound contraction results due mostly to fibroblast contraction. This contraction tends to pull the wound edges into closer proximity (Fig. 8-5).

Healing by second intention is similar to healing by first intention except that there is more cellular debris to be cleared, much more granulation tissue to be formed, and a large, often deforming scar. This type of healing is required in third-degree burns, with deep skin ulcerations, and with infected and other large wounds. Structures normally found in the scarred area are not replaced so that loss of hair follicles, sweat glands, and melanin-producing cells occurs.

Aberrant Healing

Aberrant means deviating from the normal, typical, or usual. In healing wounds, deviations from the normal may cause complications, deformity, and a decrease in function of the injured tissue. The results of aberrant healing depend on where the wound is located, the degree of the deviation, and the modifying factors present in the individual. Aberrant healing results from an abnormality in healing mechanisms that leads to formation of excess scar tissue, contracture, constrictions, or adhesions.

EXUBERANT GRANULATION AND KELOID. Exuberant granulations or keloid occurs when there is an excessive accumulation of scar tissue that may vary in size from a small to very large protrusion of tissue. Keloid scars often present a cosmetic problem and may limit function. An exuberant granulation or "proud flesh" is the protrusion of granulation tissue that blocks the epithelialization of the wound. These, once removed, do not return. A keloid is an excessive scar that extends beyond the confines of the original wound and rarely regresses. Keloid scars can occur with any wound but are more often found around the face, neck, and shoulders.

Keloid formation probably results from abnormalities in collagen synthesis and degradation. Inadequate lysis of collagen by *collagenase* may be the main defect, or elevated levels of propylhydroxylase, necessary for collagen formation, may contribute to the excess scar formation. Research has demonstrated that keloid fibroblasts in contrast to normal fibroblasts synthesize collagen at a more rapid rate possibly because of excessive histamine in the area. Keloid formation also may be a type of autoimmunity in persons demonstrating elevations in serum immunoglobulins [3].

Dark-skinned individuals have a greater incidence of hypertrophic scarring and keloid formation. Individuals below the age of 30 also have a greater propensity for development of these abnormalities. These formations tend to recur after removal.

CONTRACTURE. Wound contraction is a normal part of healing and involves migration of wound margins toward the wound center. Some wounds continue to contract after closure and a disfiguring scar and/or disability results. The ability of a wound to close a defect depends in part on the flexibility of the surrounding skin. The ability of skin to stretch on the scalp and tibial area of the leg is limited especially if little subcutaneous tissue is present. Contractures may interfere with joint mobility or with other body movements such as breathing or head movement. They can occur in any area, skin, and subcutaneous tissue, as well as following bone fractures, tendons, muscles, or nerve injuries.

DEHISCENCE AND EVISCERATION. Dehiscence refers to the disruption of the surface of a wound that results in the bursting open of a previously closed wound. This problem can occur as a result of interruption of primary or secondary healing. Dehiscence occurs when the strength of the collagen framework is not adequate to hold against the forces imposed on the wound. Poor collagen synthesis is often related to poor circulation. Evisceration refers to the internal organs moving through a dehiscence. This most frequently occurs with the abdominal organs but others may also eviscerate.

STENOSIS AND CONSTRICTION. If scar tissue forms in and around tubular areas, such as the ureter or esophagus, a stricture may develop leading to a narrowing or obstruction of an opening. Scarring may occur around an incision line or as a consequence of inflammation.

ADHESIONS. When serous or mucous membrane surfaces are inflamed, the exudate may cause scar tissue to bind or adhere to adjacent surfaces. Adhesions commonly occur in the peritoneal cavity between loops of bowel or abdominal viscera, especially following abdominal surgical procedures. Partial or complete intestinal obstruction can result from the fibrinous bands extending from organ to organ or from organ to peritoneal wall. Adhesions in the pleural space often follow pleuritis, causing dense fibrous pleural adhesions that obliterate the pleural space and restrict respiratory excursion.

REFERENCES

1. Anderson, W. A. D., and Scotti, T. *Synopsis of Pathology* (10th ed.). St. Louis: Mosby, 1980.
2. Bodel, P. Studies on the mechanism of endogenous pyrogen production. *J. Exp. Med.* 140:73, 1974.
3. Cohen, I. K., and Diegelmann, R. F. The biology of keloid and hypertrophic scar and influence of corticosteroids. *Clin. Plast. Surg.* 4:2, 1977.
4. Guyton, A. *Textbook of Medical Physiology* (6th ed.). Philadelphia: Saunders, 1981.
5. Johnston, R. B., and Lehmeyer, J. S. *Superoxide and Superoxide Dismutase*. New York: Academic, 1978.
6. Klebanoff, S. J. Antimicrobial mechanisms in neutrophilic polymorphonuclear leukocytes. *Semin. Hematol.* 12:117, 1975.
7. Robbins, S., and Cotran, R. *Pathologic Basis of Disease* (2nd ed.). Philadelphia: Saunders, 1979.

BIBLIOGRAPHY

Anderson, W. A. D., and Scotti, T. *Synopsis of Pathology* (10th ed.). St. Louis: Mosby, 1980.

Bettoli, E. J. Herpes: Facts and fallacies. *Am. J. Nurs.* 82:924, 1982.

Bodel, P. Studies on the mechanisms of endogenous pyrogen production. *J. Exp. Med.* 140:73, 1974.

Braunstein, H. *Outlines of Pathology*. St. Louis: Mosby, 1982.

Cawson, R. A., McCracken, A. W., and Marcus, P. B. *Pathologic Mechanisms and Human Disease*. St. Louis: Mosby, 1982.

Cohen, I. K., and Diegelmann, R. F. The biology of keloid and hypertrophic scar and influence of corticosteroids. *Clin. Plast. Surg.* 4:2, 1977.

Cohen, I. K., et al. Immunoglobulin, complement, and histocompatibility antigen studies of keloid patients. *Plast. Reconstr. Surg.* 63:689, 1979.

Dineen, P., and Hildick-Smith, G. *The Surgical Wound*. Philadelphia: Lea & Febiger, 1981.

Flynn, M. E. Influencing repair and recovery. *Am. J. Nurs.* 82:1550, 1982.

Flynn, M. E., and Rovee, D. T. Promoting wound healing. *Am. J. Nurs.* 82:1543, 1982.

Frobisher, M., et al., *Fundamentals of Microbiology* (9th ed.). Philadelphia: Saunders, 1974.

Giese, A. C. *Cell Physiology*. Philadelphia: Saunders, 1979.

Guyton, A. *Textbook of Medical Physiology* (6th ed.). Philadelphia: Saunders, 1981.

Ham, A. W., and Cormack, D. H. *Histology* (8th ed.). Philadelphia: Lippincott, 1979.

Hickman, C. P., et al. *Integrated Principles of Zoology*. St. Louis: Mosby, 1979.
Johnston, W. B., and Lehmeyer, J. S. *Superoxide and Superoxide Dismtase*. New York: Academic, 1978.
Junzuiera, L. C., and Carniero, J. *Basic Histology* (3rd ed.). Los Altos, Calif.: Lange, 1980.
Klebanoff, S. J. Antimicrobial mechanisms in neutrophilic polymorphonuclear leukocytes. *Semin. Hematol.* 12:1117, 1975.
Lerner, A. M. Enteric viruses. In K. J. Isselbacher, et al. (eds.), *Harrison's Principles of Internal Medicine* (9th ed.). New York: McGraw-Hill, 1980.
Lynch, J. M. Helping patients through the recurring nightmare of herpes. *Nursing 82* 12:52, 1982.
McAdams, C. W. Interferon: The penicillin of the future. *Am. J. Nurs.* 80:714, 1980.
Phaff, H. J. Industrial microorganisms. *Sci. Am.* 245:76, 1981.
Purtillo, D. T. *A Survey of Human Diseases*. Reading, Mass.: Addison-Wesley, 1978.
Robbins, S., and Cotran, R. *Pathological Basis of Disease* (2nd ed.). Philadelphia: Saunders, 1979.
Simons, K., Garoff, H., and Helenius, A. How an animal virus gets into and out of its host cell. *Sci. Am.* 246:58, 1982.
Smith, A. M. *Principles of Microbiology* (8th ed.). St. Louis: Mosby, 1977.
Taylor, D. L. Wound healing: Physiology, signs, and symptoms. *Nursing 83* 13:44, 1983.
Walter, J. *An Introduction to the Principles of Disease* (2nd ed.). Philadelphia: Saunders, 1982.
Weissman, G. (ed.). *Mediators of Inflammation*. New York: Plenum, 1974.

UNIT 5
IMMUNITY

Barbara L. Bullock

An intact, functioning immune system is essential to protect the human body from microorganism invasion and damage by foreign substances. The cells of the immune system are called immunocompetent cells and are developed during fetal life, during which time they develop self-tolerance, thus distinguishing self from nonself. Chapter 9 covers the basic immunologic response including the components of the immune system and the development of immunity. Chapter 10 describes the alterations in defense that can occur with primary or secondary immunologic deficiency. Chapter 11 describes the hypersensitivity or exaggerated immune responses. Autoimmune disease is considered to be a hypersensitive response and is discussed in this chapter.

The topic of immunity is vast and requires familiarity with much new terminology. In studying immunity the reader is encouraged to also review or study the inflammatory process. The learning objectives are helpful as a study guide outline for learning. The bibliography at the end of the unit gives some direction for further research.

CHAPTER 9
NORMAL IMMUNOLOGIC RESPONSE

LEARNING OBJECTIVES

1. Identify the functions of the organs and cells of the immune system.
2. Differentiate between T and B lymphocytes on the basis of function.
3. Trace the development of immunocompetent T and B cells.
4. Compare antibody-mediated immunity with cell-mediated immunity.
5. Define *self* and *nonself* as they are used in immunology.
6. Differentiate between primary and secondary immune responses.
7. Compare the functions of the different classes of immunoglobulins.
8. Briefly describe the role of the macrophages and the polymorphonuclear leukocytes in the immune response.
9. Explain one theory of specificity in the immune reaction.
10. Define the process of *immunosurveillance*.

The immune system consists of cells and organs that defend the body against invasion by microorganisms and damage by foreign substances. The inherent capacity to distinguish that which is foreign from that which belongs to the body is effected by particular cells called *immunocompetent* cells. These cells distinguish *self* from *nonself.* The development of *self-tolerance* involves the recognition of self proteins and is gained during fetal development. All other proteins to which the body is exposed are treated as foreign agents and are targeted for destruction.

This chapter describes the process for the development of immunity and for the recognition of foreignness. Table 9-1 lists some of the essential terminology utilized in describing this system. Knowledge in the area of immunology is expanding rapidly through research with many applications to clinical situations. The scope of immunology is broad and includes such aspects as: defense against infection, immunization, prevention of transplant rejection, and hypersensitive and defective immunologic mechanisms.

TABLE 9-1. Terms frequently used to explain immune responses

Term	Definition
Antibody	A protein produced as the result of introduction of an antigen; also called immunoglobulins; secreted from plasma cells
Antigenic determinants	Specific areas or combining sites on the surface of the cell membrane of an antigen; determines specificity
Antigens	Foreign substances, usually proteins, that are capable of stimulating an immune response
Autoimmunity	Immunity to self-antigens; loss of self-tolerance
Complement	A series of enzymes, normally inactive, circulating in the bloodstream that, when activated by an antigen-antibody reaction, participate in the inflammatory response
Immunocompetent cells	Those cells that can recognize and react with antigen; refers to T and B lymphocytes
Memory	Ability to respond to an antigenic challenge due to a previous exposure to the antigen and development of a bank of specific immunocompetent cells to that antigen
Specificity	The property of reacting with one antigen only; both the antigen and the T or B lymphocyte have surface receptors that allow them to recognize each other specifically
Tolerance	A state of unresponsiveness developed to a specific, known antigen

Source: H. H. Fudenberg, et al. (eds.), *Basic and Clinical Immunology* (3rd ed.). Los Altos, Calif.: Lange, 1980.

COMPONENTS OF THE IMMUNE SYSTEM

Lymphoid Organs and Tissues

The lymphoid organs include the lymph nodes, thymus, spleen, and tonsils. The lymphoid tissues are composed of lymphocytes and plasma cells, which are found throughout the body, especially in the gastrointestinal tract and the bone marrow. The lymphocytes travel throughout the lymphoid tissues and organs, entering and leaving the tissue spaces with ease. A network of lymphatic vessels conducts the lymph fluid to the vascular circulation and drains areas throughout the entire body.

LYMPH NODES. These encapsulated organs are distributed throughout the body, and receive the lymph circulation. A lymph node consists of an outer portion, called the *cortex*, and an inner portion, called the *medulla*. Lymphocytes are formed and/or seeded from the thymus, especially in the cortical areas. In the mid- and deep cortex is an area called the *thymus-dependent zone*, which is believed to contain chiefly T lymphocytes. The *germinal centers* contain mostly B lymphocytes but also may contain a few T lymphocytes and macrophages. The substance of the node consists of a stroma in which different types of free cells are held in place by reticular fibers and collagenic fibers. The lymph sinusoid is a thin-walled vessel through which lymph flows. The lymph sinus in the subcapsular space is like a hollow space that conducts the lymphatic flow [4]. Basically, lymph nodes serve as a series of in-line filters so that all lymph in the lymph vessels is filtered by at least one node [6]. The lymph node receives lymph from an afferent lymphatic vessel, and the lymph then passes through the cortical, paracortical, and medullary regions (see Fig. 9-1). Many lymphocytes and macrophages reside in these areas. T lymphocytes are found in the paracortical region with many plasma cells in the medullary sinuses.

THYMUS. The thymus gland, located in the mediastinal area, processes lymphocytes, and rapid production of lymphocytes occurs in this region from the early years of life until puberty. In the medullary area, lymphocytes appear to become more differentiated after which they enter the circulation (Fig. 9-2). Many of the cells that are produced by the thymus die in the gland. As the years pass, the thymus gradually begins the process of involution, beginning in the cortical zone and progressing to the medullary area. The gland never completely disappears but is seen in elderly people as a collection of reticular fibers, some lymphocytes, and connective tissue.

Regulation of lymphocyte maturation occurs through transformation of lymphocyte precursor cells into antigen-specific lymphocytes (see p. 116). This process occurs in the cortical and medullary areas under the influence of the *thymic hormones*. A group of hormones that affect cell activities have been identified, but all of the effects of these hormones are not known [2]. *Thymosin* was shown to enhance T cell immunity in certain experimental studies. The

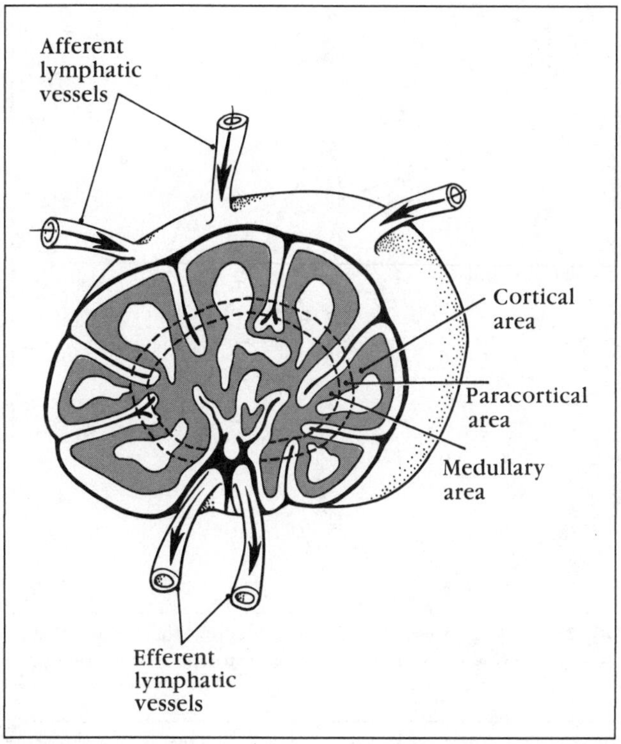

FIGURE 9-1. Regions and lymphatic vessels of a representative lymph node.

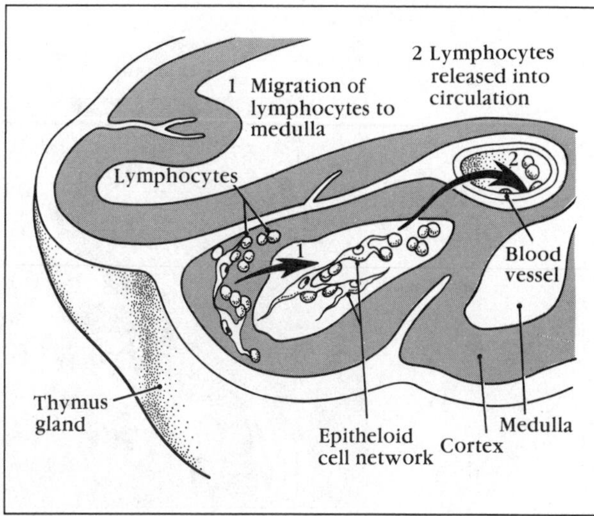

FIGURE 9-2. A thymus lobule. Note that the medulla extends into each lobule. The lymphocytes in the cortex rapidly divide and are immature. Those in the medulla are immunologically mature and are released from this area into the circulation.

other thymic hormones, thymopoietin, thymic factor, thymic humoral factor, and lymphocyte stimulating hormone, are being studied [2].

SPLEEN. This organ, the largest lymphatic organ, can function as a reservoir for blood in two areas, the venous sinuses and the pulp (Fig. 9-3). As the spleen enlarges, the quantity of red blood cells within its *red pulp* (so called because of its dark red tissue, which is rich in blood) also can increase. One of the main functions of the spleen is to process the red blood cells that squeeze through its pores. Those RBCs nearing the end of their life spans often break down here (see Chap. 14). The macrophages in the splenic tissue clear the cellular debris and process the hemoglobin.

Many phagocyte cells, especially macrophages, line the pulp and sinuses of the spleen. Groups of lymphocytes and plasma cells that can be seen with the naked eye throughout the parenchyma of the spleen are called the *white pulp*. These cells function in the process of immunity.

TONSILS. These organs are aggregations of lymphoid tissue and are named according to their location (Fig. 9-4). Those of the mouth and pharynx are called *palantine*, *lingual*, and *pharyngeal* tonsils. They are composed of lymphoid tissue and many lymphocytes.

In the intestinal area, *Peyer's patches* are accumulations of lymphoid tissue as is the vermiform appendix.

Immunocompetent Cells

The mononuclear and the polymorphonuclear leukocytes are involved in the immune response. The mononuclear T and B lymphocytes are considered to be the only immunocompetent cells. These cells provide for *specificity*, or recognition, of specific antigens by specific lymphocytes. An *antigen* is a substance recognized by the immunocompetent cells as being foreign, against which an immune reaction is initiated.

The polymorphonuclear neutrophils (PMNs) are *nonspecific* and interact with the lymphocytes to produce an inflammatory reaction (see Chap. 8). Phagocytic macrophages also play an important role in the immune response in that macrophages can be utilized for processing antigen. This role is further described in subsequent sections of this chapter.

The interaction among B cells, T cells, and macrophages with antigen provides the basis for the development of immunity.

B Lymphocytes

B lymphocytes are the cells that are responsible for *humoral-* or *immunoglobulin*-mediated immunity. These cells originate in the bone marrow and mature either there or in some other portion of the system. B lymphocytes are capable of proliferating and differentiating into *plasma cells* and *memory cells* when exposed to antigen. Plasma cells secrete large quantities of specific immunoglobulin.

Immunoglobulin secreted by plasma cells is called *antibody*. The basic unit of every immunoglobulin molecule is a symmetric arrangement of four polypeptide chains. Two of the polypeptide chains, called *heavy chains*, are iden-

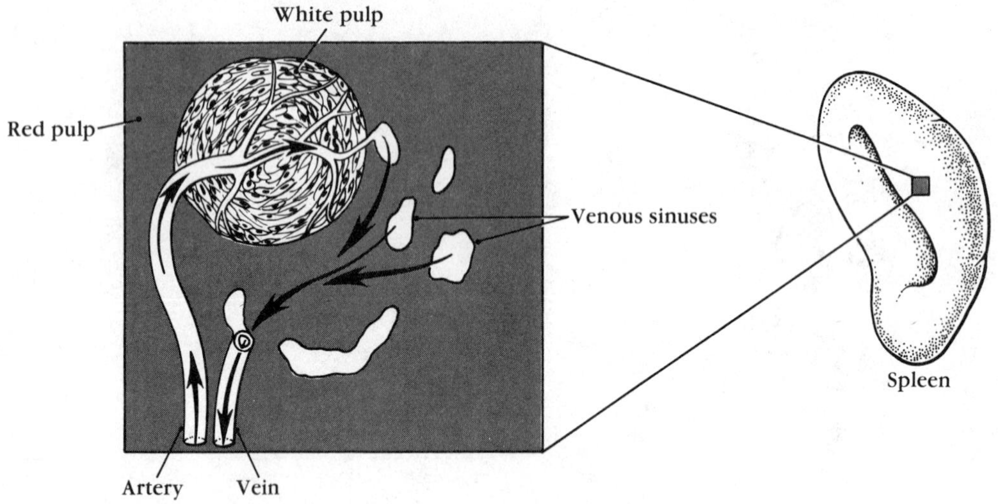

FIGURE 9-3. The structure of the spleen allows for the processing of the red blood cells and can serve as a storage area for blood.

TABLE 9-2. Immunoglobulin classification

	IgG	IgA	IgM	IgD	IgE
Serum concentration (mg/dl)	700–1500	150–400	60–170	3.0	0.03
Binds to mast cells	–	–	–	–	+
Fixes complement	++	–	+++	–	–
Percent total	80%	13%	6%	1%	0.002%
Crosses placenta	+	–	–	–	–
Function	Major ATB formed in secondary response; most common ATB in response to infection	External secretions and surfaces, saliva, tears, mucus, bile, colostrum	ATB formed in primary response	Not known; found with IgM	Reaginic ATB binds to mast cells; causes allergic symptoms

Key: – = negative; + = positive; + + = active; + + + = highly active.
Source: L. Roitt, *Essential Immunology* (3rd ed.). Oxford, England: Blackwell, 1977.

tical and have a greater molecular weight than the two *light chains*. These chains are held together by disulfide bonds. Figure 9-5 shows a representative model of an immunoglobulin. The Fab (fragment, antigen-binding) portion is the *variable* portion while the Fc (fragment, crystallizable) portion is the *constant* portion of the immunoglobulin class. The constant portion, or heavy chain, almost certainly directs the biologic activity of the antibody and perhaps the distribution or location of the immunoglobulin in the body [8]. The variable portion, or light chain, provides individual specificity for binding antigen and varies among immunoglobulin molecules. Five major classes of immunoglobulins have been identified: IgG, IgM, IgA, IgE, and IgD. The classification depends on the structure of the heavy chain portion of the molecule. Table 9-2 lists the main properties of each major classification.

IgM. Often called the macroglobulin, IgM is the first immunoglobulin produced during an immune response. It is made up of five units held together by a short peptide chain called the J chain. IgM is efficient in agglutinating antigen as well as lysing cell walls. It is found in high concentrations in the bloodstream and also is found early in the course of an infection [8].

IgG. IgG makes up about 80 percent of the antibodies found in the plasma. During the secondary response it is the major immunoglobulin to be synthesized (see p. 118). This antibody freely diffuses into the extravascular spaces to in-

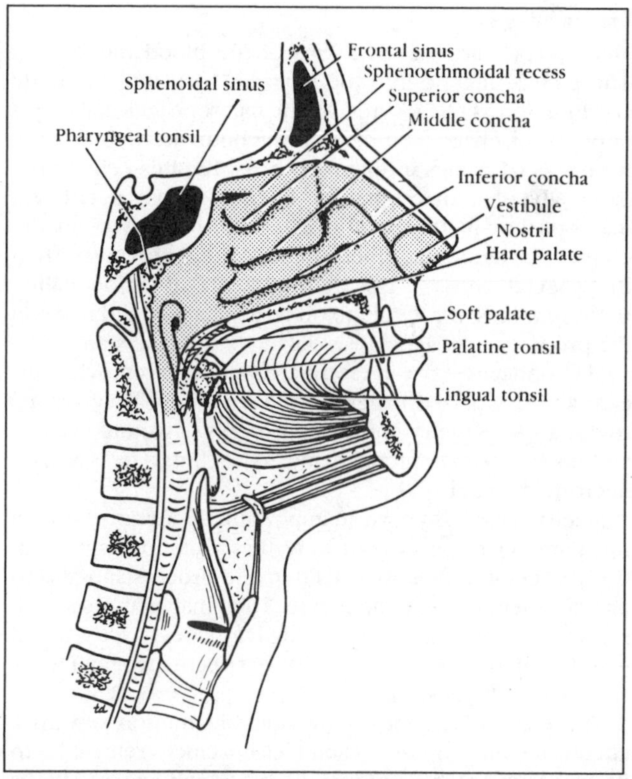

FIGURE 9-4. The tonsils of the mouth and pharynx. (From R. Snell, *Clinical Anatomy for Medical Students* [2nd ed.]. Boston: Little, Brown, 1981.)

teract with antigen. The amount of IgG synthesized is closely related to the amount of *antigenic* stimulation presented to the host. In prenatal life it diffuses across the placental barrier to provide the fetus with passive immune protection until the infant can produce an adequate immune defense. IgG has been shown to carry the major burden in neutralizing bacterial toxins and in accelerating phagocytosis [8].

IgA. IgA is selectively found in the external body secretions, such as saliva, sweat, tears, mucus, bile, and colostrum. It provides a defense against pathogens on exposed surfaces especially those entering the respiratory and gastrointestinal tracts. IgA antibodies may inhibit the adherence of pathogens to mucosal cells [8]. The structure of the IgA molecule appears to facilitate its transport into the external secretions.

IgD. IgD is found in the plasma and is readily broken down (half-life in plasma of 2–8 days). Its function is not exactly known, but the fact that it has been found on the lymphocyte surfaces together with IgM suggests that it may be the receptor that binds antigens to the cell surface [8].

IgE. IgE is called the reaginic antibody because it is involved in immediate hypersensitivity reactions. Low con-

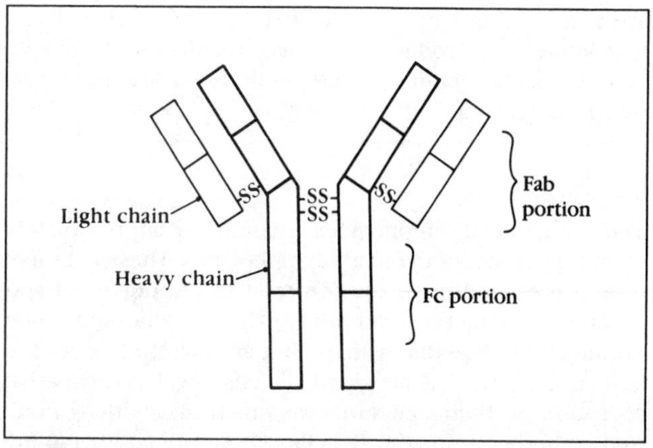

FIGURE 9-5. Schematic model of an immunoglobulin showing two light and two heavy polypeptide chains. The constant portion, or Fc, accounts for the biologic activity while the variable portion, or Fab, provides for the binding of specific antigen. SS = disulfide bonds.

centrations are found in the serum and the antibody apparently remains firmly fixed on the tissue surfaces, probably bound to mast cells. Contact with an antigen triggers the release of the cellular granules [8]. The released vasoactive amines cause the signs and symptoms seen in allergy and anaphylaxis (see Chap. 11). High serum levels of IgE are seen with allergy-prone individuals and in those infected with certain parasites, especially helminths.

Formation of Specific Antibodies

To be specific an antigen and antibody must fit together precisely, the way the right key fits into a lock. The antigen-binding or variable region of the antibody binds certain antigenic determinants strongly but does not bind others of similar structure.

An individual is confronted every day with many different kinds of antigens, both environmental and synthetic, so that the body must provide defense for a vast array of antigens.

Each immunoglobulin molecule has a constant region (C) and a variable region (V). The constant region of the immunoglobulin molecule is similar in molecules of each class. The variable region of the antibody molecule must be able to bind many different antigens and provides for specificity. Several theories have been proposed to try to explain immunoglobulin specificity.

One of these, the *selective theory*, proposes that each lymphocyte contains all the genetic information necessary to make all possible antibodies. The gene for specific antibody is activated by contact with the antigen, and large amounts of the specific antibody are formed. Expanding this theory, the *clonal selection model* assumes that large amounts of antigenic stimulation trigger the immunocompetent lymphocyte to divide and make large amounts of specific antibody [8].

When the B cell first encounters its specific antigen, it may become a *memory cell* or a *plasma cell*. Memory cells are a method of stockpiling a specific clone of B cells so that immediate production of large quantities of the specific immunoglobulins results with exposure to a particular antigen.

T Lymphocytes

These long-lived lymphocytes account for approximately 70 to 80 percent of the blood lymphocytes. These cells live from a few months to the life span of an individual and account for long-term immunity. They are thought to be produced by the bone marrow but are matured under the influence of the thymus gland. T cells develop distinctive receptors on their cell surfaces, which makes their functions different from the B cells. They proliferate rapidly in the thymus and produce large numbers of antigen-specific cells.

The T lymphocytes leave the thymus to enter special regions called thymus-dependent zones, mainly in the paracortical region of the lymph nodes and part of the white pulp of the spleen. They may remain in the lymphoid tissue, enter the blood circulation, or enter the extravascular spaces to encounter antigens that correspond to the membrane receptors on their surfaces. If a T cell encounters its specific antigen, it divides and proliferates to form a clone of T cells that can destroy the antigen. T lymphocytes can be functionally divided into three subgroups: killer, helper, and suppressor cells.

KILLER CELLS. Killer T lymphocytes bind to the surface of the invading cell, disrupt its membrane, and kill it by altering its intracellular environment. Killer T cells secrete *lymphokines,* which include such substances as chemotactic factor (CF), migratory inhibition factor (MIF), macrophage activation factor (MAF), blastogenic factor (BF), transfer factor (TF), lymphotoxin, and interferon [2]. These substances may be *chemotactic,* establishing a chemical gradient that helps to bring leukocytes and other substances into the area.

HELPER T CELLS. Helper T cells stimulate B lymphocytes to differentiate into antibody producers [2]. A message from the antigen-sensitized T lymphocyte induces the also sensitized B cell to divide and mature into a plasma cell, which begins to synthesize and secrete immunoglobulins. It has been noted that the synthesis of the class of immunoglobulin IgM seems to be the least dependent on T cell activity while IgA immunoglobulin response is the most dependent [8].

SUPPRESSOR T CELLS. These cells also function to reduce the humoral response. The production of immunoglobulins against a particular antigen can be reduced or totally abolished in the presence of suppressor T cells. The mechanism of action may be to control the production of immunoglobulins either by regulating the proliferation of B cells or by inhibiting the activity of the helper T cell.

Figure 9-6 shows the comparative formation and differentiation of T and B lymphocytes.

Macrophages

Macrophages are mature forms of the blood monocytes. These cells migrate into the different tissues of the body and function as phagocytes. Tissue macrophages make up a network of phagocytic cells throughout the body. These have special names in different areas: Kupffer cells in the liver, alveolar macrophages in the lungs, peritoneal macrophages in the peritoneal cavity, histiocytes in the connective tissue and others. In the central nervous system the special cells of the neuroglia classification called *microglia* have the ability to undergo changes and develop the property of phagocytosis during pathologic states [5].

Macrophages serve an essential function in removing foreign and devitalized material from the body. They are active at a site of injury during the process of wound healing, and in removing microorganisms, cellular debris, and necrotic material.

Macrophages also have an important, cooperative role in the immune response, but how they function is not entirely understood. These cells trap and process antigens to present them to the lymphocyte. They may play a secondary or accessory role in promoting lymphocyte activity and may function as an intermediary between specific T cells and specific B cells [8].

The macrophage moves by ameboid motion toward a chemical concentration of soluble substances released into its environment by antigens or by lymphocytes. This is called movement toward a *chemotactic gradient,* or signal, which is elicited by soluble substances such as lymphokines (see Chap. 8). The macrophage migration inhibition factor (MIF) and the macrophage activating factor (MAF), which respectively tend to retain the macrophage in an area and increase its phagocytic activity are especially important lymphokines [8].

Null Cells

Some cells cannot be classified as T or B cells or macrophages because they lack the surface markers characteristic of these cells and are not phagocytic. The cells, called null cells, resemble small or medium-sized lymphocytes. Some of these cells function to lyse opsonized antigen and function in graft rejection, lyse certain tumors, or destroy specific viruses. These cells appear to be marrow-dependent and are often called K cells or M cells according to their function.

Antigen, Immunogen, or Hapten Recognition

An *antigen* is defined as a molecule capable of inducing a detectable immune response when introduced into the body. An *immunogen* is an antigen that stimulates the immune response, denoting an active production of antibodies or sensitized cells [2]. Most antigens and immunogens are proteins, but other large molecules such as polysaccharides and nucleoproteins may also function in this way. Several characteristics appear to determine whether a molecule can stimulate an immune response and these include such aspects as size, foreignness, shape, and

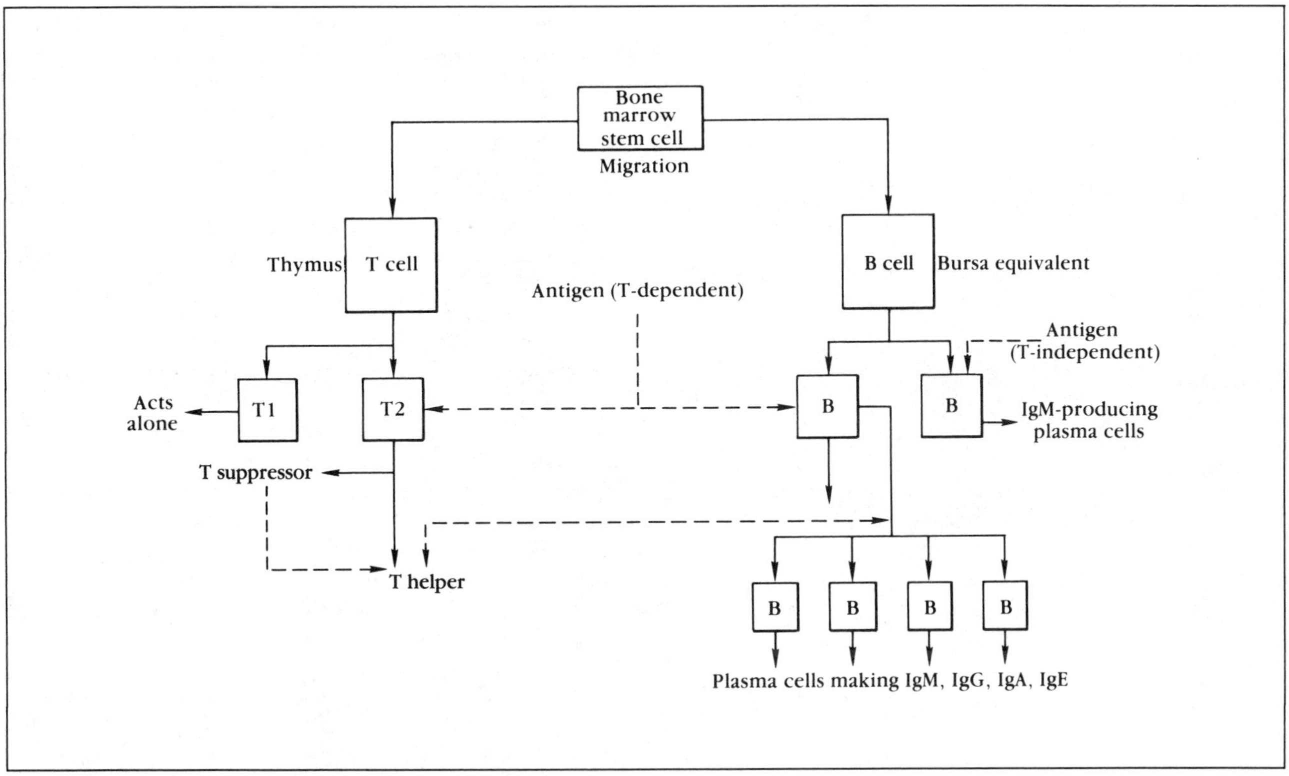

FIGURE 9-6. Both T and B lymphocytes arise from the bone marrow stem cell and migrate to the thymus gland (T cell) or to an unknown bursa equivalent area (B cell) where they mature to immunocompetent cells. T cells may act cooperatively with B cells or may act alone. Some antigens can stimulate B cells without T cell interaction, a process that imparts little or no memory.

solubility. Some molecules become antigenic only when they are combined with a carrier. Called *haptens,* these substances fail to elicit an immune response because they are small in size. These molecules cannot serve as complete antigens until they are combined with protein carriers (Fig. 9-7). An example is the contact allergens, which probably attach to proteins of the skin and stimulate the proliferation of a T cell population sensitized to the substance. Later exposure to the allergen leads to a more rapid reaction [7].

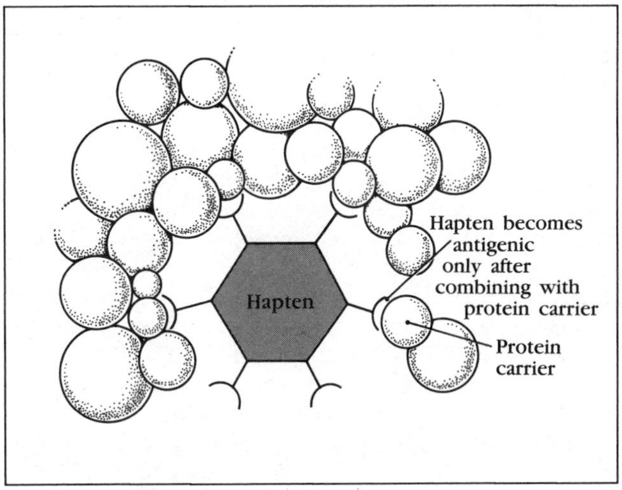

FIGURE 9-7. Some molecules become antigenic only after they have combined with a carrier, usually a protein. These molecules, called haptens, when combined with a carrier are fully antigenic.

TYPES OF IMMUNITY

Humoral Immunity

Humoral immunity refers to immunity effected by antibody synthesis or the production of specific immunoglobulin, which covers the antigen and targets it for destruction by PMNs. The interaction of antigen with antibody causes the activation of the classic pathway of the complement system (Chap. 8).

Most antigens are recognized by T helper cells, which promote the activation of specific B cells. B cells are "turned on" either by direct T cell interaction or by T cell secretions. In some cases a macrophage serves as an intermediary between the T and B cell. The B cell then divides and differentiates into a plasma cell that secretes specific immunoglobulin to target the antigen for destruction. Antigen recognition by T or B cell is often enhanced by macrophage interaction, which processes the antigen and presents it to the appropriate cell (Fig. 9-8).

Certain antigens, designated as *thymus-independent antigens,* elicit strong B cell responses without T cell interaction. Examples of these antigens include *Escherichia coli,* pneumococcal polysaccharide, dextrans, and other large polymers [2].

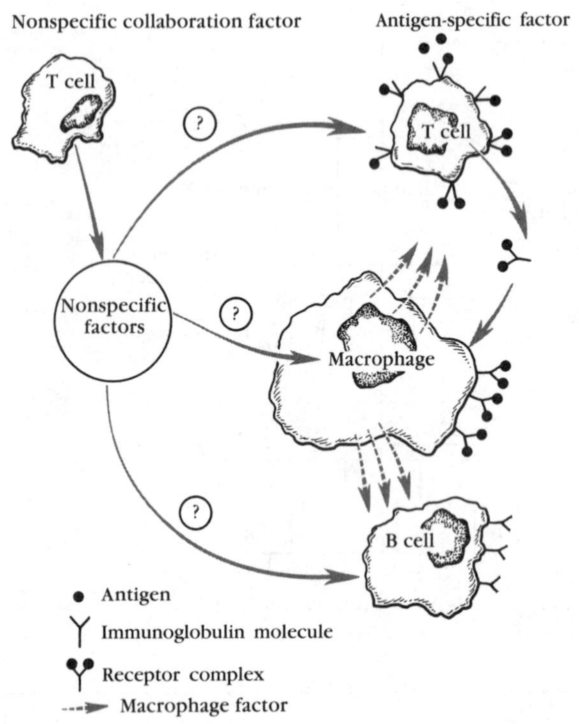

FIGURE 9-8. The macrophage often enhances antigen recognition and probably serves as an intermediary between T and B cells.

Humoral immunity is often described in terms of the *primary* and *secondary* immune response. This terminology refers to the time lapse between the introduction of antigen and the humoral or immunoglobulin response.

PRIMARY RESPONSE. The first time a particular antigen enters the body, a characteristic pattern of antibody production is induced. As the antigen binds to specific B cells, activation occurs and causes them to proliferate and differentiate into specialized antibody-producing plasma cells.

After about 6 days, antibodies specific to the antigen can be measured in the blood. The first antibodies or immunoglobulins to be produced in measurable quantities are usually IgM. IgM antibodies are produced in large quantities, increasing up to 14 days and then gradually declining in production to very little IgM production after a few weeks.

Following the initial IgM elevation, IgG immunoglobulins appear at about day 10, peak at several weeks, and maintain high levels much longer. During the course of the primary immune response, the immunoglobulins improve in their ability to bind the inducing antigen. The mechanisms responsible for this change are not known but probably more firm binding occurs because of a greater precision in the matching of surface receptors. IgG is considered to be the highest affinity antibody that binds antigenic groupings firmly [2].

SECONDARY RESPONSE. The secondary response differs from the primary response in that the production of antibodies begins almost immediately. More antibody is produced and specific IgG is produced early and in large amounts.

The secondary response is called the memory response because the immune system responds much faster to a second exposure to a particular antigen. Both T and B memory cells are involved because in the primary response lymphocytes differentiate into T and B memory cells. If the antigen is introduced into the host a second time, these cells begin immediate production of antibodies of a higher-binding capacity than in the primary response. Small amounts of antigen stimulate a highly specific response with the specific antibody [8].

COMPLEMENT ACTIVATION IN HUMORAL IMMUNITY. Complement is a system of at least 20 different proteins that circulate as functionally inactive molecules. They are capable of interacting with each other in a sequential activation cascade. They are designated by numbers with nine numbers indicating the major molecules and the components by symbols or names. Serum factors also include inactivators or inhibitors of the complement cascade.

The classic pathway for the activation of complement involves the binding of the first component, C1, with a portion of the immunoglobulin molecule. This begins the cascade of complement activation, which is essential in promoting the inflammatory process. Figure 9-9 shows the major pathway of activation and the end results of the process. The system promotes inflammation by increasing vascular permeability, chemotaxis, phagocytosis, and finally causing lysis of the foreign cell [1]. The results of the cascade tend to cause some damage to normal tissue around the foreign tissue and, in some cases, this process can be damaging to the host. In most cases, an antigen-antibody reaction is required for the activation of complement. The complement factors then can participate in the process of inflammation with the end result of foreign material destruction.

Cell-Mediated Immunity (CMI)

Cell-mediated immunity, due to T lymphocyte activity, is mediated through T cell to antigen contact with subsequent destruction of the antigen. This destruction may occur through the release of soluble chemical compounds directly into the target cell membrane or through the secretion of lymphokines (Fig. 9-10). Direct contact with an antigen is frequently termed the ***killer activity***.

The killer activity is mediated through a group of cytotoxic T cells that function in the destruction of cells with identified surface antigens. The specific recognition is through the lock-and-key approach described earlier in this chapter. The killer T lymphocyte may directly destroy the antigen by binding to the cell and producing a break in its membrane. This results in a disruption of the intracellular osmotic environment and the death of the cell. The activated killer cell may also release cytotoxic substances directly into the target cell.

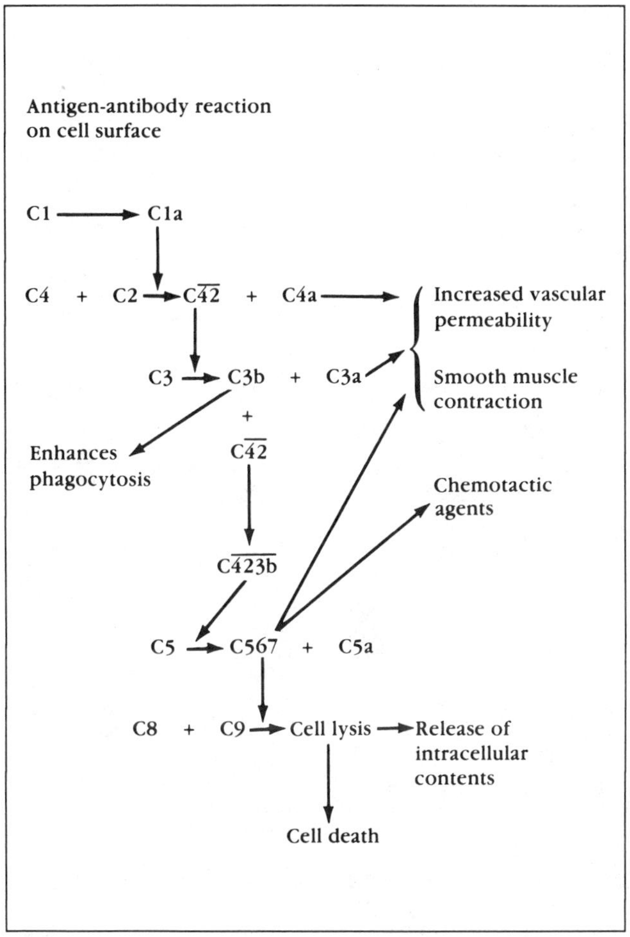

FIGURE 9-9. Classic pathway of complement activation.

The activated T lymphocytes release lymphokines, which affect other lymphocytes by enhancing or suppressing their activity. These cells also may create a chemotactic gradient that causes macrophages to accumulate in the area. The chemotactic gradient also serves to attract eosinophils, basophils, and neutrophils to the area.

Cell-mediated immunity, often termed *delayed hypersensitivity*, involves the direct intervention of T cells in a response without a corresponding humoral immunity. It results in the accumulation of mononuclear cells around the small blood vessels, resulting in destruction of vessels. This may lead to minor vascular lesions, for example, the wheal-and-flare response, or it may result in major destruction and massive necrosis. The antigen may initially react with a few specific T cells in the area, produce the chemotactic response and also macrophage inhibiting factor (MIF), which tends to keep macrophages in the area. The more antigen involved and the greater number of sensitized lymphocytes involved determine the results. The end result is cytolysis of the antigenic cell. This mechanism, which involves the T cells and associated macrophages, is responsible for transplant rejections and, in this process, is called *cell-mediated lymphocytolysis* (CML) [3].

T cells function in *immunosurveillance*, to detect cells in the host that have foreign antigens on their surface. This self-protective function prevents the transplant of tissue from one person to another unless the antigens on the surface of the cells in the tissue are similar enough for the host tissue to accept as "self."

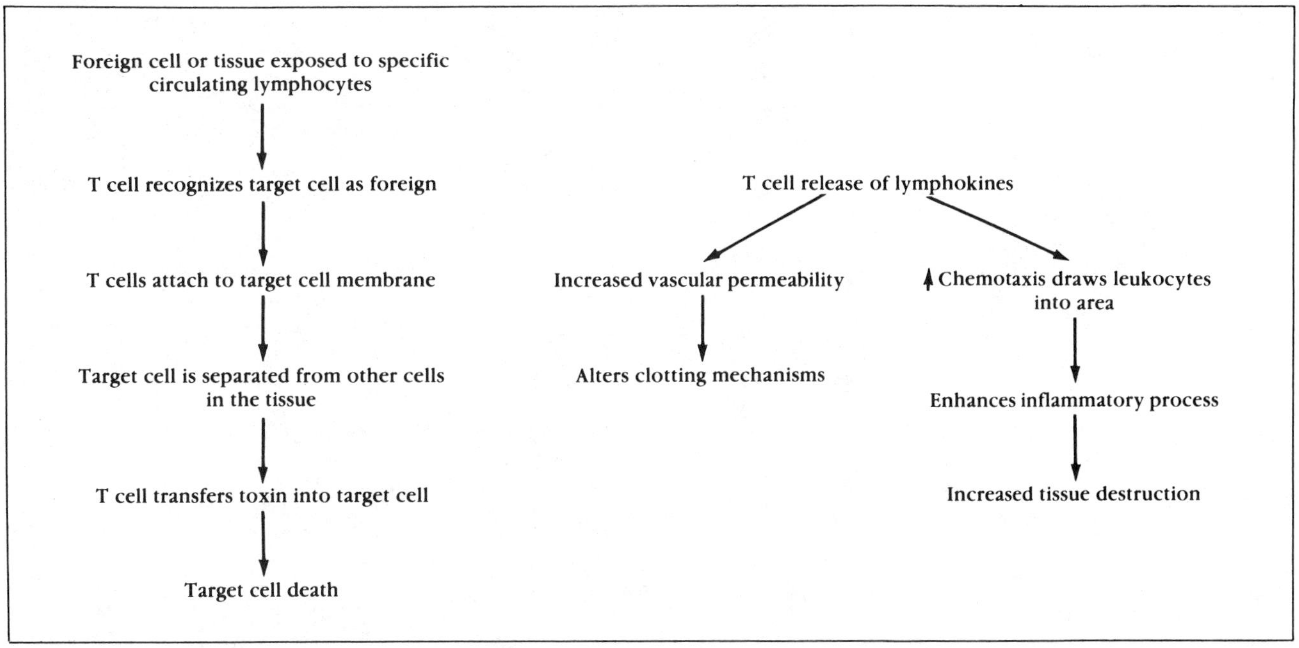

FIGURE 9-10. Cell-mediated response.

REFERENCES

1. Cooper, N. The Complement System. In H. H. Fudenberg, et al. (eds.), *Basic and Clinical Immunology* (3rd ed.). Los Altos, Calif.: Lange, 1980.
2. Fudenberg, H. H., et al. (eds.). *Basic and Clinical Immunology* (3rd ed.). Los Altos, Calif.: Lange, 1980.
3. Guttman, R. Transplantation Immunology. In B. A. Thomas (ed.), *Immunology: A Scope Monograph*. Kalamazoo, Mich.: Upjohn, 1975.
4. Ham, A. W., and Cormack, V. H. *Histology* (8th ed.). Philadelphia: Lippincott, 1979.
5. Jensen, D. *The Principles of Physiology* (2nd ed.). New York: Appleton-Century-Crofts, 1980.
6. Junquiera, L. C., and Carneiro, J. *Basic Histology* (3rd ed.). Los Altos, Calif.: Lange, 1980.
7. Robbins, S., and Cotran, R. *Pathologic Basis of Disease* (2nd ed.). Philadelphia: Saunders, 1979.
8. Roitt, I. *Essential Immunology* (3rd ed.). Oxford, England: Blackwell, 1977.

CHAPTER 10
IMMUNODEFICIENCY

LEARNING OBJECTIVES

1. Differentiate between primary and secondary immunodeficiency.
2. Differentiate between cell-mediated and humoral immunodeficiency.
3. Describe severe combined immunodeficiency (SCID).
4. Briefly identify the genetic basis for immunodeficiency.
5. Characterize the age of onset of signs and symptoms in the major described primary immunodeficiencies.
6. Explain the different symptoms that can occur according to the cell types affected.
7. Briefly describe complement abnormalities and how these affect the immune response.
8. List at least six disorders that can cause secondary immunodeficiency.
9. Describe why secondary immunodeficiency increases the risk for the host.
10. Specifically describe how stress alters the immune response.
11. Explain the effect of aging on T and B cell response.
12. List several immunosuppressive agents, giving a benefit and drawbacks for their use.
13. Describe how cancer can disrupt the immune mechanism.
14. List three causes of malnutrition and/or protein depletion and explain how these can disrupt the immune response.
15. Describe briefly the acquired immune deficiency syndrome (AIDS).

The development of an immunocompetent system is essential to protect the human organism from foreign invasion. Therefore, any deficiency in any of the components of the immune system can alter the activity of the entire defense system of the body. The effects of phagocytic dysfunction are described in Chapter 15. The major classifications of immunodeficiency are *primary and secondary immunologic deficiencies.* Primary immunologic deficiency is manifested as a developmental abnormality that results in failure of either humoral immunity, the cell-mediated response, or both of these. Complement abnormalities are briefly described as one of the categories of immune deficiency. Secondary immunologic deficiencies are acquired conditions that may be associated with disease states or produced through medical treatment.

TABLE 10-1. Classification of immunodeficiency disorders

Antibody (B cell) immunodeficiency diseases
- X-linked hypogammaglobulinemia (congenital hypogammaglobulinemia)
- Transient hypogammaglobulinemia of infancy
- Common, variable, unclassifiable immunodeficiency (acquired hypogammaglobulinemia)
- Immunodeficiency with hyper-IgM
- Selective IgA deficiency
- Selective IgM deficiency
- Selective deficiency of IgG subclasses

Cellular (T cell) immunodeficiency diseases
- Congenital thymic aplasia (Di George's syndrome)
- Chronic mucocutaneous candidiasis (with or without endocrinopathy)

Combined antibody-mediated (B cell) and cell-mediated (T cell) immunodeficiency diseases
- Severe combined immunodeficiency disease (autosomal recessive, X-linked, sporadic)
- Cellular immunodeficiency with abnormal immunoglobulin synthesis (Nezelof's syndrome)
- Immunodeficiency with ataxia-telangiectasia
- Immunodeficiency with eczema and thrombocytopenia (Wiskott-Aldrich syndrome)
- Immunodeficiency with thymoma
- Immunodeficiency with short-limbed dwarfism
- Immunodeficiency with enzyme deficiency
- Episodic lymphopenia with lymphotoxin
- GVH disease

Phagocytic dysfunction
- Chronic granulomatous disease
- Glucose 6-phosphate dehydrogenase deficiency
- Myeloperoxidase deficiency
- Chédiak-Higashi syndrome
- Job's syndrome
- Tuftsin deficiency
- "Lazy leukocyte syndrome"
- Elevated IgE, defective chemotaxis, eczema, and recurrent infections

Complement abnormalities and immunodeficiency diseases
- C1q, C1r, and C1s deficiency
- C2 deficiency
- C3 deficiency (type I, type II)
- C4 deficiency
- C5 dysfunction, C5 deficiency
- C6 deficiency
- C7 deficiency
- C8 deficiency

Source: H. H. Fudenberg, et al. (eds.), *Basic and Clinical Immunology* (3rd ed.). Los Altos, Calif.: Lange, 1980.

PRIMARY IMMUNE DEFICIENCY

A primary defect in the immunologic system results from the failure of development of an essential part of the immune system. The defect can occur at any point during the development of the immune system and may involve organ or cellular defects. Many different types of primary immunodeficiency states have been described according to the cell type affected and the developmental stage of the cellular system. Table 10-1 lists the terminology used for specific deficiencies. The more common disorders are described in the text.

Stem Cell Deficiency (Severe Combined Immunodeficiency Disease)

Severe combined immunodeficiency disease (SCID) is thought to arise from a deficiency of the stem cell population that forms the lymphocytes. It is manifested by T and B cell deficiency associated with a hypoplastic thymus. A tremendous decrease in lymphocyte numbers and lymphocyte immaturity provide for little, if any, immune response to antigen. It has been suggested that the defect is not stem cell failure, but occurs at the thymic level and at the level of B cell maturation [1]. There are several forms of this condition but the end result is a deficiency of both humoral and cell-mediated responses.

This disease causes a severely depressed ability to mount any type of immune response. The thymus is small and embryonic and the few lymphocytes present are not activated by antigen. Few plasma cells are found so that all classes of immunoglobulin are depressed resulting in the lack of production of specific antibodies.

An infant with this condition is affected from birth and is unable to cope with an environment laden with germs. The child is very vulnerable to all forms of infections and usually dies within the first year of life. The initial problem in early infancy is a failure to thrive, which is followed in the first few weeks of life by serious infections such as pneumonia and infectious diarrhea. Any type of infection may develop and none responds well to treatment. If SCID is suspected within hours of birth, the child may be placed in a germ-free environment with a later attempt to perform bone marrow and thymic transplantation [8]. These have met with relatively little success.

Deficiencies of Antibody Production

A variety of pathophysiologic defects in the immune system result in abnormal immunoglobulin synthesis or a deficiency of immunoglobulins. These can affect production of all of the immunoglobulins or of only specific classes.

X-LINKED HYPOGAMMAGLOBULINEMIA. A defect in the maturation of stem cells into B cells is found in X-linked hypogammaglobulinemia (*Bruton-type agammaglobulinemia*). This is a congenital disease that first appears in male infants at about the age of 5 to 6 months when the maternally transmitted level of antibodies has decreased. It may also be seen as an *idiopathic form* of primary immunodeficiency in adults.

Low levels of the major classes of immunoglobulins — IgM, IgG, and IgA — are found; antigens, both T cell–dependent and T cell–independent, are not cleared well from the body, causing infants with this condition to be extremely susceptible to bacterial infections, especially those caused by *Staphylococcus aureus, Streptococcus pyogenes, Hemophilus influenzae,* and the pneumococcus organisms. The result is a very high incidence of respiratory, sinus, and throat infections [8].

The cellular immune system remains competent. Allograft rejection, delayed hypersensitivity, and the ability to resist viral, fungal, and parasitic infections are apparently normal. Autoimmune diseases occur frequently, especially rheumatoid arthritis and systemic lupus erythematosus [8].

IgA DEFICIENCY. Selective IgA deficiency, which appears in apparently healthy persons who may have normal serum levels of the other immunoglobulins, is the most common immunodeficiency disorder. These persons lack IgA in the serum and the external secretions. The disease has a hereditary basis.

The presence of normal numbers of B cells with IgA expressed on their surface suggests a failure in the synthesis and release of IgA rather than an absence of IgA B lymphocytes [3]. This may be due to hyperactivity of IgA suppressor cells that prevent the differentiation of these B cells. A defect in the helper cells specific for IgA synthesis may also be present. Acquired IgA deficiency may occur in individuals treated with the drugs phenytoin and penicillamine.

The most common symptoms relate to those surfaces that are normally covered with mucosal secretions. Infections of the sinuses and respiratory tract are common. Related gastrointestinal problems include ulcerative colitis, pernicious anemia, and malsorption states. About 50 percent of persons with IgA deficiency also have some atopic disease. An increased incidence of autoimmune disease, such as systemic lupus erythematosus and rheumatoid arthritis, occurs and many persons with these diseases have anti-IgA antibodies. A high incidence of malignancies in the respiratory, gastrointestinal, and lymphoid system has been reported. The reason for this increased susceptibility to atopic disease, autoimmune disease, and malignancies is not known but a theory is that IgA normally interacts with many antigens on the mucosal surfaces of the body and prevents their entry into the body. A deficiency of IgA would allow the body to be exposed to more antigens than it can successfully combat. Because of the increased antigenic stimulation, more antigen can react with IgE and produce allergic manifestations. Increased risk of production of an antibody that will cross-react with a self-antigen increases the risk of autoimmune disease. Chronic irritation and inflammation due to the large amount of antigen could predispose the exposed tissue to malignant transformation [4].

Deficiency of Cell-Mediated Immunity (Di George's Syndrome)

Selective immunodeficiency affecting the T cell without B cells is rare. It is most frequently caused by congenital thymic hypoplasia and causes the neonate to be extremely susceptible to fungal and viral infections. If this disease is untreated, death due to overwhelming infection occurs in infancy.

The immune defect is due to the developmental failure of the thymus and parathyroid glands. The lack of the thymus gland and thus the lack of the thymic hormone result in the failure of T cell maturation.

Individuals with this problem do not exhibit any cell-mediated effects. They have an inability to reject allografts or to react to skin test antigens. There is little or no resistance to intracellular infections by viruses, fungi, and some gram-negative bacteria. A decrease of T cell helper function may depress the humoral response. The corresponding failure of parathyroid development may lead to tetany due to hypocalcemia.

The complete Di George's syndrome consists of: (1) low-set ears, slanted eyes, (2) hypoparathyroidism, (3) congenital heart defects, such as septal defects and truncus arteriosus, and (4) cellular immunodeficiency [3]. This defect has been successfully treated by transplant of the thymus gland.

Complement Abnormalities

Complement factors are necessary to promote the inflammatory process. Complement deficiency has been shown in an increased number of individuals with autoimmune disease. Various symptoms occur depending on the complement factor that is deficient. Deficiency of complement inhibitors also can result in allergic reactions; the most frequently occurring type is *hereditary angioedema* caused by a genetic deficiency of C_1 esterase inhibitor, which produces uncontrolled activation of the complement system causing angioedema in the skin, larynx, gastrointestinal, and genitourinary tracts [3].

Deficiencies of complement factors have been noted in fractions of C_1, and C_2–C_7. Most of the deficiencies result in an increased susceptibility to bacterial infections and many persons exhibit autoimmune disorders, especially lupuslike conditions (see Chap. 11).

SECONDARY IMMUNE DEFICIENCY

Secondary immune deficiency states result from the loss of a previously effective immune system. This classification includes any disorder that exhibits loss of immunocompe-

TABLE 10-2. Conditions causing secondary immunosuppression

Immunosuppressive therapy	
	Antimetabolites
	Corticosteroids
	Antibiotics
Radiation therapy	
Cancer	
	Malnutrition
	B cell lymphoproliferative disorders
	T cell deficiency
Stress	
Aging	
Systemic infections	
Renal disease	
Malnutrition	
	Cirrhosis
	Tumor cachexia
	Dietary deficiency
Burns	
Trauma	
Surgery	

tence as a result of another condition. A broad classification includes immune deficiency secondary to any of the following: stress, malnutrition, systemic infection, cancer, renal diseases, radiation therapy, immunosuppressive drugs, and aging (Table 10-2). These conditions may lead to a loss of immunoglobulins, inadequate synthesis of immunoglobulins, loss of specific lymphocytes responsible for cell-mediated immunity, loss of phagocytic inflammatory cells, or a combination of these.

Even though a decreased effectiveness of the immune system is frequently not life-threatening, it often results in a decreased ability of the organism to mount an inflammatory or immune response. Therefore, an increased susceptibility to infection by bacteria, viruses, fungi, or all three results. In some cases the loss of immunocompetence causes enough alteration in host resistance to increase morbidity and mortality.

Stress response has been the target of a great deal of research in relation to how it disrupts the physiologic functioning of the body (see Chap. 3). Stress appears to alter the immune response by neural interruption from the hypothalamus, which ultimately decreases the functioning of the thymus gland. Stress also increases the secretion of the glucocorticoids, the majority of which suppress the inflammatory response by suppression of macrophages, decreasing the number of white blood cells and causing regression of lymphatic tissue. This, then, can permit the spread of infection [5].

Aging results in immunologic deterioration, which relates to an increased rate of malignancy, increased incidence of autoimmune disease, antibody deficiency, impaired hypersensitivity response, and decreased lymphocyte regeneration [2]. Thymic involution occurs in senescence along with a decreased T and B cell–mediated immune response, resulting in an increased susceptibility to infection and increased incidence in the abnormal cell types of malignancy [7].

Immunosuppression refers to the pharmacologic suppression of the immune system. Drugs have been extensively used to decrease the rejection phenomenon in transplanted tissue, to decrease the rate of growth of malignant tumors, and to decrease the inflammation involved with autoimmune disorders. Drugs used to achieve this effect are cytotoxic drugs, such as methotrexate, and corticosteroids, such as hydrocortisone. The cytotoxic drugs are toxic to cells that are rapidly dividing. These include the T and B lymphocytes as well as the polymorphonuclear leukocytes. The corticosteroids function to suppress the inflammatory response. The result of immunosuppression is an increased sensitivity to the environmental antigens. Superimposed infections may develop and spread readily. Many pharmacologic agents cause a depression of the bone marrow formation of leukocytes and thus affect all types of white blood cells.

Systemic infections can place such a load on the defense system so that further antigenic stimulation may result in a decreased resistance. Thus, host resistance is decreased and opportunistic organisms may cause serious problems.

Cancer may cause malnutrition, due mostly to protein wasting. A decreased synthesis of lymphocytes results. Immune deficiency due to B lymphoproliferative disorders such as chronic lymphocytic leukemia (CLL) and multiple myeloma results in impairment of the antibody responses, causing secondary infections with pyogenic bacteria. Hodgkin's disease differs in that affected persons display the typical signs of T cell deficiency and this is often manifested by an increased susceptibility to tuberculosis [1].

Radiation therapy, usually instituted against malignancy, affects rapidly proliferating cells and results in a decrease in all of the cells of the inflammatory response, including the T and B lymphocytes. Opportunistic infections, especially gram-negative bacteria, viruses, and fungi occur with increased frequency [4].

Renal disease probably causes most of its immunosuppressive effects from proteinuria leading to hypoproteinemia or acid-base disruptions that can affect the formation of lymphocytes, especially T cells [1]. Many pathologic processes of the kidney are treated with corticosteroids and immunosuppression may be a result of drug therapy.

Acquired Immune Deficiency Syndrome (AIDS)

This life-threatening disease process was first described in 1978 and the reported incidence is increasing each month. By February, 1983, 1261 documented cases had been reported to the Centers for Disease Control in Atlanta [6]. Of the cases reported 75 percent have been homosexual males. Others affected include Haitian immigrants, drug abusers, and hemophiliacs. The mortality is alarming with most deaths resulting from a rare pneumonia caused by *Pneumocystis carinii* or from Kaposi's sarcoma, also a very rare cause of death. Other causes of death can be classified as opportunistic infections (OIs) from various viruses, bacteria, fungi, and protozoa. To all of these OIs the individuals have had very little ability to mount an inflammatory cell response [6].

The actual cause of the immune deficiency is unknown but it is probably transmitted by blood contamination. In most cases a history of blood or sexual contact can be elicited. The current line of research is in search of a virus or viruslike agent that could be a mutant strain introduced to a population that has no natural immunity. Demonstration of T helper cell suppression supports the inability to mount an acute inflammatory reaction. AIDS victims also demonstrate an increase or maintenance of T cell suppressors, which can further depress the defensive response.

Mortality statistics vary due to reporting procedures but a delayed mortality reported in 1980 was 90 percent [6]. With no known cure and the condition spreading rapidly, AIDS may produce a future epidemic. Further research is necessary to elucidate the cause and cure for this baffling syndrome.

REFERENCES

1. Anderson, W. A. D., and Scotti, T. *Synopsis of Pathology* (10th ed.). St. Louis: Mosby, 1980.
2. Blake, P. J., and Perez, R. C. *Applied Immunological Concepts.* New York: Appleton-Century-Crofts, 1978.
3. Fudenberg, H. H., et al. (eds.). *Basic and Clinical Immunology* (3rd ed.). Los Altos, Calif.: Lange, 1980.
4. Lawton, A., and Cooper, M. Immune Deficiency Disease. In K. J. Isselbacher, et al. (eds.), *Harrison's Principles of Internal Medicine* (9th ed.). New York: McGraw-Hill, 1980.
5. Luckmann, J., and Sorensen, K. *Medical-Surgical Nursing* (2nd ed.). Philadelphia: Saunders, 1980.
6. Much, K. AIDS: A new scourge. *The Journal* 22:4, 1983.
7. Ramsey, J. M. *Basic Pathophysiology.* Reading, Mass.: Addison-Wesley, 1982.
8. Robbins, S., and Cotran, R. *Pathologic Basis of Disease* (2nd ed.). Philadelphia: Saunders, 1979.

CHAPTER 11
HYPERSENSITIVITY AND AUTOIMMUNE REACTIONS

CLASSIFICATIONS OF TISSUE INJURY DUE TO HYPERSENSITIVITY
- **Type I: Anaphylaxis or Atopy**
  - ***Anaphylactic Shock***
  - ***Bronchial Asthma***
  - ***Atopic Eczema***
- **Type II: Cytotoxic Hypersensitivity**
  - ***Hemolytic Reactions***
  - ***Specific Target Cell Destruction***
- **Type III: Immune Complex Disease**
  - ***Serum Sickness***
  - ***Arthus' Reaction***
  - ***Other Type III Conditions***
- **Type IV: Cell-Mediated Hypersensitivity**
  - ***Delayed Hypersensitivity***
  - ***Cytotoxic Cell-Mediated Responses***
  - ***Contact Dermatitis***
- **Transplant or Graft Rejection**

CLASSIFICATION OF IMMUNE DISORDERS BY SOURCE OF ANTIGEN

AUTOIMMUNITY
- **Systemic Lupus Erythematosus (SLE)**
- **Rheumatoid Arthritis**

LEARNING OBJECTIVES

1. Define *hypersensitivity reactions.*
2. Discuss the types of agents that can elicit hypersensitivity reactions.
3. Describe the types of hypersensitivity reactions according to underlying pathophysiologic mechanisms and how they are manifested as disease conditions.
4. Differentiate between anaphylaxis and atopy.
5. Identify the mechanisms of red cell destruction seen with cytotoxic hypersensitivity reactions.
6. Describe the results of hemolysis as seen with transfusion reactions, erythroblastosis fetalis, and warm and cold antibody disease.
7. Describe Goodpasture's disease as a result of cytotoxic hypersensitivity.
8. Explain the underlying pathophysiology of immune complex disease.
9. Describe the mechanisms occurring in serum sickness.
10. Identify the pathophysiologic mechanism of Arthus' reaction.
11. Indicate an understanding of the relationship of the hypersensitivity reactions with the autoimmune disorders.
12. Describe the pathophysiologic mechanisms by which delayed hypersensitivity can result.
13. Identify the histologic pattern of contact dermatitis.
14. Describe transplant graft rejection, using the transplanted kidney as an example.
15. Describe the classification of immune disruptions according to homologous, exogenous, or autologous source of antigen.
16. List at least six conditions that are probably the result of autoimmunity.
17. Name the main clinical finding that supports diagnosis of the autoimmune phenomena.
18. Describe systemic lupus erythematosus (SLE) in terms of pathology and resultant clinical effects.
19. Specifically, list 10 of the 14 criteria issued by the American Rheumatism Association for the diagnosis of SLE.
20. Describe the basis for classifying rheumatoid arthritis as an autoimmune disease.
21. Explain the pathophysiologic results of rheumatoid arthritis on the joints and the other systems of the body.
22. Describe the signs and symptoms of rheumatoid arthritis.

Immune disorders have been classified in various ways to clarify the pathophysiologic basis of the problem encountered. Four mechanisms of immunologically mediated disorders have been described according to the manner in which tissue injury occurs [4,7]. Immune disorders also may be classified according to the source of the offending antigen. Both classifications are discussed in this chapter.

The classic term for immunologic, tissue-damaging reactions is *hypersensitivity reactions*, which refers to an exaggerated response of the immune system to an antigen. The antigen eliciting the response is frequently called an *allergen*. This allergen may produce differing responses depending on the individual genetic predisposition for an exaggerated response.

CLASSIFICATIONS OF TISSUE INJURY DUE TO HYPERSENSITIVITY

The types of hypersensitivity reactions are described in this section according to the underlying pathophysiologic mechanisms and how these manifest themselves in different disease conditions (Table 11-1).

Type I: Anaphylaxis or Atopy

Anaphylaxis refers to an acute reaction usually associated with a wheal-and-flare type of skin reaction and vasodilation that may precipitate circulatory shock. Atopy, which results from the same mechanism, chronically recurs in responses that depend on the antigen, the frequency of contact, the route of contact, and the sensitivity of the organ system to the antigen.

Atopy or anaphylactic diseases are the most common of the immediate hypersensitivity reactions. These diseases, commonly called *allergies*, occur in organs exposed to environmental antigens. The skin, the respiratory tract, and the gastrointestinal system are especially affected. Many different types of antigens or allergens can initiate the hypersensitivity state in susceptible individuals. The most common of these are the environmental allergens such as pollens, dander, foods, insect bites, and certain household cleaning agents. Drug sensitivity reactions can effect the same response. Other disease states that are classified in this group include hay fever, urticaria (hives), asthma, and atopic eczema. Susceptibility to allergy is inherited and may result from excessive IgE production.

Pathophysiologically, the immune response is activated when antigen binds to IgE antibodies attached to the surface of mast cells. Mast cells are found in profusion in connective tissue, the skin, and the mucous membranes. The reaction proceeds when the IgE molecule specific for a particular antigen becomes cross-linked on the surface of the cell and triggers the release of intracellular granules. These granules contain large quantities of histamine, slow-reacting substance of anaphylaxis (SRS-A), and other chemotactic substances. Histamine causes peripheral vasodilation and an increase in vascular permeability resulting in local vascular congestion and edema. It also causes constriction of smooth muscle in the bronchioles that accounts for the associated bronchiolar constriction often associated with the allergic reaction. SRS-A causes a slower vasodilation process and smooth muscle contraction to which the small bronchi are especially sensitive (Fig. 11-1).

ANAPHYLACTIC SHOCK. Anaphylactic shock is a systemic reaction to an antigen that occurs when the subject has been previously sensitized to the same antigen. The antigen-antibody reaction occurs on the mast cells in the connective tissue and around small blood vessels. This causes the mast cells to release histamine, SRS-A, bradykinin, and other mediators. The result is contraction of smooth

TABLE 11-1. Classification of hypersensitivity states

Type	Cause	Responsible cell or antibody	Immune mechanism	Examples of disease states
Type I Anaphylaxis Atopy	Foreign protein (antigen)	IgE	IgE attaches to surface of mast cell and specific antigen, triggers release of intracellular granules from mast cells	Hay fever Allergies Hives Anaphylactic shock
Type II Cytotoxic	Foreign protein (antigen)	IgG or IgM	Antibody reacts with antigen, activates complement, causes cytolysis	Transfusion Hemolytic drug reactions Erythroblastosis fetalis Hemolytic anemia Vascular purpura
Type III Immune complex	Foreign protein (antigen)	IgG or IgE	Ag-Ab complexes precipitate in tissue, activate complement, cause inflammatory reaction	Rheumatoid arthritis Systemic lupus erythematosus Serum sickness
Type IV Delayed cell-mediated	Foreign protein, cell,or tissue	T lymphocytes	Sensitized T cell reacts with specific antigen to induce inflammatory process by direct cell action or by activity of lymphokines	Contact dermatitis Transplant graft reaction

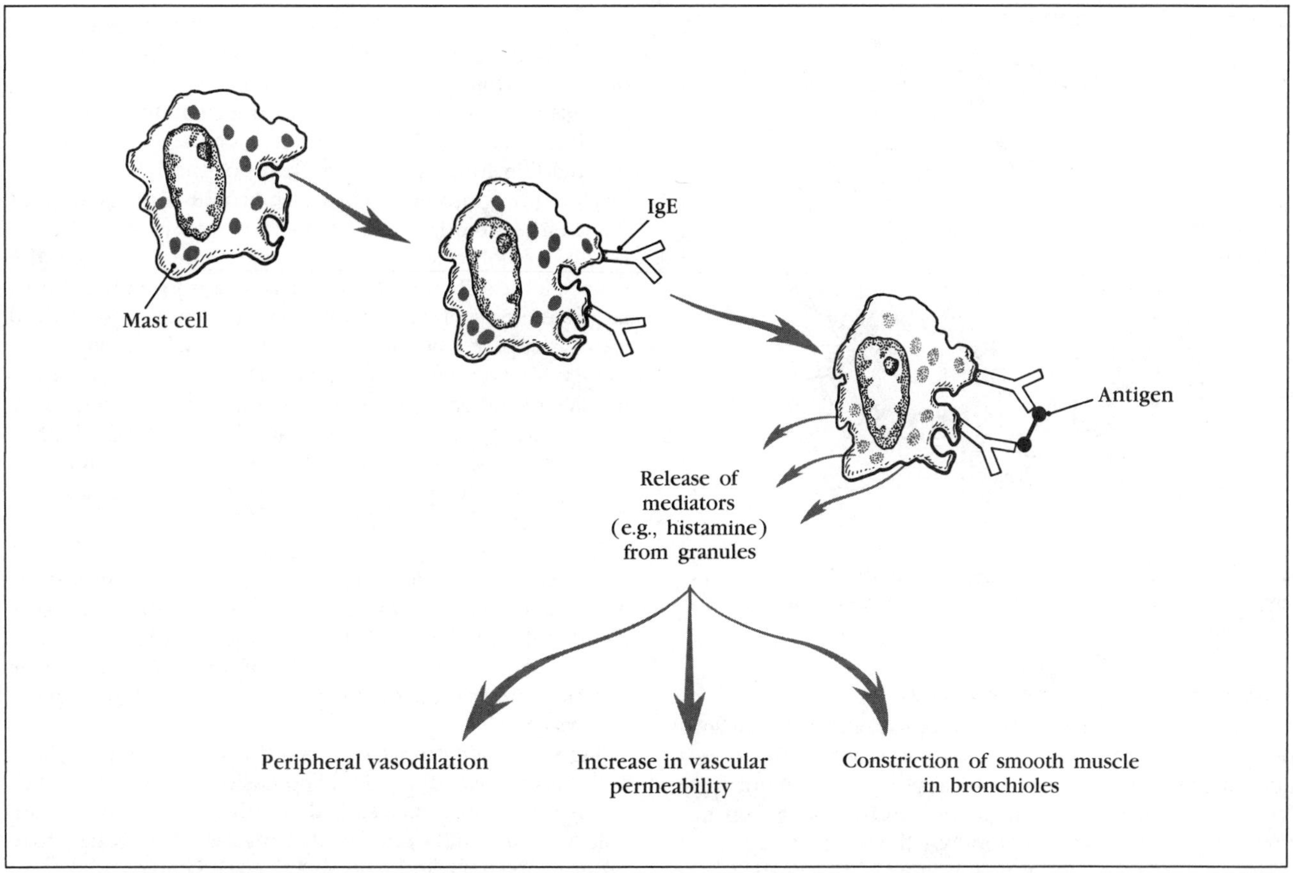

FIGURE 11-1. Type I hypersensitivity reaction. The mast cell and IgE antibody are attached by a specific antigen that causes the release of the vasoactive substances, histamine and SRS-A.

muscle and increased vascular permeability, which causes bronchospasm and the loss of intravascular fluid into the tissue spaces. Edema follows and is particularly noticeable around the eyes. This edema, called *angioneurotic edema*, may appear in the skin or mucous membranes. Laryngeal edema associated with the bronchospasm often causes acute dyspnea and air hunger.

Hives, or urticaria, may appear on any skin surface. These appear as cutaneous localized swellings.

Fluid shift from the increased vascular permeability may be significant enough to result in decreased blood pressure and shock. Signs and symptoms of anaphylaxis include urticaria, angioedema, dyspnea, hypoxia, and hypotension. Some individuals experience vascular collapse without signs of respiratory distress. Other signs that are associated with anaphylaxis include leukopenia, decreased body temperature, and bradycardia.

BRONCHIAL ASTHMA. Atopic allergy may cause bronchial asthma, frequently induced by the inhalation of environmental antigens (see Chap. 24). The mechanism for bronchial asthma, like atopy, may result from interaction of antigen with specific IgE antibodies. The inflammation produces mucosal edema, increased secretion of mucus, and bronchospasm, all of which cause narrowing of the airways and increased airway resistance. The early signs and symptoms of asthma are dyspnea and wheezing. Repeated attacks result in hypertrophy of the smooth muscle, which can exaggerate bronchoconstriction and increase the severity of each subsequent attack. Bacterial or viral infections may precipitate asthmatic attacks.

ATOPIC ECZEMA. This acute or chronic, noncontagious, inflammatory condition may occur following contact with irritants to which a person has a specific sensitivity [5]. In some cases it results from a cell-mediated reaction (see Chap. 9) and in others it is mediated by IgE with the resultant liberation of chemotactic mediators into the dermal areas.

Atopic eczema causes urticaria, or hives, and angioedema. Urticaria involves the superficial capillaries while angioedema involves the capillaries of the deeper skin layers. The wheals of urticaria have well-defined margins, erythema, and vesicles filled with clear fluid. Pruritis is frequently severe. The angioedema causes nonpitting swelling of localized areas of the skin [9]. This skin reaction to an allergen is frequently associated with respiratory hypersensitivity, especially hay fever or other types of allergy. Drug reactions may result in the same dermatologic manifestations, probably due to the same mechanisms.

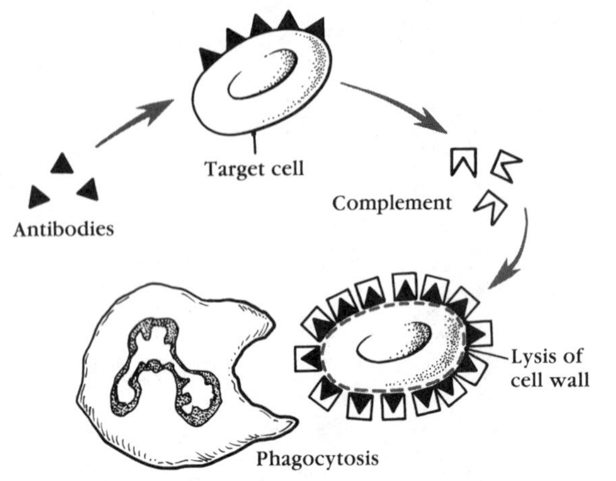

FIGURE 11-2. Type II hypersensitivity response. The target cell is covered with antibody that activates complement and sets the stage for phagocytosis.

Type II: Cytotoxic Hypersensitivity

In this type of hypersensitivity response, a circulating antibody, usually of the IgG classification, reacts with an antigen on the surface of a cell. Because individuals normally have antibodies to antigen of the ABO blood group not present on their own membranes, the antigen may be a normal component of the membrane [7]. It may also be a foreign antigen, such as a pharmacologic agent, which adheres to the surface of the host's own cells. Antibodies to one's own RBCs may produce an autoimmune hemolytic anemia. The cell is destroyed by the reaction on its surface either by phagocytosis or cell lysis. The effect on the host depends on the number and type of cells destroyed.

Some examples of this type of hypersensitivity response include autoimmune hemolytic anemia, erythroblastosis fetalis, and Goodpasture's disease. These are briefly discussed in this section following a review of some of the general pathophysiologic features.

The pathophysiology of this type of hypersensitivity usually involves the activation of complement and resultant destruction of red blood cells or specific target cells. Coating of target cells with IgG antibody sets the stage for phagocytosis by the mononuclear phagocyte system. Another mechanism involves specific IgG or IgM activation of complement with cytolysis resulting from complement activation through C$\overline{89}$ (Fig. 11-2) (see Chap. 8). Red cell destruction may be triggered by IgG opsonization and the attachment of lymphocytes or macrophages to the cell surface [6].

HEMOLYTIC REACTIONS. Examples of reactions that destroy red blood cells are transfusion reactions, erythroblastosis fetalis, autoimmune hemolytic anemia, and drug-induced hemolysis. The reaction of host antibody with the surface antigens on the red blood cells of an incompatible donor results in hemolysis. Of these, the surface antigens that make up the ABO and Rh systems are common sources of incompatibility.

Transfusion reactions result in the hemolysis of donor red blood cells with the liberation of large quantities of hemoglobin into the plasma. Some of the hemoglobin is broken down into unconjugated bilirubin. If the amount of free hemoglobin is greater than 100 mg/dl plasma, the excess hemoglobin will diffuse into the tissue or through the renal glomeruli into the renal tubules. Precipitation of large amounts of hemoglobin in the renal tubular fluid forms sharp needles in the acid urine, which can cause tubular damage and obstruction. The precipitation in the tubules of the shell of the red blood cells also frequently contributes to tubular damage and renal failure. Transfusion reactions may increase the risk of renal failure, by causing circulatory shock, renal vasoconstriction, and a decrease in renal blood flow.

The antigenic nature of mismatched blood transfusions depends on the blood type and Rh factor of the donor blood. For example, patients with type A blood possess anti-B antibodies. Therefore, the incompatible blood is coated with antibodies, usually of the IgM class. This causes agglutination of the donor cells and lysis rapidly follows [2].

Signs and symptoms of a transfusion reaction include chills, fever, low back pain, hypotension, tachycardia, anxiety, hyperkalemia, nausea and vomiting, red or port-wine colored urine, and occasionally urticaria. This process may progress to shock and irreversible renal failure.

Erythroblastosis fetalis may result if a mother without Rh antigens carries a child with Rh antigens or through ABO blood incompatibility. A mother who *lacks Rh antigens* on her red blood cells (Rh-negative) can become sensitized to the Rh antigen carried on the cells of the fetus, by mixing of maternal red blood cells with fetal red blood cells. When the mother again becomes pregnant with a fetus having Rh antigens, the maternal anti-Rh antibodies may cross the placenta and enter the fetal circulation. The result is the destruction of fetal red blood cells through a hemolytic reaction. More commonly, *ABO blood group incompatibility* causes the free passages of antibodies from the mother through the placenta to the fetus [6]. Blood types interact in different ways, but the end result is attachment and hemolysis of the fetal RBC by the maternal antibodies.

The hemolysis of fetal red blood cells results in severe *anemia*, which may lead ultimately to heart failure. Also, the release of high concentrations of bilirubin from the hemoglobin may result in brain damage, called *kernicterus*, as unconjugated bilirubin passes across the still permeable blood-brain barrier causing edematous swelling of brain parenchyma. *Hyperbilirubinemia* is common in the infant who survives more than several days and is usually manifested as jaundice, termed *icterus gravis*. The red cell activity in the bone marrow increases and extramedullary hematopoiesis begins to occur in the liver, spleen, and perhaps in other organs to compensate for lost red blood cells.

The risk of erythroblastosis fetalis in subsequent pregnancies can be reduced by the administration of anti-Rh antibodies to the mother within 72 hours after the birth of the first Rh-positive infant. ABO erythroblastosis is more difficult to predict but can be monitored when there is an awareness of blood incompatibility between parents.

Two types of hemolytic anemias with a probable autoimmune basis are classified as *warm antibody disease* and *cold antibody disease.* Warm antibody disease is called *autoimmune hemolytic anemia* and is usually due to IgG antibody, which attacks the host's own red blood cells. The disease can be life-threatening depending on the amount of hemolysis that occurs. The red blood cell develops a very limited life span and the resulting anemia can be severe. Development of autoimmune hemolytic disease may occur for no known reason or it may be associated with other autoimmune diseases, with malignancy, or with systemic infection. Cold antibody disease results when an autoantibody, usually IgM, binds to erythrocytes at temperatures below 31°C. This temperature may be reached in the fingers or toes during very cold weather. The red blood cells thusly coated with these cold antibodies reenter the general circulation, activate complement and hemolyze the red blood cells. These hemolytic attacks occur only after exposures to cold and tend to be self-limiting.

Drug-induced hemolysis may result from drug-antibody complexes that bind passively to red blood cells and initiate the complement reaction, or other drugs may act as haptens and bind to a red blood cell carrier. Antibody is formed and induces hemolysis of the red blood cell. Some drugs produce changes in the surface antigens of the red blood cells, resulting in antibody production against the host's own erythrocytes. Most drug-induced hemolytic reactions stop once the use of the drug is discontinued.

SPECIFIC TARGET CELL DESTRUCTION. The best illustration of this type of hypersensitivity reaction is *Goodpasture's disease*, which is a rapidly occurring condition characterized by the development of *antiglomerular basement membrane antibodies (anti-GBM).* These antibodies are directed at the glomerular basement membrane of the kidney as well as the basement membrane of the alveoli of the lungs. The initiator of the condition is unknown but it may progress rapidly to death due to the destruction of the basement membranes. Death is frequently due to hemoptysis or uremia. Bilateral nephrectomy has been shown in a few cases to arrest the pulmonary course of the disease [6].

Type III: Immune Complex Disease

Immune complex disease results in the formation of immune complexes as a result of antigens, antibodies, and complement activation. This results in the precipitation of complexes in vulnerable areas leading to inflammation as a consequence of the complement activation. The end result is an intravascular, synovial, endocardial, and other membrane inflammatory process affecting the vulnerable organs for a particular person.

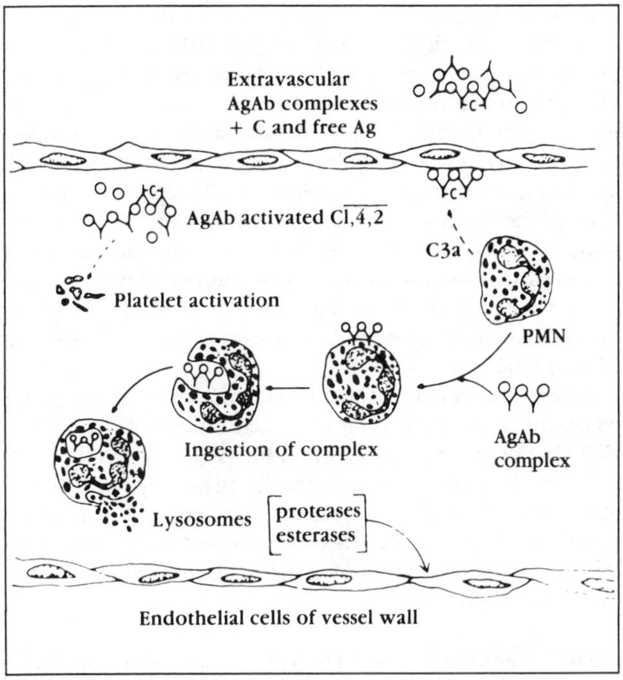

FIGURE 11-3. Type III hypersensitivity reaction showing the precipitation of antigen-antibody complexes in target tissues resulting in membrane destruction. (From Y. Hokoma and R. Nakomura, *Immunology and Immunopathology.* Boston: Little, Brown, 1982.)

Antigen-antibody complexes may be present in the plasma but may not be manifested as disease. If the complexes are not removed by the mononuclear phagocyte system, they may lodge in the tissue where they initiate an inflammatory reaction leading to tissue destruction. Frequently, the complexes are small and the size of the complexes seems to determine whether they will be cleared and whether they can lodge at a place where significant damage can occur. The antigen-antibody complexes that remain in solution cause reactions when they circulate through the body and lodge in the tissue and small vessels. Increased vascular permeability allows the complexes to be deposited in the extravascular spaces. Deposition of complexes also appears to be greater at points of high pressure, high flow, and turbulence. Once precipitated, the immune complexes initiate the inflammatory process through the activation of complement and through the release of vasoactive substances from the defensive cells (Fig. 11-3).

SERUM SICKNESS. Serum sickness results from injection of large doses of foreign material and can cause various types of arthritis, glomerulonephritis, and vasculitis. First reported after passive immunization with horse serum (equine tetanus antitoxin), which contains at least 30 different antigens, serum sickness can present as an acute reaction or as a chronic condition. Antigen-antibody complexes form in the bloodstream and precipitate into vulnerable areas.

If the antigen concentration is greater than the antibody concentrations, the resulting antigen-antibody complexes tend to be small and remain in solution for as long as 8 to 15 days after initial injection. Immune complexes are deposited throughout the vasculature of the body; complement is activated, and neutrophils and macrophages move into the area in response to chemotactic signals. Phagocytosis of the immune complexes begins with the release of lysosomal enzymes into the area that causes acute vasculitis with destruction of the elastic lamina of the arteries. Once phagocytosis of the immune complexes is complete the inflammatory process decreases leaving some scarring of the blood vessel walls [6].

Renal glomerular deposits of complexes occur even when the immune complex concentrations are not high, probably because of the efficient filtering action of the kidney. The complexes form characteristic deposits in the glomerular walls that activate complement and lead to destruction of glomerular tissue. Increased permeability of the glomerular basement membrane often produces hematuria and proteinuria.

ARTHUS' REACTION. Another type III disorder has been called *Arthus' reaction* and involves inflammation and cellular death at the site of injection of antigen into a previously sensitized person. Pathologically, it causes an acute, localized vasculitis that occurs from antibody precipitation and complement activation. It then involves all of the effects of inflammation with activation of the complement fragments through $C\overline{89}$, which destroy antigen and surrounding tissue. The vasculitis causes platelets to adhere to vessels, and thrombosis at the site of vessels. Hypersensitive pneumonitis probably is an Arthus' reaction from the inhalation of organic dusts [3]. This reaction is closely involved with the anaphylactic type I response except that IgG immunoglobulin seems to be necessary for Arthus' reaction and IgE is involved with the type I reaction. It has been postulated that some relationship exists between the two reactions [6].

OTHER TYPE III CONDITIONS. Many of the common autoimmune conditions are classified as immune complex disorders. The mechanism for inflammation and damage is the precipitation of immune complexes into vulnerable areas. Systemic lupus erythematosus, rheumatoid arthritis, and some types of glomerulonephritis are examples of these conditions. Systemic lupus erythematosus and rheumatoid arthritis are discussed more fully on pages 133–135. Glomerulonephritis is described in detail in Chapter 27.

Type IV: Cell-Mediated Hypersensitivity

This type of response is the result of specifically sensitized T lymphocytes. Two types of cell-mediated responses have been described: the delayed hypersensitivity and cell-mediated responses.

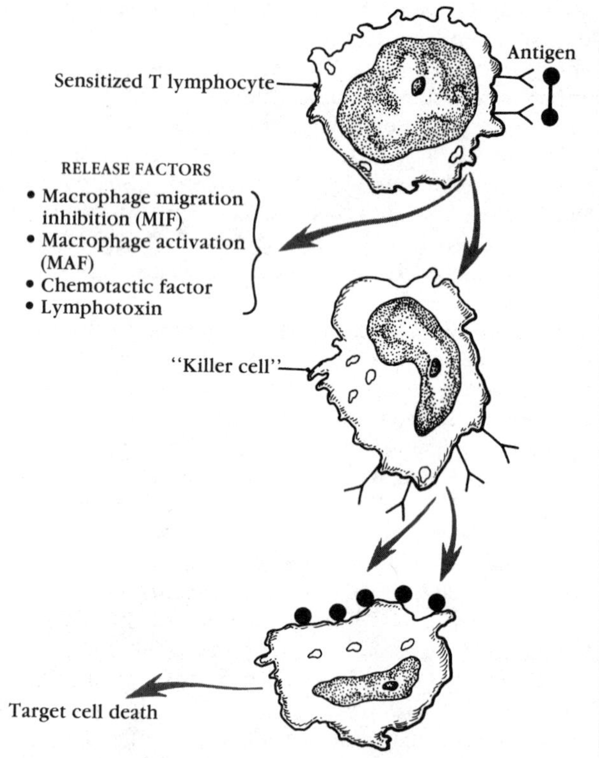

FIGURE 11-4. Type IV cell-mediated hypersensitivity. The T lymphocyte contacts the foreign material and through direct intervention or the secretion of substances toxic to the foreign material causes destruction of the foreign protein.

DELAYED HYPERSENSITIVITY. Delayed hypersensitivity responses are due to the specific interaction of T cells with antigen. The T cells react with the antigen and release lymphokines that draw macrophages into the area. The lymphokines include the macrophage migration inhibitory factor (MIF), the macrophage activating factor (MAF), chemotactic factors, lymphotoxin, transfer factor, and other factors. These substances function to enhance the inflammatory response that destroys the foreign material (Fig. 11-4). The tuberculin response is the best example of the delayed hypersensitivity response and is used to determine whether an individual has been sensitized to the disease. Reddening and induration of the site begins within 12 hours of injection of tuberculin and reaches a peak in 24 to 72 hours. This response can only by elicited when there are lymphocytes present [6].

CYTOTOXIC CELL-MEDIATED RESPONSES. Cytotoxic cell-mediated responses occur as a result of T cell contact and destruction of antigen. The surrounding cells are not damaged. The T cell may also activate macrophages and these cells may lyse tumor cells and cause destruction of tumors.

CONTACT DERMATITIS. This common allergic skin reaction seems to be a T cell response with a delayed reaction. This type of condition is seen when there is contact with certain common household chemicals, cosmetics, and plant toxins. These alter the normal skin protein so that it becomes antigenic or they may act as haptens that combine with proteins in the skin. The area of contact becomes red and indurated and vesicles begin to appear. Lymphocytes and macrophages infiltrate the area and react against the epidermal cells. Sterile, protein-rich fluid fills the blebs. If the blebs are opened, the antigen may be spread to a new area. The affected cells are destroyed, slough off, and are replaced by regenerating new cells.

Transplant or Graft Rejection

Rejection of tissue and organ transplants involves several of the hypersensitivity responses. Targeting of transplanted organs depends on whether the ***histocompatibility antigens*** are similar enough between the donor and the recipient to prevent activation of the rejection phenomenon. These surface antigens on cells distinguish them from other individuals and from other organs. These are the self-proteins to which an individual develops tolerance. Identical twins have identical histocompatibility antigens so that organs or tissue can be transplanted with ease.

Rejection is a complex reaction that involves both cell and humoral responses. Cytolytic T lymphocytes may either attack grafted tissue directly or secrete chemotactic lymphokines that enhance the activity of macrophages in tissue destruction. Humoral responses may be due to preformed circulating antibodies that were formed during previous exposure to the antigen. After transplantation, the lymphocytes become sensitized as they pass through the donor site. When antibody is involved, it appears to target the vasculature of the graft, especially the graft site [6].

The rejection phenomenon of a transplanted kidney has been studied extensively. It appears to involve both humoral and cell-mediated hypersensitivity. The sensitized lymphocytes interact with the graft proteins and release mediators that attract macrophages and PMN leukocytes to the area. The lysosomal enzymes released by these cells cause endothelial destruction, especially of the blood vessels, which leads to a decreased glomerular filtration rate and renal failure.

The T lymphocytes also are directly cytotoxic to the donor cells. They also may activate B lymphocytes to form antibodies and immune complexes that activate complement and further damage the vascular endothelium.

The process may be acute or chronic. The more adequately matched the donor and recipient, the less acute the reaction. Also, transplant patients are given immunosuppressive drugs that delay the rejection phenomenon. The chronic changes usually are vascular in nature and lead to renal ischemia and eventual failure.

Graft rejection is very common and most cadaver grafts are rejected within 5 years. Long-term survival of grafts has not been achieved except in twin or relative donors.

CLASSIFICATION OF IMMUNE DISORDERS BY SOURCE OF ANTIGEN

Immunologically mediated disorders may also be classified according to the underlying causes—exogenous, homologous, and autologous. Some antigens are basically environmental, some result from antigenic dissimilarities between individuals, and some seem to arise from loss of tolerance to self-antigens.

The *exogenous* diseases are basically atopic reactions to environmental allergens such as pollens and contact irritants. These can be prevented if there is no contact with the substance. The strength of the reaction is determined by individual sensitivity to the allergen with one person exhibiting no response and another suffering an anaphylactic reaction. The predisposition for the type of reaction elicited appears to be genetically programmed but the entire mechanism of response is not well understood.

Homologous disorders are typified by transfusion reactions, erythroblastosis fetalis, and transplant rejection. The commonality in these disorders is antigenicity among individuals, which means that the material (e.g., blood, tissue) is recognized by the recipient as foreign and the reaction is elicited to destroy the donor material. Antigenicity is a protective mechanism to ensure individual survival.

The *autologous* diseases include any of the disorders in which the body loses recognition of self-antigen and makes antibody against a self-protein. This means that there is loss of *self-tolerance* resulting in an *autoimmune* reaction.

AUTOIMMUNITY

The study of this phenomenon has been spurred by the appearance of antibodies directed toward specific cells in certain individuals. Many individuals demonstrate serum autoantibodies but show no evidence of disease. This circumstance is especially true in the elderly and much research related to the loss of self-tolerance with the aging process is being conducted. Even persons who have suffered myocardial infarctions may exhibit myocardial autoantibodies but suffer no further myocardial disruption. In juvenile diabetes mellitus, autoantibodies to the islet cells of the pancreas are often demonstrated, which leads to the theory that diabetes mellitus may be a result of an autoimmune attack on the islet cell [8].

The relationships of destructive autoimmune reactions are more clearly demonstrated in myasthenia gravis, Graves' disease, rheumatoid arthritis, systemic lupus erythematosus, and others. The possibility of autoimmunity as a causative factor has been speculated in conditions as diverse as multiple sclerosis, hepatitis, and malignancies. In the latter group, consistent demonstration of autoantibodies has not been found. The appearance of *autoantibodies* and the symptomatology of a disease process lend support for an autoimmune classification.

Observations of autoimmune phenomena have resulted in the following generalizations:

1. Specific autoimmune phenomena are seen in greater frequencies in certain families, which suggests a genetic disorder related to a fundamental disorder of thymic immune control.
2. Autoimmune diseases are more common in females than in males, which indicates a relationship between the sex hormones and the immune response.
3. Elderly persons have a greater incidence of autoantibodies, which may be the result of genetic errors due to the wearing out of the immune system through the aging process.
4. Viruses may play a role in the incidence of autoimmunity because of their ability to disrupt the immune system at any one of several levels [8].
5. Sequestered tissue (tissue and protein not normally in contact with the T and B cells) may be exposed to these cells through disease or disruption.
6. Tissue self-antigen is altered by disease or injury so that the host no longer recognizes it as "self" [1].

Systemic Lupus Erythematosus (SLE)

SLE is a multisystem, chronic rheumatic disease that may assume several forms. It is frequently fatal in persons who develop significant glomerular capillary involvement. A greater incidence of the disease is found in young women 20 to 40 years of age.

Pathologically, widespread degeneration of connective tissue especially in the heart, the glomeruli, the blood vessels, skin, spleen, and retroperitoneal tissue occurs. The skin changes involve atrophy, dermal edema, and fibrinoid infiltration. The renal glomeruli characteristically demonstrate fibrinoid changes, necrosis with scarring, and deposits of immunoglobulin and complement in the basement membrane [1]. The antinuclear antibody (ANA) is demonstrated in 80 to 100 percent of persons with SLE. These may be antibodies to DNA, to nucleoproteins, or to other nuclear components. The LE cell is positive in approximately 76 percent of cases. It is basically a mature polymorphonuclear leukocyte that has phagocytosed nuclear material. These cells may be seen to be clustered around masses of nuclear material and are then called LE rosettes [6]. The LE cell is the result of targeting by antinuclear antibodies.

The American Rheumatism Association has issued a list of 14 criteria indicative of SLE [10]. If the person exhibits four or more of these, the probable diagnosis is SLE (see Table 11-2).

Stiffness and pain in the hands, feet, or large joints are common complaints. The joints appear red, warm, and tender but do not exhibit the deformities of rheumatoid arthritis.

The exposed skin shows signs of a patchy atrophy. An erythematous rash in a butterfly pattern frequently occurs over the nose and cheeks. The dermis becomes edematous and infiltrated by lymphocytes, plasma cells, and histiocytes.

Renal involvement, a serious complication, results from the precipitation of immune complexes in the renal glomeruli. The complexes on the endothelial side of the basement membrane cause inflammatory lesions, a thickened basement membrane, tubular atrophy, and interstitial spaces filled with lymphocytes and plasma cells. The course of renal involvement is characterized by remissions and exacerbations ranging in severity from mild proteinuria to massive hematuria and proteinuria finally resulting in total renal failure.

TABLE 11-2. Criteria indicative of SLE

1. Facial erythema (butterfly rash)
2. Hemolytic anemia, leukopenia, thrombocytopenia
3. Photosensitivity
4. Chronic false-positive for syphilis
5. Alopecia
6. Psychosis or neurologic deficits or convulsions
7. Cellular casts
8. Oral or nasopharyngeal ulceration
9. Pleuritis or pericarditis
10. Arthritis without deformity
11. Discoid lupus
12. Raynaud's phenomenon
13. Proteinuria (over 3.5 gm/day)
14. LE Cell

Systemic problems including fever, fatigue, anorexia, and weight loss are common. Cardiopulmonary and neurologic manifestations are also seen. Besides antibody demonstration, hematologic abnormalities include anemia and leukopenia.

Rheumatoid Arthritis

Rheumatoid arthritis is a chronic, systemic, inflammatory disease that specifically affects the small joints of the hands and feet in its early stages, with involvement of the larger joints in later stages. It is nonsuppurative but finally results in the destruction of cartilage and joints. It may also include lesions of the heart valves, pericardium, myocardium, and pleura [1].

The pathophysiologic manifestations of rheumatoid arthritis appear to result from the development of antibody against IgG. This antibody, called rheumatoid factor (RF), is usually an antibody of the IgM class. The RF is seen in 85 to 90 percent of persons with rheumatoid arthritis and may be stimulated by a self-antigen, an antigen in the synovial cavity, or an infectious antigen. The RF continues to interact with IgG even in the absence of any specific antigen [6]. Chronic antigenic stimulation, such as that seen in chronic respiratory infections, causes the production and destruction of large amounts of antibody. The RF-IgG complexes are found in the rheumatoid lesions and apparently activate complement and/or prostaglandins or other substances that promote the inflammatory response (Fig. 11-5).

Acute attacks of rheumatoid arthritis occur as the RF-IgG complexes precipitate in the synovial fluid. Complement is activated and attracts polymorphonuclear leukocytes to the area, whose main function appears to be the phagocytosis of the complexes. The lysosomal enzymes released by

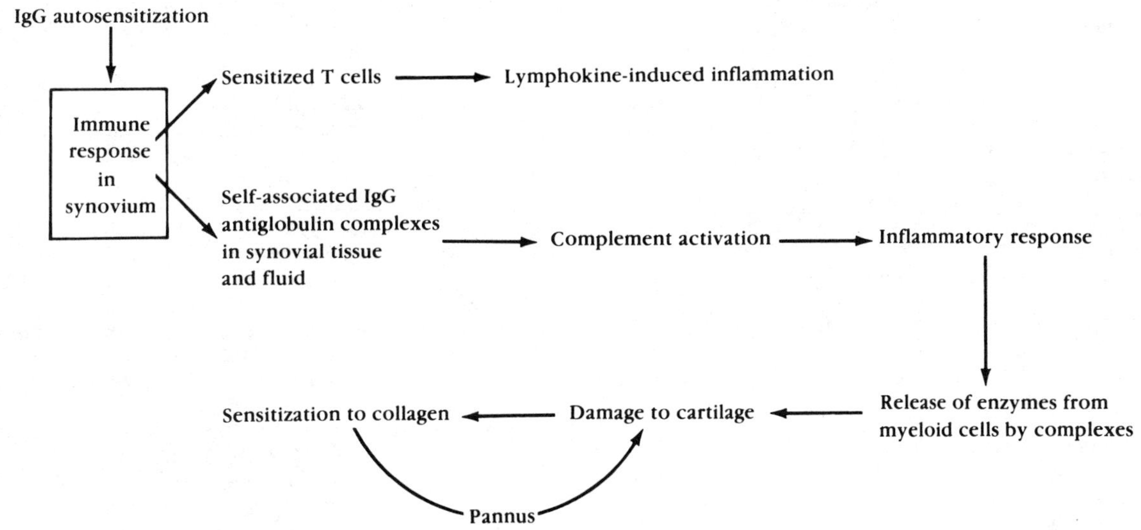

FIGURE 11-5. Hypothetical scheme showing how initial autosensitization to IgG can lead to the pathogenetic changes characteristic of rheumatoid arthritis. (From I. Roitt, *Essential Immunology* [3rd ed.]. Oxford, England: Blackwell, 1977.)

these cells intensify the inflammatory reaction and increase destruction of the articular cartilage. The granulation tissue and inflammatory cells form a mass of tissue called pannus that erodes the articular cartilage. The joint space is destroyed and the resultant scarring may completely immobilize the joint or cause bleeding and thrombosis in the area.

Rheumatoid subcutaneous nodules are often seen and are described as firm, nontender, oval masses that are up to 2 cm in diameter. These are found on the forearm and sometimes the Achilles tendon or attached to underlying periosteum or tendons.

In other systems, a necrotizing arteritis may lead to thrombosis of small arteries. Fibrinous pericarditis, cardiomyopathy, and valvular lesions may affect the heart. Pleuritis and interstitial fibrosis may affect the lungs. The rheumatoid nodules may affect the bone and other effects are seen in the nervous system and the eye.

The signs and symptoms of rheumatoid arthritis are due to both systemic and local inflammatory lesions. Fatigue, weakness, joint stiffness, and vague arthralgias are early symptoms. The individual complains of morning stiffness, which gradually improves after rising. Joints in the hands or feet may be inflamed and swollen tending to spread symmetrically so that the corresponding joint on the other extremity becomes involved.

Laboratory values, besides the positive RF, include a mild leukocytosis with eosinophilia, and an elevated erythrocyte sedimentation rate.

The course of rheumatoid arthritis is variable with remissions and exacerbations. Some patients have a relatively benign disease, while others progress rapidly to severe deformity and total disability.

REFERENCES

1. Anderson, W. A. D., and Scotti, T. *Synopsis of Pathology* (10th ed.). St. Louis: Mosby, 1980.
2. Bellanti, J. A. *Immunology* (2nd ed.). Philadelphia: Saunders, 1978.
3. Fudenberg, H. H., et al. (eds.). *Basic and Clinical Immunology* (3rd ed.). Los Altos, Calif.: Lange, 1980.
4. Gell, P. G., Coombs, R. R., and Lachmann, R. *Clinical Aspects of Immunology* (3rd ed.). Oxford, England: Blackwell, 1975.
5. Purtillo, D. *A Survey of Human Diseases.* Reading, Mass.: Addison-Wesley, 1978.
6. Robbins, S., and Cotran, R. *The Pathologic Basis of Disease* (2nd ed.). Philadelphia: Saunders, 1979.
7. Roitt, I. *Essential Immunology* (3rd ed.). Oxford, England: Blackwell, 1977.
8. Rose, N. Autoimmune disease. *Sci. Am.* 244:383, 1981.
9. Stephens, G. J. *Pathophysiology for Health Practitioners.* New York: Macmillan, 1980.
10. White, J. Systemic lupus erythematosus. *Nurs. '78* 8:26, 1978.

BIBLIOGRAPHY

Anderson, W. A. D., and Scotti, T. *Synopsis of Pathology* (10th ed.). St. Louis: Mosby, 1980.

Bach, M. K. Reagin Allergy. In B. A. Thomas (ed.), *Immunology* (3rd ed.). Kalamazoo, Mich.: Upjohn, 1975. Pp. 19–31.

Bellanti, J. A. *Immunology* (2nd ed.). Philadelphia: Saunders, 1978.

Benacerraf, B., and Unanue, E. R. *Textbook of Immunology.* Baltimore: Williams & Wilkins, 1979.

Blake, P. J., and Perez, R. C. *Applied Immunological Concepts.* New York: Appleton-Century-Crofts, 1979.

Bogolin, L., and Harris, J. Meeting the immunological challenge: Rush-Presbyterian-St. Luke's Medical Symposium. *Heart Lung* 9:643, 1980.

Bullock, W.W. ABA-T determinant regulation of delayed hypersensitivity. *Immunol. Rev* 39:3, 1978.

Cawson, R., McCracken, A., and Marcus, P. *Pathologic Mechanisms and Human Disease.* St. Louis: Mosby, 1982.

Cohen, S. The role of cell-mediated immunity in the induction of inflammatory responses. *Am. J. Pathol.* 88:502, 1977.

Cohen, S., Ward, P., and McCluskey, R. (eds.). *Mechanism of Immunopathology.* New York: Wiley, 1979.

Cooper, M.D., and Lawton, A.R. III. The development of the immune system. *Sci. Am.* 231:58, 1974.

David, J.R. Cellular Immunity and Hypersensitivity. In B.A. Thomas (ed.), *Immunology* (3rd ed.). Kalamazoo, Mich.: Upjohn, 1975. Pp. 55–67.

Edelman, G.M. Structure and function of antibodies. *Sci. Am.* 222:34, 1970.

Fahey, J.L. Antibodies and immunoglobulins: Structure and function. *J.A.M.A.* 194:41, 1965.

Fudenberg, H.H., et al. (eds.). *Basic and Clinical Immunology* (3rd ed.). Los Altos, Calif.: Lange, 1980.

Ganong, W.F. *Review of Medical Physiology.* Los Altos, Calif.: Lange, 1977.

Giese, A.C. *Cell Physiology.* Philadelphia: Saunders, 1979.

Gilbert, E., and Huntington, R. *An Introduction to Pathology.* New York: Oxford University Press, 1978.

Glasser, R. How the body works against itself. *Nurs. '77* 7:38, 1977.

Groer, M., and Shekleton, M. *Basic Pathophysiology.* St. Louis: Mosby, 1979.

Guttman, R.D., and Merrill, J.P. Transplantation Immunology. In B.A. Thomas (ed.), *Immunology* (3rd ed.). Kalamazoo, Mich.: Upjohn, 1975. Pp. 69–77.

Guyton, A. *Textbook of Medical Physiology* (6th ed.). Philadelphia: Saunders, 1981.

Hitzig, W.H. Congenital immunodeficiency disease: Pathophysiology, clinical appearance and treatment. *Pathobiol. Annu.* 6:163, 1976.

Hudgel, D., and Madsen, L. Acute and chronic asthma: A guide to intervention. *Am. J. Nurs.* 80:1791, 1980.

Isselbacher, K.J., et al. *Harrison's Principles of Internal Medicine* (9th ed.). New York: McGraw-Hill, 1980.

Jensen, D. *The Principles of Physiology* (2nd ed.). New York: Appleton-Century-Crofts, 1980.

Junqueira, L.C., and Carneiro, J. *Basic Histology.* Los Altos, Calif.: Lange, 1980.

Katz, D.H. Control of IgE antibody production by suppressor substances. *J. Allergy Clin. Immunol.* 62:44, 1978.

Koren, M.E. Cancer immunotherapy: What, why, when and how? *Nurs. '81* 11:34, 1981.

Luckmann, J., and Sorensen, K. *Medical-Surgical Nursing: A Psychophysiologic Approach* (2nd ed.). Philadelphia: Saunders, 1980.

McDuffie, F.C. Immune complexes in the rheumatic diseases. *J. Allergy Clin. Immunol.* 62:37, 1978.

Muir, B. *Pathophysiology: An Introduction to the Mechanisms of Disease.* New York: Wiley, 1980.

Notkins, A.L., and Koprowski, H. How the immune response to a virus can cause disease. *Sci. Am.* 228:22, 1973.

Parker, C. Food allergies. *Am. J. Nurs.* 80:262, 1980.

Phipps, W., Long, B., and Woods, N. *Medical-Surgical Nursing: Concepts and Clinical Practice* (2nd ed.). St. Louis: Mosby, 1983.

Purtillo, D. *A Survey of Human Diseases.* Reading, Mass.: Addison-Wesley, 1978.

Robbins, S., and Cotran, R. *Pathologic Basis of Disease* (2nd ed.). Philadelphia: Saunders, 1979.

Roitt, I. *Essential Immunology* (3rd ed.). Oxford, England: Blackwell, 1977.

Rose, N. Autoimmune diseases. *Sci. Am.* 244:80, 1981.

Ryan, G.B., and Majno, G. Acute inflammation. *Am. J. Pathol.* 86:184, 1977.

Ryan, G.B., and Majno, G. Inflammation. In B.A. Thomas (ed.), *Immunology: A Scope Monograph.* Kalamazoo, Mich.: Upjohn, 1975.

Schwartz, R.S. The immunological basis of auto-immunization. *J. Allergy Clin. Immunol.* 60:69, 1977.

Selekman, J. Immunization: What's it all about? *Am. J. Nurs.* 80:1441, 1980.

Sell, S. *Immunopathology and Immunity* (2nd ed.). Hagerstown, Md.: Harper & Row, 1975.

Sodeman, W.A., Jr., and Sodeman, W.A. *Pathological Physiology: Mechanisms of Disease.* Philadelphia: Saunders, 1978.

Stephens, G. *Pathophysiology for Health Practitioners.* New York: Macmillan, 1980.

Thaler, M.S., Klausner, R.D., and Cohen, H.J. *Medical Immunology.* Philadelphia: Lippincott, 1977.

Thomas, B.A., (ed.). *Immunology: A Scope Monograph.* Kalamazoo, Mich.: Upjohn, 1975.

Unanue, E.R. The regulation of lymphocyte functions by the macrophage. *Immunol. Rev* 40:225, 1978.

Waldmann, T.A., and Broder, S. Suppressor cells in the regulation of the immune response. *Prog. Clin. Immunol.* 3:155, 1977.

Wallach, J. *Interpretation of Diagnostic Tests* (3rd ed.). Boston: Little, Brown, 1978.

Walter, J.B. *An Introduction to the Principles of Disease* (2nd ed.). Philadelphia: Saunders, 1982.

White, J. Teaching patients to manage systemic lupus erythematosus. *Nurs. '78* 8:26, 1978.

UNIT 6
NEOPLASIA

Linda Hudson Williams
CONCEPTS OF ALTERED CELLULAR FUNCTION
NEOPLASIA

Emilie Musci
NEOPLASIA

The response of cells to the daily barrage of stimuli they receive may be growth or degeneration, alteration of normal metabolism, or even death. Cellular growth and proliferation often occur on a continuum from near normal to grossly abnormal. Neoplasia refers to an alteration in cellular growth and development. This unit examines some of the factors related to neoplasia. Chapter 12 describes cell membrane changes in neoplasia and some related alterations in cellular characteristics. Chapter 13 describes specific theories of carcinogenesis and mechanisms for growth and spread of malignant growths.

The topic of neoplasia is very inclusive and investigative studies are revealing much new, important data. The extensive bibliography at the end of this unit is an attempt to provide current and important historical documentation for this vast subject.

The reader is encouraged to study the unit by utilizing the learning objectives at the beginning of each chapter. Chapter 12 serves as a basis for Chapter 13 and should be reviewed first to facilitate understanding.

CHAPTER 12
CONCEPTS OF ALTERED CELLULAR FUNCTION

LEARNING OBJECTIVES

1. Define *neoplasia, neoplasm, benign,* and *malignant.*
2. Identify the steps in the cell life cycle.
3. Explain the physiology of each step in the cell life cycle.
4. Relate the cell life cycle to neoplasia.
5. Name three areas of potential change in the outer cell membrane that may alter cellular growth.
6. Explain the difference between neoplastic and normal cells in relationship to contact inhibition.
7. Identify the three types of intercellular connections.
8. Discuss the role of each intercellular connection in cellular adhesion.
9. Discuss alterations present in intercellular connections of neoplastic tissues.
10. Describe factors other than intercellular connections that are involved in cellular adhesion.
11. Relate electrical charge and calcium content of the outer cell membrane to cellular adhesion.
12. Define *contact inhibition.*
13. Explain the role of contact inhibition in intercellular communication.
14. Discuss the role of the gap junction in intercellular communication.
15. Explain the relationship between alterations of the gap junction and intercellular communication in neoplasia.
16. Relate second messengers in the cytoplasm of the cell to growth and neoplasia.
17. Relate the role of cytoplasmic ribosomes in protein synthesis to neoplasia.
18. Relate the role of the mitochondria in aerobic energy production to neoplasia.
19. Discuss the nucleus as the site of all hereditary information in relation to neoplasia.
20. Define *cellular differentiation.*
21. Relate cellular differentiation to neoplasia.
22. Define *anaplasia.*
23. Discuss the histologic features of an anaplastic cell.

The cell is constantly confronted by factors in its environment that either injure or stimulate it. It responds to these factors by cellular growth and proliferation, and/or cellular regression and degeneration. These two responses may occur simultaneously in a given cell population, or one may follow the other [4]. When cells are confronted with a stimulus that alters normal cellular metabolism, they may increase concentrations of normal cellular constituents, accumulate abnormal substances, change cellular size and number, and/or undergo a lethal change. The stimuli that cause these alterations may be grouped as follows: (1) physical agents, (2) chemical agents, (3) microorganisms, (4) hypoxia, (5) genetic factors, and (6) immunologic factors.

Alterations in cellular growth and proliferation may be viewed as occurring on a continuum from a near-normal cell to a grossly abnormal one; for example, from hyperplasia to anaplasia. Hypertrophy, hyperplasia, metaplasia, and dysplasia are considered to be controlled adaptive cellular responses (see Chap. 2). The cell's transition makes it vulnerable to injurious agents that can alter the normal controls on the cell's growth and development. *Anaplasia*, as a cellular change, is described in this chapter, and benign and malignant neoplasms are differentiated and discussed in Chapter 13. *Neoplasia* is defined as the development of an abnormal mass of tissue that is unresponsive to normal growth control mechanisms [13]. A *neoplasm* is a group or clump of neoplastic cells. *Benign* refers to neoplastic cells that do not invade the surrounding tissue and do not metastasize. *Malignant* refers to neoplastic cells (cancer) that grow by the invasion of surrounding tissue and metastasize to receptive tissue (see Chap. 13).

THE CELL LIFE CYCLE

The cell life cycle is composed of all the steps in the process of cellular reproduction. One complete cell life cycle, if unaltered, takes about 10 to 30 hours from reproduction to reproduction. In a normal cell population, inhibitory controls slow or stop the reproductive process. Therefore, the actual length of a cell life cycle varies. For example, the life cycle of stimulated bone marrow cells is about 10 hours, while the life cycle of a nerve cell lasts an entire lifetime. The steps of the cell life cycle are designated G0, G1, S, G2, and M (Fig. 12-1). The letter *G* is an abbreviation for "gap" and refers to the time between mitosis and synthesis (G1) and synthesis and mitosis (G2).

G0 is the symbol used to describe the cell at rest. The cell remains at rest, or dormant, until some stimulus, such as the death of other cells of the same cell population, triggers the beginning of the G1 step. Cells may remain in the G1 phase for long periods and normal cell metabolism without DNA synthesis occurs. These cells are often referred to as being in the G0 phase [14]. Cells that do not reproduce readily are said to be G0. These cells perform all metabolic activities except mitosis. Ribonucleic acid (RNA) and protein are synthesized in the G1 *interval*. The length of the G1 interval varies with each cell type. The interval is shorter in all populations with great activity. The cell may then be stimulated to begin the synthesis of deoxyribonucleic acid (DNA), and the S step is entered. DNA synthesis occurs in the S step with the replication of the chromosomes. The length of the S step varies from 6 to 8 hours. The S step is followed by a period of inactivity called G2. Very little is known about this phase except that some RNA is synthesized in preparation for mitosis [8]. Mitosis (M) occurs next, with cellular division creating two daughter cells that have identical genetic information. These daughter cells can mature and repeat the process or can enter a G1 or G0 interval until they are stimulated to reproduce (see p. 11).

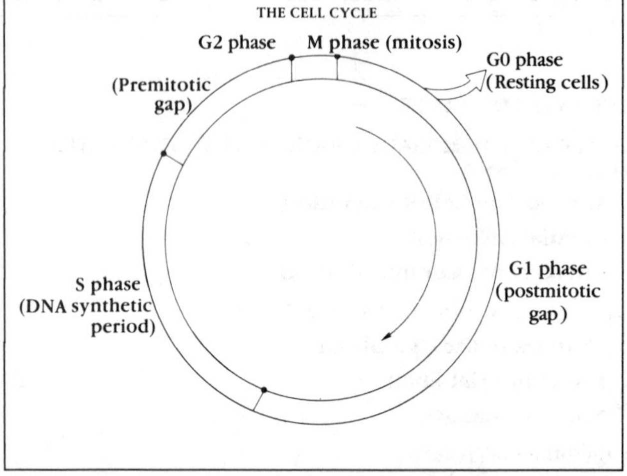

FIGURE 12-1. The cell cycle. A cell that has just completed mitosis enters the G1 phase. It may either stop cycling and enter the G0 phase or proceed to replicate its DNA in the S phase. After the entire genomic DNA has been replicated the cell is tetraploid and proceeds through the G2 phase to mitosis in the M phase. (From J. Stein (ed.), *Internal Medicine*. Boston: Little, Brown, 1983.)

An understanding of the cell life cycle has helped in beginning the understanding of the causes and effects of neoplasia. Three factors related to cell cycle are important in the actual increase in total cell numbers, or population. *Growth fraction* refers to the proportion of cells in a given cell population undergoing cell cycle activity at any given point in time. Rapidly growing neoplasms have a larger number of cells in active reproduction at any given point in time than do slow-growing neoplasms. *Cell cycle time* is usually shorter in rapidly growing neoplasms than in normal cells. *Cell loss* refers to the number of cells lost because of death or some other event. These three factors, when taken together, account for the *doubling time*, which is the rate at which a neoplasm doubles its cell population.

OUTER CELL MEMBRANE CHANGES AS AN EXPLANATION FOR NEOPLASIA

All cells are surrounded by a limiting membrane that constantly exists in a dynamic state (see Chap. 1). The parts of

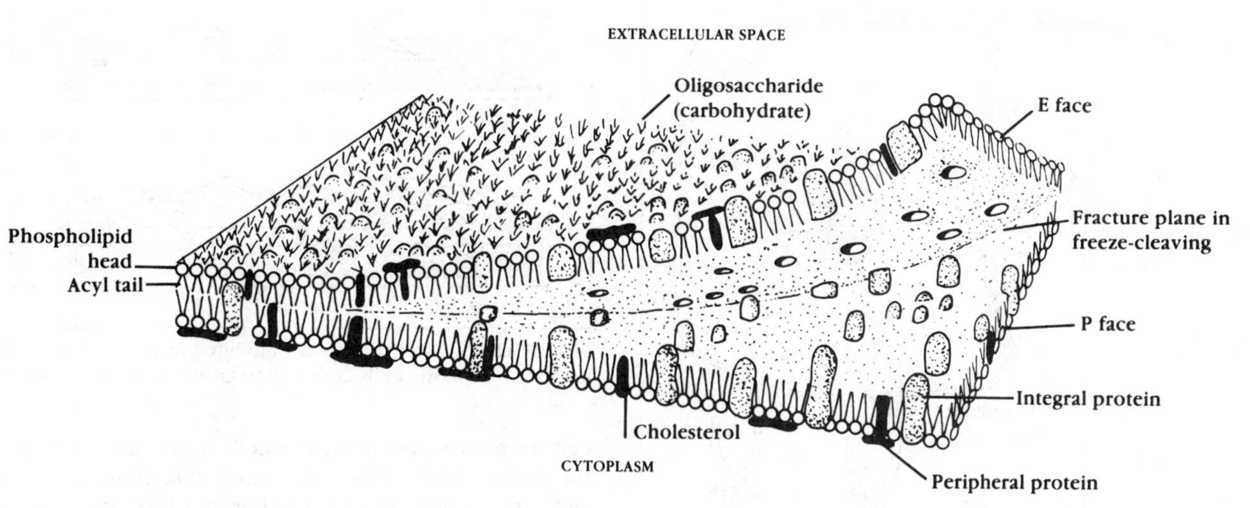

FIGURE 12-2. Outer cell membrane demonstrating integrated structures that are associated with various surface properties of the cell. (From M. Borysenko, et al., *Functional Histology* [2nd ed.]. Boston: Little, Brown, 1984.)

the membrane have the capacity to redistribute and change the cell surface properties, which may have an effect on the cell's growth, metabolism, and behavior (Fig. 12-2) [11].

The outer cell membrane is the point of contact between cells. Interactions involving the outer cell membrane function in the control of normal cellular growth. Changes in the outer cell membrane are apparent in neoplastic cells, and these changes have been implicated in the failure of the neoplastic cells to respond to normal growth control mechanisms. The membrane changes involve alterations in appropriate cell recognition, cellular adhesion, and intercellular communication.

Appropriate Cell Recognition

The mechanisms used by specific cells to recognize each other are not well defined. A mechanism for recognition can be demonstrated by mixing cells of different types in culture media; specific cells eventually segregate themselves. Membrane enzymes and surface sugar residues have been implicated in the recognition of cells, one for another. One hypothesis is that sugar-binding enzymes, glycosyltransferases, in the outer cell membrane, recognize sugar residues on glycoproteins in the membrane of neighboring cells [15]. In the neoplastic cell, glycolipids are altered (Fig. 12-3).

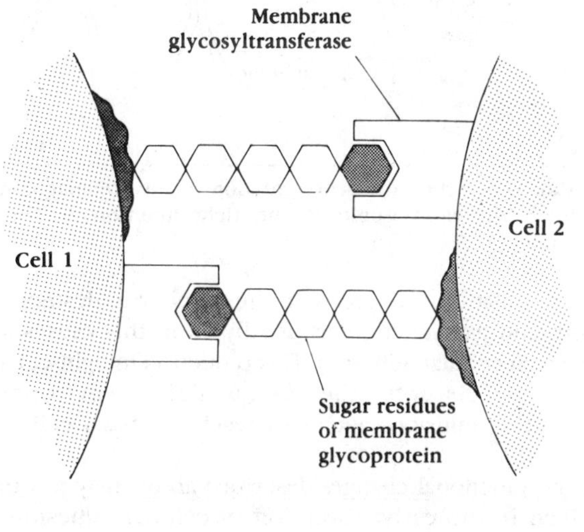

FIGURE 12-3. Cell recognition through sugar-binding enzymes and sugar residues on glycoprotein in the membrane of neighboring cells. (From M.J. Taussig, *Processes in Pathology.* Oxford, England: Blackwell, 1979.)

Cellular Adhesion

Cellular adhesion is a complex process that involves the development of connections between cells. Three types of connections have been described. (1) The *desmosome* is a mechanical way of holding cells together. Because it is composed of fibrous protein it can be destroyed by a proteolytic enzyme, such as trypsin. Once the desmosome is gone, the cells separate (see Chap. 13). (2) The *tight junction* involves the actual fusion of two cell membranes. Nothing can cross the tight junction. Hence, it is found where sharp physical separation is needed, such as in the endothelial lining of the cerebral blood vessels, forming the blood-brain barrier. (3) The *gap junction,* a pore passing through the outer cell membrane, permits the movement of low-molecular-weight substances from one adjoining cell to the next (Fig. 12-4) [12]. In the neoplastic

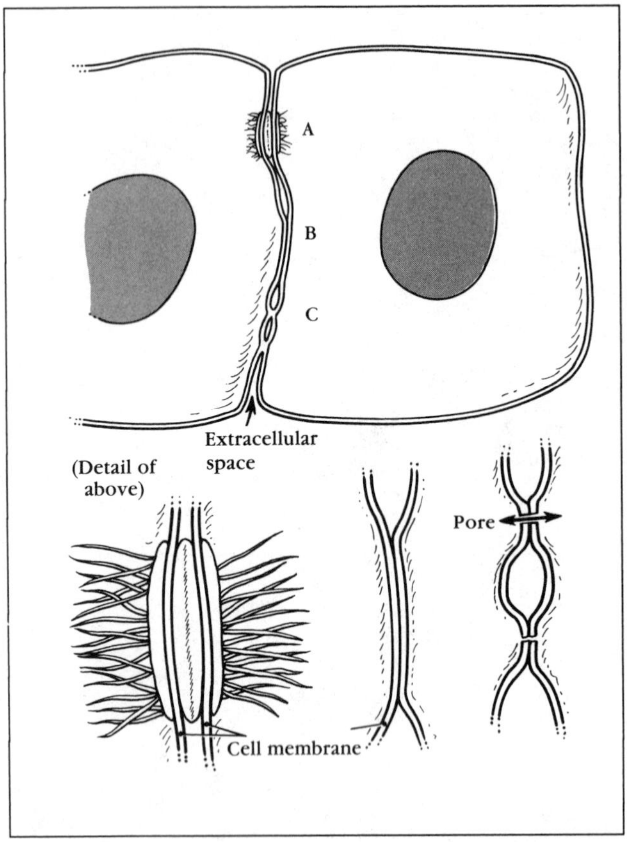

FIGURE 12-4. Schematic representation of intercellular connections. A. The desmosome. B. The tight junction. C. The gap junction.

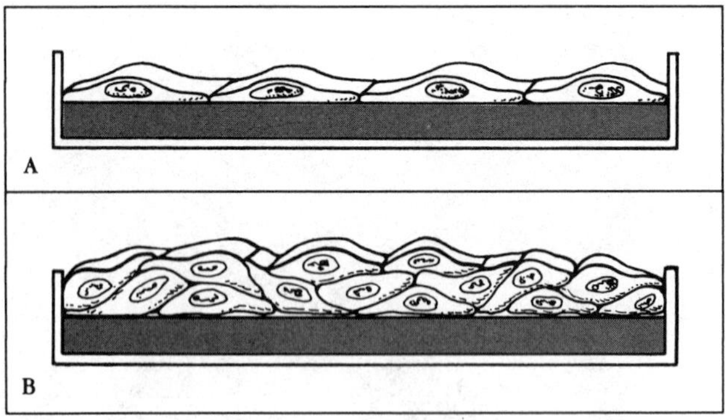

FIGURE 12-5. A. Normal cells are inhibited by a crowded environment. B. Neoplastic cells continue to grow despite cell contact.

cell population, a decrease in the number of desmosomal, tight, and gap junctions is usually seen; this causes a decrease in cellular adhesion. This reduction in tight cell connections disrupts the extracellular environment, permitting injurious agents to reach the basal cell layers [17].

The junctional changes described above may not be involved in the early disruption of cellular adhesion. Research indicates that glycosyltransferase, serum factors, cell surface proteins, cytoskeletal elements, and membrane glycoproteins all play a role in early cellular membrane changes. The role of these substances is not well understood [2, 7, 15, 17].

Other factors involved in cellular adhesion properties include the electrical charge and calcium content of the outer cell membrane. Under physiologic conditions, all mammalian cell surfaces have a negative charge, but this charge is more negative in neoplasia. The more malignant the neoplasia, the greater the increase in negativity; this tends to push cells away from each other [15]. There is also a correlation between the decreased calcium content of the neoplastic cell wall and decreased adhesion [12].

Intercellular Communication

Contact inhibition or density-dependent growth control is a phenomenon observed when normal cells are grown in culture media. Normally, the cells move around freely in the culture media until they touch one another. On contact, they adhere to one another and form parallel lines. They then grow on a single layer until they reach the edge of the culture dish. Growth then stops. The cells of neoplasm, however, respond by continuing to divide and migrate until they are several layers deep. Clearly, normal cells respond to a crowded environment, but neoplastic cells do not. Neoplastic cells have lost their ability either to receive or send the necessary information to stop growth (Fig. 12-5) [15].

In addition to contact inhibition, agglutination by lectins has been used by researchers to study both the outer cell membrane and cell growth. Using lectins (sugar-binding proteins) as molecular markers during normal and neoplastic cell growth in culture media, investigators have made the observations that normal cells, after removal of their outer layer of protein on the outer cell membrane, begin to reproduce and are agglutinated by lectin. Neoplastic cells, however, when subjected to a nonagglutinating lectin, grow to a single layer (Fig. 12-6) [15].

The use of several substances, such as serum stimulation, insulin treatment, mild proteolysis, and, in the case of nonagglutinating lectin–inhibited cells, removal of the nonagglutinating lectin, is known to cause cells that have stopped growing to reenter the growth cycle. Manio and Burger refer to this as the *go* signal [9]. All of these substances cause a quick agglutinable state in the outer cell membrane, accompanied by a quick decrease in intracellular adenosine 3′: 5′-cyclic phosphate (cyclic AMP) [3]. This signals the cell to synthesize DNA and to undergo one round of cell division.

Lectins have been used to study the cell cycle and growth signals. Normal growing cells, on entering mitosis, appear to experience an outer cell membrane change that leads to the next round of cell division via a messenger or *go* signal. Sometime after that, but before the outer cell membrane returns to the nonagglutinable state, another messenger, or *stop* signal, is received, that causes the cell to enter G0, the resting phase. If the latter is not received, the cell is committed to another round of cell division [9]. So, normal cellular growth involves signals to stop cell division that may be blocked in the neoplastic cell.

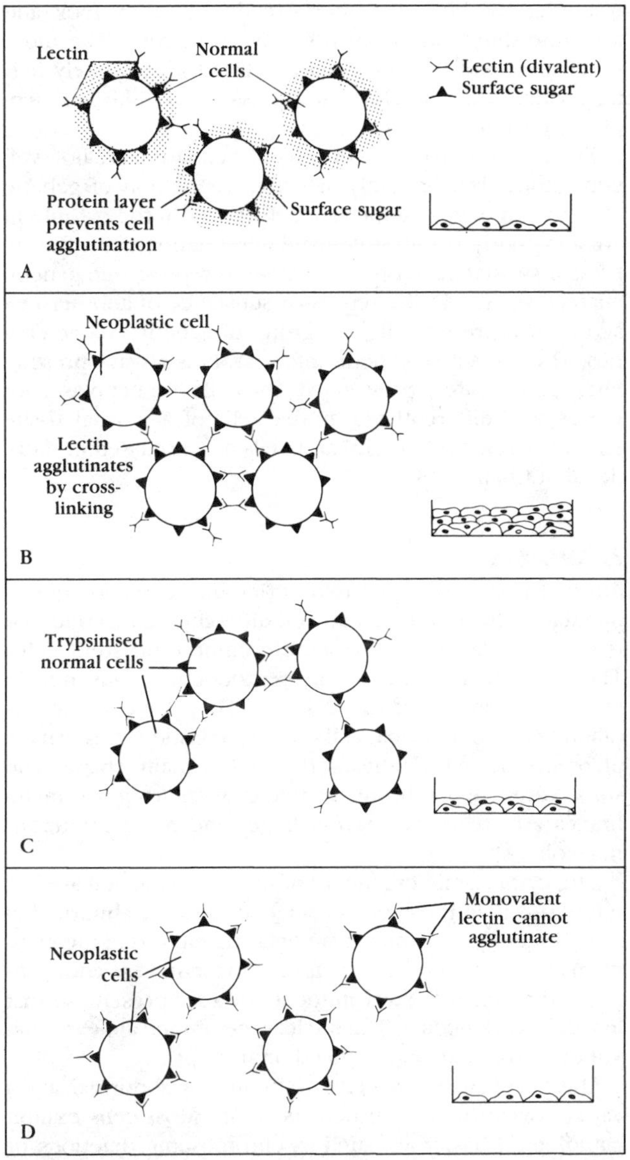

FIGURE 12-6. Effects of lectins on normal and neoplastic cells. A. Normal cells grow to monolayer in culture and are not agglutinated by lectin. B. Neoplastic cells grow as multilayers and are agglutinated by lectin. C. Normal cells after trypsin treatment enter further replication and are lectin-agglutinable. D. Neoplastic cells treated with monovalent (nonagglutinating) lectin grow to monolayer. (From M.J. Taussig, *Processes in Pathology.* Oxford, England: Blackwell, 1979.)

One other phenomenon occurs as cells are grown in culture media that relates to cell growth. Cells removed from the body and grown in culture medium can grow and reproduce indefinitely if the culture medium is constantly replenished. Growth and reproduction stops when secretions of the cells are allowed to collect in the medium. This supports the theory that substances produced by the cell provide a feedback mechanism that slows or stops growth. These substances are called *chalones.* If chalones are important to cell reproduction, then neoplasms have

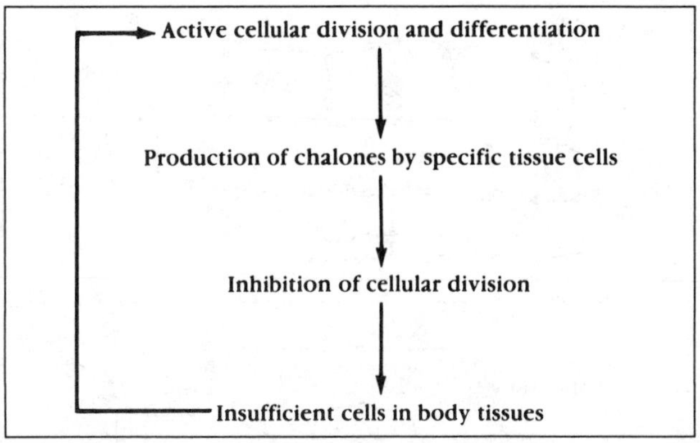

FIGURE 12-7. Negative feedback of tissue mass regulation utilizing specific chalones.

developed a way to escape their control. The neoplasm either produces no chalones or is not sensitive to them (Fig. 12-7) [15].

In summary, two mechanisms are apparently involved in cellular growth. First, cellular growth is controlled by interactions taking place on the outer cell membrane. When cell growth reaches a given density, a messenger is received by the cell that stops cell division. Second, cellular growth is controlled by a substance providing negative feedback to stop cell division. In neoplasia, one or both mechanisms may be altered.

Messengers carrying growth control information move into the cell via the gap junction. With a loss of gap junctions, as occurs as neoplasia, the cell is isolated from the growth control messengers of its normal neighboring cells, too (Fig. 12-8) [17].

INNER CELL CHANGES IN NEOPLASIA

Just as there are changes in the outer cell membrane in neoplasia, there are changes within the cell. It is difficult to tell whether these changes are a function of the neoplasia or of the increased growth rate. The changes involve the cytoplasm, cytoplasmic ribosomes, mitochondria, and the nucleus.

Changes in the Cytoplasm

The cytoplasm serves as a medium through which second messengers related to growth must move to reach the nucleus of the cell where they interact with DNA. The exact nature of the second messengers remains unclear. Protein growth factors, cyclic nucleotides (cAMP and cGMP), and ions (Ca, Mg, Na, and K) are possible second messengers. Cyclic nucleotides function mainly to activate protein kinases. A mutant cell that has no protein kinase cannot be stopped in G1. Two cAMP-dependent protein kinases that correlate with cell growth are produced during specific phases of the cell life cycle [5].

The cytoplasm also contains many enzymes active in anabolism and catabolism. Both enzyme and chromosome

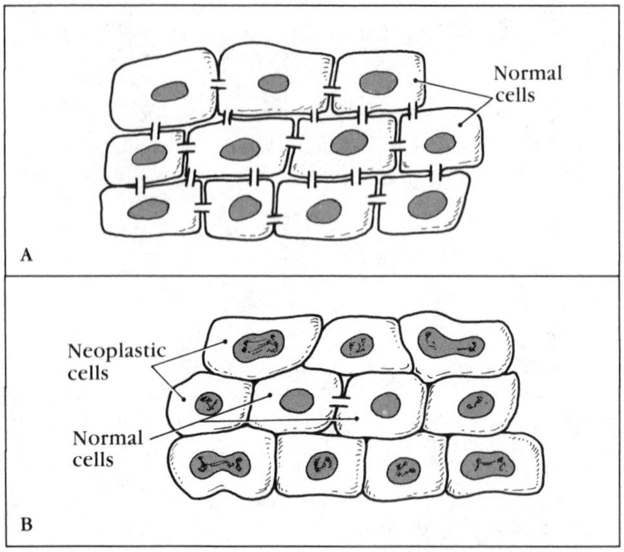

FIGURE 12-8. A. Demonstration of normal growth control information via the gap junction. B. Isolation of normal cell from neighboring cells.

changes are present in rapidly growing neoplastic cells. However, the enzyme alterations are not found in all neoplastic cells [10].

Cytoplasmic ribosomes are responsible for the synthesis of protein. In general, neoplastic cells entrap nitrogen compounds very quickly, take up amino acids, and use these acids to make new proteins through an active anabolic process. They also have key enzymes necessary for making raw products into nucleic acids [16]. The neoplastic cell makes protein more rapidly than nonneoplastic cells.

Mitochondrial Changes

The mitochondria provide for aerobic energy production. The rate of glucose utilization and lactic acid production in the presence of oxygen is increased in some neoplasms. Some neoplasms may use glucose faster than normal cells because it is moved into the cell rapidly [1].

Nuclear Changes

The nucleus is the location of the genes, the locus of all hereditary information, with the exception of the small quantity of DNA found in the organelles. Altered nuclear DNA may result from hereditary genetic information, or from carcinogenic alteration (see Chap. 13). Also, the regulation of cell growth and differentiation involves DNA [10].

DIFFERENTIATION

In the process of fetal development, cells undergo changes in their physical and structural properties as they form the different tissues of the body. This is cellular differentiation. Differentiated cells become specialized and differ from one another in physical and functional ways. Nerve cells, for example, are like other nerve cells, but they look and act quite differently from other types of cells. The more specialized and differentiated a cell is the less likely it is to divide, and, therefore, it is less susceptible to neoplastic change.

The controlling factors of cell differentiation are not well understood, but probably selective repression of genetic information occurs. Repressor substances in the cytoplasm are apparently responsible for differentiation, with the repressor substance in one cell acting to repress one genetic characteristic, and the repressor substance of another cell acting to repress a different group of genetic characteristics. The full set of genetic information is always present, but parts of it are repressed [6]. The cells of a neoplasm are not as well-differentiated as the cells of a normal tissue sample. These undifferentiated cells are discussed in more detail in Chapter 13.

ANAPLASIA

Anaplasia is a term used to describe the regression of cell population from one that is well differentiated to one that is not. Anaplastic cells resemble embryonic stem cells. They appear to function in reproduction, but not in metabolic activity of other kinds. They have numerous differences from normal cells. The anaplastic cell is usually pleomorphic, which means that it has many shapes and sizes. Large hyperchromatic nuclei with irregular membranes are exhibited, having larger and more numerous nucleoli [4].

The cytoplasmic organelles of the anaplastic cell are less numerous than those of a normal cell and are abnormal in form. Pseudopodia, microfilaments and clumps of membraneous sacs, and tubules are usually present. Less endoplasmic reticulum and fewer mitochondria are present, so that less cell work occurs. The nuclear membrane appears convoluted, irregular, and doubled on itself [4].

Mitoses of anaplastic cells are frequently abnormal, and a variety of chromosomal defects result. Most cells exhibit pathologic karyotypes, such as chromosome deletions or translocations. Few mitoses faithfully reproduce the abnormality and new aberrations occur [4].

REFERENCES

1. Bissel, M.J. Transport as a rate limiting step in glucose metabolism in virus transformed cells. *Cell Physiol.* 89:701, 1976.
2. Bosman, H.B. Cell surface enzymes effects on mitotic activity and cell adhesion. *Int. Rev. Cytol.* 50:1, 1977.
3. Burger, M., et al. Growth control and cyclic alterations of cyclic AMP in the cell cycle. *Nature* 2339:161, 1972.
4. Cheville, N.F. *Cell Pathology.* Ames, Iowa: The Iowa University Press, 1976.
5. Das, M. Mitogenic hormone-induced intracellular message: Assay and partial characterization of an activator DNA replication induced by epidermal growth factor. *Proc. Natl. Acad. Sci. USA* 77:112, 1980.
6. Guyton, A. *Textbook of Medical Physiology* (6th ed.). Philadelphia: Saunders, 1981.

7. Haddox, M. H., Magun, B. E., and Russell, D. H. Differential expression of type I and type II cyclic AMP-dependent protein kinases during cell cycle and cyclic AMP-induced growth arrest. *Proc. Natl. Acad. Sci. USA* 77:3445, 1980.
8. Isselbacher, K. J., et al. (eds.). *Harrison's Principles of Internal Medicine* (9th ed.). New York: McGraw-Hill, 1980.
9. Mannio, R. J., and Burger, M. M. Growth Control and the Mitotic Cell Surface. In A. A. Gottlief, et al. (eds.), *Fundamental Aspects of Neoplasia.* New York: Springer-Verlag, 1975.
10. Pardee, A. B. Principles of Cancer Biology: Cell Biology and Biochemistry of Cancer. In V. T. DeVita, S. Hellman, and S. A. Rosenberg (eds.), *Cancer Principles and Practice of Oncology.* Philadelphia: Lippincott, 1982.
11. Poste, G., and Weiss, L. Some Considerations in Cell Surface Alterations in Malignancy. In L. Weiss, (ed.), *Fundamental Aspects of Metasis.* New York: Elsevier North-Holland, 1976.
12. Prehn, R. T., and Prehn, L. M. Pathology of neoplasia: A teaching monography. *Am. J. Pathol.* 80:529, 1975.
13. Robbins, S. L., and Cotran, R. *Pathologic Basis of Disease* (2nd ed.). Philadelphia: Saunders, 1979.
14. Stein, J. (ed.). *Internal Medicine.* Boston: Little, Brown, 1983.
15. Taussig, M. J. *Processes in Pathology: An Introduction for Students of Medicine.* London: Blackwell, 1979.
16. Weber, G. Enzymology of cancer cells. *N. Engl. J. Med.* 296:541, 1977.
17. Weinstein, R. S., et al. The structure and function of intercellular junctions in cancer. *Adv. Cancer. Res.* 20:23, 1975.

CHAPTER 13
BENIGN AND MALIGNANT NEOPLASIA

LEARNING OBJECTIVES

1. Define *neoplasm, tumor, aberrant cellular growth, benign, malignant, cancer, carcinoma, sarcoma,* and *malignancy.*
2. Define cancer at the clinical, cellular, and molecular levels.
3. Explain the morphologic differences in the subgroups of cancer.
4. Explain staging of malignancies.
5. Describe the TMN classification.
6. Compare the characteristics of benign and malignant neoplasms.
7. Describe the somatic mutation theory of carcinogenesis.
8. Explain the two-step mutation model.
9. Differentiate between the somatic mutation theory and the aberrant differentiation theory of carcinogenesis.
10. Describe the viral theory of carcinogenesis.
11. Describe the role of DNA and RNA viruses in altering the genetic code.
12. Explain how reverse transcriptase may work to cause RNA coding of DNA.
13. Identify three viruses associated with specific human cancers.
14. Define the *cell selection theory of carcinogenesis.*
15. Define *carcinogen.*
16. Identify the two broad groups of carcinogens.
17. Classify chemical carcinogens and identify the neoplasms they are associated with.
18. Discuss radiation as a cause of malignant neoplasms.
19. List sources of irradiation and the malignant neoplasms it causes.
20. Relate dietary factors, sexuality, habits, hormones, and predisposing lesions to the development of malignant neoplasms.
21. Define *metastasis.*
22. List the five phases of metastasis.
23. Discuss the role of vascularization and collagenase IV in the ability of the malignant cell to break through the basement cell membrane.
24. Explain how malignant cells separate from the primary neoplasm.
25. Explain dissemination of malignant cells via the lymph and blood vessels.
26. Discuss the role of the immune system in the destruction of malignant cells.
27. Define *tumor-specific antigens.*

28. Explain the "sneaking through," "antigenic modulation," and "antigenic blindfolding" theories.
29. Explain the mechanisms responsible for the development of the local symptoms of neoplasms.
30. Identify symptoms that result from interference with blood supply, interference with function, and mobilization of compensatory mechanisms and immune responses.
31. Define *paraneoplastic syndromes.*
32. Briefly discuss paraneoplastic syndromes of the endocrine, nervous, hematologic, renal, and gastrointestinal systems.
33. Explain the anorexia-cachexia syndrome.

Four million cells divide every second, 350 billion divide in a day, and more than 10 to the fourteenth power divide in a year in the average adult [5]. Every time a normal cell passes through a cycle of division, the opportunity for it to become neoplastic exists. The wonder, then, is not that we have so many neoplasms, but that we have so few but still neoplastic disease causes worldwide problems of morbidity and mortality.

Malignant neoplasms constitute more than 100 distinct disease entities. Most of these are rare, but cancer of the lung, the large intestine, and the breast cause approximately one-half of the deaths that occur each year from malignant neoplasms. The three leading death-producing cancers in males are cancer of the lung, colon and rectum, and prostate. For females, the most common malignancies are those of the breast, lung, and colon and rectum. Advancing age increases the risk of developing cancer. The incidence rises sharply as age increases, with the death rate from cancer of the large intestine, for example, increasing a thousandfold between the ages of 20 and 80. Cancer follows heart diseases as the second leading cause of death in the United States, with both morbidity and mortality being greater in the black race than the Caucasian. It affects two out of three families [4].

This chapter compares benign and malignant neoplasms. Various theories of causation are discussed, and the process of metastasis is explored. The local and systemic impact of neoplasms on the individual is explained, utilizing various benign and malignant neoplasms as examples. Neoplasms of specific organs are described in the chapters relating to each system.

DEFINITIONS

Terms commonly used in discussions about abnormal cellular growth include: neoplasms, tumor, aberrant cellular growth, benign, malignant, cancer (Ca), carcinoma, sarcoma, and malignancy. *Neoplasm, tumor,* and *aberrant cellular growth* are general terms. A *neoplasm* refers to a new growth that is abnormal and the term is usually used synonomously with the term *tumor. Aberrant cellular growth* refers to an alteration in normal cellular growth. The transformation of a normal cell into one that escapes the host's usual controls on growth and differentiation is involved in all aspects of neoplasia.

Benign and *malignant* are terms used to describe the ability of abnormally dividing cells to invade normal tissues and spread to distant sites in the host. Table 13-3 indicates the commonly accepted differences between benign and malignant growths.

Cancer, often abbreviated Ca, always refers to a malignant growth and includes the following: (1) abnormal cell division, (2) invasion of normal tissues, and (3) spread to distant sites in the host. In humans, the clinical presentation of cancer is as a group of diseases with similar systemic symptoms. These can cause the death of the host if they are allowed to remain untreated. At the cellular level, cancer comprises a group of diseases caused by abnormal cellular growth resulting from defective controls on cell growth. At the molecular level, cancer is a group of diseases caused by abnormal nucleic acid and protein metabolism [3].

Cancers may be divided into three broad subgroups: carcinomas, sarcomas, and the leukemias and lymphomas. *Carcinoma* is a term often used interchangeably with cancer, but it actually refers to a group of abnormally dividing cells of epithelial origin, which invade surrounding tissues and spread to distant sites in the host. *Sarcomas* arise in connective tissues, such as the fibrous tissues and blood vessels. These also invade surrounding tissues and spread to distant sites in the host. The *leukemias* and *lymphomas* arise in the blood-forming cells of the bone marrow and lymph nodes and then invade the mononuclear phagocytic system and remaining body structures.

CLASSIFICATION OF NEOPLASMS

Neoplasms are customarily classified according to their cell of origin and whether their behavior is benign or malignant. The terminology utilized places the cell of origin as the first part of the name of the neoplasm, while "oma" forms the last portion (Table 13-1).

Squamous and basal cell kinds of epithelial benign tumors are called papillomas. Glandular epithelial benign tumors are called adenomas. Papillomas or adenomas found at the end of a stem or pedicle are referred to as polyps, but these are not necessarily neoplastic. As stated earlier, malignant neoplasms of epithelial origin are carcinomas. Those of glandular epithelial origin are termed *adenocarcinomas,* such as adenocarcinoma of the breast.

Neoplasms of muscle cell origin are named according to muscle type, for example, leiomyoma, which means "smooth muscle tumor." Malignant neoplasms of muscle cell origin are sarcomas, an example of which is leiomyosarcoma. Neoplasms of nerve cells and connective tissue cells are named in a similar manner. Neoplasms of the blood-forming cells and lymph nodes are named according to affected blood cell type.

Pigmented and embryonic cells are also significant in the nomenclature of neoplasms. Neoplasms of pigmented cells are named for their cell of origin, the melanocyte. Neoplasms of embryonic cell origin contain bits of the germinal layers, such as hair or teeth. "Terat" meaning monster, and "oma" meaning tumor (teratoma or teratocarcinoma), are used in naming these neoplasms. Neoplasms of embryonic cell origin, then, are monster tumors and are often found in the ovary or testes.

STAGING OF NEOPLASMS

Neoplasms may also be categorized by stage. Staging is an effort to describe the extent of a disease at a given point in terms that are commonly understood. The purposes of staging are to: (1) aid in determining treatment, (2) evaluate survival rates, (3) determine the relative merits of different methods of treatment, and (4) facilitate the exchange of information between treatment centers. The TMN classification varies slightly with different types of malignancy, but provides some general principles of staging. The three capital letters are used to denote the following: (1) T—the tumor or primary lesion and its extent, (2) N—lymph nodes of the region and their condition, and (3) M—distant metastasis. TIS means *tumor in situ,* or localized tumor. T_x is a term used when the extent of the tumor cannot be adequately assessed. Using the letter *T* and adding ascending numbers indicates ascending degrees of tumor size. The spread of malignancy to regional lymph nodes is indicated by N_1, referring to "few," with N_2 referring to "many" nodal metastases [10]. The presence or absence of distant metastasis is designated by a M_0, M_1, or M_2 (Table 13-2). M_x is used when the amount or extent of metastasis cannot be assessed.

TABLE 13-1. Classification of common benign and malignant neoplasms

Cell	Benign	Malignant
Epithelial		Carcinoma
Squamous	Squamous cell papilloma	Squamous cell carcinoma
Basal cell	Basal cell papilloma	Basal cell carcinoma
Glandular	Adenoma	Adenocarcinoma
Pigmented cells	Benign melanoma	Malignant melanoma
Muscle cells		
Smooth muscle	Leiomyoma	Leiomyosarcoma
Striated muscle	Rhabdomyoma	Rhabdomysarcoma
Nerve cells		
Nerve sheath	Neurilemmoma	Neurofibrosarcoma
Glial cells	Glioma	Glioblastoma
Ganglion cells	Ganglioneuroma	Neuroblastoma
Meninges	Meningioma	Malignant meningioma
Connective tissue cells		
Fibrous	Fibroma	Fibrosarcoma
Fatty	Lipoma	Liposarcoma
Bone	Osteoma	Osteosarcoma
Cartilage	Chondroma	Chondrosarcoma
Blood vessels	Hemangioma	Angiosarcoma
Lymph vessels	Lymphangioma	Lymphangiosarcoma
Bone marrow		Multiple myeloma Leukemia Ewing's sarcoma
Lymphoid cells		Malignant lymphoma Lymphosarcoma Reticulum cell sarcoma Lymphatic leukemia Hodgkin's disease
Other blood cells		
Erythrocytes	Polycythemia vera	
Granulocytes		Myelogenous leukemia
Monocytes	Mononucleosis	
Blymphocytes		Plasma cell myeloma Multiple myeloma

BENIGN NEOPLASMS

Benign neoplasms retain cells that are similar in structure to the cells from which they are derived. The cells of the

TABLE 13-2. A typical TNM classification

Stage	TNM	Extent of disease
Stage I	$T_1N_0M_0$	Mass limited to organ of origin Lesion is operable and resectable No nodal or vascular spread Affords best chance for survival (70–90%)
Stage II	$T_2N_1M_0$	Mass has spread into surrounding tissue and first-station lymph nodes Lesion is operable and resectable, but there is doubt about complete removal, due to extent of disease Specimen shows evidence of microinvasion into capsule and lymphatics Good chance of survival (45–55%)
Stage III	$T_3N_2M_0$	Mass is extensive, with fixation to deeper structures, bone invasion, and lymph nodes involvement Lesion is operable but not resectable, so disease is left behind Some chance of survival (15–25%)
Stage IV	T_4N_3M+Mx	Evidence of distant metastasis beyond local site Lesion is inoperable Little or no chance of survival (0–5%)

Source: P. Rubin, Statement of the Clinical Oncologic Problem. In P. Rubin (ed.), *Clinical Oncology For Medical Students and Physicians: A Multidisciplinary Approach.* Rochester, N.Y.: American Cancer Society, 1978.

benign neoplasm are more cohesive than those of a malignant neoplasm. Growth of the benign mass occurs evenly from the center of the neoplasm, usually resulting in a well-defined border. The edges of the benign neoplasm move outward, smoothly pushing adjacent cells out of the way (Fig. 13-1). As this occurs, most benign neoplasms become encapsulated. The capsule, composed of connective tissue, separates the tumor from surrounding tissues. The growth of a benign neoplasm is usually slow and limited to one area. The blood supply of the benign neoplasm is less profuse than that of malignant neoplasms. A benign neoplasm rarely recurs after surgical removal and rarely ulcerates, undergoes necrosis, or causes systemic effects, unless it is a secreting endocrine neoplasm.

MALIGNANT NEOPLASMS

Malignant neoplasms are atypical in cell structure, with abnormal nuclear divisions and chromosomes. The malignant cell loses its resemblance to the cell of origin. It is not cohesive and, consequently, its pattern of growth is irregular; no capsule is formed, and distinct separation from surrounding tissues is difficult (Fig. 13-2). Malignant cells invade adjacent cells, rather than pushing them aside. They have varying growth rates and develop a greater blood supply than normal tissues or benign neoplasms. The hallmark of a malignant neoplasm is its ability to metastasize or spread to distant sites. It does frequently recur after surgical removal and can cause systemic problems. Table 13-3 summarizes the differences between benign and malignant neoplasms.

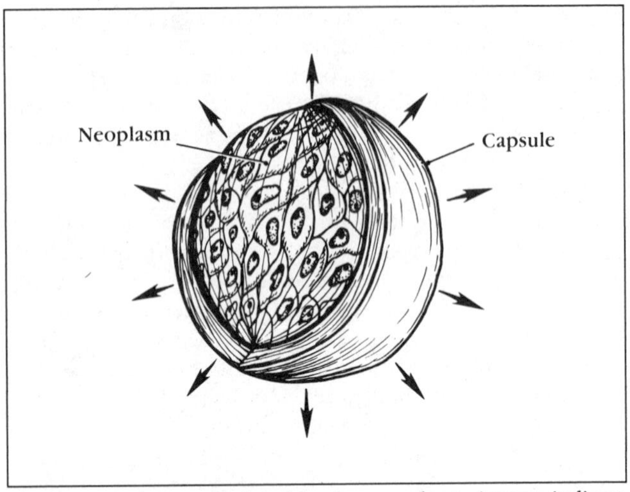

FIGURE 13-1. An encapsulated benign neoplasm. Arrows indicate equal expansion from the center.

THEORIES OF CAUSATION

Most research related to the etiology of neoplasia relates to malignant neoplasms. Because cancer is not one disease, but rather, more than 100 distinct disease entities, it probably has a phenomenal number of etiologies. None of the theories that attempt to explain the pecularities of the cancer cell has successfully provided a complete explanation. The current theories are grouped by the mechanisms they invoke: (1) somatic mutation, (2) aberrant differentiation, (3) virus activation, and (4) cell selection [12].

Somatic Mutation Theory

In 1928 Bauer formulated the somatic cell mutation theory of cancer. Abnormalities in the genes result from mutational changes that may be induced by carcinogenic agents and hereditary susceptibility. This theory can be used to explain the irreversible character of cancer, a wide variety of causes, and the tendency of a cancer to reproduce the same kind of cancer. It does not explain the long latent period that usually is seen between cell mutation and the development of a mass [2].

There is evidence to suggest that in persons who have specific chromosomal disorders, certain kinds of neo-

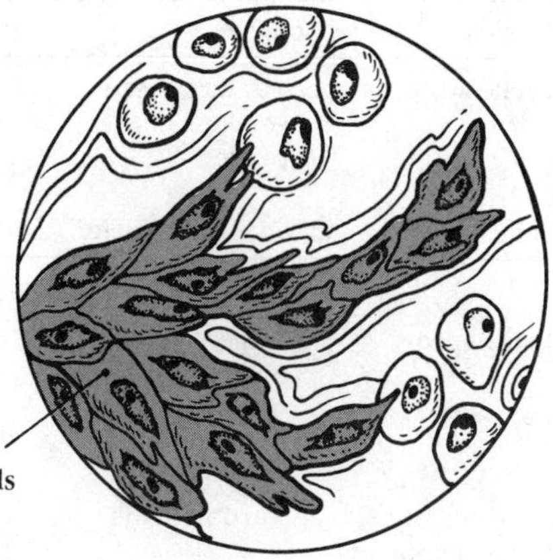

FIGURE 13-2. A malignant neoplasm with irregular borders, indistinct from surrounding tissues.

TABLE 13-3. A comparison of benign and malignant neoplasms

Benign	Malignant
Similar to cell of origin	Dissimilar from cell of origin
Edges move outward smoothly (encapsulated)	Edges move outward irregularly
Compresses	Invades
Slow growth rate	Rapid to very rapid growth rate
Slight vascularity	Moderate to marked vascularity
Rarely recurs after removal	Frequently recurs after removal
Necrosis and ulceration unusual	Necrosis and ulceration common
Systemic effects unusual unless it is a secreting endocrine neoplasm	Systemic effects common

plasms are likely to develop [12]. For example, the incidence of leukemia is greater in individuals with the trisomies, especially trisomy 21. Retinoblastoma occurs with a high frequency in individuals with D-deletion syndrome, a disorder in which there is deletion of part of chromosome 13. Individuals with chronic myelocytic leukemias (CML) have a Philadelphia chromosome (translocation of chromosome 22) in up to 90 percent of cases [12].

Some of the Mendelian recessive diseases also have an associated high incidence of malignant neoplasms, with a notable example being xeroderma pigmentosum, a disorder associated with a high incidence of skin cancers. Mendelian dominant patterns are linked with such malignant disorders as Wilms' tumor of the kidney and neurofibromatosis.

A *two-step mutation model* is necessary in most cases that involve *initiation* and *promotion*. These steps were first demonstrated in experiments conducted by Berenblum in the 1940s. The description of the process is frequently referred to as *Berenblum's theory*. The stage of initiation occurs rapidly and does not appear to be reversible. The substances that initiate the process and cause the mutations are called *carcinogens*, which may be grouped as physical, living, or chemical substances. An example of a physical carcinogen is radiation. Living carcinogens include viruses and aflatoxin, a fungal contaminate. Some chemical carcinogens are coal tars, diethylstilbestrol, polyvinyl chloride, and sodium nitrite. The cells produced during this initiation stage do not appear as malignant, neoplastic cells. The development of malignancy appears to be dose-related and related to individual susceptibility to the carcinogen. The second stage of carcinogenesis, *promotion*, changes the mutated gene to a rapidly growing malignant neoplasm. The mechanism for this change is not well understood. The promotion stage of carcinogenesis occurs over a long period of time and in its early phases may be partially reversible [6].

Aberrant Differentiation or Epigenetic Theory

The aberrant differentiation theory of carcinogenesis states that neoplastic change may result from a disturbance in the regulation of normal genes, through abnormal repression of adult differentiated tissue, or through the turning on of normally inactivated embryonic genes [10]. Because changes in the regulation of the genes is the problem, carcinogenesis alters established normal genes. Studies support the idea that normal genes are intact in the malignant cell and that these can appropriately be expressed under the right conditions. Carried further, the data suggest that the malignant process can be reversed. In other words, a permanent mutation may not have occurred [13].

The incidence of malignant neoplasms often increases during periods of alterations in growth and development. Dermoid cysts, hamartomas, and teratomas are neoplasms that result from altered embryonic growth and development. Cohnheim's theory, one of the oldest theories of neoplasms, relates growth, alterations in germinal layers, and differentiated development as embryologic developmental problems. This theory is somewhat outdated but is supported in some cases by demonstration of a neoplastic cell type that is embryologic in appearance.

Viral Theory

Viruses have been implicated as possible causes of human malignant neoplasms and have been directly associated with tumor induction in animals. Viruses that have been implicated in human cancers are called *oncogenic viruses*. Current evidence favors the view that viruses alter the genome of the infected cell, which then alters the progeny (offspring) of the host cell [12].

The two kinds of oncogenic viruses are deoxyribonucleic acid (DNA) and ribonucleic acid (RNA) viruses.

TABLE 13-4. Viruses implicated in malignant neoplasia

Virus	Associated malignancy
C type RNA virus	Leukemia
B type RNA virus	Breast cancer
Herpesvirus II	Cancer of cervix
Epstein-Barr virus	Burkitt's lymphoma Nasopharyngeal cancers

TABLE 13-5. A summary of chemical carcinogens and their sites of action

Carcinogen	Source	Site of action
Polycyclic aromatic amines	Soots, tars, cigarette smoke, benz-pyrene	Lip, tongue, oral cavity, head, neck, larynx, lung, bladder
Aromatic amines	Dyes, Naphthylene, 2-acetylamino-fluorine	Bladder
Alkylating agents	Nitrogen mustard and mustard gas, drugs (cyclophos-phamide and melphalan)	Lung, larynx, bladder, hemo-poietic system
Nitrosamines and nitrosocompounds	4-Nitrobiphenyl	
Naturally occurring products	Aflatoxin B Betel nut	Liver Oral cavity
Drugs	Griseofulvin, hycanthone, metronidazole, diethylstilbestrol	Cancers in rats, vagina, bladder, hemopoietic system

The *DNA viruses* are incorporated into the genes of the host and are then transmitted to subsequent generations. The gene is then expressed without the usual symptoms that accompany infections [12]. The *RNA viruses,* or oncornaviruses, also contribute genetic information to the host cell. The mechanism for this viral transmission is not entirely clear, but it appears to involve a reversal of normal processes, the transcription and synthesis of DNA from an RNA template, using an enzyme called reverse transcriptase [10]. This explanation clarifies the process by which genes are expanded and new DNA sequences are developed without alteration of the parent structures. As part of the genome of the host cell, the provirus is not attacked and destroyed by the immune system. Present evidence favors the view that reverse transcriptase acts to accomplish reverse transcription, to degrade RNA in the new DNA-RNA complex, and to form the new DNA double strand [10].

Some viruses associated with human malignant neoplasms are the C-type RNA viruses (oncornavirus), the B-type RNA viruses, and certain DNA viruses. Although the mechanism is not clear, the C-type RNA viruses are implicated as a causative agent in the development of leukemia; the B-type RNA viruses may be a factor in breast cancer; and herpesviruses may be associated with cervical cancer. The Epstein-Barr virus, a DNA virus of the herpes type, has been closely associated with Burkitt's lymphoma and nasopharyngeal carcinoma [10]. The unit bibliography includes a number of studies relating to the above associations. Table 13-4 summarizes the viruses most closely implicated in the development of malignant neoplasia.

Cell Selection Theory

The cell selection theory explains neoplasms as developing through a step-by-step mutational process. This theory is used mainly to explain the fact that certain substances, although not carcinogens in themselves, support and promote carcinogenic growth. The process may stop or reverse itself if there is no stimulus.

Immunodeficiency, either spontaneous or induced, increases the risk of developing a neoplastic growth. Involved in this is impairment of immune surveillance, with a weak immunologic reaction enhancing the survival and growth of malignant tumors.

CARCINOGENS

Since Sir Percival Pott's linking, in 1775, the incidence of scrotal cancer in chimney sweeps and their exposure to soot, it has been known that certain substances are capable of inducing neoplastic growth. These substances are *carcinogens* or *oncogens.* Carcinogens are substances that are known to increase the likelihood that exposed individuals will develop a neoplasm. *Cocarcinogens* increase the activity of carcinogens, but in and of themselves do not cause neoplasms. Some substances in higher doses and exposure rates are carcinogenic, while at lower doses and exposure rates the same substances may be cocarcinogenic. Many carcinogens in their original form cannot induce cellular changes, but require metabolic activation in the body. Carcinogens can be divided into two groups: (1) chemical and (2) physical.

Chemical Carcinogens

Between 1971 and 1977, the International Agency for Research on Cancer evaluated more than 350 chemicals and found that most were capable of causing neoplasms either in humans (a total of 26) or animals (a total of 221) [1]. Chemical carcinogens can be grouped as polycyclic aromatic hydrocarbons, aromatic amines, alkylating agents, nitrosamines and other nitrosocompounds, naturally occurring products, drugs, metals, and industrial carcinogens (Table 13-5).

Polycyclic aromatic hydrocarbons are some of the most powerful carcinogens. They are found in the condensates of tobacco smoke, automobile exhaust, and other products of combustion. Cancers of the lip, tongue, oral cavity, head, neck, larynx, lung, and bladder are associated with exposure to polycyclic aromatic hydrocarbons.

Aromatic amines are another significant group of carcinogens. These include certain foods, naphthalene (a coal tar found in moth repellents and insecticides), and 2-acetyl-amino-fluorine, an insecticide. The aromatic amines are linked with cancer of the bladder [11].

Alkylating agents in controlled circumstances are used for therapeutic purposes but can be carcinogenic. Two common alkylating agents are nitrogen mustard (cyclophosphamide) and mustard gas. Cancers of the lung, larynx, bladder, and hemopoietic system are associated with alkylating agents [11].

Nitrosamines and other nitrosocompounds develop under physiologic conditions from chemical interactions between nitrites and other secondary amines. Nitrites are found in foods as additives. A number of drugs and nicotine may supply the amines for the process.

Naturally occurring products implicated in the causation of malignant neoplasm include aflatoxin and the betel nut. Aflatoxin B is a mold, *Aspergillus flavus,* found on corn, barley, peas, rice, soybeans, fruit, some nuts, milk, and cheddar cheese. It has been linked to liver cancer in humans. In animals, aflatoxin B has been shown to cause liver, stomach, colon, and kidney cancer [11]. Chewing the betel nut has been implicated in the causation of cancer of the oral cavity.

Several drugs besides the alkylating agents are known to have carcinogenic effects. Griseofulvin, an antifungal agent used to treat mycotic disease of the skin; hycanthone, an antischistosomal agent; and metronidazole, an antiprotozoal used to treat *Trichomonas vaginalis* and *Entamoeba histolytica* have been found to cause cancer in rats. Diethylstilbestrol, used to prevent spontaneous abortion, increased the incidence of cancer of the vagina in the daughters of women who received this treatment.

Asbestos, cadmium, chromium, and nickel are some of the metals involved in carcinogenesis. All are associated with cancer of the lung. Chromium and nickel are also involved in nasal cavity tumors. Cadmium may be associated with cancer of the prostate. Asbestos may cause pleural cavity and gastrointestinal tract malignancies.

Industrial compounds have been implicated in carcinogenesis. One example of these is polyvinyl chloride, which is used in the manufacture of plastics and may cause angiosarcomas of the liver [11].

Physical Carcinogens

Ionizing radiation is a recognized cause of cellular mutations. Damage to DNA may be direct or indirect. Direct damage results from interaction of the electron itself with the DNA of the cell. Indirect damage occurs as a secondary electron interacts with a water molecule, giving rise to a free radical, OH, which then damages DNA. A long latent period often exists between exposure and the development of clinical disease. Firm evidence links exposure to large doses of radiation to leukemia.

Even low doses of irradiation may cause cancer in susceptible individuals. The incidence of breast cancer increases with small, widely spread doses of irradiation, and the incidence of thyroid cancer increases with head and neck x rays during childhood. X rays of the fetus in utero increase its chances of developing childhood cancer.

Ultraviolet radiation from the sun is a major cause of skin cancers. Fair-complexioned individuals are more likely to develop skin cancers than their darker-complexioned counterparts, because of the lack of melanin, which acts to protect darker-complexioned individuals from the injurious effects of the sun (see Chap. 40).

Overexposure to radiation from atomic bomb detonation has been extensively studied in survivors of Hiroshima and Nagasaki. The high incidence of leukemia in these persons supports the relationship between leukemia and radiation. Plastic films implanted at various body sites in rodents have been shown to be carcinogenic. A profuse foreign body reaction occurs before the tumor develops. Sarcomas have been observed in relation to foreign body reactions in humans, but no conclusive evidence is available regarding cancer and prosthetic insertions in humans.

Schistosoma haematobium infestations, common in inhabitants of the Nile Valley, Mozambique, and Rhodesia, are associated with squamous cell carcinoma of the bladder. The development of this cancer is also preceded by chronic inflammation and fibrosis of the bladder wall.

Injections of mineral oil into the peritoneal cavity of mice is known to cause a granulomatous inflammation of the peritoneum, followed by plasma cell tumors [9]. This seems to support the role of chronic inflammation or foreign body reactions in the development of neoplasms [12].

OTHER FACTORS IN CARCINOGENESIS

Epidemiologic studies have revealed other factors in the occurrence of neoplasms besides chemical and physical carcinogens. These other factors are primarily related to habits of daily living and religious or cultural traditions. Some predispose persons to the development of neoplasms, while others serve a protective function. For example, cancer of the stomach is more common in Japan than in the United States, while cancers of the intestine, breast, and prostate are less common. These differences are lost within a generation or two after Japanese individuals take residence in the United States.

Diet

Dietary customs have been the subject of a great deal of research. Under certain circumstances, carcinogenesis can be enhanced by high-fat diets, although the evidence seems to support low-fiber diets as a cause of cancer of the colon. Food preservation seems to play a role in carcinogenesis. Foods preserved by salting, drying, or charring increase the consumer's risk of cancer of the stomach [15].

Sexuality

Customs and religious beliefs involving sexuality seem to have a role in carcinogenesis. Cancer of the cervix is more likely to occur in women who begin having sexual intercourse at a young age and who have many sexual partners. The incidence of cervical cancer is lowest in nuns, virgins, and Jewish women. This latter is thought to be due to hygiene practices and circumcision. Cancer of the penis is also lowest among Jewish men who are circumcised after birth. Cancer of the breast is more prevalent in women who have no children, who begin menses early, or who enter menopause late [15].

Habits

A person who consumes 6 oz of eighty-proof alcohol a day over a period of time increases the risk of developing cancer of the esophagus 2 to 3 times. The risk is even greater for those who also smoke cigarettes. A person who smokes cigarettes increases the risk of lung cancer fourfold by smoking 9 to 10 cigarettes a day, or 10 or more times by smoking a pack or more a day. There also seems to be a relationship between polluted air, cigarette smoking, and the development of cancer [15].

Hormones

Alterations in hormonal balance resulting in increased hormonal levels over a prolonged time may cause neoplasms in the target cells. Cancer of the breast, endometrium, vagina, prostate, thyroid, and adrenal cortex are thought to be related to altered hormonal influences.

Predisposing Lesions

There are many neoplastic changes in tissues that are known to be precancerous. For example, chronic cystic disease of the breast predisposes the individual to cancer of the breast. Adenomatous polyps of the colon and rectum remain questionably precancerous.

METASTASIS

The ability of a malignant neoplasm to spread to distant sites is termed *metastasis.* A clump of malignant cells, no longer attached to the original neoplasm, travels to and becomes established at a new site. The original malignant neoplasm is the primary neoplasm, tumor, or site. Metastasis involves the release of many malignant cells, only some of which are able to survive the defense mechanisms and hostile environment. Five phases are involved in the process of metastasis: (1) invasion, (2) cell separation, (3) dissemination, (4) initial establishment, and (5) proliferation (Fig. 13-3) [14].

Invasion

To invade normal adjacent cells, the malignant cells grow out from their original location into the neighboring location. To infiltrate a body cavity or blood vessel, the malignant cells must break through the basement cell membrane. Vascularization usually follows penetration of the basement membrane. Malignant cells may escape into the bloodstream through gaps between endothelial cells as rapidly growing capillary tubes penetrate the basement membrane [5]. A major structural component of the basement cell membrane is type IV collagen. When high levels of collagenase IV exist, neoplastic cells may metastasize. Greatly damaged endothelium has high levels of collagenase IV, which may be significant as malignant cells select invasion sites [12].

Cell Separation

After invading the neighboring tissues, body cavities, and blood vessels, malignant cells separate from the primary neoplasm so that they can travel to distant sites. Degenerative products such as lysosomal enzymes that favor cell separation are released as the neoplasm outgrows its blood supply. Focal necrosis then occurs.

Dissemination

The most common route that malignant cells take to distant sites from the primary neoplasm is through the lymphatic and blood vessels. Malignant cells move from lymphatic to blood vessels and vice versa. A malignant neoplasm of just a few grams may shed several million cells into the circulation each day. A very large proportion of these circulating malignant cells die, and few possess the factors necessary for survival in the hostile, turbulent circulatory system. To survive in the circulatory system and to effect arrest in the endothelium, malignant cells undergo a variety of cellular interactions involving immunity and adherence.

To survive in the circulation or, in fact, to survive anywhere, the malignant cell must resist the host's defense system. Tumor-specific antigens can be found on the surface of the outer cell membrane of almost all malignant cells. These tumor-specific antigens are thought to be composed of protein and carbohydrate synthesized inside the malignant cell and then moved into the cell coat. Tumor-specific antigen should provoke an immune response by B lymphocytes and T lymphocytes. This response includes B lymphocytes and T lymphocytes. B lymphocytes interact with the tumor-specific antigen and then synthesize and secrete antibodies. The antibodies then bind to the antigen and release a toxic substance that destroys the cell. T lymphocytes, once exposed to the tumor-specific antigen, seem to synthesize antibodylike molecules on their outer cell membrane. These antibodylike molecules recognize the antigen on the next encounter with it and act to destroy the cell with the recognized antigens. T lymphocytes also release substances that control interactions between B lymphocytes, T lymphocytes, and macrophages (large scavenger cells). While the T lymphocyte is probably more important

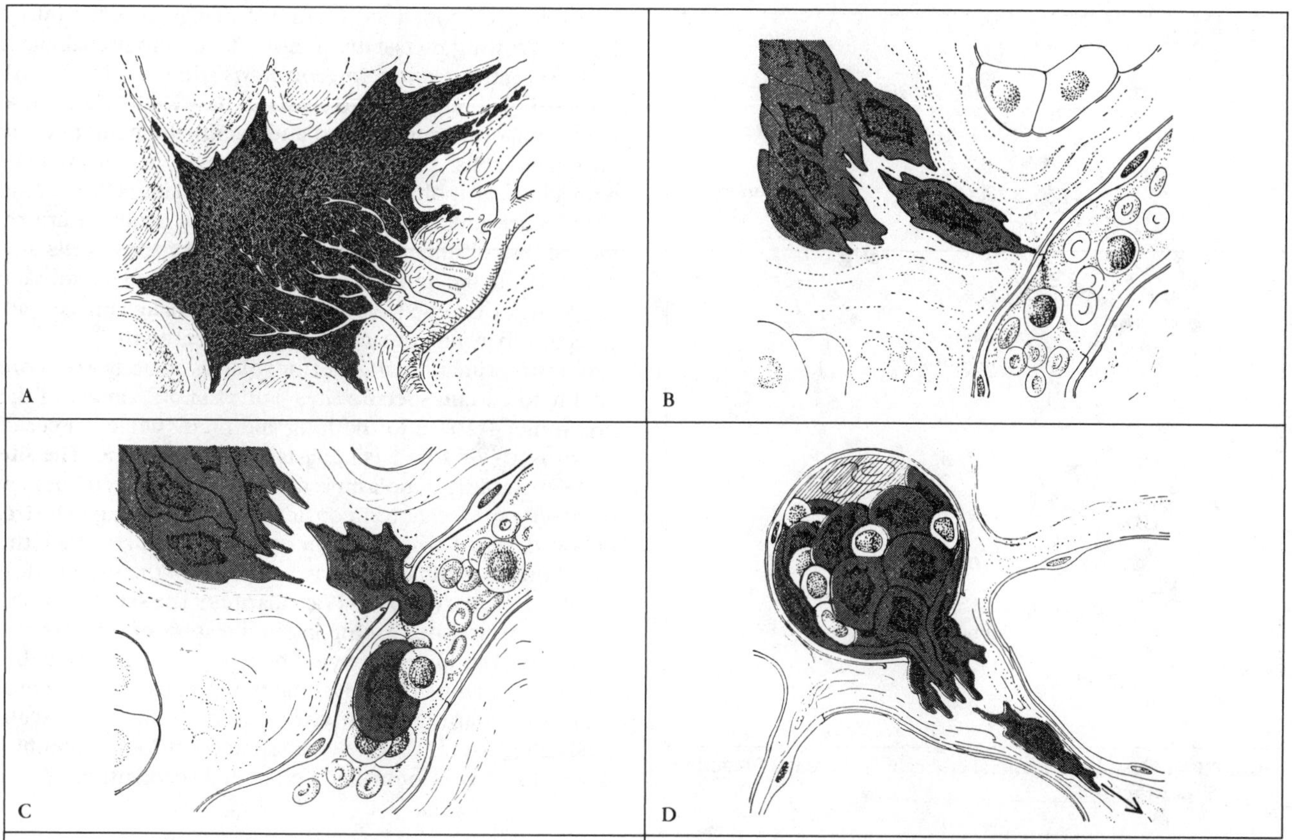

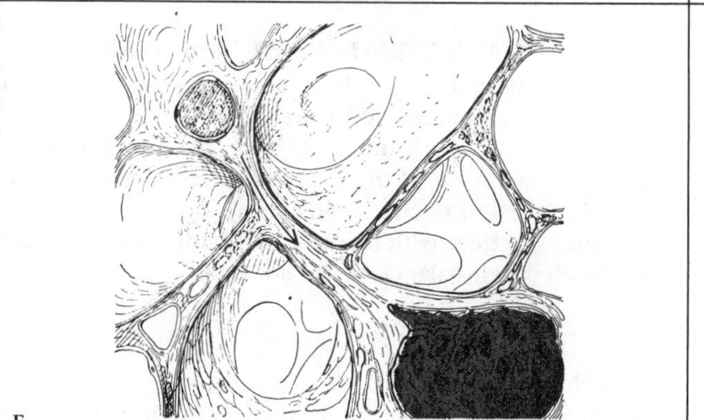

FIGURE 13-3. Stages of bloodborne metastasis are diagrammed. A. The primary tumor enlarges as the malignant cells proliferate, but it grows rapidly only after vascularization provides an adequate blood supply. B. The tumor invades the surrounding tissue. C. A few cells, singly or in groups, penetrate the basement membrane of a capillary, squeeze between the endothelial cells, and enter the bloodstream, where they may interact with blood cells such as lymphocytes. D. In this case, the tumor cells are carried through the heart to the lung, where they are arrested in a capillary; tumor cells penetrate the capillary wall. E. The cells then enter the alveolar tissue and proliferate to establish a new tumor colony. (From G. L. Nicolson, Cancer metastasis. *Sci. Am.* 240:70, 1979.)

in neoplastic immunity, both humoral and cellular immunity are involved (Fig. 13-4) (see Chap. 9). A few malignant cells do manage to avoid the destructive forces of the human body.

Several theories have been advanced to explain the malignant neoplasm's ability to overcome the immune response of the individual. The *sneaking through theory* very simply states that at the onset, when individual cells are involved, the immune system is not alerted, and then later, when it is, the malignant neoplasm is already too large to be controlled. The *antigenic modulation theory* explains that the malignant cell has the ability to hide or lose antigens when attacked by the immune system. The *antigenic blindfolding theory* discusses flooding of the body with tumor antigens. The antigens then bind to antibodies or receptors on the lymphocytes. This, in turn, prevents the antibodies or lymphocytes from destroying the malignant cells. Because immune responses are under genetic control, it is possible that individuals with a normal immune system do not have the necessary genes to recognize certain tumor-specific antigens. The complement system, a series of blood proteins, is also involved in immune responses. It is possible that a person could produce adequate levels of antibody but lack complement, so that the antibody fails to destroy the malignant cell [8]. The ability of the malignant cell to avoid the defensive mechanisms of the person, then, may involve the tumor-specific antigens, the antibodies, or neither.

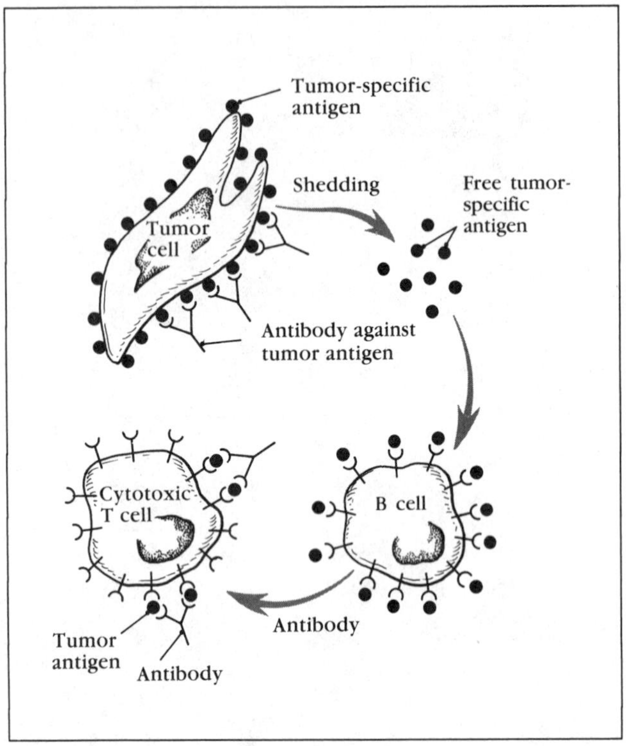

FIGURE 13-4. Postulated humoral and cellular immunity reactions in tumor destruction.

Adherence is also involved in the survival of the malignant cell in the circulatory system, as well as its arrest in the endothelium of the capillary. Malignant cells adhere to other malignant cells and to other normal cells to form clumps. As they enter the capillary bed, they adhere to endothelial cells lining the capillary and tend to become entrapped or arrested in the capillary, as they embolize into the smaller capillary network. After arrest in the endothelium of the capillary, the clump of malignant cells surrounds itself with fibrin, which offers protection during growth.

Initial Establishment and Proliferation

After entrapment in the small vessels of the arteries or veins, the aberrant clump of malignant cells must break through the vessel into the interstitial spaces in order to continue to grow. Cell-free spaces in the endothelial lining of the capillary appear to be induced by the malignant cells, a process that involves alterations in cellular adhesion and consequent retraction of the endothelial cells. A new environment conducive to cellular growth must be established, once the malignant cells are in the interstitial spaces.

Once the growth of the clump of malignant cells exceeds about 2 cm in diameter, it can no longer supply its nutritional needs by diffusion. The development of its own blood supply becomes essential for further development. The establishment of a blood supply is the factor that changes a self-contained clump of malignant cells into a rapidly growing metastatic tumor. The clump of malignant cells secretes *tumor angiogenesis factor* (TAF). TAF causes the blood vessels to send out new capillaries. These new capillaries grow toward and eventually penetrate the malignant cells, providing the clump of malignant cells with a blood supply. As a result the malignant cells become pink, nourishment is provided, and waste products are removed. Establishment and proliferation of these cells also depends on the immunologic and outer cell membrane properties discussed earlier. Thus, the malignant cell adjusts its environment to further its own growth.

Certain primary malignant neoplasms metastasize more readily to certain specific sites. For example, cancer of the breast metastasizes to the lung and brain, while cancer of the prostate or adrenals metastasizes to the bone. The site of the metastatic neoplasm is not randomly chosen but may be based on mechanical considerations involving cell size, pressure, vessel size, and other physical features. Also, the site chosen for metastasis may be similar to the site that fostered the primary growth. Vascularity of the secondary site is a well-established factor in the location of a metastatic neoplasm. The lungs may well be a popular site simply because malignant cells entering the venous system enter their first capillary network there. Other less well-established factors include differences in local immunity and cell surface–controlled cell-to-cell recognition.

CLINICAL MANIFESTATIONS OF NEOPLASMS

In their earliest stages of development, benign and malignant neoplasms are asymptomatic. The mass of cells simply is not large enough to interfere with any bodily function. However, as the size of the neoplasm increases, local alterations in function occur. As malignant neoplasms metastasize, they interfere with function at distant sites and disrupt the biochemical balance of the body.

Local Manifestations

The nature and development of local symptomatology depends on the location of the neoplasm and on the size and distensibility of the space containing the neoplasm. A neoplasm located in the abdomen, which is a large distensible space, may grow to considerable size without producing symptoms. However, a neoplasm the size of a pea located in the cranial vault, a rigid space containing vital sensory and motor functions, may cause major symptoms.

The mass of cells that makes up a primary or a metastatic neoplasm occupies space and compresses surrounding tissues, organs, and their blood supply. The resulting symptomatology is related to interference with blood supply, interference with function, and with mobilization of compensatory mechanisms and immune responses.

Interference with the blood supply to the tissues and/or organs compressed by the neoplasm decreases their oxygen and nutrient supply, resulting in ischemia and necrosis. In addition, waste products are not removed, and lactic acid accumulates. As lactic acid accumulates and blood vessels are eroded the individual experiences pain and bleeding. Ischemic necrotic tissues may become sites of secondary infections.

The symptomatology produced by interference with the function of the organ varies with the organ involved and the degree of interference. A carcinoma of the lung that obstructs a bronchus may cause atelectasis, abscess formation, bronchiectasis, or pneumonitis distal to the site. The obstruction produced by the neoplasm inhibits removal of secretions and bacteria from that area of the bronchus distal to the obstruction. The person experiences coughing, which may or may not be productive, along with signs and symptoms of infection. Infection is a common occurrence in structures obstructed by a neoplasm. Neoplasms of the colon obstruct the bowel. If the obstruction is incomplete, the individual experiences pencil-thin bowel movements, constipation, and cramping. Activated function, rather than an altered function, may occur. For example, compression of nerves or stretching of a nerve-rich membrane by a tumor stimulates the nerve and produces pain.

Compensatory mechanisms also vary with the organ involved. The cramping associated with obstruction of the bowel is the result of increased peristalsis in an attempt to force the fecal mass past the obstruction. Mobilization of the immune system awakens the inflammatory response. As a result, the individual experiences increased pulse rate, increased temperature, and increased white blood cell count.

Systemic Manifestations

Neoplasms have systemic as well as local effects. Systemic symptoms may be the first indication that a person has a neoplasm, or they may accompany the more advanced metastatic aspect of the disease. Some of the systemic symptoms experienced are anorexia, nausea, weight loss, and malaise, as well as signs and symptoms of anemia and infection. These signs and symptoms occur away from either the primary or metastatic neoplasm and are not a direct effect of the neoplasm. The term used to describe them is *paraneoplastic syndromes* [10]. Up to 75 percent of all persons with a malignant neoplasm experience a paraneoplastic syndrome sometime during the time of their illness. Significant features of paraneoplastic syndromes related to the endocrine, nervous, hemotologic, renal, and gastrointestinal systems are explored in this chapter.

Only those hormones produced by nonendocrine neoplastic tissues are paraneoplastic. The symptoms that occur as a result of endocrine paraneoplastic syndromes vary with the hormone produced. For example, all types of lung cancer and small-cell lung cancer can produce adrenocorticotropic hormone (ACTH), causing the person to experience symptoms of Cushing's syndrome, that is, moon face, salt retention, water retention, and so on. Another example is the hypercalcemia or hypocalcemia that can be caused either by the production of a parathormonelike agent or calcitonin by ectopic neoplastic tissues. This type is commonly found in multiple myeloma, breast, and lung cancer [7].

Persons with malignant neoplasm frequently experience neurologic difficulties that most frequently are due to direct effects of the neoplasm, its metastasis, or endocrine, fluid, and electrolyte alterations. However, a small group of neurologic symptoms are paraneoplastic and may be the primary symptom of a malignant neoplasm. The possible neurologic symptoms the person may experience can be grouped or related to the area involved, as cerebral, spinal cord, or peripheral nerve. Some examples of cerebral symptoms are ataxia, dysarthria, hypotonia, pendular reflexes, and dementia. Some examples of spinal cord symptoms are muscular weakness, atrophy, spasticity, hyperreflexia, extensor plantar responses, paralysis. The syndromes associated with the spinal cord may resemble amyotrophic lateral sclerosis. Some examples of peripheral nerve symptoms are sensory loss, weakness, wasting, and areflexia.

Hematologic alterations also most frequently result from the direct effects of the malignant neoplasm, its metastasis, or therapy. Some of the hematologic alterations may be paraneoplastic, and these include an increase in red blood cells (associated with an erythropoietin-secreting tumor), anemia, increase in granulocytes, decrease in granulocytes, increase in thrombocytes, and a decrease in thrombocytes [7]. Symptoms related to the specific alteration are experienced. For example, in the presence of anemia, the person may experience fatigue, cold feet, increased respirations, and palpitations. Coagulation alterations also occur frequently in individuals with malignant neoplasm resulting in either hemorrhage or thrombosis. Disseminated intravascular clotting (DIC) often results from tumor secretions (see Chap. 16). Nonbacterial thrombotic endocarditis, in either the presence or absence of DIC, is another cause of thrombosis or hemorrhage.

Renal paraneoplastic syndromes result from lesions of the glomeruli and obstructions that are caused by neoplasm products. The nephrotic syndrome with proteinuria may be experienced. Hodgkin's disease is the most common neoplastic cause of the nephrotic syndrome. Tumor antigens and other products of the immune response have also been identified in the glomeruli.

Gastrointestinal paraneoplastic syndromes include loss of protein into the gut, malabsorption, liver dysfunction, and anorexia-cachexia. In over 90 percent of advanced cases, afflicted persons have a low serum albumin. Loss of albumin into the gastrointestinal tract occurs as a result of: (1) inflammation and ulceration of the mucosa, (2) intestinal lymph channel abnormalities (usually neoplastic obstruction), (3) congestive heart failure, and (4) a group of unknown origin. The hypoalbuminemia causes edema. The liver may enlarge in the absence of metastatic involvement. Other abnormalities, such as elevated alkaline phosphatase, hyperglobulinemia, hypocholesterolemia, and prolonged prothrombin time may occur. Anorexia, cachexia, weight loss, and taste changes are experienced by most individuals with advanced malignant neoplasia.

The anorexia-cachexia syndrome may occur either early or late in the history of the malignant process. This condition may be the diagnostic manifestation of an undiagnosed malignancy. A wide range of other events may cause anorexia-cachexia, such as chemotherapy, radiation therapy, obstruction of the gastrointestinal tract, and toxicity. About one-third of persons with malignant neoplasms experience negative nitrogen balance. The person experiencing the anorexia-cachexia syndrome has anorexia, loss of strength, loss of body fat, protein, and other nutrients, anemia, water and electrolyte imbalance, and increased metabolic rate and energy utilization.

Taste plays an important role in appetite. Persons with malignant neoplasms may have altered taste perception. A dislike for meats and other protein foods correlates with a lower threshold for bitter taste, while satisfaction with sweets indicates an elevated threshold for sugars. Besides taste, hunger and satiety are controlled by other complex mechanisms, such as the satiety center and feeding center of the hypothalamus, insulin, glucagon, and amino acid levels. The cause of the anorexia-cachexia syndrome is likely to involve alterations in these mechanisms as a result of the impact of the neoplasm.

Paraneoplastic syndromes are seen in all organ systems. Other paraneoplastic phenomena may not be related to an organ system and include lactic acidosis, hyperlipidemia, amylase elevation, and various muscle and joint pains [12]. Fever occurs frequently; paraneoplastic fever refers to an unexplained temperature elevation that subsides with destruction of the malignant neoplasm but recurs with reappearance of the malignancy. It occurs with a variety of neoplasms, for example, Hodgkin's disease, myxomas, hypernephroma, and osteogenic sarcoma.

REFERENCES

1. Althouse, R., Huff, J., and Tomatis, L. An evaluation of chemicals and industrial processes associated with cancer in humans based on human and animal data: SARC monographs. *Cancer Res.* 40:1, 1980.
2. Berenblum, I. Theoretical and Practical Aspects of the Two Stage Mechanism of Carcinogenesis. In A. D. Griffin and C. R. Shaw (eds.), *Carcinogens: Identification and Mechanisms of Action.* New York: Raven Press, 1979.
3. Calman, K. C., and Paul, J. *An Introduction to Cancer Medicine.* New York: Wiley, 1978.
4. *Cancer Facts and Figures, 1982.* Rochester, N. Y.: American Cancer Society, 1981.
5. Folkman, J. The vascularization of tumors. *Sci. Am.* 234:58, 1976.
6. Miller, E. C., and Miller, J. A. Mechanisms of chemical carcinogenesis. *Cancer* 47:1055, 1981.
7. Minna, J. D., and Bunn, P. A. Paraneoplastic Syndromes. In V. T. DeVita and S. Hellman (eds.), *Cancer: Principles and Practice of Oncology.* Philadelphia: Lippincott, 1982.
8. Old, L. J. Cancer immunology. *Sci. Am.* 236:62, 1977.
9. Potter, M., and Cancro, M. Plasmacytomagenesis and the Differentiation of Immunoglobulin Producing Cells. In C. F. Saunders (ed.), *Cell Differentiation and Neoplasia.* New York: Raven Press, 1978.
10. Robbins, S., and Cotran, R. *Pathological Basis of Disease* (2nd ed.). Philadelphia: Saunders, 1979.
11. Tomatis, L., Agtha, C., and Bartsch, H. Evaluation of the carcinogeneity of chemicals: A review of the monograph program of the International Agency for Research on Cancer. *Cancer Res.* 38:877, 1978.
12. Upton, A. C. Principles of Cell Biology: Etiology and Prevention of Cancer. In V. T. DeVita and S. Hellman (eds.), *Cancer: Principles and Practice of Oncology.* Philadelphia: Lippincott, 1982.
13. Weinstein, I. B., Yamaguchi, N., and Gebert, N. Use of epithelial cell cultures for studies on the mechanism of transformation by chemical carcinogens. *In Vitro* 2:130, 1975.
14. Weiss, L. Introduction. In L. Weiss (ed.), *Fundamental Aspects of Metastasis.* New York: American Elsevier, 1976.
15. Whelan, E. M. What is your cancer risk? What factors increase your risk of cancer? How can you protect yourself? *Med. Times* 105:96, 1977.

BIBLIOGRAPHY

Abercrombie, M., and Turner, A. Contact reactions influencing cell locomotion of a mouse sarcoma in culture. *Med. Biol.* 56:299, 1978.

Allison, A. C. Immunological surveillance of tumors. *Cancer Immunol. Immunother.* 2:1, 1977.

Althouse, R., et al. An evaluation of chemicals and industrial processes associated with cancer in humans based on human and animal data: SARC monographs, volumes 1 to 20: Report of an ARC working group. *Cancer Res.* 40:1, 1980.

Baltimore, D. Tumor viruses. *Cold Spring Harbor Symp. Quant. Biol.* 39:23, 1975.

Barrett, J. C., and Ts'o, P. O. Evidence for the progressive nature of neoplastic transformation in vitro. *Proc. Natl. Acad. Sci. USA* 75:3761, 1978.

Barrett, J. C., and Ts'o, P. O. Relationship between somatic mutation and neoplastic transformation. *Proc. Natl. Acad. Sci. USA* 75:3297, 1978.

Berenblum, I. Sequential Aspects of Chemical Carcinogenesis: Skin. In F. F. Becker (ed.), *Cancer: A Comprehensive Treatise* (vol. I). New York: Plenum, 1975.

Berenblum, I. Theoretical and Practical Aspects of the Two Stage Mechanism of Carcinogenesis. In A. D. Griffin and C. R. Shaw (eds.), *Carcinogens: Identification and Mechanisms of Action.* New York: Raven Press, 1979.

Bjekle, E. Epidemiology of Colorectal Cancer with Emphasis on Diet. In W. Davis, K. R. Harrup, and G. Stathopoulos (eds.), *Human Cancer: Its Characterization and Treatment.* Proceedings of the Eighth International Symposium on the Biological Characterization of Human Tumors. Amsterdam: Excerpta Medica, 1980.

Blackman, M. R., et al. Ectopic hormones. *Adv. Intern. Med.* 23:85, 1978.

Blumberg, B. S., et al. Primary Hepatic Carcinoma and Hepatitis B Infection: A Summary of Recent Work. In H. E. Nieburg (ed.), *Prevention and Detection of Cancer* (vol. 2). *Cancer Detection in Specific Sites.* New York: Marcel Dekker, 1980.

Bosmann, H. B. Cell surface enzymes: Effects on mitotic activity and cell adhesion. *Int. Rev. Cytol.* 50:1, 1977.

Brand, K. G. Foreign Body Induced Sarcomas. In F. F. Becker (ed.), *Cancer: A Comprehensive Treatise* (vol. 7). New York: Plenum, 1975.

Brooks, R. F., et al. Mammalian cell cycles need two random transitions. *Cell* 19:493, 1980.

Brunson, K. W., Beattie, G., and Nicholson, G. L. Selection and altered tumor cell properties of brain-colonizing metastatic melanoma. *Nature* 272:543, 1978.

Burch, P. R. J. *The Biology of Cancer: A New Approach.* Baltimore: University Park Press, 1976.

Cairns, J. Review article: Mutation selection and the natural history of cancer. *Nature* 255:197, 1975.

Cairns, J. The cancer problem. *Sci. Am.* 233:64, 1975.

Calman, K. C., and Paul, J. *An Introduction to Cancer Medicine.* New York: Wiley, 1978.

Cancer Facts and Figures 1982. New York: American Cancer Society, 1981.

Carney, D. H., and Cunningham, D. D. Cell surface action of thrombin is sufficient to initiate division of chick cells. *Cell* 14:811, 1978.

Cheville, N. F. *Cell Pathology.* Ames, Iowa: The Iowa University Press, 1976.

Chu, E. H. Y., et al. Mutational approaches to the study of carcinogenesis. *J. Toxicol. Environ. Health* 2:1317, 1977.

Clayson, D. B. Nutrition and experimental carcinogenesis: A review. *Cancer Res.* 35:3292, 1975.

Cleaver, J. E. Human Diseases with In Vitro Manifestations of Altered Repair and Replication of DNA. In J. J. Mulvihill, R. W. Miller, and J. F. Fraumeni, Jr. (eds.), *Progress in Cancer Research and Therapy* (vol. 3). *Genetics of Human Cancer.* New York: Raven Press, 1977.

Clifton, K. H., and Sridharan, B. N. Endocrine Factors and Tumor Growth. In F. F. Becker (ed.), *Cancer: A Comprehensive Treatise* (vol. 3). New York: Plenum, 1975.

Coffino, P., et al. Molecular mechanisms of cyclic AMP action: A genetic approach. *Recent Prog. Horm. Res.* 32:669, 1976.

Cohen, A. J., et al. Hereditary renal-cell carcinoma associated with chromosomal translocation. *N. Engl. J. Med.* 301:592, 1979.

Council on Scientific Affairs. Carcinogen regulation. *J. A. M. A.* 246:253, 1981.

Cronin, R. E., et al. Renal cell carcinoma: Unusual systemic manifestations. *Medicine* (Baltimore) 55:291, 1976.

Cryer, P. E., and Kissane, J. M. Clinicopathologic conference: Malignant hypercalcemia. *Am. J. Med.* 67:486, 1979.

Curatalo, L., et al. Evidence that cells from experimental tumours can activate coagulation factor X. *Br. J. Cancer* 40:228, 1979.

Das, M. Mitogenic hormone-induced intracellular message: Assay and partial characterization of an activation of DNA replication induced by epidermal growth factor. *Proc. Natl. Acad. Sci. USA* 77:112, 1980.

Das, M., and Fox, C. F. Molecular mechanism of mitogen action: Processing of receptor induced by epidermal growth factor. *Proc. Natl. Acad. Sci. USA* 75:2644, 1978.

De Fronzo, R. A. Renal function in patients with multiple myeloma. *Medicine* (Baltimore) 57:151, 1978.

DeLeo, A. B., et al. Detection of a transformation related antigen in chemically induced sarcomas and other transformed cells of the mouse. *Proc. Natl. Acad. Sci. USA* 76:2420, 1979.

Del Regato, J. A. Pathways of metastatic spread of malignant tumors. *Semin. Oncol.* 4:33, 1977.

DeWys, W. D. Abnormalities of taste as a remote effect of neoplasm. *Ann. N. Y. Acad. Sci.* 230:427, 1974.

DeWys, W. D. Working conference on anorexia and cachexia of neoplastic disease. *Cancer Res.* 30:2816, 1970.

Diamond, L., O'Brien, T. G., and Bard, W. M. Tumor promoters and the mechanism of tumor promotion. *Adv. Cancer Res.* 32:1, 1980.

Doll, R. The epidemiology of cancer. *Cancer* 45:2475, 1980.

Drezner, M. K., and Lebovitz, H. E. Primary hyperparathyroidism in paraneoplastic hypercalcemia. *Lancet* 1:1004, 1978.

Easty, G. C., and Easty, D. M. Mechanisms of Tumor Invasion. In T. Symington and R. L. Carter (eds.), *Scientific Foundations of Oncology.* London: William Heinemann, 1976.

Elgjo, K. Epidermal Chalone in Experimental Skin Carcinogenesis. In J. C. Houck (ed.), *Chalones.* New York: Elsevier North-Holland, 1976.

Everson, T. C., and Cole, W. H. *Spontaneous Regression of Cancer.* Philadelphia: Saunders, 1966.

Fidler, I. J. Tumor heterogeneity and the biology of cancer invasion and metastasis. *Cancer Res.* 38:2651, 1978.

Fidler, I. J., Gerstein, D. M., and Hart, I. R. The biology of cancer invasion and metastasis. *Adv. Cancer Res.* 28:149, 1978.

Fidler, I. J., Gerstein, D. M., and Riggs, C. W. Relationship of host immune status to tumor cell arrest, distribution, and survival in experimental metastasis. *Cancer* 40:46, 1977.

Fidler, I. J., and Kripke, M. L. Metastasis results from preexisting variant cells within a malignant tumor. *Science* 197:893, 1977.

Fogel, M., et al. Differences in cell surface antigens of tumor metastasis and those of the local tumor. *J. Natl. Cancer Instit.* 62:585, 1979.

Folkman, J. The vascularization of tumors. *Sci. Am.* 234:58, 1976.

Folkman, J., and Cotran, R. Relation of vascular proliferation to tumor growth. *Int. Rev. Exp. Pathol.* 16:207, 1976.

Foulds, L. *Neoplastic Development.* New York: Academic, 1969 (vol. I), 1975 (vol. II).

Gaddy, D. S. Nursing care in childhood cancer. *AJN* 82:415, 1982.

Gallo, R. C. Terminal transferase and leukemia. *N. Engl. J. Med.* 292:804, 1975.

Garfinkel, L., et al. Cancer in Black Americans. *CA* 30:39, 1980.

Gelfant, S. A new concept of tissue and tumor cell proliferation. *Cancer Res.* 37:3845, 1977.

Gershman, H., Katzin, W., and Cook, R. T. Mobility of cells from solid tumors. *Int. J. Cancer* 21:309, 1978.

Gold, J. Cancer cachexia and gluconeogenesis. *Ann. N. Y. Acad. Sci.* 230:103, 1974.

Gonda, M. A., et al. Ultrastructural studies of surface features of human normal and tumor cells in tissue culture by scanning and transmission electron microscopy. *J. Natl. Cancer Inst.* 56:245, 1976.

Gorden, P., et al. Epidermal growth factor: Morphological demonstration of binding, internalization and lysosomal association in human fibroblasts. *Proc. Natl. Acad. Sci. USA* 75:5025, 1978.

Gospodarowicz, D., and Ill, C. R. Do plasma and serum have different abilities to promote cell growth? *Proc. Natl. Acad. Sci. USA* 77:2726, 1980.

Graham, S., et al. Diet in the epidemiology of cancer of the colon and rectum. *J. Natl. Cancer Instit.* 61:709, 1978.

Gropp, C., Havermann, K., and Scheuer, A. Ectopic hormones in lung cancer patients at diagnosis and during treatment. *Cancer* 46:347, 1980.

Guyton, A. C. *Textbook of Medical Physiology* (6th ed.). Philadelphia: Saunders, 1981.

Haddox, M. K., Magun, B. E., and Russell, D. H. Differential expression of type I-type II cyclic AMP-dependent protein kinases during cell cycle and cyclic AMP-induced growth arrest. *Proc. Natl. Acad. Sci. USA* 77:3445, 1980.

Hall, T. C. (ed.). Paraneoplastic syndromes. *Ann. N. Y. Acad. Sci.* 230:565, 1974.

Hamlin, J. L., and Pardee, A. B. Control of DNA synthesis in tissue culture cells. *In Vitro* 14:119, 1978.

Harris, H. Some thoughts about genetics, differentiation, and malignancy. *Somatic Cell Genet.* 5:923, 1979.

Herberman, R. B., and Holden, H. T. Natural cell-mediated immunity. *Adv. Cancer Res.* 27:305, 1978.

Herberman, R. B., et al. Natural killer cells: Characteristics and regulation of activity. *Immunol. Rev.* 44:43, 1979.

Herbst, A. L., et al. Adenocarcinoma of the vagina: Association of maternal stibesterol therapy with tumor appearance in young women. *N. Engl. J. Med.* 284:878, 1971.

Hitayama, T. Epidemiology of breast cancer with special reference to the role of diet. *Prev. Med.* 7:173, 1978.

Hoeg, J. M., and Slatopolsky, E. Cervical carcinoma and ectopic hyperparathyroidism. *Arch. Intern. Med.* 140:569, 1980.

Holtz, G., Johnson, T. R., Jr., and Schrock, M. E. Paraneoplastic hypercalcemia in ovarian tumors. *Obstet. Gynecol.* 54:483, 1979.

Hoover, R. G., et al. Menopausal estrogens and breast cancer. *N. Engl. J. Med.* 295:401, 1976.

Houck, J. C. (ed.). *Chalones.* New York: Elsevier North-Holland, 1976.

Huberman, M., et al. Herpes zoster and small cell bronchogenic carcinoma. *Am. J. Med.* 68:214, 1980.

Hynes, R. O., et al. LETS Glycoprotein Arrangement and Function at the Cell Surface. In R. A. Lerner and D. Bergsma (eds.), *The Molecular Basis of Cell-Cell Interactions.* White Plains, N. Y.: March of Dimes, 1980.

Isselbacher, K. J., et al. *Harrison's Principles of Internal Medicine* (9th ed.). New York: McGraw-Hill, 1980.

Johnson, P. C., et al. Paraneoplastic vasculitis of nerve: A remote effect of cancer. *Ann. Neurol.* 5:437, 1979.

Kahan, B. Ovarian localization by embryonal teratocarcinoma cells derived from female germ cells. *Somatic Cell Genet.* 5:763, 1979.

Kelsey, J. L. A review of the epidemiology of human breast cancer. *Epidemiol. Rev.* 1:74, 1979.

Kerbel, R. S. Implications of immunological heterogeneity of tumours. *Nature* 280:358, 1979.

Kersey, J. H., and Spector, B. D. Immune Deficiency Diseases. In J. F. Fraumeni, Jr. (ed.), *Persons at High Risk of Cancer.* New York: Academic, 1975.

Klein, G. Lymphoma development in mice and humans: Diversity of initiation is followed by convergent cytogenetic evolution. *Proc. Natl. Acad. Sci. USA* 76:2442, 1979.

Knudson, A. G., Jr., and Meadows, A. T. Sounding board. Regression of neuroblastoma IV-S: A genetic hypothesis. *N. Engl. J. Med.* 302:1254, 1980.

Kopelouich, L., Blas, N. E., and Helson, L. Tumor promoter alone induces neoplastic transformation of fibroblasts from humans genetically predisposed to cancer. *Nature* 282:619, 1979.

Labarthe, D., et al. Design and preliminary observations of National Cooperative Diethylstilbesterol Adenosis (DESAD) Project. *Obstet. Gynecol.* 51:453, 1978.

Liotta, L. A., et al. Degradation of basement membrane by murine tumor cells. *J. Natl. Cancer Instit.* 58:1427, 1977.

Liotta, L. A., et al. Metastatic potential correlates with enzymatic degradation of basement membrane collagen. *Nature* 284:67, 1980.

Lojek, M. A., et al. Cushing's syndrome with small cell carcinoma of the uterine cervix. *Am. J. Med.* 69:140, 1980.

Lowenstein, W. R. Junctional intercellular communication and the control of growth. *Acta Biochim. Biophys.* 560:1, 1979.

Maclure, K. M., and MacMahon, B. An epidemiologic perspective of environmental carcinogenesis. *Epidemiol. Rev.* 2:19, 1980.

Magee, P. N. The Relationship Between Mutagenesis, Carcinogenesis and Teratogenesis. In D. Scot, B. A. Bridges, and F. Sobels (eds.), *Progress in Genetic Toxicology* (vol. 2). New York: Elsevier North-Holland, 1977.

McCormack, R. M., et al. Skin Cancer. In P. Rubin (ed.), *Clinical Oncology for Medical Students and Physicians: A Multidisciplinary Approach.* Rochester, N. Y.: American Cancer Society, 1978.

McKeehan, W. L., and McKeehan, K. A. Serum factors modify the cellular requirement for Ca^{2+}, K^{+}, Mg^{2+}, phosphate ions and 2-oxocarboxylic acids for multiplication of normal human fibroblasts. *Proc. Natl. Acad. Sci. USA* 77:3417, 1980.

Melief, C. J. M., and Schwartz, R. S. Immunocompetence and Malignancy. In F. F. Becker (ed.), *Cancer: A Comprehensive Treatise.* New York: Plenum, 1975.

Merrill, J. M., and DeWys, W. The Paraneoplastic Syndromes. In P. Rubin (ed.), *Clinical Oncology for Medical Students and Physicians: A Multidisciplinary Approach.* Rochester, N. Y.: American Cancer Society, 1978.

Miller, D. G. On the nature of susceptibility to cancer. *Cancer* 46:1307, 1980.

Miller, E. C., and Miller, J. A. The Mutagenicity of Chemical Carcinogens: Correlations, Problems, and Interpretations. In A. Hollaender (ed.), *Chemical Mutagens: Principles and Methods for Detection* (vol. 1). New York: Plenum, 1971.

Miller, E. C., and Miller, J. A. Mechanisms of chemical carcinogenesis. *Cancer* 47:1055, 1981.

Miller, J. A. Naturally Occurring Substances That Can Induce Tumors. In F. M. Strong (ed.), *Toxicants Occurring Naturally in Foods.* Washington, D.C.: National Academy of Science, 1973.

Miller, J. A. Concluding Remarks on Chemicals and Chemical Carcinogenesis. In A. C. Griffin and C. R. Shaw (eds.), *Carcinogens: Identification and Mechanisms of Action.* New York: Raven Press, 1979.

Miller, J. A., and Miller, E. C. Ultimate Chemical Carcinogens as Reactive Electrophiles. In A. H. Hiatt, J. D. Watson, and J. A. Winsten (eds.), *Origins of Human Cancer.* New York: Cold Spring Harbor Laboratory, 1977.

Miller, R. W. The Discovery of Human Teratogens, Carcinogens and Mutagens: Lessons for the Future. In A. Hollaender and F. J. de Serres (eds.), *Chemical Mutagens.* New York: Plenum, 1978.

Minna, J. D., and Bunn, P. A., Jr. Paraneoplastic Syndromes. In V. T. DeVita and S. Hellman (eds.), *Cancer Principles and Practice of Oncology.* Philadelphia: Lippincott, 1982.

Mintz, B. Gene expression in neoplasia and differentiation. *Harvey Lect.* 71:193, 1978.

Mintz, B. Genetic Mosaicism and In Vivo Analyses of Neoplasia and Differentiation. In G. F. Saunders (ed.), *Cell Differentiation and Neoplasia.* New York: Raven Press, 1978.

Modan, B. Role of diet in cancer etiology. *Cancer* 49:1887, 1977.

Moore, D. H. The Mammary Tumor Virus. In A. A. Gottlieb, et al. (eds.), *Fundamental Aspects of Neoplasia.* New York: Springer-Verlag, 1975.

Moses, H. L., et al. Comparisons of RNA metabolism in G_1 arrested and stimulated nontransformed and chemically transformed mouse embryo cells in culture. *Cancer Res.* 39:4516, 1979.

Mulvihill, J. J. Genetic Repertory of Human Cancer. In J. J. Mulvihill, R. W. Miller, and J. F. Fraumeni, Jr. (eds.), *Progress in Cancer Research and Therapy* (vol. 3). *Genetics in Human Cancer.* New York: Raven Press, 1977.

Murray, G. C., and Persellin, R. H. Metastatic carcinoma presenting as monarticular arthritis: A case report and review of the literature. *Arthritis Rheum.* 23:95, 1980.

Nery, R. Carcinogenic mechanisms: A critical review and a suggestion that oncogenesis may be adaptive ontogenesis. *Chem. Biol. Interact.* 12:145, 1976.

Nicolson, G. L. Cancer metastasis. *Sci. Am.* 240:66, 1979.

Nicolson, G. L., et al. Cell Interactions in the Metastatic Process: Some Cell Surface Properties Associated with Successful Blood-Borne Tumor Spread. In M. M. Burger and J. Lash (eds.), *Cell and Tissue Interactions.* New York: Raven Press, 1977.

Nicolson, G. L., Brunson, K. W., and Fidler, I. J. Specificity of arrest, survival and growth of selected metastatic variant cell lines. *Cancer Res.* 38:4105, 1978.

Nicolson, G. L., and Poste, G. The cancer cell: Dynamic aspects and modifications in cell-surface organization. *N. Engl. J. Med.* 295:197, 1976.

Nowell, P. C. The clonal evolution of tumor cell populations. *Science* 194:23, 1976.

O'Brien, P. C., et al. Vaginal epithelial changes in young women enrolled in the National Cooperative Diethylstilbesterol Adenosis (DESAD) Project. *Obstet. Gynecol.* 53:300, 1979.

Odell, W. D., and Wolfsen, A. R. Humoral syndromes associated with cancer. *Annu. Rev. Med.* 29:379, 1978.

Old, L. J. Cancer immunology. *Sci. Am.* 236:62, 1977.

O'Neill, F. J. Differential in vitro growth properties of cells transformed by DNA and RNA tumor viruses. *Exp. Cell Res.* 117:393, 1978.

Osterland, C. K., and Espinoza, L. R. Biological properties of myeloma proteins. *Arch. Intern. Med.* 135:32, 1975.

Patterson, M. C. Environmental Carcinogenesis and Imperfect Repair of Damaged DNA in Homo Sapiens Causal Relation Revealed by Rare Hereditary Disorders. In A. C. Griffin and C. R. Shaw (eds.), *Carcinogens: Identification and Mechanisms of Action.* New York: Raven Press, 1979.

Pierce, G. B., and Cox, W. F. Neoplasms as Caricatures of Tissue Renewal. In G. F. Saunders (ed.), *Cell Differentiation and Neoplasia.* New York: Raven Press, 1978.

Pierce, G. B., Shikes, R., and Fink, L. M. *Cancer: A Problem of Developmental Biology.* Englewood Cliffs, N.J.: Prentice-Hall, 1978.

Pitot, H. C. *Fundamentals of Oncology.* New York: Marcel Dekker, 1978.

Pitot, H. C., Barsness, L., and Kitagawa, T. Stages in the Process of Hepatocarcinogenesis in Rat Liver. In T. J. Slaga, A. Sivale, and R. K. Boutwell (eds.), *Carcinogenesis: A Comprehensive Survey* (vol. 2). *Mechanisms of Tumor Promotion and Cocarcinogenesis.* New York: Raven Press, 1978.

Poste, G., and Fidler, I. J. The pathogenesis of cancer metastasis. *Nature* 283:139, 1979.

Poste, G., and Weiss, L. Some Considerations on Cell Surface Alterations in Malignancy. In L. Weiss (ed.), *Fundamental Aspects of Metastasis.* New York: Elsevier North-Holland, 1976.

Pott, P. *Chirurgical Observations Related to the Cataract, the Polypus of the Nose, the Cancer of the Scrotum, the Different Kinds of Rupture, and the Mortification of Toes and Feet.* London: Hawes, Clarke, and Collins, 1775.

Potter, M., and Concro, M. Plasmacytomagenesis and the Differentiation of Immunoglobulin-Producing Cells. In G. F. Saunders (ed.), *Cell Differentiation and Neoplasia.* New York: Raven Press, 1978.

Rapp, F. Viruses as an etiologic factor in cancer. *Semin. Oncol.* 3:49, 1976.

Recklies, A. D., et al. Secretion of proteinases from malignant and nonmalignant human breast tissue. *Cancer Res.* 40:550, 1980.

Reif, A. Evidence for Organ Specificity of Defenses Against Tumors. In H. Waters (ed.), *The Handbook of Cancer Immunology* (vol. 1). New York: Garland STPM Press, 1978.

Reimer, R. R., et al. Precursor lesions in familial melanoma: A new genetic preneoplastic syndrome. *J. A. M. A.* 239:744, 1978.

Rinkus, S. J., and Legaton, M. S. Chemical characterization of 465 known or suspected carcinogens and their correlation with mutagenic activity in the *Salmonella typhimurium* system. *Cancer Res.* 39:3289, 1979.

Rodgers, J. E. Catching the cancer strays. *Science 83* 4:42, 1983.

Rotkin, I. D. Sexual characteristics of a cervical cancer population. *Am. J. Public Health* 57:815, 1967.

Rubin, P. Statement of the Clinical Oncologic Problem. In P. Rubin (ed.), *Clinical Oncology for Medical Students and Physicians: A Multidisciplinary Approach.* Rochester, N.Y.: American Cancer Society, 1978.

Sandberg, A. A. *The Chromosomes in Human Cancer and Leukemia.* New York: Elsevier North-Holland, 1980.

Schoental, R. The role of nicotinamide and of certain other modifying factors in diethylnitrosamine carcinogenesis. *Cancer* 40:1833, 1977.

Siracky, J. An approach to the problem of heterogeneity of human tumor-cell populations. *Br. J. Cancer* 39:570, 1979.

Slaga, T. J., et al. Inhibition of Tumor Promotion by Anti-Inflammatory Agents: An Approach to the Biological Mechanism of Promotion. In T. J. Slaga, A. Sivale, and R. K. Boutwell (eds.), *Carcinogenesis: A Comprehensive Survey* (vol. 2). *Mechanisms of Tumor Promotion and Cocarcinogenesis.* New York: Raven Press, 1978.

Slaga, T. J., Sivale, A., and Boutwell, R. K. *Mechanisms of Tumor Promotion and Cocarcinogenesis* (vol. 2). *Carcinogenesis: A Comprehensive Survey.* New York: Raven Press, 1978.

Smets, L. A. Cell transformation as a model for tumor induction and neoplastic growth. *Acta Biochim. Biophys.* 605:93, 1980.

Spratt, J. S. The primary and secondary prevention of cancer. *J. Surg. Oncol.* 18:219, 1981.

Stiles, C. D., and Kawahara, A. A. The Growth Behavior of Virus-Transformed Cells in Nude Mice. In J. Fogh and B. Giovanella (eds.), *The Nude Mouse in Experimental and Clinical Research.* New York: Academic, 1978.

Surgeon General's Advisory Committee on Smoking and Health. *A Report of the Surgeon General* (U.S. Department of Health, Education and Welfare; Public Health Service [PHS] 79-50066). Washington, D.C.: Government Printing Office, 1979.

Sylven, B. Biochemical and Enzymatic Factors Involved in Cellular Detachment. In S. Garattini and G. Franchi (eds.), *Chemotherapy of Cancer Dissemination and Metastasis.* New York: Raven Press, 1973.

Tao, T. W., and Burger, M. M. Nonmetastasizing variants selected from metastasizing melanoma cells. *Nature* 270:437, 1977.

Taussig, M. J. *Processes in Pathology: An Introduction for Students of Medicine.* Oxford, England: Blackwell, 1979.

Temin, H. M. On the origin of RNA tumor viruses. *Harvey Lect.* 69:173, 1975.

Todaro, G. J. RNA Tumor Virus Genes (Virogenes) and the Transforming Genes (Oncogenes): Genetic Transmission, Infectious Spread and Modes of Expression. In H. H. Hiatt, et al. (eds.), *Origins of Human Cancer.* New York: Cold Springs Harbor Laboratory, 1977.

Tomatis, L., et al. Evaluation of the carcinogeneity of chemicals: A review of the monograph program of the international agency for research on cancer. *Cancer Res.* 38:877, 1978.

Upton, A. C. Principles of Cancer Biology: Etiology and Prevention of Cancer. In V. T. De Vita and S. Hellman (eds.), *Cancer Principles and Practice of Oncology.* Philadelphia: Lippincott, 1982.

Varani, J., Orr, W., and Ward, P. A. Hydrolytic enzyme activities, migratory activity and in vivo growth and metastatic potential of recent tumor isolates. *Cancer Res.* 39:7, 1979.

Viola, M. V., et al. Reverse transciptase in leukocytes of leukemic patients in remission. *N. Engl. J. Med.* 294:74, 1976.

Warren, B.A., Chaurin, W.J., and Philips, J. Blood-Borne Tumor Emboli and Their Adherence to Vessel Walls. In S. B. Day, (ed.), *Cancer Invasion and Metastasis: Biologic Mechanisms and Therapy.* New York: Raven Press, 1977.

Wattenburg, L. W. Inhibitors of Carcinogenesis. In A. C. Griffin and C. R. Shaw (eds.), *Carcinogens: Identification and Mechanisms of Action.* New York: Raven Press, 1979.

Weber, G. Enzymology of cancer cells. *N. Engl. J. Med.* 296:541, 1977.

Weinstein, I. B., Yamaguchi, N., and Gebert, R. Use of epithelial cell cultures for studies on the mechanism of transformation by chemical carcinogens. *In Vitro* 2:130, 1975.

Weiss, L. Introduction. In L. Weiss (ed.), *Fundamental Aspects of Metastasis.* New York: Elsevier North-Holland, 1976.

Yalow, R. S., et al. Plasma and tumor ACTH in carcinoma of the lung. *Cancer* 44:1789, 1979.

SECTION III

ORGAN AND SYSTEM MECHANISMS

Adaptation and Alterations

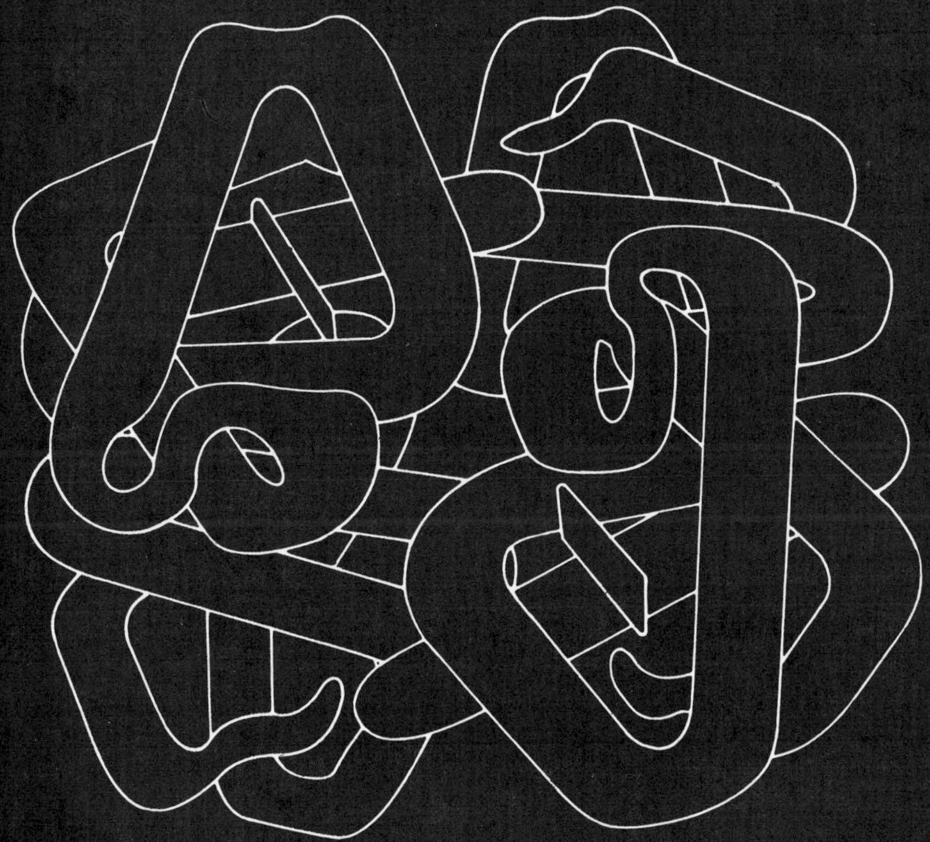

UNIT 7
HEMATOLOGY

Gloria Anderson
ERYTHROCYTE FUNCTION

Marilyn Pase
LEUKOCYTE FUNCTION
COAGULATION

This unit consists of three chapters that deal with the major functions of blood cells. Some of the white blood cells were previously discussed in Units 4 and 5.

Chapter 14 details the erythrocytic activities with special emphasis on the pathologic processes of erythrocytosis and anemia. Descriptions of crucial hematologic studies are included in all three chapters. Chapter 15 expands on leukocyte function and emphasizes nonmalignant and malignant white blood cell disorders. Blood coagulation is explained in Chapter 16, providing a basis for understanding the normal clotting process and coagulation deficiency disorders. The detailed nature of this unit provides for increased understanding of pathologic processes involving blood cell disorders.

The reader is again encouraged to utilize the specific learning objectives as study guides. The unit bibliography presents resources for further study.

CHAPTER 14
NORMAL AND ALTERED ERYTHROCYTE FUNCTION

LEARNING OBJECTIVES

1. Describe the composition of whole blood.
2. List three physical characteristics of blood.
3. List four factors that affect blood volume.
4. Give five primary functions of blood.
5. Explain the stem cell theory.
6. Describe the development of erythrocytes.
7. Explain the structure and function of hemoglobin.
8. List five substances needed for erythropoiesis.
9. Review energy production in the erythrocyte.
10. Give two factors thought to influence erythropoiesis.
11. Explain the meaning of the terms *AB blood, Rh negative.*
12. Describe the process of red blood cell destruction.
13. Describe the factors that may cause erythrocytosis.
14. Differentiate between physiologic erythrocytosis and polycythemia.
15. Contrast erythrocytosis and hemoconcentration.
16. List and differentiate between the morphologic characteristics of five types of anemia.
17. Describe how aplastic anemia can develop.
18. Explain the difference between intrinsic (intracorpuscular) and extrinsic (extracorpuscular) hemolytic anemias.
19. Specifically describe the precipitating etiology and environment that produce sickle cell anemia.
20. Explain why iron deficiency anemia is a common malady in children and young women.
21. Trace the relationship of lack of iron to the morphologic characteristics of iron deficiency anemia.
22. Explain the relationship of intrinsic factor deficiency to the development of pernicious anemia.
23. Differentiate between the etiologies of pernicious anemia and folic acid anemia.
24. Briefly explain why posthemorrhagic anemia may not be seen immediately after an acute hemorrhage.
25. Briefly describe the laboratory findings and diagnostic tests that are helpful in diagnosing red blood cell disorders.

All living cells require materials to survive and to perform functions that are necessary to maintain life. The blood and interstitial fluid provide the means by which essential substances are delivered to the cells and materials not needed by the cells are removed. The transportation of cellular and humoral messages by the blood provides for integration of body processes, thus enabling the body to function as a unified whole.

Since ancient times there has been much interest in and curiosity about the blood and its relationship to life. The blood was known to be essential to human existence. Loss of large amounts of blood became associated with loss of life.

The first description of red blood cells (RBCs) came with the discovery of the microscope by Leeuwenhoek (1632–1723). He examined the blood and described the red corpuscles [14]. Sophisticated and advanced technology of today makes it possible to examine and describe blood components and their functions in minute detail.

The primary role of the blood is to integrate body functions and to meet the needs of specific tissues. Some of the functions basic to meeting this overall goal are the transportation and distribution of numerous substances, for example, respiratory gases to and from the tissues, hormones to body tissues or other organs, and nutrients to the cells; in addition, blood is involved in the regulation of acid-base balance, thermoregulation, and electrolyte distribution. As detailed in Chapter 15, the leukocytes provide a defense mechanism for the body against invading microorganisms. The platelets also help in body defense by attaching themselves to foreign bodies such as bacteria, and in the coagulation process by playing a role in clot formation (see Chap. 16).

Blood is made of a clear yellow fluid called plasma in which cells and many other substances are suspended. Plasma proteins are the major solutes in plasma and consist primarily of albumins, globulins, and fibrinogen. The composition of plasma is very similar to that of interstitial fluid, with the exception of the protein concentration, which is greater in the plasma. This higher concentration of proteins in the blood holds fluid within the capillary by exertion of colloid osmotic pressure. In addition to holding water within the intravascular spaces, the plasma proteins also bind insoluble substances such as lipids, transport iron, and other metals; contribute to viscosity of blood; and provide for coagulation of the blood (see Chap. 16). Plasma proteins also play a role in the regulation of acid-base balance and in immune defense (see Chap. 9).

Blood accounts for about 8 percent of the total body weight [9]. The total blood volume is divided into two main categories, plasma and cells, of which 99 percent are red blood cells. Table 14-1 summarizes the substances suspended in the plasma.

The blood volume is the sum of volumes of plasma and formed elements of the blood within the vascular system. It can be calculated from either the plasma volume or the cell volume, which in the normal adult male averages 45 ml/kg body weight and 30 ml/kg respectively [9].

TABLE 14-1. Some compounds present in human blood

Compound[a]	Concentration and fraction[b]
Acetoacetic acid + acetone ("ketone bodies")	0.2–2.0 mg/100 ml (S)
Adenosine diphosphate	100 μM (E)
Adenosine monophosphate	13 μM (E)
Adenosine triphosphate	1 μM (E)
Aldosterone	3–10 mg/dl (P)
Alpha amino acid nitrogen	3.0–5.5 mg/dl (P)
Amino acid (total)	300 mg/dl (P); 120 mg/dl (E)
Ascorbic acid	0.4–1.5 mg/dl (Fasting B)
Bicarbonate	25 mM
Bilirubin	Direct: 0.1–0.3 mg/dl (S); Indirect: 0.2–1.2 mg/dl (S)
Calcium	8.5–10.5 mg/dl; 4.3–5.3 mEq/L (S)
Carbon dioxide	26–28 mEq/L (S)
Carotenoids	0.08–0.4 μg/ml (S)
Ceruloplasmin	27–37 mg/dl (S)
Chloride	100–106 mEq/L (S); 102 mM (P); 78 mM (E)
Cholesterol	150–280 mg/dl (S)
Cholesterol esters	≅60–75% of total cholesterol (S)
Cobalt	17 μM (E)
Copper (total)	100–200 μg /dl (S); 17 μM (E)
Cortisol (17-hydroxy-corticoids)	5–18 μg/dl (P)
Creatine	40 μM (P); 600 μM (E)
Creatinine	0.7–1.5 mg/100 ml (S); 450 μM (P); 160 μM (E)
2,3-Diphosphoglycerate (DPG)	4 mM (E)
Glucose (Folin)	80–120 mg/dl (Fasting, B)
Glucose (true)	70–100 mg/dl (B)
Iodine (protein bound)	3.5–8.0 μg /dl (S)
Iron	50–150 μg/dl (S)
Lactic acid	0.6–1.8 mEq/L (B); 1 mM (P)
Lead	3 μM (E)
Lipase	Below 2 units/ml (S)
Lipids, total	450–1000 mg/dl (S)
Magnesium	1.5–2.0 mEq/L; 1–2 mg/dl (S)
Nonprotein nitrogen	15–35 mg/dl (S)
Phosphatase, acid, total[c]	Male: 0.13–0.63 sigma units/ml (S); female: 0.01–0.56 sigma units/ml (S)
Phosphatase, alkaline[c]	2.0–4.5 Bodansky units/ml (S)
Phospholipids	145–225 mg/dl (S)
Phosphorus, inorganic	3.0–4.5 mg/dl (adult, S); 0.9–1.5 mM/L (adult, S)
Potassium	4 mM (P); 111 mM (E)
Protein	
Total	6.0–8.0 gm/dl (S)
Albumin	3.5–4.5 gm/dl (S)
Globulin	2.0–3.0 gm/dl (S)
Pyruvic acid	0–0.11 mEq/L (P)
Riboflavin	500 nanomolar (E)
Sodium	136–145 mEq/L; 310–340 mg/dl (S); 140 mM (P); 6 mM (E)
Sulfate	0.5–1.5 mEq/L (S)
Transaminase (serum glutamic oxaloacetic transaminase [SGOT])[c]	10–40 units/ml (S)

TABLE 14-1. (continued)

Compound[a]	Concentration and fraction[b]
Urea nitrogen (blood urea nitrogen, BUN)	8–25 mg/dl (B)
Uric acid	3.0–7.0 mg/dl (S)
Vitamin A	0.15–0.6 μg/ml (S)

[a]The substances and the values listed for them in this table give an indication of the biochemical complexity of blood and are not to be construed as absolute. Blood levels of specific components can vary among normal individuals or in the same individual at different times. Furthermore, the normal values for specific blood constituents can differ greatly among different laboratories, depending on the technique used for their determination.
[b]Abbreviations used for the several blood fractions are: B = whole blood; P = plasma; S = serum; E = erythrocytes.
[c]Activities of over 50 specific enzymes have been detected in various blood fractions, only 3 of which are listed here.
Source: D. Jensen, *The Principles of Physiology* (2nd ed.). New York: Appleton-Century-Crofts, 1980.

A wide variation in normal blood volumes exists because of the following factors:

1. *Weight.* Since fatty tissue contains little water, the total blood volume correlates more closely with lean body mass than with total body weight.
2. *Sex.* Because females usually have a higher ratio of fat tissue to lean tissue the blood volume per kilogram for females is generally lower than that for males.
3. *Pregnancy.* There is a gradual rise in total blood volume as a pregnancy progresses with the greatest increase occurring primarily in plasma volume.
4. *Posture* or *position.* Volume tends to increase when a person is in bed for a period of time and decreases when he or she assumes the erect position. This blood volume change may result from capillary pressure changes that lead to changes in glomerular filtration.
5. *Age.* Total blood volume is higher in the newborn and decreases with increasing age.
6. *Nutrition.* Lack of nutrients may cause a decrease in RBCs or plasma formation, thus decreasing the total blood volume.
7. *Environmental temperature.* The volume of blood increases when the environmental temperature is increased.
8. *Altitude.* At high altitudes the environmental oxygen pressure is greatly decreased and greater numbers of red blood cells are produced for oxygen transport.

Although there are a number of factors that affect the blood volume, it remains relatively stable in each normal person. A number of compensatory mechanisms contribute to this stability; for example, decreased RBC volume is followed by an increased plasma volume, thus returning the total blood volume to its normal level. Capillary dynamics and renal mechanisms play major roles in maintaining plasma volume.

TABLE 14-2. Physical characteristics of blood

Characteristic	Normal	Example of alterations
Color	Arterial: bright red Venous: dark red or crimson	Anemia
pH	Arterial: 7.35–7.45 Venous: 7.31–7.41	Below 7.40 (acidosis); i.e., diabetic acidosis Above 7.40 (alkalosis)
Specific gravity	Plasma: 1.026 RBC: 1.093	
Viscosity	3.5–4.5 times that of water	Increases in polycythemia; decrease in anemia
Volume	5000 ml (70 kg/male) Approximately 3 L in plasma 2 L blood cells	Decrease in dehydration Increase in pregnancy

General physical characteristics of the blood are summarized in Table 14-2. The oxygenated arterial blood is bright red in color, changing to a dark red or crimson color when oxygen is lost and carbon dioxide is added. The pH is regulated within the narrow limits of 7.35 to 7.45 (see Chap. 6). The relatively high viscosity of blood is primarily due to the suspension of cells and plasma components, which causes it to flow more slowly than water.

The circulation of the blood provides for maintenance of a steady state for individual body cells. The constituency of the blood rapidly and continuously changes but the overall concentration of substances remains relatively constant. This constancy in the environment of individual body cells is essential for life.

HEMATOPOIESIS

Bone Marrow

In the adult the bone marrow produces all of the blood cells and platelets. At birth, *red marrow* is found in all bone but much of the skeleton is still cartilage. In the first 3 years of life there is only enough red marrow to keep an adequate production of red cells. After the age of 3 the red marrow becomes more extensive and can accommodate an increased demand for red blood cells. After approximately the age of 5 there is so much reserve that the red marrow begins to change to fat and is called *yellow marrow.* By the age of 20 to 25, red marrow is found in the cranial bones, the vertebrae, sternum, ribs, clavicles, scapulae, pelvis, and the proximal ends of the femora and humeri. In the aged person red marrow begins to leave the cranial bones and lower vertebrae [5]. The marrow then contains mostly blood, hematopoietic cells, and fat. The blood supply to the marrow comes from large-lumened, thin-walled arteries that branch into a network of capillaries to become a bed of sinusoids. Between the sinuses lies the hematopoietic tissue in which the blood cells are formed. The new cells then enter the sinuses through small openings in

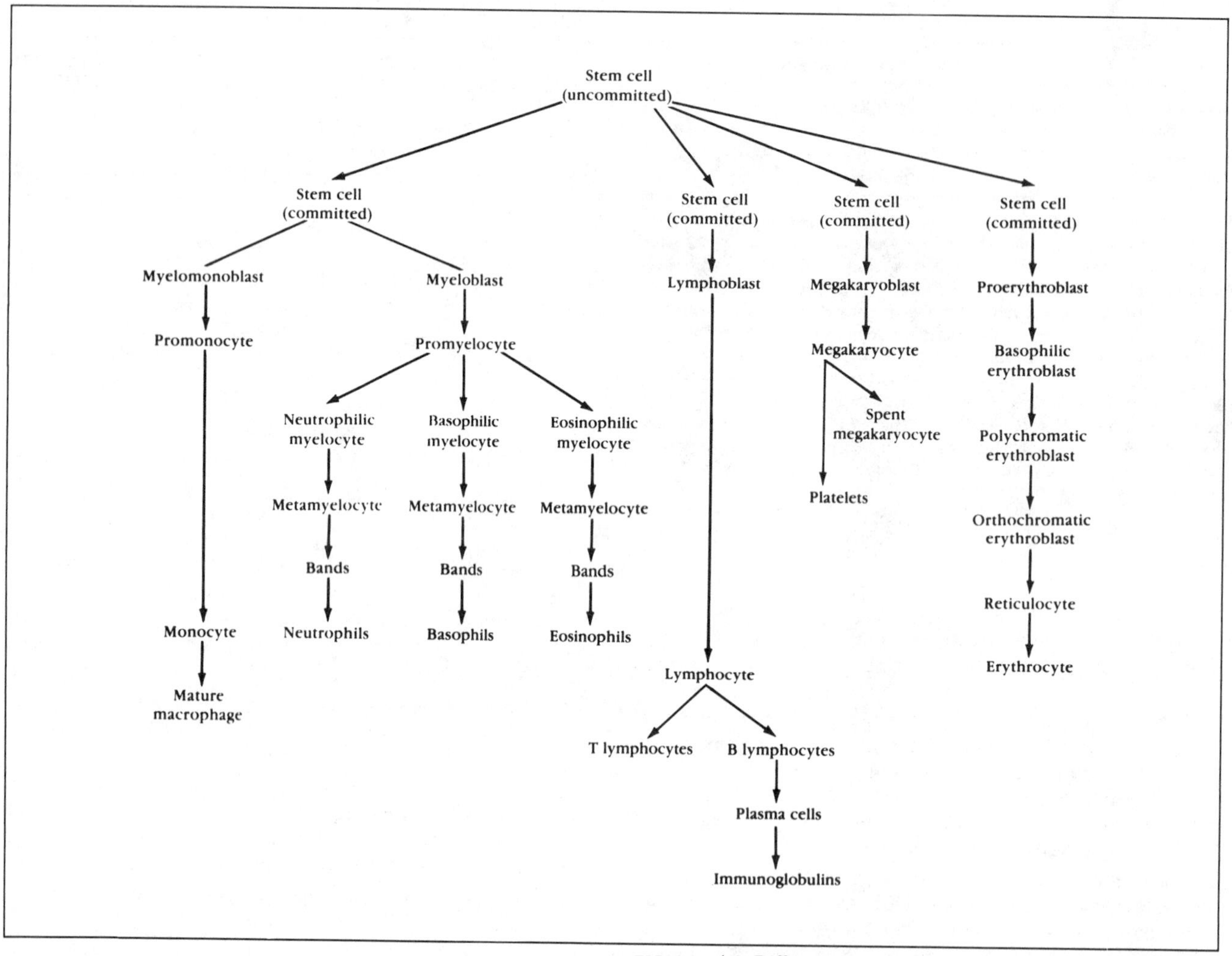

FIGURE 14-1. Differentiation of stem cells in the bone marrow.

the walls. The blood cells gain access to the sinusoids at a critical moment in their maturation phase, and maturation is completed in the circulatory system and tissues. Loss of integrity of the sinus walls may allow the release of immature cells into the circulation.

Hematopoiesis is a dynamic ongoing process with a rapid turnover of blood cells and a constant need for new cells. The bone marrow can meet the body's changing needs for various types and numbers of cells. It maintains a reserve supply of cells for stressful and unexpected situations that create an increased demand for hematopoietic cells.

Stem Cell Theory

Most of the formed elements of the blood have a limited life span. Erythrocytes live approximately 120 days while granulocytes circulate in the blood for an average of 6 hours, then move into the tissues where they may live for several days. Other cells, such as macrophages and lymphocytes, may live months or years. A continual supply of cells is needed to replace lost hematopoietic cells. The original derivation of cells that develop into mature erythrocytes, leukocytes, and platelets has been investigated for many years. The results of study have led to the *stem cell theory,* which helps to explain the various stages of cell differentiation in the bone marrow [6]. Two theories have evolved from the investigations: (1) the *unitarian* or *monophyletic* theory, which assumes that all blood cells are derived from a common stem cell that gives rise to granulocytes, monocytes, platelets, and erythrocytes; and (2) the *polyphyletic* theory, which favors more than one precursor cell for the blood cell lines, from only two stem cells (myeloid and lymphatic) to a primitive stem cell for each type of blood cell [14].

Stem cells may be defined from a morphologic, kinetic, or operational standpoint. *Morphologically,* they have been described as being small mononuclear cells resembling lymphocytes. A small number are normally found in the blood. The ***kinetic*** definition recognizes the stem cell pool (compartment) as able to maintain itself and to pro-

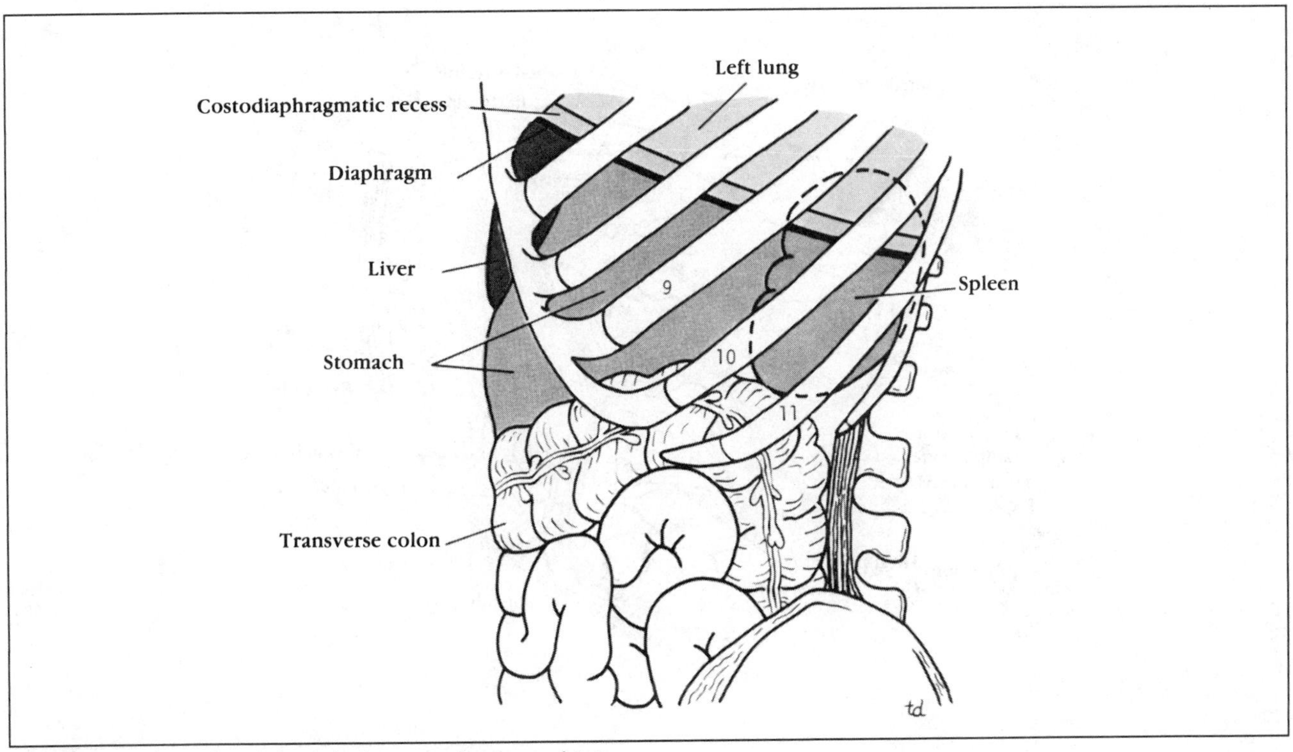

FIGURE 14-2. Spleen, showing notched anterior border, and its relation to adjacent structures. (From R. Snell, *Clinical Anatomy for Medical Students* [2nd ed.]. Boston: Little, Brown, 1981.)

duce differentiated cells. The *operational* definition regards the stem cell as a colony forming unit (CFU). Marrow cells have been injected intravenously into irradiated mice in which the spleen and marrow were reduced to stroma, hematologically empty. Colonies developed in the spleen and later specific differentiation took place. These colonies contained cells for erythrocytes, neutrophils, and megakaryocytes [2].

The stem cell maintains its pool and apparently can recover if it is not lethally damaged [15]. The explanation for this continual supply of cells is unknown. A summary of the stem cell theory is given in Figure 14-1, which is based on the theory that the primitive stem cell is pleuripotential; that is, it gives rise to all mature blood cells. The production and function of the erythrocytes is considered in greater detail in this chapter. The reader is referred to Chapters 9, 15, and 16 for the other blood cells.

Spleen

The spleen is a large, highly vascular organ with lymphoid and mononuclear phagocyte system elements. It is located in the left upper abdominal cavity, directly beneath the diaphragm, above the left kidney and behind the fundus of the stomach (Fig. 14-2). The spleen is covered by peritoneum and held in position by the peritoneal folds. It has a connective tissue capsule from which trabeculae (supporting strands) extend inside the organ and form a framework. Splenic pulp is found in the small spaces of this framework (Fig. 14-3). The major areas found in the spleen are:

1. *White pulp* sequesters lymphocytes, macrophages, and antigen and permits them to interact. Mature plasma cells are found in the marginal zone.
2. *Red pulp* stores and tests the viability of red cells, granulocytes, and platelets.
3. *Marginal zone* lies between the white pulp and the red pulp and receives the terminal branches of most of the arterial vessels. A large blood flow and meshwork structure make this area the major filtration site of blood in the spleen [4].

The blood supply to the spleen is brought by the splenic artery, which divides into several branches before entering the concave side of the spleen; a small portion of the splenic blood passes directly into the sinusoids. This is called the *rapid-transit pathway* because it goes almost unobstructed to the venous collecting system. The greatest portion of the splenic circulation travels the *slow-transit pathway,* which brings it into close contact with the marginal zone, the red pulp, and the phagocytic cells of the white pulp. Much of the plasma and leukocytes is diverted into right-angle branches that lead to the white pulp. Therefore, the blood that reaches the marginal zone and the red pulp becomes concentrated. The arterial capillaries empty their contents into the vascular spaces of the reticular meshwork of the marginal zone and the red pulp. In the red pulp, the capillaries are quite permeable so that blood, including erythrocytes, passes from the capillaries into and

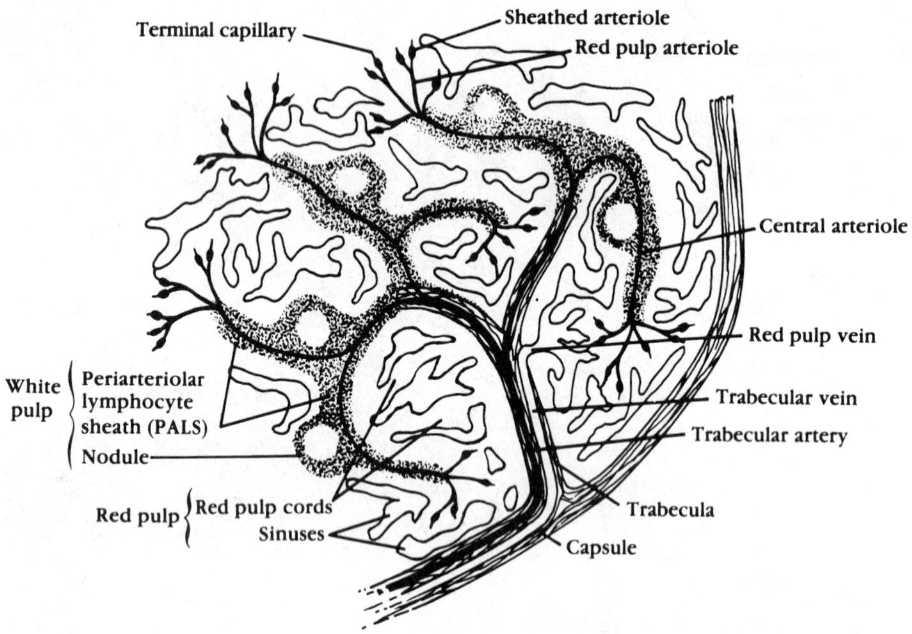

FIGURE 14-3. A schematic representation of part of the spleen showing the relationship of the vasculature to the red and white pulp. (From M. Borysenko, *Functional Histology* [2nd ed.]. Boston: Little, Brown, 1984.)

through the venous sinuses. The capillaries empty into thin-walled veins that finally terminate in the splenic vein, which itself terminates in the portal vein.

Although the spleen is not necessary for survival, four general functions have been attributed to this organ: (1) production of lymphocytes in the white pulp, (2) destruction of erythrocytes in the red pulp, (3) filtration and trapping of foreign particles in both areas, destroying bacteria and viruses, and (4) storage of blood [7]. In fetal life the spleen is active in hematopoiesis, an activity that mostly ends at or before birth. The stasis of blood flow through the marginal zone and the red pulp provides an opportunity for phagocytosis by the phagocytic cells. The destruction of old and imperfect red blood cells is sometimes referred to as "culling." Reticulocytes and many platelets are stored in the spleen. The normal adult spleen holds about 150 to 200 ml of blood, but this volume can increase in pathologic states such as congestive heart failure.

The spleen is a nonmuscular organ and consequently does not contract in times of stress. The storage and release of blood is thought to be related to passive dilatation of the organ, and/or dilatation and constriction of vessels within the spleen.

ERYTHROPOIESIS

Description of Erythrocytes

Erythrocytes are nonnucleated biconcave disks. This shape provides a large surface-to-volume ratio that permits distortion of the cell without stretching of the membrane. The red blood cell has the ability to traverse very small capillaries and the normal cells adapt to the sinusoids of the spleen, escaping without being trapped and destroyed. The unique shape of the erythrocyte is also conducive to gas exchange. The membrane is made of lipids and proteins with the lipid layer located between the two protein layers. The erythrocyte contains hemoglobin, which binds loosely with oxygen and carbon dioxide to carry essential gases to and away from the tissues.

Development of Erythrocytes

Erythrocytes are formed in the blood islands of the yolk sacs during the first several prenatal weeks of life. During the second trimester of pregnancy fetal RBC production occurs in the liver, spleen, and lymph nodes. After birth the bone marrow becomes the principal site of RBC production. After adolescence the red marrow of the membranous bones, especially the pelvic bone, sternum, ribs, and vertebrae, take over the major erythropoietic function. This marrow cell pool provides a constant supply of peripheral red blood cells.

The forerunner of the mature RBC is derived from a stem cell, which proceeds through several divisions and differentiations prior to reaching the final stage of maturity (Fig. 14-4). During the process of maturation the nucleus decreases in size, the total size of the cell shrinks, the

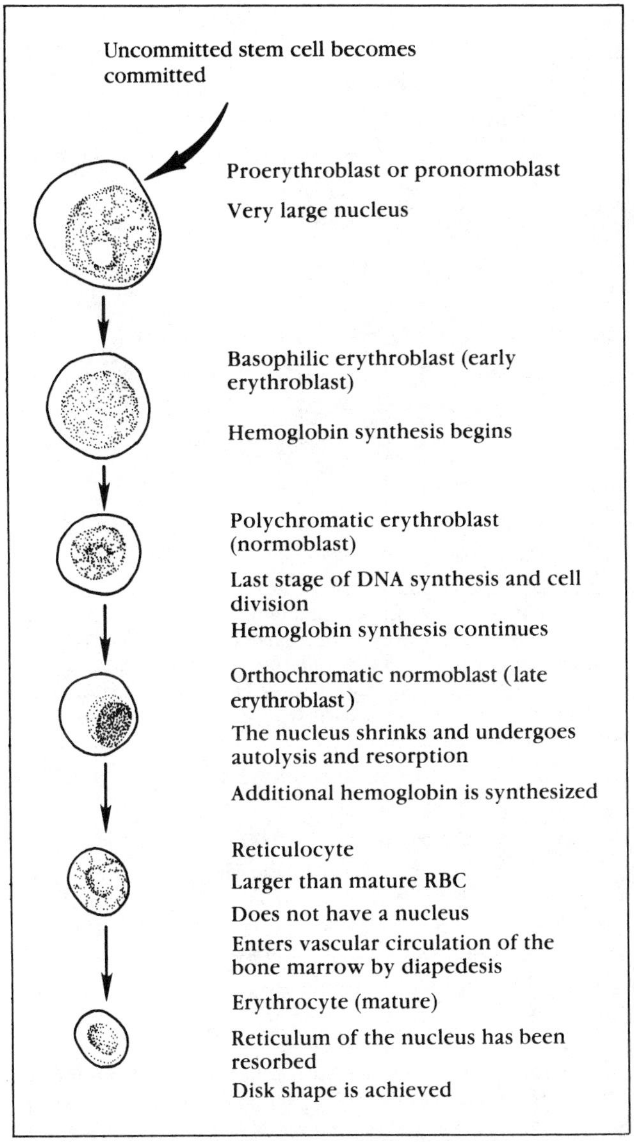

FIGURE 14-4. Development of red blood cells.

amount of ribonucleic acid (RNA) lessens, and hemoglobin synthesis increases.

The maturational process of the RBC appears to follow the following sequence:

1. *Proerythroblast.* This is the most immature cell of the erythropoietic developmental process and is formed from the stem cell located in the bone marrow. The nucleus occupies the greatest portion of this cell; it is large, centrally located, and contains from one to five nucleoli that are not clearly separated from the rest of the nucleus.
2. *Basophilic erythroblast.* The nucleus becomes smaller and the synthesis of hemoglobin is begun. These cells contain small pinocytic vesicles that are thought to be involved in the uptake of ferritin.
3. *Polychromatic erythroblast.* The nucleus becomes even smaller and more dense. This cell contains a mixture of basophilic material and red hemoglobin, giving it the name *polychromatic.*
4. *Late orthochromatic normoblast.* Hemoglobin synthesis is almost complete, reaching a concentration of 34 percent of the cell volume. The nucleus continues to shrink and often assumes an odd shape before being lost. The nucleus migrates into a pseudopodlike protrusion from the cytoplasm. It is surrounded by a cytoplasmic membrane, which degenerates; the freed nucleus is ingested by surrounding macrophages.
5. *Reticulocyte.* This is a large, nonnucleated immature cell with basophilic reticulum scattered among the hemoglobin in the cytoplasm. It remains in the marrow approximately 1 day and then in the bloodstream 1 day before becoming a mature RBC.
6. *Erythrocyte.* This cell follows the resorption of the reticulum found in the reticulocyte. It is shaped like a biconcave disk that is capable of altering its shape without damage to the membrane.

Hemoglobin

Hemoglobin is a conjugated protein with a molecular weight of approximately 64,500. The synthesis of hemoglobin begins in the erythroblast and continues through the normoblast stage. Small amounts of hemoglobin are formed for a day or so by the reticulocytes. There are two parallel processes involved in hemoglobin synthesis, the formation of the porphyrin structure (heme) that contains iron, and formation of the polypeptide chains that make up globin (Fig. 14-5). The adult hemoglobin molecule (HbA) is composed of a globin (made of two alpha and two beta large polypeptide chains) with four heme (iron porphyrin) complexes. One iron atom is present for each heme molecule. Each of the four iron atoms of the molecule combines reversibly with an atom of oxygen. When oxygen concentration is high, as in the lungs, the oxygen combines with hemoglobin, but when oxygen concentration is lower, as in the tissues, the oxygen is released. In the lungs about 95 percent of the hemoglobin becomes saturated with oxygen. The high density of hemoglobin in each red blood cell allows the transport of a large amount of oxygen. The disk shape of the erythrocytes provide a good surface area per unit mass of hemoglobin, enhancing gas exchange.

Substances Needed for Erythropoiesis

A number of substances are essential for the proper formation of the red blood cell and the hemoglobin. Among these are amino acids, iron, copper, pyridoxine, cobalt, vitamin B_{12}, and folic acid. Iron is essential for the production of heme, and approximately 65 percent of iron is found in hemoglobin. The total amount of iron in the body equals about 4 gm with 15 to 30 percent of this amount being stored as ferritin, primarily in the liver. This stored iron is readily available for hemoglobin synthesis when needed through the aid of a beta globulin called *transferrin.*

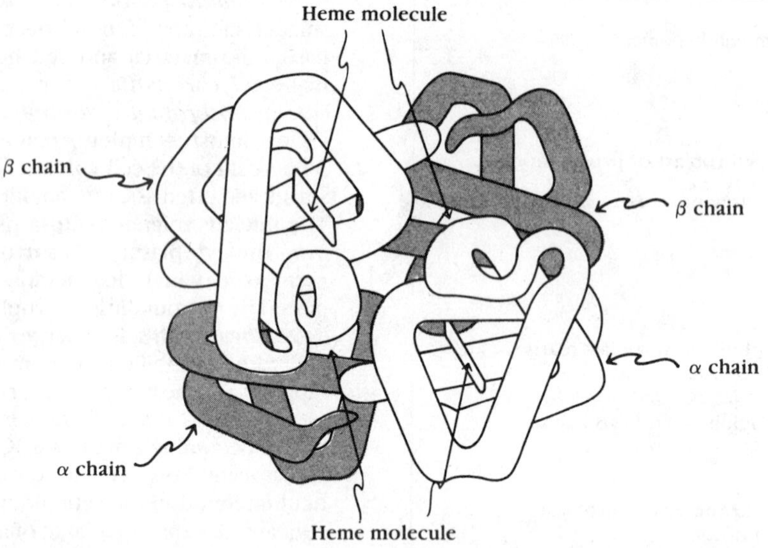

FIGURE 14-5. Structure of the hemoglobin molecule. The hemoglobin molecule is made up of four polypeptide chains. Two identical chains are called α-chains, and the other two identical chains are called β-chains. Each chain encloses a heme molecule. (From G. Schmid, *The Chemical Basis of Life: General, Organic, and Biological Chemistry for the Health Sciences.* Boston: Little, Brown, 1982.)

Transferrin has specific binding capabilities that facilitate the transfer of iron across the membrane of immature erythrocytes. Transferrin also carries the iron released from worn-out erythrocytes to the bone marrow reused for hemoglobin synthesis.

Daily losses of iron are replaced by dietary intake. It is absorbed mostly in the duodenum by an active process that apparently continues until all of the transferrin is saturated. When the transferrin can accept no more iron, absorption of iron almost entirely ceases in the duodenum. Conversely, if the stores are depleted larger amounts of iron are absorbed. The result is a feedback mechanism that keeps a stable level of iron for hemoglobin synthesis [5]. Lack of iron in the diet or poor absorption of iron leads to an iron deficiency anemia (see p. 179).

Vitamin B_{12} (cyanocobalamin) is essential for the synthesis of deoxyribonucleic acid (DNA) molecules in the forming RBCs. This large molecule does not easily penetrate the mucosa of the gastrointestinal tract but must be bound to a glycoprotein known as the *intrinsic factor* (IF) for its absorption. The IF is secreted by the parietal cells of the gastric mucosa and functions by binding to vitamin B_{12} to protect it from the digestive enzymes. After absorption from the gastrointestinal tract, vitamin B_{12} is stored in the liver and is available for the production of new erythrocytes. Long-standing lack of B_{12} leads to maturation failure anemia (pernicious anemia) (see p. 179).

Folic acid (pteroylglutamic acid) is also needed for the synthesis of DNA and promotes red cell maturation. Lack of folic acid causes a folic acid anemia, a type of maturation failure that readily responds to dietary replacement.

Energy Production in the Erythrocyte

Immature erythropoietic cells are comparable to other tissue cells in their metabolic activity but the mature erythrocytes cannot synthesize nucleic acids, complex carbohydrates, lipids, or proteins. Because there are no mitochondria for oxidative metabolism, the energy of the mature red blood cell is generated from the metabolism of glucose by the Embden-Meyerhof (anaerobic) and at least three other pathways that utilize oxygen in different ways. The erythrocyte needs energy to provide for three major functions:

1. Retaining the integrity of the cell. Cationic gradients are needed to balance flow of iron and water across the membrane; for example, maintenance of intracellular potassium and extracellular sodium.
2. Maintenance of hemoglobin iron in the ferrous form.
3. Regulation of oxygen attraction to hemoglobin.

Function of the Red Blood Cell in Oxygen and Carbon Dioxide Transport

Most of the oxygen that crosses the alveolocapillary membrane to the blood combines with the heme portion of the hemoglobin. This combination is in a loose bond called *oxyhemoglobin.* This hemoglobin saturation with oxygen is usually 97 percent in arterial blood, and oxygen is rapidly released when it reaches the tissues, which have an oxygen pressure (PO_2) of about 40 mm Hg. In normal venous blood the PO_2 is approximately 40 mm Hg with a hemoglobin saturation of approximately 70 percent (see Chap. 22).

Transport of carbon dioxide from the tissues on the red blood cell occurs in two major ways: (1) in combination

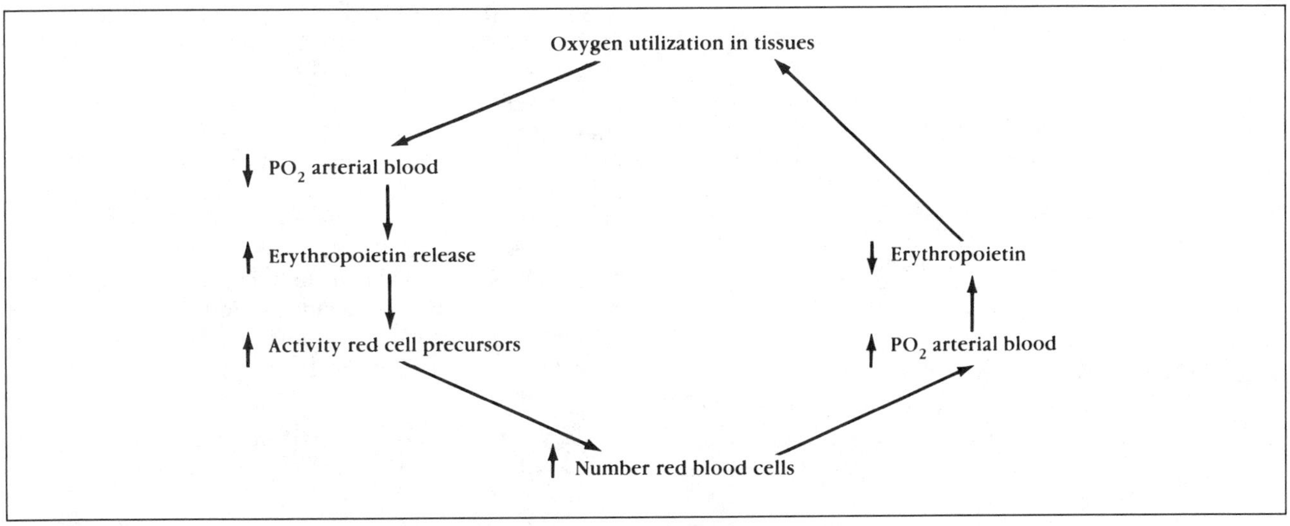

FIGURE 14-6. Feedback mechanism for maintenance of red blood cell population.

with hemoglobin as carbaminohemoglobin (20–25%), or (2) in the dissolved form of bicarbonate (70%). When carbon dioxide is released from the tissue cell it diffuses into the RBC and combines with water with carbonic anhydrase as the catalyst to form carbonic acid. Carbonic acid (H_2CO_3) dissociates into free hydrogen ion and bicarbonate ion. The free hydrogen attaches to hemoglobin and the bicarbonate is free to diffuse into the plasma or attach to a positive ion within the RBC. When it diffuses into the plasma it is usually replaced by chloride in the *chloride shift* (see pp. 306–308).

Factors Influencing Erythropoiesis

The normal life span of adult red blood cells is 120 days. Aged red blood cells are continuously destroyed, and new erythrocytes are regenerated daily for replacements. There is normally little variation in the rate of destruction and production and the total red blood cell mass in the body remains relatively constant. Control of erythropoiesis is affected by the number of circulating red blood cells. Decreased numbers of circulating erythrocytes stimulate the activity of the bone marrow to increase the RBCs. Erythropoiesis also is stimulated by a decrease in the oxygen tension (PO_2) of arterial blood. Over a long period of time, hypoxemia produces an increase in the number of circulating red blood cells.

Erythropoietin, a hormonelike substance, is thought to stimulate the bone marrow through a negative feedback mechanism. (Fig. 14-6). Hypoxia to renal tissue is thought to stimulate the kidneys to release an enzyme called the renal erythropoietic factor (erythrogenin), which acts on a plasma protein (erythropoietinogen) that is produced by the liver to make erythropoietin [7]. The erythropoietin is carried by the blood to the bone marrow where it increases the differentiation of stem cells into erythroblasts and increases the rate of erythrocyte maturation. Erythrocytes are then released into the circulation and hypoxia to the renal tissue is alleviated. Consequently, the stimulus for erythropoietin synthesis decreases and the rate of erythropoiesis is decreased. Conversely, if the volume of circulating red blood cells is increased, erythropoiesis is delayed.

Androgenic hormones also increase the production of erythrocytes and the total blood volume. This seems to account for the occurrence of a higher RBC count in men than women.

Antigenic Properties of Erythrocytes

More than 100 red blood cell antigens have been identified with at least 15 different blood group classifications. The distinct RBC antigenic properties are genetically determined. The antigens found in the blood of one person may react with plasma or cells of another, a situation that often results after a blood transfusion. The antibody to the RBC antigen attaches to the antigenic sites and may cause hemolysis or agglutination of the RBCs. Blood types are classified according to the antigens present on the red cell membrane. Antigens most commonly found on RBC membranes are antigens A, B, and Rh. These make up the O-A-B system of antigens and the Rh system (Table 14-3). A person may inherit neither of these antigens (type O), or may inherit one (A or B) or both (A and B). Type O blood is commonly referred to as the universal donor but the recipient's plasma may contain other agglutinins, which makes cross-matching of blood necessary. Type AB blood, commonly referred to as the universal recipient, contains neither anti-A nor anti-B antibodies but may contain other agglutinins. A person normally develops no antibodies against his or her own cellular antigens but plasma contains antibodies against antigens other than red cell antigens. Rh type is determined by the presence or absence of particular antigens on the red blood cell. Rh negative refers to the absence of these antigens while Rh positive refers to the inherited presence of three dominant mendelian traits.

TABLE 14-3. Blood types

Percent of population	Type
47	O: neither antigen A nor B
41	A: antigen A on RBC; no anti-A antibodies; contains anti-B antibodies
9	B: antigen B on RBC; no anti-B antibodies; contains anti-A antibodies
3	AB: both antigen A and antigen B on RBC; no anti-A; no anti-B antibodies in plasma

Destruction of Erythrocytes

When red blood cells are released into the circulation from the bone marrow they have a limited life span. The metabolism of glucose begins to fail in the aging erythrocytes, causing a gradual decrease in the amount of available adenosine triphosphate (ATP). Without an adequate supply of ATP the cell is no longer able to maintain functions that are essential for life. The fragile cell membrane may rupture when passing through a tight spot in the circulation such as the spleen, or it may be phagocytized by cells in the spleen, liver, or bone marrow. Following lysis of the RBC, the hemoglobin is reduced releasing iron, which is then recycled. After the removal of iron, the remainder of the components in the heme molecule are converted to bilirubin. Bilirubin is taken to the liver to be conjugated with glucuronide (see Chap. 36).

A few RBCs undergo intravascular destruction. When the RBC membrane is damaged the hemoglobin moves out of the cell and quickly becomes bound with a plasma globulin called *haptoglobin*. The resulting complex prevents the renal excretion of the hemoglobin. The complex is then taken up by the phagocytic cells in the liver and processed. Hemoglobin *dimers* that are not combined with haptoglobin rapidly pass through the kidneys and are resorbed by the tubules. When the amount presented to the uptake exceeds capacity, free hemoglobin and methemoglobin appear in the urine [12]. The membranous remains of the RBCs are called "ghosts" when they appear in blood samples.

ERYTHROCYTOSIS

No general agreement has been reached regarding the use of the term *erythrocytosis* versus the term *polycythemia* [13]. Some authorities use the terms interchangeably while others make the clear distinction stating that polycythemia implies an excess of *all* types of blood cells, while erythrocytosis refers to an increase in erythrocytes only. The latter of these two approaches is utilized in this presentation.

The most commonly recognized causes of erythrocytosis are:

1. *Hypoxemia.* A decrease in oxygen availability to the tissue cells causes an increase in blood levels of erythropoietin, stimulating the marrow to produce more red blood cells and causing release of increased numbers of reticulocytes. In the process of acclimatization to high altitudes a reduction in plasma volume, a slow rise in red cell volume, and increased total hemoglobin are seen, resulting in an increase in total blood volume. Hypoxemia is frequently found in persons with pulmonic disease, and many of these affected persons have an associated erythrocytosis. Heavy smokers often have an increased hematocrit level, which is probably due either to an increase in red cell mass or a decrease in plasma volume, or both. This probably results from the high carbon monoxide levels of the cigarette smoke that displace oxygen from the hemoglobin and reduce oxygen content.

2. *Overproduction of erythropoietin.* An inappropriate production of erythropoietin has been associated with renal disease, tumors, or other conditions where there is a disturbance of renal blood flow.

The elevated RBC count seen with dehydration and with burns results from loss of plasma and returns to normal with reexpansion of the plasma volume. This is more properly termed *hemoconcentration* rather than erythrocytosis.

Polycythemia Vera

Polycythemia vera is considered to be a myeloproliferative disorder in which there is an increased production of all the formed elements (RBCs, granulocytes, and platelets) of blood. The etiology of this condition is unknown. It is a relatively rare disease that is found more frequently in males between the ages of 40 and 60.

The abnormal proliferation often initially involves both white and red elements of the marrow. Thrombocytosis and erythrocytosis may be double the normal value. Current evidence supports the belief that the disease is a neoplastic stem cell disorder that suppresses the normal stem cells [12].

The result of the proliferating cellular elements is an increase in RBC count, increased blood viscosity, and increased blood volume. The liver and spleen become congested and packed with RBCs. The thick blood causes stasis and thrombosis in many areas, which may lead to infarction in any area. The course of the disease may change, resulting in aplastic, fibrotic, or even leukemic bone marrow [12]. The leukemic change has been questioned and some authorities doubt the conversion of polycythemia vera to chronic granulocytic leukemia [13].

The onset of signs and symptoms of polycythemia vera is insidious. Most symptoms appear to be related to the increased blood volume and changes in cerebral blood flow. Light-headedness, visual disturbances, headaches, and vertigo may be described. A ruddy cyanosis of the face is usually apparent. Pruritus is a common complaint and may be the reason for seeking medical advice. Thrombophlebitis and thrombosis of digital arteries, accompanied by gangrene, may occur. Associated laboratory values are increased hematocrit, hemoglobin, red cell mass, leukocytes, thrombocytes, leukocyte alkaline phosphatase, serum B_{12} and B_{12}-binding protein, and uric acid. The RBC count may be 7 to 9 million/μl or higher; sedimentation rate is decreased and the blood volume is elevated.

ANEMIAS

Anemia ordinarily refers to a decrease in hemoglobin concentration, a decrease in the number of circulating RBCs, or a decrease in volume of packed cells (hematocrit) compared to a normal group. Anemias are generally categorized according to etiology and/or morphology (Table 14-4). The etiologic approach is to first determine the underlying mechanism of the disease, for example, decreased production, abnormal maturation, or early destruction of RBCs. The reticulocyte count is of primary importance in diagnosis. Size, shape, color, and hemoglobin content of RBCs as determined on blood smear is the primary means of diagnosis used in the morphologic approach. Morphologic characteristics of red blood cells are usually used in the classification of anemias. The terms used include the following:

1. *Normocytic/normochromic*—normal size and color imparted from hemoglobin concentration
2. *Microcytic/hypochromic*—small red blood cells with decreased color due to inadequate hemoglobin concentrations
3. *Macrocytic*—large red blood cells
4. *Anisocytosis*—variations in red blood cell sizes
5. *Poikilocytosis*—variations in red blood cell shapes

Alterations in RBC size or hemoglobin content are commonly seen in anemias related to deficiencies of iron, folate, or vitamin B_{12}. The shape of the RBC cells gives valuable clues in diagnosis of inherited membrane abnormalities, hemolytic anemias, and hemoglobinopathies. In addition, the blood smear provides information regarding red cell inclusions. Increased stimulus for erythrocyte production is indicated by an increased number of reticulocytes (polychromomatophilia) or normoblasts in the peripheral blood.

Aplastic Anemia

Aplastic anemia occurs as a result of a reduction in bone marrow function and causes a decline in all of the blood elements. The blood-forming cells do not mature. A severe anemia results with the formed RBCs in the blood being normocytic and normochromic.

The cause of aplastic anemia is poorly understood. Genetic failure of bone marrow development or injury to the stem cells may prohibit their reproduction and differentiation. Physical agents such as whole-body radiation have been implicated. Chemical agents that may cause aplastic anemia include cytotoxic drugs used for treatment of malignant disease, antimicrobial agents such as chloramphenicol, anticonvulsants, and anti-inflammatory drugs. Aplastic anemia may also occur as a complication of infections, for example, viral hepatitis.

TABLE 14-4. Classification of anemias

Type	Morphologic characteristics	Causes
Aplastic anemia	Normocytic, normochromic RBCs, depletion of leukocytes and platelets	1. Drug toxicity 2. Genetic failure 3. Radiation 4. Chemicals 5. Infections
Hemolytic anemia	Normocytic, normochromic, number reticulocytes	1. Mechanical injury 2. RBC antigen-antibody reaction 3. Complement binding 4. Chemical reactions 5. Hereditary membrane defects
Macrocytic or megaloblastic; pernicious or folic acid anemia	Macrocytic with variation in size (anisocytosis) and shape (poikilocytosis) of RBC	1. Inadequate diet 2. Lack of intrinsic factor for pernicious anemia 3. Impaired absorption
Microcytic anemia; iron deficiency; chronic blood loss	Microcytic, hypochromic	1. Inadequate diet 2. Blood loss-chronic 3. Increased need
Posthemorrhagic; acute hemorrhage	Normocytic, normochromic, ↑ number reticulocytes within 48–72 hours	1. Loss of blood leading to hemodilution from interstitial fluid within 48–72 hours 2. Internal or external hemorrhage leading blood volume depletion

Key: ↑ = increased.

A routine blood examination followed with marrow aspiration and biopsy provide essential information regarding bone marrow function. The marrow is hypocellular or, in rare cases, hypercellular. The marrow biopsy reveals large areas of fat with clusters of lymphocytes, reticular cells, and plasma cells. There is decreased uptake of iron by the marrow and serum iron is increased. RBC smears show normocytic, normochromic cells that are profoundly decreased in number.

The onset of symptoms is variable and usually develops gradually. Symptoms are usually associated with the progressive anemia and the concomitant decrease in oxygen transport. Weakness, dyspnea, headaches, and syncope are common. Symptoms resulting from leukopenia include decreased immunologic defense and recurrent infections. The thrombocytopenia is variable with bleeding tendencies ranging from formation of small petechiae to severe bleeding.

Bone marrow transplantation may be a practicable option for the younger individual if a compatible family donor is available. Blood components may be replaced by use of blood transfusions to allow time for recovery of the bone marrow in situations of transient bone marrow failure. Drugs and other chemical agents should be discontinued. Splenectomy may be indicated if active hemolysis is associated. The prognosis of aplastic anemia varies with the causative agent. Gradual recovery of the hematopoietic function can occur once the agent has been discontinued. Severe, progressive anemia is a poor prognostic sign, although infection and hemorrhage are the most frequent causes of death.

Hemolytic Anemia

The life span of the RBC may be shortened by intrinsic or extrinsic factors that adversely affect the cell; the shortening may be compensated for by an increase in erythrocyte production. However, when erythrocyte survival is shortened to 20 days or less, hemolytic anemia results [11]. Increased erythropoiesis becomes unable to compensate for the rapid RBC destruction.

There are a number of ways to classify hemolytic anemias. Categories often overlap and no classification seems to be completely satisfactory. The most commonly used classification is the extrinsic (extracorpuscular) group that is usually acquired and the intrinsic (intracorpuscular) group that is usually inherited. Another useful classification from a clinical standpoint is antibody-mediated and non-antibody-mediated hemolytic anemias. Coombs' test is used to determine the presence or absence of antibody mediation [11]. A third classification utilizes the primary mechanisms of red cell injury to separate each group [1]. The intracorpuscular and extracorpuscular classification will be used in this presentation.

INTRACORPUSCULAR (INTRINSIC) DEFECTS. This classification of hemolytic anemias represents those primarily inherited disorders of the red cell membrane, abnormalities of red cell enzymes, and abnormalities of hemoglobin. The two major disease processes included in this group are sickle cell anemia and the group of thalassemias.

Sickle syndromes. Two related genetic disorders are described as sickle syndromes; sickle cell trait and sickle cell anemia. These syndromes are found almost exclusively in the black race and are demonstrated by the bizarre shape assumed by the RBC when it is exposed to a decreased oxygen tension. About 10 percent of American blacks carry the gene HbS with approximately 0.2 percent exhibiting the actual disease [12]. The sickle cell trait is carried by heterozygous individuals; sickle cell anemia occurs when the individual is homozygous.

Persons having the sickle cell trait usually exhibit no symptoms unless they suffer a hypoxic episode during which some hemolysis and anemia may be exhibited. The heterozygous red blood cells require a very low oxygen tension to precipitate the characteristic sickling effect so that RBC life span is usually not affected.

Sickle cell anemia causes a shortened life expectancy with symptoms beginning at approximately 6 months of age. It involves the substitution of an amino acid on the beta chain of the globin molecule. The resulting hemoglobin, called *HbS,* when deoxygenated undergoes gelation or crystallization, which distorts the red blood cell into a sickled or holly-leaf shape. When there is a significant disparity between the oxygen needed by the cells and the amount of oxygen available, the cells become rigid and take on bizarre shapes. Small blood vessels become blocked by aggregates of these sickle cells and blood supply to all parts of the body may be compromised. The damaged RBCs are trapped in the spleen and eventually the entire organ may become infarcted.

Infections or hypertonic plasma greatly enhances the chances of sickling. As the RBCs obstruct blood flow to the tissues further deoxygenation and more sickling occurs. The characteristic sickle shape usually returns to normal when oxygen again becomes available.

Hemolysis occurs when the RBCs assume the sickled form and average RBC survival time becomes 10 to 15 days. Bilirubin is released from the hemoglobin during hemolysis and jaundice may become evident when increased conjugated and unconjugated bilirubin accumulates in the plasma.

The bone marrow often becomes hyperplastic with evidence of increased erythropoiesis. Reticulocytes and even normoblasts may be released into the circulating blood.

The signs and symptoms of sickle cell anemia vary in severity from sickle crisis in acute hemolysis to impairment of growth and maturity. Susceptibility to infections, especially those caused by pneumococci, causes repeated episodes of painful crisis. These result from microinfarcts from the vasoocclusive phenomenon [3]. Anemia is usually severe with most of the hemolysis occurring in the extravascular spaces. Chronic leg ulcers, attacks of abdominal pain, and neurologic complications of sudden onset are common. Joint pains may mimic osteomyelitis and joint effusions are frequent. Chronic organ damage may affect any organ. The splenic function is markedly impaired. Renal isosthenuria characteristically contributes to the dehydration and sometimes leads to frank renal failure (see Chap. 29). The prognosis for sickle cell anemia is improving with more individuals surviving to adulthood with supportive care.

THALASSEMIAS. These intrinsic, congenital disorders result from defects in the synthesis of hemoglobin and cause a hypochromic, microcytic anemia. Both beta and alpha chain defects are known. Those involving defect of beta chain synthesis are found most frequently in inhabitants of the Mediterranean areas, Central Africa, Asia, the South Pacific, and parts of India [3]. Defects in alpha chain synthesis are found most frequently among southern Orientals. The effects vary markedly depending on whether they are heterozygous or homozygous in presentation. Severe forms exhibit ineffective erythropoiesis and peripheral hemolysis, which stimulates enlargement of the red marrow to increase RBC formation. Sometimes the liver also becomes involved in erythropoiesis resulting in hepatomegaly [3]. Clinical manifestations include anemia, wasting, jaundice, hepatomegaly, and characteristic "chipmunk" faces (due to enlargement of marrow of molar bones of jaws).

Extracorpuscular (Extrinsic) Defects

Extracorpuscular (extrinsic, acquired) hemolytic anemias result from a wide range of causes, such as infections, transfusion reaction, systemic disease, trauma, liver or renal disease, snake or spider venom, or drugs. Many of these conditions are discussed in other sections of this book.

Trauma to circulating RBCs has been reported from prolonged exercise, artificial cardiac valves, extracorporeal circulation devices, and conditions in which fibrin deposited in the microvasculature causes fragmentation of RBCs. The results include mild to severe hemolysis and bilirubinemia. The degree of the hemolysis is related to the severity of the symptomatology; for example, artificial cardiac valves may be replaced if significant hemolysis continues.

Maturation Failure

PERNICIOUS ANEMIA. Vitamin B_{12} deficiency may occur as a result of decreased dietary intake or of malsorption factors. *Pernicious anemia*, which results from this deficiency, is most frequently seen in persons over the age of 60 who have fair complexions and a family history of the disease. It is currently thought to result from an autoimmune reaction against the gastric parietal cells [1].

Normally, vitamin B_{12} binds chemically with the intrinsic factor that enhances its absorption. In certain conditions, such as atrophy of the gastric mucosal cells, lack of secretion of the intrinsic factor leads to malsorption of vitamin B_{12}. Normal erythrocyte maturation is dependent on adequate amounts of vitamin B_{12} for the synthesis of deoxyribonucleic acid (DNA) molecules. Without the B_{12} a macrocytic or megaloblastic anemia results with marked anisocytosis and poikilocytosis. Ineffective erythropoiesis and enhanced erythroblast destruction result in hyperbilirubinemia. Although the most pronounced changes are seen in the RBCs, a mild neutropenia and thrombocytopenia may also be seen.

The onset of symptoms is usually insidious but the onset may be hastened by conditions such as infection. Persons with pernicious anemia do not secrete hydrochloric acid (on gastric analysis) even after parenteral stimulation with histamine. Many of the signs and symptoms of pernicious anemia are common to any of the anemic states. Anorexia, fatigue, shortness of breath, and irritability are common. Soreness of the tongue characteristically occurs early in the illness and progressively gets worse. The soreness is quickly relieved after adequate vitamin B_{12} treatment. Numbness and tingling of the toes and fingers are fairly common and indicate early neurologic disease. Neurologic symptoms may not entirely remit following treatment.

FOLIC ACID ANEMIA. A deficiency of folic acid produces anemia with characteristics similar to those of pernicious anemia. The anemia of folate deficiency is also probably attributable to impaired DNA synthesis, and it results in a macrocytic or megaloblastic form of the disease. Dietary deficiency can result in rapid onset of anemia along with a smooth, red tongue and stomatitis. Folic acid anemia usually responds well to dietary replacement unless there is a malsorption problem.

Microcytic Hypochromic Anemia

IRON DEFICIENCY ANEMIA. This anemia is characterized by deficient hemoglobin synthesis due to a lack of iron. With severe deficiencies the RBCs become microcytic and hypochromic because of low concentrations of hemoglobin. This type of anemia is the most common type and occurs in all geographic locations and in all age groups. The main causes of iron deficiency are an increase in the loss of iron, as in chronic or acute bleeding, and a decrease in dietary intake. The intermittent blood loss during menstruation accounts for a high incidence of iron deficiency in women. Iron deficiency is common among preschool children presumably because of increased dietary need and poor dietary supply.

Because iron is absorbed mostly in the duodenum and its ionization and absorption are enhanced by gastric hydrochloric acid, iron deficiency anemia may accompany pernicious anemia or gastrectomy. Also, malsorption syndromes impair absorption of iron along with other nutrients.

Laboratory values reflect a decreased serum iron and apoferritin (iron-binding protein produced by the liver) in the early stages. Anemia, characterized by microcytic, hypochromic RBCs, is a relatively late manifestation.

Clinical manifestations are nonspecific and insidious. Fatigue, tachycardia, irritability, and pallor with epithelial abnormalities such as sore tongue or stomatitis may be seen. Thinning or spooning of the nails (koilonychia) is encountered occasionally. Pica may be striking with affected individuals craving dirt, starch, or ice [8]. Late manifestations may include cardiac murmurs, congestive heart failure, loss of hair, and pearly sclera.

Posthemorrhagic Anemia

Posthemorrhagic anemias may follow acute or chronic blood loss, although chronic blood loss usually results in iron deficiency anemia. Plasma and red blood cells are both lost during a hemorrhage so that laboratory values may reveal a normal hemoglobin level and red blood cell count immediately following a hemorrhage.

Blood volume is restored by the movement of fluid from the interstitial spaces into the capillaries, causing a dilution of the remaining red blood cells (dilutional anemia). This dilute blood carries too few RBCs to be an efficient oxygenator of the tissues. Anemia of a normocytic and normochromic type becomes apparent. The bone marrow is stimulated to produce increased numbers of red blood cells, but this process requires a period of time that varies according to the amount of blood lost. In acute massive bleeding, this compensatory effect may not occur in time to be lifesaving without transfusions of whole blood.

LABORATORY OR OTHER DIAGNOSTIC TESTS

Hematologic Studies

Examination of the blood provides valuable information in the diagnosis and treatment of blood disorders. Normal hematologic values are summarized in Table 14-5. Normal values are based on the examination of statistically significant numbers of healthy persons. Normal values vary with age differences, environment, sex, genetics, and physiologic state. The most important erythrocyte studies are explained in this section.

HEMOGLOBIN. The primary function of hemoglobin is to carry oxygen in the form of oxyhemoglobin; therefore, the oxygen-combining capacity of blood is directly proportional to the hemoglobin concentration. Decreased levels of hemoglobin may be seen in anemia or circulatory overload. Increased levels of hemoglobin are found in persons with polycythemia.

RED BLOOD CELLS (ERYTHROCYTES). The erythrocyte is the mature circulating red blood cell whose primary function is the transport of oxygen and carbon dioxide. Increases and decreases in red cell counts usually vary in the same direction as the hemoglobin as previously mentioned.

PACKED CELL VOLUME (PCV) OR HEMATOCRIT (HCT). The packed cell volume is the ratio of packed cells to total volume in a sample that has been centrifuged. The packed cell volume is used in determining red blood cell indices, in calculating blood volume and total red blood cell mass, and in roughly measuring the concentration of red blood cells [10]. Increased levels are seen in conditions associated with hemoconcentration (burns, shock, and trauma), hypovolemia, and polycythemia. A decreased hematocrit is seen in hypervolemic states (cardiac failure, overhydration with intravenous fluid), hemorrhage, and hemolysis.

SEDIMENTATION RATE (SED RATE OR ESR). Blood is a suspension of formed elements in plasma; therefore, when it is mixed with an anticoagulant and stands, the heavier red blood cells sink to the bottom. The rate at which the settling of the red blood cells occurs is a function of fibrinogen and globulin. These proteins enhance clumping of erythrocytes, thus increasing the rate at which the cells fall. Other factors that affect the rate are alterations in the positive charge of the plasma, the ratio of plasma protein fractions to each other, and changes in the erythrocyte surface.

The ESR is a nonspecific test but because the sedimentation rate is increased in many inflammatory conditions it can serve differential diagnosis in such conditions as acute myocardial infarction and angina pectoris, or rheumatoid arthritis and osteoarthritis.

MEAN CORPUSCULAR VOLUME (MCV). The MCV measures the volume of each red blood cell. An increased MCV is found in megaloblastic anemias (large cells) while decreased MCV is seen in iron deficiency (small cells).

MEAN CORPUSCULAR HEMOGLOBIN (MCH). The MCH gives the amount of hemoglobin by weight in the average red blood cell. Macrocytic cells with large volume of hemoglobin show increased levels as seen in macrocytic anemia. Decreased levels of MCH are found in conditions related to hemoglobin deficiency as seen in iron deficiency anemia.

TABLE 14-5. Normal hematologic values

Red blood cells	
Infant, first day	5.1 ± 1 millions/μl
Child, 1 year	4.5 ± 1 millions/μl
Child, 6–10 years	4.7 ± 1 millions/μl
Adult	
Female	4.8 ± 0.6 millions/μl
Male	5.4 ± 0.8 millions/μl
Hemoglobin	
Infant, first day	19.5 ± 5.0 gm/dl
Child, 1 year	11.2 ± 2.3 gm/dl
Child, 6–10 years	12.9 ± 2.3 gm/dl
Adult	
Female	14.0 ± 2.0 gm/dl
Male	16.0 ± 2.0 gm/dl
Volume-packed RBC (hematocrit)	
Infant, first day	54 ± 10 ml/dl
Child, 1 year	35 ± 5 ml/dl
Child, 6–10 years	37.5 ± 5 ml/dl
Adult	
Female	42 ± 5 ml/dl
Male	47 ± 5 ml/dl
Sedimentation rate (ESR)	
Males	0–15 mm/hour
Females	0–20 mm/hour
Mean corpuscular volume (MCV)	
Males and females	87 ± 5 cuμ
Mean corpuscular hemoglobin (MCH)	
Males and females	29 ± 2 μμg
Mean corpuscular hemoglobin concentration (MCHC)	
Males and females	34 ± 2%
Reticulocyte count	0.5–1.5% of erythrocytes

Source: J. Wallach, *Interpretation of Diagnostic Tests* (3rd ed.). Boston: Little, Brown, 1978.

MEAN CELL HEMOGLOBIN CONCENTRATION (MCHC). This measurement gives the average percent hemoglobin saturation or the concentration of hemoglobin in the average red cell. Decreased levels are found in hemoglobin deficiency.

RETICULOCYTE COUNT. The reticulocyte is a young, nonnucleated cell of the erythrocyte line. An elevated reticulocyte count is indicative of increased bone marrow activity with early release of increased numbers of reticulocytes as is seen in hemolytic anemias.

BONE MARROW STUDIES. Bone marrow may be obtained for purposes of examination by bone marrow aspiration or biopsy. Data obtained from bone marrow examination are very useful in the diagnosis, progression, and prognosis of blood disorders.

Diagnostic Tests

SCHILLING TEST. This test measures the absorption of vitamin B_{12}. Radioactive B_{12} is administered orally and a 24-hour urine collection is begun. The presence of radioactivity in the urine indicates gastrointestinal absorption of vitamin B_{12}. Above 8 percent excretion of the radioactive dose is normal. This test is used in the diagnosis of pernicious anemia.

REFERENCES

1. Babior, B., and Bunn, H. F. Megaloblastic Anemias. In K. J. Isselbacher, et al. (eds.), *Harrison's Principles of Internal Medicine* (9th ed.). New York: McGraw-Hill, 1980.
2. Beck, W. S. *Hematology* (2nd ed.). Cambridge, Mass.: The M.I.T. Press, 1977.
3. Bunn, H. F. Disorders of Hemoglobin Structure, Function and Synthesis. In K. J. Isselbacher, et al. (eds.), *Harrison's Principles of Internal Medicine* (9th ed.). New York: McGraw-Hill, 1980.
4. Dietschy, J. M., et al. (eds.). *Hematology and Oncology.* New York: Grune & Stratton, 1980.
5. Guyton, A. *Textbook of Medical Physiology* (6th ed.). Philadelphia: Saunders, 1981.
6. Jensen, D. *The Principles of Physiology* (2nd ed.). New York: Appleton-Century-Crofts, 1980.
7. Junqueira, L. C., and Carneiro, J. *Basic Histology* (3rd ed.). Los Altos, Calif.: Lange, 1980.
8. Lee, G. R., Wintrobe, M., and Bunn, H. F. Iron Deficiency Anemia and the Sideroblastic Anemias. In K. J. Isselbacher, et al. (eds.), *Harrison's Principles of Internal Medicine* (9th ed.). New York: McGraw-Hill, 1980.
9. Mountcastle, V. B. (ed.). *Medical Physiology* (14th ed.). St. Louis: Mosby, 1980.
10. Platt, W. R. *Color Atlas and Textbook of Hematology.* Philadelphia: Lippincott, 1979.
11. Reich, P. R. *Hematology: Physiopathologic Basis for Clinical Practice.* Boston: Little, Brown, 1978.
12. Robbins, S., and Cotran, R. *Pathologic Basis of Disease* (2nd ed.). Philadelphia: Saunders, 1979.
13. Thompson, R. B. *Disorders of the Blood.* New York: Churchill Livingstone, 1977. P. 713.
14. Wintrobe, M. M. *Blood, Pure and Eloquent.* New York: McGraw-Hill, 1980.
15. Wintrobe, M. M., et al. *Clinical Hematology* (7th ed.). Philadelphia: Lea & Febiger, 1974.

CHAPTER 15
NORMAL AND ALTERED LEUKOCYTE FUNCTION

LEARNING OBJECTIVES

1. List the five types of leukocytes and describe their general characteristics.
2. Differentiate between the leukocytes on the basis of morphology and function.
3. Define the normal white cell count per microliter of blood and explain its significance.
4. Describe the differential white count and list the relative proportion of each cell type.
5. Describe phagocytosis and discuss the significance of this property of leukocytes with respect to the destruction of microorganisms and immunologic integrity.
6. Differentiate between pinocytosis and phagocytosis.
7. Compare the average life span of the five types of leukocytes.
8. Explain the phagocyte properties of locomotion, diapedesis, degranulation, killing, chemotaxis, and opsonization with respect to phagocytosis and immunologic integrity.
9. Explain the function of the mononuclear phagocyte system.
10. Compare quantitative and qualitative alterations of granulocytes and list several examples of conditions that influence these alterations.
11. Compare qualitative and quantitative alterations of monocytes and lymphocytes. List several examples of conditions that influence these alterations.
12. Describe the characteristics of a myeloproliferative disorder.
13. Differentiate between malignant and nonmalignant disorders in leukocytes.
14. Describe the qualitative and quantitative alterations of leukocytes found in leukemia.
15. Explain the basis of classification for leukemia.
16. Differentiate between acute and chronic leukemia.
17. Differentiate generally between reactive lymphadenopathies and malignant lymphomas.
18. Differentiate between Hodgkin's disease and other lymphomas on the basis of laboratory findings.
19. Describe the qualitative and quantitative alterations of leukocytes found in a person with infectious mononucleosis.
20. Discuss the causative agent of infectious mononucleosis and its significance with respect to malignancy and immunosuppression.
21. Explain the significance of the Reed-Sternberg cell with respect to Hodgkin's disease.
22. Discuss the clinical features and pathologic alterations found in a person with multiple myeloma.
23. Explain the significance of Bence-Jones proteinuria.

Leukocytes, larger and less numerous than the erythrocytes, play a key role in the defense mechanisms of the body. As the name implies, the leukocytes are almost white. Examination of a centrifuged tube of whole blood reveals a fuzzy gray-white layer between the packed red cells and the clear yellow plasma. This layer, called the "buffy coat," contains the leukocytes and the platelets. The white buffy color is due to the leukocytes and is responsible for their name. It is this fraction of the blood that plays the key role in the defense mechanisms of the body.

The most important function of the leukocytes is to defend the body against invasion by foreign organisms and to produce, transport, and distribute defensive elements such as antibodies or other factors that are necessary for the immune response. The various types of leukocytes work together in an integrated system. Each type performs different functions in the defense mechanisms of the body, but each function is necessary for a total integrated and effective defense.

NORMAL LEUKOCYTE FUNCTION

Characteristics of Leukocytes

There are normally about 5000 to 10,000 leukocytes/μl of adult human blood [2]. Of these, the *granulocytes* (polymorphonuclear leukocytes, or polys) occupy the largest percentage of the total number. These cells have large granules and horseshoe-shaped nuclei that differentiate and become multilobed with two to five distinct lobes connected by thin strands. The background cytoplasm stains blue to pink with Wright's stain, which enhances their morphologic identification (Table 15-1).

The polymorphonuclear leukocytes are subdivided into three cell types: neutrophils, eosinophils, and basophils. The *neutrophils* are the most numerous, making up 50 to 70 percent of the total white cell count. They have small, fine, light-pink or lilac acidophilic granules, when stained, and a segmented irregularly lobed purple nucleus.

The *eosinophils* constitute approximately 1 to 5 percent of the normal white cell count. They have large round granules that contain red-staining basic mucopolysaccharides and multilobed purple blue nuclei.

Like the eosinophils, the *basophils* also constitute a small percentage of the total white cell count, which can range from 0 to 1 percent of the total count. The coarse basophilic blue granules often conceal the segmented nucleus. The content of these granules includes histamine, heparin, and acid mucopolysaccharides.

Lymphocytes and monocytes are the remaining white blood cell types found normally in peripheral blood. They are often called *agranulocytes* because they were originally thought to be without granules. Their granules are very small and stain quite differently than the large granules of the granulocytes. Lymphocytes and monocytes are also called mononuclear leukocytes because they do not have the multilobed nucleus as the granulocytes do.

TABLE 15-1. Staining characteristics of leukocytes

Leukocyte	Cytoplasm	Cytoplasmic granules	Nucleus
Neutrophils	Blue to pink	Lilac	Purple blue
Eosinophils	Blue to pink	Red	Purple blue
Basophils	Blue to pink	Blue black	Purple blue
Lymphocytes	Pale blue		Dark blue
Monocytes	Gray blue	Pink	A blue lighter than lymphocytes

Lymphocytes are cells with large, round, deep-staining nuclei and very little cytoplasm. The cytoplasm is slightly basophilic and stains a pale blue. They make up approximately 20 to 40 percent of the total white cell count.

The mature *monocyte* is about 20 to 30 μ in diameter with a prominent multishaped nucleus that is sometimes kidney-shaped. The chromatin in the nucleus has the characteristics of lace due to the small chromatin particles tied together by fine strands. The chromatin is less clumped than in the mature granulocyte or lymphocyte. The gray-blue cytoplasm is filled with many fine lysosomes that stain pink with Wright's stain. Monocytes constitute about 1 to 6 percent of the total white cell count. Figure 15-1 illustrates the appearance of the different types of white blood cells.

White Cell Count

The white cell count is determined by counting cells in a diluted blood sample. The procedure can be done manually, but usually an electronic enumerator counts the leukocytes suspended in a dilute fluid that lyses the erythrocytes to prevent interference. Normal values range between 5000 and 10,000 white cells/μl. The white count is important as a diagnostic tool in cases of infection, malignancy, and other disorders that cause alterations of the white blood cells. Significant increases or decreases of the white blood cell count are known quantitative alterations.

Differential White Cell Count

Each of the leukocytes has a specific function in the defense of the body. An attack by a specific foreign agent often elicits a specific response by a certain type of leukocyte. For example, a pyogenic bacterial infection may elicit an increase in neutrophils, or a parasitic infection might elicit an increase in eosinophils. Therefore, an increase or decrease in the normal proportion of leukocytes may have significant diagnostic value. The relative proportion of leukocyte cell types is called the *differential count.*

The differential count is determined on a smear of blood one cell-layer thick. This layer has been stained with a polychrome solution containing both basic and acidic dyes. Wright's stain is usually used. The leukocyte cellular structure will absorb the dye differentially and permit an evalua-

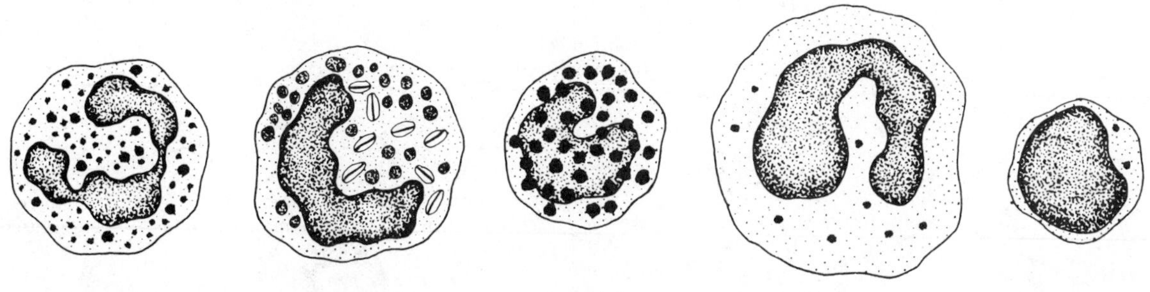

FIGURE 15-1. Characteristics of different types of leukocytes (From M. Borysenko, *Functional Histology* [2nd ed.]. Boston: Little, Brown, 1984.)

TABLE 15-2. Normal differential count of leukocytes

Neutrophils, segmented	50–70%
Neutrophils, bands or stabs	0–5%
Eosinophils	1–4%
Basophils	0–1%
Lymphocytes	20–40%
Monocytes	1–6%

tion not only of the relative proportions of the white cells, but also of leukocyte cellular elements and platelets. Differentials may be done manually or electronically (Table 15-2).

Normal differential white cell proportions vary with age. The neutrophils, for example, are significantly increased at birth, but fall below the normal adult level by 2 weeks of age. Lymphocytes, higher at birth and early childhood, decrease in numbers until adult levels are reached. The relative proportion, however, is higher from 4 weeks to 4 years (Table 15-3) [11].

Often an *absolute count* of a particular leukocyte is necessary for diagnosis. The absolute number of a specific type of leukocyte can be obtained by using a special diluting fluid that lyses the erythrocytes and either lyses or does not stain the other white cells present. The specific leukocyte type can then be counted without interference from the other cells.

Genesis of Leukocytes

The multipotential or uncommitted stem cells in the bone marrow are essentially responsible for blood cell and platelet formation. These cells will differentiate into unipotential or committed stem cells that will ultimately become the white blood cells, the platelets and erythrocytes (Fig. 15-2).

TABLE 15-3. Normal age-related leukocyte differential count in peripheral blood

Cell type	Percent	Number per microliter
Segmental neutrophils		
Infant, first day	47 ± 15	8870/μl
Child, 1 year	23 ± 10	2600/μl
Child, 10 years	46 ± 15	3700/μl
Adult, over 21	51 ± 15	3800/μl
Band neutrophils		
Infant, first day	14.2 ± 4	2580/μl
Child, 1 year	8.1 ± 3	990/μl
Child, 10 years	8.0 ± 3	645/μl
Adult, over 21	8.0 ± 3	620/μl
Eosinophils		
Infant, first day	2.4	450/μl
Child, 1 year	2.6	300/μl
Child, 10 years	2.4	200/μl
Adult, over 21	2.7	200/μl
Basophils		
Infant, first day	0.5	100/μl
Child, 1 year	0.4	50/μl
Child, 10 years	0.5	40/μl
Adult, over 21	0.5	40/μl
Lymphocytes		
Infant, first day	31 ± 5	5800/μl
Child, 1 year	61 ± 15	7000/μl
Child, 10 years	38 ± 10	3100/μl
Adult, over 21	34 ± 10	2500/μl
Monocytes		
Infant, first day	5.8	1100/μl
Child, 1 year	4.8	550/μl
Child, 10 years	4.3	350/μl
Adult, over 21	4.0	300/μl

Source: J. Wallach, *Interpretation of Diagnostic Tests* (3rd ed.). Boston: Little, Brown, 1978.

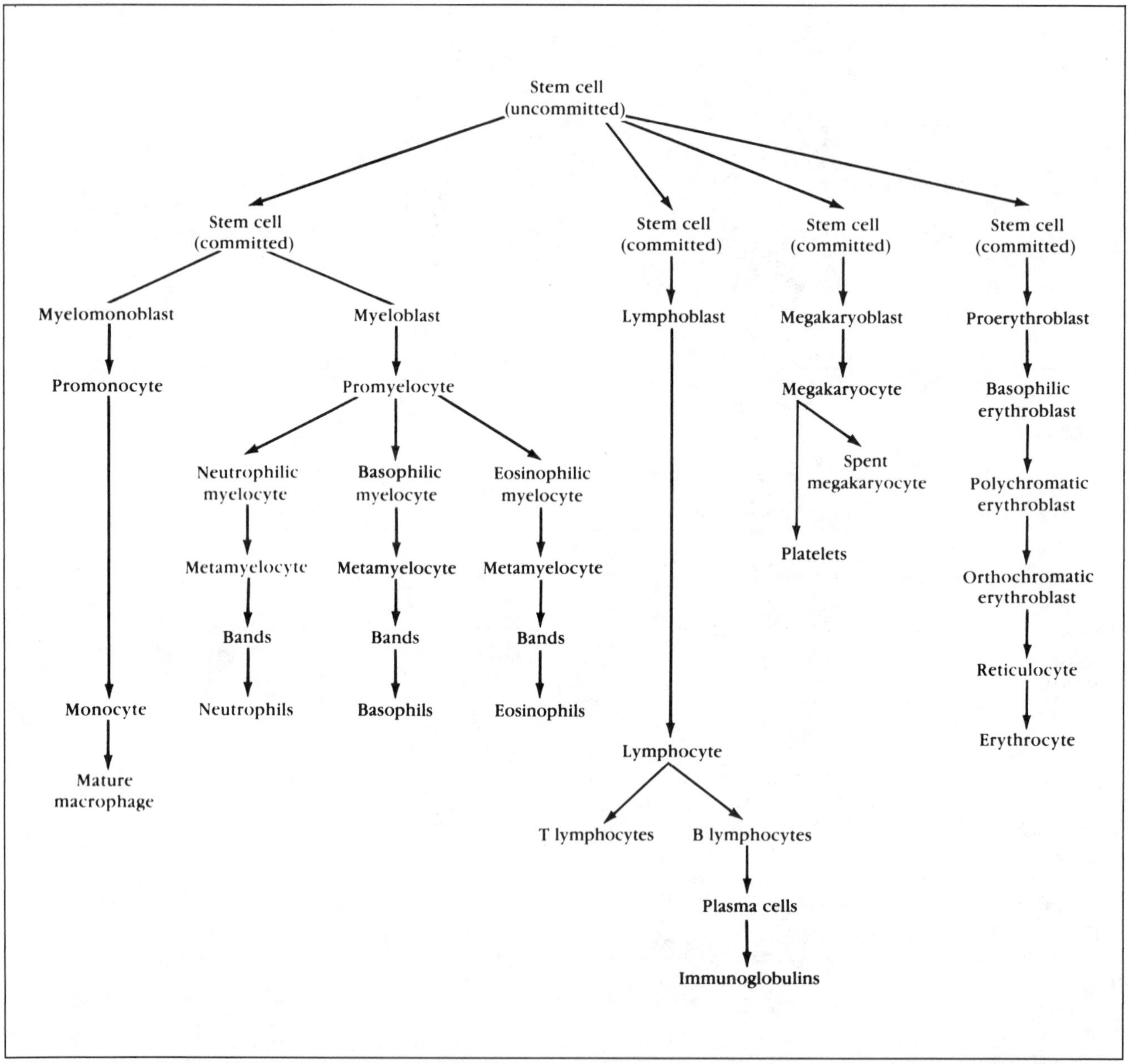

FIGURE 15-2. Differentiation of stem cells in the bone marrow.

Neutrophils, basophils, and eosinophils are formed in the bone marrow and can be stored there until needed. If the need is greater than the supply, immature forms may be released.

The granulocytes and monocytes are thought to be derived from a common committed stem cell. The promonocyte is also formed and differentiated in the bone marrow. It is then released into the circulation as a mature monocyte. The monocyte can leave the blood for the tissues where it enlarges and is transformed or matured into a lysosome-filled macrophage. The macrophage may have a diameter of 50 μ or more [1]. This large size is important for the phagocytosis of large particles and debris. Both granulocytes and monocytes have phagocytic properties.

The lymphocytes are thought to be formed from a separate committed stem cell in the bone marrow. In the fetus, proliferating stem cells migrate from the yolk sac to the liver, which functions as a major blood-forming organ during gestation [6]. Unlike the granulocytes and monocytes, most lymphocytes are not differentiated in the bone marrow. This process usually takes place in the lymphoid tissue, thymus, or spleen. Only large and small lymphocytes and plasma cells can be identified by morphology. B and T lymphocyte identification involve such laboratory techniques as cell marker studies and cytochemistry. The differentiation of the B and T lymphocytes in the lymphoid tissue is an important aspect of the immunologic response (see Chap. 9).

Life Span of White Blood Cells

The life span of the white blood cell in the circulating blood is generally short. The average half-life of a neutrophil in the blood is approximately 6 hours [3]. During a serious infection, granulocytes often live 2 hours or less until they are used or destroyed. Granulocytes mature in the bone marrow. After myelocytes (the precursors of the granulocytes) stop dividing, the maturing granulocytes accumulate as a reserve in the bone marrow. Under normal conditions, there is about a 5-day supply of granulocytes in this reserve. Once the granulocytes leave this reserve, they will spend an average of 12 hours in the circulation and about 2 to 3 days in the tissues before they are destroyed.

The monocytes spend less time in the bone marrow pool than the granulocytes. The life span of the monocyte in the circulation is approximately 36 hours or about 3 times as long as that of granulocytes [1]. After the monocyte has been transformed into a mobile or fixed macrophage in the tissues its life is long, ranging from months to years.

The life span of the lymphocytes varies tremendously. A small population of extremely long-lived cells may survive for many years. These cells are necessary for maintaining the immunologic memory and have the special ability to reenter cell division through specific stimulation by an antigen.

Most of the T lymphocytes of the peripheral lymphatic tissue recirculate about every 10 hours [1]. They follow a path from the blood to the lymphatic tissue, through the lymphatic channels, and back to the blood through the thoracic duct. The survival rate of the T lymphocytes ranges from a few days to months and years. In general, most T lymphocytes have slow replacement rates and a long survival time.

The B lymphocytes are largely noncirculating. They remain mainly in the lymphoid tissue and can differentiate under appropriate stimulation into plasma cells. Mature plasma cells, which have the ability to secrete specific antibodies, have a survival rate of about 2 to 3 days (see Chap. 9). Table 15-4 summarizes the life span of the various white blood cells.

TABLE 15-4. Life span of white blood cells

Cell type	In circulating blood	Tissue life
Granulocytes	6–8 hours; time shortened in acute infection	2–3 days
Monocytes	Short transit time, often less than 36 hours	Months or years as tissue macrophages
T lymphocytes	Remain in the blood a few hours but recirculate about every 10 hours	Life span varies from a few days to years
B lymphocytes	Few circulate	Most remain in lymphoid tissue; when they become secreting plasma cell, they survive 2–3 days
Platelets	Most circulate; are totally replaced every 10 days	

Properties of the Leukocytes

FUNCTIONAL CLASSIFICATION. The properties of the leukocytes can be best understood by the separation of the leukocytes into two major functional groups: the *phagocytes* and the *immunocytes*. As discussed in the previous section, immunocytes and phagocytes are thought to be derived from a common stem cell in the bone marrow. The immunocytes or lymphocytes may undergo a differentiation phase outside the bone marrow. The phagocytes undergo maturation in the bone marrow, which results in the release of mature granulocytes and monocytes into the circulation. Granulocytes and monocytes are classified as phagocytes. Monocytes must enter the tissues and differentiate into macrophages to exhibit the property of phagocytosis.

PHAGOCYTOSIS. The most important property of the phagocytes (granulocytes and macrophages) is phagocytosis. Phagocytosis is a process similar to that used by an ameba to ingest and digest its nourishment. The phagocyte can change its shape by sending out processes from its protoplasm. Microorganisms, old cells, or foreign particles can then be enveloped or engulfed in a vacuole, or *phagosome*, formed by the fusing of the processes of protoplasm. Associated with ingestion of the foreign or devitalized material is a rapid increase in cellular energy and the generation of hydrogen peroxide (Fig. 15-3).

DEGRANULATION. Phagocytosis not only involves ingestion of a microorganism or particle but also the digestion or destruction of this foreign body. After the material has become engulfed in the phagosome, degranulation occurs. This process involves attachment of lysosomes (granules) that fuse with the internal membrane of the phagosome and empty their contents into its vacuole. The biochemical events of this morphologic phenomena are incompletely understood. The granules contain hydrolytic enzymes that cause the dissolution of the phagosome contents and eventually the lysis of the phagocyte itself.

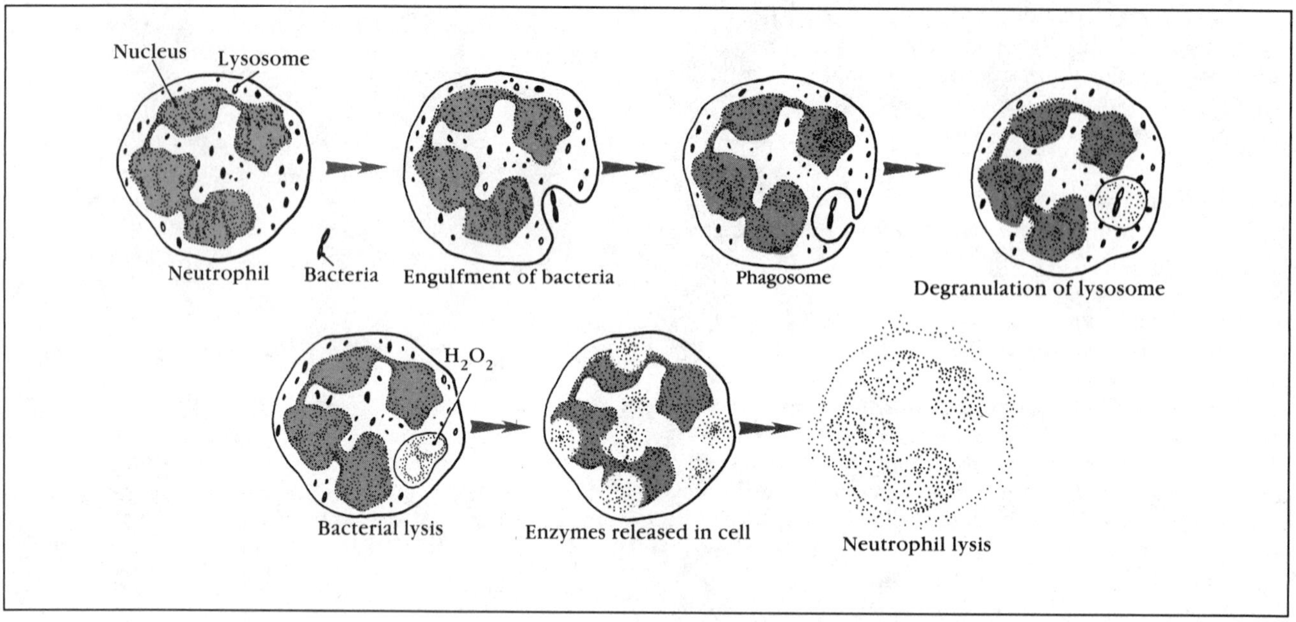

FIGURE 15-3. Process of phagocytosis of bacteria.

KILLING. Killing is the process by which the phagocytosed microorganism contained within the membrane-bound phagosome is actually killed. The majority of the hydrolytic enzymes contained in the granules serve a digestive function and are not directly involved in the killing process [8]. The process that actually kills the microorganism involves peroxidation of hydrogen peroxide, which, in the presence of iodide, can destroy the microbial membrane. Most bacteria can be killed by this process. However, some organisms such as the acid-fast bacilli causing tuberculosis and leprosy are able to survive within the phagocyte.

Dissolution is a complex process that involves the integrated action among many hydrolytic enzymes. The phagocyte as well as the foreign invader is often lysed by its own enzymes and becomes part of the degradation products (see Fig. 15-3).

The degradation products after phagocytosis usually intensify the inflammatory process to varying degrees. The released lysosomal enzymes of the degranulation process or toxins released by the bacteria may cause damage to the surrounding tissues. Degradation products include thromboplastic products that lead to vascular clotting (see Chap. 16).

Phagocytosis is promoted by other factors such as temperature and electrical charge. Higher body temperatures or increased heat at the site of infection enhances phagocytosis. Fever during an infection may serve as a protective mechanism within limits. The electrical charge on antigen surfaces may also enhance phagocytosis, since the charge on dead or foreign particles is different from the charges on living tissues and is considered to be a dominant factor in specificity [6].

Increased glucose metabolism and cellular oxygen consumption is needed for phagocytosis as increased energy is necessary for the production of large amounts of hydrogen peroxide used for the peroxidative killing of bacteria. The energy adenosine triphosphate (ATP) is supplied by glycolysis in the white blood cell itself.

DIAPEDESIS. Phagocytes have the ability to accumulate at the site of invasion or injury. Like the ameba, they are able to form pseudopodialike processes that allow for locomotion through avenues of the body. Granulocytes and monocytes can leave the circulation and enter tissue by a process called diapedesis. Diapedesis refers to the ability of the phagocyte to slip through the walls of the capillary vessel by ameboid motion. A small portion of the phagocyte slides through at a time until the entire phagocyte leaves the circulation. Some of these cells may slip into the gastrointestinal system and be excreted from the body. Diapedesis allows for phagocytic accumulation at the invasion site (see Chap. 8).

CHEMOTAXIS. The phagocytes must be able to find the site of a bacterial invasion or recognize that infection has taken place. Necrotic material is also broken down and digested by specific phagocytes. Chemical substances called chemotactic agents or mediators are released from the infected or necrotic tissues and provide a signal for the leukocytes. These chemical substances cause the leukocytes to move toward the source of the chemical. This process, called chemotaxis, is dependent on a concentration gradient. A greater concentration of the chemical causes more leukocytes to move toward the source. Other chemotactic agents include the complement system, plasminogen, the fibrinolytic system, kallikrien (the kinin system), and substances released from the phagocytes.

PINOCYTOSIS. Pinocytosis involves the cellular engulfment by the phagocyte of tiny particles included in a droplet of fluid [1]. It differs from phagocytosis in that in phagocytosis the membrane sends out processes to grasp a relatively large particle using a biochemical mechanism similar to muscle action. In pinocytosis, macrophages can ingest and break down macromolecules. The role of pinocytosis in many macrophage activities is not totally understood [6].

RECOGNITION OF THE PARTICLE. Before a phagocyte can ingest a bacterium or particle, recognition of the particle must occur. Recognition of the particle or foreign invader is achieved through mediation in one of two ways: (1) opsonization, or (2) surface properties [5].

Opsonization of the antigenic surface is needed for the attachment of the phagocyte to the antigen. Opsonization is mediated by activation of the complement protein system or by specific antibodies. Activation of complement results in C3b attachment to the surface of the particle, which, with specific antibody, allows it to be recognized and phagocytosed by the leukocyte [8].

Some particles have special *surface properties* that result in adherence to the phagocyte and subsequent phagocytosis. These physiochemical properties allow adhesion of the particle to the cell membrane of the phagocyte while pseudopodia surround and engulf the particle. This type of phagocytosis is seen in the early phases of an illness and is more effective with tightly packed leukocytes. The exact mechanism of attachment of the phagocyte to the antigen before antibody formation, complement activation, or cell devitalization, is not known.

Function of the Phagocytes

The functions of the granulocytes and monocyte-macrophages overlap but, in general, the granulocytes function as the first line of defense against microbial invasion. The neutrophils are adept at recognizing, ingesting, and killing pyogenic bacteria. The monocyte-macrophages are important in the final removal or cellular cleanup of debris after phagocytosis and cellular lysis. They are able to ingest bigger particles and larger amounts of debris because of their larger size. Inert materials as large as wood or steel fragments can be engulfed by macrophages and removed from the site of inflammation. If a particle is very large, large multinucleated foreign-body giant cells may be produced. The characteristic foreign-body giant cell may represent fusion of several macrophages. Macrophages not only provide the final removal of microorganisms, but also clear the body of its own aged and damaged cells. Some macrophages possess the ability to break down and recycle old red blood cells. A type of tissue macrophage possesses heme oxidase activity, which enables it to break down hemoglobin that can be recycled. Macrophages of the liver, spleen, and bone marrow can return iron to transferrin to be transported to the erythroid marrow for red blood cell synthesis.

Phagocytes contain antibacterial substances, peroxidase, and lysosomal enzymes necessary for phagocytosis and other activities. Macrophages are thought to kill tumor cells that have been processed by the lymphocytes. Monocytes and granulocytes also interact with other biologically active substances such as complement.

In order for the phagocytes to accomplish their defensive purpose, the following must occur: (1) They must accumulate in sufficient numbers at the right place. (2) They must attach to the foreign material or agent. (3) They must envelop or engulf the agent. (4) They must dispose of the debris [8]. Alterations in any of these functions results in defective phagocytosis, which then results in a defective defensive response.

Function of Basophils and Eosinophils

The precise function of the basophils and eosinophils is not well understood but some properties and functions are known. These cells participate in the inflammatory and allergic reactions.

BASOPHILS. The blood basophil contains histamine, heparin, and small quantities of bradykinin and serotonin. It is found in small numbers in the blood but larger numbers are found in the connective tissue and pericapillary areas. The function seems to be largely in the prevention of clotting in the microcirculation and in chemical mediation of allergic reactions [7]. It has been noted that persons with allergies often have elevated immunoglobulin E (IgE). IgE receptor sites have been found on the basophils. When these receptor sites are attached, histamine and other substances are released that increase chemotaxis and also enhance the allergic response (see Chap. 11). An increase in basophils is found in some of the myeloproliferative diseases, such as polycythemia vera.

EOSINOPHILS. These cells exhibit the properties of phagocytosis and chemotaxis weakly [7]. They are found in large numbers in the mucosa of the intestinal tract and of the lungs. Because of this they probably function to detoxify foreign proteins. The circulating level of eosinophils is increased in persons with allergies and may be the result of removal and digestion of the antigen-antibody complex by the eosinophil. Eosinophilia is associated with worm infestation or parasitic infections. In trichinosis the numbers of eosinophils can increase 25 to 50 percent. The relationship of basophils and eosinophils to allergy or hypersensitivity is discussed in Chapter 11.

Mononuclear Phagocyte System

The *mononuclear phagocyte system* is a term used to describe the large system of stationary and mobile macrophages. Important in the body's defense system, it is considered to be mainly a functional rather than an anatomic system. It includes all the fixed and mobile phagocytic cells in the liver, spleen, lymph nodes, and gastrointestinal tract. The fixed macrophages in these organs seem to exist in dynamic equilibrium with mobile macrophages. All tissue macrophages, including the Kupffer's cells of the liver and alveolar macrophages in the lungs, originate from the mobile circulating macrophages. This system is important in preventing the spread of infection, removing cellular debris and products of metabolic degradation. Many of the metabolic products are conserved and recycled.

Unlike monocytes and granulocytes, the lymphocytes do not possess phagocytic capabilities but function to protect the body against specific antigens. This specific immunity, discussed in Chapter 9, is integrated with other general immune responses. The lymphocytes occupy the same anatomic area, the lymphoid tissues, as the macrophages.

NONMALIGNANT WHITE BLOOD CELL DISORDERS

Quantitative Alterations of Granulocytes

Quantitative alterations of granulocytes result from a number of conditions that cause a significant increase or decrease in the number of leukocytes. This is usually measured by calculating the number of leukocytes in the blood. Each cell type is often considered and counted individually in order to identify the causative condition.

NEUTROPHILS. A normal physiologic shift in the number of neutrophils can be influenced by a number of conditions. Leukocytosis can be caused by exercise, emotional stress, menstruation, sunlight, cold, and anesthesia. During pregnancy there is a consistent increase in polymorphonuclear leukocytes or neutrophils. This increase is even more exaggerated during labor and the first postpartum week. The newborn infant also has increased neutrophil levels.

Neutrophilic leukocytosis is defined as an absolute neutrophil count greater than 7500 per μl blood [2]. The total white count in this condition is usually greater than 10,000 per μl blood [2]. A *shift to the left* occurs when there is an increase in the number of leukocytes of nonsegmented neutrophils in the circulating blood. Because of the release of increased numbers of neutrophils in an inflammatory process, some of those released may be in immature forms called bands or stabs, which have a very short life span. An increased number of these cells in the peripheral blood is often a good indicator of an inflammatory process, especially an acute bacterial infection. If the percentage of immature forms is decreasing in the peripheral blood smear, it is said that there is a *shift to the right*. Generally it can be said that a leftward shift indicates progression of infection while a rightward shift indicates a subsiding infection [8]. Neutrophilic leukocytosis occurs in such pathologic conditions as acute pyogenic infections, hemorrhage, hemolysis, tissue necrosis, or metabolic chemical toxic poisonings.

Neutrophilic leukopenia occurs when the absolute neutrophil count is less than 2500 per μl of blood [2]. Radiation, anaphylactic shock, and systemic lupus erythymatosus are specific causes of this decrease. Chemical agents that affect the *hematopoietic* system will cause a decrease in the neutrophils. Antithyroid drugs, phenothiazines, and chemotherapeutic agents are only a few of the many drugs that can cause *neutropenia*. Disorders that affect the *hematopoietic* system, such as aplastic anemia and acute leukemia, cause a neutrophilic leukopenia.

Nonpyogenic bacterial, viral, and rickettsial infections cause a decrease in the neutrophil count. Any overwhelming bacterial infection can cause a neutrophilic leukopenia because the vast numbers of cells used to fight the infections is much greater than the reserve supply.

EOSINOPHILS. Eosinophilic leukocytosis, also known as eosinophilia, is defined as an absolute eosinophil count exceeding 500 per μl of blood and is often associated with allergy [2]. It is believed that this increase with the allergic condition is due to the tissue reactions associated with allergy-released products that specifically increase the production of the eosinophils in the bone marrow.

Eosinophilic leukocytosis also occurs in response to parasitic infection. This is probably the most common cause of extremely large numbers of eosinophils in the blood. The mechanism by which the parasitic infections cause the increased eosinophil count is not known, but if the main function of the eosinophils is to detoxify proteins then the parasitic proteins are a constant source of stimulation to the bone marrow for increased production of eosinophils.

Eosinophilic leukocytosis can also be caused by hemopoietic disorders, myeloid leukemia, collagen disease, and malignancy. It can also be idiopathic.

Eosinophilic leukopenia, or *eosinopenia*, occurs when there is an absolute eosinophil count of less than 50 per μl of blood [2]. The decrease may be due to severe infection, shock, or adrenocortical stimulation.

BASOPHILS. Basophilic leukocytosis, or *basophilia*, is defined as an absolute basophil count exceeding 50 to 100 per μl of blood [2]. This is usually greater than 2 percent of the white cell differential and is associated with myeloproliferative disorders, ulcerative colitis, chronic granulocytic leukemia, and certain skin diseases.

Basophilic leukopenia, or *basopenia*, occurs when there is an absolute basophil count less than 20 per μl of blood [2]. Causes include severe infection, shock, and adrenocortical stimulation.

Qualitative Alterations of Granulocytes

When granulocytes display defective physical and chemical functions, they are said to have qualitative abnormalities. Most of these defective functions are related to the process of effective phagocytosis. The defects may be in phagocyte locomotion or in the phagocyte itself, such as that seen in the "lazy leukocyte" syndrome. There may be deficient chemotaxis generation and complement abnormalities. Complement abnormalities are associated with collagen vascular disorders and occasionally with bacterial infections.

Normal human serum contains a low concentration of heat-stable globulin that impairs both chemotaxis and phagocytosis in vitro. This inhibitor has been found to be elevated in the sera of the majority of patients with cancer.

Ethanol has been shown to cause a significant decrease in the leukocyte migration and chemotaxis during acute intoxication. Chemotaxis can also be decreased by the use of some antibiotics such as gentamicin in therapeutic doses [8].

Granulomatous disease refers to qualitative defects of the granulocytes, especially neutrophils, and results in defective bactericidal activity. In chronic granulomatous disease (CGD), there is an inherited absence of neutrophil oxidase. This enzyme is necessary for the actual killing of the bacteria, without which the leukocyte is unable to oxidize or destroy certain bacteria. Diagnosis can be made by the nitroblue tetrazolium (NBT) reduction test. Normally, NBT is reduced to a blue-black material called blue formazan but in CGD this reduction is not seen. CGD results in severe recurrent infections of skin, lymph nodes, lungs, liver, and bones [5].

There are several inherited qualitative abnormalities of the granulocytes. The nuclear structure and appearance may be altered, excessive granulation of the cytoplasm may occur, and hypersegmentation of the neutrophils may be seen. These alterations may affect the process of phagocytosis or it may have no clinical implications.

Monocyte Abnormalities

Monocytosis infers an absolute monocyte count greater than 750 per μl in children and 500 to 600 per μl of blood in adults [2]. This disorder is seen in nonpyogenic bacterial infections such as active tuberculosis, subacute bacterial endocarditis, syphilis, and brucellosis. It is associated with recovery from such disorders as agranulocytosis, hematologic disorders, malignancy, and collagen disease.

Monocytopenia refers to a decrease in the blood monocyte counts. It is frequently seen secondarily to acute stress reactions and/or glucocorticoid administration. Overwhelming infections or immunosuppressive agents will also decrease the monocyte count.

Lymphocytic Disorders

Lymphocytosis must be defined according to the developmental stage of the individual. The absolute lymphocyte count from birth to 3 years is 9000 per μl of blood. From 4 to 12 years it is 7000 per μl and it is 4000 per μl in the adult [2]. Disorders that produce lymphocytosis include such viral disorders as mumps, rubella, rubeola, hepatitis, and varicella. Lymphocytosis also occurs in pertussis and chronic lymphocytic leukemia with an increase of the small lymphocytes. Also, increased numbers of atypical lymphocytes are seen with infectious mononucleosis, cytomegalic inclusion disease, and toxoplasmosis. Only infectious mononucleosis is considered in detail in this section.

INFECTIOUS MONONUCLEOSIS. Infectious mononucleosis, a disease often seen in young adults, is characterized by the development of cervical lymphadenopathy, fever, sore throat, and splenomegaly. An exudative tonsillitis is common.

The designation *mononucleosis* is misleading because the proliferating cells found in the lymph nodes, spleen, tonsils, and other organs are lymphocytes and monocytes. The serologic findings show an increase in lymphocytes and monocytes with 10 to 20 percent of these being abnormal.

Mononucleosis is caused by the Epstein-Barr virus (EBV). This is the same herpesvirus that causes the malignant Burkitt's lymphoma found in some areas in Africa. It has been found that if cultured infectious mononucleosis lymphocytes are transplanted into immunosuppressed animals, a malignant lymphoproliferative disorder results. Genetically determined defects in the immune response may be the key to this malignancy [3].

The Epstein-Barr virus subclinically infects from 50 to 80 percent of the world's population [10]. Large epidemiologic studies have shown that only persons without antibodies against EBV are at risk for developing infectious mononucleosis. The active disease is associated with the brief appearance of IgM antibodies against the Epstein-Barr virus. Since the IgM antibody increase represents a primary response, this would indicate a recent exposure to the virus.

Infectious mononucleosis affects particularly the adolescent and young adult age groups. Epstein and Achong [9] postulated that, in low socioeconomic groups, exposure to the Epstein-Barr virus occurs early in life and is almost entirely asymptomatic. If the person is exposed later in adolescence or young adulthood, infectious mononucleosis may result in up to two-thirds of the exposed population.

Hematologic changes are characteristic of mononucleosis. At first there may be a mild leukopenia, but by the second week the white cell count reaches 15,000 to 30,000 per μl of blood. Atypical lymphocytes make up 15 to 60 percent of the white cells in the second through the fourth week. The atypical lymphocyte may take one of several forms, but the most common picture includes nuclear chromatin that is finely divided or clumped. The nucleolus is usually absent and vacuoles are often present in the cytoplasm. If atypical lymphocytes are present in large numbers, the hematologic picture may resemble acute leukemia.

The Epstein-Barr virus induces an increase in antibody formation by the B lymphocyte. This antibody formation forms the basis for laboratory diagnostic testing. The heterophil antibody titer test, the monoscreening, monodiff, and the monospot test are used for differential diagnosis. No correlation has been found between the levels of EBV or antibody titer and severity of the disease [5].

Clinical symptoms of infectious mononucleosis disappear before the abnormal hematologic findings disappear. Clinical characteristics of mononucleosis include fever, malaise, sore throat, and weakness. Splenomegaly and hepatic dysfunction may be present. Gradual recovery usually occurs in 2 to 4 weeks with no residual effects.

Lymphopenia is defined as an absolute lymphocyte count of less than 1400 per μl in the child and less than 1000 per μl in the adult [2]. This condition may be caused by such factors as stress, adrenocortical stimulation, alkylating agents, and irradiation. It is associated with Hodgkin's disease, lymphosarcoma, terminal uremia, and acute tuberculosis.

LYMPHADENOPATHY. Lymphadenopathies are characterized by enlarged lymph nodes. The enlarged nodes may be classified as tender or nontender and movable or fixed. Nodes involved by lymphomas or leukemias tend to be large, firm, and movable while those of metastatic spread of malignancy tend to be adherent to surrounding structures. In acute infections the nodes tend to be asymmetric with associated redness and edema.

Localized lymphadenopathy usually indicates drainage of an inflammatory process that may be due to infection, neoplasm, or an early lymphoma. Generalized lymphadenopathy is less frequently caused by infection in the adult and may be caused by a malignant or nonmalignant process.

Lymph node enlargement may be due to reactive follicular hyperplasia of nonspecific origin. There is usually hyperplasia of follicular center cells, which may be due to stimulation of B cells in viral diseases, in syphilis, or in autoimmune diseases such as rheumatoid arthritis or systemic lupus erythematosus.

Lymphadenopathies show individual pathologic features depending on the causative agent. Suppurative lymphadenitis is characterized by neutrophils in the sinusoids of the lymph nodes. These nodes serve as the filtration units for the regions infected by pyogenic bacteria. Many other conditions may be associated with lymph node enlargement. The following is a representative list:

Autoimmune diseases
Hyperthyroidism
Addison's disease
Metastatic carcinomas of lung, breast, and larynx
Any type of infection and hypersensitivity responses

MALIGNANT WHITE BLOOD DISORDERS

Leukemia

Leukemia is the designation for a group of malignant diseases characterized by both qualitative and quantitative alterations in the circulating leukocytes. It is associated with diffuse abnormal growth of leukocyte precursors in the bone marrow. The word *leukemia* is derived from the Greek words *leukos* and *haima* meaning white blood, referring to the abnormal increase in leukocytes. This uncontrolled increase in abnormal leukocytes eventually leads to anemia, infection, thrombocytopenia, and in some cases, death.

TABLE 15-5. Classification of leukemia

Acute leukemia
- Acute lymphoblastic or lymphocytic (ALL)
  - L_1: small cell, homogenous, some with T lymphocyte markers
  - L_2: larger cell, more heterogenous, some with T lymphocyte markers
  - L_3: large cell, homogenous, B lymphocyte markers
- Acute myelogenous or acute myeloid (AML)
  - M_1: myeloblastic without maturation, nongranular
  - M_2: myeloblastic with maturation to promyelocyte stage or beyond
  - M_3: hypergranular, abnormal promyelocytes
  - M_4: granulocytic and monocytic differentiation
  - M_5: monocytic or monoblastic
  - M_6: abnormal erythroblasts, myeloblasts, promyelocytes

Chronic leukemia
- Chronic granulocytic (CGL): chromosome marker (Philadelphia chromosome) in marrow and peripheral blood
  - Myeloproliferative, intermediate maturity, thrombocytosis; WBC count: 150,000/μl; may convert to AML
- Chronic lymphocytic (CLL): proliferation of mature appearing, nonfunctional lymphocytes; B lymphocyte proliferation with hypogammaglobulinemia; WBC count: usually 100,000/μl

Source: S. Robbins and R. Cotran, *Pathological Basis of Disease* (2nd ed.). Philadelphia: Saunders, 1979. P. 781.

CLASSIFICATION. Classification of leukemia is usually based on (1) *the course and duration of the illness,* and (2) *the abnormal type of cells and tissue involved.* The course of the illness has been subclassified into acute and chronic leukemia (Table 15-5). *Acute leukemia* is associated with a rapid onset, a massive number of immature leukocytes, rapidly progressive anemia, severe thrombocytopenia, high fever, infective lesions of the mouth and throat, bleeding into vital areas, accumulation of leukocytes in vital organs, and severe infection. Laboratory studies usually show some degree of anemia and thrombocytopenia. Demonstration of leukemic cells in the peripheral blood cannot always be relied on. Open surgical biopsy of the bone marrow will usually demonstrate the abnormal cells.

Chronic leukemia is characterized by a gradual onset and leukocytes that are more mature. This disease usually strikes an older age group. The clinical course progresses more slowly but can end with the onset of acute leukemia. Laboratory analysis usually reveals a well-differentiated leukemic cell that can be classified into lymphocytic or granulocytic types.

Leukemia is further classified by the type of tissue and abnormal cell involved. Three broad classification categories based on tissue origin are (1) *myeloid*, which includes the granulocytes (neutrophils, eosinophils, or basophils), (2) *monocytic*, and (3) *lymphocytic*. If abnormal proliferation of granular leukocytes or their precursors are found in the blood or bone marrow the leukemia may be labeled granulocytic, myelocytic, or myelogenous. With abnormal proliferation of lymphocytes or monocytes the leukemia would be labeled lymphocytic or monocytic, respectively.

If the majority of cells are immature, the suffix -blastic is used instead of -cytic. For example, lymphoblastic, myeloblastic, or monoblastic are designations to indicate the immature condition of the leukocyte.

Classification of the chronic leukemias has not been a diagnostic problem because there are usually sufficient abnormal mature cells present from which to make a diagnosis. Diagnosis and classification of acute leukemia presents a greater challenge. Because of the immature nature of the cell, it is sometimes difficult to identify the cellular type. Research and technologic advances have led to a more sophisticated identification and classification system. This includes the use of cell marker studies, cell secretory activity, and cytochemistry as well as morphology and response to therapy.

Many factors are thought to influence the development of leukemia. These can be generally divided into three groups: (1) genetic factors, (2) acquired diseases, and (3) chemical and physical agents.

Genetic factors that pose a high risk are (1) an identical twin with leukemia, and (2) Bloom's syndrome. Bloom's syndrome is caused by an autosomal recessive trait characterized by dwarfism, photosensitivity, and butterfly telangiectatic erythema of the face with numerous defects of the skin pigment and keratin development. A sibling of a person with leukemia and a person with Down's syndrome are also at significant risk for developing leukemia.

Acquired diseases with high-risk factors for leukemia include myelofibrosis, polycythemia vera, and sideroblastic refractory anemia. Multiple myeloma and Hodgkin's disease also represent increased risk for development of the disease.

Physical and chemical agents that pose significant risk for leukemia include radiation and long-term exposure to benzene. There is also some risk associated with the chemotherapeutic agents chloramphenicol and the alkylating agents.

CLINICAL MANIFESTATIONS. Pathologic alterations due to the disease process create characteristic signs and symptoms. Infection due to marrow failure and granulocytopenia is the most common cause of fatality. It may appear in any organ or area and may be manifested by fever, chills, inflammation, and weakness. Bleeding of the skin, gingivae, or viscera often occurs due to thrombocytopenia. Disseminated intravascular coagulation (DIC), due to reduced platelets and coagulation factors, may cause a significant hemorrhage (see Chap. 16). DIC is probably triggered by proteolytic enzymes or factors released by the leukemic cells that activate the clotting process [4].

Reduced appetite and hypermetabolism result in weight loss, weakness, fatigue, and pallor associated with anemia. Calcium and magnesium abnormalities can be seen in serologic laboratory tests.

Leukemic infiltration of the meninges, central nervous system, and cranial nerves results in such clinical manifestations as headache, visual disturbances, nausea, and vomiting. Bone infiltration results in bone tenderness and pain. Hepatosplenomegaly and infiltration of other viscera are manifested by abdominal tenderness and anorexia. Lymphadenopathy and neoplastic masses are due to local infiltration.

PROGRESSION OF THE DISEASE. Chemotherapy in the treatment of leukemia has markedly increased the survival rates for acute leukemia. Untreated acute lymphoblastic leukemia (ALL) is usually fatal in 3 months. Studies show over 50 percent of children treated with chemotherapy living after 5 years [4]. Acute myeloblastic leukemia (AML) has a poorer record, even with treatment, with an average survival of 1 to 2 years.

The chronic leukemias have a variable course that can be controlled by oral alkylating agents or radiation. The progressive anemia and susceptibility to infection are hazards, and CML may terminate by transforming into AML.

Malignant Lymphomas

Malignant lymphomas are solid neoplasms containing cells of lymphoreticular origin. *Lymphoreticular organs* include the lymph nodes, spleen, bone marrow, thymus, liver, and the submucosa of the gastrointestinal and respiratory tracts.

Pathologically, lymphadenopathy is characteristic with eventual involvement of the liver, spleen, and viscera. Diffusely diseased nodes are gray in appearance with capsular infiltration occurring later in the process. The enlarged nodes may become adherent to each other and to surrounding organs and tissues [10].

CLASSIFICATION. The classification of malignant lymphomas is usually based on the predominant cell type and its degree of differentiation. The classification may be further divided into nodular and diffuse types depending on the predominant pattern of cell arrangement.

Table 15-6 shows examples of two common methods for the classification of malignant lymphoma according to cell type. Also included is the widely used Ann Arbor staging classification.

TABLE 15-6. Classification of lymphomas

Non–Hodgkin's (Rappaport)	Malignant lymphomas (Lukes and Collins)	Ann Arbor staging classification
Nodular	*B cell*	
Lymphocytic, poorly differentiated (NPDL)	Small lymphocyte	I: Single node or region involvement
	Plasmacytoid lymphocytic	
Mixed lymphocytic, histiocytic (NMC)	Follicular center cell	II: Two or more node regions, same side of diaphragm
	Immunoblastic sarcoma	
Histiocytic (NH)	Hairy-cell leukemia	
Diffuse	*T cell*	
Lymphocytic, well differentiated (DWDL)	Small lymphocyte	III: Involvement of lymph node regions, both sides of diaphragm
	Convoluted lymphocyte (undifferentiated)	
Lymphocytic, poorly differentiated (DPDL)		IV: Diffuse or disseminated involvement; extralymphatic organs involved
	Immunoblastic sarcoma	
Mixed lymphocytic, histiocytic (DMC)		
Histiocytic (DHL)	*U cell*	
Lymphoblastic	Undefined cell systems	
Undifferentiated		

Key: NPDL = neoplastic, poorly differentiated, lymphocytic; NMC = neoplastic, mixed cellularity; NH = neoplastic, histiocytic; DWDL = diffuse, well differentiated, lymphocytic; DPDL = diffuse, poorly differentiated, lymphocytic; DMC = diffuse, mixed cellularity; DHL = diffuse, histiocytic, lymphocytic.
Source: J. Ultmann and V. DeVita, Hodgkin's Disease and Other Lymphomas. In K. J. Isselbacher, et al. (eds.), *Harrison's Principles of Internal Medicine* (9th ed.). New York: McGraw-Hill, 1980.

The diffuse lymphomas are more invasive than the nodular lymphomas. The higher the stage the greater the involvement, and the prognosis is worse. The more undifferentiated the cell, the more aggressive the tumor becomes. As with leukemia, most individuals with lymphomas develop immunodeficiencies that are followed by infection.

HODGKIN'S DISEASE. *Hodgkin's disease* is a malignant lymphoma that occurs in various distinct forms. It is characterized by proliferation of malignant cells of unknown origin. Peculiar giant cells called Sternberg-Reed cells are produced. Infiltration of the nodes with eosinophils and plasma cells occurs and this infiltration is associated with necrosis and fibrosis.

The histologic criteria in malignancy of Hodgkin's disease are similar to those in non-Hodgkin's lymphomas. The Sternberg-Reed cell, which is a multinucleated bizarre giant cell with a prominent nucleolus, must be present to confirm the diagnosis. Hodgkin's disease appears to involve a defect in the T cell. The total lymphocyte count is depressed and infection often causes major complications.

Hodgkin's disease has been classified into four types: (1) lymphocyte predominant, in which there is diffuse replacement by lymphocytes; (2) mixed type, which shows several distinct cell patterns, both lymphocytic and histiocytic; (3) lymphocyte depletion, showing a predominant pattern of large malignant cells; and (4) nodular sclerosing, which shows extensive scarring [10].

Staging of Hodgkin's disease uses the same classification as other lymphomas (see Table 15-6). Bone marrow examination and examination of the spleen for pathology following a splenectomy are often used as the basis for staging. As with other lymphomas, the higher the stage number the poorer the prognosis.

Common clinical manifestations of Hodgkin's disease are enlarged, palpable lymph nodes, fever, weight loss, and loss of energy. The enlargement of the nodes may cause compression on the spinal cord or other organs. The tumor may invade the vasculature or the lung parenchyma.

Anemia and immunodeficiency with lymphocytopenia occur in the later stages. Biopsy may demonstrate the Sternberg-Reed cells. The immunodeficiency, enhanced by chemotherapy, leads to ineffective control of microbial invasion, especially fungal and protozoal. Infection is a common complication both of the disease and of the tumor.

Treatment with chemotherapy and radiation therapy has markedly improved the prognosis for Hodgkin's disease with 90 to 100 percent remission rates being reported.

Multiple Myeloma

Multiple myeloma or plasma cell myeloma is a malignant neoplasm of plasma cells that causes damage to the bone marrow and skeletal structure. The aberrant myeloma cells arise from a single clone of plasma cells that are B-cell derived and secrete anomalous circulating immunoglobulins, also called paraproteins. These immunoglobulins are of the IgG class but also may be IgA, IgM, or, rarely, IgD or IgE [10].

Laboratory examination of the bone marrow shows a proliferation of both mature and immature plasma cells with about 20 percent or over having multinucleated forms. These cells often completely replace the bone marrow. There is abnormal serum protein electrophoresis and immunoelectrophoresis. Bence-Jones proteinemia and proteinuria, which are proliferations of light chains of immunoglobulin molecules, are present in about 50 percent of the individuals. A higher incidence of renal failure correlates with the amount of protein found in the urine [6]. About 1 percent of the affected plasma cells do not secrete antibodies.

The malignant neoplasm that arises in the bone usually does not metastasize outside the bone. The destructive bone lesions erode the bone and cause punched-out lytic lesions observable on x ray. These lesions can be visualized in any bone but are most frequently seen in the vertebral column, ribs, skull, pelvis, femur, clavicle, and scapula [10]. The bones can become so fragile that simple movements can cause fractures.

Calcium metabolism is often abnormal, causing some persons to have elevated serum calcium levels. There is often a normocytic, normochromic anemia, with variable depression of the white cell and platelet count.

Bone or back pain is the most common presenting symptom. Pallor and weakness due to secondary anemia may occur.

The pathology usually results in pathologic fractures due to the bone lesions especially of the weight-bearing regions.

In some cases, myeloma nephrosis occurs, due to the infiltration and precipitation of the light chains (Bence-Jones protein) in the distal tubules as the urine is concentrated. The laminated, crystalline casts in the distal tubules damage the kidney cells and obstruct the tubules. Pathologic interstitial inflammation and fibrosis further impair kidney function, leading to uremia and a poor prognosis for the affected individual.

Anemia, thrombocytopenia, which leads to bleeding, and neutropenia, resulting in infection, are common results of the disorder. Vascular insufficiency may occur in the peripheral areas and is apparently related to an increased blood viscosity due to the high levels of circulating immunoglobulins. Survival statistics remain poor and depend largely on the person's response to the chemotherapeutic regimen, with 1 to 4 years as the norm.

REFERENCES

1. Allan, E.T., and Gabuzda, T.G. *Pathophysiology of Blood* (2nd ed.). Philadelphia: Saunders, 1979.
2. Braunstein, H. (ed.). *Outlines of Pathology.* St. Louis: Mosby, 1982.
3. Brinkhous, K.M. (ed.). *The Year Book of Pathology and Clinical Pathology.* Chicago: Year Book, 1981.
4. Clarkson, B. The Acute Leukemias. In K.J. Isselbacher, et al. (eds.), *Harrison's Principles of Internal Medicine* (9th ed.). New York: McGraw-Hill, 1980.
5. Dale, D. Abnormalities of Leukocytes. In K.J. Isselbacher, et al. (eds.), *Harrison's Principles of Internal Medicine* (9th ed.). New York: McGraw-Hill, 1980.
6. Fudenberg, H.H., et al. *Basic and Clinical Immunology* (3rd ed.). Los Altos, Calif.: Lange, 1980.
7. Guyton, A.C. *Textbook of Medical Physiology* (6th ed.). Philadelphia: Saunders, 1981.
8. Ham, A.W., and Cormack, D.H. *Histology* (8th ed.). Philadelphia: Lippincott, 1979.
9. LoBuglio, A.F. (ed.). *The Medical Clinics of North America: Symposium on Hematologic Disorders.* Philadelphia: Saunders, 1980.
10. Robbins, S.L., and Cotran, R. *Pathologic Basis of Disease* (2nd ed.). Philadelphia: Saunders, 1979.
11. Wallach, I. *Interpretation of Diagnostic Tests* (3rd ed.). Boston: Little, Brown, 1978.

CHAPTER 16
NORMAL AND ALTERED COAGULATION

LEARNING OBJECTIVES

1. Define *hemostasis* and list the four major events included in this process.
2. Explain the role of vasoconstriction in the hemostatic process and the mechanism of stimulation.
3. State the purpose of hemostasis and coagulation.
4. Describe the function of the platelets and explain their role in the hemostatic process.
5. Describe the sequence of events in the coagulation process.
6. Briefly describe the essential clotting factors, where they are formed, and how they act.
7. Explain the common pathway of blood coagulation.
8. Differentiate between the intrinsic pathway and the extrinsic pathway to prothrombin activation.
9. Define a zymogen and describe its role in the cascade activation process.
10. Diagram the interrelationships of the major components involved in hemostasis.
11. Describe the composition of the blood clot.
12. Explain the action of the fibrinolytic system.
13. List several factors normally present in the blood that inhibit the clotting process.
14. Differentiate between factors enhancing coagulation and factors inhibiting coagulation in normal blood.
15. Explain the basis of common laboratory tests used to determine coagulation problems.
16. Briefly explain the role of liver function with respect to normal coagulation.
17. Differentiate between the factor deficiencies that cause the various types of hemophilia.
18. Explain how uncontrolled bleeding occurs in disseminated intravascular coagulation (DIC).
19. Differentiate between thrombocytosis and thrombocytopenia. List some causative conditions for each.
20. Describe some platelet disorders that are associated with hypercoagulability.

Coagulation is an essential, protective part of hemostasis that prevents blood loss when a vessel is damaged. Coagulation, the ability of the blood to change from a fluid to a semisolid mass, involves the conversion of *fibrinogen*, a soluble macromolecule composed of three polypeptide chains, to *fibrin* monomers by action of the proteolytic enzyme *thrombin*. Polymerization of the monomers follows and spontaneously bonds fibrin monomers together. A fibrin stabilizing factor acts on the fibrin to cause crosslinkage bonding, which forms an insoluble threadlike mesh on which a clot forms. This mechanism for clot initiation and clot formation involves a series of sequential cascadelike reactions that employ multiple factors in the blood and injured tissues.

HEMOSTASIS

Hemostasis, which refers to arrest of bleeding or circulation of the blood, is often divided into four main events: (1) vasoconstriction, (2) hemostatic platelet plug formation, (3) blood coagulation, and (4) clot formation. The interaction of all four events is essential for normal blood hemostasis. The general dynamic interaction of these events is illustrated in Figure 16-1.

Vasoconstriction

Vasoconstriction is the result of many events that occur during an injury. Immediately after the wall of a vessel is injured, there is a contraction of the vessel that acts to decrease the flow of blood entering or leaving the vessel. This contraction is due mainly to two factors: (1) nervous reflexes, and (2) local myogenic spasms [2]. Nervous reflexes are probably initiated by pain impulses created by the tissue or vascular trauma. Local myogenic spasm is initiated by direct damage to the vascular wall and by the release of serotonin from platelets.

The greater the portion of vessel traumatized, the greater the degree of spasm. A sharply cut vessel will bleed longer than a crushed one [2]. A clean cut by a sharp razor

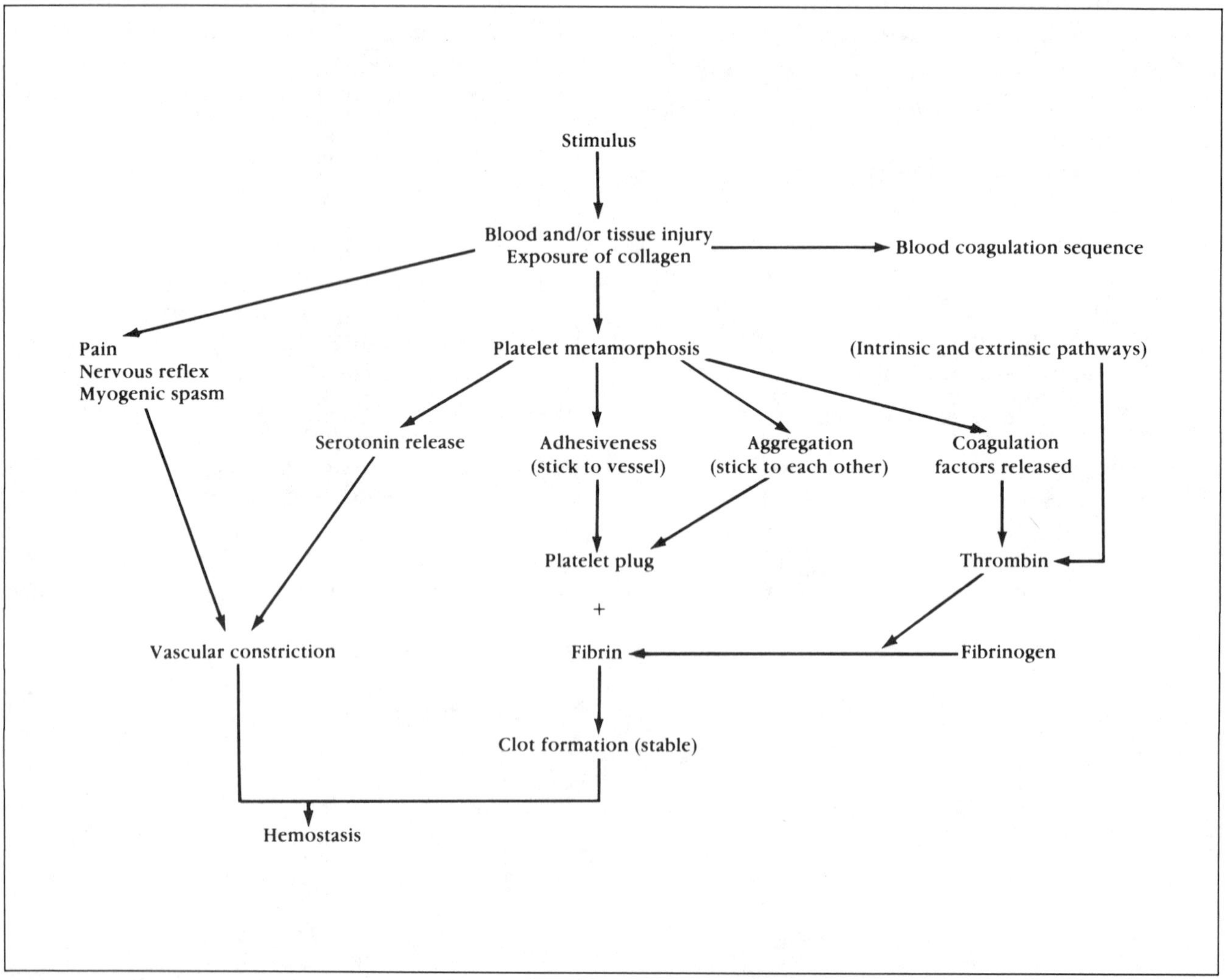

FIGURE 16-1. Homeostatic mechanisms.

blade, for example, will bleed longer than a scrape or jagged cut.

Hemostatic Platelet Plug Formation

When a blood vessel is damaged, the endothelial lining is disrupted, allowing the exposure of underlying collagen. When platelets are exposed to collagen or other foreign surfaces such as antigen-antibody complexes, thrombin, proteolytic enzymes, endotoxins, or viruses, they undergo a dynamic change, which has been described as *viscous metamorphosis.* They begin to swell and form irregular shapes with processes protruding from their surfaces. They become sticky and adhere to the collagen and basement membrane of the vessel. The platelets release adenosine diphosphate (ADP), which attracts other platelets and aids in platelet adhesion and aggregation. ADP also is released from disrupted red blood cells and damaged tissue. Enzymes released from the platelets cause the formation of thromboxane A in the plasma. ADP and thromboxane A activate nearby platelets that stick to the original platelets, thus creating a cycle of activation of platelets. The platelet plug results, causing adherence to the collagen fibers of the damaged endothelial vessel wall. This plug is loose and arrests circulation only if the tear in the vessel is small. Later, a tight plug is formed by fibrin threads that result from the process of coagulation.

Hundreds of minute ruptures occur in the capillaries each day. The platelet plug is important because it can stop bleeding completely if the damage to the vessel is small. A significant decrease in the number of platelets can lead to small hemorrhagic areas under the skin and in the internal tissue [2]. Usually the platelet plugging mechanism seals the tear in the vessel rather than occluding the lumen of the vessel.

Characteristics and Physiology of Platelets

Platelets are fragments of megakaryocytes formed in the bone marrow and released into the circulation. The normal platelet concentration in the blood is about 140,000 to 340,000 per μl [7]. Adequate numbers of platelets must be present for normal hemostasis and clotting.

Each platelet has four major functional regions called the peripheral, sol-gel, organelle, and membrane systems zones (Fig. 16-2) [8]. The *peripheral zone* includes the cell membrane and closely associated structures in which are found the receptors for the various stimuli that trigger platelet activation, the substrate for adhesion and aggregation reactions, and a surface for coagulant protein interaction. Adhesion and aggregation do not mean the same thing. Adhesion involves the platelet-collagen interaction that results in the platelets sticking to the site of injury on the blood vessel. Aggregation is a calcium-requiring process of platelet-platelet association. The peripheral zone translates the signals of stimuli into chemical messages and initiates the physical alterations required for platelet activation. *The solgel zone* is composed of the platelet cytoplasm matrix. Here are found the fiber systems that support the disklike shape of the unstimulated platelets and provide the con-

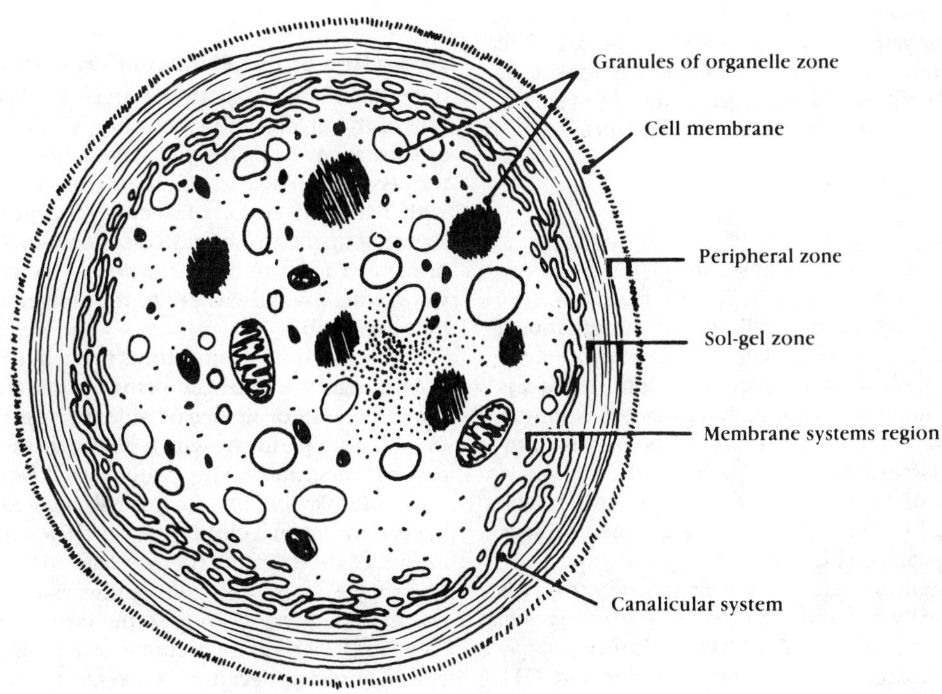

FIGURE 16-2. Major functional regions of the platelet.

tractile systems that allow the platelets to change shape, form pseudopods, and perform contraction and secretion functions. *The organelle zone* contains the cellular organelles, which are imbedded in the sol gel matrix and serve metabolic purposes. This zone is an important storage area for enzymes, serotonin, calcium, and protein constituents. The fourth region is called the *membrane systems region* and is comprised of canalicular systems or tiny surface-connected canallike structures, which have access to the interior. In this region plasma substances are able to enter and cellular products may be released or secreted. Products stored in secretory organelles are extruded to the outside through an energy-dependent process [8].

Contractile physiology dominates the platelet response and is critical to the development of the hemostatic plug. The contractile ability allows shape changes and internal transformation. It facilitates the process of secretion and converts loosely clumped platelets into tightly packed masses that can seal a vascular rent. Contraction of the platelets provides the force for contraction of the platelet fibrin meshwork and allows for retraction of a clot.

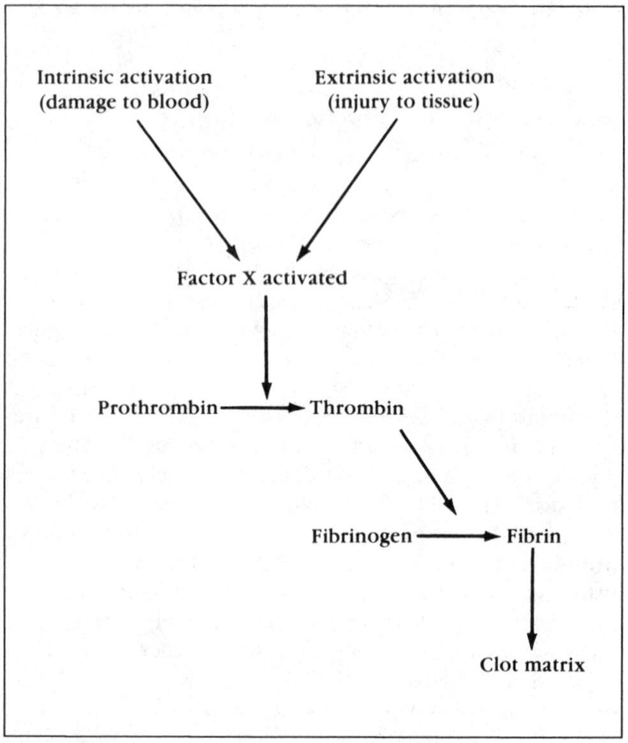

FIGURE 16-3. Common pathway of blood coagulation.

GENERAL MECHANISM OF BLOOD COAGULATION

Three basic reactions constitute the sequential pathway for blood coagulation. (1) A prothrombin activator is formed via the intrinsic or extrinsic pathway in response to tissue or endothelial damage. (2) Prothrombin activator catalyzes the conversion of prothrombin to thrombin. (3) Thrombin then catalyzes the conversion of soluble fibrinogen to solid fibrin polymer threads. These fibrin threads form the meshwork on which plasma, blood cells, and platelets aggregate to form the clot (Fig. 16-3). Before these three reactions can occur, a series of reactions must take place. A group of reactants, called clotting factors, effect the process that terminates in the formation of the blood clot.

Clotting Factors

The clotting factors are a series of plasma proteins that are generally inactive forms of proteolytic enzymes. Table 16-1 summarizes these factors and indicates the international nomenclature utilized for each. The enzymatic proteolytic actions cause successive reactions of the clotting process in a cascadelike sequence. One activated factor is important for the activation of the next factor. The inactive precursor enzyme is activated by peptide-bond cleavage. A low level or lack of even one of these inactive proteolytic enzymes can lead to abnormal bleeding and hemorrhage [6]. Fibrinogen, prothrombin, and factors VII, IX, and X are essential procoagulation factors. *Fibrinogen* (factor I) is synthesized in the liver at a rate that usually corresponds to the rate of utilization or need. The levels of fibrinogen may be increased by adrenocorticotropic hormone (ACTH), growth hormone, endotoxin, pregnancies, and occlusive arterial disease. *Prothrombin* (factor II) and factors VII, IX, and X are also synthesized exclusively in the liver by a process that requires vitamin K. These factors are affected by pregnancy, oral contraceptives, and diethylstilbestrol [10].

Formation of the Prothrombin Activator

Initiation of the coagulation process begins with the formation of the prothrombin activator, a substance or complex of substances [2]. The mechanism begins with trauma to the tissues, trauma to the blood, or contact of the blood with damaged endothelial cells, collagen, or other substances outside the blood vessel endothelium. This injury or contact leads to the formation of the prothrombin activator, which will then lead to the conversion of prothrombin to thrombin.

The prothrombin activator is formed in one of two ways: (1) through the extrinsic pathway, initiated by trauma to the vessel wall or tissues outside the vessel, or (2) through the intrinsic pathway, which begins with trauma to blood components, altering the platelets and factor XII.

An interplay of both the intrinsic and extrinsic systems is needed for normal clotting. A deficiency of a single protein in one of these pathways may lead to a clotting disorder. The intrinsic and extrinsic pathways converge on a final common pathway leading to the formation of a fibrin clot (see Fig. 16-3). Each precursor protein is important in the clotting process because it is necessary for the activation of the next protein.

The clotting process occurs by a cascade of zymogen

TABLE 16-1. Blood coagulation factors

Factor (international nomenclature)	Common synonyms	Remarks
I	Fibrinogen	Soluble macromolecule Synthesized in liver Fibrin precursor
II	Prothrombin	Synthesized in liver Vitamin K required for formation
III	Tissue thromboplastin Thrombokinase	Phospholipid Involved in activation of extrinsic pathway
IV	Calcium	Involved in several complexes in the coagulation process
V	Proaccelerin Labile factor Ac-globulin; Ac-G	Synthesized in liver Modifier protein, not enzyme Required in prothrombin activator complex
(VI)	Obsolete term	Same as factor V
VII	Proconvertin Stable factor Serum prothrombin conversion accelerator	Part of enzyme complex in extrinsic pathway Synthesized in the liver Vitamin K required for formation
VIII	Antihemophilic globulin (AHG); antihemophilic factor (AHF); antihemophilic factor A	Required for intrinsic pathway function Possibly synthesized in liver, spleen, RES, or kidney
IX	Plasma thromboplastin component (PTC) Christmas factor Antihemophilic factor B	Synthesized in liver Requires vitamin K Needed for intrinsic pathway function
X	Stuart-Prower factor Stuart factor	Synthesized in the liver Requires vitamin K Needed for both intrinsic and extrinsic pathways
XI	Plasma thromboplastin antecedent (PTA) Antihemophilic factor C	Substrate in intrinsic activator enzymatic complex Needed for intrinsic system activation Area of synthesis unknown
XII	Hageman factor Contact factor Antihemophilic factor D	Involved in first step of activation of intrinsic system Area of synthesis unknown
XIII	Fibrin stabilizing factor (FSF) Plasma transglutaminase	Causes amide cross linkage fibrin Stabilizes clot formation Synthesized by platelets and possibly other proteins, may be activated by liver

activations. A *zymogen* is an inactive precursor that is converted to an active enzyme by the action of another enzyme. The activated form of one factor sequentially catalyzes the activation of the next factor in cascadelike fashion leading to clot formation.

Intrinsic Pathway

Joseph Lister, in 1863, noted that blood stayed fluid longer in the excised veins of an ox than in a glass container [6]. When the blood was put in a glass container it clotted rapidly. The abnormal surface of the glass activated components that were already in the blood. This means of activation was called the intrinsic pathway because the clotting was triggered by substances that were normally present in the blood.

The intrinsic mechanism for initiating clotting begins inside the vessel. When the blood comes into contact with collagen or damaged endothelium, an intrinsic activator enzymatic complex is formed. An important part of this complex is the Hageman factor (activated factor XII), a proteolytic enzyme. This complex acts enzymatically to activate factor XI. Sequential events continue in cascade fashion. Activated factor XI acts enzymatically to activate factor IX. Factor IX acts to form factor X activation complex, which consists of activated factor IX, factor VIII, calcium, and phospholipids. Activated factor X then combines with factor V, calcium, and phospholipids to form a complex called the prothrombin activator. The prothrombin activator initiates within seconds the proteolytic cleavage of the prothrombin bonds to form thrombin. The amount of thrombin formed is closely related to the amount of prothrombin activator present. Once thrombin is formed, the final clotting process is set in motion (Fig. 16-4).

If factor VIII or the platelets are not at an adequate level, activation of factor X is impaired. Decreased factor VIII is the major problem in classic hemophilia and decreased platelets result in bleeding disorders such as thrombocytopenia (see p. 207). All of the clotting factors are essential to the normal coagulation sequence.

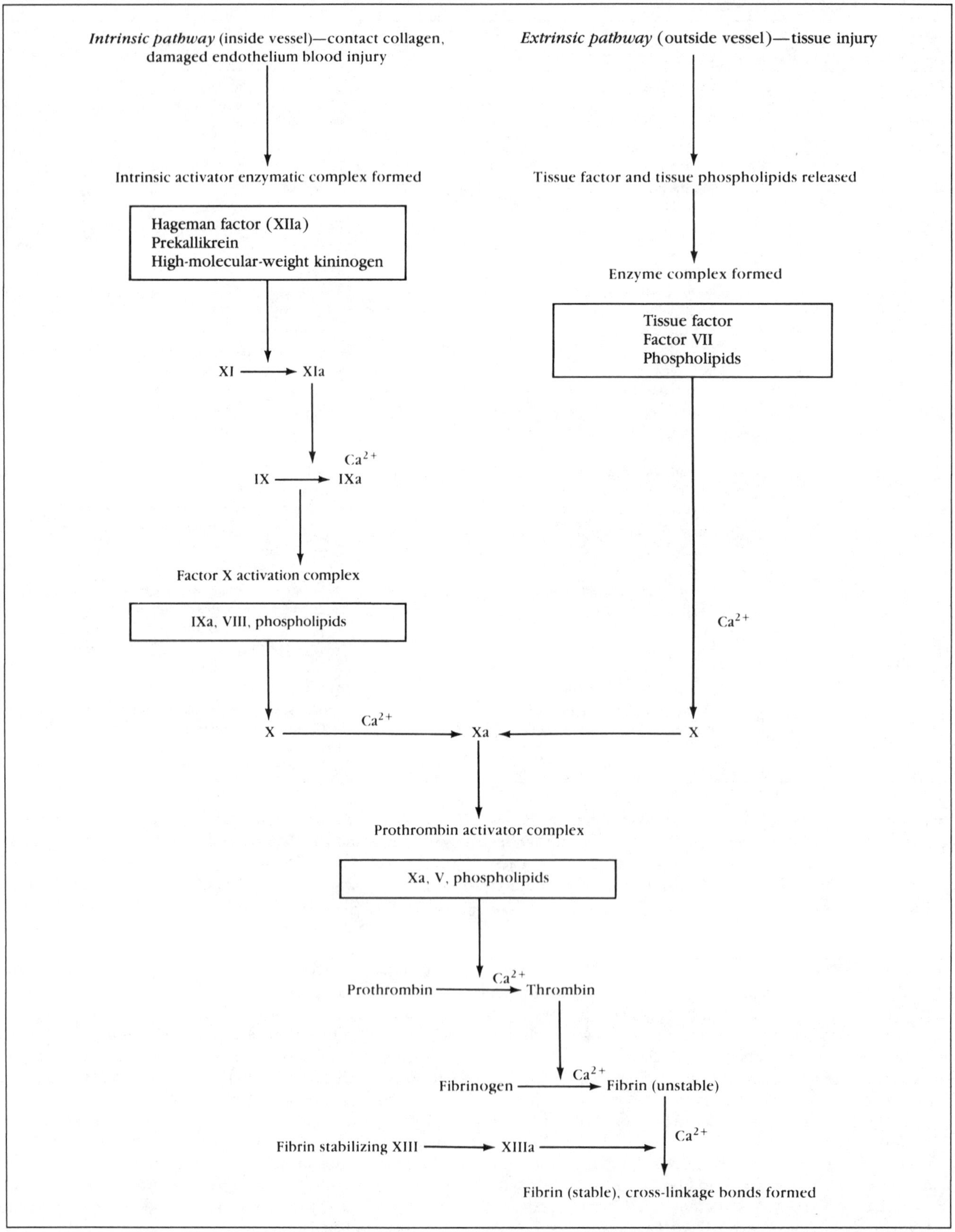

FIGURE 16-4. Blood coagulation sequence. Key: a = activated enzyme; Ca^{2+} = calcium, necessary in several reactions.

Extrinsic Pathway

The extrinsic pathway for coagulation is triggered by substances not normally present in the blood, such as extracts from damaged tissues or other foreign materials. When the blood comes in contact with a traumatized vascular wall or extravascular tissue, there is a release of what have been called tissue factor and tissue phospholipids. The tissue factor is a proteolytic enzyme with cleavage ability, and the tissue phospholipids are mainly the phospholipids of the tissue cell membrane.

The tissue factor, factor VII, calcium, and phospholipids form a complex. This complex acts enzymatically on factor X to form an activated factor X. Activated factor X then becomes part of the prothrombin activator complex, which acts enzymatically to convert prothrombin to thrombin. Thrombin in turn acts enzymatically to convert fibrinogen to fibrin (see Fig. 16-4).

Enzymatic Complexes

The "cascade hypothesis" used to describe the relationships among the protein constituents associated with the blood coagulation process has been the object of much study over the years. Most of the enzymes involved in the process and their precursors have been isolated and identified. The nature of the specificity of the proteolytic cleavages and activation processes in the coagulation transformations is quite well understood. Recently, progress has been made in the isolation and understanding of nonenzyme cofactor proteins, which are necessary for the blood coagulation process. Four principal enzymatic complexes involving these cofactors have been isolated [3]. They include:

1. The "intrinsic" activator, which includes the Hageman factor (factor XII), prekallikrein, high-molecular-weight kininogen, and the substrate for the reaction factor XI
2. Factor VII, tissue factor, calcium, and phospholipids
3. Factor X activation, which is composed of activated factor IX, cofactor, factor VIII, calcium, and phospholipids
4. The "prothrombinase" complex, which includes activated factor X, activated factor V, calcium, and phospholipids

The significance of the cofactors and complex formation may be illustrated by the "prothrombinase" complex. The cofactors in this complex at physiologic concentrations lead to an amplification of the reaction rate by 300,000 times [3]. It is obvious that without these cofactors and the interactions of the components in the complex, prothrombin conversion to thrombin would be slowed tremendously.

Final Common Pathway to Clot Formation

With the activation of factor X and the formation of the prothrombin activator complex, the final common pathway for clot formation begins. Prothrombin activator complex causes the conversion of prothrombin to thrombin. Thrombin, in turn, enzymatically converts fibrinogen to fibrin. These reactions constitute the final coagulation pathway for both the intrinsic and extrinsic systems. The rate of the blood coagulation reaction is generally related to the amount of prothrombin activator formed and the amount of activation of factor X. If either is inhibited or stopped because of the absence of a clotting factor or other reasons, the coagulation process becomes altered and excess bleeding results (see Fig. 16-3).

Clot Formation

Blood coagulation occurs faster with severe trauma to the vascular wall than with minor trauma. The general sequence of physical events takes place in a comparatively short time. After the vessel is severed, the platelets agglutinate and fibrin appears. A fibrin clot can form in as little as 15 seconds up to 6 minutes. Clot retraction follows and may take 30 minutes to an hour. After the clot is formed, either dissolution or fibrous organization of the blood clot occurs.

BLOOD CLOT COMPOSITION. The blood clot is composed of a meshwork of the polymerized fibrin threads with blood cells, platelets, and plasma products that have become attached in the meshwork. The fibrin threads adhere to the damaged vessel surface holding the clot in place and preventing blood loss. The meshwork is produced by spontaneous aggregation of fibrin monomer to form polymer threads. Transglutaminase (factor XIII) acts on the fibrin to form covalent cross-links. This stabilizes the clot and makes it resistant to dissolution [6].

CLOT RETRACTION. The contractile physiology of the platelet response is critical in the clot retraction process. Failure of clot retraction often indicates a decrease in the number of platelets. The platelets entrapped in the clot continue to release the fibrin stabilizing factor. Stronger bonding of the fibrin threads occurs and causes the threads to contract. Clot retraction pulls the edges of a broken vessel closer together, which allows the vascular wall to mend. After contraction of the clot is completed, blood serum, which includes plasma and the clotting factors, is expressed from the clot.

LYSIS OF BLOOD CLOTS

Plasmin or fibrinolysin, a proteolytic enzyme that resembles trypsin, is formed from inactive circulating plasminogen by the action of thrombin and substances in the tissues. It digests fibrin threads and causes lysis of the clot along with destruction of blood clotting factors. Large amounts of the inactive enzyme, plasminogen, are incorporated in the clot and activated by vascular endothelial factors, thrombin, activated factor XII, and lysosomal enzymes in damaged tissue [2]. Plasmin largely mediates the fibrinolytic system. This built-in, self-destructing system for clots functions to break down and limit excessive clot formation.

The degradation products produced from fibrinolysis are called fibrinogen degradation products (FDP). These products inhibit the formation of thrombin and limit the formation of the clot. A balance between the formation of thrombin and plasmin must be present for normal coagulation and clotting to occur.

OTHER ANTICOAGULATION FACTORS IN NORMAL BLOOD

Anticoagulants inhibit the process of coagulation and are important in keeping the blood fluid. Factors that aid in the prevention of clotting include the smooth endothelial lining of the vessel, rapid blood flow through an area, negatively charged proteins on the endothelial surface, and anticoagulants in the blood.

Smoothness of the endothelium and a monomolecular layer of negatively charged proteins adsorbed on the endothelium are two essential conditions for maintaining the fluid state of the blood. Rapid blood flow dilutes the factors that promote coagulation, thus preventing the initiation of the clotting process. An intact, smooth endothelium prevents contact activation of the intrinsic pathway, and the layer of negatively charged proteins repels clotting factors and platelets that might stick to the vessel wall.

Several plasma proteins can dampen the activity of proteolytic enzymes generated in the coagulation and fibrinolytic systems. These include antiplasmin, activated protein C inhibitor, antithrombin III, and alpha$_2$ macroglobulin [5]. These plasma proteins serve to localize the coagulation action at the site of injury and prevent propagation of the coagulation effect throughout the vascular system.

Anticoagulation processes act to remove thrombin from the blood mostly by adsorption to fibrin threads that are formed during the clotting process. Excess thrombin not adsorbed combines with the plasma protein antithrombin III, which blocks the effect of thrombin on fibrinogen and inactivates the thrombin.

Vitamin K deficiency will prolong or prevent the clotting process. The normal production of prothrombin by the liver requires an adequate supply of vitamin K. Lack of vitamin K or liver disease can decrease the normal production of prothrombin so severely that bleeding and even hemorrhage can result.

Heparin, a potent anticoagulant, is found in the granules of the circulating basophils and the tissue mast cells. Heparin acts as an anticoagulant mainly by inhibition of factor IX, factor X, and thrombin. It reacts with factors in both the intrinsic and extrinsic pathways.

LABORATORY TESTS FOR COAGULATION PROBLEMS

Clotting or Coagulation Time

One of the oldest tests for normal coagulation is based on the amount of time drawn blood takes to clot. This can be done by simply observing the clotting time of blood in a test tube. Increased time needed for clotting indicates that a problem exists, but a normal clotting time does not rule out a hemostatic abnormality. The normal coagulation time (Lee-White) is 6 to 17 minutes in a glass tube or 19 to 60 minutes in a siliconized tube [7].

Causes of prolonged clotting time include deficiencies of any factor in the intrinsic clotting system or in the common pathway, fibrinogen deficiency, or excessively rapid fibrinolysis. This test has long been used for persons receiving heparin therapy but is now being replaced by the partial thromboplastin time (PTT), which is a more sensitive measurement of the coagulation factors.

Table 16-2 lists the laboratory tests for coagulation problems.

TABLE 16-2. Normal blood coagulation values

Clotting or coagulation time	6–17 minutes (glass tube) 19–60 minutes (siliconized tube)
Prothrombin time	11–16 seconds
Partial thromboplastin time (PTT)	60–90 seconds
Activated partial thromboplastin time (APTT)	22–37 seconds
Platelet count	140,000–340,000/μl (Rees-Ecker) 200,000–350,000/μl (Coulter Counter model B)
Bleeding time	4 minutes (Ivy method) 1–4 minutes (Duke method)
Clot retraction	Begins: 30–60 minutes Complete: 12–24 hours

Source: J. Wallach, *Interpretation of Diagnostic Tests* (3rd ed.). Boston: Little, Brown, 1978.

Prothrombin Time

Animal tissue extract and calcium are added to freshly drawn and separated citrated plasma. The time the mixture takes to clot is given in seconds. The purpose of the tissue extract is to bypass the intrinsic clotting system so that only factors VII, X, V, prothrombin, and fibrinogen affect the test. Normal prothrombin time (11–16 seconds) is increased if any of the above factors is deficient [7]. Deficiencies of factors XII, XI, IX, and VIII do not affect the prothrombin time.

The prothrombin time is often used to monitor the effects of the coumarin anticoagulants. Coumarin depresses the synthesis of factors VII, IX, X, and prothrombin.

Partial Thromboplastin Time (PTT)

Partial thromboplastin time is a relatively simple test for mild to moderate deficiencies of the intrinsic clotting factors. A phospholipid with moderate clot-promoting activity is added to the plasma. The phospholipid and plasma mixture normally take about 60 to 90 seconds to clot [9]. Deficiencies of all the factors will prolong the partial thromboplastin time with the exception of factor VII. A person with a factor VII deficiency will have a normal partial thromboplastin time and a prolonged prothrombin time. Activated partial thromboplastin time (APTT), a variation of the PTT, is used to detect deficiencies in thromboplastin formation and normally is 22 to 37 seconds [7].

Partial thromboplastin time can be used to demonstrate circulating anticoagulants in plasma. If a mixture of test plasma mixed with normal plasma has a longer PTT than normal plasma alone, it indicates that something in the test plasma has inhibited coagulation.

Tests for Specific Deficiencies

Special tests can be designed to determine the absence of specific clotting factors. Small amounts of blood are added to samples of plasma known to be deficient in a particular factor. If, for example, the added plasma corrects the partial thromboplastin time to normal for the plasma known to be deficient in a particular factor, then that factor is not deficient in the sample. The process is repeated until the tested plasma does not correct the PTT. This identifies the missing factor in the plasma of the individual being tested. There are several special tests for coagulation factors based on this laboratory method.

Platelet Count

One of the most common laboratory tests, the complete blood count (CBC), usually includes the platelet count. Platelets normally range from about 140,000 to 340,000 per μl (Rees-Ecker) or 200,000 to 350,000 per μl (Coulter Counter Model B) [7]. Platelets are difficult to count because of the inherent nature of the platelets to clump, adhere to the vessel, and aggregate. Electronic means of counting platelets offers the greatest accuracy.

Bleeding Time

Bleeding time involves an incision made either on the earlobe (Duke method) or on the inner surface of the forearm (Ivy method). The time needed for active bleeding from a clean, superficial wound to stop is called the bleeding time. Normal bleeding time is less than 4 minutes by the Ivy method and 1 to 4 minutes by the Duke method [7]. The variables involved are vascular contractility and platelet aggregation.

Secondary bleeding time can be measured by noting how long it takes for bleeding to cease after a scab is removed. Secondary bleeding time is prolonged in persons with deficiencies of factors in the intrinsic pathway or factor XIII, the fibrin-stabilizing factor.

Clot Retraction

Clot retraction time consists of observation of the degree and time in which a clot retracts and expresses serum. Whole blood is left in a test tube at 37° centigrade. Clot retraction normally begins in about 30 minutes and by 4 hours there is a well-defined clot surrounded by clear serum. Complete retraction requires about 12 to 24 hours if measured at room temperature [9]. If the platelet function or number is decreased, clot retraction is impaired.

DEFICIENCIES IN BLOOD COAGULATION

Deficiency of any of the clotting factors can result in a defect or impairment of blood coagulation. This impairment may result from genetic deficiencies of clotting factors, suppression of clotting components, or consumption of the major clotting components. The process of coagulation does not occur as an isolated, independent event, but continually interacts with other mechanisms of the body such as the inflammatory process. Alterations in the process can result in injury, hemorrhage, or death.

Single Coagulation Factor Deficiencies

Single coagulation factor deficiencies are usually hereditary. The most common deficiencies are of factor VIII, IX, and XI. All cause bleeding that may involve any of the soft tissues or the joints.

HEMOPHILIA. *Hemophilia* is a term used to loosely define several different hereditary deficiencies of coagulation factors of the intrinsic pathway. The most common cause of this coagulation disorder is a deficiency in factor VIII, accounting for about 83 to 85 percent of cases of hemophilia [1, 2]. Usually a factor VIII is produced but it is abnormal and will not promote the coagulation process. The classic factor VIII deficiency is genetically transmitted through a sex-linked recessive gene. It affects only males; females are asymptomatic carriers. This type of hemophilia is called *classic hemophilia* or *hemophilia A* and is characterized by spontaneous or traumatic subcutaneous and intramuscular hemorrhages. Hematuria and bleeding from the mouth, gums, lips, and tongue are common manifestations. Joint hemorrhages cause extreme pain and deformity. Transfusion of normal factor VIII or fresh plasma relieves the bleeding tendency for a short time.

Von Willebrand's disease is characterized by a quantitative and qualitative deficiency of factor VIII dysfunction. This condition, thought to be hereditary in nature, has also been shown to be associated with some of the autoimmune or lymphoproliferative conditions.

Factor IX deficiency, hemophilia B or Christmas disease, is sex-linked and accounts for about 10 to 15 percent of cases of hemophilia [1]. Bleeding tends to be severe with crippling joint deformities.

Factor XI deficiency, hemophilia C or Rosenthal's disease, is a mild bleeding disorder manifested by bruising, epistaxis, and menorrhagia [10]. It is transmitted as an autosomal recessive trait and accounts for about 2 percent of hemophiliacs.

Rare deficiencies of prekallikrein, kininogen, and factor VII have been reported. Factor VII deficiency is an autosomal recessive disorder.

Vitamin K Deficiency

Many disorders can lead to deficiencies of multiple coagulation factors. One example is the fat-soluble vitamin K, which is required for the synthesis of factors VII, IX, X, and II. These vitamin K–dependent factors can be monitored by prothrombin time. Factor VII has a very short half-life and will prolong the prothrombin time more quickly than the other factors. Deficiencies of vitamin K may result from several conditions. A newborn infant is normally deficient in vitamin K due to an immature liver and lack of the intestinal bacteria that are important for the synthesis of vitamin K. The newborn is often given injections of vitamin K to help prevent any possible bleeding disorder that might occur.

Obstructive liver disease and malsorption disorders can also cause a deficiency in vitamin K. Obstructive liver disease blocks the flow of bile necessary for the absorption of fat-soluble vitamins and malsorption disorders do not allow enough vitamin K to be absorbed into the circulation.

Coumarin anticoagulants act as competitive inhibitors of vitamin K. Vitamin K can be injected as an antidote in case of excessive bleeding or possible hemorrhage due to overdose of these drugs.

Many coagulation factors are synthesized in the liver. Cirrhosis and other severe liver diseases seriously affect the coagulation of the blood, often leading to hemorrhage and death.

Disseminated Intravascular Coagulation (DIC)

This condition involves both bleeding and clotting. It occurs as a complication of a variety of clinical conditions. The mechanism of the process begins with activation of the coagulation sequence causing coagulation, usually throughout the small vessels. The widespread coagulation activation leads to a consumption of clotting factors, such as platelets and fibrin. Also secondary activation of the fibrinolytic system occurs. Table 16-3 indicates some of the diverse factors that can initiate the coagulation sequence.

Persons who develop DIC are often critically ill as a result of the underlying pathology. DIC then often develops insidiously so that widespread bleeding becomes the initial sign of the problem.

The clotting sequence is triggered either by endothelial damage that activates the intrinsic coagulation cascade or by release of thromboplastic substances. The resultant clotting causes occlusion of a large proportion of the small peripheral blood vessels. The clotting sequence activates the fibrinolytic system and thus causes diffuse fibrinolysis. The conversion of plasminogen to plasmin in the fibrinolytic system inhibits the proteolysis of fibrinogen by the thrombin and may inhibit platelet aggregation. *Fibrin degradation products* are formed by the lysis of plasmin, and the lysis of fibrinogen and fibrin. These end products form a complex with the fibrin monomer, which prevents the laying down of the fibrin thread and platelet aggregation. Therefore, despite widespread clotting, the major problem is bleeding.

TABLE 16-3. Etiology of disseminated intravascular coagulation

Causative agent or condition	Probable massive coagulation stimulus
Infection	
Gram-negative bacteria	Endotoxemia; endothelial damage
Gram-positive bacteria	Fulminating sepsis; endothelial damage
Rickettsia rickettsii (Rocky Mountain spotted fever)	Parasitization of endothelial cells; rupture walls of small vessels
Plasmodium falciparum (falciparum malaria)	Injury to red cells and platelets; possible antigen-antibody reaction
Complications of pregnancy	
Amniotic fluid embolism	Circulating/thromboplastins absorbed
Saline abortions	
Dead fetus	
Hydatidiform mole	
Puerperal sepsis	Vascular damage
Toxemia	
Large hemangiomas	Turbulence of blood, stasis Endothelial damage
Disseminated carcinoma	Circulating tissue thromboplastins from malignant tissue
Hemolytic transfusion RX, anaphylaxis, hemolytic-uremic syndrome	Antigen-antibody reactions
Tissue damage	
Massive trauma	Thromboplastins released
Heat stroke	
Extensive burns	
Snake bites	
Extracorporeal circulation	Blood injury

Uncontrolled bleeding occurs because of the consumption of the clotting factors. Normal hemostasis of blood is prevented so that varying degrees of ecchymosis, petechiae, and bleeding from any opening may occur. The onset may be acute, such as that following acute obstetric emergencies, or it may gradually develop, as is seen with disseminated cancers. Bleeding problems usually predominate and venipuncture sites or incisions may bleed profusely. Acrocyanosis is often seen in the digits, being indicated by cold, mottled fingers and toes. Hypoxemia may cause dyspnea, cyanosis, and air hunger. Neurologic or renal symptoms may result from microthrombi that occlude the small vessels.

Laboratory tests that are helpful include the prothrombin time, partial thromboplastin time, fibrinogen level, and platelet count. Both the PT and PTT are prolonged while fibrinogen and platelet levels are depressed. The fibrin split products (FSP) are elevated.

Primary Fibrinolysis

Primary fibrinolysis results when massive amounts of plasminogen activator are released into the system. The activator, such as streptokinase, may be administered therapeutically to try to dissolve pulmonary emboli. Plasminogen activators can also be released by activator-rich neoplastic tissue such as prostatic carcinoma. Severe anoxia, shock, or surgical procedures may also precipitate their release.

Disseminated intravascular coagulation and primary fibrinolysis reactions are similar. Both are associated with increased fibrinolytic activity, but primary fibrinolysis results in increased amounts of plasminogen activator in the plasma, while fibrinolysis in DIC is a secondary response to the coagulation process.

Antibody Anticoagulants

Antibodies to various coagulation factors have been observed in many disease states. About 10 percent of the treated hemophilia A patients develop an anti-factor antibody to factor VIII [1]. Antibodies to paraproteins in patients with multiple myelomas and antibodies to multiple coagulation factors in patients with systemic lupus erythematosus are other examples of antibodies that act as circulating anticoagulants. The development of antibodies to coagulation factors then results in an increased risk of hemorrhage.

Platelet Disorders

THROMBOCYTOPENIA. This quantitative platelet disorder involves the presence of a very low quantity of platelets in the circulatory system. If the platelet number falls below 50,000 there is a potential for hemorrhage associated with trauma such as surgery or accidents. A platelet count of about 20,000 is associated with petechiae, ecchymoses, and sometimes bleeding from mucous membranes. With a count below 5000, a great risk exists for fatal hemorrhage through the intestinal tract or central nervous system [1].

An abnormal decrease in the number of platelets may occur in a number of disorders. These include defective platelet production, increased platelet destruction, sequestration of platelets, and loss of platelets from the system. The two major types of thrombocytopenia are idiopathic thrombocytopenic purpura (ITP) and secondary thrombocytopenia.

Idiopathic thrombocytopenia purpura is apparently an autoimmune condition that causes an increased rate of destruction of platelets. The result is either an acute destruction of platelets, which often follows a viral infection, or chronic ITP, which may be associated with another autoimmune disease such as autoimmune hemolytic anemia. The pathogenesis appears to involve the production of autoantibodies directed against the platelets. Clinical manifestations include diffuse petechiae, ecchymosis, epistaxis, hemorrhages into the soft tissues, melena, or hematuria.

Secondary thrombocytopenia may be seen in association with drug hypersensitivity, viral infections, and some of the autoimmune conditions. The platelet count is depressed as a result of a superimposed hemorrhagic problem caused by the underlying condition. Drugs that may induce secondary thrombocytopenia include chlorothiazide derivatives, quinidine, sulfonamides, chloramphenicol, antimetabolites, and antihistamines.

THROMBOCYTOSIS. *Thrombocytosis* is defined as an increased number of platelets in the peripheral blood. Counts of 400,000 to 1,000,000 per μl are usually asymptomatic, but counts greater than 1,000,000 per μl may result in thrombosis, bleeding, or other malfunctions of platelets [1]. Physiologic thrombocytosis occurs in response to infection, trauma, and other conditions. It is almost always seen after splenectomy when all of the platelets are circulated in the blood because pooling in the spleen is no longer possible. Idiopathic thrombocythemia refers to a sustained platelet count of greater than 800,000 per μl. The condition is generally regarded as one of the myeloproliferative disorders, which is supported by the fact that it is responsive to chemotherapy, seen with splenic enlargement, and may be associated with other myeloproliferative disorders such as chronic myelogenous leukemia and polycythemia vera. Affected individuals often exhibit peripheral thrombosis and episodes of spontaneous bleeding.

QUALITATIVE PLATELET DISORDERS. Qualitative platelet disorders include those alterations that have a prolonged bleeding time with a normal platelet count in most instances. The disorders are due to a variety of defects of platelet function such as a platelet adhesion defect as in von Willebrand's disease, or a defect in platelet aggregation as in thromboasthenia, a congenital disorder. Qualitative platelet disorders can also be acquired. Drugs such as aspirin may impair the aggregation of platelets, while in uremia a dialyzable factor is formed that inhibits platelet aggregation.

HYPERCOAGULATION. Hypercoagulation may involve accelerated rates of coagulation, hyperviscosity, and increased platelet activity or antithrombin III deficiency. Atherosclerosis associated with vascular clotting and myocardial infarction has been found to involve increased platelet turnover and increased platelet release of factor IV and beta thromboglobulin [4]. Giant hemangiomas have an increased platelet and fibrinogen turnover, which is thought to be the result of massive blood turbulence and stasis in the large bed of vascular tissue. A very extensive hemangioma may lead to a pattern of disseminated intravascular coagulation, thrombocytopenia, and low levels of circulating fibrinogen, factor V, and factor VII, with an increase in fibrin degradation products [4]. *Thrombotic thrombocy-*

topenic purpura, a rare disorder, is characterized by thrombocytopenia, anemia, neurologic deficits, and renal failure. Endothelial cell damage may be the activator in the disorder with an immune vasculitis affecting the endothelial cells. Platelet adhesion and aggregation leads to the obstruction of the vessel and ischemia of the surrounding tissues [4].

Blood stasis in the small vessels is enhanced when the blood is more viscous. Polycythemia increases the viscosity and affects the rate of blood flow. An increased number of any of the formed blood elements may increase the viscosity of blood.

Hyperfunction of platelets in the absence of thrombocytosis has been postulated as a mechanism for various pathologies. It has been postulated that strokes and transient ischemic attacks in younger patients who have no evidence of arterial abnormalities or degenerative changes could be the result of hyperfunction of the platelets. Platelet clumping in small vessels may result in alterations of blood supply [4].

Platelet activation and release of thromboxane A_2 may lead to coronary artery spasm, ischemia, and infarction. Platelet function in these cases can be examined by laboratory means for increased platelet sensitivity to aggregating agents and increased release of thromboxane A_2 and other platelet factors.

Several cases of sudden deafness have been associated with an increased platelet sensitivity. A single artery supplies the cochlea and may constrict, causing obstruction to the blood flow. The sudden deafness is often preceded by an acute viral infection. Myxoviruses, under experimental conditions, have been shown to cause platelet damage and acceleration of the release of platelet factor III. The viral action may be the mechanism responsible for initiating this deafness syndrome [4].

Antithrombin III deficiency is an inherited familial disorder that results in thrombosis. The antithrombin III inactivates most of the active proteases involved in thrombin formation. A modest decrease in this inhibitor allows the proteases to remain active for a longer period, which results in the rapid formation of thrombi. Antithrombin III deficiency can also occur as an acquired disorder and is associated with liver disease or disseminated intravascular coagulation. Birth control pills and heparin also reduce antithrombin III levels.

REFERENCES

1. Braunstein, H. *Outlines of Pathology.* St. Louis: Mosby, 1982.
2. Guyton, A. C. *Textbook of Medical Physiology* (6th ed.). Philadelphia: Saunders, 1981.
3. Mann, K. G. Complex formation in blood-clotting reactions. *Clin. Chem.* 27:721, 1981.
4. Penner, J. A. Hypercoagulation and thrombosis. *Med. Clin. North Am.* 64:542, 1980.
5. Rosenberg, R. D. Inhibition of clotting. *Clin. Chem.* 27:879, 1981.
6. Stryer, L. *Biochemistry.* San Francisco: Freeman, 1975.
7. Wallach, J. *Interpretation of Diagnostic Tests* (3rd ed.). Boston: Little, Brown, 1978.
8. White, J. G. Calcium prostaglandins and granules in platelet function. *Clin. Chem.* 27:618, 1981.
9. Widmann, F. K. (ed.). *Goodale's Clinical Interpretation of Laboratory Tests.* Philadelphia: Davis, 1973.
10. Williams, W. J., et al. *Hematology* (3rd ed.). New York: McGraw-Hill, 1983.

UNIT 8

CIRCULATION

Barbara L. Bullock
NORMAL CIRCULATORY DYNAMICS
RHEUMATIC FEVER
HYPERTENSION

Leah Oakley
COMPROMISED PUMPING ABILITY OF THE HEART
ALTERATIONS IN SYSTEMIC CIRCULATION

Betty Norris
CORONARY ARTERY DISEASE
HYPERTENSION

Donna Packa
Joan M. Vitello
VALVULAR HEART DISEASE
PERICARDITIS
ENDOCARDITIS

Jules Constant
Pearl Rosendahl
HEART SOUNDS
MURMURS

The study of circulation requires an understanding of both normal circulatory dynamics and alterations of circulatory structures that lead to the effects of compromised tissue perfusion.

Chapter 17 examines the anatomy of the heart and vessels. The physiology of the system is reviewed in sufficient depth to support the content in subsequent chapters. An attempt has been made to relate the electrophysiology of the heart to electrocardiography without delving into all of the arrhythmias that may occur. The reader is referred to the bibliography for further information especially regarding electrophysiology. Chapter 18 details heart failure, an end result of many other problems. In an attempt to simplify the concept, the author has classified heart failure into left heart failure and right heart failure on the basis of the clinical manifestations. It must be emphasized that both left and right heart failure are interrelated and that which affects one side of the heart will ultimately affect the other. Chapter 19 details specific disease conditions of the heart and pericardium. Chapter 20 classifies and clarifies hypertension. Chapter 21 discusses the often neglected subject of peripheral vascular disease, both arterial and venous.

It is suggested that the reader utilize the learning objectives in each chapter and the bibliography at the end of the unit to enhance learning.

CHAPTER 17
NORMAL CIRCULATORY DYNAMICS

LEARNING OBJECTIVES

1. Locate the major structures of the heart, including the chambers, the valves, and the vessels.
2. List the three layers that compose the atrial and ventricular walls.
3. Show the position of the trabeculae carnae, the papillary muscles, and the chordae tendineae.
4. Differentiate between the structures of the atrioventricular valves and the semilunar valves.
5. Locate the origin and the branches of both the right and left coronary arteries.
6. Locate the conduction system of the heart.
7. Describe the P cells and intermediate cells.
8. Differentiate, structurally, a myocardial muscle cell from a skeletal muscle cell.
9. Define *intercalated disk* and *syncytium.*
10. Review the general mechanism for skeletal muscle contraction.
11. Compare skeletal and cardiac muscle contraction.
12. Define *absolute* and *relative refractory periods* in cardiac muscle.
13. Describe cardiac metabolism and cardiac work.
14. Clearly describe the properties of the heart: automaticity, rhythmicity, excitability, and conductivity.
15. Define *diastolic depolarization* in the sinoatrial node and indicate why the SA node is considered to be the pacemaker of the heart.
16. Relate the events of the cardiac cycle to the wave forms seen on an ECG tracing.
17. Describe the four interrelated factors of cardiac contraction: preload, afterload, contractility, and heart rate.
18. Define *ventricular compliance.*
19. Define *inotropic* and *chronotropic effects.*
20. Describe the events of the cardiac cycle.
21. Differentiate between isovolumic contraction, ejection, and isovolumic relaxation as phases in ventricular systole.
22. Explain how a different stroke volume between the ventricles is compensated for or equalized.
23. List the pressures and oxygen saturations normally found in the chambers of the heart and in the vessels.
24. Describe the factors responsible for generating the heart sounds.
25. Explain sympathetic and parasympathetic influence on the heart.
26. Locate and define the function of the chemoreceptors and the baroreceptors.

27. Differentiate between the elastic and nutrient arteries.
28. Define *exchange vessel* and *capacitance vessel.*
29. Describe the structure and function of the lymphatic system.
30. Describe the generation of the Korotkoff sounds.
31. List some factors that can affect the pulse pressure.
32. Clearly describe the four direct determinants of blood pressure.

Understanding the dynamics of the normal cardiac contraction provides the basis for understanding the effects of alterations to structures within the heart, the myocardial muscle, or the vessels. The first part of this chapter is devoted to normal cardiac anatomy and physiology; the second part deals with the dynamics of circulation.

ANATOMY OF THE HEART

The heart is a double pump that pumps its blood to the lungs and to the systemic arteries. It provides for oxygenation and nutrition to all of the tissues of the body.

The heart is composed of four pumping chambers, the right and left atria and the right and left ventricles. The right atrium and ventricle receive blood from the systemic veins and pump it to the lungs via the pulmonary artery. The left atrium and ventricle pump blood received from the pulmonary veins to the systemic arteries through the aorta. Figure 17-1 shows the general anatomy of the heart and blood vessels.

Atria

The *right atrium* is a low-pressure, thin-walled chamber that receives blood from the superior and inferior vena cava and from the veins draining the heart. The *left atrium* is a slightly smaller chamber than the right and receives its blood from the four pulmonary veins that carry oxygenated blood from the lungs back to the heart.

The atrial walls are composed of three layers: (1) *epicardium,* a thin outer layer that is continuous with the outer layer of the ventricles; (2) *myocardium,* the middle, or muscular, layer of the atria, discontinuous with that of the ventricles; and (3) *endocardium,* a thin, continuous inner layer that covers the inner surface of the atria, the valves, the ventricles, and the vessels entering and leaving the heart. The muscular layer of the atria is much thinner than that in the ventricles and accounts for the lower pressures maintained in these chambers. The atria serve mostly as storage reservoirs and conductive passageways for the movement of blood to the ventricles.

Dividing the atria is the membranous atrial septum, a separation that prevents the communication of blood between the atria. This septum houses the fossa ovalis, which was a fetal communication, the foramen ovale.

Ventricles

The ventricular walls are also composed of three layers, epicardium, myocardium, and endocardium (Fig. 17-2). The *right ventricle* has been described as having a bellows appearance with a myocardial layer that is thicker than that in the atrial walls, but thinner than that of the left ventricle. The *left ventricle* has a more circular appearance than the right. Its myocardial muscle layer is much thicker than the right ventricle, which allows it to achieve the high pressures required for systemic arterial circulation.

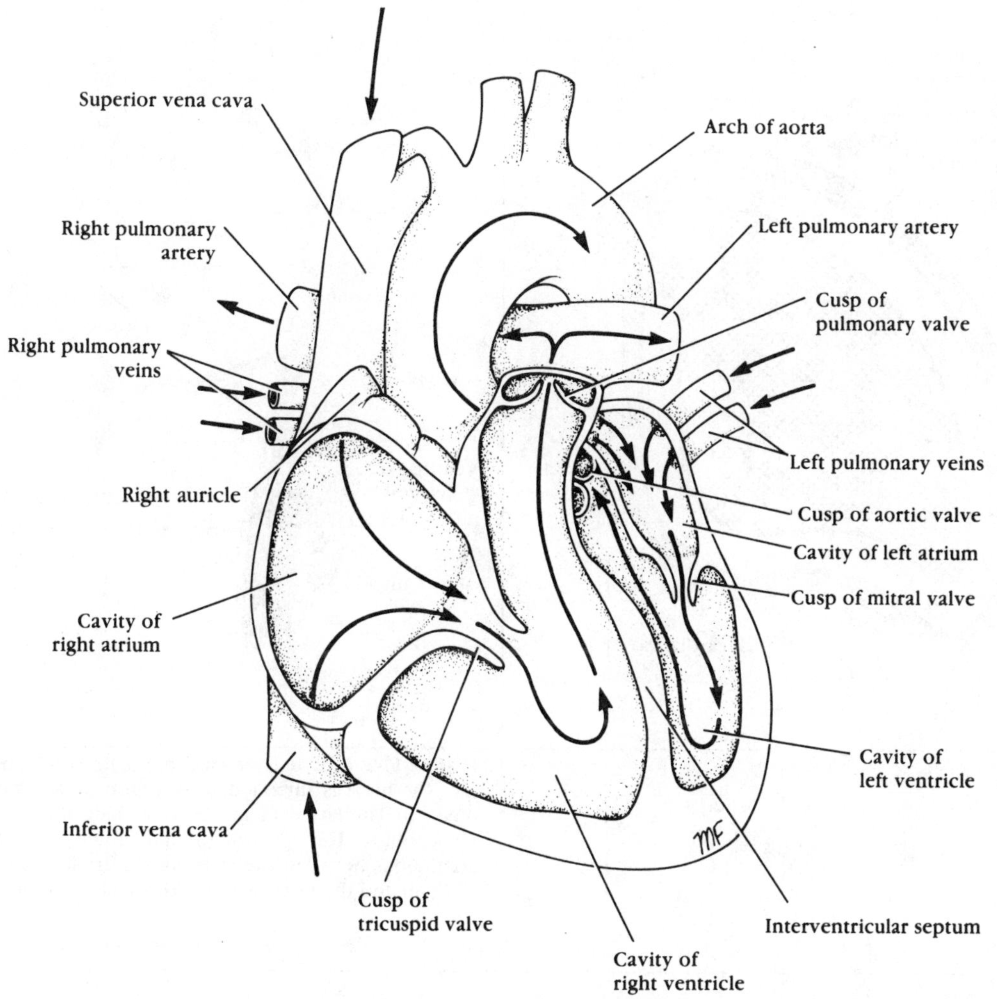

FIGURE 17-1. Anatomy of the heart and great vessels. *Arrows* show flow of blood through the heart. (Figs. 17-1, 17-8, 17-9, 17-10, 17-15, 17-16, 17-21, from R. S. Snell, *Clinical Histology for Medical Students.* Boston: Little, Brown, 1984.)

Separating the ventricles is the ventricular septum, which is a thick muscular area that becomes membranous as it nears the atrioventricular valves (Fig. 17-3). This septum houses the branches of the conduction tissue and provides an important fulcrum during contraction of the ventricles.

The inner surface of the ventricles contains areas of raised muscle bundles that are undercut by open spaces. These muscle bundles are called the *trabeculae carnae* (Fig. 17-4). The papillary muscles project from the trabeculated surface, yielding two groups of papillary muscles in the left ventricle and three groups in the right. These muscles give off strong fibrous strands called *chordae tendineae,* which attach to the margins of the atrioventricular valves.

Atrioventricular Valves

The mitral or bicuspid valve lies between the left atrium and the left ventricle (see Fig. 17-4). It is composed of two leaflets of fibroelastic tissue, which slightly overlap each other when the valve is in the closed position (Fig. 17-5). The margins of the valve are attached to the fibrous chordae tendineae. The tricuspid valve is composed of three leaflets and lies between the right atrium and the right ventricle. The leaflets, also composed of fibrous tissue, are thinner than those of the mitral valve. These are also attached to chordae tendineae that project from the right ventricular papillary muscles.

Semilunar Valves

The aortic and pulmonary valves are called semilunar valves because they have three cusps that are cuplike in appearance (Fig. 17-6). The margins of the valve cusps meet when the valves are in the closed position. Two coronary

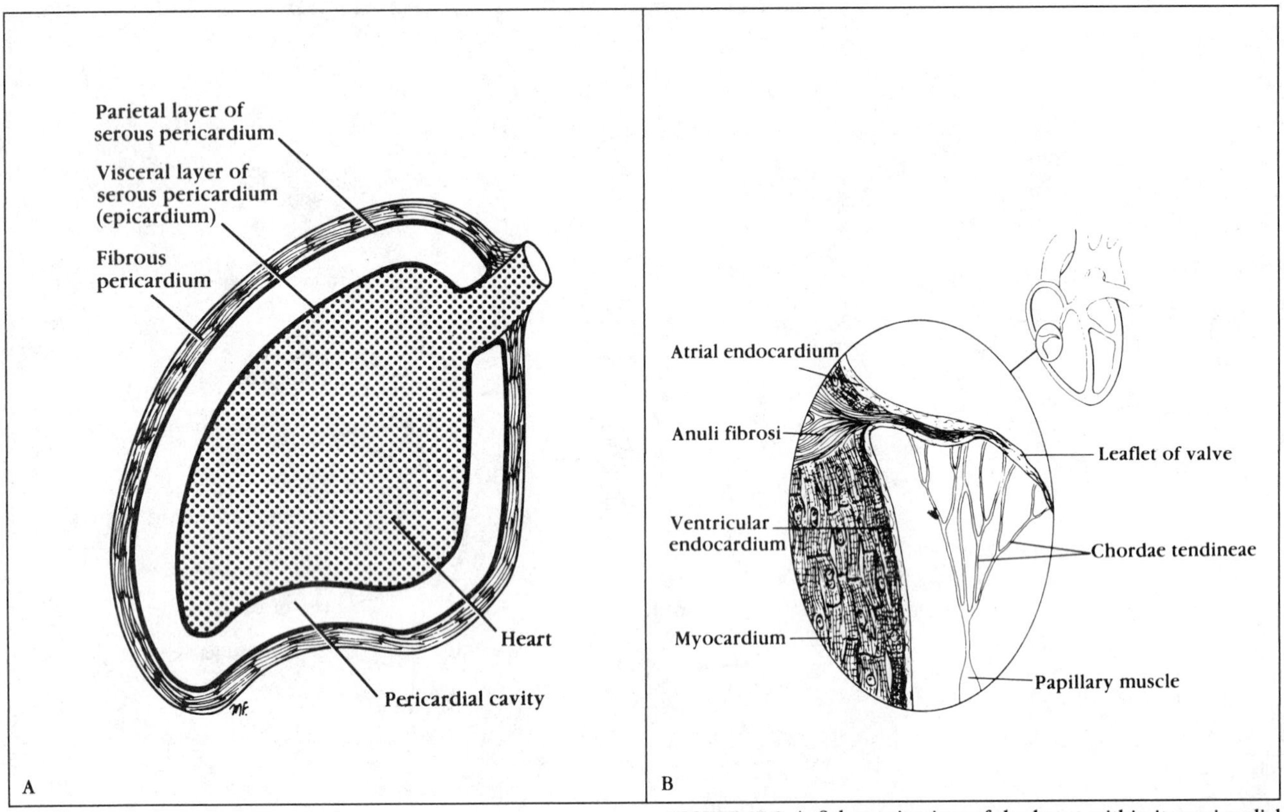

FIGURE 17-2. A. Schematic view of the heart within its pericardial sac. The heart is surrounded by a fibrous sac called the pericardium. B. The layers of the heart include the endocardium and myocardium. The epicardium (not shown) is a thin outer layer continuous between the atria and ventricles. Between the pericardium and the heart is the pericardial space or cavity.

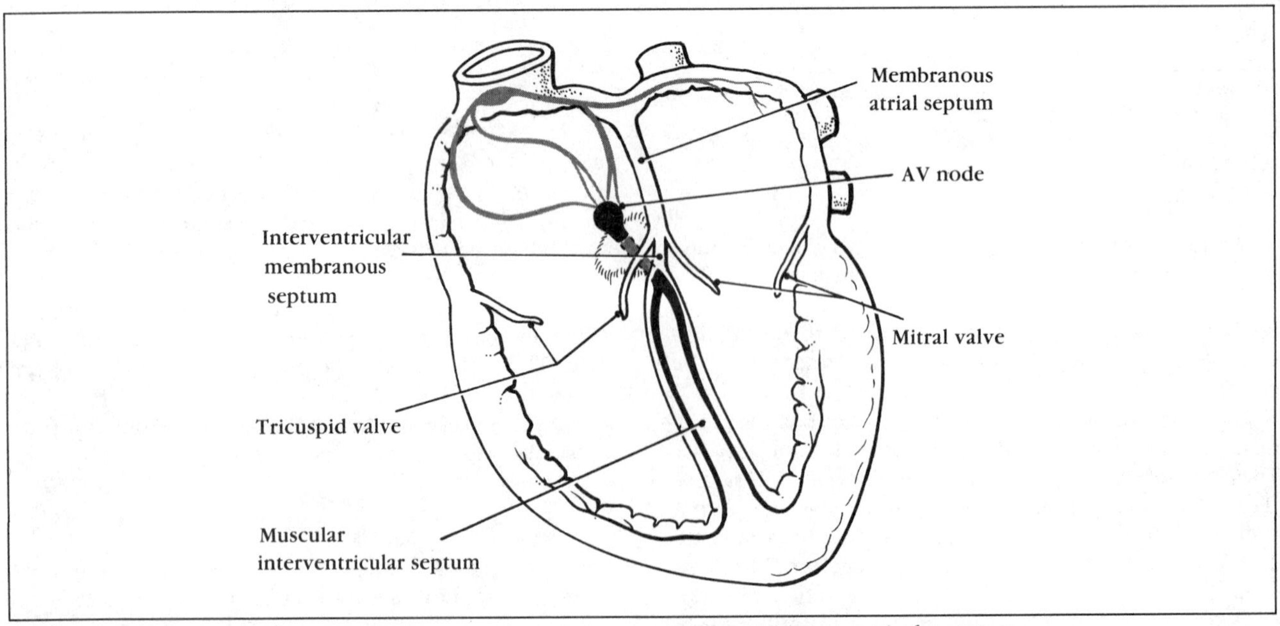

FIGURE 17-3. Interventricular septum.

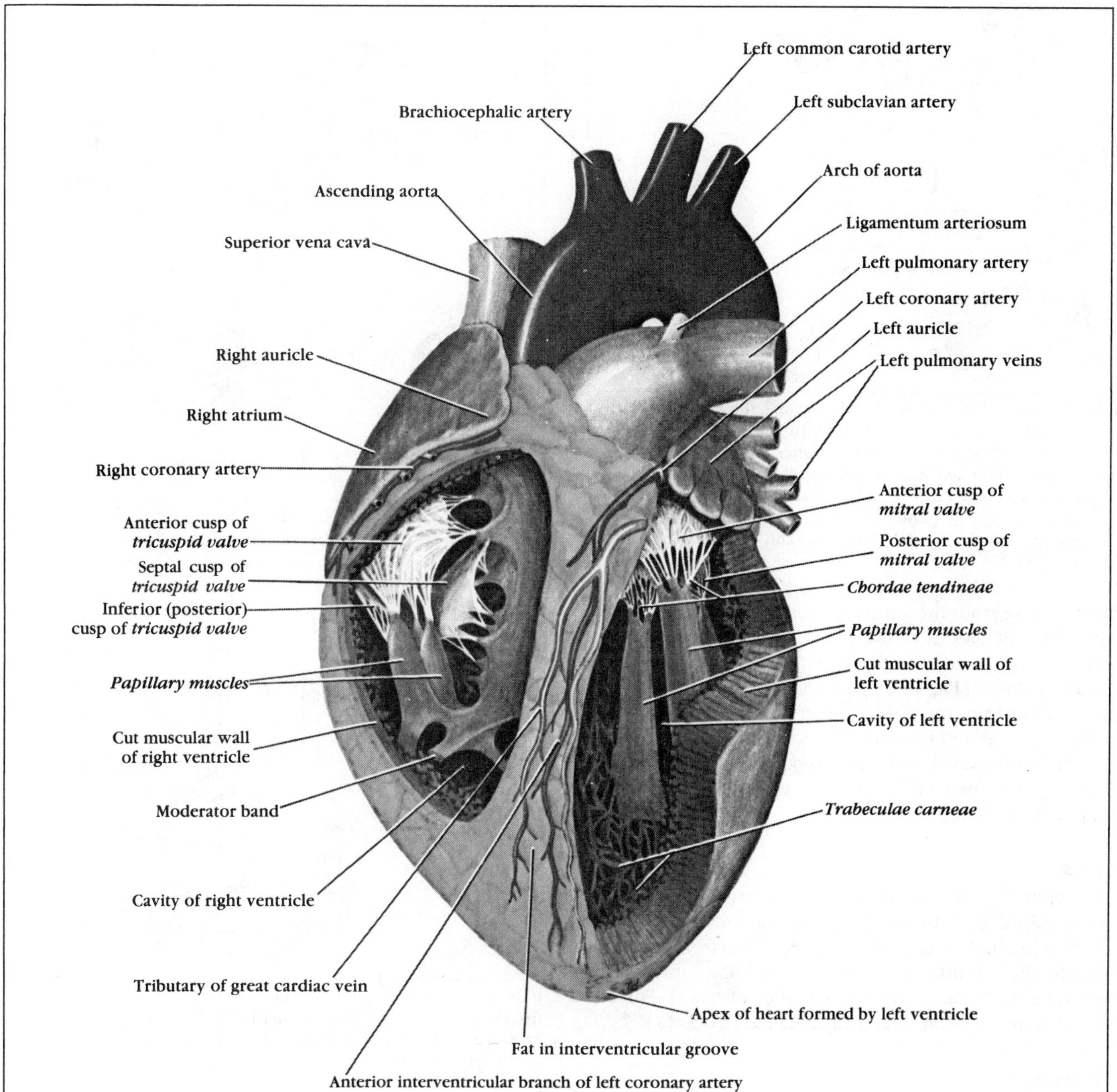

FIGURE 17-4. The heart viewed from the left side. The anterior wall of the right ventricle and posterior wall of the left ventricle have been removed. Note the *trabeculae carnae* or raised muscle bundles, more prominent in the left ventricle than the right. (From R. Snell, *Atlas of Clinical Anatomy.* Boston: Little, Brown, 1978.)

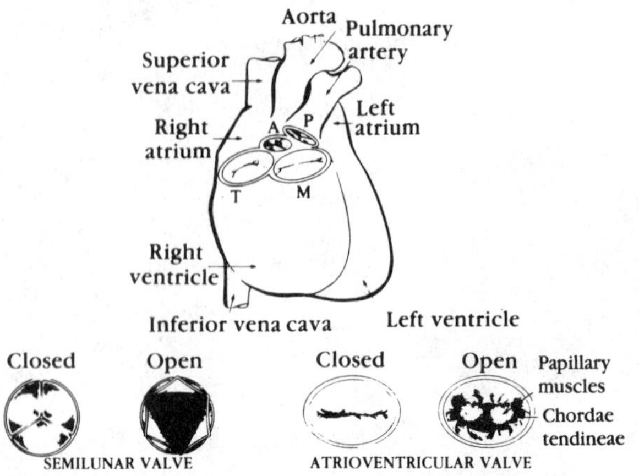

FIGURE 17-5. Outline of the heart showing the fibrous skeleton containing the four major valves. Inferiorly, the ventricles are suspended from this fibrous skeleton; superiorly are the atria and great vessels. Opened and closed appearance of the two valve types is also shown. (Key: T = tricuspid valve, M = mitral valve, A = aortic valve, P = pulmonic valve) (From E. E. Selkurt, *Basic Physiology for the Health Sciences* [2nd ed.]. Boston: Little, Brown, 1982.)

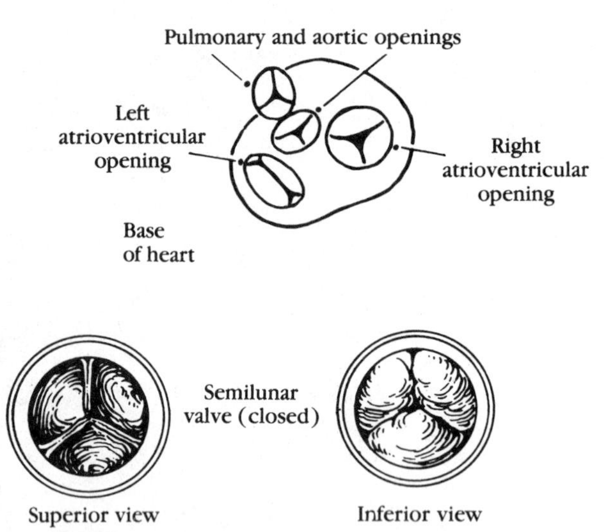

FIGURE 17-6. Appearance of the semilunar valves from superior and inferior position, in the closed position. (From J. Kernicki, B. Bullock, and J. Matthews, *Cardiovascular Nursing*. New York: Putnam, 1971.)

arteries arise from the aortic sinuses of Valsalva, which are pouchlike dilatations of the cusps. The coronary ostia, or openings, are located in the upper one-third of the aortic coronary cusps (Fig. 17-7). Occasionally a third coronary artery arises from the right coronary sinus.

The aortic and pulmonary valves are similar in structure except that the aortic valve is composed of slightly thicker fibrous cusps than the pulmonary valve. Both valves are supported by strong fibrous tissue, or valve rings.

Veins

The superior and inferior venae cavae bring the systemic venous blood back to the heart. The pulmonary veins, usually four in number, carry oxygenated blood from the lungs back to the left atrium. Veins are distensible, thin-walled structures that can hold large volumes of blood. For this reason veins are often called capacitance vessels [1].

Arteries

The two major arteries leading from the heart are the pulmonary artery and the aorta. The pulmonary artery leads from the right ventricle to the lungs. It branches into smaller and smaller vessels that finally become the pulmonary capillary bed where oxygen and carbon dioxide exchange occurs. The pulmonary artery opening from the right ventricle is guarded by the pulmonary valve. The aorta is the main systemic artery and carries oxygenated blood to all of the tissues of the body. It leads away from the left ventricle and is guarded by the aortic valve. The aorta and pulmonary arteries are composed of three layers: a tunica intima, or endothelial layer or coat; a tunica media, or muscular layer; and tunica externa, or outer, adventitial coat. The aorta gives off numerous branches for the supply of the systemic tissues.

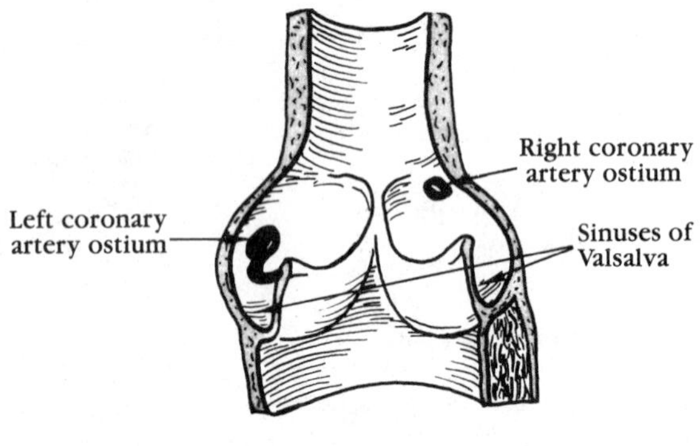

FIGURE 17-7. A coronal section of the origin of the aorta viewed from the posterior and diagrammatically illustrating the sinuses of Valsalva. (From J. Kernicki, B. Bullock, and J. Matthews, *Cardiovascular Nursing*. New York: Putnam, 1971.)

Coronary Arteries

Anatomically, two main coronary arteries arise from the sinuses of Valsalva of the aortic valve. The *right coronary artery* (RCA) arises from the right coronary sinus and the *left coronary artery* (LCA) arises from the left coronary sinus (Fig. 17-8A). The right coronary artery usually arises as a singular vessel from the right coronary ostium, but two vessels may arise from this position. This second vessel is usually called the *conus artery*. When a single coronary artery arises on the right side, the conus artery is the first branch off the right main coronary artery. The RCA travels in the atrioventricular groove or sulcus and turns downward in the posterior surface to the posterior interventricular sulcus. Smaller arterial vessels branch off the main

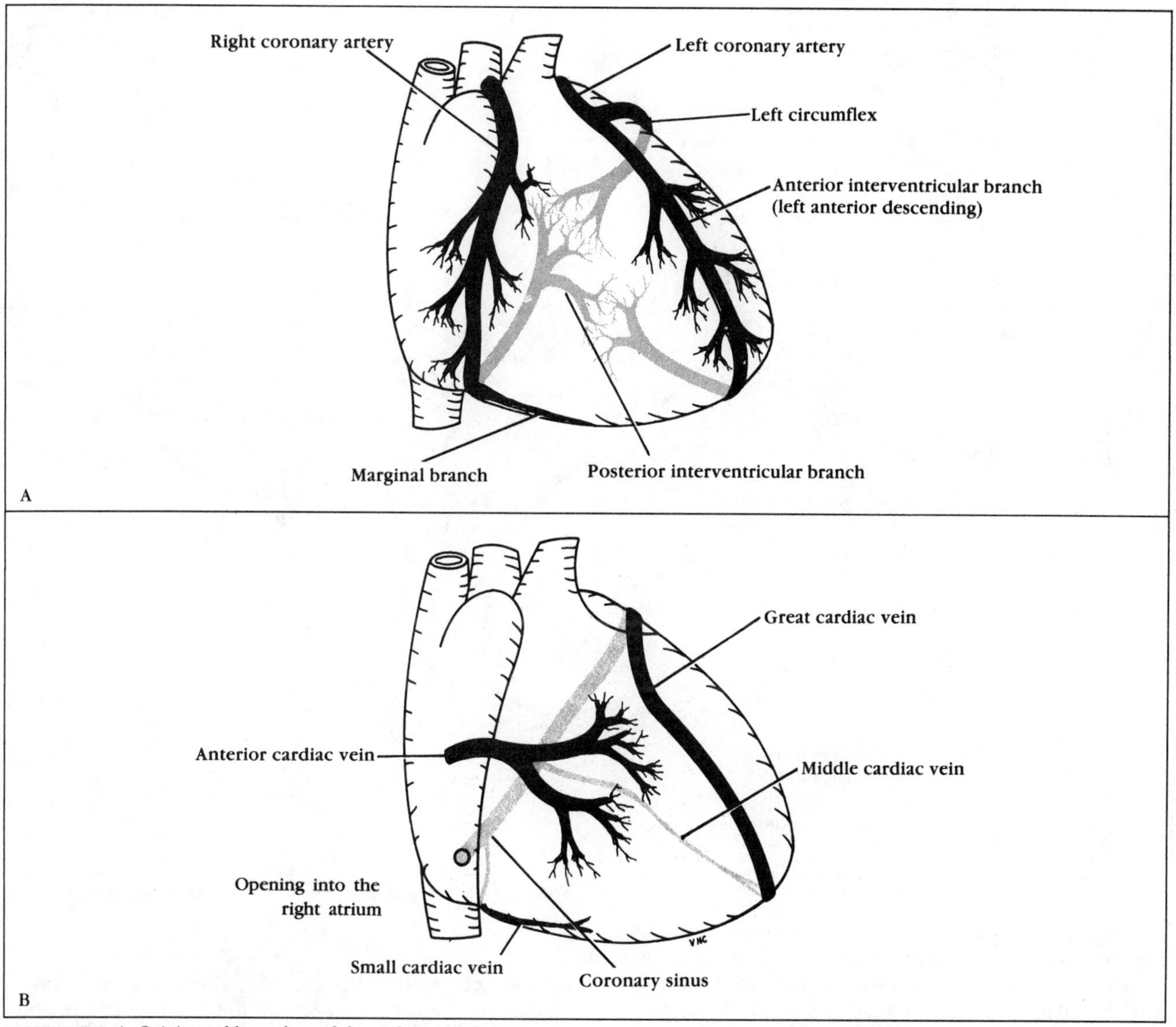

FIGURE 17-8. A. Origin and branches of the right and left coronary arteries. B. Origin of the coronary veins.

artery. In about 55 percent of human hearts, the RCA supplies blood to the sinoatrial node (SA) and in about 90 percent it supplies the atrioventricular node (AV). In some hearts the right coronary artery supplies the posterior surface of the right and left ventricles and the posterior interventricular septum. It may extend to supply part of the lateral and apical surfaces of the heart. A variance in the amount of myocardial tissue supplied by the right coronary artery accounts for the difference in myocardial pathology when there is coronary artery disease involving the RCA.

The left main coronary artery arises from a single ostium in the left coronary sinus. It travels in the atrioventricular sulcus to the left for a few millimeters to a few centimeters and then divides, or bifurcates, into the left anterior descending coronary artery (LAD) and the left circumflex. At the point of the bifurcation other branches, called *diagonal arteries,* may branch off. The diagonal arteries, one to four in number, supply the anterior surface of the left ventricle. The LAD descends in the anterior interventricular sulcus and supplies blood to the anterior left ventricle, the anterior interventricular septum, and the apex of the heart. The circumflex artery comes off the main left coronary artery at a sharp angle and travels in the left atrioventricular sulcus to the posterolateral surface of the left ventricle. Its branches supply blood to the lateral left ventricle and various amounts of posterior wall. In a small percentage of persons the circumflex is dominant and supplies the entire left ventricle and interventricular septum [5]. The circumflex also supplies the SA node in approximately 45 percent of persons and usually supplies blood to the left atrium.

The coronary arteries divide into smaller and smaller branches that penetrate deep into the myocardial muscle. These form a network of capillaries that supply the myocardial cells. Numerous functional and nonfunctional

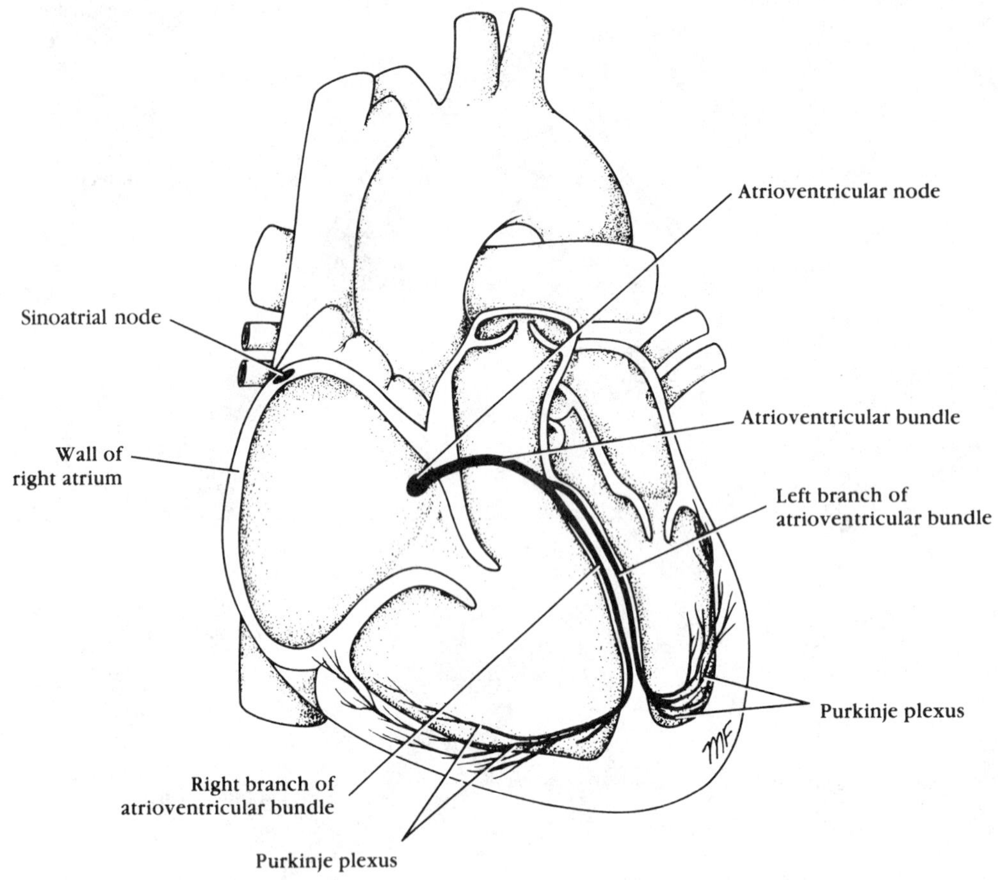

FIGURE 17-9. Position and appearance of conduction system of the heart.

anastomoses exist between the coronary vessels, and these have been shown to enlarge when the flow in one arterial branch is decreased. Enlargement of anastomoses can improve blood flow to myocardial segments [5]. The endocardial layer of the heart is the only portion of the heart that receives oxygen and nutrients from the blood that circulates within the chambers.

Coronary Veins

The coronary veins provide for the venous drainage of the myocardium and empty into the right atrium (Fig. 17-8B). The majority of drainage from the left ventricle is received by the coronary sinus and its branches. The coronary sinus is basically an extension of the great coronary vein. The anterior cardiac veins drain the right ventricle and usually empty directly into the right atrium. The remaining venous blood empties into the heart via the small thesbian veins.

Conduction System

The normal contraction of the heart is initiated by specialized conductive tissues, which are actually myocardial muscle cells with fewer myofibrils than the other myocardial cells. Figure 17-9 shows the location of the conductive structures within the heart. The structures include the sinus node (SA node), the atrial internodal tracts, the atrioventricular (AV) node, the bundle of His, the right and left bundle branches, and the terminal or Purkinje network.

The sinus node is a small mass of cells located near the entrance of the superior vena cava into the right atrium. It normally serves as the pacemaker of the heart because of its ability to generate an impulse through automatic diastolic depolarization (see p. 222). It is composed of P cells and intermediate cells. The P cells are so-named because of their pale cytoplasm. In the sinus node these cells are more numerous in the center of the node. No nerve endings from the autonomic system terminate directly in the P cell, but the basement membrane around the P cell lies close to terminal nerve endings. The intermediate cells appear more like the ordinary cardiac muscle cells and are thought to conduct the impulse from the SA node [5].

The atrial internodal tracts extend from the SA node and are difficult to distinguish from the surrounding cardiac muscle. These tracts travel to the left atrium, through the right atrium, and through the atrial septum to merge at the AV node.

The atrioventricular node and bundle of His form an interconnecting structure between the atria and ventricles that functionally joins the two units. The AV node lies in the right atrium at the juncture of the atrial septum. This node is composed of dense fibrous tissue that continues into the bundle of His. The AV node and bundle of His pathway is the only muscular and functional connection between the atrial and ventricular muscles [8]. The AV node also contains P cells that are less numerous than in the SA node. The slow conduction in the AV node may be partly due to the unspecialized structure of these P cells. The bundle of His directly connects with the AV node and crosses into the membranous portion of the ventricular septum (see Fig. 17-3). It is composed of fibrous tissue with a few myofibrils and terminates in the bifurcation of the common bundle into the right and left bundle branches.

The right and left bundle branches travel down the interventricular septum to terminate in the Purkinje network. The right bundle branch descends superficially in the endocardium of the right ventricular septum. It divides into numerous branches that penetrate the walls of the right ventricle. The left bundle divides into *three fascicles*: the *posterior*, the *anterior*, and the *septal* fascicles, which travel in the left interventricular septum for varying distances. The posterior fascicle sends its branches to the lateral and posterior wall and papillary muscle. The anterior fascicle primarily goes to the anterior and lateral wall of the left ventricle. The septal fascicle travels to the interventricular septum and the apex of the left ventricle [5]. The fascicular branches subdivide into smaller and smaller divisions and terminate in the Purkinje network.

The Purkinje network is composed primarily of Purkinje cells but P cells are found in scattered portions. Purkinje cells have few myofibrils and are joined end-to-end by intercalated disks that aid in the property of accelerated conduction of the impulse [5]. A Purkinje fiber is composed of many Purkinje cells in a series. These fibers penetrate about one-third of the way into the myocardial muscle, thus facilitating the excitation of the right and left ventricles.

Myocardial Cellular Structure

The cardiac muscle cell is similar to skeletal muscle cells in many ways but has some fundamental differences. Cardiac muscle cells have a single central nucleus while skeletal cells have peripheral nuclei. The muscle cells are closely approximated so that impulses generated in one myocardial cell can be passed easily to the next.

The myofibril is the contractile unit of the myocardial muscle cell. Its action occurs through the movement of actin on myosin in the sarcomere unit. The thin actin filament also contains two other inhibitory proteins called *tropomyosin* and *troponin*. The activity of these proteins in muscle contraction is described in detail in Chapter 38.

The myocardial muscle cell has a poorly developed sarcoplasmic reticulum but a highly developed transverse tubular system. This tubular system probably contributes to the intracellular release of calcium [1]. The cardiac cell also contains a large number of mitochondria that also have been shown to store calcium. Glycogen and lipid are also stored within the cells.

Cardiac muscle cells reside in close proximity to one another. The end of one cell very closely approximates the next. The junction of one cell with the next is through intercalated disks, which form a tight junction from cell to cell and allow for the rapid passage of an impulse from one cardiac cell to the next (Fig. 17-10). The myocardial cellular structure allows the entire myocardial unit to contract when one cell is stimulated to threshold level. The heart behaves as a syncytium; that is, if one cell is stimulated the entire unit contracts. The heart is composed of two functional syncytiums, the atrial and the ventricular.

PHYSIOLOGY OF THE HEART

The physiology of the heart will be considered in some detail in terms of the electrical and mechanical activity of the myocardial muscle. The cellular aspects are briefly outlined and greater detail can be found in the bibliography. Table 17-1 summarizes some of the commonly used terms in the cardiac cycle.

Contraction of Cardiac Muscle

Cardiac contraction occurs in much the same way as skeletal muscle except that cardiac muscle functions as a syncytium. This means that if one cardiac muscle cell is stimulated to threshold and contracts, the impulse spreads to all of the muscle cells and the entire unit contracts. There are two separate syncytial units in the myocardium, the atrial and ventricular, which are functionally joined by the AV node and the bundle of His.

The mechanism for contraction is similar to that described in Chapter 38. The action potential generated causes the release of calcium from the sarcoplasmic reticulum (SR) into the sarcoplasm. The calcium binds with the inhibitory proteins troponin and tropomyosin allowing actin to slide on myosin. Actin and myosin are the contractile proteins that make up the sarcomere units of the myocardial muscle cell. The calcium ion apparently has two major roles in excitation-contraction. It functions as the trigger substance or initiator and as the regulator of contraction [10]. When the action potential is initiated there is a rapid influx of sodium. The traversing of the action potential down the extensive T tubular system puts it in close proximity with the terminal cisternae of the SR. The SR releases large amounts of free calcium that bind with troponin, and thus inhibit both troponin and tropomyosin. Energy for the contraction is obtained from adenosine triphosphate (ATP), which is split by an adenosine triphosphatase (ATPase) site on the myosin filament when it interacts with actin [10].

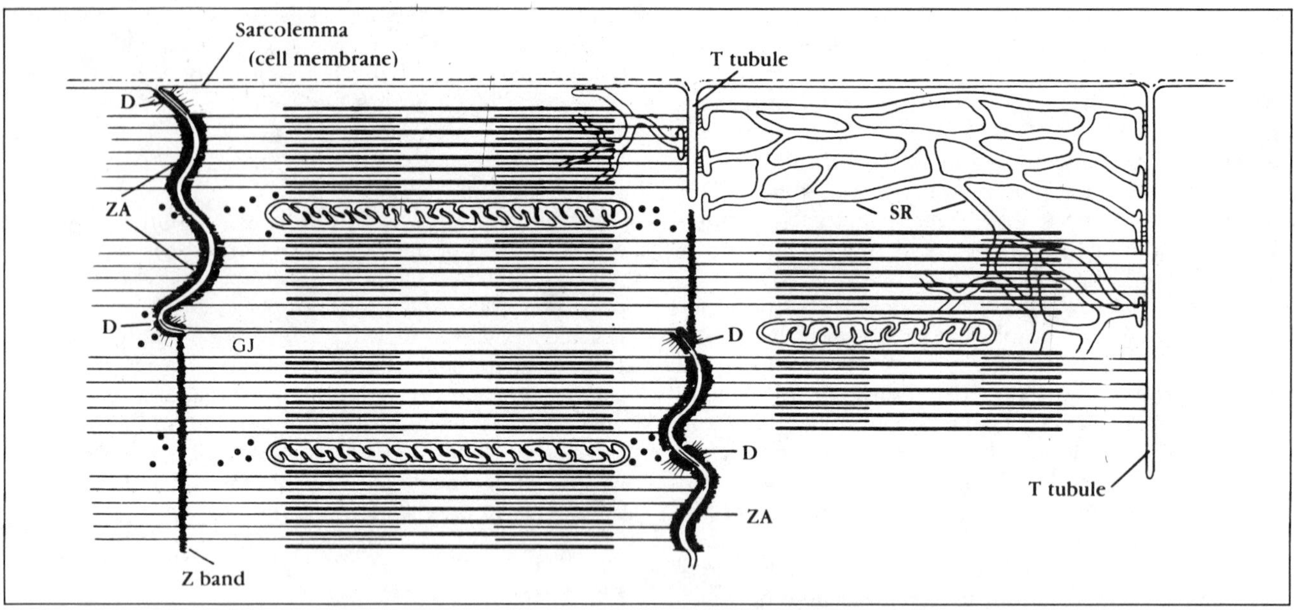

FIGURE 17-10. A thin section through cardiac muscle as it might appear with electron microscopy. Portions of two cardiac muscle fibers are depicted in the area where their plasmalemmas associate to form the interrelated disk. Desmosomes (*D*) provide structural integrity to the disk. Thin filaments insert into the zascia adherentes (*ZA*) of the disk. The gap junctions (*GJ*) are located in the horizontal part of the disk. The disk occurs where a Z band would have been. T tubules occur at the Z lines. The sarcoplasmic reticulum (*SR*) forms a sleeve around the myofibrils, but here it is depicted alone to show its pattern more clearly. (From M. Borysenko, et al., *Functional Histology* [2nd ed.]. Boston: Little, Brown, 1984.)

TABLE 17.1. Terms used in the cardiac cycle

Cardiac output Amount of blood pumped from the heart per minute. Cardiac output = stroke volume × heart rate.

Stroke volume Amount of blood ejected from each ventricle per beat. This is not all of the blood in each ventricle but is about 60–75% of the volume and is called the *ejection fraction.*

End diastolic volume Amount of blood in the ventricle just prior to systole.

End systolic volume Amount of blood in the ventricle following ventricular systole.

Isovolumic contraction Period of ventricular pressure rise prior to opening of the semilunar valves.

Ejection Period of time when ventricular pressure exceeds the arterial pressure and blood is ejected from the heart.

Incisura Inscription of a pressure recording that occurs when the aortic valve closes and is due to a momentary reversal of pressures between the aorta and left ventricle.

Isovolumic relaxation Rapid drop of pressure in the ventricles toward the diastolic pressure. This occurs prior to the opening of the atrioventricular valves and ventricular filling.

Systole Contraction of the heart.

Diastole Relaxation of the heart.

The amount of calcium available to inhibit troponin is directly related to the rate and amount of myocardial tension developed [10]. It is also possible that competition between sodium and calcium for binding sites affects myocardial contractility. Calcium then must be returned to the sarcoplasmic reticulum through an unknown stimulus that decreases the free calcium and allows inhibition of actin and myosin by the troponin-tropomyosin complex.

When the myocardial muscle cell is at rest, the resting membrane potential is approximately −85 to −95 mV. When an action potential occurs it changes the membrane potential from the negative to a slightly positive value. The action potential in cardiac muscle remains in plateau longer than in other excitable cells, which allows for a longer contraction in cardiac muscle. Following the action potential or depolarization, contraction occurs, which is followed by repolarization or a return to the resting state. During this period, restimulation may not cause the muscle to contract again. This is called the refractory period of the heart and occurs in both atrial and ventricular muscle. The *absolute refractory period* is the period during which the membrane is completely depolarized and/or contracting and no stimulus can cause it to respond or contract again. The *relative refractory period* occurs when the muscle membrane is repolarizing and a strong stimulus will cause it to contract.

Metabolism of Cardiac Muscle

The cardiac muscle requires a high-yield production of ATP. There is little reserve for this energy and it must be constantly produced. ATP is produced mostly in the numerous myocardial mitochondria using fatty acids and other nutrients, especially lactate and glucose. If one substance is not available, cardiac muscle can efficiently use another.

The amount of ATP produced is equivalent to the work needed to pump incoming blood into the arteries with sufficient pressure to maintain vital body functions.

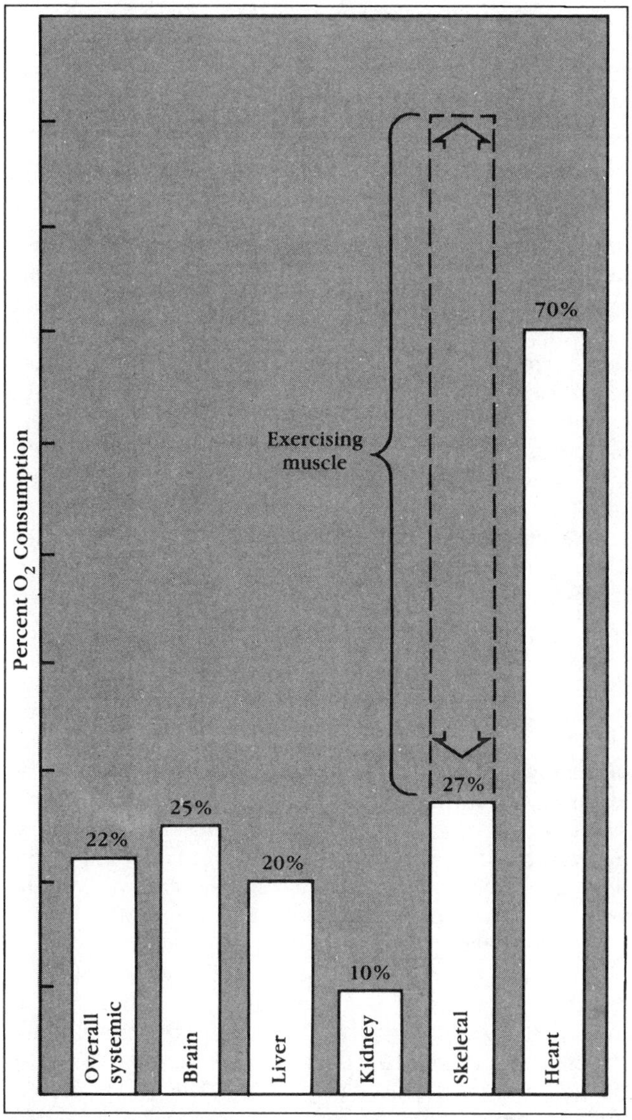

FIGURE 17-11. Oxygen extraction by the heart and other organs. (From M. Jackle and M. Halligan, *Cardiovascular Problems.* Bowie, Md.: Brady, 1980.)

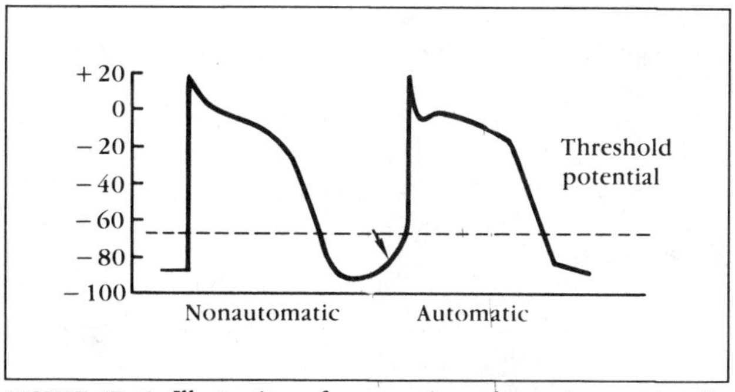

FIGURE 17-12. Illustration of automatic and nonautomatic cells. The automatic slides toward threshold potential at regular intervals.

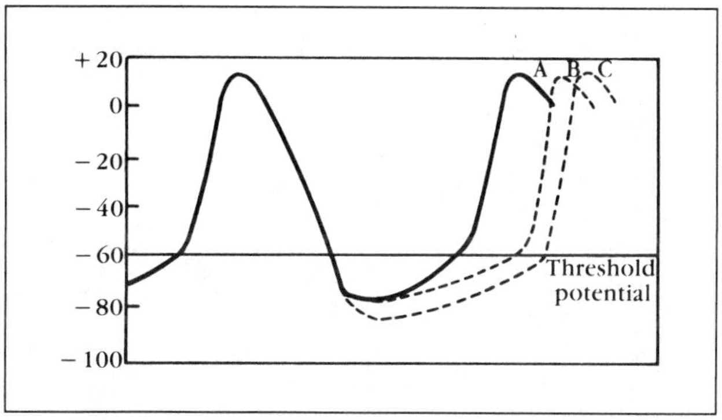

FIGURE 17-13. Changes in rhythmicity can result from: A. changes in threshold, B. reduced diastolic depolarization, or C. hyperpolarization.

Myocardial work is generated by the ventricular wall tension during systole and diastole. The wall tension generated during systole creates the pressure to eject blood into the arteries. Cardiac work is often expressed in terms of myocardial oxygen consumption. The amount of oxygen consumed is closely related to the amount of stress developed in the ventricular wall. The major factors that affect oxygen consumption include the amount of myocardial muscle mass, the contractile or inotropic state, the heart rate, and the intramyocardial tension generated [10]. The oxygen supply for this work is totally delivered from the coronary arteries. Increased oxygen is needed in stress situations because of the enhanced contractility and tachycardia induced by the catecholamines.

The myocardial muscle takes up a large amount of the oxygen delivered to it from the coronary arteries. The oxygen extraction of up to 70 percent leaves little oxygen reserve. Increased energy needs can only be met by increasing the heart rate (Fig. 17-11).

Automaticity

The spontaneous property of generating an action potential by the conduction tissue is termed *automaticity.* This occurs through a slow, sliding depolarization that creeps toward threshold. When the threshold level is reached spontaneous depolarization occurs. The action potential usually arises in the SA node where there is an inward leakage phenomenon that allows sodium to drift into the cell. If this is not offset by an electrically equal positive ion drifting out, then self-initiation of the action potential or diastolic depolarization occurs [11]. Figure 17-12 shows how this phenomenon normally occurs. The importance of this phenomenon is further illustrated by Figure 17-13, which shows how the action potential can be affected by altering the threshold at which the cell can respond. Enhanced automaticity usually refers to increased irritability of cells of the conduction tissue outside the SA node.

Pharmaceutical agents, hypoxemia, and injury are examples of factors that can alter the threshold for myocardial response. Some drugs, for example, raise the threshold for generation of the action potential and thus decrease the rate of diastolic depolarization. This is especially effective if ectopic impulses are causing ventricular arrhythmias.

Parasympathetic influences through the vagus nerve slow the rate of diastolic depolarization and decrease the rate of SA nodal automaticity. Sympathetic influences increase the automaticity and the rate of the diastolic depolarization.

Rhythmicity

This important property of the conduction tissue is characteristic of all of the potential pacemakers of the heart. It refers to the rhythmic or regular generation of an action potential. The leakage phenomenon described above remains regular, allowing for the same amount of time from one depolarization to the next. Therefore, the discharge of the action potential occurs regularly. This rhythmicity also may be affected by the sympathetic nervous system and the parasympathetic system. A cyclic increase and decrease in cardiac rate due to respiratory influences on the vagus nerve result in an increased cardiac rate on inspiration and a decreased rate on expiration in certain persons. Rhythmicity may be interrupted by enhanced automaticity of ectopic influences, nervous system stimulation, electrolyte imbalances, and pharmaceutic agents.

Excitability

This property of cardiac muscle refers to the ability of the cell to respond to stimulation. In the heart there are fast and slow conductors. The fast conductors include atrial and ventricular muscle cells and the Purkinje fibers, while the slow responses are those seen in the SA node and the AV node. However, Purkinje and muscle fibers have been shown to have both fast and slow channels [11].

CONDUCTIVITY. Impulse transmission in cardiac muscle is affected mostly by the structure of the intramyocardial cells, which allows the current to flow easily from one cell to the next. Therefore, threshold current from one cell rapidly passes to and depolarizes the adjacent cell. The property of conductivity is effected through the intercalated disk or the tight junctions between the myocardial muscle cells.

Electrical Events of the Cardiac Cycle

As stated earlier, the initiation of the cardiac cycle occurs through the specialized conduction tissue. These pacemaker cells spontaneously depolarize in a rhythmic fashion. The critical threshold is gradually reached; spontaneous depolarization occurs and is followed by repolarization.

The pacemaker of the heart is the sinus node because spontaneous depolarization occurs more frequently here than in the other potential pacers. This depolarization probably causes the discharge of the other potential pacers, a mechanism sometimes called *overdrive suppression* [11]. The conduction tissue has been referred to in the literature as a cascade of potential pacers that fire at different rates and can take over pacemaker function if the more rapid pacemaker is not operational [8]. Figure 17-14 shows the approximate potential rates of inherent cardiac pacemakers.

The process of excitation of cardiac muscle normally follows a strict sequential pattern. The sinus node begins the excitation. This is due to the less negative resting membrane potential (-55 to -60 mV) in the sinus node than in the other cardiac muscle fibers, and to increased membrane permeability to sodium. The impulse or action potential occurs and sends the excitation wave through the internodal pathways causing depolarization of the atrial muscle and excitation of the AV node. At the AV node, the impulse is slowed as it passes through the dense fibrous tissue. This allows time for the atria to complete contraction before the depolarization wave is sent to the ventricles. The impulse is then sent down the bundle of His, the bundle branches, and to the Purkinje network, which causes rapid depolarization and contraction of the ventricles.

The electrocardiogram shows the electrical events of the heart by inscribing waveforms as impulses are passing through the conduction tissue. Figure 17-15 shows the appearance of the ECG in relation to the electrical activities occurring in the heart. This activity of the heart creates an electrical field, which is distributed to the body surfaces. Therefore, if two electrodes (one of positive and one of negative polarity) are placed on different areas, the potential difference between the areas can be obtained. The QRS wave, showing ventricular depolarization, indicates the impulse passage from endocardium to epicardium. If the exploring electrode is placed on the epicardial surface, the resulting waveform will be upright or positive (+) as the impulse travels toward it. The greater the muscle mass the impulse traverses, the larger will be the positive deflection in the epicardial leads (Fig. 17-16). The final portion of the QRS wave occurs from activation of the posterobasal segments of the left ventricle and upper interventricular septum [11]. Repolarization is indicated on the ECG by the T waves. T waves on the ECG are generally positive if the heart is without ischemia. The repolarization takes longer than the QRS. The fact that the T wave is usually the same polarity or direction as the QRS in most leads is due to the fact that repolarization occurs in a reverse fashion from depolarization. In other words, it starts later and lasts longer in the endocardial area than on the epicardial surface.

Mechanical Events of the Cardiac Cycle

The mechanical events of cardiac contraction are regulated by the following four interrelated factors: (1) preload, (2) afterload, (3) contractility, and (4) heart rate [10]. These factors are described in this section and related to the events occurring in the heart.

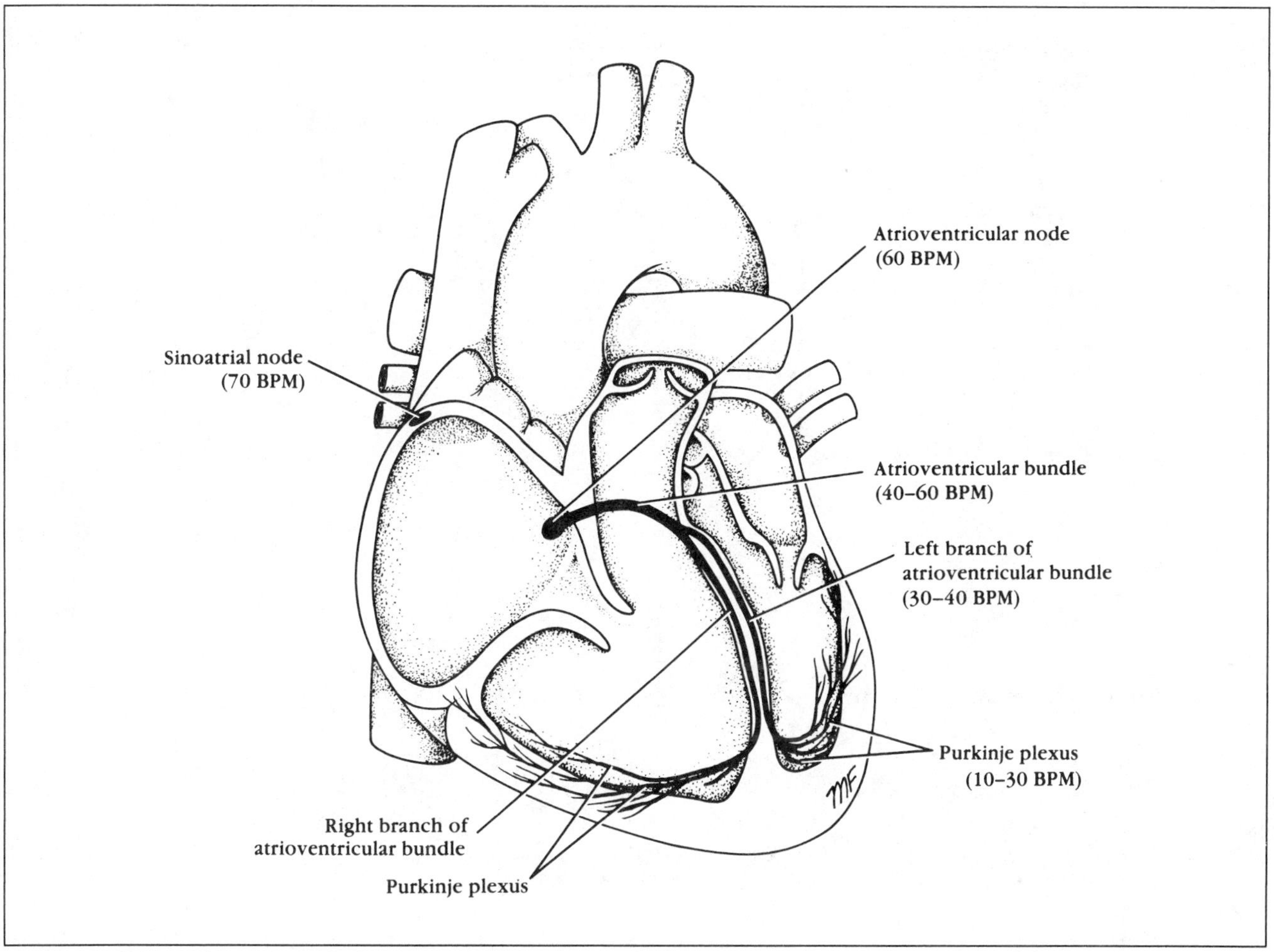

FIGURE 17-14. Approximate rates of inherent cardiac pacemakers.

PRELOAD. This term refers to the degree of stretch or myocardial muscle length prior to contraction. The property of cardiac muscle that allows for an increased force of contraction due to increased initial fiber length is called the *Frank-Starling law of the heart.* The increased fiber length is related to an increased volume of blood, which causes the initial stretch. When the fiber is stretched it will respond with an increased force of contraction. This has been related to the all or nothing law of the heart, which has come to mean that despite the strength of stimulus applied, the cardiac muscle responds either to its fullest or not at all.

In the normal, compliant ventricle, changes of volume can be accommodated quite readily. Ventricular compliance or distensibility refers to the ability of the ventricle to accept more diastolic volume. Normally, the right ventricular output equals that of the left even though the stroke volumes may vary. Respiratory excursion, for example, may cause a temporary increase in right ventricular output, but when this increased volume is received by the left ventricle it increases its output to balance the minute cardiac output. Ischemia, pericardial restriction, and hypertrophy are examples of factors that can affect this compliance by limiting venous inflow or limiting the contractility that normally would be seen. Increased ventricular distensibility without effective contraction may be seen in heart failure.

AFTERLOAD. This factor refers to the resistance that is normally maintained by the aortic and pulmonary valves, the condition and tone of the aorta, and the resistance offered by the systemic and pulmonary arterioles. Increased blood viscosity and added preload also contribute to the afterload. Pathologic states, such as hypertension and aortic stenosis, significantly increase the afterload. As afterload increases so does cardiac work and oxygen consumption. Greater muscle mass is required to maintain cardiac output against the increased resistance.

CONTRACTILITY. Contractility refers to the force of contraction generated by the myocardial muscle. This may be expressed in terms of the *inotropic state,* which is referred to as positive (+) if the force of contraction is increased and

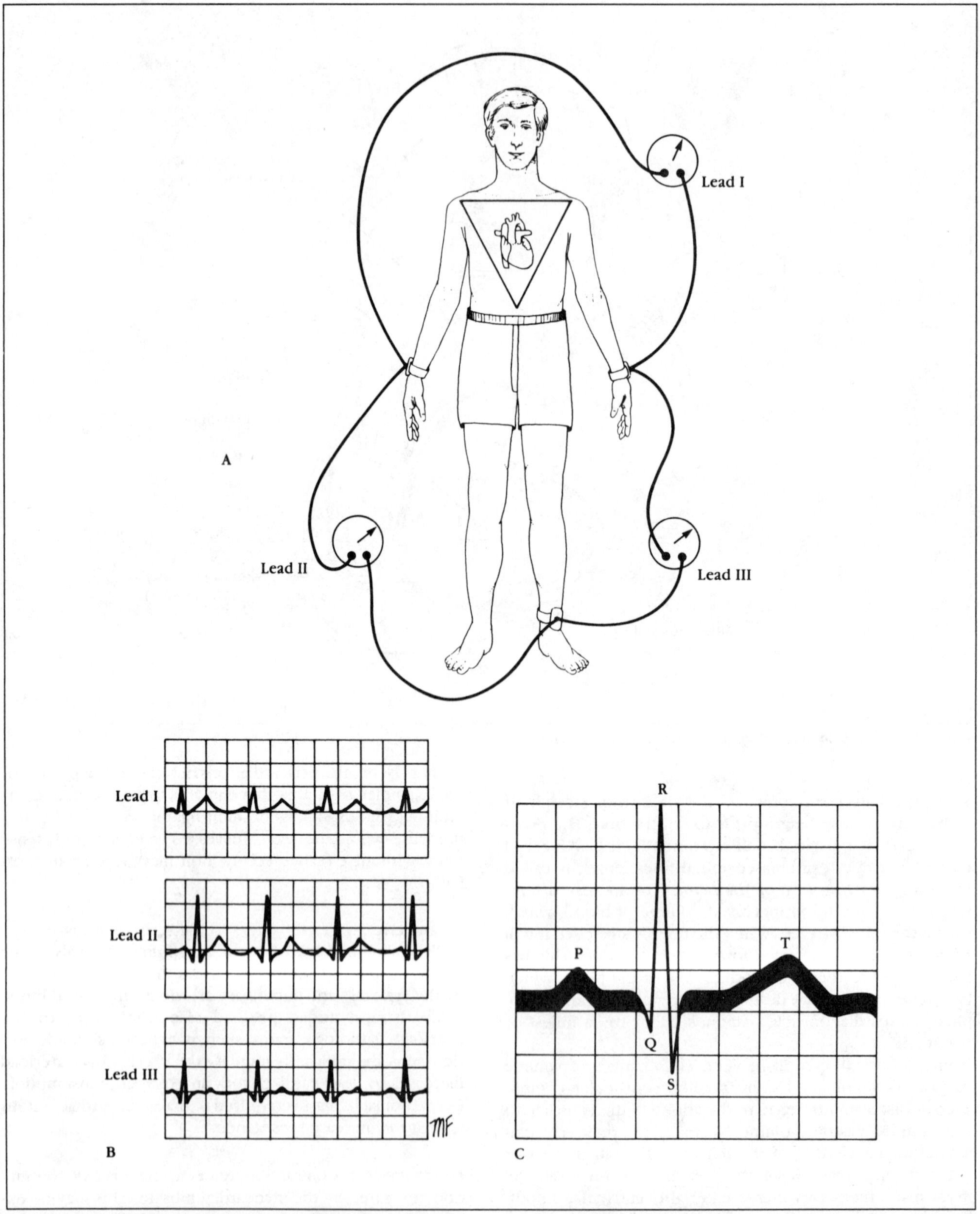

FIGURE 17-15. A. The standard electrocardiographic leads with their attachments to the body. B. Electrocardiograms recorded with leads I, II, and III. C. The normal electrocardiogram from lead II. Each small square represents 0.04 seconds in time on the horizontal plane. Measurements are made of time required for impulse passage through different portions of the conduction system. The P wave indicates SA node initiation of the impulse. The QRS indicates ventricular depolarization, and the T wave reflects ventricular repolarization.

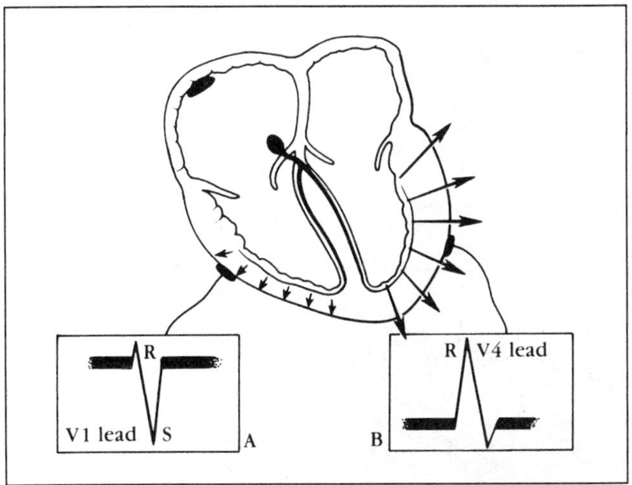

FIGURE 17-16. A. As the depolarization wave spreads from endocardium to epicardium in the right ventricle, the small muscle mass produces a small positive wave in the V1 or right ventricular lead of the 12-lead ECG. The deep S wave reflects left ventricular depolarization, which is seen as moving away from the V1 lead. B. Endocardial to epicardial depolarization produces a tall R wave in V4 because of the thick muscle mass of the left ventricle.

negative (−) if the force of contraction is decreased. This factor is influenced by both preload and afterload but it may also occur independently of these influences. The sympathetic nervous system, through the influence of catecholamines, causes an increase in the cardiac rate and force of contraction. Also, by increasing the recoil of the ventricular muscle on diastole, diastolic ventricular pressure is decreased. This allows for greater filling, greater fiber stretch, and therefore a stronger contraction [10].

HEART RATE. Stress, in any form, causes stimulation of the sympathetic nervous system, which leads to an increased cardiac rate. This increased rate leads to an increased cardiac output and increased ventricular contractility. Rate changes are often called the *chronotropic effect,* with a positive (+) chronotropic effect referring to an increased rate and a negative (−) chronotropic effect referring to the decreased rate.

Phases of the Cardiac Cycle

There are two major phases of cardiac activity termed *systole* and *diastole.* Systole refers to contraction and generally refers to the ventricular events. Diastole refers to relaxation, usually of the ventricles. The events of the cardiac cycle, from the atria through the ventricles, relating systole and diastole are discussed in this section.

ATRIAL FILLING AND CONTRACTION. As the atria receive blood from the incoming veins, the blood accumulates in these structures until the ventricular pressures fall below atrial pressures. As the atrial pressure rises, the flow of blood passively opens the atrioventricular valves and blood flows into the ventricles. Approximately 70 percent of blood flow from the atria to the ventricles occurs passively. Atrial contraction, which follows atrial depolarization from the sinoatrial pathways, provides the "atrial kick" to move the remaining atrial blood to the ventricles.

VENTRICULAR FILLING AND CONTRACTION. Rapid ventricular filling occurs after the atrioventricular valves open. Blood moves into the ventricles passively and then actively through the atrial kick. Ventricular depolarization and ventricular contraction occur from the conduction pathways and Purkinje activation of the muscle. Ventricular systole occurs in discrete phases:

1. Ventricular pressure begins to rise, causing an increased tension around the AV valve structures and closure of the mitral and tricuspid valves. This period of time is called the *isovolumic contraction* period and occupies that period of time between onset of ventricular contraction and opening of the semilunar valves.

2. Ejection of blood from the ventricles happens when the pressures in the ventricles exceed the diastolic pressures maintained in the aorta and the pulmonary artery. This increased pressure opens the semilunar valves and blood flows into the arteries.

3. Following ejection of the stroke volume, the pressure in the ventricles begins to fall. At a certain point the pressure falls below the arterial diastolic pressure and closure of the semilunar valves results. On a pressure tracing, the closure of the aortic valve is indicated by the *incisura* or *aortic dicrotic notch.* The *isovolumic relaxation phase* occurs as the pressure continues to descend in the ventricles toward the low diastolic pressure. This lasts until the pressure in the ventricles falls below the atrial pressure when rapid ventricular filling begins again.

The mechanical events occur at the same time in both the right and left sides of the heart. Figure 17-17 shows some significant differences between the chambers in terms of pressures and oxygen saturations. It can be readily seen that left-sided pressures exceed the right. While both arteries maintain a diastolic pressure, the aortic pressure is much higher than the pulmonary. The diastolic pressure in the ventricles is normally very low, nearing zero. Oxygen saturations differ between the two sides of the heart.

HEART SOUNDS. There are two major distinct sounds produced in the normal heart; the first, S1, often called the mitral sound, and the second, S2, which occurs with the closure of the semilunar valves. The S1 occurs when the ventricles begin contraction or during cardiac systole. It has always been attributed to the closure of the atrioventricular valves, but the closure of these valves may or may not be a component of the production of the sound. The S1 is probably produced by the acceleration and deceleration of blood with tensing of the valve structures and cardiac vibrations [7]. This sound is best heard in the fifth intercostal space, in the midclavicular line. The second heart sound, or S2, is mainly due to closure of the semilunar valves. It has two components, the aortic and the pul-

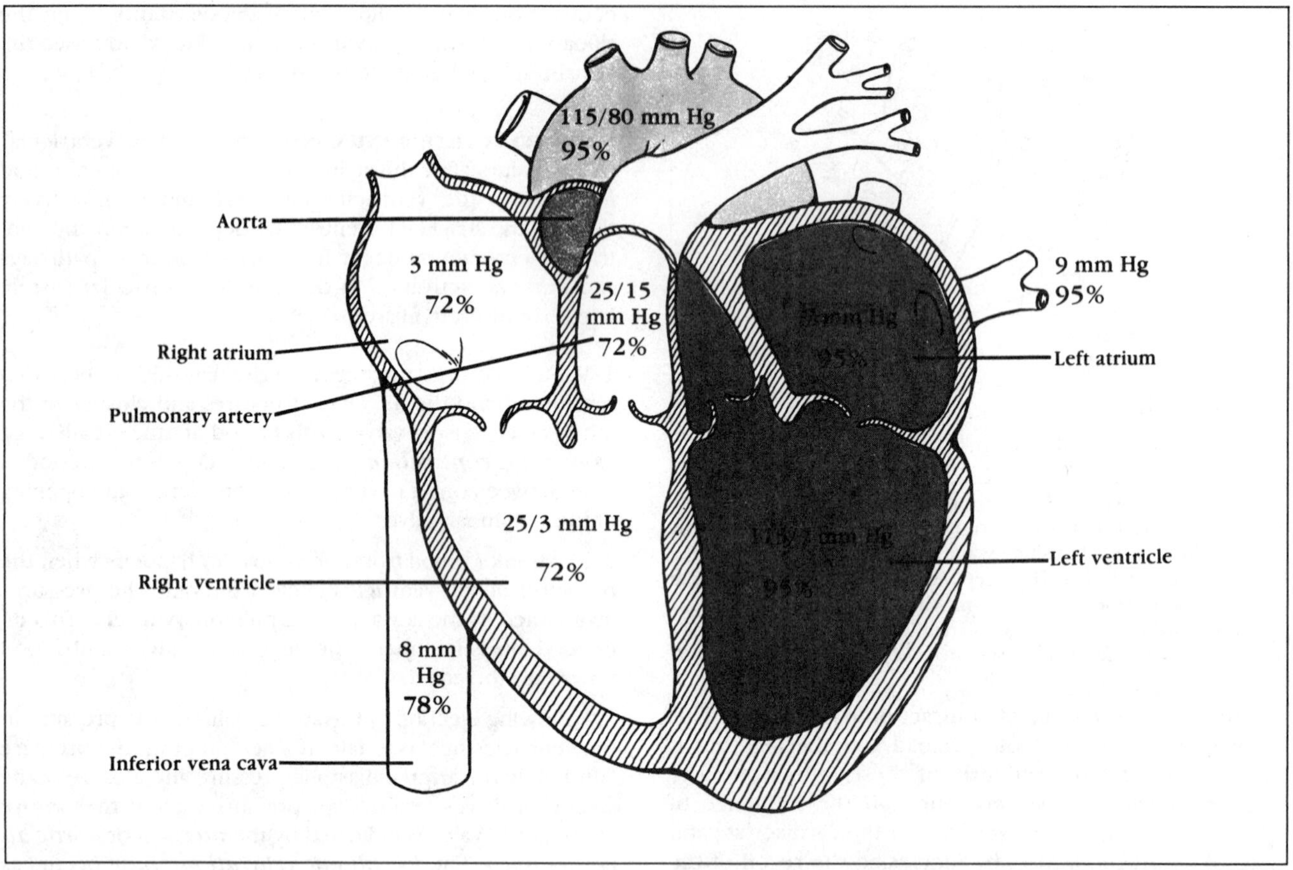

FIGURE 17-17. The normal central circulation. Oxygenated blood is depicted in red. Blood pressures (in torr) and oxygen saturations (in %) are average normal values. (From R. Judge, G. Zuidema, and F. Fitzgerald, *Clinical Diagnosis.* Boston: Little, Brown, 1982.)

monary closure sound. During the inspiratory phase of respiration there is an increase in the venous return to the right side of the heart, which increases the volume in the right ventricle, thereby increasing ejection time; the pulmonary valve closes slightly after the aortic valve. This split is more obvious in young persons and when a person is hyperventilating. This sound is best heard in the aortic and pulmonary areas at the second intercostal spaces (Fig. 17-18).

The third heart sound, S3, is a sound normally heard with young children but it is usually pathologic in adults. When heard it occurs after the second sound. It results from the tensing of the chordae and atrioventricular ring during the end of the rapid filling phase [7]. This sound is more frequently heard when there is a dilated ventricle or volume overload.

The fourth heart sound, S4, occurs with increased ventricular pressure during atrial contraction. It is heard immediately before the first sound and may be associated with hypertension or decreased ventricular compliance. S3 and S4 are heard best at the apex with the bell portion of the stethoscope.

Figure 17-19 shows the relationship of the S1 and S2 heart sounds to cardiac events and pulse waveforms. Also shown are the times of ventricular systole and diastole.

Autonomic Influences on Cardiac Activity

The autonomic nervous system (ANS) provides an external influence on myocardial contractility and rate. This influence involves adjusting the heart rate and contractility to the demands of the body. The ANS has an enhancing or restraining effect on the inherent pacemaker system of the heart and can alter the automaticity of abnormal pacemaker systems.

SYMPATHETIC NERVOUS SYSTEM (SNS). Fibers from the SNS are found in the atrial wall, the ventricles, and the SA and AV nodes (Fig. 17-20). When stimulated these fibers release norepinephrine, which stimulates the rate of depolarization and the rate of impulse transmission through the conduction tissue. Therefore, increased sympathetic tone increases the cardiac rate and the contractility of the myocardial muscle. The predominant effect is usually on the sinus node and causes a sinus tachycardia such as a response to exercise or fear. SNS stimulation also can increase the irritability of ectopic cells, causing abnormal or early depolarization, such as with premature atrial or

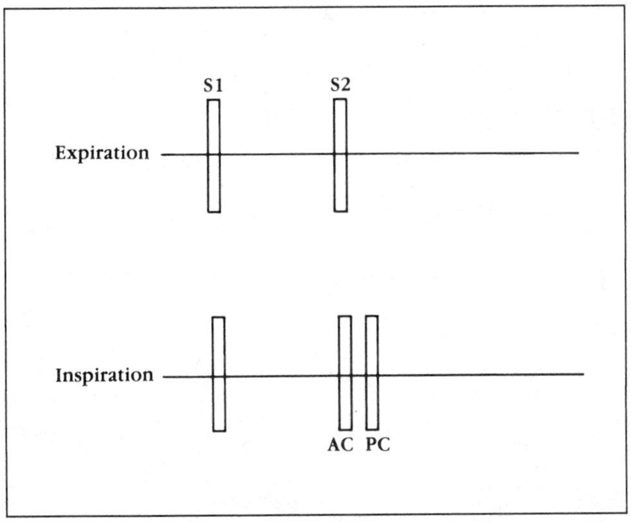

FIGURE 17-18. Illustration of splitting of the second heart sound on inspiration. Note that aortic closure (*AC*) occurs first; pulmonic closure (*PC*) follows. On inspiration two separate sounds may be heard.

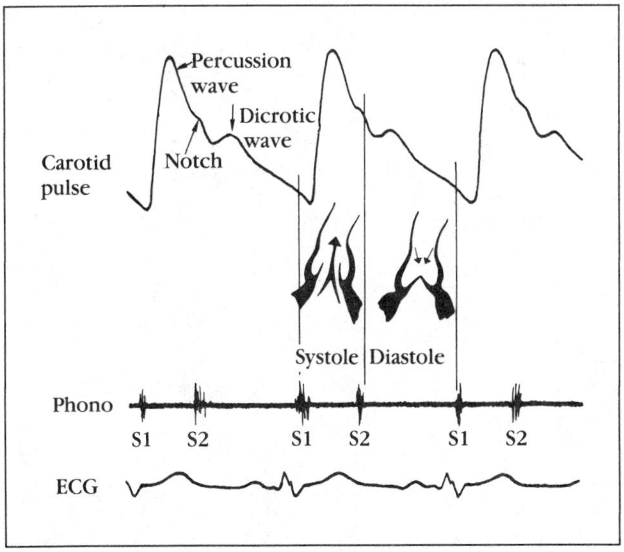

FIGURE 17-19. Characteristic normal arterial pulse wave with simultaneous recordings of a phonocardiogram and electrocardiogram. (From J. Sana and R. Judge, *Physical Assessment Skills for Nursing Practice.* Boston: Little, Brown, 1982.)

ventricular contractions. The effects of the SNS on the coronary arteries are somewhat more complex. Norepinephrine has been shown to cause coronary artery vasoconstriction and causes increased oxygen extraction by the myocardial cell. Some individuals have a hyperactive response to norepinephrine and exhibit coronary artery vasospasms during stressful situations. Ischemia results and causes the liberation of metabolites that, in turn, can cause vasodilation. Epinephrine, most of which is released from the adrenal gland, has a secondary dilating action on the coronary arteries. Prostaglandins, which may be stimulated secondarily in the stress response, are synthesized by the myocardial cells and arteries and may dilate or constrict the coronary arteries.

In the normal person autoregulation of coronary blood flow appears to counteract the effects of neural stimulation. Studies by Berne and associates relate that an increased release of fluid adenosine, a powerful coronary artery vasodilator, results from increase in myocardial oxygen need [1]. When ANS stimulation induces coronary vasoconstriction, coronary autoregulation usually overrides the mechanism and ischemia is prevented [6]. This mechanism seems to affect the small coronary arteries but is ineffective in the larger vessels.

PARASYMPATHETIC NERVOUS SYSTEM (PSNS). The PSNS is mediated through the chemical transmitter, acetylcholine, which is released from the vagal fibers. The major effect of vagal stimulation is on the sinoatrial node, the atrial muscle, and the atrioventricular node. The result of stimulation is a restraining influence on the conduction tissue with only a slight decrease in ventricular contractility. Vagal stimulation slows the heart rate by restraining the rate of diastolic depolarization in the conduction tissue.

Baroreceptors

These receptors are pressure-sensitive structures found mostly in the carotid sinus and the aortic arch. A decreased systolic blood pressure causes a reflex sympathetic response with increased pulse, increased contractility, and vasoconstriction. An increase in pressure causes stimulation of stretch receptors and a reflex vagal response, which results in a decreased heart rate and passive vasodilation in the systemic arterioles.

Chemoreceptors

The major chemoreceptor of the body is the medulla oblongata, but special receptors are located in the carotid and aortic bodies. Chemical changes in the blood, especially of pH, carbon dioxide, and oxygen cause alterations in cardiac activity. A decreased pH or PO_2 causes a reflex sympathetic discharge that results in tachycardia, vasoconstriction, and increased myocardial contractility. A decreased PCO_2 and increased pH reduce the vasoconstrictor effect leading to passive vasodilatation [8].

ANATOMY OF THE ARTERIES, CAPILLARIES, VEINS, AND LYMPHATICS

Arteries

The arteries are composed of three layers: the tunica intima, the tunica media, and the tunica externa or adventitia (Fig. 17-21). The layers contain variable amounts of collagen and muscle fibers according to the type of artery, but basically the outer coat serves to support or give shape to the vessel, the middle or muscular coat regulates the diameter of the vessels, and the inner coat provides a smooth

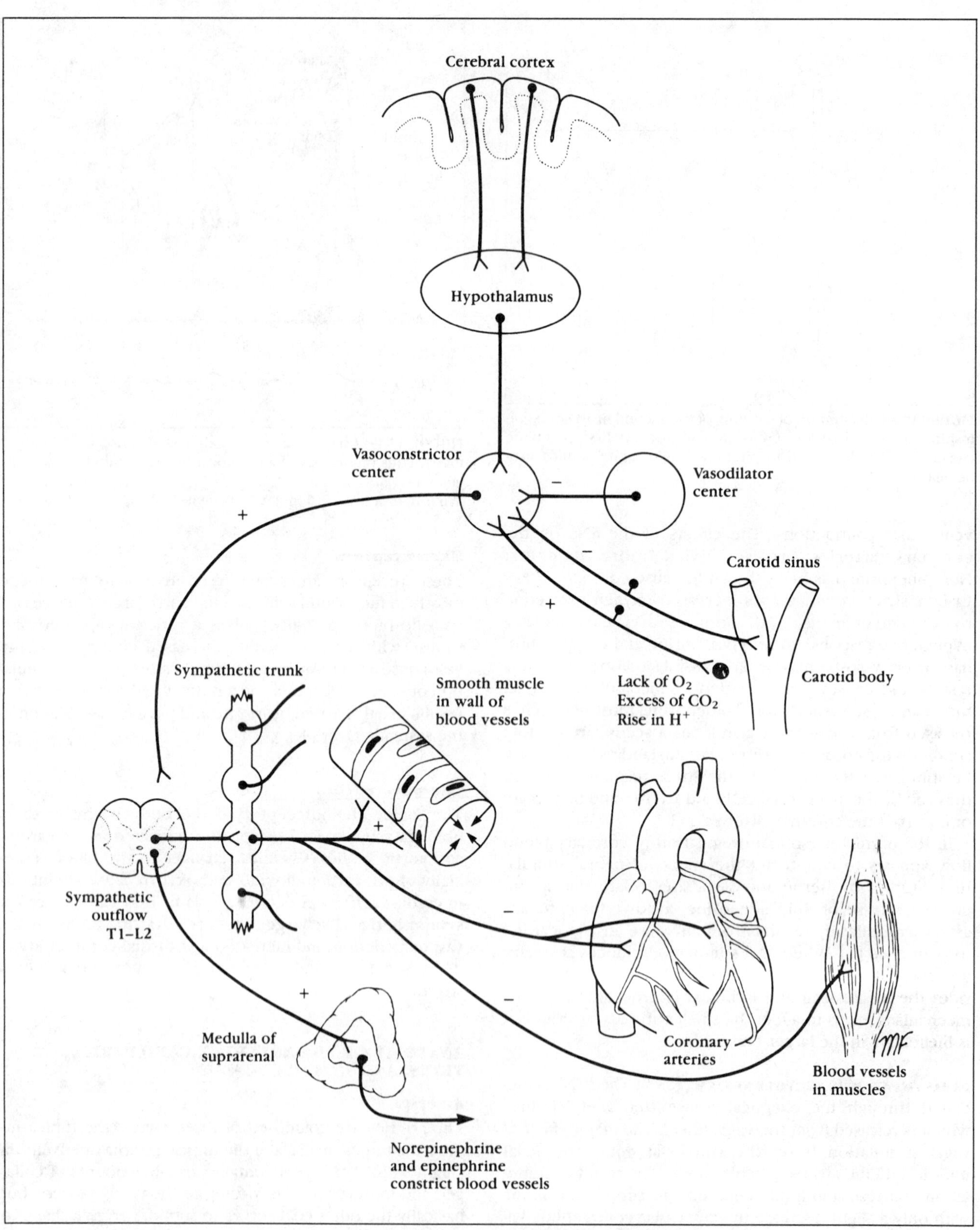

FIGURE 17-20. Effect of SNS stimulation.

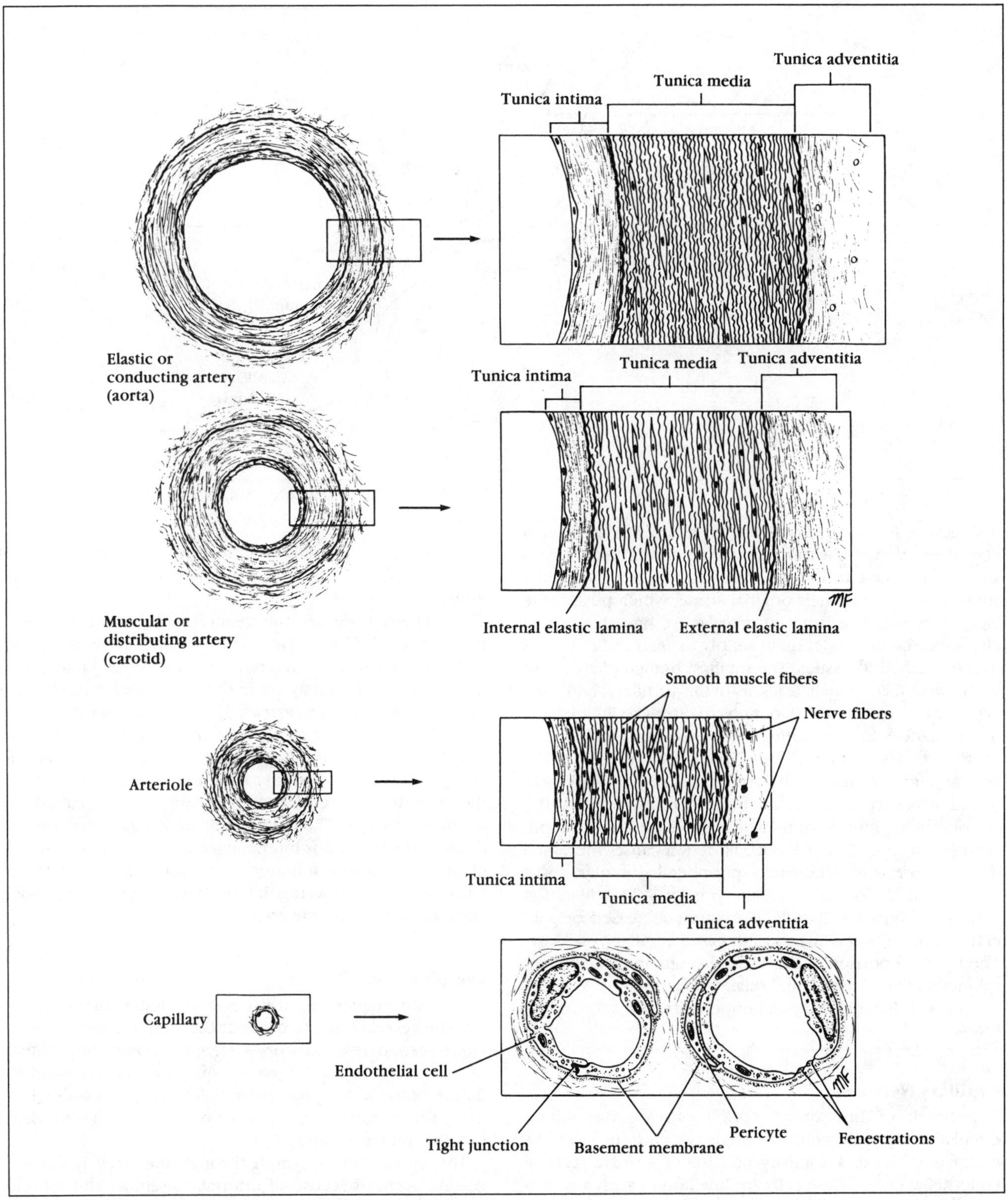

FIGURE 17-21. Layers of the aorta, artery, arterioles, and capillary.

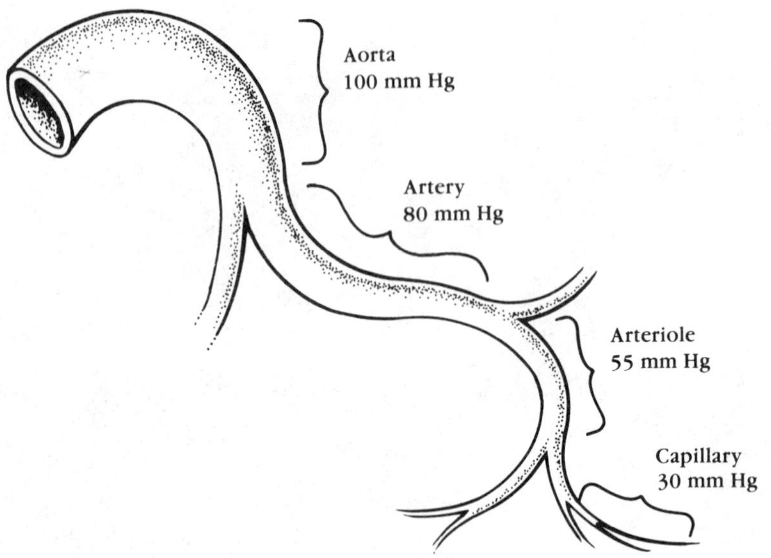

FIGURE 17-22. Blood pressure changes in the arteries.

passageway for blood flow. The large arteries are called *elastic vessels* because they can stretch or increase their diameter to receive the stroke volume of the heart and then contract or resume their original shape, which pushes the blood forward. The *nutrient arteries* are branches of the elastic vessels and function to supply oxygen and nutrients to the organs and tissues. The smallest branch of an artery is the *arteriole,* which leads into the capillary bed (see Fig. 17-21). The arteriole functions to offer varying degrees of resistance to circulating blood by constriction or dilation of its diameter. This mechanism regulates the volume and pressure in the artery and the capillary bed. Blood pressure changes as blood courses down the arteries, being highest in the aorta and lowest in the capillary system (Fig. 17-22). Vasoconstriction causes increased diastolic pressure (increased peripheral vascular resistance) and decreased capillary pressure. Vasodilatation causes a decreased diastolic pressure (decreased peripheral vascular resistance) and increased capillary pressure. The terminal portion of the arteriole contains precapillary sphincters that constrict and relax with autonomic stimulation or with local changes in temperature, pH, and oxygen levels.

Capillary Network

A network of tiny blood vessels provide the microcirculation through which materials can enter or leave the circulating blood. A capillary consists of a single layer of endothelial cells. These cells are lined up in such a way as to allow for the exchange of fluids, dissolved gases, and small molecules [8]. Large molecules, such as the plasma proteins, are held back in the capillaries and provide an osmotic pressure. Capillary pressures differ in different organs and systems.

Veins

The smallest veins are the venuoles, which receive their blood from the capillaries. These vessels have very thin walls through which some nutrients and oxygen may leave and waste products may enter. Capillaries and venuoles are often called *exchange vessels* [8]. Venuoles join together to form the veins. Many more veins than arteries are formed. These vessels contain approximately 75 percent of circulating blood volume at any one time. Because they have the capability to stretch and hold blood, they are called *capacitance vessels.* The larger veins have valves that are endothelial flaps or folds interspersed along the inner surface of the veins. These function to prevent the back flow of blood and are numerous in the lower extremities, especially in skeletal muscle areas.

Lymph Vessels

These important structures begin as blind-ended capillaries. The vessels serve to connect the lymph nodes and provide a secondary circulatory system. Approximately 2 liters of fluid is left in the interstitial spaces every day and this diffuses into the lymph capillaries. The lymph vessels effectively remove any excess plasma proteins that have leaked into the interstitial area.

The movement of lymph through the large lymphatic vessels occurs because of arterial pulsations and muscle movement. Backflow is prevented by the lymphatic vessel valves. Lymph flow in the thoracic duct is approximately 1.3 ml/kg of body weight per hour [8]. If the lymphatic circulation is decreased or blocked, *lymphedema* (an edema of high protein content) occurs.

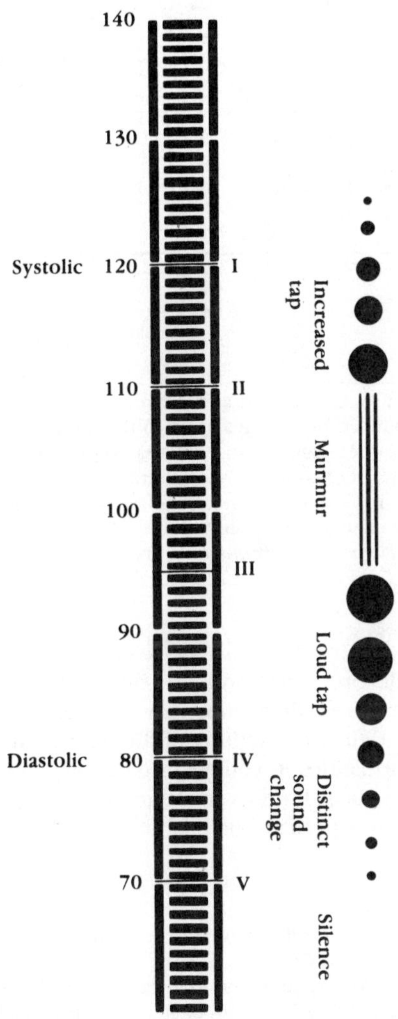

FIGURE 17-23. Korotkoff sounds. (From C. Kenner, C. Guzzetta, and B. Dossey, *Critical Care Nursing: Body-Mind-Spirit.* Boston: Little, Brown, 1981.)

FACTORS CONTROLLING ARTERIAL PRESSURE AND CIRCULATION

Arterial Blood Pressure

Arterial blood pressure is determined by the cardiac output and the resistance to blood flow. The highest pressure is called the *systolic pressure,* which is that achieved by the contracting left ventricle in the ejection of its stroke volume. The *diastolic pressure* maintained or stored as potential energy in the aorta during diastole permits a continuous forward flow of blood. The difference between these two pressures is called the *pulse pressure.* The sounds described in auscultating the blood pressure are called *Korotkoff sounds* (Fig. 17-23). These sounds are generated after a cuff is placed around an extremity and pressure sufficient to occlude the blood flow is applied. As the cuff pressure is released the beating sounds begin when the pressure falls below the systolic blood pressure. As the cuff pressure is continually released the sounds become muffled and disappear at the point of the diastolic pressure. It is generally appreciated that an error of 8 to 10 mm Hg (systolic pressure underestimated by 4 to 5 mm Hg and diastolic pressure overestimated by the same amount) occurs with this indirect measurement [8].

Pulse Pressure

Pulse pressure changes are affected by changes in the systolic or diastolic pressure levels. High systolic and low diastolic pressures increase or widen the pulse pressure. Low systolic and high diastolic pressures decrease or narrow the pulse pressure (Fig. 17-24). Either component can be altered with a net effect of pulse pressure alteration. Increased pulse pressure is usually the result of an increased stroke volume, a decreased peripheral volume, or a decreased peripheral vascular resistance, factors that might be seen during exercise, fever, with aortic insufficiency, or sometimes with atherosclerosis. A narrowed pulse pressure can occur with increased peripheral vascular resistance, decreased cardiac output, hypovolemia, or other conditions; this often indicates a pathologic condition [9].

The pulse pressure normally decreases as the pressure waves pass into the small arteries. In normal subjects it averages 1 mm Hg at the capillary but this difference can be increased in conditions such as aortic insufficiency, patent ductus arteriosus, and wide dilatation of the arterioles [4].

Direct and Indirect Determinants of Blood Pressure

The contraction of the left ventricle moves its stroke volume into the aorta. The left ventricle pumps against the elastic resistance of the aortic wall, the resistance offered by the arterioles, and the residual volume in the aorta. Therefore, direct determinants of arterial blood pressure include the cardiac output, vascular resistance, aortic impedance (resistance to flow), and diastolic arterial volume [3]. Indirect determinants of blood pressure include the activity of the autonomic nervous system and the renin angiotensin-aldosterone system.

CARDIAC OUTPUT. The amount of blood ejected from the heart is partly determined by the end-diastolic fiber length or the Frank-Starling mechanism. Changes in stroke volume vary in normal persons and increased ventricular volume at the end of diastole will of itself produce a stronger ventricular contraction. However, if an individual is hypovolemic the decreased end-diastolic fiber length will lead to a decrease in the force of ventricular contraction and subsequently a decrease in cardiac output [2].

VASCULAR RESISTANCE. Vascular resistance is often called *peripheral vascular resistance* (PVR) and refers to the impedance offered to blood flow by the arterioles. Constriction of the arterioles increases the resistance against which

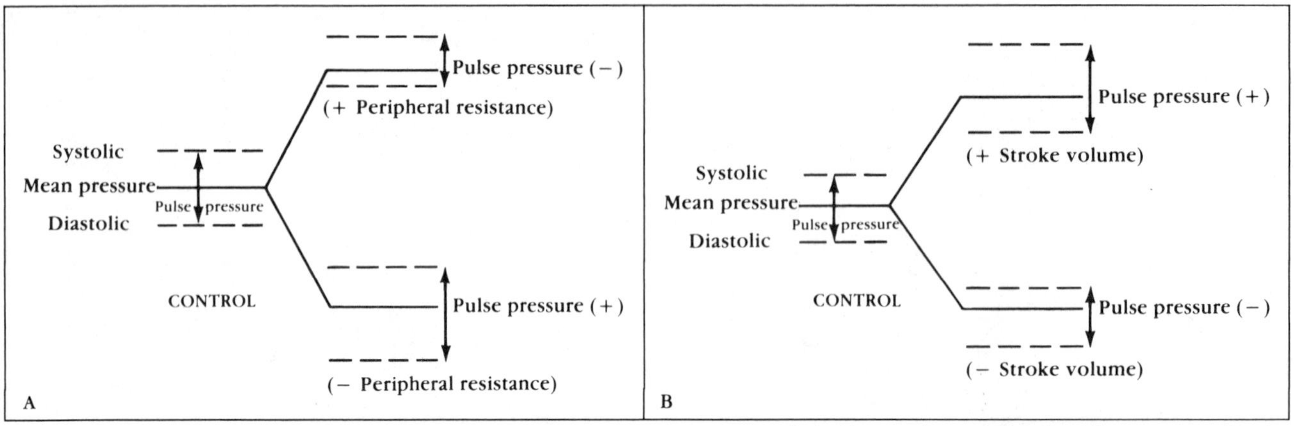

FIGURE 17-24. A. Changes in systolic, diastolic, mean, and pulse pressure produced by changes in peripheral resistance. Increased (+) peripheral resistances cause decreased pulse pressure and increased mean. Decreased (−) peripheral resistance gives the opposite effect. B. Changes in systolic, diastolic, and mean pressure produced by changes in stroke volume. (From R. C. Little, *Physiology of the Heart and Circulation* [2nd ed.]. Chicago: Yearbook, 1981.)

the heart has to pump and raises the blood pressure. Dilatation of the arterioles decreases the impedance offered and decreases the blood pressure. Stimulation of the adrenergic nerves causes vasoconstriction, a mechanism that is important in blood pressure elevations with exercise or fear. Humoral mechanisms can cause an increased or decreased PVR. Prostaglandins, renin, kinins, and many other substances are under study in relation to their regulation of PVR.

The control of blood flow by the tissues is called *autoregulation* and probably occurs with selective opening and closing of capillary sphincters. Hyperemia occurs when the channels are open and increased blood flows to an area.

AORTIC IMPEDANCE. Aortic impedance is offered by the elastic aortic wall and the aortic valve. The aortic valve normally remains closed until the pressure in the left ventricle exceeds the pressure maintained in the aorta. After this occurs, the valve opens and the ventricle must pump against the resistance offered by the elastic aortic wall. When elasticity decreases, such as with aging, more aortic impedance is offered to the left ventricle. Also, with narrowing of the aortic valve, impedance requires an increased ventricular force to eject its contents.

DIASTOLIC ARTERIAL VOLUME. The amount of blood remaining in the aorta on diastole is related to all of the factors mentioned in the previous paragraph. If cardiac output is increased and peripheral vascular resistance is also elevated, increased amounts of blood will remain in the arterial circuit during diastole. This usually increases the diastolic pressure and the resistance against which the ventricle has to pump. If cardiac output is increased and the peripheral vascular resistance is decreased, the "run-off" will decrease the diastolic volume and volume resistance against which the heart is pumping.

FACTORS AFFECTING THE VENOUS CIRCULATION

Blood in the veins does not normally pulsate as does arterial blood. Movement of blood through the systemic veins is due to pressure differences, skeletal, thoracic, and visceral muscle pressures, and the valves that prevent the backflow of blood. Pulsations may be seen in the jugular veins; these reflect the activity of the right atrium and ventricle. Abnormalities in venous circulation can result from such conditions as fluid overloading, venous insufficiency, and constrictive pericarditis.

REFERENCES

1. Berne, R. M. The role of adenosine in the regulation of coronary blood flow. *Circ. Res.* 47:807, 1980.
2. Cohn, J. N. Recognition and Management of Shock and Acute Pump Failure. In J. W. Hurst, et al. (eds.), *The Heart* (5th ed.). New York: McGraw-Hill, 1982.
3. Dustan, H. P. Pathophysiology of Hypertension. In J. W. Hurst, et al. (eds.), *The Heart* (5th ed.). New York: McGraw-Hill, 1982.
4. Guyton, A. *Textbook of Medical Physiology* (6th ed.). Philadelphia: Saunders, 1981.
5. James, T. N., et al. Anatomy of the Heart. In J. W. Hurst, et al. (eds.), *The Heart* (5th ed.). New York: McGraw-Hill, 1982.
6. Kirk, E. S., and Jennings, R. B. Pathophysiology of Myocardial Ischemia. In J. W. Hurst, et al. (eds.), *The Heart* (5th ed.). New York: McGraw-Hill, 1982.
7. Leatham, A., et al. Auscultation of the Heart. In J. W. Hurst, et al. (eds.), *The Heart* (5th ed.). New York: McGraw-Hill, 1982.
8. Little, R. C. *Physiology of the Heart and Circulation* (2nd ed.). Chicago: Year Book, 1981.
9. Nutter, D. O. Measurement of the Systemic Blood Pressure. In J. W. Hurst, et al. (eds.), *The Heart* (5th ed.). New York: McGraw-Hill, 1982.
10. Schlant, R. C., and Sonnenblick, E. H. Pathophysiology of Heart Failure. In J. W. Hurst, et al. (eds.), *The Heart* (5th ed.). New York: McGraw-Hill, 1982.
11. Wallace, A. G. Electrical Activity of the Heart. In J. W. Hurst, et al. (eds.), *The Heart* (5th ed.). New York: McGraw-Hill, 1982.

CHAPTER 18
COMPROMISED PUMPING ABILITY OF THE HEART

LEARNING OBJECTIVES

1. Differentiate between cardiac and circulatory failure.
2. Describe the terms *preload* and *afterload.*
3. Discuss compensatory mechanisms of cardiac failure.
4. Describe cause and effect of dilatation of the heart chambers.
5. List the underlying factors that can precipitate heart failure.
6. Describe the pathophysiology of right and left heart failure.
7. Describe the basis for the clinical manifestations of left heart failure.
8. Describe the basis for the clinical manifestations of right heart failure.
9. Discuss radiologic changes in heart failure.
10. Identify the purposes of the Swan-Ganz catheter in monitoring congestive heart failure.
11. Identify blood tests used to aid in the diagnosis of congestive heart failure.
12. List causes of cardiogenic shock.
13. Discuss the mechanism of compensated shock.
14. Identify clinical signs and symptoms of cardiogenic shock.
15. Discuss irreversible or decompensated shock.
16. Define *cardiomyopathy.*
17. Differentiate between primary and secondary cardiomyopathies.
18. Describe congestive, restrictive, and hypertrophic cardiomyopathy.

Many conditions may lead to impairment of myocardial contractility. The end result of this impairment is congestive heart failure. This chapter examines heart failure, its sequelae, cardiogenic shock, and the entity of cardiomyopathy.

CONGESTIVE HEART FAILURE

Heart failure refers to a constellation of signs and symptoms that result from an inability of the heart to pump enough blood to meet the metabolic demands of the body. The *pump* itself is impaired and unable to adequately supply blood to meet the cellular needs. Cardiac failure is one type of *circulatory failure,* a term that also includes hypoperfusion resulting from extracardiac conditions such as hypovolemia, peripheral vasodilatation, and inadequate oxygenation of the hemoglobin.

The clinical result of heart failure includes *circulatory overload* or *congestive heart failure* (CHF). CHF is a clinical syndrome characterized by abnormal sodium and water retention resulting from renal compensation for the decreased cardiac output. The circulatory overload is enhanced by the resulting excess blood volume and increased venous return.

The causes of heart failure are varied and include intrinsic myocardial disease, malformation or injury, and secondary abnormalities (Table 18-1). Myocardial failure is often the cause of death in terminal illness of a noncardiac etiology.

TABLE 18-1. Intrinsic and secondary causes of heart failure

Intrinsic*	Secondary
	Pulmonary embolism
Cardiomyopathy	Anemia
Myocardial infarction	Thyrotoxicosis
Myocarditis	Systemic hypertension
Ischemic heart disease	Arteriovenous shunts
Congenital heart defects	Blood volume excess
Pericarditis/cardiac tamponade	Metabolic/respiratory acidosis
	Drug toxicity
	Cardiac arrhythmias

**Intrinsic* refers to myocardial, endocardial, and pericardial disease, and congenital malformations that increase ventricular volume load and ischemia or infarction of the ventricular myocardium.

Pathophysiology of Heart Failure

The onset of heart failure may be acute or insidious. It is often associated with systolic or diastolic overloading and with myocardial weakness. As the physiologic stress on the heart muscle reaches a critical level, the contractility of the muscle is reduced and the cardiac output declines, but the venous input to the ventricle remains the same. The responses to the decreasing cardiac output are predictable and include (1) reflex increase in sympathetic activity, (2) release of renin from the juxtaglomerular cells of the kidney, (3) anaerobic metabolism by affected cells, and (4) increased extraction of oxygen by the peripheral cells. The responses of the heart to the increased volume of blood in the ventricles are also predictable and include both short- and long-term mechanisms: (1) In *acute* or *short-term mechanisms,* as the end-diastolic fiber length increases, the ventricular muscle responds with dilatation and an increased force of contraction (Frank-Starling effect). (2) In *long-term mechanisms,* ventricular hypertrophy increases the ability of the heart muscle to contract and push its volume into the circulation. The pathology of the predisposing condition determines whether heart failure is acute or insidious in onset, as compensation often occurs for long periods of time before the manifestations of heart failure develop. An example of long-term compensation is that which results from *systemic hypertension.* Because the ventricle must pump against increased pressure (increased afterload), the ventricular myocardium hypertrophies, the heart pumps with more force, and the heart rate is often elevated. These mechanisms may effect normal cardiac output for years prior to the onset of failure. Symptoms of CHF signal that the pump can no longer keep up with the cellular demands. Gradually, the manifestations of heart failure become apparent. An example of the acute onset of heart failure is that seen with a large myocardial infarction, which causes direct impairment of cardiac contractility, a sudden decrease in cardiac output, and insufficient available time for the development of hypertrophy.

SYMPATHETIC RESPONSE TO HEART FAILURE. A decrease in the cardiac output results in a decreased blood pressure, which causes a reflex stimulation of the sympathetic nervous system (SNS). The SNS causes an increase in the rate and force of the contraction of the ventricles both through the conduction system and through an increase in ventricular irritability. It also results in vasoconstriction of the arterioles throughout the body. The SNS activity is mediated through epinephrine and norepinephrine. Epinephrine mostly functions to increase the rate and force of cardiac contractions, while norepinephrine functions mainly in arteriolar vasoconstriction.

RENIN RELEASE FROM THE KIDNEY. When the blood pressure decreases the decline is perceived by the renal juxtaglomerular cells, which release renin. Renin acts on angiotensinogen, a plasma protein produced by the liver, to form angiotensin I. Angiotensin I is converted to angiotensin II by an enzyme found mostly in the lungs (Fig. 18-1). Angiotensin II is a potent vasoconstrictor that constricts renal arterioles, stimulates the thirst center in the brain, and stimulates the secretion of aldosterone by the adrenal gland [3]. These actions cause vasoconstriction, which leads to increased blood pressure and expansion of the blood volume through the aldosterone effect of sodium preservation. Angiotensin II is rapidly destroyed by *angiotensinase,* a term used for various blood tissue enzymes [3].

ANAEROBIC METABOLISM. When cells do not receive adequate circulation or oxygen, metabolism decreases and

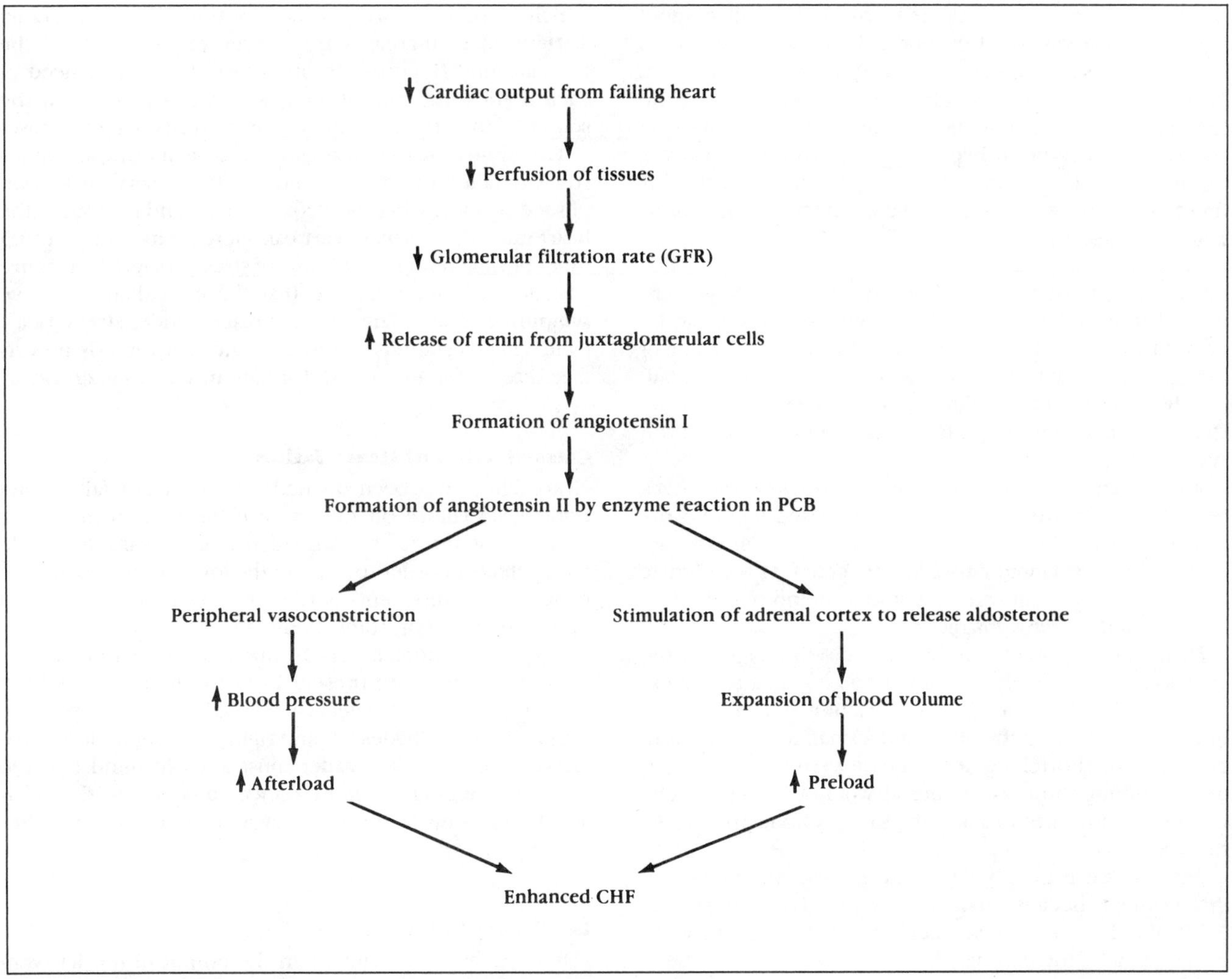

FIGURE 18-1. Renin-angiotensin-aldosterone (RAA) system in CHF. Note the positive feedback created as the body attempts to adjust to the decreased cardiac output.

alternate methods of energy production are utilized. The major alternate method is the anaerobic production of adenosine triphosphate (ATP), which is an inefficient process but accomplishes the purpose of keeping cells alive for a limited period of time. This compensatory mechanism is utilized only in severe circulatory failure and shock.

OXYGEN EXTRACTION FROM THE RED BLOOD CELLS. Oxygen extraction from the red blood cells (RBCs) to the tissues increases when the circulation is inadequate and perfusion is diminished. Normally about 30 percent of oxygen is extracted from the RBC by the peripheral tissue, but greater amounts are extracted during periods of poor perfusion. Unfortunately, this mechanism is not very useful to the myocardium because myocardial muscle normally extracts 65 to 75 percent of the oxygen it receives [1].

FRANK-STARLING LAW OF THE HEART. When the heart is not pumping all of its contents out, increased amounts of blood are left within the organ. This residual volume increases diastolic fiber length. The inherent compensatory mechanism is an increase in the force of recoil so that the heart responds with increased stroke work and volume. In the failing heart diastolic fiber, length is continually increased, causing enlargement of the heart size. With activation of the renin-angiotensin-aldosterone (RAA) system, blood volume is increased adding to this diastolic preload (Fig. 18-1).

HYPERTROPHY OF THE MYOCARDIUM. When increased stress is placed on any chamber of the heart hypertrophy can result. This stress response is due to a chronic increased workload. The individual myocardial muscle cells increase in size but not in number. Hypertrophy probably results when the wall tension of the chamber must continuously increase on systole to eject the contents of the chamber. Atrial hypertrophy may be seen in mitral stenosis or tricuspid stenosis but ventricular hypertrophy is more common. It may be classified as *concentric* or *eccentric*. Concentric hypertrophy reveals a thickened ventricular wall without apparent enlargement of the heart. This is often seen with aortic stenosis and sometimes with systemic hypertension. Eccentric hypertrophy exhibits a proportionate increase in left ventricular wall size and in the diameter of the ventricle [7]. This type of hypertrophy is often seen in conditions associated with increased preload. Hypertrophy functions to maintain or increase contractility until heart failure ensues.

DILATATION OF THE HEART. Dilatation refers to enlargement of cardiac chamber size. It often occurs because of an increased volume of blood that enters the heart. Dilatation of the ventricle is always seen in acute congestive heart failure. It often coincides with hypertrophy especially if the stressful event causing the failure is chronic, such as with systemic hypertension.

X-ray enlargement of the cardiac shadow characterizes heart failure. In the normal heart, increased input to the ventricle results in increased ventricular force of contraction, but no permanent enlargement occurs. As the cardiac reserve fails, the ventricle is unable to pump out all of its contents and thereby enlarges.

Dilatation imposes a mechanical disadvantage on the ventricle. As ventricular volume increases, a large portion of the mechanical energy of contraction is expended in imparting tension to the fibers and a smaller portion for fiber recoil or shortening. If one heart were twice as big in its linear dimensions as another, it would take 4 times the contractile power to produce the same systolic pressure in the larger heart.

A heart that is greatly dilated also works at a metabolic disadvantage because its need for oxygen is increased. More blood to the myocardium is needed, which may not be supplied by the coronary arteries.

Dilatation is characteristic of cardiomyopathy in which separation of the trabeculae carnae may be seen along with fibrosis of the myocardium. Usually, the greater the dilatation the more ineffective the cardiac contraction. Ineffective left ventricular contraction is often called *hypokinesis* of the left ventricle.

In persons with valvular insufficiency, septal defects, or other abnormal communications, the diastolic inflow to one or both ventricles is permanently augmented. In such conditions, dilatation of cardiac chambers occurs to maintain a normal or near normal circulation even if a defect is quite large.

The compensatory mechanisms previously described may preserve the life of the individual but they usually aggravate the underlying condition.

The sympathetic regulation tends to preserve circulation to the brain and heart, but it increases the cardiac workload by increasing the afterload, which may work to depress the effectiveness of the cardiac contraction. Activation of the RAA system also increases afterload because of the peripheral vasoconstriction produced. The aldosterone effect increases blood volume and thus increases the preload. Anaerobic metabolism causes metabolic acidosis, which depresses myocardial contractility. The Frank-Starling effect increases the energy requirements of the myocardium. Hypertrophy increases the oxygen need of each myocardial muscle cell, which is a problem if the source of the original pathology is coronary artery disease.

The ability of the heart to increase its output under stress is called the *cardiac reserve*. This reserve is accomplished by increasing the stroke volume and increasing the heart rate. The normal heart can increase its output 4 to 5 times normal under conditions of stress [3]. As heart failure ensues, the reserve falls so that the individual may have symptoms of heart failure when placed under stress. Heart failure manifestations at rest indicate that there is no cardiac reserve for any stressful situation, such as exercise.

Classification of Heart Failure

Heart failure has been divided into left heart failure and right heart failure on the basis of the clinical manifestations. It has further been divided into forward and backward effects in order to explain the low output and venous congestion components of CHF. In some cases the forward or low-output syndrome dominates while in others the congestive phenomenon is the major manifestation. In reality, both features are present in heart failure just as both left- and right-sided effects necessarily must be present. This discussion divides left and right heart failure into separate entities, but the reader must keep in mind that the heart and lungs are an interconnected system so that what affects one side of the heart eventually affects the other (Fig. 18-2).

Left Heart Failure (LHF)

Left-sided failure occurs when the output of the left ventricle is less than the total volume of blood received from the right side of the heart via the pulmonary circulation. As a result, the pulmonary circuit becomes congested with blood that cannot be moved forward and the systemic blood pressure falls.

CAUSES OF LEFT HEART FAILURE. The most common cause of predominantly left ventricular failure is myocardial infarction. Other causes include systemic hypertension, aortic stenosis or insufficiency, and cardiomyopathy. Mitral stenosis and mitral insufficiency also cause the symptoms of left heart failure [8].

PATHOPHYSIOLOGY OF LEFT HEART FAILURE. Because the left ventricle cannot pump out all of its blood, blood dams back from the left ventricle to the left atrium, into the four pulmonary veins and the pulmonary capillary bed (PCB). As the volume of blood in the lungs increases the pulmonary vessels enlarge. The pressure of blood in the PCB increases and when it reaches a certain critical point (approximately 25–28 mm Hg), fluid passes across the pulmonary capillary membrane into the interstitial spaces around the alveoli and finally into the alveoli (Fig. 18-3). Acute pulmonary

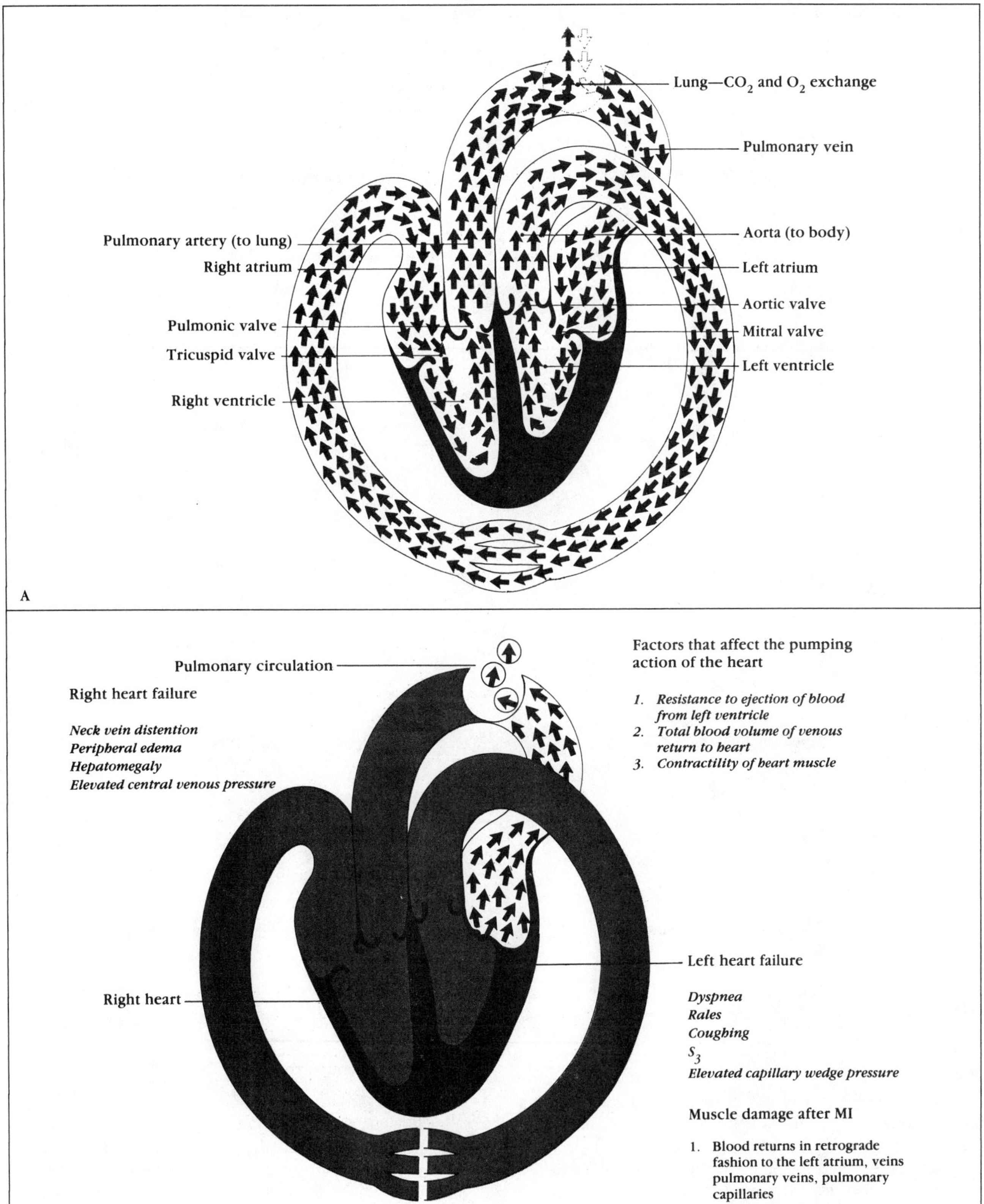

FIGURE 18-2. A. Normal circulation. B. Congestive heart failure. (From C. V. Kenner, C. E. Guzzetta, and B. M. Dossey, *Critical Care Nursing: Body-Mind-Spirit.* Boston: Little, Brown, 1981.)

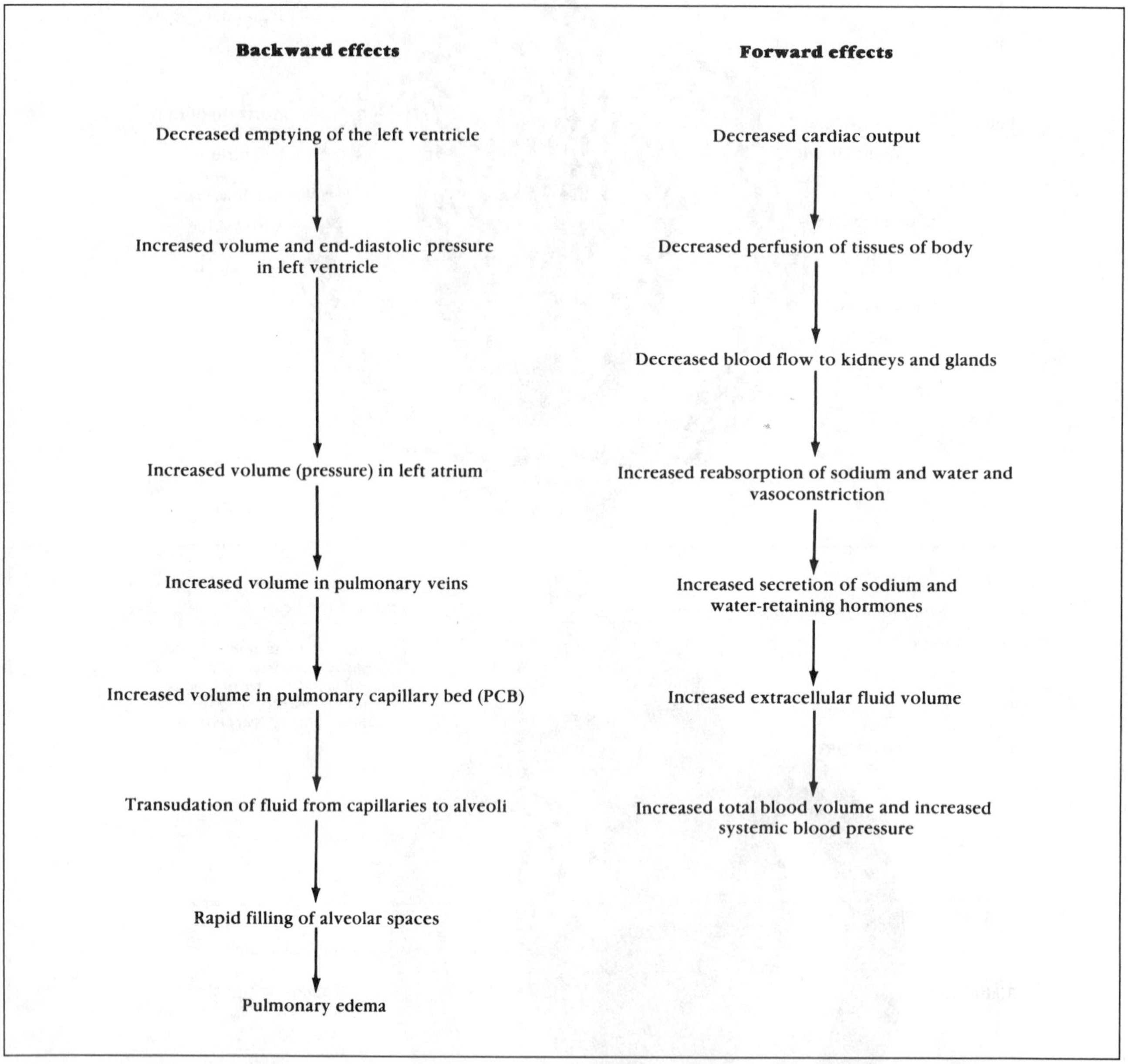

FIGURE 18-3. Pathophysiology of left heart failure.

edema (APE) results, which impairs gas exchange and can be life-threatening. Higher PCB pressures may cause rupture of the capillary membranes leaking small or large amounts of blood into the alveolar sacs. All of these changes are called the *backward effects of LHF.*

The left ventricle also cannot pump its normal stroke volume out the aorta. Thus, the systemic blood pressure decreases. This decreased blood pressure is sensed by the pressoreceptors that cause a reflex stimulation of the SNS. The result of this is increased heart rate and peripheral vasoconstriction. The RAA system is stimulated, leading to further vasoconstriction along with sodium and water retention (see Fig. 18-3). These are the main manifestations of the *forward effects of LHF.*

Chronic left heart failure is often seen in mitral valve disease and it may progressively occur in cardiomyopathy and postmyocardial infarction. In this situation, pulmonary congestion may be evidenced but APE does not occur unless additional stress increases the cardiac demand. Individuals with mitral stenosis, for example, have been shown to have a pulmonary pressure greater than 30 mm Hg without symptoms of APE. However, in conditions of sudden onset, this level would cause acute manifestations.

SIGNS AND SYMPTOMS OF LEFT HEART FAILURE. In the early stages of LHF, the symptoms of dyspnea are exhibited when the cardiac reserve is exceeded. As fluid begins to accumulate in the PCB, the formation of interstitial edema causes a defect in oxygenation. The oxygen saturation of blood decreases causing the chemoreceptors to stimulate the respiratory center. The respiratory rate increases at first during exercise and later even at rest.

Because of the decreased cardiac output and decreased oxygen saturation of the blood, hypoxia of the body tissues occurs, which results in easy fatigue, weakness, and dizziness. The dizziness occurs due to hypoxia to the brain. As failure and the resulting hypoxia worsen, disorientation, confusion, and ultimately unconsciousness can occur. Loss of potassium induced by increased levels of aldosterone also causes muscle weakness.

The inability to breathe in a supine position is called *orthopnea.* In chronic left heart failure, interstitial and alveolar pulmonary edema may be present all of the time and the upright position is assumed so that fluid will gravitate to the bases of the lungs.

Paroxysmal nocturnal dyspnea (PND) refers to the onset of an acute episode of dyspnea at night. This condition is thought to result from improved cardiac performance at night, which causes increased resorption of fluid into the systemic circuit. This increased fluid overloads the left ventricle causing acute pulmonary congestion until the individual assumes the orthopneic position. Acute breathlessness and a feeling of smothering are described.

Pulmonary edema is an acute, life-threatening condition that usually results from left heart failure but may also result from abnormal permeability of the alveolocapillary membrane. Signs and symptoms of APE include dyspnea of sudden onset, basal rales, gasping respirations, extreme anxiety, rapid weak pulse, increased venous pressure, and decreased urinary output. The skin is cool and moist to the touch, ashen-gray, or cyanotic. A cough accompanied by expectoration of frothy, pink-tinged, or bloody sputum is usually present.

Right Heart Failure (RHF)

Right-sided failure occurs when the output of the right ventricle is less than the input from the systemic venous circuit. As a result, there is congestion of the systemic venous circuit and a decreased output to the lungs.

CAUSES OF RIGHT HEART FAILURE. The major cause of RHF is LHF; the right ventricle fails because of the excessive pulmonary pressures generated by failure of the left heart. Other causes include chronic obstructive lung disease (COPD), pulmonary embolus, and congenital heart defects, especially those that involve pulmonary overloading and pulmonary hypertension.

PATHOPHYSIOLOGY OF RIGHT HEART FAILURE. In RHF the right ventricle cannot pump all of its contents forward, so blood dams back from the right ventricle to the right atrium causing an increased pressure in the systemic venous circuit. The increased volume and pressure are transmitted to distensible organs such as the liver and spleen. The increased pressure in the peritoneal vessels leads to transudation of fluid into the peritoneal cavity. Increased pressure at the capillary line causes fluid to move into the interstitial space and systemic edema results (see Fig. 18-4). The cardinal signs of RHF are jugular venous distention, hepatomegaly, splenomegaly, and peripheral, dependent edema. These are considered the *backward,* or *congestive,* effects of RHF.

The right ventricle also cannot maintain its output to the lungs. This results in a decreased pulmonary circulation and decreased return to the left side of the heart. These *forward effects of RHF* cause all of the forward effects of LHF (Fig. 18-4).

SIGNS AND SYMPTOMS OF RIGHT HEART FAILURE. The signs and symptoms of RHF reflect both forward and backward effects. Dependent, pitting edema is characteristic and may be noted in the sacrum or sternum of a bedridden patient as well as the feet and legs of an individual in the sitting position.

Enlargement of the spleen and liver can cause pressure on surrounding organs, respiratory impingement, and organ dysfunction. Inadequate deactivation of aldosterone by the liver may lead to further fluid retention. Jaundice and coagulation problems may result with severe, decompensated RHF. Ascites also occurs when the RHF is severe and may cause respiratory embarrassment and abdominal pressure.

Jugular venous distention occurs with RHF and can be measured at the bedside. The amount of distention is measured in centimeters when the head is elevated to a 30- to 45-degree or a 90-degree angle (Fig. 18-5).

Diagnosis of Congestive Heart Failure

RADIOLOGIC CHANGES. X-ray evidence of pulmonary congestion usually precedes the development of audible rales in LHF. Cardiac enlargement is noted by an increased size of the left ventricular shadow. The left ventricle extends past the midclavicular line and fluid effusion may be seen throughout the lung fields (Fig. 18-6). In RHF the right ventricular shadow can be seen extending out from the right sternal border. Pulmonary markings may be decreased (Fig. 18-7).

HEMODYNAMIC MONITORING. The balloon-tipped flow-directed catheter (Swan-Ganz) is an invaluable monitoring system for assessing pulmonary and systemic circulations. The Swan-Ganz catheter is threaded into the pulmonary artery where it finally impacts in a vessel slightly smaller than the inflated balloon tip, blocking the flow of blood from the right ventricle [9]. A pressure reading at this time reflects the diastolic pressures of the left ventricle if there is no concomitant mitral valve disease. This pulmonary artery wedge pressure (PAWP) reflects its pressures because of the continuous circuit to the left heart. Pressure measurements, then, reflect the left ventricular end-diastolic pres-

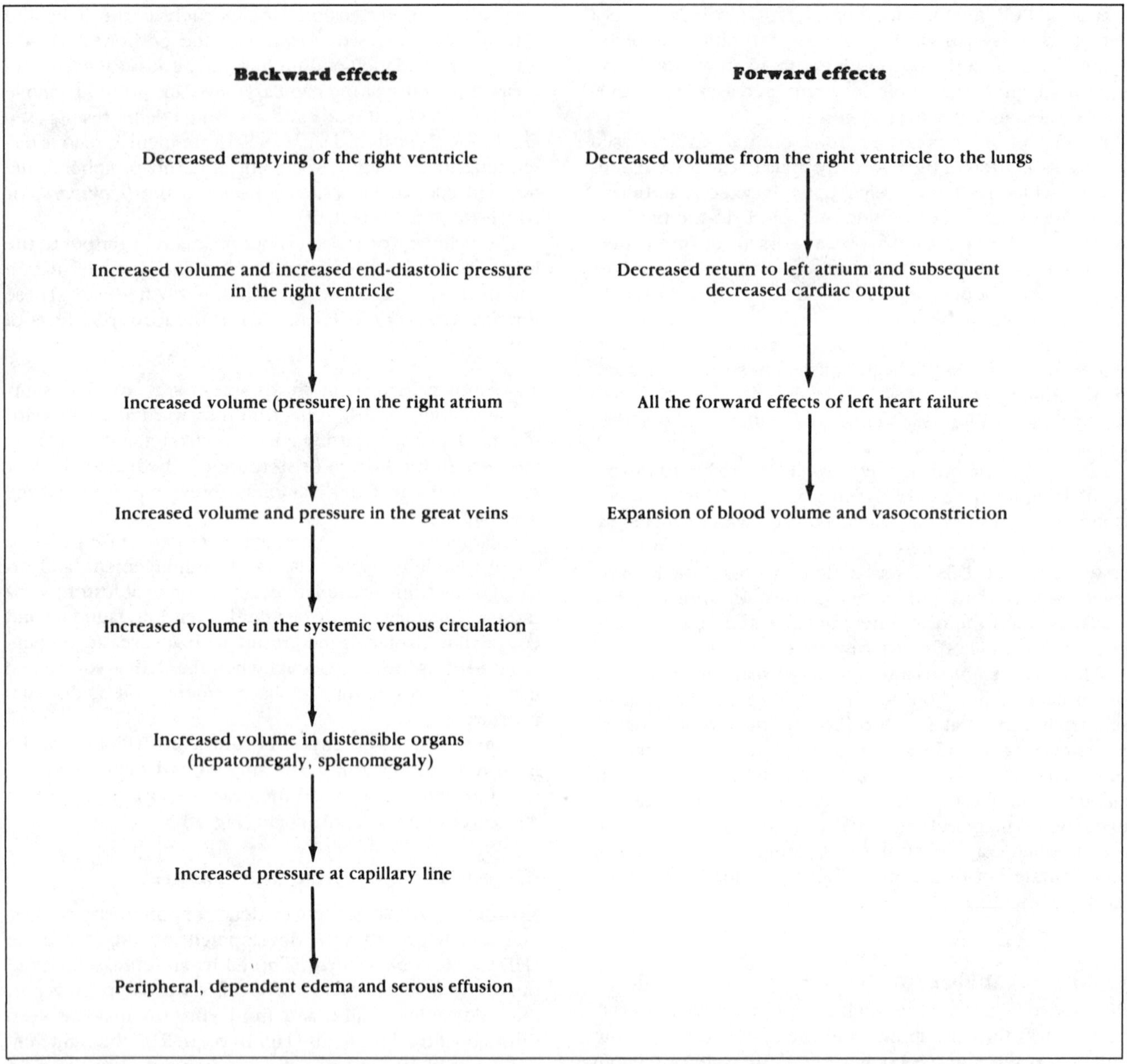

FIGURE 18-4. Pathophysiology of right heart failure.

sure (LVEDP). When the balloon tip is deflated, the catheter tip usually locates in the right or left main pulmonary artery [9]. The Swan-Ganz catheter also measures central venous pressure (right atrial pressure) and pulmonary artery pressure. Most Swan-Ganz catheters also can be used to obtain cardiac output measurements by the thermodilution method. This method utilizes a computer analysis of temperature differential between two points on the catheter. The normal cardiac output is approximately 4 to 8 liters/minute. The level of the decreased cardiac output in persons with CHF helps to determine the necessary treatment. Levels of 2.2 to 3.0 liters/minute or below may indicate cardiogenic shock depending on the size and age of the individual.

ARTERIAL BLOOD GASES. The normal arterial and venous blood gases are presented in Table 18-2. Hypoxemia ($\downarrow PO_2$) is often the only change that is noted. The O_2 saturation often remains normal until decompensation is severe. PCO_2 may be low due to hyperventilation.

OTHER LABORAORY TESTS. *Serum sodium* levels are often low in CHF even though body sodium is almost always elevated. *Serum potassium* may also be low due to the aldosterone effect and potassium-depleting diuretics (see Chap. 5).

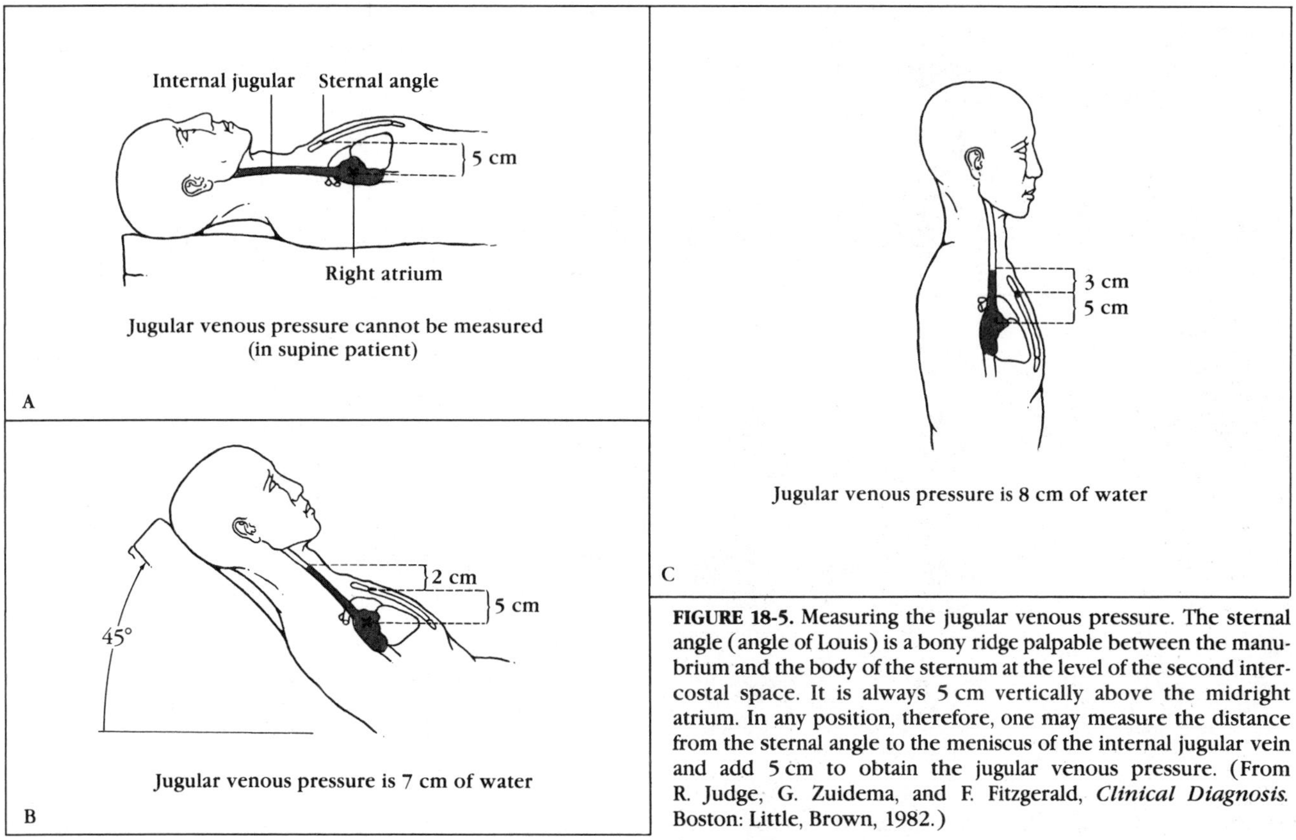

FIGURE 18-5. Measuring the jugular venous pressure. The sternal angle (angle of Louis) is a bony ridge palpable between the manubrium and the body of the sternum at the level of the second intercostal space. It is always 5 cm vertically above the midright atrium. In any position, therefore, one may measure the distance from the sternal angle to the meniscus of the internal jugular vein and add 5 cm to obtain the jugular venous pressure. (From R. Judge, G. Zuidema, and F. Fitzgerald, *Clinical Diagnosis.* Boston: Little, Brown, 1982.)

TABLE 18-2. Arterial and venous blood gas studies (normal values in healthy adults)

	Arterial blood	Mixed venous blood
pH	7.40* (7.35–7.45)	7.36* (7.30–7.41)
PO_2	80–100 mm Hg	35–40 mm Hg
O_2 Sa	95%	70–75%
PCO_2	35–45 mm Hg	41–51 mm Hg
HCO_3	22–26 mEq/L	22–26 mEq/L
Base excess (BE)	−2–+2	−2– +2

*Mean.

CARDIOGENIC SHOCK

Causes of Cardiogenic Shock

Heart failure may lead to cardiogenic shock with either a low-output component or with the addition of the congestive phenomena. The most common cause of cardiogenic shock is myocardial infarction, but cardiomyopathy, arrhythmias, cardiac tamponade, pulmonary embolism, or any factor that can depress myocardial function may also precipitate this syndrome.

Cardiogenic shock always carries a grave prognosis. If it develops after myocardial infarction (MI), the mortality is approximately 60 to 80 percent, which correlates well with the amount of ventricular mass lost. A 30 to 40 per-

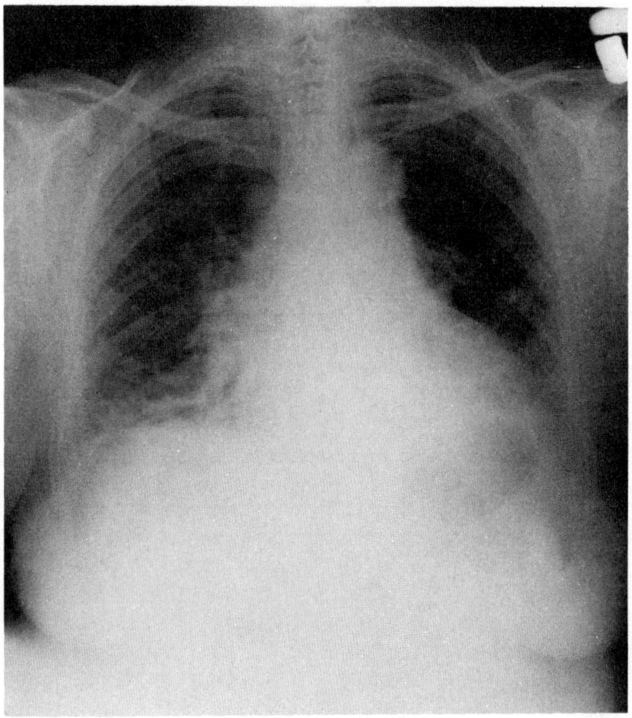

FIGURE 18-6. Radiologic changes seen in LHF. Note left ventricular enlargement and fluid effusion in lung fields.

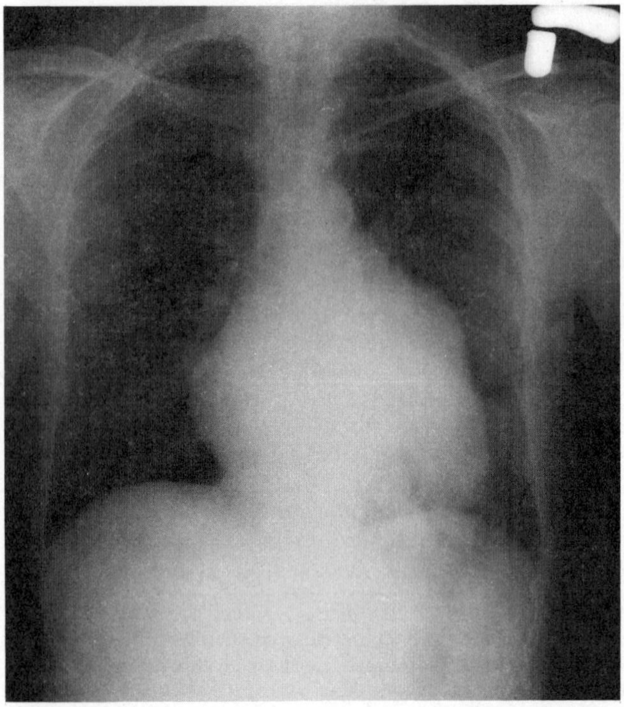

FIGURE 18-7. Radiologic changes in RHF. Note right ventricular shadow extending out from the right sternal border.

cent loss of left ventricular mass by infarctions, both new and old, is often correlated with cardiogenic shock [1].

Pathophysiology of Cardiogenic Shock

Cardiogenic shock results from a decreased ability of the left or right ventricle to maintain adequate cardiac output. This results in a decreased systolic blood pressure with reduced peripheral perfusion manifested by cold, clammy skin; diaphoresis; tachycardia; mental confusion; and decreased urinary output. The cold, clammy skin and tachycardia result from sympathetic stimulation. The effects of SNS stimulation increase the taxation on an already overtaxed heart but serve to enhance cerebral and coronary blood flow.

Anaerobic metabolism begins in peripheral cells as vital oxygen deprivation occurs. The effect of this energy production is to keep cells viable but the production of lactic acid as a by-product can lead to metabolic acidosis (see Chap. 6).

Cardiogenic shock is often described in stages. If the compensatory mechanisms can restore the arterial pressure and urinary output, the shock is termed *compensated shock*. If the underlying cause of the shock is not corrected, the response of the body to the poor tissue perfusion results in continuation of the shock state, which is called *progressive shock*. When arteriolar tone is finally destroyed and peripheral pooling occurs, death becomes inevitable; this condition is called *irreversible* or *decompensated* shock. Pooling is enhanced by loss of arteriolar tone prior to loss of venular tone, which encourages fluid movement into the interstitial spaces. The anaerobic energy production and lactic acidosis eventually cause cellular failure and death [6].

Diagnosis of Cardiogenic Shock

Diagnosis of cardiogenic shock is often one of exclusion. Sometimes hypovolemic shock must be ruled out. The physical examination reveals gallop rhythms, sometimes venous engorgement, and the effects of acute hypotension. ECG recordings often show cardiac arrhythmias and evidence of myocardial infarction. The Swan-Ganz catheter reveals elevated pulmonary wedge pressures and decreased cardiac outputs.

DISEASES AFFECTING MYOCARDIAL CONTRACTILITY

The term *cardiomyopathy* refers to a group of myocardial diseases that primarily affect the pumping ability of the heart. *Myocarditis* is the term used for myocardial disease that is associated with inflammation of the myocardium.

Cardiomyopathy

Primary or idiopathic myocardial disease refers to those conditions affecting the ventricular muscle that have no known origin. *Secondary cardiomyopathy* designates those conditions in which the causative factors are known. The cardiomyopathies have been classified as congestive, restrictive, and hypertrophic [2].

CONGESTIVE OR DILATED CARDIOMYOPATHY. Congestive or dilated cardiomyopathy is usually of unknown etiology, but it has been described in association with beriberi, thyrotoxicosis, alcoholism, childbirth or the postpartum period, diabetes mellitus, drug toxicity (especially from daunorubicin), cobalt therapy, and certain neuromuscular disorders. The striking effect of this type of cardiomyopathy is immense cardiomegaly. The enlargement is a combination of dilatation and hypertrophy of the heart. This dilatation leads to a hypokinetic myocardium with the usual onset of biventricular CHF. Symptoms include exertional dyspnea, fatigue, paroxysmal nocturnal dyspnea, and pulmonary edema with symptoms of RHF in the later course of the disease. Atrial and ventricular gallops may be noted on auscultation. Peripheral edema and hepatomegaly are signs of RHF.

RESTRICTIVE CARDIOMYOPATHY. Restrictive cardiomyopathy describes the clinical picture of a person with constrictive pericarditis but the underlying cause is actually myocardial. The usual etiology of this condition is unknown but the condition has been described in association with such diverse conditions as amyloidosis, hemosiderosis, and glycogen storage disease. The myocardial muscle becomes infiltrated with abnormal substances that apparently cause dysfunction of the ventricle.

Congestive and restrictive cardiomyopathy are mostly differentiated on the basis of the presence or absence of cardiomegaly. Symptoms of biventricular failure are common. Ventricular filling is impeded and the end-diastolic pressure of the ventricles usually becomes exceedingly high. The prognosis for survival is poor and death often results from CHF.

HYPERTROPHIC CARDIOMYOPATHY. Hypertrophic cardiomyopathy usually refers to an asymmetric increase in ventricular muscle mass. It has also been termed *idiopathic hypertrophic subaortic stenosis* (IHSS) and *hypertrophic obstructive cardiomyopathy.*

The etiology of this condition is unknown. A familial incidence is noted with no predominance for one sex or another. Certain studies support a prenatal disorder of myocardial development [4]. The pathologic features include greater hypertrophy of the ventricular septum than of the ventricular chambers. Small or normal ventricular chamber size and disorganization of septal muscle cells, especially of the myofibrils, may be seen.

Other significant abnormalities associated with this condition include fibrous plaque on the endocardium, abnormal septal arteries, and mitral valvular insufficiency [2].

Because of the septal hypertrophy, the left ventricular cavity is misshapen and, on contraction, the hypertrophied septum causes obstruction to the flow of blood from the ventricle. Any condition that enhances contractility increases the degree of obstruction. The associated left ventricular hypertrophy causes impairment of ventricular filling during diastole and a reduction of ventricular compliance [5].

The signs and symptoms are mainly those of LHF including exertional dyspnea, angina, periods of syncope, and orthopnea. Right-sided effects occur later in the course of the disease.

Myocarditis

Inflammation of the myocardium may result from an infectious process or such conditions as radiation therapy or chemical agents. Viruses, especially the coxsackieviruses, have been implicated in etiology. Myocarditis is often a self-limiting condition that is manifested by tachycardia, symptoms of heart failure, and auscultation of a gallop rhythm. Many types of myocarditis resolve with bed rest, fluid restriction, and limited drug therapy. A small percentage of cases become progressive and develop all of the manifestations of dilated, congestive myocardiopathy.

REFERENCES

1. Braunwald, E., Alpert, J., and Ross, R. Acute Myocardial Infarction. In K.J. Isselbacher, et al. (eds.), *Harrison's Principles of Internal Medicine* (9th ed.). New York: McGraw-Hill, 1980.
2. Goodwin, J.F., Roberts, W.C., and Wenger, N.K. Cardiomyopathy. In J.W. Hurst, et al. (eds.), *The Heart* (5th ed.). New York: McGraw-Hill, 1982.
3. Guyton, A.C. *Textbook of Medical Physiology* (6th ed.). Philadelphia: Saunders, 1981.
4. Manasek, F.J. Histogenesis of the embryonic myocardium. *Am. J. Cardiol.* 25:149, 1970.
5. Martin, L.B., and Cohen, L.S. Cardiomyopathy. *DM* 28:13, 1981.
6. Messer, J.V. Cardiogenic shock: Etiological and pathophysiological considerations, monitoring and management. *Cardiol. Pract.* 86:283, 1978.
7. Robbins, S., and Cotran, R. *Pathologic Basis of Disease* (2nd ed.). Philadelphia: Saunders, 1979.
8. Schlant, R.C., and Sonnerblick, E.H. Pathophysiology of Heart Failure. In J.W. Hurst, et al. (eds.), *The Heart* (5th ed.). New York: McGraw-Hill, 1982.
9. Swan, H.J. Technique of Swan-Ganz Catheterization. In J.W. Hurst, et al. (eds.), *The Heart* (5th ed.). New York: McGraw-Hill, 1982.

CHAPTER 19
ALTERATIONS IN SPECIFIC STRUCTURES IN THE HEART

LEARNING OBJECTIVES

1. Describe the following diagnostic procedures: coronary arteriogram, thallium scan, exercise ECG, multigated blood pool scan, cardiac catheterization, and echocardiography.
2. Differentiate between the pathologic and clinical manifestations of angina and myocardial infarction.
3. Describe the development of an atherosclerotic plaque in a coronary artery.
4. Identify the most common sites of coronary artery lesions.
5. List the risk factors for coronary atherogenesis.
6. Describe the process of healing after a myocardial infarction.
7. List and explain the significance of the characteristic ECG changes of angina and myocardial infarction.
8. Briefly describe why heart pain occurs and why it radiates to other areas.
9. Explain how a myocardial infarction impairs myocardial contractility.
10. Differentiate between the significant changes of *each* of the cardiac enzymes.
11. Describe at least four common complications of myocardial infarction.
12. Relate the pathophysiologic consequences of acute rheumatic fever to chronic valvular disease.
13. State the major pathophysiology and compensatory mechanisms that are utilized in mitral stenosis, mitral insufficiency, mitral valve prolapse, aortic stenosis, aortic regurgitation.
14. Describe the clinical manifestations of mitral stenosis, mitral insufficiency, mitral valve prolapse, aortic stenosis, and aortic regurgitation.
15. Describe how pulmonary hypertension can develop from mitral stenosis.
16. Briefly describe the major characteristics of cardiac murmurs produced by valvular defects.
17. Identify the pathophysiologic alterations in and clinical manifestations of infective endocarditis.
18. State the pathophysiologic alterations in and clinical manifestations of pericarditis.

CORONARY ARTERY DISEASE: ISCHEMIC HEART DISEASE (IHD)

Atherosclerosis of the coronary arteries is the leading cause of coronary artery disease in the United States. Between 1968 and 1976 the mortality from IHD declined about 20 percent. This may reflect widespread application of cardiopulmonary resuscitation, better medical control of emergencies, control of hypertension, lower cholesterol diets, or numerous other reasons [19].

There are multiple theories of the pathogenesis of atherosclerosis with most agreeing that it begins early in life and progresses over a period of decades (see Chap. 21). Many factors probably interact to accelerate the atherogenic process. These have been identified as risk factors in epidemiologic studies since they seem to reflect an increase in the incidence of the development of coronary atherosclerosis in a person but do not predict the severity or extent of an atherosclerotic lesion [19].

The risk factors that cannot be altered include age, sex, race, and genetic heritage. Susceptibility to coronary artery disease (CAD) increases with age; especially noted is the protection of women from the disease during the childbearing years. After the menopausal years, women become as susceptible as men to atherosclerosis of the coronary arteries. The likelihood of premature atherosclerotic heart disease is increased in persons who have a positive family history and in those afflicted with diabetes mellitus. Risk factors that can be altered by life-style changes include: (1) elevated serum lipids, (2) hypertension, (3) cigarette smoking, (4) diets high in saturated fats, (5) sedentary life-style, (6) stressful life-style, and (7) obesity. Modifying these risk factors has the potential of retarding the atherogenic process. A considerable time lag exists between the time of occurrence of pathologic coronary artery narrowing and the appearance of symptomatic disease. During this latent period modification of risk factors can have a preventive effect. Geographic differences seem to markedly affect the predisposition to CAD. For example, in men between the ages of 35 to 64, the mortality for myocardial infarction is 4 to 5 times higher in the United States than in Japan [14]. The effect of the geographic differences appears to be environmentally rather than genetically induced. Perhaps diet, physical activity, and life-style differences are determinative of CAD incidence.

Pathogenesis of Coronary Artery Disease

The lesions of coronary atherosclerosis develop progressively in much the same manner as those of atherosclerosis of the other major arteries (see Chap. 21). The initial change is seen early in life and consists of a fatty streak that may develop into a fibrous plaque or atheroma. This atheromatous plaque is white in appearance, becomes elevated, and partially occludes the lumen of the artery. The cores of the atheromatous plaques become necrotic and hemorrhage, and calcification may result. Thrombosis on or around the plaque may also occur partially or completely occluding the lumen of the vessel (Fig. 19-1).

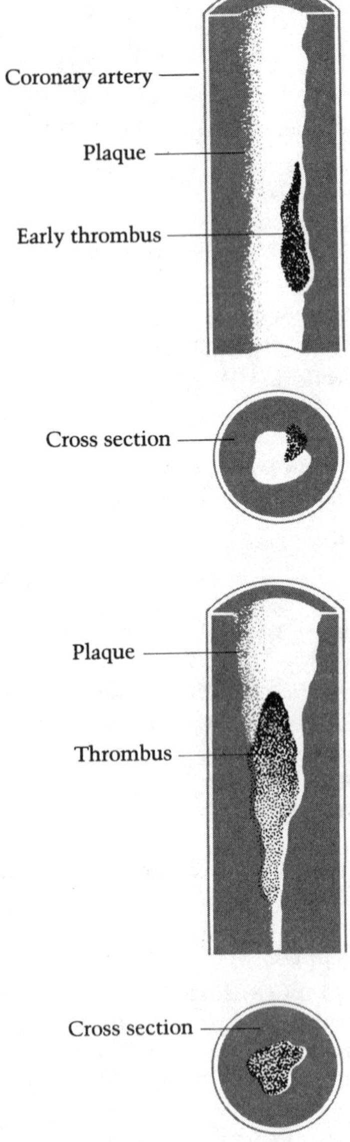

FIGURE 19-1. The arterial thrombus most frequently begins at the areas of luminal narrowing caused by atherosclerotic plaques. The chief thrombus components are platelets, and then platelets and fibrin. (From C. V. Kenner, C. E. Guzzetta, and B. M. Dossey, *Critical Care Nursing: Body-Mind-Spirit.* Boston: Little, Brown, 1981.)

Lesions do not usually cause symptoms until the atherosclerotic process is well advanced, occluding 60 percent or more of the vascular supply to an area. Sometimes total occlusion of a vessel does not cause ischemia to a supplied area because of the development of collateral circulation.

Atherosclerotic plaques tend to appear at bifurcations, curvatures, and tapering of arteries. The right and left main coronary arteries branch sharply off the aorta and thus become a prime target for the development of atheromas.

The vessels then bifurcate and taper rapidly so that these areas also can become affected quickly.

As the coronary artery lumen narrows with increasing plaque formation, resistance to blood flow increases and myocardial muscle blood supply is compromised. As was noted in Chapter 17, normal myocardial oxygen uptake is quite efficient, taking 60 to 75 percent of the oxygen supplied for myocardial muscle utilization. As the amount of blood flow through the vessel decreases, the oxygen uptake cannot increase significantly, resulting in compromise of the oxygen supply to the tissues. When this compromise causes myocardial ischemia angina pectoris results. Further compromise or lack of blood supply may cause necrosis of the myocardial muscle.

A considerable latent period usually exists between the onset of arterial lumen narrowing and symptomatic disease. This period can span 2 to 4 decades and symptoms begin when the lumen is obstructed over 75 percent. The final event that produces infarction may be sudden and involve hemorrhage into an atherosclerotic plaque, thrombosis on an established plaque, or coronary artery spasm.

Angina Pectoris: Myocardial Ischemia

Myocardial ischemia is manifested by angina pectoris, which is a squeezing, substernal pain described as a feeling of tightness or fullness. The pain results from an imbalance between myocardial oxygen supply and myocardial demand for oxygen. In other words, insufficient oxygen is supplied to the myocardial cell for its effective functioning. This condition is almost always related to atherosclerotic coronary artery narrowing. Ischemia suggests, however, that the changes are reversible and cellular function can be restored with restoration of oxygen to the affected muscle. Anaerobic metabolism is utilized to produce adenosine triphosphate (ATP) during the oxygen insufficiency, but the resulting accumulation of lactic acid causes impairment of left ventricular function. This results in a decreased strength of cardiac contraction and impaired wall motion. The degree of impairment depends on the size of the ischemic area and the general contractility of the left ventricular myocardium. Depression of left ventricular function may lead to decreased stroke volume and systemic blood pressure changes.

The heart is unique in that it can be manipulated or operated on without the occurrence of heart pain. However, ischemic cardiac muscle causes intense pain. The cause for this pain is not known but ischemic myocardial muscle releases acidic substances (lactic acid) that may then stimulate the nerve endings in the muscle, conducting pain through the sympathetic nerves to the middle cervical ganglia and through the thoracic ganglia to the spinal cord. The referred nature of the pain (to the left or right arm or neck) probably has to do with nervous interconnections in the sympathetic nerves. These nerve fibers enter the cord all the way from C3 to T5 [9]. When the ischemia is very severe cardiac pain may be also described as crushing, substernal pain. The source of this pain also is not entirely understood but may be from sensory nerve endings from the heart to the pericardium that reflect pain to the great vessels [9].

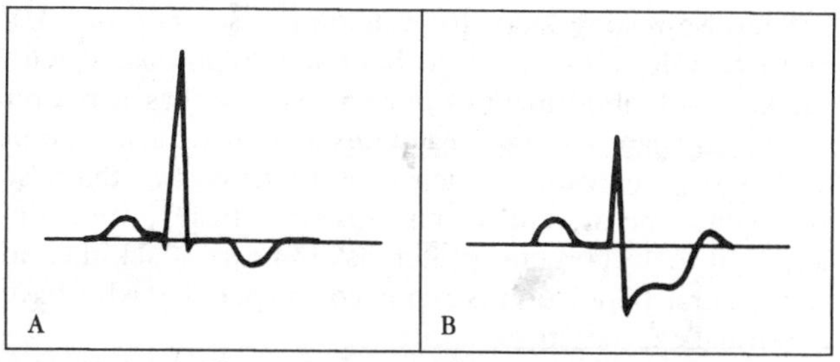

FIGURE 19-2. A. T wave inversion. B. S–T segment depression.

The ischemic episodes causing the chest pain of angina pectoris usually subside in minutes if the imbalance is corrected. Ischemia is totally reversible and a return to normal metabolic, functional, and hemodynamic balance occurs.

CLINICAL MANIFESTATIONS. The clinical picture of angina pectoris is related to the pain experienced and the physiologic response to that pain. The pain is typically described as substernal, a feeling of tightness or fullness, or oppression. It may radiate down one or both arms or into the neck and jaws. Characteristically, the person suffering the pain will become immobile and also may exhibit pallor, profuse perspiration, and dyspnea. The dyspnea may be a compensatory result of temporary cardiac failure induced by left ventricular hypokinesis (see Chap. 18). Classically, angina is precipitated by activity (physical or emotional stress) and is relieved within minutes by rest or the administration of a coronary vasodilator, such as nitroglycerin. During the anginal attack typical electrocardiographic changes are seen. These include T wave inversion and S–T segment depression (Fig. 19-2). Approximately 50 to 70 percent of persons with angina pectoris who have had no previous myocardial infarction have normal electrocardiograms at rest. Cardiac enzymes drawn during or after an anginal attack are usually normal.

DIAGNOSTIC TESTS. The electrocardiogram, cardiac enzymes, and other routine tests may be used to differentiate angina pectoris from a myocardial infarction. Other tests are also used for differential diagnosis and to determine the degree of cardiac impairment. These include the exercise ECG, myocardial imaging, and cardiac catheterization, with a coronary arteriogram.

EXERCISE ECG OR GRADED EXERCISE TEST (GXT). The exercise test with a treadmill or stationary bicycle allows for the evaluation of exercise-induced symptoms and electrocardiographic changes. Exercise-induced S–T segment displacement is the only reliable ECG change of diagnostic significance in myocardial ischemia. S–T segment shifts are probably recorded on the ECG because the injury current can only be interpreted at that phase when the action potentials are at their isoelectric plateau [8].

Exercise testing helps to evaluate the severity of CAD. For example, a person who becomes hypotensive with marked S–T abnormalities during exercise has a poorer prognosis than one who maintains a good cardiac output with less significant S–T changes on exercise. Exercise testing may be used to screen apparently healthy individuals. A 10 to 15 percent greater risk of heart attack than in the general population is reported for persons who have abnormal exercise tests.

NUCLEAR CARDIOLOGY. These techniques detect, define, and quantify radiation that emanates from cardiac structures [18]. The procedures are basically noninvasive and involve the injection of short-lived radionuclides. The purpose of these procedures is to determine myocardial metabolism, perfusion, and viability. One of the more common procedures utilizes the thallium 201 radionuclide tracer. This substance has the ability to substitute for ionic potassium so that it rapidly accumulates in viable myocardial cells [18]. The nuclear camera records an image of the thallium distribution in the myocardium following injection of the substance. The thallium may be injected at peak exercise or at rest. With normal myocardial perfusion, the radioisotope will distribute equally throughout the myocardium. If there is a significant decrease in coronary blood flow, the thallium fails to localize in that segment of the myocardium. This is called a *perfusion defect,* which is a negative image. Positioning of the individual is crucial in localizing defects, especially if the areas affected are small.

CORONARY ARTERIOGRAM. The coronary arteriogram is the most specific test for diagnosing the presence, location, and extent of coronary artery atherosclerosis. The procedure involves the injection of a radiopaque substance into each coronary artery followed by sequential x-ray pictures of up to 12 per second. Cineangiography may be used and involves the filming of the procedure from dye injection through the movement of the dye through the vessels. The x-ray picture usually is more detailed but the cinematography provides a dynamic picture. The procedure reveals (1) the location of lesions, (2) the degree of obstruction, (3) the status of the vessels distant to a point of obstruction, and (4) the presence of collateral circulation. The decision to perform coronary artery bypass surgery is usually made on the basis of the results of this test. The grades of stenosis commonly used are (1) normal, (2) less than 50 percent reduction, (3) 50 to 74 percent reduction, (4) 90 percent reduction, (5) greater than 90 percent reduction, and (6) total obstruction [7]. Because of differences in techniques, *cross-sectional reduction* (the measurements indicated above) is not equivalent to the *diameter method* of classification so that choice of the method to be used is crucial.

During the coronary arteriogram procedure, injection of contrast material into the left ventricle also can be performed. This permits visualization of left ventricular wall motion and chamber size. Pressure readings and oxygen saturations also give valuable information.

Unstable or Preinfarctional Angina

As atherosclerotic disease progresses in the coronary arteries, symptoms of pain may become more severe and occur with increasing frequency. An impending myocardial infarction is often forewarned by increasing severity of anginal attacks. The ECG often shows continual signs of ischemia and injury.

Myocardial Infarction (MI)

PATHOPHYSIOLOGY OF MI. Myocardial infarction, or ischemic necrosis of the myocardium, results from prolonged ischemia to the myocardium with irreversible cell damage and muscle death. The time between onset of ischemia and myocardial muscle death is approximately 15 to 20 minutes, although this varies with the individual and the vessel that is occluded. Myocardial infarction almost always occurs in the left ventricle and often significantly depresses left ventricular function. The larger the infarcted area the greater the loss of contractility. Functionally, myocardial infarction causes (1) reduced contractility with abnormal wall motion, (2) altered left ventricular compliance, (3) reduced stroke volume, (4) reduced ejection fraction, and (5) elevated left ventricular end-diastolic pressure (LVEDP).

The alterations in function depend not only on size but on the location of an infarct. An anterior left ventricular infarct often results from occlusion of the left anterior descending coronary artery. Posterior left ventricular infarcts often arise from right coronary artery obstruction, while lateral wall infarcts usually arise from circumflex artery obstruction (Table 19-1). This distribution varies because of individual variations in coronary artery supply. The infarct is also described in terms of where it occurs on the myocardial surface. Figure 19-3 shows the commonly used terms for different types of infarcts. The transmural infarct extends from endocardium to epicardium. The subendocardial type is found on the endocardial surface while the subepicardial is found on the epicardial surface. The intramural infarction is often seen in patchy areas of the myocardium and is usually associated with long-standing angina pectoris. The relative frequency of different types of myocardial infarctions according to arterial involvement has been documented as follows: left anterior descending 40 to 50 percent; right coronary artery 30 to 40 percent; and left circumflex artery 15 to 20 percent [14].

All myocardial infarctions have a central area of necrosis or infarction that is surrounded by an area of injury; the area of injury is surrounded by a ring of ischemia (Fig. 19-4). Each of these emits characteristic ECG patterns that help to localize and determine the extent of the infarct on the 12-lead recording.

When the myocardial muscle cells die they liberate the intramyocardial cellular enzymes. These enzymes can be utilized to date an infarct and partially to judge its severity. Because the affected myocardial muscle is dead, tissue regeneration is not seen after an infarction. Healing requires the

TABLE 19-1. Relationship between myocardial lesion and infarction produced

Coronary artery affected	Percent of cases	Areas of infarction
Left anterior descending	40–50	Anterior left ventricle Anterior interventricular septum
Right coronary artery	30–40	Posterior wall of left ventricle Posterior interventricular septum
Left circumflex	15–20	Lateral wall of left ventricle

Source: S. L. Robbins and R. Cotran, *Pathologic Basis of Disease* (2nd ed.). Philadelphia: Saunders, 1979. P. 655.

TABLE 19-2. Morphologic changes of transmural myocardial infarction

Time postinfarct	Morphologic appearance
0–6 hours	Usually inapparent
6–12 hours	Pallor of affected area
18–24 hours	Pale, gray brown appearance
2–4 days	Necrotic focus with hyperemic border Central portion is yellow brown and soft
4–10 days	Yellow gray to bright yellow (fatty change) Central necrotic area, often contains areas of hemorrhage Margins intensely red and highly vascularized
10–14 days	Progressive replacement of necrotic muscle by fibrous, vascularized scar tissue
Up to 6 weeks	Usually total replacement by scar tissue

Source: S. L. Robbins and R. Cotran, *Pathologic Basis of Disease* (2nd ed.). Philadelphia: Saunders, 1979.

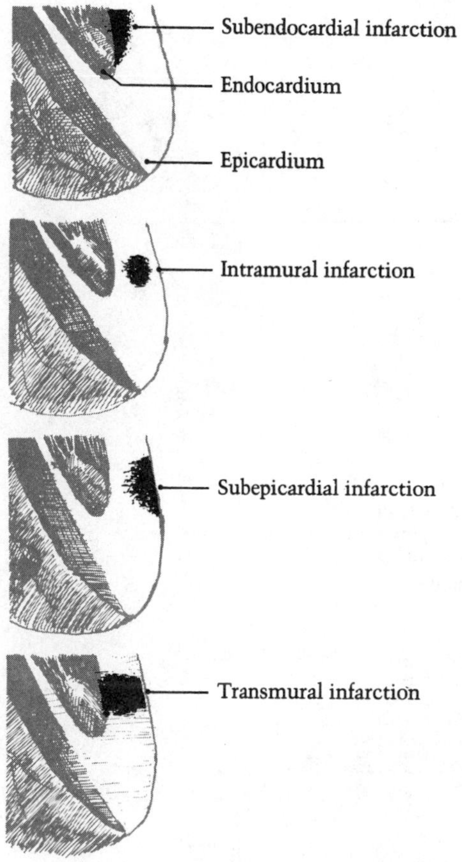

FIGURE 19-3. Location of various types of infarction in the ventricular wall. (From C. V. Kenner, C. E. Guzzetta, and B. M. Dossey, *Critical Care Nursing: Body-Mind-Spirit.* Boston: Little, Brown, 1981.)

formation of scar tissue that replaces the necrotic myocardial muscle. This involves a series of morphologic changes from no apparent cellular change in the first 6 hours to the total replacement by scar tissue. Table 19-2 outlines these changes.

Scar tissue may inhibit contractility. As contractility fails, the compensatory mechanisms described in Chapter 18 begin to be utilized in an attempt to maintain cardiac output. Arteriolar vascular constriction, heart rate increase, and renal retention of sodium and water all help to regulate the cardiac output. Ventricular dilatation is commonly seen. If a large amount of scar tissue is present contractility may be greatly compromised and congestive heart failure or cardiogenic shock may ensue.

The clinical manifestations of myocardial infarction depend on the severity of the infarct, the previous physical condition of the individual, and whether previous infarcts have occurred. The manifestations can range from sudden death, due to arrhythmias or ventricular rupture, to no symptoms whatsoever. Acute, substernal radiating chest pain is often described. Diaphoresis, dyspnea, nausea and vomiting, extreme anxiety, and any type of arrhythmia may be noted. Often the clinical manifestations reveal associated complications (see pp. 251–252).

DIAGNOSTIC TESTS. Laboratory studies are often very helpful in the diagnosis of acute myocardial infarction. The complete blood count (CBC) often reveals an elevated leukocyte count; the sedimentation rate and cardiac enzymes elevate because of cellular damage. The cardiac enzymes, normally present in myocardial muscle, are available in abnormally large amounts in the blood as a result of cellular death. These enzymes include creatinine phosphokinase (CPK), glutamic oxaloacetic transaminase (SGOT), and lactic dehydrogenase (LDH) (Fig. 19-5). Their values elevate and return to normal in a characteristic pattern after a myocardial infarction. Because the enzymes are found in other tissues, coexisting disease processes can produce misleading enzyme elevation measurements. Isoenzymes provide more specific accuracy. The isoenzyme CPK-MB is usually considered diagnostic of myocardial infarction especially in the presence of an in-

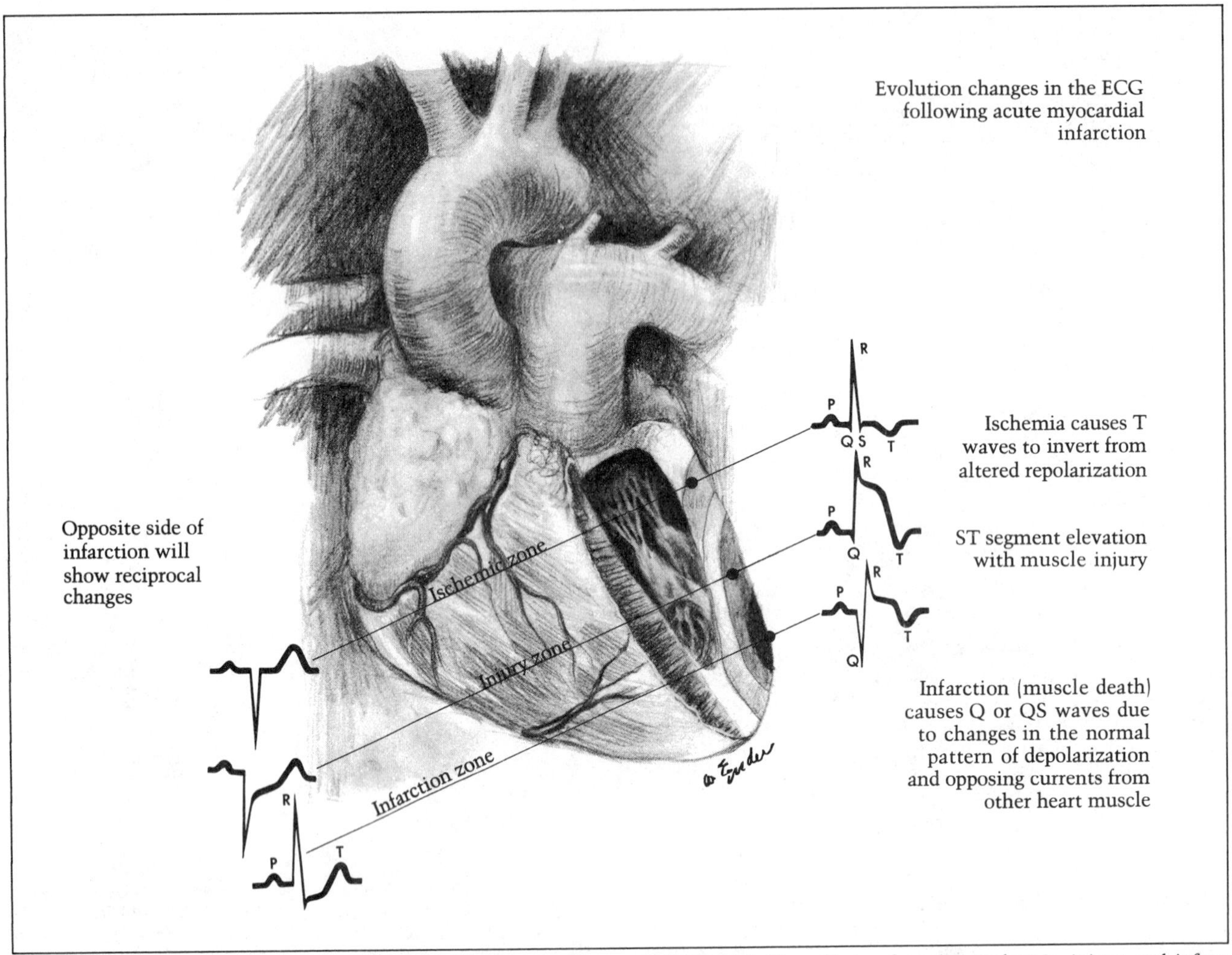

FIGURE 19-4. The effects of cardiac ischemia, injury, and infarction. (From C. V. Kenner, C. E. Guzzetta, and B. M. Dossey, *Critical Care Nursing: Body-Mind-Spirit.* Boston: Little, Brown, 1981.)

creased LDH_1. Table 19-3 lists the cardiac enzymes with their normal distribution in the body.

Electrocardiographic changes of acute myocardial infarction consist of pronounced Q waves and S–T elevation. These changes are reflected in the leads overlying the area of injury so that the location of the infarction can be generally determined by the ECG. Over time, the S–T segment and T wave changes return to normal, but the Q wave persists as evidence of an old infarction and can be used to localize the defect throughout life.

Bedside techniques to measure pulmonary artery pressures and cardiac output are invaluable in evaluating left ventricular function following myocardial infarction. The insertion of the Swan-Ganz catheter intravenously through the right heart into the pulmonary artery allows for continuous monitoring of pulmonary artery pressures that are a reflection of left ventricular function. The catheter also permits periodic calculations of cardiac output (see Chap. 18). A myocardial infarction that results in significant alteration of left ventricular contractility will result in an increased left ventricular end-diastolic pressure (LVEDP). This is reflected as an increased pulmonary artery pressure and a decrease in cardiac output.

MYOCARDIAL INFARCTION IMAGING. Technetium pyrophosphate myocardial imaging has proved to be a sensitive indicator of acute myocardial damage. Following infarction there is an efflux of calcium out of damaged cells. The technetium pyrophosphate will combine with the calcium and show up as a *hot spot.* Normally the technetium is not visualized in the myocardium when images are taken after intravenous injection. This procedure is most beneficial in determining the presence of myocardial infarction in the acute situation but its usefulness is limited to specific instances [18]. Multigated blood pool scan is another procedure that utilizes the injection of pyrophosphate, which has an affinity for red blood cells. Twenty minutes after the injection of the pyrophosphate, technetium is injected and it then attaches to the pyrophosphate-tagged red blood

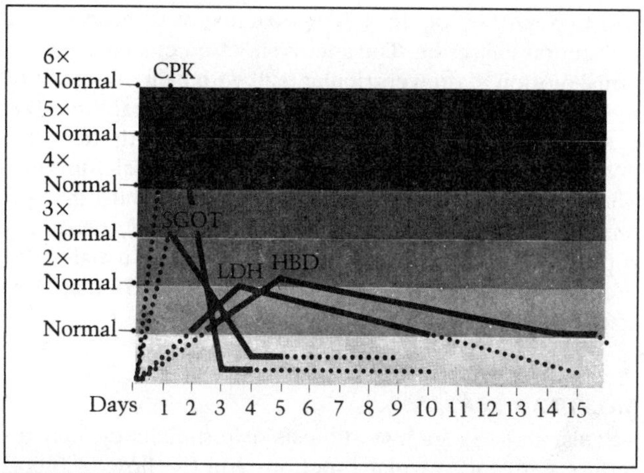

FIGURE 19-5. Time sequence of serum-enzyme elevations in acute myocardial infarction. (From C. V. Kenner, C. E. Guzzetta, and B. M. Dossey, *Critical Care Nursing: Body-Mind-Spirit.* Boston: Little, Brown, 1981.)

cells. The pooling or accumulation of the blood in the heart allows for visualization of technetium by special nuclear cameras. The computerized camera allows multiple images to be taken during the cardiac cycle. The computer then can calculate multiple measurements that include the end-diastolic volume, end-systolic volume, ejection fraction, and stroke volume. This procedure is of particular benefit in evaluating the effects of the infarction on myocardial function. With this test, myocardial function can be monitored noninvasively in a variety of situations.

COMPLICATIONS OF MYOCARDIAL INFARCTION. *Dysrhythmias.* The most common complication of acute myocardial infarction is a disturbance in cardiac rhythm. Ninety percent of affected individuals have some disturbance in rhythm. Myocardial infarction itself produces multiple predisposing factors to account for this high incidence including: (1) tissue ischemia, (2) hypoxemia, (3) sympathetic and parasympathetic nervous system influences, (4) lactic acidosis, (5) hemodynamic abnormalities, (6) drug toxicity, and (7) electrolyte imbalance. The two basic mechanisms for cardiac rhythm abnormalities include abnormal *automaticity* and abnormal *conduction* or both of these together. The most common arrhythmias associated with myocardial infarction are listed in Table 19-4. Dysrhythmias may cause a decline in cardiac output, increased cardiac irritability, and further compromise of myocardial perfusion. The most common cause of death outside of the hospital in individuals with MI is probably ventricular fibrillation.

Congestive heart failure and cardiogenic shock. Congestive heart failure is a state of circulatory congestion produced by myocardial dysfunction. Myocardial infarction compromises myocardial function by reducing contractility and producing abnormal wall motion. As the ability of the ventricle to empty becomes less effective, stroke volume falls and residual volume increases. The fall in stroke volume elicits compensatory mechanisms to maintain the cardiac output (see Chap. 18).

Cardiogenic shock results from profound left ventricular failure, usually from a massive myocardial infarction. This pump failure shock follows myocardial infarction in 10 to 15 percent of cases and the mortality is approximately 80 to 95 percent [3].

Thromboembolism. Mural thrombi are common in postmortem examinations of individuals who die of myocardial infarction. In a study of 924 fatalities due to acute MI,

TABLE 19-3. Serum enzyme changes in myocardial infarction

Enzyme	Elevates	Peaks	Period of elevation	Site of formation
CPK (creatinine phosphokinase)	4–8 hours	12–36 hours	72 hours	
Isoenzymes				
CPK I (BB)	0	0	0	Produced mostly by brain
CPK II (MB)	4–8 hours	12–36 hours	72 hours	Produced mostly by heart
CPK III (MM)	0	0	0	Produced mostly by skeletal muscle
SGOT (serum glutamic oxalacetic transaminase); also called asparate aminotransferase (AST)	6–12 hours	36–48 hours	4–6 days	Found mostly in heart, liver, and muscle tissue
LDH (lactic dehydrogenase)	12–24 hours	24–96 hours	8–14 days	Found in heart, liver, muscles, and erythrocytes
Isoenzymes				
LDH1	12–24 hours	24–96 hours	8–14 days	Produced mostly by heart and erythrocytes
LDH2	0	0	0	Produced mostly by RES
LDH3	0	0	0	Produced mostly by lungs and tissues
LDH4	0	0	0	Produced by placenta, kidney, and pancreas
LDH5	0	0	0	Produced by liver and skeletal muscle

TABLE 19-4. Common dysrhythmias after myocardial infarction

Ventricular	
	Premature ventricular contractions (PVCs)
	Ventricular tachycardia
	Ventricular fibrillation
Atrial	
	Premature atrial contractions
	Atrial flutter
	Atrial fibrillation
Conduction defects	
	Bundle branch blocks, either right or left
	Second-degree heart block
	Third-degree or complete heart block
Sinus	
	Sinus tachycardia
	Sinus bradycardia
	Sinus arrythmia

44 percent were found to have mural thrombi attached to the endocardium [14]. These thrombi are usually associated with large infarcts and therefore probably occur more frequently in nonsurvivors than survivors. Mural thrombi adhere to the endocardium overlying an infarcted area. Fragments, however, can produce systemic arterial embolization. Autopsy studies reveal that 10 percent of individuals who die of myocardial infarction also have arterial emboli to the brain, kidney, spleen, or mesentery.

Almost all pulmonary emboli originate in the veins of the lower extremities. Bed rest and heart failure predispose to venous thrombosis and pulmonary embolism. Both of these occur in individuals with acute myocardial infarction. When prolonged bed rest was standard therapy for all cases of MI, the incidence rate of pulmonary embolus was 20 percent. With early mobilization and widespread use of prophylactic anticoagulation therapy, pulmonary embolus has become a rare cause of death as a complication of MI.

Pericarditis. This syndrome associated with MI was first described by Dressler and is often called Dressler's syndrome. It usually follows a transmural infarction but may follow subepicardial infarction. The incidence is very common, affecting 50 percent of individuals after transmural infarction. The pericarditis is usually transient, appearing in the first week after infarction. A pericardial friction rub is common but often the syndrome is not recognized. The symptoms of chest pain and low-grade fever may be confused with extension of the myocardial infarct.

Myocardial rupture. Rupture of the free wall of the left ventricle accounts for 10 to 15 percent of deaths in the hospital due to acute myocardial infarction [10]. This causes an immediate cardiac tamponade and death. Rupture of the interventricular septum is less common, occurs with extensive myocardial damage, and produces a ventricular septal defect.

Ventricular aneurysm. This event is a late complication of myocardial infarction that involves thinning, ballooning, and hypokinesis of the left ventricular wall following a transmural infarction. The aneurysm often creates a paroxysmal motion of the ventricular wall with ballooning out of the aneurysmal segment on ventricular contraction. The dysfunctional area often becomes filled with necrotic debris and clot and sometimes is rimmed by a calcium ring. The debris or clot may fragment and be sent into the systemic arterial circulation. Occasionally these aneurysms rupture causing tamponade and death, but usually the problems that result are due to declining ventricular contractility or embolization.

VALVULAR DISEASE

Valvular disease, such as stenosis or insufficiency, may interfere with the valvular functions and the flow of blood through the heart. In valvular stenosis there is a narrowing of the valve orifice (opening), and the valve leaflets (cusps) become fused together in such a way that the valve cannot open freely. This narrowing of the opening causes obstruction of blood flow and, as a result, the chamber behind the affected valve must build up more pressure to overcome resistance. The muscle fibers in that chamber must thicken in order to do more work to push the blood through the narrowed opening [11]. Over a period of time, the muscle hypertrophies in response to the added work load. With valvular insufficiency (regurgitation), the valve cannot close completely. The incomplete closure results from scarring and retraction of the valve leaflets. As a result, blood is permitted to flow backward (retrograde) through the opening. The heart chamber, which receives the additional retrograde flow, is then forced to pump the added regurgitant volume along with the volume being received. As a response to the increased volume present in the chamber behind the regurgitant valve, the muscle fibers lengthen or stretch. This dilatation of the muscle fiber increases the surface area in order to accommodate the additional volume. Both hypertrophy and dilatation are referred to as compensatory mechanisms that occur in the presence of specific valvular defects.

When stenosis and regurgitation occur simultaneously, the defect is called a mixed lesion, and usually occurs in advanced disease. In the clinical setting, the classification of the lesions is in terms of the predominant mechanical load that is placed on the heart. This then leads to the classification of valvular defects as predominant or "pure" stenosis, regurgitation, or mixed stenosis and regurgitation. In addition to having a mixed lesion on one valve, there may also be disease on another valve at the same time. This is known as combined valvular disease, which may present a rather complex clinical picture depending on the number of valves involved and the types of lesions [16].

Diagnostic Tests

CHEST X RAY. The chest x ray (roentgenogram) is utilized in the recognition of abnormalities in cardiac size and in cardiac failure as a result of certain valvular lesions. The car-

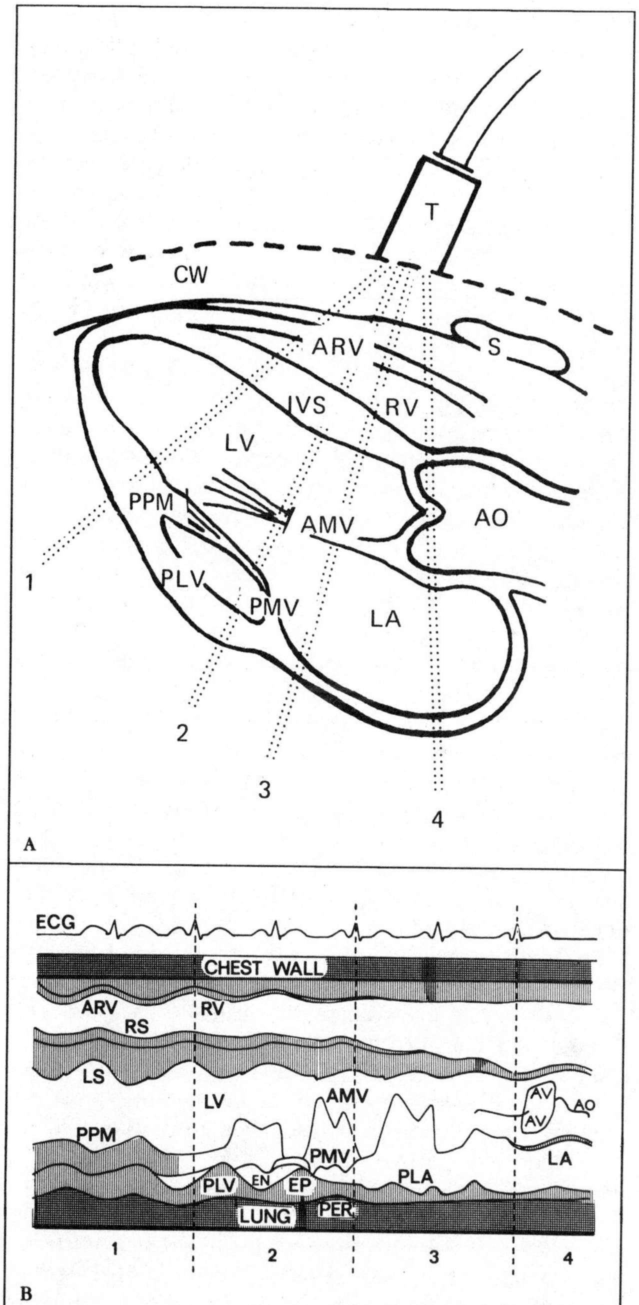

FIGURE 19-6. A. Schematic representation of the course of the ultrasonic beam to achieve the echo represented in B. CW = chest wall; T = transducer; S = sternum; ARV = anterior right ventricular wall; RV = right ventricle; IVS = interventricular septum; LV = left ventricle; PPM = posterior papillary muscle; AMV = anterior mitral valve leaflet; AO = aorta; PLV = posterior left ventricular wall; PMV = posterior mitral valve leaflet; LA = left atrium. B. Schematic representation of an echocardiogram from the four transducer positions. RS = right side of interventricular septum; LS = left side of interventricular septum; EN = endocardium; EP = epicardium; PER = pericardium; PLA = posterior left atrial wall; AV = aortic valve cusps. (From H. Feigenbaum, Clinical application of echocardiography. *Prog. Cardiovasc. Dis.* 14:531, 1972. Reprinted with permission.)

diac silhouette enlarges, for instance, in the presence of aortic regurgitation (insufficiency) because of the dilatation of the chamber and hypertrophy of the muscle. Cardiac failure as a sequela of mitral stenosis can be seen on the chest x ray as accumulation of fluid in the interlobular spaces of the lung, the result of blood damming back into the pulmonary area.

ELECTROCARDIOGRAM. The electrocardiogram, which records the electrical current produced by the excitable cells of the myocardium, is useful in diagnosing atrial, ventricular, or biventricular hypertrophy related to valvular disease. Chamber hypertrophy usually causes an increase in amplitude of the QRS complex, and characteristic S–T and T wave changes.

The electrocardiogram can also be affected in the presence of acute pericarditis. S–T segments may be elevated or depressed in many leads; T wave inversion may or may not accompany these changes. In addition, if pericardial effusion is present, there may be low voltage in both the QRS complex and T wave in all leads.

ECHOCARDIOGRAPHY. Echocardiography uses sound waves to identify intracardiac structures using the principle of sonic reflection [6]. When a sound wave passes through a medium such as blood, it is reflected backward or echoed when it comes in contact with a medium of different density or elasticity such as the muscle of the heart. Intracardiac structures have different densities, which are referred to as interfaces. In echocardiography, an ultrasound wave (beam) is transmitted from the transducer to the cardiac interfaces, and these waves are reflected back to the transducer as an echo. The sonic energy is then transformed into electrical energy that can be displayed in graphic form (Fig. 19-6). The recording depends on the transducer's angle and on the intracardiac structures that lie within the beam's pathway [6].

Used as a noninvasive tool at the bedside, echocardiography is employed to assess valvular motion and pumping action of the heart, and to measure cardiac chamber size [4]. Because it assesses valvular motion, the echocardiogram can be used to diagnose such valvular abnormalities as stenosis, regurgitation, mitral valve prolapse, and ruptured chordae tendineae. Fluid inside the pericardial membrane (pericardial effusion) can also be detected. In addition, echocardiography is useful in the assessment of abnormal thickening of the ventricular walls and septum or abnormal dilatation of the cardiac chambers.

CARDIAC CATHETERIZATION. Cardiac catheterization is an invasive diagnostic procedure that can yield important information regarding the chambers of the heart. A catheter is passed either to the right or left side of the heart; pressure and oxygen are recorded throughout the process. In left heart catheterization, assessment of left ventricular and aortic function is made along with assessment of the mitral and aortic valves. In right heart catheterization, assessment of right atrial and ventricular function is made along with assessment of the tricuspid and pulmonic valves. In right heart catheterization, the catheter is normally inserted into the antecubital or saphenous vein and guided sequentially into the right atrium, the right ventricle, the pulmonary artery, and the pulmonary arterial wedge position. With left heart catheterization, the catheter is inserted into the femoral artery or the brachial artery and is advanced retrograde through the aorta into the left ventricle. Another method of insertion is the transseptal approach. This is accomplished by inserting a long, curved needle through a catheter positioned in the right atrium in order to puncture the intact interatrial septum. This approach may be employed when mitral disease is suspected [15].

Once a catheter is in place in either the left or right heart, the chambers may be visualized by injecting a radiopaque substance (dye) through the catheter into the specific chamber under investigation. This is known as cardiac angiography. During the injection of the dye, abnormalities in valvular motion such as stenosis or regurgitation may be detected.

Cardiac catheterization is also useful in determining pressure differences between chambers as in valvular stenosis in which a pressure gradient may be present. This procedure helps to assess the severity of the disease process and to determine whether surgical intervention is necessary. Quantitative measurements of volumes, pressures, ejection fraction, and cardiac output are recorded during cardiac catheterization.

Because of its invasive nature, the procedure has inherent risks to the individual. Right heart catheterization is rarely associated with morbidity or mortality; however, left heart catheterization can produce serious complications [15]. These complications include cardiac perforation, major arrhythmias, hypotension, hemorrhage, vascular thrombosis, acute myocardial infarction, and cerebral embolism as well as death.

Acute Rheumatic Fever: A Major Cause of Valvular Disease

Rheumatic fever is a delayed inflammatory disease that occurs in *susceptible* persons following untreated pharyngeal infection with the group A beta-hemolytic streptococcus. It appears to be an individual "immune" reaction to the streptococcal organism. Rheumatic fever causes inflammation of the joints, heart, skin, and nervous system [17]. The attack rate of rheumatic fever is 1 to 3 percent in the individual with untreated streptococcal sore throat. Effective treatment with penicillin virtually eliminates the disease. The most common age of onset is 5 to 15 years of age, and incidence is greater in crowded, substandard living conditions. Recurrent attacks of rheumatic fever are common in susceptible, untreated individuals with a greater risk of valvular disease with each recurrence.

PATHOPHYSIOLOGY. The joints are affected with an exudative, synovitis with associated subcutaneous nodules. A characteristic acute carditis is noted with the diagnostic lesion, the *Aschoff body,* being found in the myocardium. *Verrucae,* which are small warty vegetations produced by fibrin or ground substance, appear on the valve leaflets. These apparently cause inflammation and exudation causing interadherence of the leaflets (Fig. 19-7). These also may line up on the chordae tendineae producing scarring and shortening of these structures over a long period of time. During the acute phase the valves and endocardial surface are inflamed and edematous. The nervous system involvement is manifested by chorea, which is rapid, jerky involuntary movements of the arms and legs [14]. No diagnostic CNS lesion has been found to explain this manifestation. Erythema marginatum may be noted and is described as a pink, erythematous rash on the trunk and extremities. It often appears in concentric circles that fade and enlarge in minutes to hours. Rheumatic arteritis, pneumonitis, and pleuritis are other relatively rare manifestations of the disease.

CLINICAL MANIFESTATIONS. The onset of the disease may be acute or subacute. The acute form causes migratory polyarthritis, which refers to joint inflammation that moves from joint to joint. Fever is characteristic. A tachycardia out of proportion to the level of the fever may be associated with mitral or aortic murmurs, cardiac enlargement, and congestive heart failure. Chorea is uncommon and may begin up to 3 months after the streptococcal infection. It is characterized by aimless, irregular movements, and emotional instability [17].

Chronic rheumatic carditis may occur and run a fatal course over a few months. Fortunately, this manifestation is rare and cardiac involvement is subsequently expressed through valvular defects, often years after the initial disease.

Laboratory tests are not diagnostic but the antistreptolysin O titer (ASO) is increased after streptococcal infection. The erythrocyte sedimentation rate (ESR) is increased indicating an inflammatory process. Most cases of rheumatic fever abate within 12 weeks. The onset in later years of valvular dysfunction is hard to predict but treatment of later streptococcal infections, thus preventing rheumatic fever, has led to few reported cases of valvular stenosis or regurgitation in the United States. A significant number of cases still are reported from the Middle East, Southeast Asia, and Third World countries.

Mitral Stenosis

Stenosis of the mitral valve causes impairment of blood flow from the left atrium to the left ventricle (Fig. 19-8). The impairment of blood flow is due to an abnormality in the structure of the valve leaflets that prevents the valve from opening completely in diastole. The most common

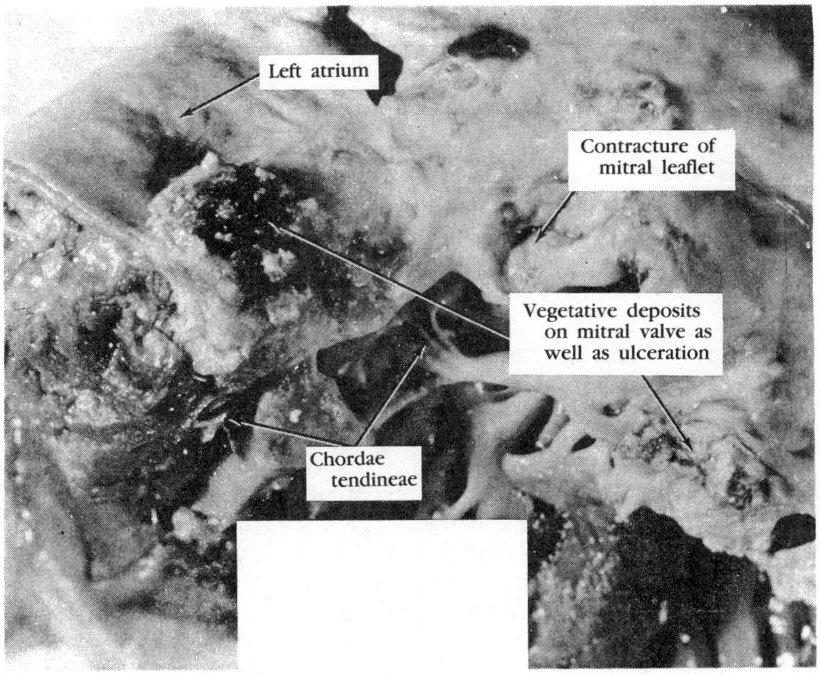

FIGURE 19-7. Mitral valve viewed from above showing vegetative deposits, ulceration of valve leaflets, and fusion of commissures. (From J. Kernicki et al., *Cardiovascular Nursing.* New York: Putnam, 1971.)

cause of mitral stenosis is rheumatic endocarditis. In pure mitral stenosis (without regurgitation), about one-half of patients will describe a history of known rheumatic fever. Mitral stenosis is more common in women than in men [13].

PATHOPHYSIOLOGY AND COMPENSATORY MECHANISMS. The basic alteration in mitral stenosis is the decrease in blood flow from the left atrium to the left ventricle. As a result of the rheumatic process, the commissures (junctional areas between the leaflets) become fibrous and fused, the chordae become shortened, and the valve becomes funnel-shaped in appearance. As the valve becomes more stenotic, the leaflets thicken with scar tissue and become calcified at the valve ring and at the leaflet margins. There are rarely any symptoms until the mitral valve orifice decreases in size from the normal 4 to 6 cm to 1.5 to 2.5 cm [13]. As the orifice further decreases in size, pulmonary symptoms appear. Mitral valve orifice (opening) size correlates relatively well with symptoms. Since the orifice size usually decreases very gradually over a period of years, symptoms are often first noted in the fourth or fifth decade of life.

In the normal heart, there is no functional pressure gradient between the left atrium and left ventricle in diastole. A pressure gradient is the difference in pressures in two chambers when the valve dividing them is open. In mitral stenosis, the gradient is determined by the size of the mitral valve orifice and the flow across the valve. The flow is determined by the duration of diastole (during which filling occurs), and by the cardiac output [13]. The stenotic mitral valve does not permit increases in blood flow and so left atrial pressure must increase to discharge its contents into the left ventricle. Because of the constant increase in left atrial volume and pressure, the left atrium dilates and hypertrophies. As the atrial size increases the risk for developing various atrial arrhythmias also increases. Atrial fibrillation commonly develops, further compromising the blood flow to the ventricle because of the ineffective atrial contraction. Constant increased pressure and volume in the left atrium cause an increase in pressure in the pulmonary veins and capillary bed. If the pressure in the pulmonary capillaries becomes greater than the plasma oncotic pressure, transudation of fluid into the interstitial spaces and eventually the alveoli occurs.

The chronic elevation of left atrial pressure causes the onset of the pulmonary hypertension. The pulmonary hypertension results from chronic elevation of pulmonary capillary pressure. This excessive pulmonary pressure can rise to nearly systemic values, causing an increased pressure load against which the right ventricle must pump. Chronic pulmonary edema (congestion) in the interstitial spaces occurs and right ventricular failure is the end result of the process. The classic manifestations of mitral stenosis include pulmonary congestion and all the signs of right heart failure [13].

CLINICAL MANIFESTATIONS. Dyspnea as a result of the pulmonary congestion is the most common symptom. Dyspnea is increased by any condition that increases the heart rate, such as exercise, stress, fever, or atrial fibrillation with a rapid ventricular response. Paroxysmal nocturnal dyspnea

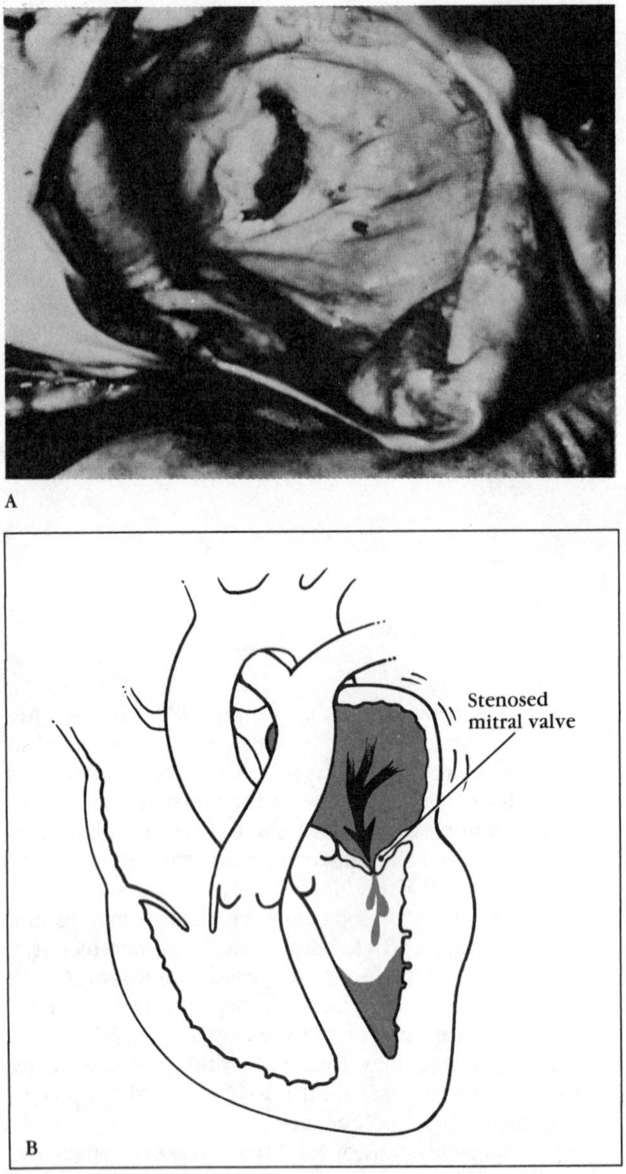

FIGURE 19-8. A. Stenotic mitral valve as seen from the left atrium. (From J. E. Dalen and J. S. Alpert, *Valvular Heart Disease.* Boston: Little, Brown, 1981). B. Mitral stenosis as viewed during atrial contraction.

may be reported by persons with some degree of right heart failure. Fatigue is also common and is related both to the pulmonary hypertension and right ventricular failure. Hemoptysis may be seen as a result of frank pulmonary hemorrhage from a ruptured pulmonary vein, as frothy-pink, blood-tinged sputum of pulmonary edema, or as a result of pulmonary infarction [16]. Palpitations may be reported, especially in the presence of atrial fibrillation. Palpation of the precordium may reveal a parasternal lift with the development of right ventricular hypertrophy [13].

Auscultation reveals (1) a loud first heart sound, (2) an opening snap, and (3) a diastolic rumble (Fig. 19-9). The loud first heart sound is due to the closure of the mitral valve apparatus when it remains deep in the left ventricle at the time of contraction. The changes in leaflet mobility also contribute to the production of the loud first heart sound [13]. The opening snap heard on auscultation is thought to result from the sudden cessation of the opening of the valve leaflets. It also may be due to calcification of the valve leaflets.

The diastolic rumble of mitral stenosis is a loud, long, rumbling murmur that begins just after the opening snap and has a decrescendo pattern. It results from the movement of the valve leaflets toward the closed position in mid-diastole despite the continuing blood flow across the mitral valve produced by the pressure gradient [13].

DIAGNOSTIC TESTS. The appearance of the cardiac silhouette in mitral stenosis on the chest x ray is characteristic. In the posteroanterior (PA) view the left heart border is straightened, the pulmonary artery is enlarged, and there is a double density due to left atrial enlargement. In the lateral view the enlarged left atrium and right ventricle are seen.

The electrocardiogram characteristically shows a broad, notched P wave in lead II, called *P mitrale.* This probably reflects the atrial enlargement. As many as 40 percent of patients with mitral stenosis develop atrial fibrillation [13]. As pulmonary hypertension develops, right ventricular hypertrophy may be noted.

Loss of posterior leaflet movement, left atrial enlargement, changes suggestive of pulmonary hypertension, and right ventricular enlargement may be seen on the echocardiogram. If mitral stenosis is complicated by the presence of mitral valve incompetence, left ventricular enlargement is also noted on the echocardiogram [13].

Direct measurements of a gradient across the mitral valve cannot be made by conventional means but can be assessed by simultaneous measurement of the pulmonary artery wedge pressure and left ventricular diastolic pressure. Correlation of the pressure gradient with the cardiac output, heart rate, and diastolic filling time provides the examiner with data to calculate the mitral valve area [16].

COURSE AND COMPLICATIONS. The uninterrupted course of mitral stenosis is long and progressively downhill. Atrial fibrillation adds an additional burden to the already compromised hemodynamics. Systemic emboli complicate the course of mitral stenosis and relate to onset of atrial fibrillation. Pulmonary hypertension is associated with permanent vascular changes. The development of right heart failure from the pulmonary hypertension complicates the clinical course of the disease. Fatigue is a major complaint and is often associated with peripheral edema, ascites, liver enlargement, and an enlarged right ventricle.

Mitral Regurgitation or Insufficiency

Mitral regurgitation is described as the backflow of blood from the left ventricle across the mitral valve to the left

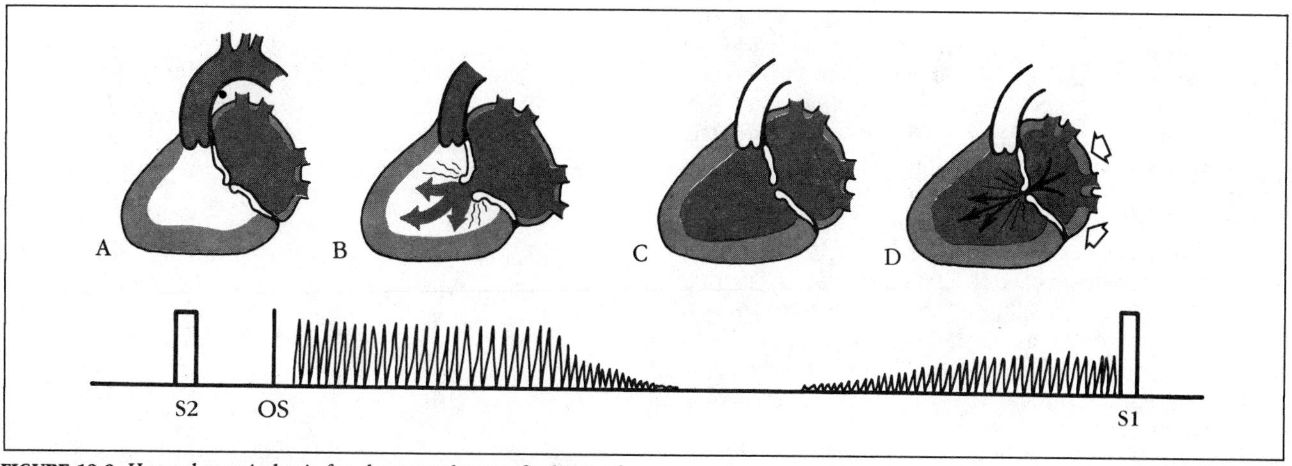

FIGURE 19-9. Hemodynamic basis for the auscultatory findings of mitral stenosis. A. Aortic valve closes; second heart sound (*S2*) is generated. B. Mitral valve opens and opening snap (*OS*) occurs; early diastolic component is generated. C. Flow from left atrium to left ventricle diminishes, and murmur decreases in mid-diastole. D. Atrial systole increases flow across mitral valve, resulting in presystolic increase in intensity of murmur. Ventricular systole then causes closure of thickened mitral valve, resulting in loud first heart sound (*S1*). (From R. Judge, G. Zuidema, and F. Fitzgerald, *Clinical Diagnosis.* Boston: Little, Brown, 1982.)

atrium during ventricular systole. Regurgitation occurs when the mitral valve fails to close completely. The most common cause of mitral regurgitation is rheumatic endocarditis.

PATHOPHYSIOLOGY AND COMPENSATORY MECHANISMS. The same basic processes that lead to mitral stenosis contribute to the production of mitral regurgitation. When the changes on the valve leaflets and chordae cause the leaflets to stay in a closed position stenosis results. When the changes cause the valve to stay in the open position regurgitation results. The scarring and retraction of the mitral leaflets extend from one leaflet to another, crossing one or more commissures.

In mitral regurgitation the cardiac output is divided into regurgitant and systemic flow (Fig. 19-10). The amount of regurgitant flow is determined by the degree of mitral valve incompetence and the resistance to flow through the aortic valve. The regurgitant flow increases proportionately to the mitral valve orifice size. Any factor that increases resistance at the aortic valve, such as aortic stenosis, will decrease the systemic flow and increase the regurgitant flow.

The left ventricle responds to the increased volume from the left atrium with dilatation and hypertrophy so that sufficient systemic cardiac output is maintained [13]. The regurgitant volume entering the left atrium gradually increases and the left atrium gradually dilates, sometimes to aneurysmal size to accommodate the increased volume. As a result of left atrial enlargement, there is stretching of the valve anulus with displacement of the posterior leaflet of the mitral valve, which leads to further mitral regurgitation. As mitral regurgitation progresses, there is a decrease in contractility of the left ventricle leading to a decrease in systemic flow and the onset of left ventricular failure.

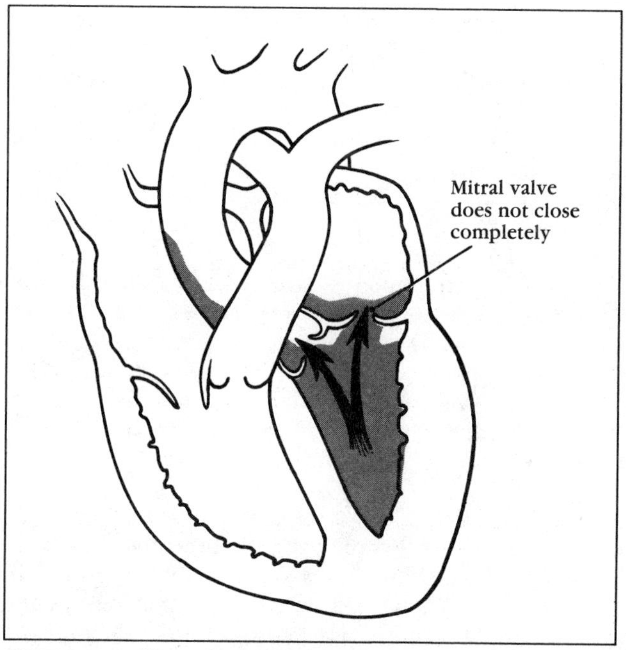

FIGURE 19-10. View of mitral insufficiency during systole.

CLINICAL MANIFESTATIONS. Many people who have mitral regurgitation have no symptoms for several years. However, when symptoms appear, dyspnea and fatigue are common presenting symptoms. These symptoms are due to a decreased cardiac output and increased pulmonary venous pressure. Other common symptoms include orthopnea, paroxysmal nocturnal dyspnea, and palpitations.

The person with mitral regurgitation can better tolerate the onset of atrial fibrillation than one with mitral stenosis. Atrial fibrillation occurs in about 75 percent of persons with mitral regurgitation.

The general appearance of the person is normal but there may be signs of congestive heart failure if the disease is long-standing. In chronic mitral regurgitation the apex impulse is often displaced laterally and is larger than normal. This finding is related to left ventricular dilatation. The systolic murmur characteristic of mitral regurgitation is almost always present [13]. The murmur is loud, high-pitched, holosystolic (of constant intensity throughout systole), and is heard best at the apex (Fig. 19-11). Radiation of the murmur to the axilla or back may be noted. The first heart sound is usually diminished in mitral regurgitation. A third heart sound that is associated with the rapid phase of ventricular filling may also be present. If present, the third heart sound indicates some degree of cardiac decompensation.

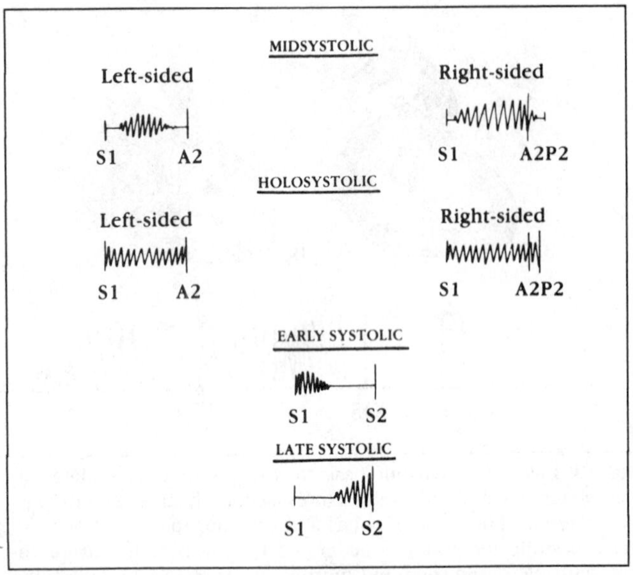

FIGURE 19-11. All possible shapes of mitral regurgitation murmurs.

DIAGNOSTIC TESTS. Left atrial and ventricular enlargement are frequent findings on the chest x ray in patients who have mitral regurgitation. As in mitral stenosis, there may be a greatly enlarged left atrium. Pulmonary venous changes on the chest x ray may be present but the occurrence of these is less frequent than in mitral stenosis [13].

The usual findings of chronic mitral regurgitation on the electrocardiogram are atrial and ventricular hypertrophy. Atrial fibrillation is common. Right ventricular hypertrophy, however, is less common in mitral regurgitation than in mitral stenosis [13].

Cardiac catheterization provides data to describe the amount of mitral regurgitation and the pumping ability of the left ventricle. The amount of mitral regurgitation can be quantitatively measured during the catheterization. The ejection fraction is measured and is useful in determining the pumping ability of the left ventricle. Cardiac output is usually decreased in symptomatic individuals.

COURSE AND COMPLICATIONS. The course of mitral regurgitation is long and slowly progressive, but the point at which left ventricular contractility is significantly compromised correlates with the time of development of pulmonary congestion [13]. Atrial fibrillation causes a further decrease in the cardiac output.

Mixed Mitral Stenosis and Regurgitation

A mitral valve that has both fused commissures and structures that fail to close properly exhibits a mixture of mitral stenosis and regurgitation. The course of these mixed lesions depends on which of the processes is predominant. If there is a greater degree of stenosis than incompetence, there is a smaller amount of backflow of blood across the mitral valve during systole and a smaller amount of forward flow of blood across the valve in diastole. If there is greater incompetence then stenosis, there is more backflow of blood across the valve in systole, and more forward flow of blood across the valve in diastole [16].

Dyspnea is the most common symptom and may be of acute onset when atrial fibrillation ensues. Palpitations are also common and are frequently found to be related to rapid atrial arrhythmias. The heart is usually enlarged. The first heart sound may be loud and there may be an opening snap. Often, a third heart sound will be present in addition to, or instead of, the opening snap. The characteristic pansystolic murmur of mitral regurgitation and the diastolic murmurs of mitral stenosis are usually present [16]. Pulmonary congestion in mixed stenosis and regurgitation may lead to pulmonary edema, especially with the onset of atrial fibrillation.

DIAGNOSTIC TESTS. Diagnostic procedures as with mitral stenosis and insufficiency are helpful in determining the extent of decompensation from the valvular lesions. The course and complications depend on the extent of the lesions.

Mitral Valve Prolapse

Mitral valve prolapse is a common condition that is due to a posterior displacement of the posterior cusp of the mitral valve. This condition is probably a congenital abnormality of the valve tissues in which the large posterior leaflet bulges back into the left atrium during systole [16]. As the ballooning of the leaflet into the left atrium continues, the chordae and papillary muscles become stressed. Contraction of the papillary muscles decreases and mitral regurgitation occurs. The amount of this regurgitation is usually hemodynamically insignificant but may produce symptoms. More frequently, the symptoms produced are the result of an atrial arrhythmia.

Most persons with mitral valve prolapse are completely free of symptoms. For this reason it is commonly diagnosed during a routine physical examination. A nonanginal type of chest pain may be present along with palpitations, fatigue, and dyspnea.

Mitral valve prolapse is most commonly diagnosed in women in the second to fourth decade of life [13]. There may be a familial tendency toward development of the condition. Auscultation at the apex reveals a late systolic murmur that is crescendo in nature, loud and musical. The murmur may be preceded by one or more clicks in systole.

Mitral valve prolapse is associated with extracardiac defects including bony abnormalities such as scoliosis, pectus excavatum, pectus carinatum, and kyphosis.

Diagnostic procedures reveal a normal cardiac shadow on x ray. The electrocardiogram often reveals multiple arrhythmias, especially sinus arrhythmias, atrial fibrillation, premature ventricular contractions, and ventricular tachycardia. Other ECG changes include S-T–T wave abnormalities and prolongation of the Q–T interval. The echocardiogram is useful in diagnosis and helps to determine the presence and amount of insufficiency.

Complications are rare but may include bacterial endocarditis or acute mitral insufficiency from chordae rupture or stretching.

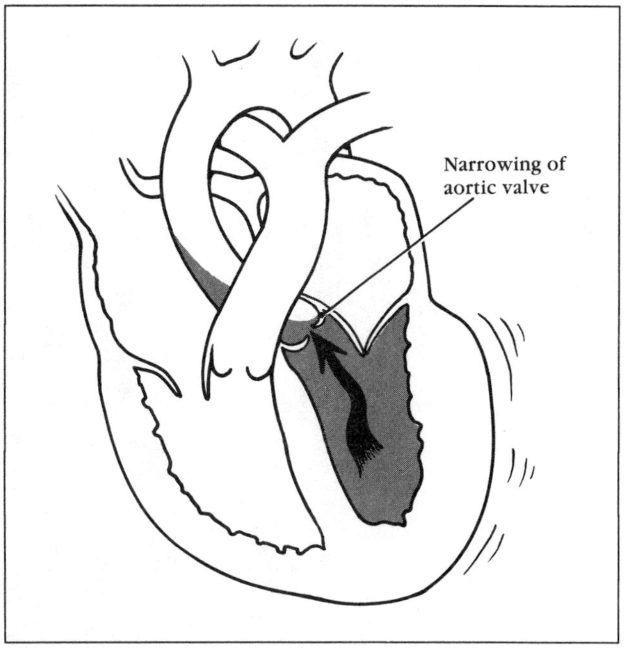

FIGURE 19-12. View of aortic stenosis during systole.

Aortic Stenosis

There are several causes of aortic stenosis. Among these are rheumatic fever, congenital aortic stenosis with a bicuspid or a unicuspid valve, degenerative calcific disease found in the elderly, and idiopathic hypertrophic subaortic stenosis [13]. The most frequent cause for those under 30 years of age is a congenital stenotic aortic valve. Between 30 and 70 years of age, rheumatic heart disease is the usual underlying cause but in individuals over 70 years of age, the degenerative calcific type is predominant.

PATHOPHYSIOLOGY AND COMPENSATORY MECHANISMS. Significant narrowing of the valve orifice leads to a decrease in blood flow from the left ventricle to the aorta. The obstruction of outflow from the left ventricle leads also to a strain or pressure load on the left ventricle that occurs as the left ventricle tries to push blood through the narrowed opening (Fig. 19-12). This resistance to ejection is reflected by an increase in pressure in the left ventricle to force more blood through the stenotic valve during systole. A systolic pressure gradient develops between the left ventricle and aorta and is called an *aortic valve gradient.* These hemodynamic consequences will not be manifested until the valve orifice, which is normally 2.6 to 3.5 sq cm, has narrowed to approximately one-third of normal. The left ventricle is capable of compensating for increasing pressure demands through hypertrophy for a long period of time (Fig. 19-13). This mechanism allows for increasing systolic pressures to maintain an adequate systemic blood pressure. The increased muscle mass requires increased oxygen supply that may or may not be supplied by the coronary arteries. If the stenosis becomes increasingly severe, the persistent pressure overload (strain) leads to myocardial failure.

CLINICAL MANIFESTATIONS. The classic clinical manifestations that accompany severe aortic stenosis are chest pain, syncope, and heart failure. The chest pain and syncope are related to the reduction in cardiac output, increased perfusion needs, and decreased perfusion of the coronary arteries and brain. Congestive heart failure results from chronic strain on the left ventricle.

The chest pain is usually manifested after physical exertion as a result of the inability of the heart to increase coronary blood flow during exercise [16]. This type of angina can occur in up to 70 percent of those with severe aortic stenosis [13].

Syncopal episodes, "grey outs" or periods of confusion associated with severe aortic stenosis, are dangerous signs. Without surgical intervention, the prognosis is poor.

The chronic strain imposed on the left ventricle eventually leads to heart failure and may terminate in pulmonary edema. Left ventricular failure is the cause of death in over one-half of those who have severe stenosis.

Auscultation may reveal a paradoxical splitting of the second heart sound, which results when the aortic valve closes after the pulmonic valve. In addition, a diamond-shaped (crescendo-decrescendo) systolic ejection murmur begins after the first heart sound, increases in intensity to reach a plateau toward the middle of the ejection period, and fades progressively to end just before the aortic valve closes (Fig. 19-14). There may also be an ejection click that occurs during systole as the calcified stiff valve leaflets try to open.

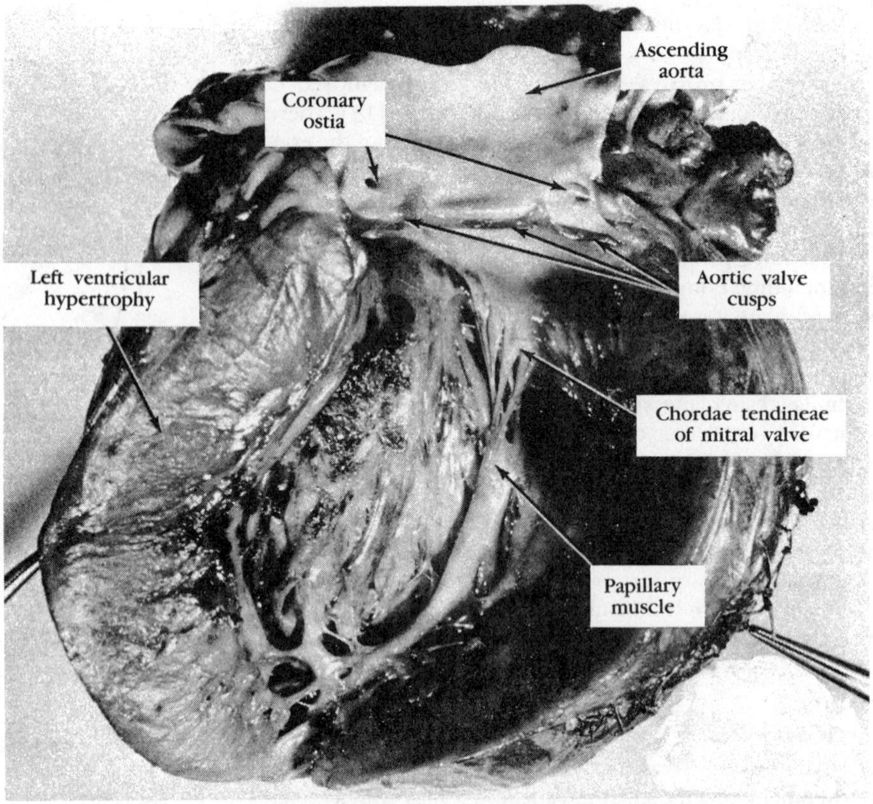

FIGURE 19-13. Marked thickening of the left ventricular myocardium showing a normal aorta and medial leaflet of the mitral valve. (From J. Kernicki, et al., *Cardiovascular Nursing*. New York: Putnam, 1971.)

DIAGNOSTIC TESTS. A chest x ray may show apical bulging if hypertrophy is present. Calcification of the valve ring may be seen. In the presence of left ventricular failure, pulmonary vascular enlargement may be noted.

Electrocardiographic abnormalities include left ventricular hypertrophy and strain. Left ventricular hypertrophy produces changes in the amplitude of the QRS complex and S–T segment displacement (strain pattern) in the precordial leads particularly [13]. Conduction system disturbances such as heart block may be manifested.

The echocardiogram is useful in assessing valve structure and motion along with providing information regarding ventricular function. Changes in the thickness, calcification, and mobility of the aortic valve can be recorded, and ventricular wall thickness can be evaluated.

Cardiac catheterization is useful in determining the systolic gradient across the valve as well as the valve orifice size. The gradient may be as much as 100 mm Hg, which means, for example, that in order to attain a systemic systolic pressure of 100 mm Hg, the left ventricle must attain a systolic pressure of 200 mm Hg.

Aortic Regurgitation, Insufficiency, or Incompetence

Aortic regurgitation is incomplete closure of the aortic valve. It can occur as a chronic or an acute lesion. Causes of chronic lesions include rheumatic fever, syphilis, hypertension, connective tissue disorders, and atherosclerosis [5]. The acute lesion can result from dissecting aneurysm of the aorta, infectious endocarditis, and occasionally from rheumatic fever.

PATHOPHYSIOLOGY AND COMPENSATORY MECHANISMS. The pathologic process in aortic regurgitation differs with each cause. For example, with rheumatic aortic insufficiency, there is fibrosis and unequal contracture of the leaflets leading to malalignment of the leaflets [13]. Perforation or destruction of one or more of the leaflets with infectious endocarditis may occur. In syphilitic aortic regurgitation, dilatation of the ascending aorta creates a stretching of the individual leaflets rendering them too short to close completely during diastole. Dissecting aortic aneurysm dilates the valve ring and prevents aortic closure.

The hemodynamic alterations of aortic insufficiency depend on the size of the leak, the diastolic pressure gradient across the valve, and the duration of diastole [13]. During systole, blood is ejected out of the left ventricle through the aortic valve and into the aorta, but some of it flows back into the ventricle during diastole when the pressure in the aorta exceeds that in the left ventricle. Likewise, during diastole blood is flowing into the ventricle from the left

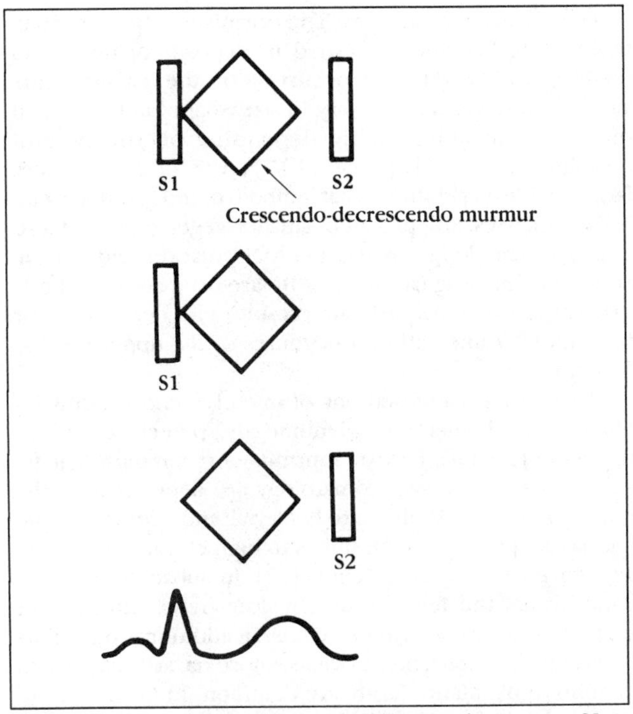

FIGURE 19-14. Sound of a crescendo-decrescendo murmur. Note the relationship of the sounds to the ECG recording below. The examiner should concentrate on each component. The S1 is followed by a sound of increasing intensity that stops just prior to the S2.

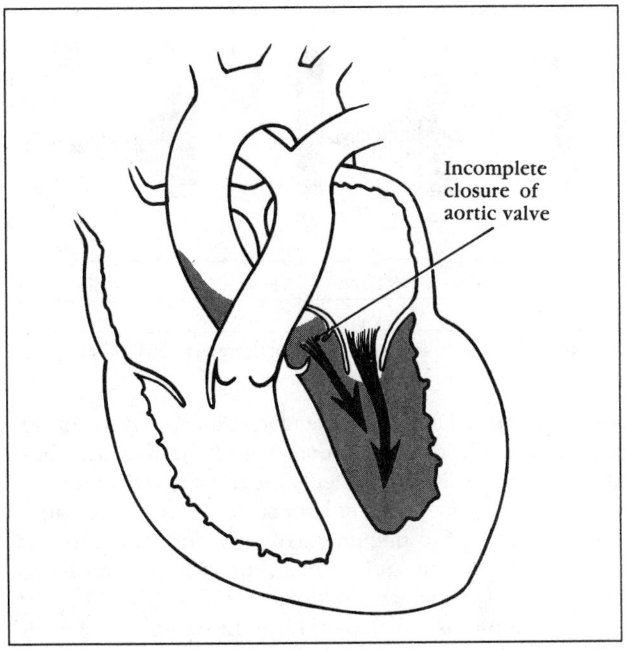

FIGURE 19-15. View of aortic insufficiency during early ventricular diastole.

atrium (Fig. 19-15). The left ventricle then becomes volume-overloaded by receiving blood from the left atrium through the regurgitant valve. An increase in the left ventricular end-diastolic volume results.

If the increase in end-diastolic volume in the left ventricle occurs over a period of time (chronically), the left ventricle gradually dilates as a compensatory mechanism. In other words, the myocardial fibers stretch to increase the surface area to accommodate this extra volume. This dilatation permits the left ventricle to eject a larger stroke volume (Starling's law) in order to maintain the cardiac output.

Long-standing hypertrophy is associated in this case with dilatation and often results in myocardial fibrosis so that cardiac muscle cells become unable to resume their normal shape after surgical replacement of the diseased valve [16]. As a result, the left ventricle fails causing acute pulmonary edema.

In *acute aortic regurgitation,* the time factor does not permit the compensatory mechanisms to develop. The volume overload in this case is so sudden that acute dilatation occurs and the left ventricle cannot maintain stroke volume and cardiac output. In acute aortic regurgitation there is a sudden increase in the left ventricular end-diastolic pressure. This is reflected to the pulmonary capillary bed causing pulmonary edema. Death often rapidly ensues unless heroic measures are instituted.

CLINICAL MANIFESTATIONS. In chronic aortic insufficiency with the compensatory mechanisms functioning, symptoms may not develop for many years. Palpitations may be described, especially when the person lies on the left side. A prominent apical impulse and an observable left ventricular lift on the precordium are often noted [13]. The onset of heart failure is indicated by increasing fatigue, dyspnea, chest pain, orthopnea, and paroxysmal nocturnal dyspnea.

Auscultatory findings in chronic aortic regurgitation depend on the severity of the regurgitation. In mild regurgitation, there is a decrescendo diastolic murmur beginning shortly after S2 and ending before S1 (Fig. 19-16). With moderate regurgitation, there may be another type of murmur called an *Austin Flint murmur.* This murmur is a diastolic rumble heard at the apex. It is caused by the premature closure of the mitral valve during rapid filling of the ventricles and corresponds to the severity of the aortic regurgitation.

The diastolic murmur of acute aortic regurgitation differs from those heard in chronic aortic regurgitation. The diastolic murmur can be cooing or coarsely vibrating. The first heart sound may be diminished or absent because of the premature closure of the mitral valve [13].

In the presence of severe regurgitation there is also a marked increase in the amplitude of the pulse when it is palpated. This is noted as a sudden sharp pulse followed by a rapid collapse of the diastolic pulse and is referred to as a *water-hammer* or *Corrigan's pulse.* A widening of the pulse pressure reflects the inability of the aortic valve to exert its influence on maintenance of the aortic diastolic

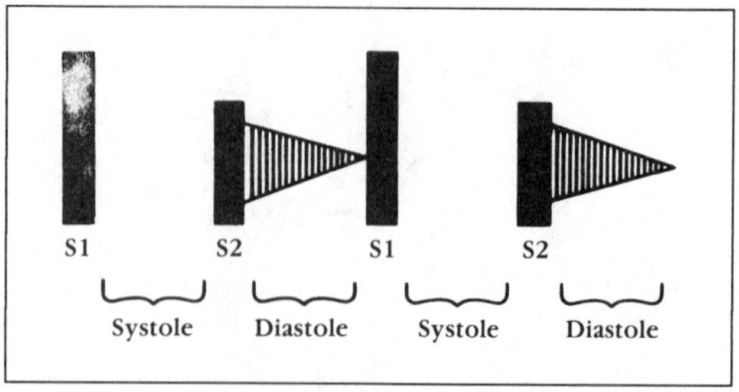

FIGURE 19-16. Diastolic murmur of aortic regurgitation.

blood pressure [16]. The electrocardiogram reflects left ventricular hypertrophy, especially in the precordial leads, and the echocardiogram reflects the increased chamber dimensions that may occur in later stages [1]. Cardiac catheterization is used to document the severity and extent of aortic regurgitation and to make quantitative measurements of left ventricular function.

Once symptoms develop, in both the acute and chronic forms, a fairly swift deterioration occurs and, if left untreated, severe aortic regurgitation will eventually lead to heart failure and death.

Mixed Aortic Stenosis and Regurgitation

When aortic stenosis and regurgitation are both present, the condition is referred to as a mixed lesion. It has been reported that the majority of individuals with aortic valve disease have mixed lesions. One of the lesions usually predominates over the other hemodynamically.

INFECTIVE ENDOCARDITIS

Infective endocarditis affects the lining of the heart and is caused by an invading microorganism. The causative agents include bacteria, fungus, rickettsiae, and, rarely, viruses and parasites [16]. Infective endocarditis has been described by a variety of terms: (1) subacute bacterial endocarditis (SBE), (2) acute bacterial endocarditis (ABE), (3) prosthetic valve endocarditis (PVE), and (4) native valve endocarditis (NVE) [5]. Subacute and acute bacterial endocarditis are included in this discussion.

With subacute bacterial endocarditis, the invading organism is usually of low virulence and the process can develop gradually over weeks and months [5]. SBE usually affects an already damaged heart such as one with congenital or rheumatic heart disease. The most common causative organism is the *Streptococcus viridans* [8]. ABE is often found in persons with normal hearts but can affect damaged hearts. Because the organism is of high virulence, the process usually progresses very rapidly. The most common organism in causation is the *Staphylococcus aureus.*

The organism traveling in the bloodstream attaches to the endocardial lining of a normal heart or to the area of defect of an abnormal heart. The organisms, after attaching themselves, become enmeshed in deposits of fibrin and platelets with vegetations occurring on the leaflets of the valves. These vegetations vary in size, shape, and color and may become quite friable depending on the type of invading organism [2] (Fig. 19-17). ABE often produces large friable vegetations that embolize and produce embolic abscesses. SBE produces smaller vegetations that also embolize and lodge in the microcirculation and spleen. Some precipitating factors for ABE are drug abuse and cardiac surgery whereas SBE often results after dental work or through instrumentation procedures of the upper respiratory tract.

The clinical manifestations of infective endocarditis include fever, hematuria, splenomegaly, petechiae, Osler's nodes, and anemia. Cardiac murmurs are common. The fever and its related symptomatology are dependent on the type of infection. With acute bacterial endocarditis the fever has a rapid onset with spikes to high elevations that are accompanied by shaking chills [12]. In subacute bacterial endocarditis the fever is usually low-grade, intermittent with elevations, and without chills. In addition, complaints of weakness, fatigue, night sweats, anorexia, arthralgias, and exhibition of splenomegaly are common. In both types of infective endocarditis there may be Osler's nodes, which are painful, tender, red subcutaneous nodules in the pads of the fingers; Janeway's lesions, which are flat, small, irregular, nontender red spots found on the palms and soles; and Roth's spots, which are retinal hemorrhages that appear with a white or yellow center surrounded by a red, irregular halo [5].

The vegetations produced by the infectious process settle on the cardiac valves and invade the leaflets. These vegetations prevent normal alignment of the cusps and may, therefore, cause incomplete closure or regurgitation leading to cardiac murmurs. The murmurs produced correspond to the affected valve. For example, with mitral insufficiency a systolic murmur results, and with aortic insufficiency the murmur is an early diastolic murmur.

If the vegetations grow and infiltrate the downstream side of the valve, small fragments may break off as blood is pushed through the valve orifice. These fragments, if located on the left side of the heart, may cause embolization to the cerebral and systemic circulation and, if on the right side, may embolize to the lungs. In addition, heart failure may ensue with severe hemodynamic alterations that occur from severe valvular regurgitation [12].

The diagnosis of infective endocarditis is based on positive blood cultures, which are present in the majority of cases. Also, a normocytic, normochromic anemia and an elevated sedimentation rate may be noted.

Treatment measures are aimed at identifying the causative microorganism followed by antibiotic therapy that requires effective penetration of the vegetation in order to reach the microorganism and kill it. Recovery from untreated infective endocarditis is rare and death often results [5].

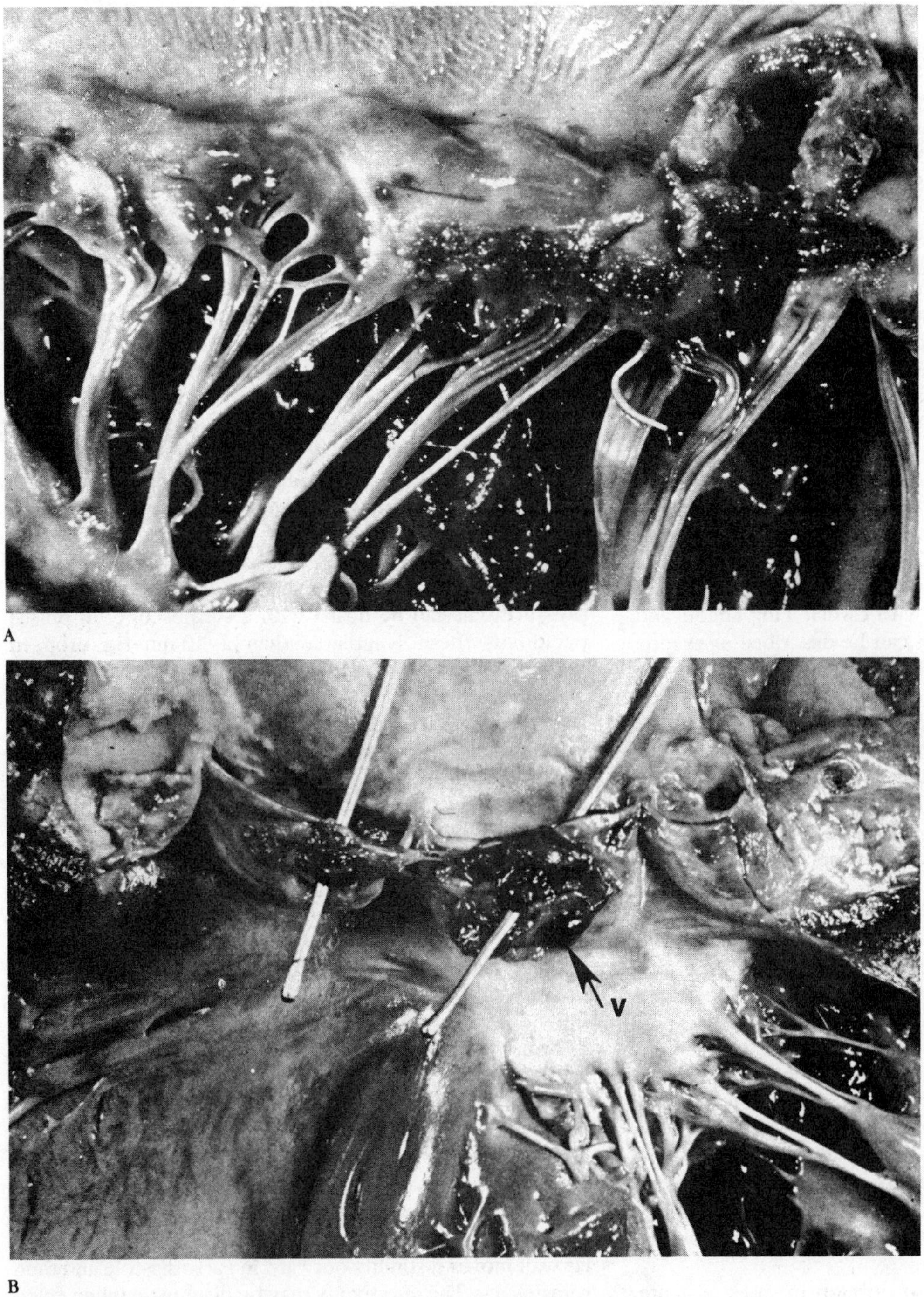

FIGURE 19-17. Infective endocarditis. A. The vegetations are massive, crumbly, and hemorrhagic. Top and to the right, the valve has been perforated by the infective process. B. The aortic valve cusps are distorted and perforated. Vegetations (*V*) are present on the ventricular aspect of the valve. (From R.A. Cawson, A.W. McCracken, and P. R. Marcus, *Pathologic Mechanisms and Human Disease.* St. Louis: Mosby, 1982.)

PERICARDITIS

The pericardium is the fibrous sac surrounding the heart that acts to protect the heart and secretes a lubricant for cardiac movement. It also prevents dilatation of the chambers of the heart during exercise and hypervolemia, and contains the heart in a fixed position. In addition, it provides a barrier to infections from the lungs and pleural cavities.

Pericarditis is an inflammation of the pericardium that may be caused by open heart surgery (the leading cause), uremia, myocardial infarction, viral or bacterial infections, tumors, anticoagulants, or trauma [1].

As the pericardium becomes inflamed, it may become thickened and fibrotic. If it does not heal completely after an acute episode, the pericardium may calcify over a period of time and form a firm scar surrounding the heart. This interferes with diastolic filling of the ventricles. This condition is then referred to as chronic constrictive pericarditis. Pericarditis may be classified as either acute or chronic (constrictive).

In acute pericarditis, some of the clinical manifestations are pain, pericardial friction rub, electrocardiographic changes, pericardial effusion with cardiac tamponade, and a paradoxical pulse. The pain can be described as severe, sharp, and aching; it is usually precordial or substernal in location; and it may radiate to the left or right shoulder, arm, and elbows. On occasion, the pain may spread to the jaw, throat, and ears. It may be intensified by deep breathing, sneezing, coughing, moving, or changing position. The pain may be relieved when the person sits up and leans forward. It is often confused with the pain of myocardial ischemia, which may lead to misdiagnosis of this condition [15].

In addition to pain, one of the most important physical signs of pericarditis is a friction rub that is heard best at the apex and at the lower left sternal border. It is an intermittent, transitory sound that imitates the sound of sandpaper rubbing together. This loud "to and fro" leathery sound may disappear on one day and reappear on the next.

Acute pericarditis can produce the following changes on the ECG: (1) S–T elevation occurs in two or three standard limb leads and V2–V6; (2) reciprocal depressions occur in AVR and V1; and (3) several days to weeks after the early stage, the S–T segments return to normal and the T waves invert. Low voltage is characteristic and no Q waves develop; this helps to distinguish acute pericarditis from an acute myocardial infarction.

Pericardial effusion may also develop in cases of acute pericarditis. This is fluid that accumulates between the pericardium and myocardium. If the fluid accumulates rapidly it can cause cardiac compression and tamponade. With pericardial effusion the heart sounds are faint and apical impulse may disappear. On chest x ray, there is enlargement of the cardiac silhouette. The heart may appear as a "water bottle" configuration (Fig. 19-18). The echocardiogram detects the presence of pericardial fluid.

When fluid accumulates rapidly or in an amount large enough to impair cardiac function, the condition is referred to as cardiac tamponade. The amount of fluid that can cause tamponade varies according to the rate of fluid accumulation. In rapid accumulation of fluid, 250 ml may produce significant obstruction. When an effusion develops slowly, 1000 ml or more may accumulate before significant symptoms develop. As fluid collects in the pericardium, the pressure rises in the pericardial cavity. The pressure rises to a level equal to the pressures in the heart during diastole. The first structures to be compressed are the right atrium and ventricle because they have the lowest diastolic pressures. This compression causes increased venous pressure with decreased right atrial filling. Systemic venous congestion with edema and hepatomegaly result. There is also a decrease in the diastolic filling of the ventricles, which leads to a decrease in stroke volume and cardiac output. This can be a life-threatening complication of pericarditis, and death may occur from circulatory collapse [1].

A characteristic sign of cardiac tamponade is *pulsus paradoxus.* This is a large inspiratory reduction in arterial pressure that can be heard with a stethoscope. In pulsus paradoxus there is greater than a 10-mm Hg drop in the systolic blood pressure during inspiration. If the tamponade is severe, pulsus paradoxus may be palpated as a weakness or disappearance in the arterial pressure during inspiration.

Chronic constrictive pericarditis results from the healing of acute pericarditis, and formation of granular tissue that gradually contracts to form a firm scar surrounding the heart. This scar causes a constriction of the heart and interferes with filling of the ventricles; this complication is similar to the physiologic abnormality that results from cardiac tamponade except that it develops slowly.

Clinical manifestations of chronic constrictive pericarditis are weakness, fatigue, weight loss, anorexia, and edema. Individuals may complain of abdominal discomfort due to systemic venous congestion. This discomfort may be related to hepatic congestion and swelling of the abdomen. A characteristic sign of constrictive pericarditis is jugular neck vein distention, which is indicative of elevated venous pressure.

The echocardiogram may show pericardial thickening and paradoxical septal motion in constrictive pericarditis. Also noted on the echocardiogram is that the left ventricular wall moves distinctly outward in early diastole and then remains flat. The chest x ray may be diagnostic when calcification appears in the pericardium.

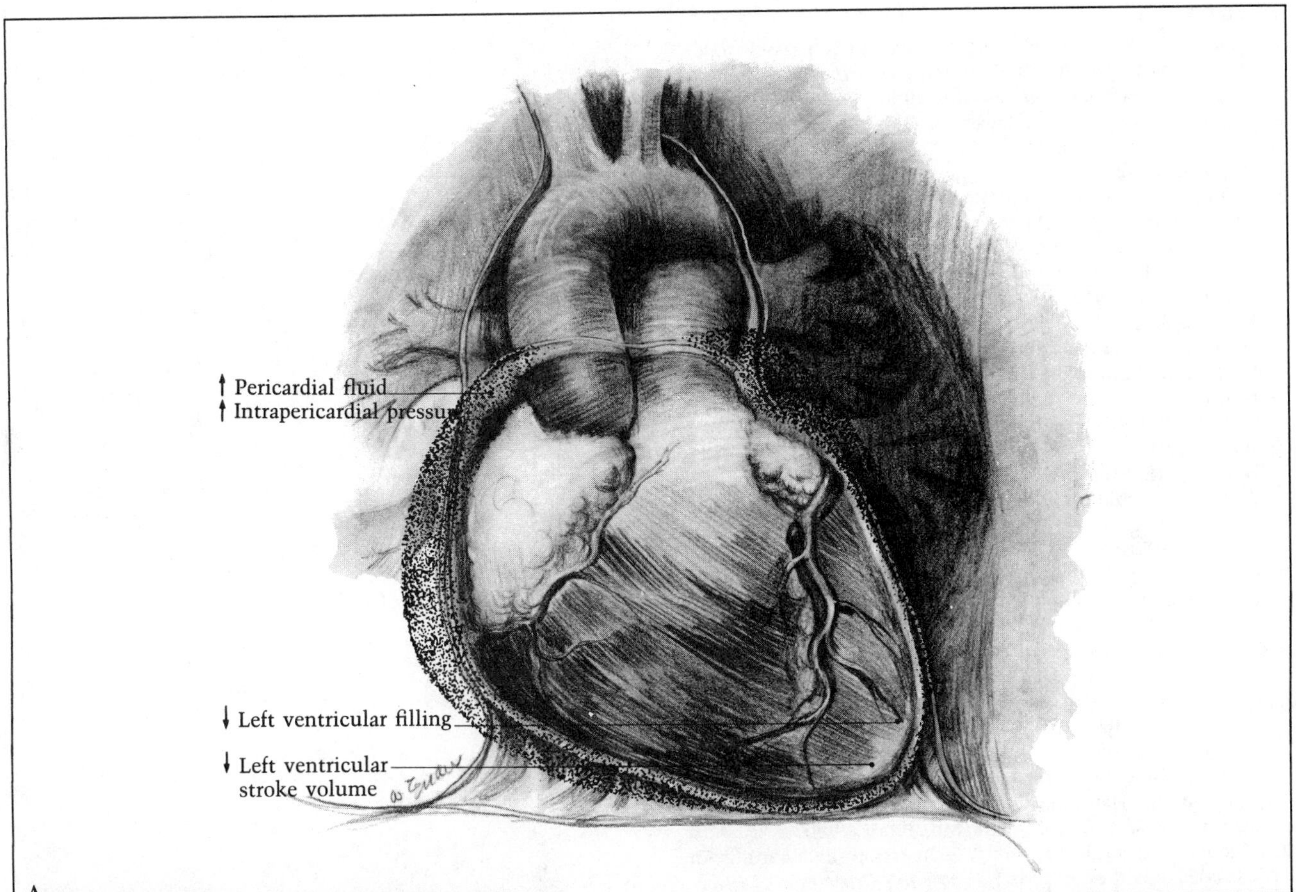

A

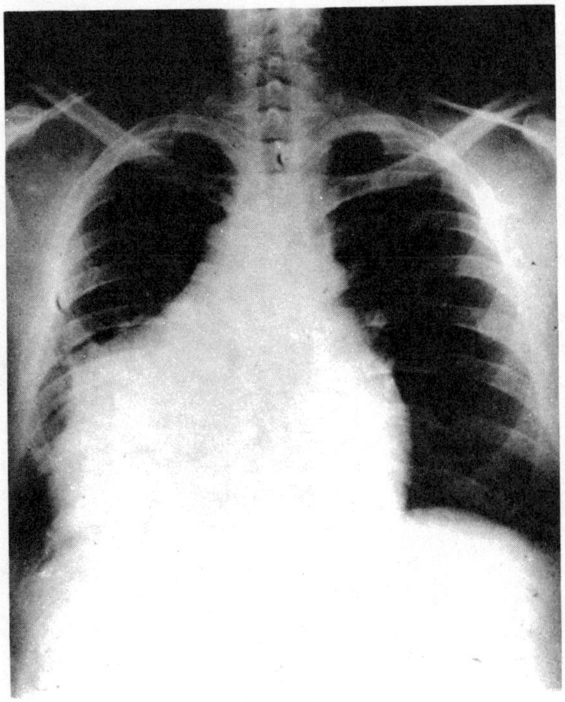

B

FIGURE 19-18. A. Pericardial effusion and cardiac tamponade. The following hemodynamic effects may result following pericardial effusion: (1) accumulation of pericardial fluid resulting in intrapericardial pressure, (2) elevation of right atrial pressure, (3) elevation of left ventricular end-diastolic pressure, (4) reduction in left ventricular end-diastolic volume and cardiac output, (5) elevated venous pressure. B. Chest x ray from a patient with a large pericardial effusion that resulted in pericardial tamponade. (From C. V. Kenner, C. E. Guzzetta, B. M. Dossey, *Critical Care Nursing: Body-Mind-Spirit.* Boston: Little, Brown, 1981.)

REFERENCES

1. Braumwald, E. Valvular Heart Disease. In K.J. Isselbacher, et al. (eds.), *Harrison's Principles of Internal Medicine* (9th ed.). New York: McGraw-Hill, 1980.
2. Christopherson, P.J., and Swarajan, E.S. Infective Endocarditis. In S.L. Underhill (ed.), *Cardiac Nursing*. Philadelphia: Lippincott, 1982.
3. Cohn, J.N. Recognition and Management of Shock and Acute Pump Failure. In J.W. Hurst, et al. (eds.), *The Heart* (5th ed.). New York: McGraw-Hill, 1982.
4. Disch, J.M. Diagnostic Procedures for Cardiovascular Disease Series II. *Surgical Aspects of Cardiovascular Disease*. New York: Appleton-Century-Crofts, 1979.
5. Durack, D.T. Infective and Noninfective Endocarditis. In J.W. Hurst, et al. (eds.), *The Heart* (5th ed.). New York: McGraw-Hill, 1982.
6. Fortium, M.J. Echocardiography: How it works. *Med. Times* 108:120, 1980.
7. Franch, R.H., King, S.B., and Douglas, J.S. Techniques of Cardiac Catheterization Including Coronary Arteriography. In J.W. Hurst, et al. (eds.), *The Heart* (5th ed.). New York: McGraw-Hill, 1982.
8. Froelicher, V.F. Techniques of Exercise Testing. In J.W. Hurst, et al. (eds.), *The Heart* (5th ed.). New York: McGraw-Hill, 1982.
9. Guyton, A. *Textbook of Medical Physiology* (6th ed.). Philadelphia: Saunders, 1981.
10. Hurst, J.W., et al. Atherosclerotic Coronary Heart Disease, Angina Pectoris, Myocardial Infarction, and Other Manifestations of Myocardial Ischemia. In J.W. Hurst, et al. (eds.), *The Heart* (5th ed.). New York: McGraw-Hill, 1982.
11. Jackle, M., and Halligan, M. *Cardiovascular Problems: A Critical Care Nursing Focus*. Bowie, Md.: Brady, 1980.
12. Pelletier, L.L., and Petersdorf, R.G. Infectious Endocarditis. In K.J. Isselbacher, et al. (eds.), *Harrison's Principles of Internal Medicine* (9th ed.). New York: McGraw-Hill, 1980.
13. Rackley, C.E., et al. Aortic Valve Disease and Mitral Valve Disease. In J.W. Hurst, et al. (eds.), *The Heart* (5th ed.). New York: McGraw-Hill, 1982.
14. Robbins, S., and Cotran, R. *Pathologic Basis of Disease* (2nd ed.). Philadelphia: Saunders, 1979.
15. Ross, J., and Peterson, K.L. Cardiac Catheterization and Angiography. In K.J. Isselbacher, et al. (eds.), *Harrison's Principles of Internal Medicine* (9th ed.). New York: McGraw-Hill, 1980.
16. Sokolow, M., and McIlroy, M.B. *Clinical Cardiology* (2nd ed.). Los Altos, Calif.: Lange, 1979.
17. Stollerman, G.H. Acute Rheumatic Fever and Its Management. In J.W. Hurst, et al. (eds.), *The Heart* (5th ed.). New York: McGraw-Hill, 1982.
18. Zaret, B.L., and Berges, H.J. Techniques of Nuclear Cardiology. In J.W. Hurst, et al. (eds.), *The Heart* (5th ed.). New York: McGraw-Hill, 1982.
19. Zelis, R.F., and Werger, W.K. Prevention of Coronary Atherosclerosis. In J.W. Hurst, et al. (eds.), *The Heart* (5th ed.). New York: McGraw-Hill, 1982.

CHAPTER 20
HYPERTENSION

LEARNING OBJECTIVES

1. Define *hypertension* as it relates to different age groups.
2. Compare the definitions of *borderline, labile, benign,* and *malignant hypertension.*
3. List and briefly describe the factors that are related to the causation of hypertension.
4. Briefly describe the significance of the serum lipoproteins in hypertension.
5. Explain how the blood pressure levels are normally maintained in the arterial system.
6. Describe the abnormal renin theory in the production of essential hypertension.
7. Compare the pathophysiology of essential and secondary hypertension.
8. List the typical symptoms of hypertension.
9. Explain the four major morbid sequelae of hypertensive disease.
10. List the diagnostic tests used in hypertensive disease.

Hypertension is the most common disease in the United States, affecting an estimated 23 million Americans. It is a direct risk factor contributing to the incidence of myocardial infarction and cerebrovascular accidents. The incidence of sudden death is markedly increased among hypertensive persons.

DEFINITIONS

Hypertension is defined as an abnormal elevation of the systolic arterial blood pressure. The levels that are considered to be hypertensive vary with the age of the person. Blood pressure (BP) levels fluctuate within certain limits depending on the body position, age, and stress levels (Table 20-1). *Borderline hypertension* in adults is considered to be consistent readings between 140/90 and 160/95 with readings above 160/95 considered to be definitely hypertensive [3]. Hypertension is also frequently classified as mild, moderate, or severe on the basis of the diastolic pressure. Mild hypertension is in the range of 95–104, moderate 105–114, and severe 115 or greater. Persons who have occasional elevation of the blood pressure have *labile hypertension.*

The most frequent form of hypertension is that which exhibits mixed systolic and diastolic blood pressures. Occasionally, the diastolic pressure is elevated without a significant increase in systolic pressure. This indicates an increase in the peripheral vascular resistance (PVR) and is more frequently seen in the younger person. Increase in the systolic pressure without diastolic elevation may be found in elderly persons, with hyperdynamic circulation, such as with hyperthyroidism, or with aortic insufficiency. Systolic hypertension is defined as a systolic pressure above 160 and a diastolic pressure less than 95.

Other definitions of hypertension include essential or idiopathic hypertension, which has no specific etiologic basis and is the most common form. Secondary hypertension is that due to a known cause (Table 20-2). *Benign* and *malignant hypertension* refer to the course of the disease and either may result from essential or secondary hypertension. Benign hypertension is a misnomer because it causes permanent damaging effects even though it has a gradual onset and begins with blood pressure levels slightly above normal. Malignant hypertension is a rapidly progressive form of uncontrollable blood pressure that causes a high incidence of complications including renal failure, cerebrovascular accident, retinal hemorrhages, congestive heart failure, and encephalopathy.

ETIOLOGY OF HYPERTENSION

Age

There is a positive relationship between age and the incidence of hypertension. The incidence and prevalence increase as the individual ages. Hypertension in those below the age of 35 markedly increases the incidence of heart disease (coronary artery disease [CAD]) and premature death.

TABLE 20-1. Hypertension as it relates to different age groups

	Normal	Hypertensive
Infants	80/40	90/60
Children		
7–11 years old	100/60	120/80
Teenagers		
12–17 years old	115/70	130/80
Adults		
20–45 years old	120–125/75–80	135/90
45–65 years old	135–140/85	140/90–160/95
Over 65 years old	150/85	160/90 (borderline)

Sex

Overall, men have a higher incidence than women, but at middle age and beyond, the prevalence begins to change and the incidence in women exceeds that in men at the older ages (over the age of 65).

Race

Blacks have at least twice the incidence of hypertension as whites. The consequences of the disease are usually more severe in the black race. For example, at diastolic levels of 115 or over mortality for black men is 3.3 times that of similarly hypertensive white men and 5.6 times that of white women [4].

Life-Style

Factors such as education, income, and other life-style factors have been studied with inconclusive results. Low

TABLE 20-2. Causes of hypertension

ESSENTIAL, IDIOPATHIC OR PRIMARY HYPERTENSION

Related to obesity, hypercholesteremia, atherosclerosis, high-sodium diet, diabetes, stress, type A personality, familial history, smoking, and lack of exercise

SECONDARY HYPERTENSION

Renovascular
- Parenchymal disease, such as acute and chronic glomerulonephritis
- Narrowing, stenosis of renal artery—due to atherosclerosis or congenital fibroplasia

Cushing's disease or syndrome
- May be due to increased secretion of glucocorticoids as the result of adrenal disease or pituitary dysfunction

Primary aldosteronism
- Increased aldosterone secretion, often as a result of an adrenal tumor

Pheochromocytoma
- Tumor of adrenal medulla causing increased secretion of adrenal catecholamines

Coarctation of the aorta
- Congenital constriction of aorta usually at the level of the ductus arteriosus with increased blood pressure above the constriction and decreased pressure below the constriction

income, low educational levels, and stressful lives or occupations seem to be related to a higher incidence of hypertension. A familial history of hypertension has always been considered a risk factor; however, this relationship may be related more to life-style than to a straight genetic link, especially with essential hypertension. Obesity is considered to be a major risk factor. When weight reduction is achieved, the blood pressure often returns to the normal range. Finally, cigarette smoking is implicated as a high-risk factor for both hypertension and CAD. Persons who have a blood pressure of greater than 130 systolic have twice the frequency of myocardial infarction than the normal population. Hypercholesteremia and hyperglycemia are both major factors in the development of atherosclerosis, which is closely associated with hypertension. The lipoproteins responsible for hypercholesteremia have been studied in terms of atherogenesis. These will be briefly described.

SERUM LIPOPROTEINS. Five families of lipoproteins have been identified: (1) chylomicron, (2) very-low-density lipoprotein (VLDL), (3) intermediate-density lipoprotein, (4) low-density lipoprotein (LDL), and (5) high-density lipoprotein (HDL) [4]. Each group of lipoproteins performs different functions in the body. Chylomicrons transport most of the dietary substances and VLDL carry most of the triglycerides. Much of the plasma cholesterol is carried by LDL. HDL apparently serves as a reservoir for lipoproteins involved in triglyceride transport and in the esterification of cholesterol. HDL is usually higher in women than in men and may encourage the storage of cholesterol in the liver in women [4]. Research continues into the role of HDL in protection from CAD.

Diabetes Mellitus (DM)

The relationship between DM and hypertension is obscure, but the statistics support a definite link between hypertension and CAD. The main cause of death with diabetes mellitus is cardiovascular disease, especially with early onset and poor control. The main cause of death with diabetes mellitus is cardiovascular disease, especially with early onset and poor control of the diabetic condition. Hypertension associated with diabetes causes increased mortality. Diabetics without hypertension have a mortality 2.47 times that of normal subjects. Hypertensive diabetics (BP 150/95) have a mortality 13.52 times normal. This mortality difference declines with age so that at the age of 50 hypertensive diabetics have 2.96 times normal mortality compared to nonhypertensive diabetics who have 2.21 times normal mortality for age [1].

Secondary Hypertension

As is described on p. 271, hypertension can develop secondarily to known diseases. These are listed in Table 20-2.

PATHOPHYSIOLOGY

To understand the pathophysiology of hypertension a review of normal arterial pressure determinants is necessary. In the normal person, the blood pressure is maintained within rather narrow limits. However, during sleep the blood pressure may fall to 60/40 mm Hg or less, and during exercise marked increases may be noted that often correspond to changes in heart rate and cardiac output. Total peripheral resistance is an important factor in the regulation of the arterial blood pressure. It is the sum of all resistances offered by the vascular beds of the body. These vary with different organs but the systemic peripheral resistance has the greatest effect on the mean arterial blood pressure. Very small changes in *arteriolar diameter,* also called the *precapillary sphincter diameter,* cause significant effects on both systemic arterial pressure and blood flow. Mean arterial pressure can be calculated by using the following formula:

$$\text{Cardiac output (CO)} \times \text{total peripheral resistance (TPR)} = \text{mean arterial pressure (MAP)}$$

One other factor that affects systolic and diastolic pressure is aortic impedance, which is regulated by the aortic valve and the elasticity of the aortic wall. The diastolic arterial ***volume*** and consequently the pressure is regulated largely by the tone of the arterioles and the precapillary sphincters.

Other factors have an influence on the arterial pressure, especially by affecting the cardiac output and the peripheral resistance. The sympathetic nervous system (SNS) causes an increased peripheral vascular resistance and increased cardiac contractility, which, in turn, increases the blood pressure. The SNS also influences the renin-angiotensin-aldosterone (RAA) system, which causes arteriolar constriction through angiotensin II and increased blood volume through the liberation of aldosterone. The role of the SNS and RAA system in producing hypertension is described in the following discussion.

Essential Hypertension

There is no real agreement as to the etiology of essential hypertension. Ninety percent of all hypertension has no definite identifiable cause. It is known that the arterioles offer an abnormally increased resistance to blood flow. This increases peripheral vascular resistance, causes a decreased capillary flow, and results in an increased resistance against which the heart must pump. Numerous theories have been offered to explain hypertension. These include: (1) changes in the arteriolar bed itself causing chronically increased resistance; (2) abnormally increased tone of the SNS from the vasomotor centers causing increased PVR; (3) increased blood volume resulting from renal or hormonal dysfunction; and (4) a genetic increase in arteriolar thickening causing the abnormal PVR.

One theory that has been studied extensively is the *abnormal renin theory.* It has been demonstrated that when blood flow to the kidney is decreased, the juxtaglomerular cells release renin, which reacts with angiotensinogen (a plasma protein formed by the liver) to form angiotensin I,

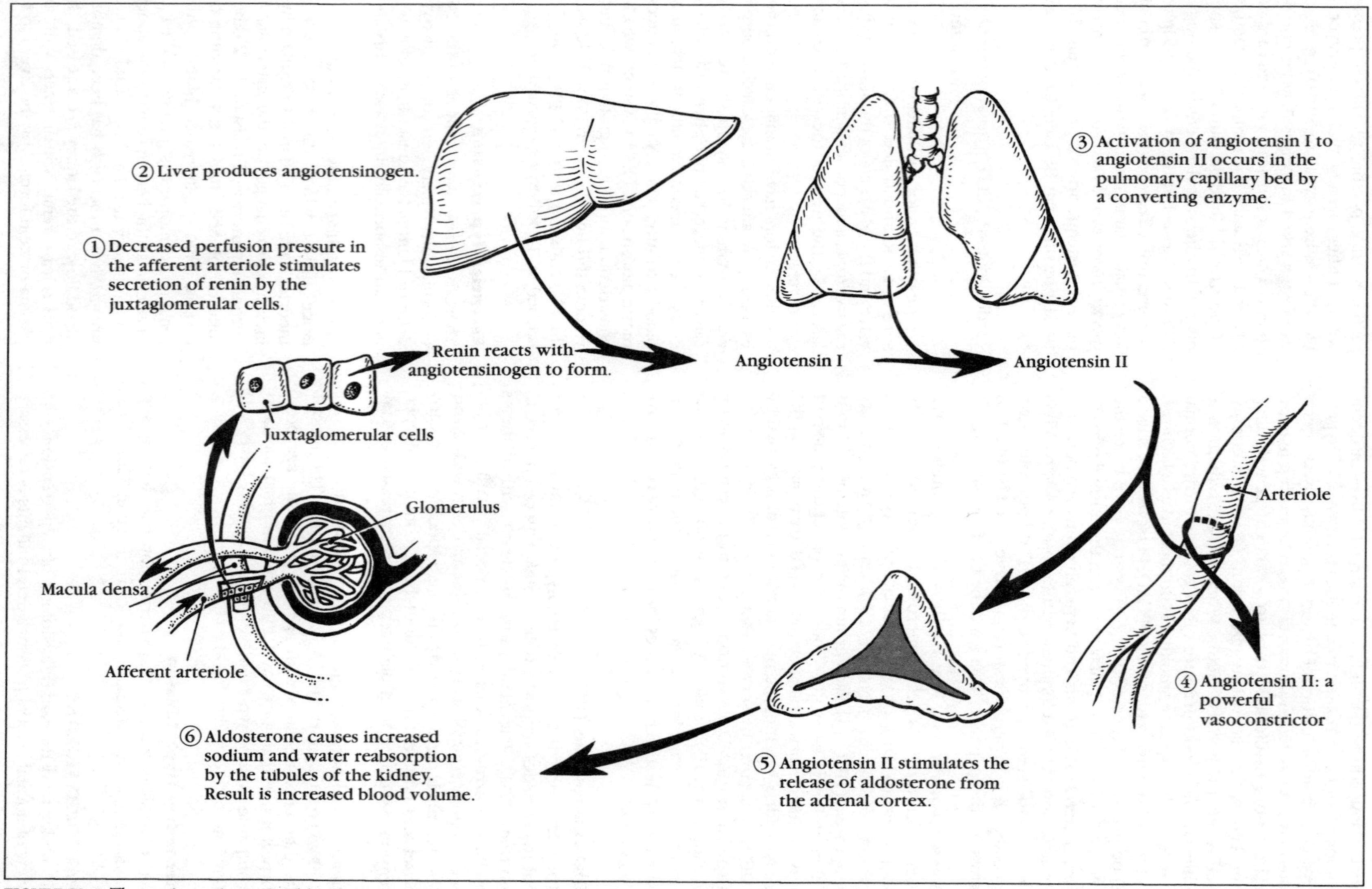

FIGURE 20-1. The renin-angiotensin-aldosterone system.

which is then converted to angiotensin II in the lungs. Angiotensin I is an intermediate step in the process that exhibits no physiologic activity, but angiotensin II is a potent vasoconstrictor. The target for angiotensin II effect is the arterioles. Circulating angiotensin II also works in some unknown manner to stimulate aldosterone secretion, which, in turn, increases the blood volume by conserving sodium and water (Fig. 20-1).

Serum renin elevation is not seen in every form of hypertension but it correlates well with some types and also with the malignant form. Classifying hypertension into categories according to plasma renin activity (PRA) is quite helpful in determining the course of the disease. High renin activity (HRA) is often associated with increased aldosterone levels and malignant hypertension. Low renin activity (LRA) accounts for 30 percent of cases, 55 percent have normal renin activity (NRA), and 15 percent have HRA. Therapy is now being based on PRA. For example, propranolol (Inderal) is an effective drug for cases of HRA but not of LRA. Studies have shown that an absolute or relative excess of renin and angiotensin II is involved with essential hypertension in 50 to 70 percent of cases [1, 4].

Secondary Hypertension

This type of hypertension develops from a specific underlying cause. Table 20-2 lists some causes of secondary hypertension and some factors related to primary hypertension.

Renovascular hypertension has been studied extensively. It results from atherosclerotic or fibrous dysplastic stenosis of one or both renal arteries [3]. The resultant decrease in renal perfusion causes activation of the RAA system. The degree of the hypertension is closely related to the amount of renal ischemia produced by the obstruction. Serum renin levels are usually elevated but the amount of aldosterone secreted in relation to the amount of angiotensin II present is inappropriately increased for no known reason [3]. The end result of this type of hypertension is a marked increase in the peripheral vascular resistance and cardiac output with the production of very high levels of systemic blood pressure.

Renal parenchymal disease, such as glomerulonephritis and renal failure, often causes a renin- or sodium-dependent type of hypertension. The pathophysiology varies depending on the extent of renal insufficiency and the type of renal disease. A hypervolemic picture with normal PVR may appear or a normal or diminished circulation with a very increased PVR or both increased volume and PVR may result.

Cushing's disease causes an increase in the blood volume and thus in the blood pressure. *Primary aldosteronism* also is volumic, or salt- and water-dependent.

Pheochromocytoma is a secreting tumor of chromaffin cells, usually of the adrenal medulla. This tumor causes hypertension as a result of increased secretion of epinephrine and norepinephrine. Epinephrine functions mainly to increase cardiac contractility and rate while norepinephrine functions mainly to increase PVR. The hypertension produced by a pheochromocytoma is usually severe, running a very malignant course.

Coarctation of the aorta is a congenital constriction of the aorta, often at the level of the ductus arteriosus. This produces a syndrome of markedly elevated pressures in the upper extremities and a decrease in perfusion of the lower extremities. Sometimes the PRA is seen to be increased but this finding is not consistent and PVR may not be elevated [3].

Clinical Manifestations of Hypertension

When symptoms do occur, the disease is usually far advanced. The classic symptoms of headache, epistaxis, dizziness, and tinnitus thought to be associated with high blood pressure are no more common in hypertensive than in normotensive individuals. However, the symptoms of unsteadiness, waking headache, blurred vision, depression, and nocturia have been shown to be increased in untreated hypertension [2].

The triad of hypertension was first described by Richard Brighton in 1863 and George Johnson in 1873. Dr. Brighton described the symmetrically contracted kidneys with fibrotic lesions in the nephrons, and the concentric hypertrophy of the left ventricle. Dr. Johnson described the arteriolar hyaline sclerosis of the systemic vessels [8]. These have been accepted as the pathologic sequelae of hypertension regardless of the cause. These pathologic sequelae can cause the death of the affected person.

Four major morbid sequelae are associated with hypertensive disease: (1) stroke, (2) myocardial infarction, (3) renal failure, and (4) encephalopathy [8].

STROKE. Vascular lesions may cause either a hemorrhagic or an ischemic stroke. The increasing pressures may cause dilatation of the small, sometimes nonelastic, and aged vessels. This, in turn, causes breaks in the vessel and hemorrhage into the brain parenchyma. The dilatations of the smaller intracerebral arteries are called *Charcot-Bouchard aneurysms.* These microaneurysms may rupture and cause signs of intracerebral hemorrhage; they have also been noted in the eye grounds of the eyes [8]. In the process of aneurysm formation, the vessels undergo some repair, which eventually leads to thickening and tortuosity of the endothelium.

Ischemic infarcts often occur from associated atherosclerosis of the extracranial vessels (carotids and vertebrals). The thickened endothelium of the small vessels decreases or obstructs the blood flow to an area.

MYOCARDIAL INFARCTION. Myocardial infarction may result from atherosclerosis of the coronary arteries or from the same type of hyaline sclerosis previously described in relation to arterioles of the brain. It is believed that hypertension accelerates atherosclerosis because it causes injury to the endothelium, which increases lipid accumulation and atheroma formation [8].

RENAL FAILURE. Renal failure from primary hypertension frequently results from progressive damage to the arcuate arteries and the afferent arterioles. Progressive hyaline sclerosis leads to ischemic death of nephrons, and to fibrosis, which leads to contracted kidneys. With significant loss of nephrons, renal failure ensues. This process is markedly accelerated with fibroid necrosis of the larger arteries when it is associated with malignant hypertension.

ENCEPHALOPATHY. This ominous manifestation results from leakage of water and electrolytes from the brain capillaries into the tissues of the brain. The leakage produces cerebral edema and is often associated with papilledema (optic disk swelling). Encephalopathy is more common in malignant hypertension or when a hypertensive state assumes a malignant pattern. This condition may be heralded by agitation, convulsions, or coma, and frequently causes death.

Unlike many other diseases, hypertension is usually asymptomatic and the disease may not be recognized for years unless the person seeks medical attention for another health problem or has a routine blood pressure reading.

Pathophysiology in Target Organs

Untreated hypertension damages the small arterioles, which, in turn, cause *target organ dysfunction.* The organs most acutely affected by vascular damage are the brain, eyes, kidneys, and heart. Problems that may result in the target organs are summarized in Table 20-3. The effects on the target organs has been termed the *morbid sequelae* of prolonged systemic blood pressure elevation.

The blood pressure remains consistently above the normal level for the age of the person. Many affected persons complain of angina pectoris especially on exertion or during stressful situations. Headache is occasionally described, especially an occipital type that may be present on waking and may be associated with nausea, vomiting, and mental confusion. Renal dysfunction may be the first sign with nocturia or hematuria being described. Symptoms of left ventricular failure are common, especially of dyspnea on exertion.

With the malignant form of hypertension, the rapid onset of renal failure, heart failure, or hypertensive encephalopathy may occur. Cerebrovascular accident may be indicated by intense headache followed by neurologic deficits. Death often ensues without immediate appropriate treatment.

TABLE 20-3. Hypertensive effects on target organs

Organ	Effect	Manifested by
Heart	Myocardial infarction	ECG changes; enzyme elevations
	Congestive failure	Decreased cardiac output S3 or summation gallop auscultated; cardiomegaly on x ray
	Myocardial hypertrophy	Increased voltage R wave in V3–V6; increased incidence of angina; left ventricular strain, manifest by S–T, T wave changes
	Arrhythmias	Usually ventricular arrhythmias or conduction defects
Eyes	Blurred or impaired vision	Nicking arteries and veins; hemorrhages and exudates on visual exam
	Encephalopathy	Papilledema
Brain	Cerebrovascular accident	Severe occipital headache, paralysis, speech difficulties, coma
	Encephalopathy	Rapid development of confusion, agitation, convulsions, death
Kidney	Renal insufficiency	Nocturia, proteinuria, elevated BUN, creatinine
	Renal failure	Fluid overload, accumulation of metabolites, metabolic acidosis

DIAGNOSIS OF HYPERTENSION

Correct and accurate measurement of the blood pressure is the key element of the physical examination for hypertension. The blood pressure should be measured after at least 5 minutes of rest and in several positions. The usual recommended positions for recording blood pressures include the right and left arm sitting, right arm supine, and right leg prone position.

Examination for vascular insufficiency, including peripheral pulses, is essential. Evidence of cardiac involvement may be revealed by gallop rhythms on auscultation or displacement of the point of maximal impulse (PMI) indicating cardiomegaly. Changes in the vascular bed of the eye may be noted on ophthalmic examination (see Table 20-3).

A complete health history should be taken and tests, including an electrocardiogram, intravenous pyelogram, blood urea, and creatinine should be made. Sometimes an electroencephalogram may also be indicated. All of the tests are to determine presence and extent of target organ damage.

The prognosis for uncontrolled hypertension is dismal. Statistics of premature death correlate with levels of blood pressure elevation. The risk of cerebrovascular accident, for example, is 5 times higher for hypertensive than for normotensive individuals. Better case finding and proper treatment has improved the outlook for victims of systemic hypertension.

REFERENCES

1. Alderman, M. H. *Hypertension: The Nurse's Role in Ambulatory Care.* New York: Springer, 1977.
2. Bullpitt, C. J., Dollery, C. T., and Carne, S. Change in symptoms of hypertensive patients after referral to hospital clinic. *Br. Heart J.* 38:121, 1976.
3. Dustan, H. P. Systemic Arterial Hypertension. In J. W. Hurst, et al. (eds.), *The Heart* (5th ed.). New York: McGraw-Hill, 1982.
4. Gotto, A. M. Diagnosis and Management of Risk Factors for Atherosclerosis. In A. M. Gotto, et al. (eds.), *Atherosclerosis.* Kalamazoo, Mich.: Upjohn, 1972.

5. Hall, W. D., Wollam, G. L., and Tuttle, E. P. The Diagnostic Approach to the Patient with Hypertension. In J. W. Hurst, et al. (eds.), *The Heart* (5th ed.). New York: McGraw-Hill, 1982.
6. Laragh, J. H. Trends: Research and Treatment in High Blood Pressure. In M. H. Alderman (ed.), *Hypertension: The Nurse's Role in Ambulatory Care.* New York: Springer, 1977.
7. McGurn, W. C. *People with Cardiac Problems: Nursing Concepts.* Philadelphia: Lippincott, 1981.
8. Santos-Buch, C. A. The Pathology of High Blood Pressure. In M. H. Alderman, (ed.), *Hypertension: The Nurse's Role in Ambulatory Care.* New York: Springer, 1977.

CHAPTER 21
ALTERATIONS IN SYSTEMIC CIRCULATION

LEARNING OBJECTIVES

1. Define *atherosclerosis* and *arteriolosclerosis.*
2. Describe the clinical effects of atherosclerosis in the abdominal aorta; aorta-iliac, femoral, carotid, and cerebral arteries; and the renal and mesenteric arteries.
3. Explain how a thrombus can become an embolus.
4. Describe the pathologic process of arteriosclerosis obliterans.
5. List the symptoms and signs that are characteristic of arteriosclerosis obliterans.
6. Differentiate among the pain of intermittent claudication, rest pain, ulceration, and gangrene.
7. Describe the etiology, site, and signs and symptoms of the major types of aneurysms.
8. Differentiate between Raynaud's phenomenon and Raynaud's disease.
9. Describe the typical color changes in Raynaud's disease.
10. Describe thromboangiitis obliterans (Buerger's disease).
11. Describe the pathologic characteristics of thromboangiitis.
12. Enumerate the signs and symptoms of arterial insufficiency to a limb.
13. List the three major predisposing factors in venous thrombosis.
14. Differentiate between the types of thrombophlebitis.
15. Compare superficial and deep thrombophlebitis with respect to signs, symptoms, and complications.
16. Describe the mechanism that causes chronic venous insufficiency.
17. Describe the etiology of varicose veins.
18. List at least three contributing factors that lead to the development of varicosities.
19. Describe the pathologic physiology of venous insufficiency.
20. Identify the skin changes that may be associated with venous insufficiency.
21. Define *lymphedema, lymphangitis,* and *lymphadenitis.*
22. Differentiate between primary and secondary lymphedema.
23. Describe the following diagnostic procedures that are useful in the detection of peripheral vascular disease: arteriography, Doppler ultrasound, translumbar aortography, and peripheral arteriography.

Peripheral vascular disease is a term that, in its broadest sense, applies to disease of any of the blood vessels outside of the heart and to disease of the lymph vessels. This chapter includes diseases of the arteries, veins, and lymphatics.

Peripheral vascular disease is a general term that literally means hardening of the arteries but is used to describe a group of arterial disorders that exhibit thickening and loss of elasticity of the walls of the arteries. Generally included in this group are atherosclerosis, arteriolosclerosis, and Monckeberg's medial calcific sclerosis. Many of the changes in the vessels are closely related to advancing age but the onset of changes has been accelerated, probably by diet and other environmental factors.

PATHOLOGIC PROCESSES OF ARTERIES

Atherosclerosis

Atherosclerosis is a disease of the large and medium-sized arteries, which begins as a *fibrofatty plaque* on the intimal surface of the vessel (Fig. 21-1). It usually causes no symptoms until the impedance of arterial blood flow causes ischemia or infarction of the affected organ.

Many factors have been studied in the production of atherosclerosis. While not totally explanatory for every case, these factors have statistically been correlated to atherosclerotic plaque development (Table 21-1). All of the factors correlate, with multiple factors usually interacting to cause the pathology of the disease. Most of the statistics regarding atherosclerosis are related by myocardial infarction mortality, so that the actual incidence of extracardiac occlusive or nonocclusive atherosclerotic disease can only be surmised.

PATHOLOGY OF ATHEROSCLEROSIS. The possible precursor of the lesion of atherosclerosis is the *fatty streak* that is found beginning at about the age of 1 year in children. This streak is composed of lipid material that is deposited on the intima of arteries. When the atherosclerotic lesion forms, it is often referred to as an *atheroma* or an *atheromatous plaque*. It is composed of fatty and fibrofatty material with a white to yellow appearance; it protrudes into the artery and may combine with other localized atheromas to form a large mass [7]. The atheroma alone rarely causes arterial obstruction but does so when thrombosis and hemorrhage of the plaque occur (Fig. 21-2). Sometimes the atheromatous lesion causes medial weakening and aneurysmal dilatation of the artery [7]. Calcification of long-standing lesions is common and contributes to stiff, noncompliant vessels.

Because atherosclerosis can be induced in most animals by feeding them a diet high in cholesterol and because the disease process rarely occurs in humans unless the cholesterol is greater than 160 mg/dl, hyperlipidemia can be considered as a major causative factor. The lipid in the atheroma is derived from serum lipoproteins [7].

TABLE 21-1. Factors implicated in the development of atherosclerosis

Age	Increased incidence occurs with advancing age
Weight	Probably related to diet, obesity correlates with increased incidence of MI
Heredity	Increased incidence at an early age within certain families points to a familial predisposition that also may reflect dietary habits
Diet	Diets high in saturated fats with incidence of hyperlipidemia increases ischemic heart disease
Sex	Significantly increased in males until ages of 75 or greater when it approaches equality
Diabetes	Almost twofold increase as compared to nondiabetics; also, relates with obesity
Cigarette smoking	Correlates with amount of cigarettes smoked and decreases when smoking stopped
Hypertension	Correlates with degree of hypertension; diastolic pressure the most important figure
Occupation or life-style	Behavior pattern (type A or B personality) inconclusive but risk appears to be twofold with type A personality

TABLE 21-2. Clinical and pathologic effects of atherosclerosis in different anatomic sites

Site	Clinical and pathologic effect
Abdominal/terminal aorta	Ischemic effects in lower extremities; gangrene of toes, feet; effects of fusiform abdominal aneurysm; embolism of atherosclerotic debris to smaller arteries
Aortoiliac and femoral arteries	Intermittent claudication; gangrene of toes, feet; aneurysmal formation of iliac arteries
Coronary arteries	Angina pectoris; conduction disturbances; myocardial infarction
Carotid and vertebral arteries	Transient ischemic attacks; cerebrovascular accident (CVA) or stroke
Renal artery	Hypertension; renal ischemia (hematuria proteinuria)
Mesenteric arteries	Intestinal ischemia (ileus, bowel perforation with peritonitis)

Even though any vessel in the body may be affected by atherosclerosis, the aorta, the coronary, the carotid, and iliac arteries are affected with the greatest frequency. A wide range of clinical effects may result from the ischemia and infarction of specific areas. Table 21-2 summarizes some of the common clinical and pathologic effects.

Embolization from a thrombosed atheroma causes the characteristic signs of arterial occlusion: (1) diminished or absent pulses, (2) skin pallor and/or cyanosis, (3) pain, and (4) muscle weakness. A large embolus may arise from

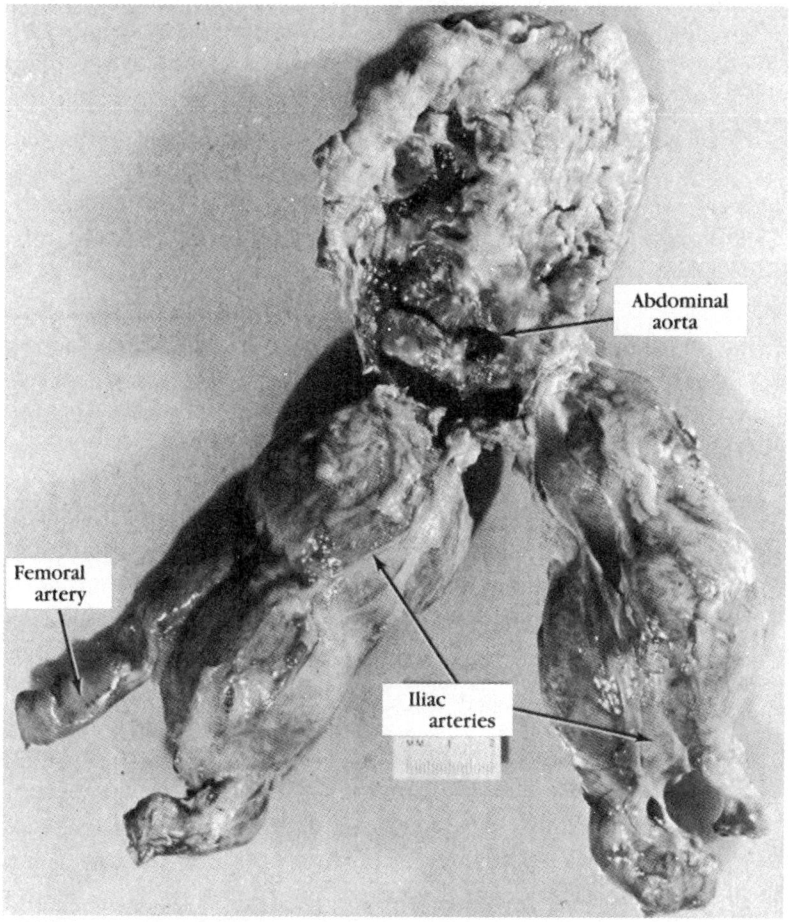

FIGURE 21-1. Abdominal aorta opened showing diffuse atherosclerotic plaques with ulceration. There are aneurysms of both common iliac arteries as viewed from the posterior aspect. (From J. Kernicki, B. Bullock, and J. Matthews, *Cardiovascular Nursing.* New York: Putnam, 1971.)

a thrombosed atheroma in the descending aorta and may travel to the terminal aorta. If the embolus occludes the iliac arteries and terminal aorta, it is known as a *saddle embolus.* The source of this embolus is usually the heart, either from a subendocardial infarction or from mitral valve disease.

Arteriosclerosis Obliterans

PATHOGENESIS OF ARTERIOSCLEROSIS OBLITERANS. A gradual occlusion of an atherosclerotic terminal aorta or of other large vessels can cause symptoms and signs of ischemia to the part supplied. In the terminal aorta these clinical manifestations include intermittent claudication, loss of peripheral hair, shiny skin, and impotence. The term *arteriosclerosis obliterans* is used to describe chronic occlusive arterial disease of the large arteries. It most commonly affects the terminal portion of the aorta and the large and

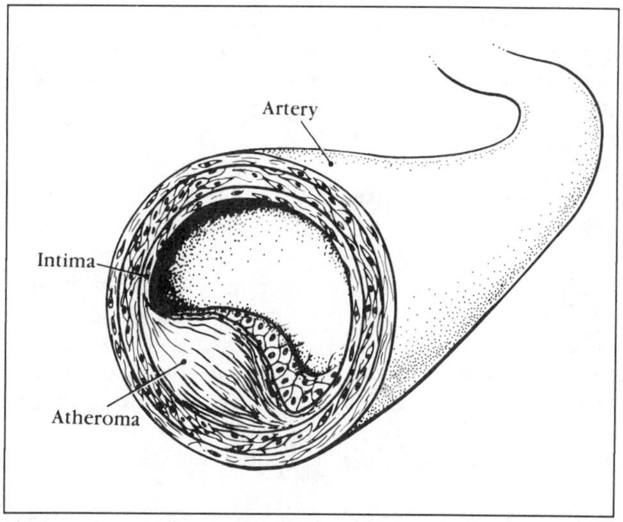

FIGURE 21-2. Schematic representation of an atheromatous plaque. A central area of necrosis and hemorrhage into the area both impinge on the lumen of the vessels.

medium arteries, especially those of the lower extremities. Arteriosclerosis obliterans is predominantly seen in men between the ages of 50 and 70. Diabetes mellitus increases the prevalence and severity of this disorder.

When a large artery is obstructed the pressure in the smaller arteries distal to the obstruction decreases and the blood flow declines. Thrombosis of the small arteries may follow and lead to gangrene if the cellular deprivation of oxygen is critical enough to cause cellular death. Gangrene may also occur if the ischemic area becomes infected, further increasing the need for blood supply.

PAIN. Various types of pain are described that are related to the degree of impairment of circulatory supply. ***Intermittent claudication*** is an aching, persistent, cramplike, and squeezing pain that occurs after a certain amount of exercise of the affected extremity. It is relieved by rest without change of position. This condition is a common complaint that occurs in almost all cases at some stage of the disease. It is frequently the first symptom noticed and often begins in the arch of the foot or calf of the leg. ***Rest pain*** is usually localized in the digits. It is described as a severe ache or a gnawing pain, often occurring at night, and persisting for hours at a time. Rest pain is caused by severe ischemia of tissues and sensory nerve terminals. Its onset may herald the onset of gangrene. It is aggravated by elevation of the extremity and often relieved by dependency. *Pain of ischemic neuropathy* usually occurs late in the course of progressive arteriosclerosis obliterans with severe ischemia. This severe pain is often associated with various types of paresthesias. It may be described as a lightening, shocklike sensation that usually occurs in both the foot and leg and follows the distribution of the peripheral sensory nerves. The pain of ulceration and gangrene is usually localized to the areas adjacent to ulcers or gangrenous tissue. It is severe, persistent, and usually worse at night. The pain is described as an aching sensation and sometimes may be associated with sharp, severe stabs of pain.

COLDNESS OR COLD SENSITIVITY. Coldness or sensitivity to cold is a frequent symptom of arteriosclerosis obliterans. Complaints of coldness in the digits or feet on exposure to a cold environment may be associated with color changes such as blanching or cyanosis.

IMPAIRED ARTERIAL PULSATIONS. Pulsation in the posterior tibial (PT) and dorsalis pedis (DP) arteries is impaired or absent in the majority of lower-extremity occlusions. Impairment of pulsations in the popliteal and femoral arteries is less frequent.

COLOR CHANGES. Affected extremities may be of a normal color but in advanced cases, cyanosis or an abnormal red color, called *rubor*, may be seen, particularly when the extremity is placed in a dependent position. Postural color changes are often asymmetric and affected extremities or digits become abnormally blanched after being elevated for a few minutes. When the extremity is placed in a dependent position a delay of 5 to 60 seconds may be required for color to return to the skin. The part first becomes abnormally red and then gradually the rubor lessens. The rubor is due to maximal dilatation of the arterioles and capillaries of the part [3]. The amount of color change relates to the severity of the vascular occlusion. The changes range from no postural change to a delay of up to 60 seconds for assumption of normal color.

ULCERATION AND GANGRENE. These lesions may occur spontaneously on an ischemic extremity or they may occur as a result of trauma such as pressure on the toenails from shoes. Gangrene may also result from bruises, nicks, or cuts in the skin; freezing; burning; or application of strong, irritating medicines or chemicals. Gangrene is usually confined to one extremity at a time. The lesion may be manifested by small spots on a digit or it may involve a whole extremity. Ulcers may develop on the tips of digits, between the toes, or at the base of the flexor surface of the toe. The area around the ulcer is painful and may be swollen or exhibit redness at the margin. Secondary infections are common and lead to abscess formation, cellulitis, and spread of infection.

EDEMA. In severe cases of arteriosclerosis obliterans edema of the feet and legs may occur. This edema is more evident when the legs are in a dependent position. Associated ischemic skin lesions, capillary atony, deep venous thrombosis, and lymphangitis contribute to the edema.

OTHER TROPHIC CHANGES. As a result of moderate to severe chronic ischemia small scars, depressions, or pitting on the tips of the digits may form. Nail growth is slow and the nail may become thickened and deformed. Paper-thin nails also may be seen. The digits or an entire foot may appear shrunken due to absorption of fat. The muscles atrophy and, therefore, the calf or thigh may decrease in size.

SUPERFICIAL THROMBOPHLEBITIS. At some stage of the disease superficial nonvaricose veins are involved in a type of thrombophlebitis. This occurs in approximately 40 percent of cases of arteriosclerosis obliterans. The smaller veins are usually involved with lesions or are red, raised, indurated, tender, cordlike veins that measure approximately 0.5 to 3.0 cm in length. The lesions usually cause permanent occlusion of the veins but the redness and symptoms of thrombophlebitis subside, usually in 1 to 3 weeks.

Aortic Aneurysms

An aneurysm is a localized dilation of the wall of an artery. It develops at a site of weakness of the medial layer of the artery. The majority of aneurysms are atherosclerotic in nature but they also may result from congenital defects, infections such as syphilis, and trauma.

Fusiform aneurysms produce circumferential dilatation of the vessel. The wall balloons out on all sides (Fig. 21-3). As the process is occurring the aneurysmal sac fills with

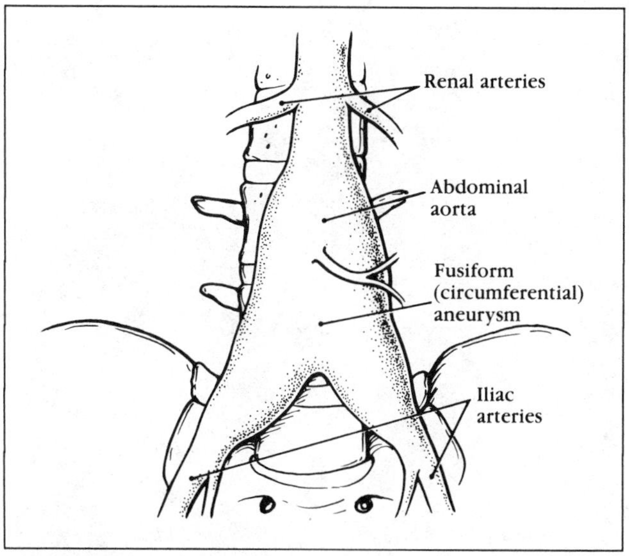

FIGURE 21-3. Fusiform aneurysm of the aorta.

necrotic debris and thrombus. Calcium infiltrates the area. The sac dilates because of a weakened medial layer. The dangers of this type of aneurysm include rupture, embolization to a peripheral artery, pressure on surrounding structures, and obstruction to blood flow of organs supplied by the tributary arteries.

ABDOMINAL AORTIC ANEURYSMS (AAA). Almost all AAAs are atherosclerotic and occur distal to the branchings of the renal arteries. They often extend to and include the iliac arteries. Clinical manifestations are usually nonexistent. Occasionally, the person will discover a pulsatile abdominal mass. More frequently, the aneurysm is discovered on physical examination for some other reason. Vague abdominal symptoms or poor peripheral circulation may cause the person to seek medical advice. Rupture may cause the initial symptoms with bleeding frequently occurring into the retroperitoneal space. This locality tends to prevent exsanguination due to the space limitation of the hemorrhage. The initial symptoms of this type of hemorrhage include abdominal pain and symptoms of hemorrhagic shock. Pressure from a large or enlarging AAA on surrounding abdominal organs along with lack of blood supply to the intestines can precipitate ileus or intestinal obstruction.

THORACIC ANEURYSMS. Thoracic aneurysms may be caused by atherosclerosis, necrosis of the medial layer, and syphilis. Atherosclerotic aneurysms are usually fusiform and are located in the arch and descending segments (see Fig. 21-3). Aneurysms that result from medial necrosis and syphilis are discussed later in this chapter. The most common clinical manifestation of thoracic aneurysm is deep, aching pain. This may be associated with erosion of the ribs or the pain may be an indication that expansion of the aneurysm is occurring and that rupture may be imminent [3]. Compression of respiratory structures and of the recurrent laryngeal nerve may cause dyspnea, hoarseness, and coughing. Rupture as the initial manifestation is usually fatal.

DISSECTING ANEURYSMS. This condition is not a true aneurysm and is often termed a *dissecting hematoma.* It requires an intimal tear and degeneration of the medial layer to allow blood to separate the intimal layer from the adventitial layer (Fig. 21-4). Aortic dissection most frequently occurs in the ascending aorta. Eighty percent of individuals having this problem also have systemic hypertension. It also may be associated with the hereditary disorder called *Marfan's syndrome.* Marfan's syndrome causes degeneration of the elastic fibers of the aortic media, usually beginning at the aortic root and spreading segmentally throughout the aorta. It is characterized by long extremities, thin hands and feet, lax ligaments, and deformities of the thoracic cage [4] (Fig. 21-5).

The clinical manifestations of dissection often present a striking change in appearance. External rupture may lead to exsanguination but, more frequently, the process involves dissection from the initial point away from the heart. As it dissects through the aortic segment it often causes obstruction to vessels branching off the aorta. If it occurs across the arch of the aorta, color changes and cerebral ischemia may be noted suddenly. Aortic regurgitation may result if the dissection occurs through the aortic valve.

Mortality for dissecting hematomas is very high. The initial 24-hour period after dissection has a 38 percent mortality with continuing high mortality in the first and second weeks following. One of the main factors that determine the mortality is the place of origin of dissection and whether the process is self-limiting.

SACCULAR ANEURYSMS. This type of aneurysm is frequently associated with syphilis or congenital malformations rather than atherosclerosis. These aneurysms are characterized by an outpouching on one side of an artery (Fig. 21-6). Common congenital saccular aneurysms are described as *berry aneurysms* when they occur on the arteries of the circle of Willis. The danger of the intracerebral aneurysms is intracranial rupture and bleeding, which often has a fatal outcome.

Saccular syphilitic aneurysms most frequently arise on the ascending and descending thoracic aorta. These can compress the mediastinal structures, cause pressure on the surrounding skeletal structures, thrombose, or rupture. Syphilitic or luetic aneurysms are rarely reported in the United States because of improved treatment measures for the control of syphilis.

Mönckeberg's Sclerosis

This type of arterial hardening causes focal calcification of the medial layer, especially in the medium-sized arteries. It is usually seen past the age of 50; the vessels become very hard because of the extensive calcification. In some cases atherosclerosis is associated with the calcification process but the process is not atherosclerotic in nature.

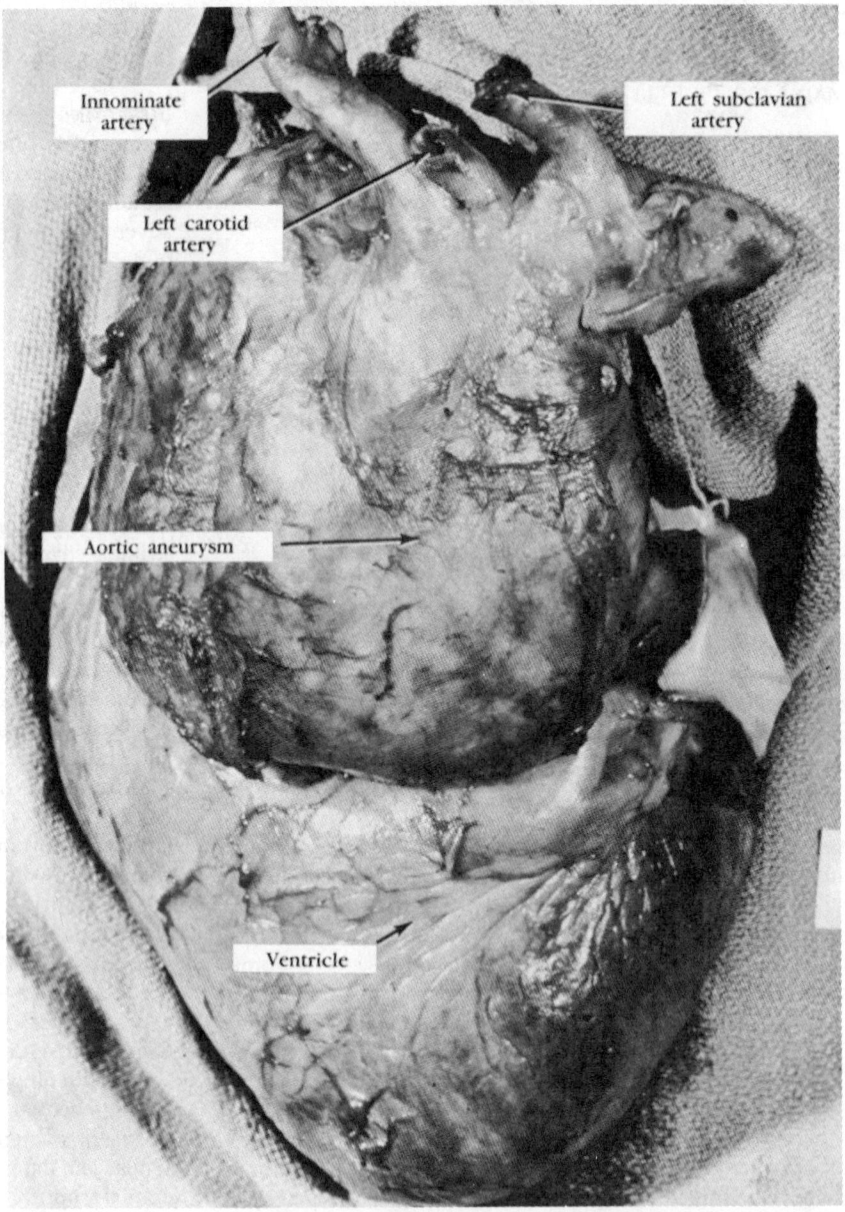

FIGURE 21-4. External view of the heart showing aneurysmal dilation of the ascending aorta and involvement of the arch. (From J. Kernicki, B. Bullock, and J. Matthews, *Cardiovascular Nursing*. New York: Putnam, 1971.)

Arteriolosclerosis

This condition, as its name implies, involves degeneration of the intima and media of small arteries and arterioles. When this affects the kidney hypertension results, but hypertension often is the initiator of the problem (see Chap. 19). This condition also may be seen in the peripheral arteries and arterioles of the aged and is considered by some to be a part of the process of aging.

Raynaud's Disease

Raynaud's phenomenon is defined as an episode of constriction of the small arteries or arterioles of the extremities, resulting in intermittent pallor and cyanosis of the skin of the extremities. After an episode of constriction, hyperemia may produce a red color (rubor). Raynaud's phenomenon may occur in association with a number of conditions and diseases. Raynaud's phenomenon, then, is a vasospastic disorder that produces temporary changes in skin color and often has no underlying pathologic basis.

Raynaud's disease occurs predominantly in women and heredity may play a role in its development. Onset of symptoms usually begins between the ages of 20 and 40. Because investigators rarely are able to examine sections of the blood vessels in cases of early Raynaud's disease, little is known of the pathologic changes in the early stages. In

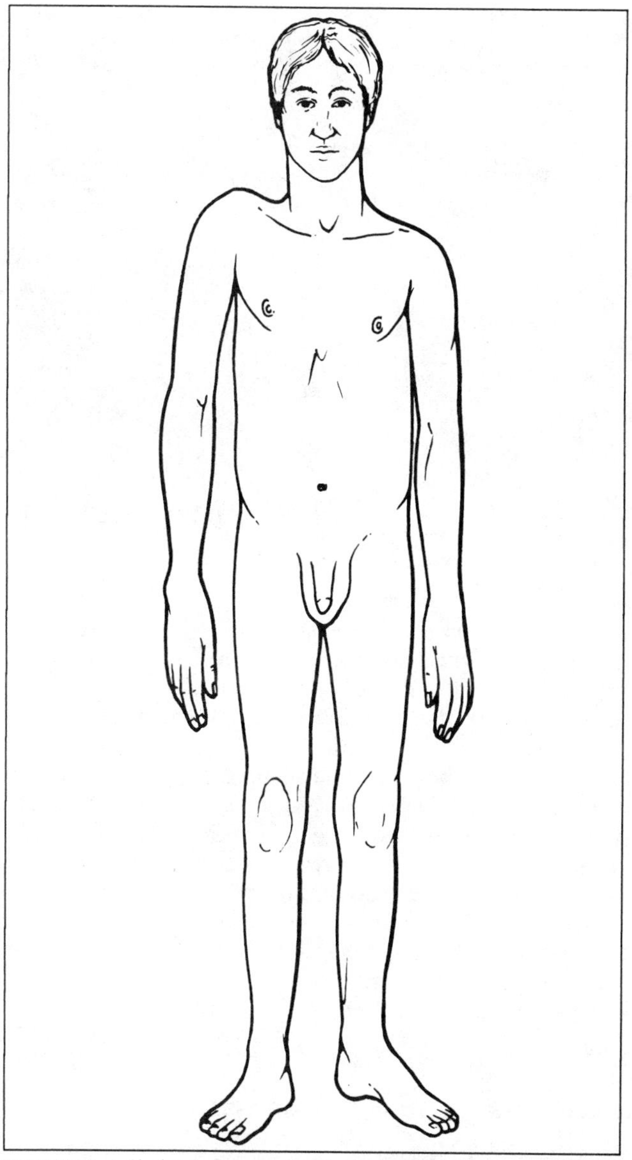

FIGURE 21-5. Skeletal changes in Marfan's syndrome.

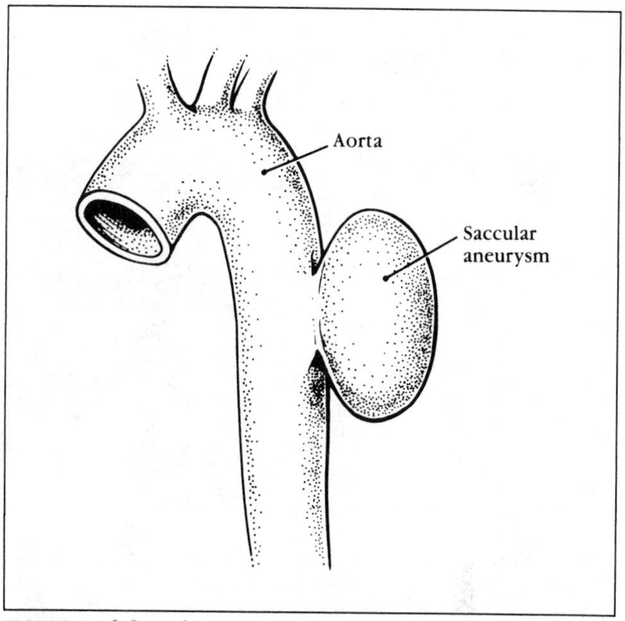

FIGURE 21-6. Saccular aneurysm of the descending aorta.

advanced stages the intima of the digital arteries is thickened.

The typical clinical picture of Raynaud's disease is color changes on exposure to cold. At first only the tips of the fingers are involved but later the more proximal parts also exhibit color changes. All of the fingers of both hands are usually involved with the color changes that include pallor, cyanosis, and rubor. The sequential color changes from pallor to cyanosis and finally rubor is a characteristic of the disease. Pallor is caused by spasm of the arterioles and possibly the venules. During this time blood flow into the capillaries is decreased or absent causing a dead white appearance in the affected part. Cyanosis results from capillary dilatation, which occurs later in the course of the disease. The blood flow becomes sluggish with extraction of more oxygen. Rubor indicates excessive hyperemia due to reactive vasodilatation. Exposure to emotional or thermal (cold) stimuli initiate color changes in the digits. Pain becomes associated when the disease is far advanced and often is associated with ulceration on the tips of the digits (Fig. 21-7). Paresthesias such as numbness, tingling, throbbing, and a dull ache may be present. During an actual attack, coldness of the digits is evident, sensory acuity is decreased, and swelling of the involved digits may occur.

Thromboangiitis or Buerger's Disease

Buerger's disease affects the medium-sized arteries and medium-sized, mostly superficial, veins of the extremities. It frequently results in arterial occlusion causing ischemia and gangrene to the extremities. This nonatherosclerotic lesion consists of microabscesses that have a central focus of polymorphonuclear leukocytes usually surrounded by mononuclear cells [4]. Histopathologic evidence indicates that Buerger's disease has some of the characteristics of a collagen or autoimmune disease.

Clinical manifestations include: invariable use of tobacco, frequent coexisting migratory phlebitis, early tenderness over the involved vessels, upper extremity involvement, absence of heart disease, marked early venospasm, and generally a low serum cholesterol concentration.

Pathologically, the disease has certain outstanding characteristics that may be stated as follows:

1. Thromboangiitis is primarily a disease of the blood vessels of the extremities. It involves the lower extremities more commonly and usually more severely than the upper extremities.
2. The disease almost always develops in medium-sized or small arteries. Arteries commonly involved are the pos-

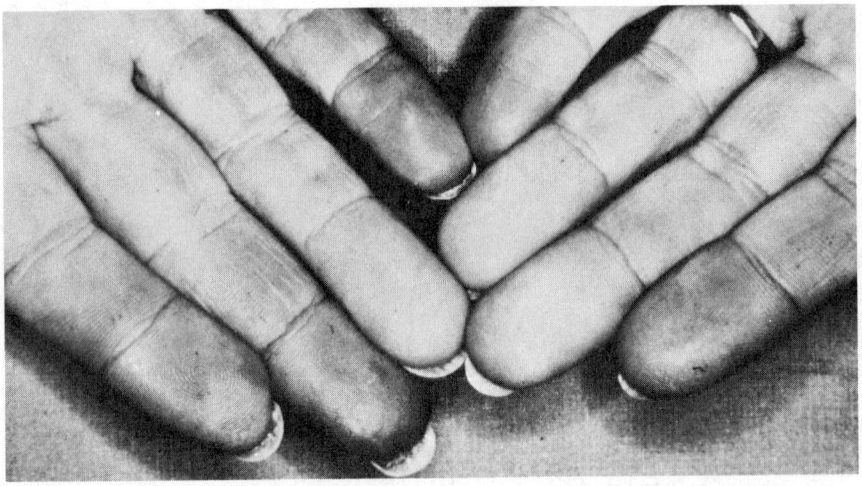

FIGURE 21-7. Cyanosis of the fingers in Raynaud's phenomenon. (From R. Judge, G. Zuidema, and F. Fitzgerald, *Clinical Diagnosis.* Boston: Little, Brown, 1982).

terior tibial, anterior tibial, radial, ulnar, plantar, palmar, and digital. Larger arteries, such as the femoral and brachial, are affected late and only when the disease is severe. Small and medium-sized veins are affected less commonly and large veins are rarely affected.
3. The lesions are focal or segmental and not diffuse.
4. The lesions appear to be of different ages, but in general the disease throughout a single affected segment seems to be of essentially the same age.
5. The disease produces occlusions of the vessels, followed by development of collateral and anastomotic vessels. The secondary anatomic effects of the disease are the result of ischemia of tissues [8].

The gross characteristics of the vessels affected by thromboangiitis obliterans vary depending on the ages of the lesions at the time they are examined. The vessels appear contracted at the site of destruction. The occluded segments are indurated but not brittle. The arteries are more frequently obliterated than their accompanying veins. In the diseased vessel the occlusion may extend for variable lengths and then stop abruptly. Occlusions may occur at two different levels in the same vessel and between these sites the vessel may be completely patent.

The most striking physiologic change is the impairment of arterial blood flow. There is reduced blood flow through peripheral arteries in the extremities, particularly in more distal portions. Another factor that contributes to ischemia is arteriolar spasm. The degree of spasm varies in different cases and may vary with the stage of the disease.

The degree of arterial insufficiency in the affected extremities depends on two factors: (1) the amount of arterial occlusive disease, and (2) the tone of the arterioles, which may vary from a normal tone to conditions of moderate or severe spasm.

Venous obstruction, the result of thrombophlebitis, may be an associated factor in the circulatory disturbance in thromboangiitis obliterans. The obstruction is often minor because in the venous circulation there is a great capacity for the development of collateral venous circulation. In some cases venous obstruction contributes to malnutrition of capillaries and a tendency to develop edema in the affected extremity if it remains in a dependent position for a long time.

Dependent rubor (an abnormal red color) is caused by the presence of numerous dilated capillaries in skin that contain blood of a high oxygen content [2]. This rubor is seen in cases of thromboangiitis associated with chronic and moderately severe arterial insufficiency. One explanation, supported by studies of the oxygen content of the venous blood, is that capillaries suffer from malnutrition and become atonic and their capacity for the interchange of oxygen and other metabolic products becomes impaired.

PATHOLOGIC PROCESSES OF VEINS

Obstructive Disease of Veins

Obstructive lesions of the veins may be permanent or temporary, partial or complete. Obstruction to some portion of the main trunk causes the distal large veins to become dilated with incompetent valves, and the small veins and venules may be damaged permanently as a result of pressure, stretching, hypoxemia, and malnutrition. Permanent impairment in interchange of fluid may result from disruption of small vessels. Damaged venous capillaries may function normally when the person is in a recumbent position but may show inadequacy in a standing position. This inadequacy is due to increased hydrostatic pressure and sometimes to associated incompetent valves.

VENOUS THROMBOSIS. Lesions in veins may produce localized thrombi in small veins or extensive thrombi in the larger veins. Venous thrombosis may develop as a result of an inflammatory or traumatic lesion of the endothelium of the vein wall. In the majority of cases, however, there is no evidence of either. An inflammatory reaction may develop in the wall of the vein as a reaction to primary thrombosis so that phlebitis may ensue several hours after the thrombus is formed.

Lesions of the endothelium, relative stasis of venous blood flow, and hypercoaguability of the blood are the three factors that precipitate venous thrombosis. One or a combination of these factors may produce a thrombus. A venous thrombus develops as a result of slowed flow in the venous bloodstream and is associated with platelet aggregation. It forms as a white thrombus at the head with red and white material at the tail. This represents fibrin, erythrocytes, platelets, and leukocyte components. The platelets accumulate in the slower moving periphery of the bloodstream and stick to the endothelium. Platelet aggregation is mediated by adenosine diphosphate (ADP), which is released by platelets. The platelets adhere to the site of a preexisting lesion of the endothelium. Platelets then tend to disintegrate, leukocytes are attracted, and a small amount of fibrin is precipitated. These events are followed by layered deposits of more platelets, fibrin, and leukocytes that may or may not occlude the lumen of the vein. The body and tail of the thrombus develop in the proximal direction (toward the heart). Probably increased coaguability of the blood is responsible for the development of the tail of the thrombus. The body and tail may develop rapidly. The tail may float free in the bloodstream for a short time but eventually it tends to adhere to the endothelium. When the tail adheres to the endothelium, organization by fibroblasts from the endothelium follows rapidly and the adhesion is complete [6].

As the body and tail of any thrombus extend, a portion or all of it may detach and become an embolus. Detachment may occur as the body or tail propagates past a juncture with a tributary vein or as it propagates into a larger trunk. The current from the tributary or larger trunk breaks the projecting portion or even the entire thrombus from its attachment. The tail of a thrombus may extend as far as the juncture of a large tributary vein and then stop. After several days and after development of a secondary reaction in the wall of the thrombosed vein, there may be a sudden proximal extension from the end of the original organizing thrombus. Emboli may develop at this time from the sudden proximal extension, or the new clot may stick and become organized. Emboli may be small or large and tend to lodge in the vessels of the pulmonary circulation (see Chap. 25) [6].

Thrombi organize from the outer margins centrally. In some veins the entire thrombus becomes organized with complete and permanent occlusion of the lumen. In a large thrombus, involution usually occurs by a process of partial fibrosis and partial lysis, which is probably due to the action of naturally occurring fibrinolysins in the blood. In most cases the center disappears and a varying portion of the periphery may organize on a fibrous ring. In other instances, bands of fibrous tissue extend across the old lumen of the vein and divide it into many small lumina. The ultimate result is usually some restoration of function of the vein, but the lumen is partially obstructed by the remaining fibrous tissue and decrease of its circular diameter [5].

The degree of inflammatory reaction in the different layers of the veins varies in different cases. In some the thrombus causes minimal reaction, while in others an intense reaction extends throughout all layers. Inflammatory cells, leukocytes, lymphocytes, and fibroblasts accumulate and cause a congestion of capillaries in and around the venous wall. Venous thrombosis causes obstruction to venous blood flow and relates to the size and location of the involved vein. If the thrombosis occurs in superficial veins and in short segments, collateral circulation will compensate. This may also be true in obstruction of the saphenous vein of the leg, or a larger vein of the arm, (such as the median basilic or cephalic) because of the numerous anastomoses that occur. Collateral channels may become evident even following obstruction of the superior or inferior vena cava [5].

When thrombosis occurs in the iliofemoral or axillary veins, the collateral circulation compensates only partially and venous pressure increases in the veins distal to the thrombosis. This increased pressure results in distention of all veins and even venules of the limb. The increased venous pressure in the venules and capillaries causes intense congestion of these areas. Pressure changes result in inhibition of normal resorption of fluid and electrolytes from the tissues in the venous end of the capillaries. Edema of the affected limb then occurs.

Thrombophlebitis and Phlebothrombosis

Thrombophlebitis refers to an inflamed vein as a result of a thrombus. Phlebothrombosis is probably the same entity but does not exhibit a marked inflammatory component. Thrombosis in a vein will ultimately cause inflammatory changes [6].

Idiopathic thrombophlebitis is a recurrent entity that produces segmental lesions in the small and medium-sized veins. The thrombus may be recanalized and the lumen restored but more frequently the vein becomes completely obliterated. *Suppurative thrombophlebitis* differs in that it usually results from bacterial invasion. The wall of the vein becomes markedly inflamed with leukocyte infiltration. Bacteria found within the thrombus and portions of the endothelium ultimately lead to abscesses. The abscesses may rupture into the bloodstream. *Chemical thrombophlebitis* may result from venous irritation from drugs (e.g., antibiotics or potassium) or other chemicals that gain access to the venous circulation. The thrombus becomes adherent and completely organized resulting in a vein that is contracted, fibrotic, and cordlike.

The symptoms and signs of thrombophlebitis develop acutely and usually persist for 1 to 3 weeks. With small or medium-sized vein involvement, acute thrombophlebitis rarely produces systemic reactions. With involvement of

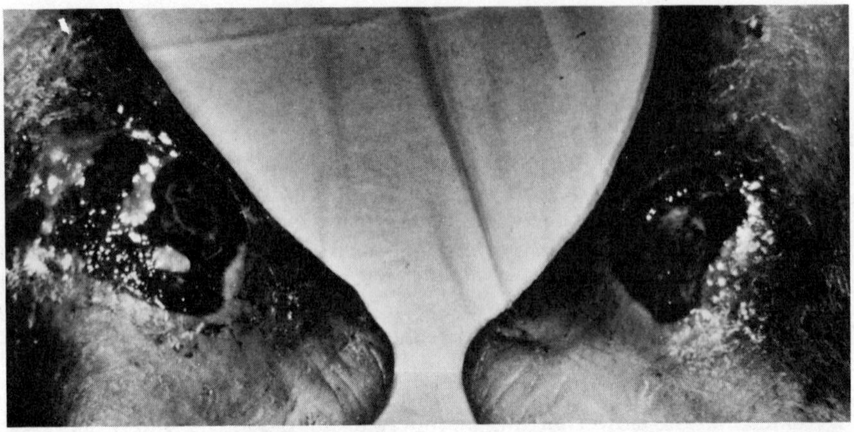

FIGURE 21-8. Bilateral stasis ulcers with surrounding dermatitis. (From R. Judge, G. Zuidema, and F. Fitzgerald, *Clinical Diagnosis*. Boston: Little, Brown, 1982.)

the larger vessels, a temperature rise to as high as 102°F (39°C) may be noted. Thrombosis of superficial veins often involves redness, pain, tenderness, and localized edema.

Thrombophlebitis of the deep veins of the legs produces calf pain and tenderness in the calf muscles. Enlargement of the calf and a positive Homan's sign may result. Thrombosis of the iliofemoral vein usually produces a typical acute clinical picture. Moderate to severe pain in the thigh and groin with diffuse pain throughout the limb is described. Superficial veins of that limb may be prominent and distended with an enlarged limb. The skin of the leg and thigh may be slightly cyanotic. Thrombosis is manifested by impaired or absent pulses from associated arterial spasm. Fever and tachycardia may also be associated. Pitting edema is characteristic with onset occurring a few days after the obstruction ensues. As the edema becomes chronic it may be associated with skin changes and brawny edema (thick, hardened skin with nonpitting edema).

Thrombosis of the axillary and subclavian veins produces a clinical picture similar to that produced in the leg by iliofemoral thrombosis. The axillary vein becomes tender, prominent, and enlarged with pitting edema being noticed in the forearm and hand. Superficial veins of the entire arm are prominent and superficial veins of the pectoral region of the affected side may be distended.

Venous Insufficiency and Stasis

Chronic venous insufficiency results from stasis of venous blood flow, especially of the iliofemoral veins. Old iliofemoral thrombophlebitis leaves behind a thickened inelastic vein wall, damaged venous valves, and a partially or sometimes completely obstructed lumen. In the lower extremity the three groups of veins — the deep, the communicating, and the superficial — normally have thin, elastic walls and segmentally spaced valves of the bicuspid type. Venous flow against gravity in the lower limbs is made possible by action of the calf muscle and the competent valves. Muscular compression of the elastic veins forces blood upward and the valves prevent retrograde flow. This mechanism fails in chronic venous insufficiency usually because of extensive damage from thrombophlebitis. Ambulatory venous pressure is high and this upsets the normal equilibrium of capillary fluid exchange causing development of congestion and edema. Stasis also results from the high ambulatory pressures as is manifested by changes in the skin and subcutaneous tissues around the distal third of the leg and around the ankle. Changes that may occur include edema, hyperpigmentation, dermatitis, induration, stasis cellulitis, and ultimately, venostasis ulcers (Fig. 21-8). Pain may or may not be present. A dull ache in the affected leg may develop after the individual has been standing for variable periods. Pain is usually described as being more severe when standing still rather than when walking. The pain usually disappears within 5 to 30 minutes after the assumption of a recumbent position with the leg elevated. Nocturnal muscular cramps may be reported.

Varicose Veins: Venous Varicosities

Varicosities are dilated, elongated, and tortuous veins. These occur most frequently in the lower extremities where they are manifested as dilated or incompetent superficial veins (Fig. 21-9). Varicose veins probably develop because of an inherent weakness in the structure of the vein. Superficial veins dilate when normal resistance against intraluminal pressure is lacking. Primary varicose veins may develop from hereditary predisposition, pregnancy, standing for long periods of time, and marked obesity. Prolonged periods of standing in certain occupations favor development of varicosities because of the high gravitational pressure within the veins. Obesity tends to place external pressure on the veins, especially the iliofemoral veins.

Deep thrombophlebitis often gives rise to secondary varicosities. Loss of valve sufficiency produces unusual strain on the superficial veins. A frequent finding in vari-

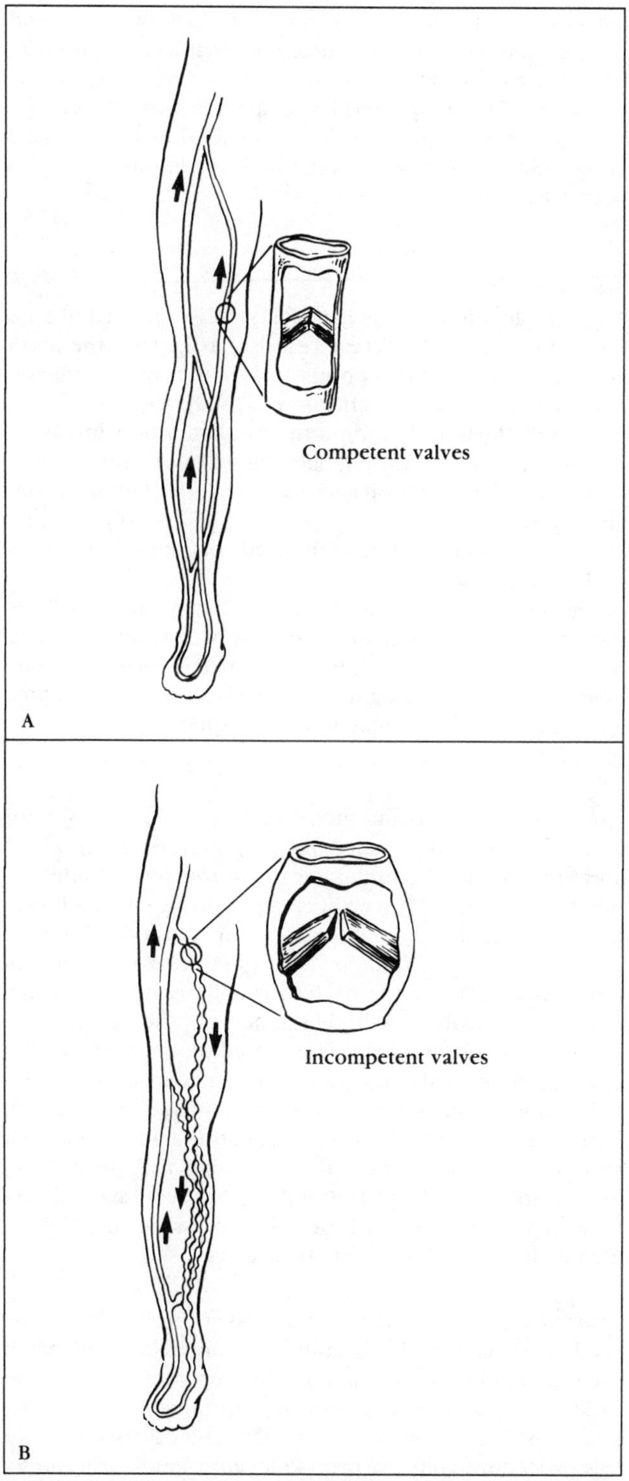

FIGURE 21-9. Chronic venous insufficiency. A. Competent valves, nondilatated vessel. B. Incompetent valves, dilatated vessel. In the leg varicose veins, B, there is retrograde flow due to incomplete closure of valves. (From E. A. Hincker and L. Malasanos [eds.], *The Little, Brown Manual of Medical-Surgical Nursing*. Boston: Little, Brown, 1983.)

cose veins is the presence of localized dilatations just distal to the venous valves. Valve incompetency is due primarily to extreme dilatation in the affected veins, which causes separation of the valve cusps. In primary varicose veins the incompetency tends to progress downward in the saphenous main channel as well as in its tributaries. In secondary varicose veins, which arise because of deep vein insufficiency, the incompetency tends to progress upward from incompetent perforating veins in the lower third of the leg [1].

Varicose veins can lead to chronic venous insufficiency. In the early stages localized pain and heat may be noticed after prolonged standing. Persistent edema may develop along with trophic skin changes and stasis ulcers. The varicose ulcers heal slowly and often become infected.

Diagnosis of venous insufficiency can be made by assessment of physical findings, and occasionally phlebography. *Phlebography* involves the injection of radiopaque material into the venous system with x-ray views of the injected area. It is utilized to localize deep vein thrombosis or to evaluate varicosities.

PATHOLOGIC PROCESSES OF THE LYMPHATIC SYSTEM

The lymphatic system serves the essential function of draining excess fluids and proteins from the interstitial space. It provides the only means for returning plasma proteins that have leaked into this space to the general circulation. Whenever the tissue fluid increases, lymphatic drainage also increases. In this way, lymphatic flow is an essential method for control of tissue fluid volume. Venous obstruction and congestive heart failure have been identified as factors that can alter capillary pressure and produce edema. In situations where there is chronic escape of fluids into the interstitial spaces, edema may not be noted because of compensation by the lymphatic system.

Obstruction of the lymph vessels interferes with this control mechanism and may precipitate or contribute to edema. Multiple etiologic factors may cause lymphedema and these may be categorized as inflammatory or noninflammatory. *Lymphangitis* is the term utilized for inflammation of the lymph vessels, usually by bacterial organisms. *Lymphadenitis* refers to inflammation that involves the lymph nodes. *Lymphedema* is a term utilized for edema resulting from lymphatic obstruction.

Primary or idiopathic lymphedema is rare. Milroy's disease, a congenital lymphedema noticeable at birth, is usually caused by faulty development of lymphatic channels. *Lymphedema praecox* affects females predominantly between the ages of 9 and 25. It is characterized by swelling of one or both feet that becomes progressive and unremitting. The lymphatic channels are noted to be dilated with incompetence of the lymph valves.

Secondary lymphedema is much more common than the primary form. Obstruction to the lymph channels may result from malignant metastatic infiltration of the lymph nodes and channels. Hodgkin's disease, which primarily affects the lymphatic system, also may cause obstruction to the channels. Inflammation or infection of the channels may result in fibrosis and obstruction. A final, very common cause of lymphedema is the surgical removal or irradiation of lymph nodes to prevent the spread of a malignant process.

Lymphedema is essentially the result of stasis. Chronic stasis often leads to *brawny* edema, which describes the appearance of the skin subjected to continual stretch. The skin becomes thick, hardened, infiltrated with plasma proteins, and often "orange-peel" in appearance. The edema produced differs from cardiac edema in that it does not pit on digital pressure.

Inflammatory lymphedema usually follows an acute infection of the lymphatic system. Lymphangitis is characterized by painful red streaks following the lymph vessels, which may eventually involve the lymph nodes as well. The most common agent for causation of lymphangitis is the β-hemolytic streptococcus organism but any virulent pathogen may initiate it. The systemic effects include a marked temperature elevation, malaise, and chills. Localized edema occurs and may become progressive if attacks are recurrent. *Chronic lymphangitis* may follow causing fibrosis of the affected area, further edema, skin changes, and sometimes ulcerations.

Diagnosis of lymphedema is primarily to differentiate this form of edema from edema of venous origin. Lymphangiography involves the injection of radiopaque dye into the affected lymph vessel and radiologic inspection. This procedure may localize the source of the lymphatic obstruction.

DIAGNOSTIC PROCEDURES FOR VASCULAR LESIONS

Physical Examination

Diagnosis of vascular system problems is usually based on the signs and symptoms of arterial occlusion or of venous insufficiency. Palpation of the peripheral pulses is important in estimating the blood flow in the peripheral arterial circuit. Systolic bruits over the abdominal area and femoral artery are common and in association with other signs may indicate peripheral arterial disease. Tenderness to palpation or tenderness with the inflation of a blood pressure cuff over the calf or thigh (Lowenberg's cuff sign) gives high suspicion for deep vein thrombosis. Pain on stretching of the gastrocnemius muscle (Homan's sign) also may be present [5]. Ankle edema, especially unilateral, may be seen. Many procedures may be performed to clearly diagnose vascular lesions. Several of these are discussed in this section.

Doppler Ultrasound

This procedure involves the use of a Doppler recorder to hear flow over the larger veins. It is normally increased by distal compression of the vein, decreased by the Valsalva maneuver, and varies with respiration. Lack of flow sound may indicate venous thrombosis. Arterial lesions also may be evaluated by Doppler studies. The proximal and distal pressures of the suspected lesion are auscultated to determine the pressure gradient. The Doppler flowmeter is used at the ankle to compare arterial pressure in the ankle with brachial systolic pressure.

Angiography

Angiography involves the use of a contrast material of high opacity to outline the great vessels, particularly the aorta and its branches. The contrast material may be injected into an artery, vein, or a chamber of the heart.

In individuals with symptoms of obstruction involving the superior vena cava, angiography will show the site and extent of the obstruction and may give important data concerning the nature of the obstructing lesion. Angiography also may be of great value in the study of known aneurysms of the thoracic aorta.

Specific procedures used for visualizing special vessels include (1) translumbar aortography, which is used mainly to study aortoiliofemoral thromboocclusive disease, (2) renal arteriography, (3) visceral arteriography, and (4) inferior venacavography, especially to identify caval thrombosis.

TRANSLUMBAR AORTOGRAPHY. In the presence of severe atherosclerosis the translumbar puncture method of aortography may be preferable to retrograde catheterization from a femoral artery because of the hazards: injuring the arterial wall and embolization from a dislodged thrombus or plaque; perforations; and aggravation of thrombus formation. Because arteriosclerosis obliterans of the lower extremities involves multiple segments of the vascular system it is important to evaluate the inflow proximal to the diseased artery. This procedure carries the main risk of retroperitoneal bleeding from direct puncture of the aorta. Careful assessment of blood coagulation and blood pressure are necessary prior to performing this procedure. Aortography can detail the entire peripheral arterial system. Renal arteries can be evaluated for stenosis by injecting dye at the level of these arteries.

PERIPHERAL ARTERIOGRAPHY. Femoral arteriography can be used when aortic visualization is unnecessary and when the lesion is limited to the leg. This approach also may be used to pass a catheter retrograde up the aorta to the desired position for dye injection. The clinical usefulness of this procedure is in the precise localization of atherosclerotic disease and sometimes in thromboangiitis obliterans and aneurysms.

REFERENCES

1. Fairbairn, J. F. II, Juergens, J. L., and Spittell, J. A., Jr. *Peripheral Vascular Diseases* (4th ed.). Philadelphia: Saunders, 1972. P. 606.

2. Fairbairn, J. F. II, Juergens, J. L., and Spittell, J. A., Jr. *Peripheral Vascular Diseases* (4th ed.). Philadelphia: Saunders, 1972. P. 336.
3. Lindsay, J., DeBakey, M. E., and Beall, A. C. Diseases of the Aorta. In J. W. Hurst, et al. (eds.), *The Heart* (5th ed.). New York: McGraw-Hill, 1982.
4. McKusick, V. A., et al. Buerger's disease: A distinct clinical and pathologic entity. *J.A.M.A.* 181:5, 1962.
5. Perdue, G. D., and Smith, R. B. Diseases of the Peripheral Veins and the Venae Cavae. In J. W. Hurst, et al. (eds.), *The Heart* (5th ed.). New York: McGraw-Hill, 1982.
6. Robbins, S., and Cotran, R. *Pathologic Basis of Disease* (2nd ed.). Philadelphia: Saunders, 1979.
7. Ross, R. Factors Influencing Atherogenesis. In J. W. Hurst, et al. (eds.), *The Heart* (5th ed.). New York: McGraw-Hill, 1982.
8. Young, J. R., and de Wolfe, V. G. Diseases of the Peripheral Arteries. In J. W. Hurst, et al. (eds.), *The Heart* (5th ed.). New York: McGraw-Hill, 1982.

BIBLIOGRAPHY

Alderman, M. H. *Hypertension: The Nurse's Role in Ambulatory Care.* New York: Springer, 1977.

Alpert, J. S., and Francis, G. S. *Manual of Coronary Care.* (2nd ed.). Boston: Little, Brown, 1980.

Berne, R. M. The role of adenosin in the regulation of coronary blood flow. *Circ. Res.* 47:807, 1980.

Berne, R. M., and Levy, M. D. *Cardiovascular Physiology* (4th ed.). St. Louis: Mosby, 1981.

Borg, N., et al. *Care Curriculum for Critical Care Nursing* (2nd ed.). Philadelphia: Saunders, 1981.

Braunwald, E. *Heart Disease.* Philadelphia: Saunders, 1980.

Chang, S. *Echocardiography: Techniques and Interpretation.* Philadelphia: Lea & Febiger, 1981.

Christopherson, D. J., and Sivarajan, E. S. Infective Endocarditis. In S. L. Underhill, et al. (eds.), *Cardiac Nursing.* Philadelphia: Lippincott, 1982.

Chung, E. K. *Principles of Cardiac Arrhythmias.* Baltimore: Williams & Wilkins, 1982.

Davis, M. J. *Pathology of Cardiac Valves.* Woburn, Mass.: Butterworth, 1980.

Dawber, T. R. *The Framingham Study Series: Commonwealth Fund.* Cambridge, Mass.: Harvard University Press, 1980.

deFaire, U., and Theorell, T. *Life Stress and Coronary Heart Disease.* St. Louis: Warren Green, 1982.

Disch, J. M. *Diagnostic Procedures for Cardiovascular Disease. Series 2: Surgical Aspects of Cardiovascular Disease.* New York: Appleton-Century-Crofts, 1979.

Doroghazi, R. M., and Slater, E. E. *Aortic Dissection.* New York: McGraw-Hill, 1983.

Dresdak, R. J. DD and management of cardiogenic shock. *Med. Times* 104:50, 1976.

Durack, D. T. Infective and Non-Infective Endocarditis. In J. W. Hurst, et al. (eds.), *The Heart* (5th ed.). New York: McGraw-Hill, 1982.

Eich, R. *Introduction to Cardiology.* Hagerstown, Md.: Harper & Row, 1980.

Feigenbaum, H. *Echocardiography* (3rd ed.). Philadelphia: Lea & Febiger, 1981.

Felner, J. M. Techniques of Echocardiography. In J. W. Hurst, et al. (eds.), *The Heart* (5th ed.). New York: McGraw-Hill, 1982.

Fortuin, N. J. Echocardiography: How it works. *Med. Times* 108, 120, 1980.

Foster, S. B. Pump failure following myocardial infarction: An overview. *Heart Lung* 9:293, 1980.

Fowler, N. O. *Cardiac Diagnosis and Treatment* (3rd ed.). Hagerstown, Md.: Harper & Row, 1980. Pp. 186–317.

Fowler, N. *Cardiac Disease and Treatment.* Hagerstown, Md.: Harper & Row, 1980.

Friedman, S. A. *Vascular Diseases: A Concise Guide to Diagnosis, Management, Pathogenesis and Prevention.* Littleton, Mass.: Wright-PSG Publishing, 1982.

Genest, J., et al. *Hypertension: Physiopathology and Treatment* (2nd ed.). New York: McGraw-Hill, 1983.

Goldberger, E. *Textbook of Clinical Cardiology.* St. Louis: Mosby, 1982.

Gotto, A. M., et al. *Atherosclerosis: A SCOPE Publication.* Kalamazoo, Mich.: Upjohn, 1977.

Gröer, M. E., and Shekleton, M. E. *Basic Pathophysiology: A Conceptual Approach.* St. Louis: Mosby, 1979. Pp. 217–253.

Guyton, A. C. *Textbook of Medical Physiology* (5th ed.). Philadelphia: Saunders, 1981.

Heller, L. J., and Mohrman, D. E. *Cardiovascular Physiology.* New York: McGraw-Hill, 1981.

Holling, H. E. *Peripheral Vascular Diseases: Diagnosis and Management.* Philadelphia: Lippincott, 1972. Pp. 38–56.

Honig, C. *Modern Cardiovascular Physiology.* Boston: Little, Brown, 1981.

Jackle, M., and Halligan, M. *Cardiovascular Problems: A Critical Care Nursing Focus.* Bowie, Md.: Brady, 1980.

Johnson, R., Haber, E., and Austen, W. (eds.). *The Practice of Cardiology.* Boston: Little, Brown, 1980.

Jones, R. J. An overview of cardiogenic shock: Approaches. *Primary Cardiol.* 9:38, 1976.

Juergens, J. L. Thromboangitis Obliterans (Buerger's Disease). In J. Fairbairn, II, J. L. Juergens, and J. A. Spittell, Jr. (eds.), *Peripheral Vascular Diseases* (4th ed.). Philadelphia: Saunders, 1972. Pp. 327–349.

Juergens, J. L., et al. *Peripheral Vascular Disease* (5th ed.). Philadelphia: Saunders, 1980.

Karassi, A. *Acute Myocardial Infarction.* New York: McGraw-Hill, 1980.

Kelman, G. R. *Applied Cardiovascular Physiology.* Woburn, Mass.: Butterworth, 1977.

Levine, H. *Clinical Cardiovascular Physiology.* New York: Grune & Stratton, 1976.

Little, R. *Physiology of the Heart and Circulation* (2nd ed.). Chicago: Year Book, 1982.

MacIver, A. G., et al. The pathology of arterial disease. *Br. J. Anaesth.* 53:675, 694, 1981.

Marcus, M. L. *The Coronary Circulation in Health and Disease.* New York: McGraw-Hill, 1983.

Martin, L. B., and Cohen, L. S. Cardiomyopathy. *DM* 28:13, 1981.

Mason, D. T. *Congestive Heart Failure: Mechanisms, Evaluation and Treatment.* New York: Yorke, 1976.

McGurn, W. C. *People with Cardiac Problems: Nursing Concepts.* Philadelphia: Lippincott, 1981.

Messen, J. V. Cardiogenic shock: Etiological and pathophysiological considerations, monitoring and management. *Pract. Cardiol.* 6:86, 1978.

Miller, D. C., and Roon, A. J. *Diagnosis and Management of Peripheral Vascular Disease.* Reading, Mass.: Addison-Wesley, 1982.

Moore, H. D., and Rinehart, J. F. Histogenesis of coronary arteriosclerosis. *Circulation* 6:481, 1952.

Mudge, G. H. *Manual of Electrocardiography.* Boston: Little, Brown, 1981.

Price, S. A., and Wilson, L. M. *Pathophysiology Clinical Concepts of Disease Processes* (2nd ed.). New York: McGraw-Hill, 1982.

Rackley, C. E., et al. Aortic Valve Disease. In J. W. Hurst, et al. (eds.), *The Heart* (5th ed.). New York: McGraw-Hill, 1982.

Resnikow, L., and Desmond, Y. (eds.). *Friedberg's Diseases of the Heart* (4th ed.). London: Churchill-Livingstone, 1982.

Rias, J. *Clinical Electrocardiographic Correlations.* Philadelphia:

Davis, 1977.
Robbins, S. L., and Cotran, R. S. *Pathologic Basis of Disease* (2nd ed.). Philadelphia: Saunders, 1979.
Ross, J., and Peterson, K. L. Cardiac Catheterization and Angiography. In K. J. Isselbacher, et al. (eds.), *Harrison's Principles of Internal Medicine* (9th ed.). New York: McGraw-Hill, 1980.
Rushmer, R. F. *Structure and Function of the Cardiovascular System.* Philadelphia: Saunders, 1976.
Russek, H. I., and Zohman, B. L. *Coronary Heart Disease.* Philadelphia: Lippincott, 1971.
Shamroth, L. *The Disorders of Cardiac Rhythm* (2nd ed.). St. Louis: Blackwell/Mosby, 1980.
Shoenberg, B. S. *Precursors of Stroke: Etiologic, Preventive and Therapeutic Implications.* New York: Oxford University Press, 1982.
Silverman, M. D., et al. *Electrocardiography: Basic Concepts and Clinical Application.* New York: McGraw-Hill, 1983.
Smith, L., and Thier, S. *Pathophysiology.* Philadelphia: Saunders, 1981.
Sodeman, W., and Sodeman, W. *Pathologic Physiology.* Philadelphia: Saunders, 1979.
Sokolow, M., and McIlroy, M. B. *Clinical Cardiology* (2nd ed.). Los Altos, Calif.: Lange, 1979.
Sonnerblick, E., and Lisch, M. *Valvular Heart Disease.* New York: Grune & Stratton, 1974.
Tilkian, S. M., Conover, M. B., and Tilkian, A. G. *Clinical Implications of Laboratory Tests* (2nd ed.). St. Louis: Mosby, 1979. Pp. 61–101.
White, B. B. *Therapy in Acute Coronary Care.* Chicago: Year Book, 1972.
Williams, R. C. Bacterial Endocarditis: An Analysis of Immunopathology. In E. Kaplan and A. Taranta (eds.), *Infective Endocarditis.* Dallas: American Heart Association, 1977.
Woodcock, J. P. Special ultrasonic methods for the assessment and imaging of systemic arterial disease. *Br. J. Anaesth.* 53:719, 1981.
Yu, P. N., and Goodwin, J. F. *Progress in Cardiology* (vol. 10.). Philadelphia: Lea & Febiger, 1982.

UNIT 9
RESPIRATION

Barbara L. Bullock
NORMAL RESPIRATORY FUNCTION
RESTRICTIVE AND OBSTRUCTIVE ALTERATIONS

Joseph Andrews
OXYGEN–CARBON DIOXIDE EXCHANGE
HYPOXIA-HYPERCAPNEA

Eileen Sjoberg
LUNG CLEARANCE AND DEFENSE

Carol Stephenson
VENTILATION/DIFFUSION/PERFUSION

This unit has been divided into four chapters, each of which deals with aspects of the pulmonary system. Chapter 22 emphasizes the normal anatomy and physiology of the pulmonary system. The content is intended as a review that provides the basis for the subsequent chapters relating to the pathophysiologic process of the pulmonary system. Chapters 23, 24, and 25 deal with various aspects of pathophysiology of the pulmonary system.

Diseases of the pulmonary system have been categorized as restrictive, obstructive, and other pulmonary alterations. There is necessarily some overlap between these categories but an attempt to classify them according to functional impairments has been made. The chapters contain discussion of pathologic, clinical, and diagnostic aspects of pulmonary disease, but discussion of treatment and therapeutic care of the individual have been excluded.

The reader is encouraged to utilize the learning objectives as study guides and to supplement the material with references found in the unit bibliography.

CHAPTER 22
NORMAL RESPIRATORY FUNCTION

LEARNING OBJECTIVES

1. Describe the normal basic pulmonary anatomy.
2. Describe the action of the pulmonary pumping mechanism.
3. Identify the mechanisms of nervous control in the respiratory tract.
4. Compare the concepts of compliance and elasticity in the normally functioning pulmonary system.
5. Describe the importance of the anatomic dead space in pulmonary function.
6. Identify the major muscles of respiration and their function.
7. Compare tissue resistance and airway resistance.
8. Relate the concept of work of breathing to oxygen consumption and carbon dioxide production.
9. Describe the major patterns of airway resistance.
10. Describe the anatomy and dynamics of pulmonary perfusion.
11. Compare normal ventilation and perfusion from the apex to the base of the lung.
12. List factors that alter ventilation and perfusion.
13. List the normal pressures in the heart and pulmonary vascular system.
14. Relate the oxyhemoglobin dissociation curve to tissue oxygenation.
15. Outline the pattern of normal gas exchange.
16. Describe the function of surfactant in the alveoli.
17. Describe the function of alpha$_1$ antitrypsin in the lung.
18. Identify deposition sites of particulates in the airway.
19. List the major protective reflexes of the lung.
20. Explain the function of the mucociliary transport system in the defense of the lungs.
21. Trace the clearance of particulates from the alveoli.
22. Distinguish between humoral and cell-mediated immunity in the lung.
23. Describe the role of the macrophages in the lung.
24. Explain the probable activity of interferon.

To delineate clearly the pathophysiology of respiratory diseases, the material presented in this chapter will review the anatomy and physiology of the pulmonary system including an in-depth discussion of the following essential concepts: compliance, elasticity, resistance, ventilation, perfusion, diffusion, and alveolar airway clearance in health. A description of pulmonary function tests is also included.

To live is to breathe. Between a newborn's first breath, inspiration, and the last expiration is a lifetime of respiration. Breathing is the only bodily function that occurs automatically and can be controlled voluntarily as well. It is also the only bodily function that immediately interacts with the environment whatever it may be: a fresh ocean breeze, stale cigarette smoke, a noxious automobile exhaust, a damp cellar, or a dusty workplace. Normally, breathing occurs below the level of consciousness, rhythmically and inconspicuously, unless some kind of physical stress interferes, such as breathlessness after running, swimming, or climbing a mountain, or when the lungs are impaired by diseases such as asthma, emphysema, bronchitis, pneumonia, or fibrosis.

The human body must adapt itself continually to an unfriendly environment. The lungs, as one of the body's frontiers, are constantly attacked by irritants, noxious gases, and microorganisms. Consequently, the respiratory apparatus has developed an elaborate defense system to protect itself and the body from these inhalants.

The lungs take oxygen from the air and deliver it across the alveolar-capillary membrane to the hemoglobin. It is transported on the hemoglobin by the circulation of blood to the tissues. At the tissue line it diffuses across the cellular membrane to the mitochondria to aid in energy production to support the metabolic processes of life. As a result of these metabolic processes, carbon dioxide is produced that is transported through a reverse pathway and expelled into the air.

ANATOMY OF THE PULMONARY TREE

Airways

Air normally enters the body through the nose or the mouth. Here, and in the pharynx, it is warmed, moistened, and filtered. Even though air has been filtered in the upper respiratory tract, it is not sterile when it reaches the lower respiratory tract. Much debris remains, as evidenced by autopsies of the lungs of smokers or those exposed to heavy air pollution.

The air passes through the larynx and into the respiratory tree, which is a series of successively smaller, branching tubes (Fig. 22-1). Immediately below the larynx is the trachea, which divides at a point called the carina into the right and left main stem bronchi. The right main stem bronchus is shorter and wider than the left, coming off the trachea in a nearly straight line (Fig. 22-2). This explains why aspirated objects and fluids lodge more frequently in the

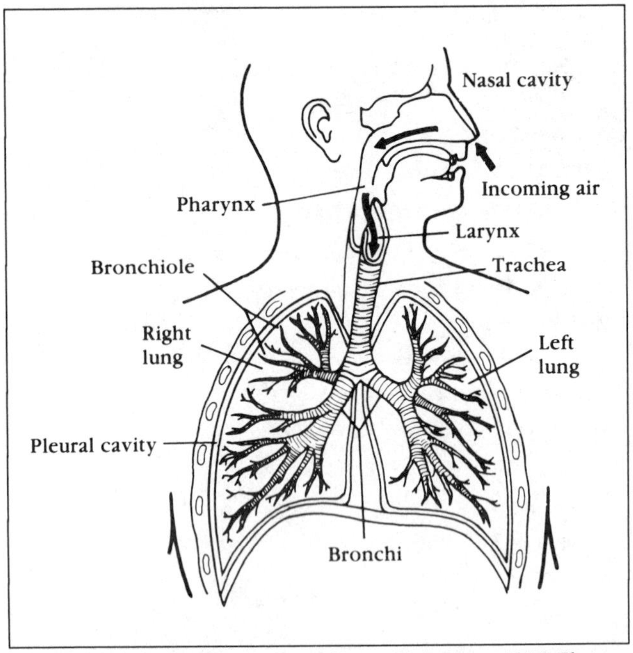

FIGURE 22-1. Respiratory system. (From H. A. Braun, F. W. Cheney, Jr., and C. P. Loehnen, *Introduction to Respiratory Physiology* [2nd ed.]. Boston: Little, Brown, 1980.)

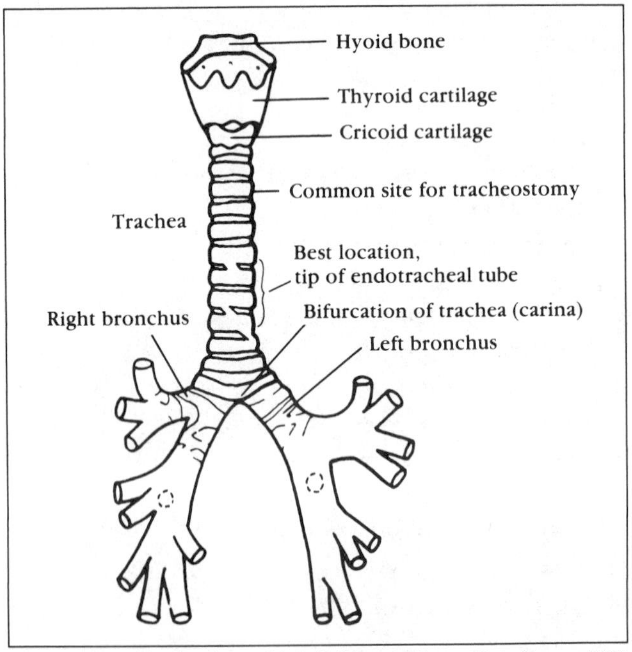

FIGURE 22-2. Tracheobronchial divisions. (From H. A. Braun, F. W. Cheney, Jr., and C. P. Loehnen, *Introduction to Respiratory Physiology* [2nd ed.]. Boston: Little, Brown, 1980.)

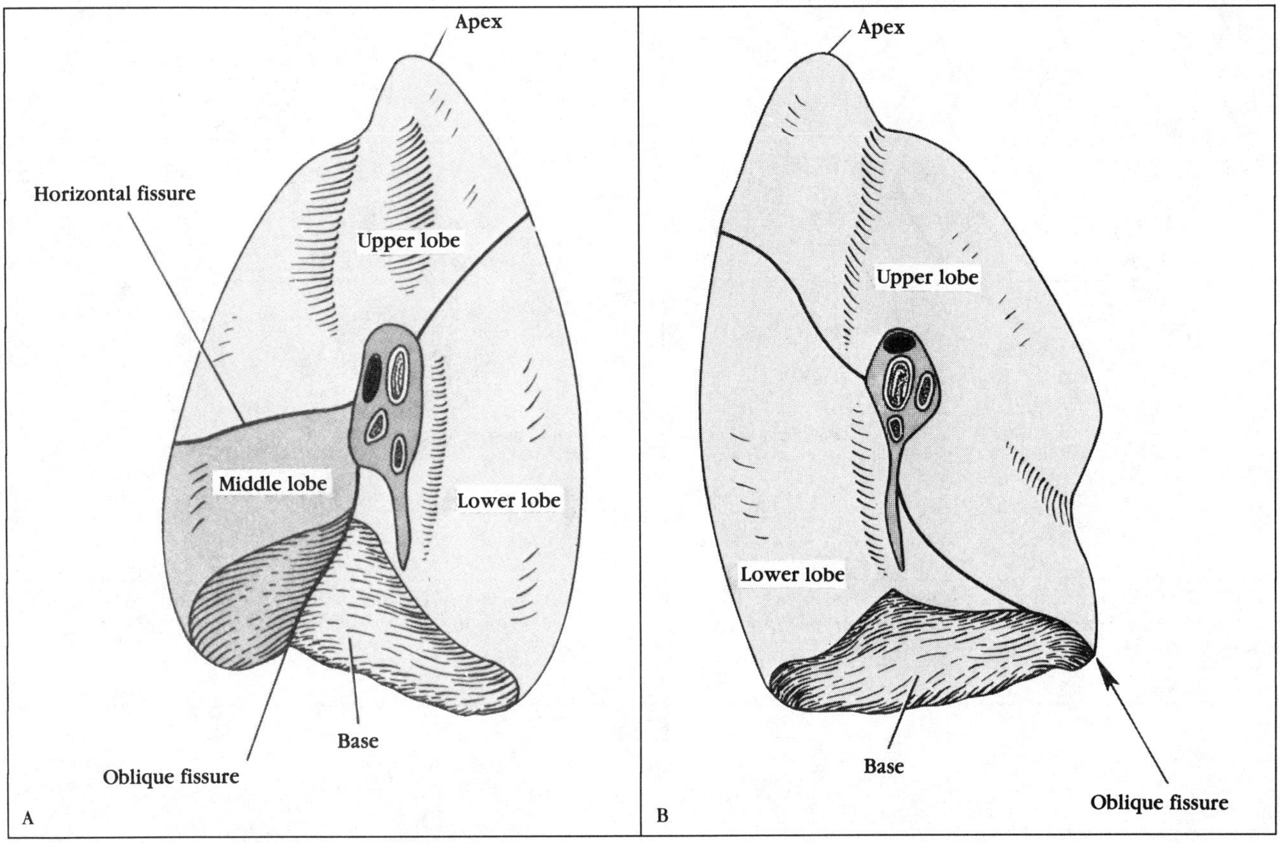

FIGURE 22-3. A. Lateral and medial surfaces of right lung. B. Lateral and medial surfaces of left lung. (From R. S. Snell, *Clinical Anatomy for Medical Students* [2nd ed.]. Boston: Little, Brown, 1981.)

right lung than in the left. It also makes suctioning of the left main stem bronchus difficult.

The right and left main stem bronchi divide into the lobar bronchi, which divide into the segmental bronchi. The segmental bronchi then divide into the terminal bronchioles. The diameter of each of these successive segments is smaller than the last, but the number of airways in the smaller segments is greater than in the larger ones, providing a broader surface area. This anatomic division, called the *generations of bronchi*, ends at approximately the sixteenth generation from the trachea.

The terminal bronchioles branch into the respiratory bronchioles. Occasional alveoli can be found in the walls of these latter structures.

Anatomy of the Lungs

The lungs lie in the thoracic cavity, separated from each other by the mediastinum. The lungs are cone-shaped in appearance with the narrow ends, or *apices*, directed upward, and the wide *bases* at the lower portion. Each lung is composed of lobes, three on the right and two on the left (Fig. 22-3). The lobes are divided into smaller compartments called *lobules*. The lobules then are further divided into smaller segments terminating finally in the alveolar sacs.

Surrounding the lungs is the pleural membrane, which provides for a covering over the lungs and lines the thoracic wall. The layer overlying the lung parenchyma is called the *visceral pleura* while the outer layer is termed the *parietal pleura* (Fig. 22-4). Between these two layers is a thin film of serous fluid that allows for the movement of the visceral layer on the parietal layer without friction during normal ventilation. Between the two layers is a potential space called the *intrapleural* or *pleural* space.

Parenchyma of the Lungs

The alveolar ducts, the final generation, are totally lined with alveoli (Fig. 22-5). Respiratory gas exchange takes place only in the alveoli; therefore, these structures are designated collectively as the respiratory zone of the lung. Because of their tiny size and sheer numbers, the alveoli have a volume of about 2500 ml in the adult. They have a diffusing area (surface area) about the size of a tennis court, or approximately 70 sq m. Each terminal bronchiole supplies its own unit of several alveoli called the *acinus.* The alveoli within the acinus do not have separate connections with the terminal bronchiole but are of various shapes and are interconnected. The individual alveolus is

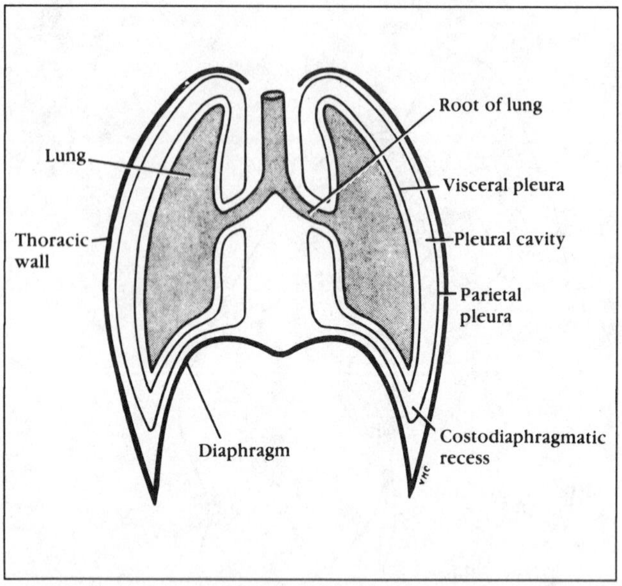

FIGURE 22-4. Position of visceral and parietal pleura with the pleural space. (From R.S. Snell, *Clinical Anatomy for Medical Students* [2nd ed.]. Boston: Little, Brown, 1981.)

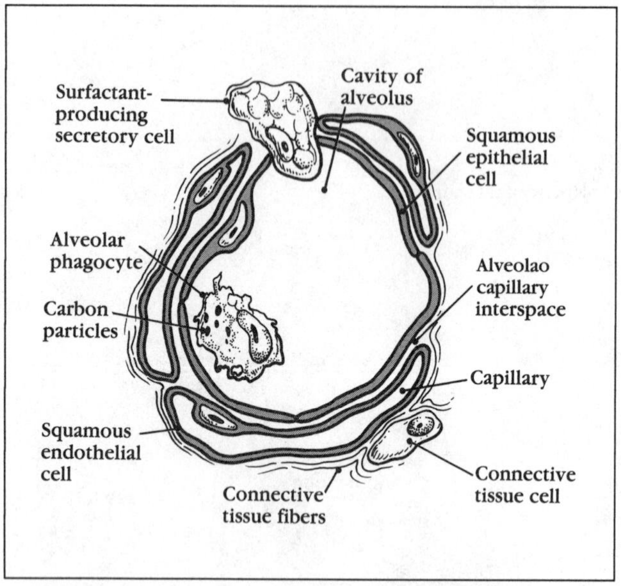

FIGURE 22-6. Representation of a single alveolus with surrounding capillaries and other cells. Note alveolocapillary interspace.

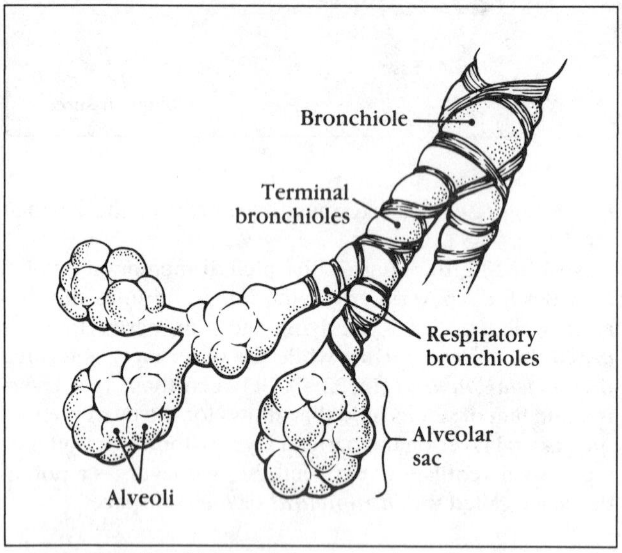

FIGURE 22-5. Termination of the generations of respiratory tubes in alveolar sacs and individual alveoli.

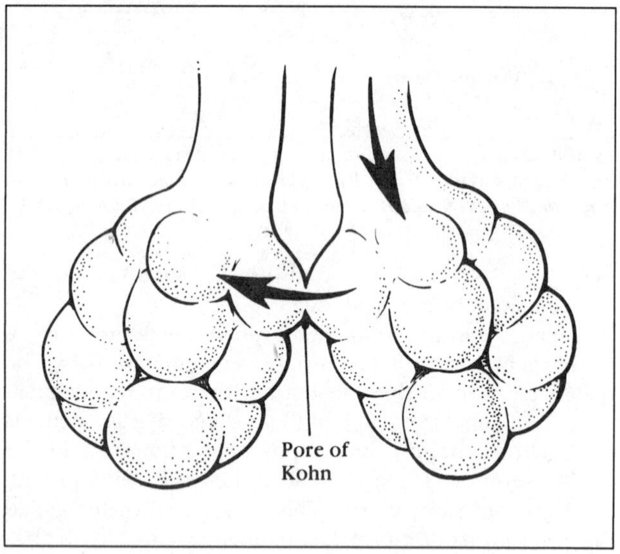

FIGURE 22-7. Demonstration of collateral communication between the alveoli through pores of Kohn.

one layer of cells in thickness and is built on a structure of elastin and muscle fibers. Each alveolus communicates with the pulmonary capillary bed to move gases by the process of diffusion across the *alveolocapillary interspace* (Fig. 22-6). Interconnecting the alveoli are tiny openings called the *pores of Kohn* (Fig. 22-7), which function to allow air to circulate among the alveoli, so that within a second or less after inspiration all alveoli within an acinus have the same gas concentration. In young children, the pores of Kohn are few in number and poorly developed, but with age these structures increase in number and size.

The pores of Kohn are helpful in the event of an obstruction of a small airway. In a process called *collateral ventilation*, if an airway smaller than a lobar bronchiole is obstructed, the alveoli that the airway normally supplies can continue to be ventilated by the pores of Kohn [4]. Collateral ventilation appears to be more effective in adults than in young children.

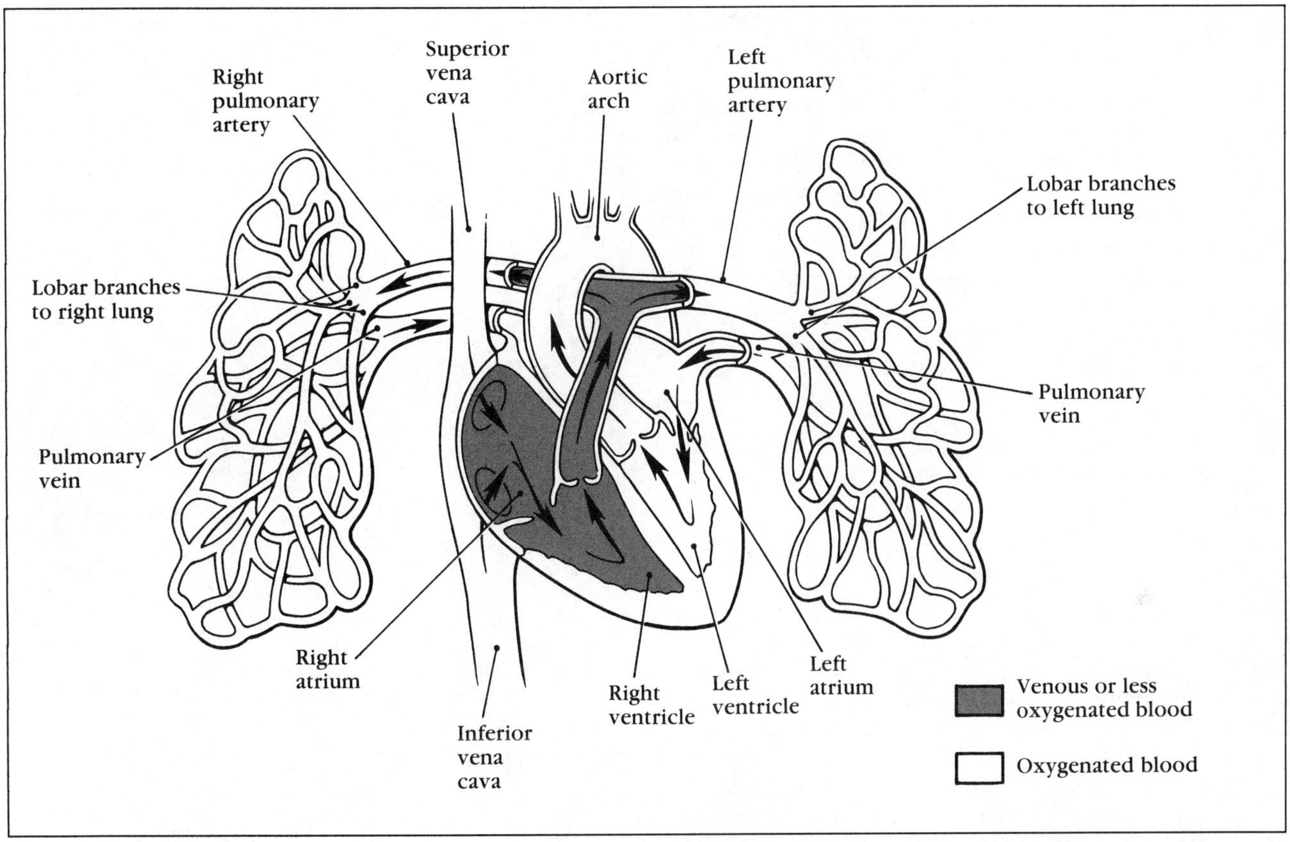

FIGURE 22-8. Circulation from the right heart to the lungs to the left heart.

THE PULMONARY CIRCULATION

The lung has two blood supplies, consisting of the *bronchial* and the *pulmonary circulations*. The first consists of the bronchial arteries, which arise in the thoracic aorta and upper intercostal arteries. As a part of the systemic blood supply, these arteries nourish the trachea and bronchi to the level of the respiratory bronchioles. After forming capillary plexuses, some of the bronchial circulation returns through a pulmonary vein to the left atrium, while some empties into the bronchial vein that terminates in the azygos system.

The bronchial circulation supplies the lung's supporting tissues, its nerves, and the outer layers of the pulmonary arteries and veins; normally, it supplies neither the alveolar walls and ducts nor the respiratory bronchioles. In the event of interruption of the pulmonary circulation, the bronchial circulation can support the metabolic needs of these tissues, but the tissues lose the ability to participate in gas exhange.

The second blood supply to the lungs is the pulmonary circulation. From the pulmonary artery, the lungs normally receive the entire output of the right ventricle. This blood circulates through the pulmonary capillary bed and then returns to the left heart by way of the pulmonary veins (Fig. 22-8).

MAJOR MUSCLES OF VENTILATION

The major muscle of ventilation, which acts to enlarge the chest cavity, is the *diaphragm*. Innervated by the phrenic nerves, this flat, dome-shaped muscle will lower approximately 1 cm in quiet respiration. In forced inspiration, however, it may descend as much as 10 cm. This diaphragmatic movement temporarily compresses the abdominal contents. Consequently, the movement of the diaphragm can be impeded by abnormalities in the abdominal cavity such as ascites and hepatomegaly. If abdominal pain is present, diaphragmatic action is reduced because of the *splinting effect*. The splinting effect is a voluntary limitation of ventilatory movements because of abdominal or thoracic pain.

Thoracic cavity enlargement is further aided by an upward and outward motion of the lower ribs accomplished by the *external intercostal muscles*. The upper ribs also move in an outward fashion. The ribs are attached to the vertebrae in such a way as to rotate on an axis as they are moved by these muscles.

While inspiration normally is an active effort, expiration is a passive one in which the muscles relax and allow the lungs and chest wall structures to seek their resting size. The pressure in the thorax gradually rises and air moves out of the lungs.

The *internal intercostal muscles* are used in forced expiration to stiffen the intercostal spaces during straining. The *muscles of the abdominal wall* are also powerful aids to forced expiration. Normally, they are used only to generate the explosive pressure that is necessary for coughing. They also contract at the end of forced inspiration in synchrony with glottic closure to abruptly limit and stop the inspiration. The *accessory muscles*, the scalene and sternomastoids, are used during labored breathing to raise the first two ribs and sternum and increase the size of the thoracic cavity.

NERVOUS CONTROL OF RESPIRATION

Nerve Supply

The major nerve supply to the diaphragm is through the two *phrenic nerves*. Each half of the diaphragm is innervated by one of these nerves, each of which originates mainly from the fourth cervical nerve of the respective side. The eleventh cranial nerve, the accessory, functions to innervate most of the larynx and pharynx.

Bronchial muscle is innervated by both *parasympathetic (vagus) and sympathetic nerve supply.* An increased vagal influence causes bronchoconstriction while an increased sympathetic stimulation causes bronchodilation. Any factor that decreases the caliber of the airway increases resistance and work of breathing whereas an increased caliber of the airway has the opposite effect [15].

The vagus nerve also transmits the appropriate signal to limit inspiration when an overstretch signal is received from the lungs. This reflex, called the *Hering-Breuer reflex*, serves as a protective mechanism to limit lung inflation.

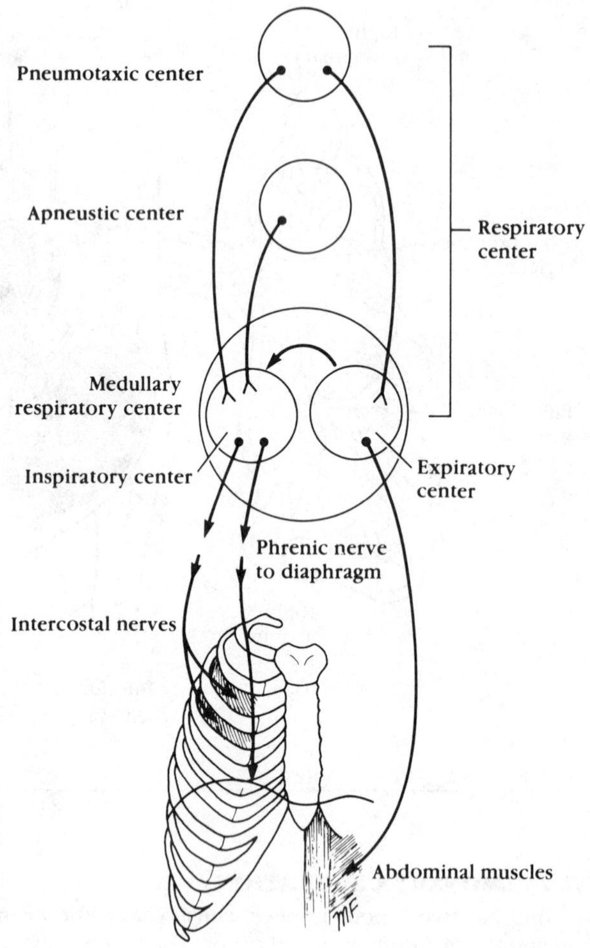

FIGURE 22-9. The medullary inspiratory and expiratory centers. (From R. S. Snell, *Clinical Histology for Medical Students.* Boston: Little, Brown, 1984.)

Respiratory Centers

The nervous system functions to adjust alveolar ventilation to the demands of the body. This occurs through the *respiratory centers* that are located in the medulla oblongata and the pons. Normally, these areas function to regulate ventilatory rate and depth through the chemical signals of carbon dioxide and hydrogen ion levels.

Central Chemoreceptors

Respiratory neurons located in the medulla oblongata are the major chemosensitive areas (chemoreceptors). The areas demonstrated in Figure 22-9 show separate areas responsible for inspiration and expiration. The major stimulus for the *inspiratory area* is the carbon dioxide concentration of the blood, but this area also transmits input from the peripheral chemoreceptors. The regular rhythm for the ventilatory effort is generated in the inspiratory area. The effort continues below the conscious level although the conscious control of breathing always overrides the unconscious.

The *expiratory* area is located in a separate area of the medulla but is usually not active unless there is some respiratory distress. When pulmonary ventilation becomes excessive, the expiratory muscles become activated to aid the expiratory effort. How the interaction occurs between the inspiratory and expiratory area is not known [7].

The *pneumotaxic center* is located in the pons and participates continually in the inspiratory effort through direct effect on the inspiratory effort to limit the tidal volume of air inspired. Activation of this center serves to increase rate of respiration while decreased stimulation decreases the respiratory rate. Another center in the pons, the *apneustic center,* functions in some brain pathology to cause excessive inflation of the lungs with occasional expiratory efforts.

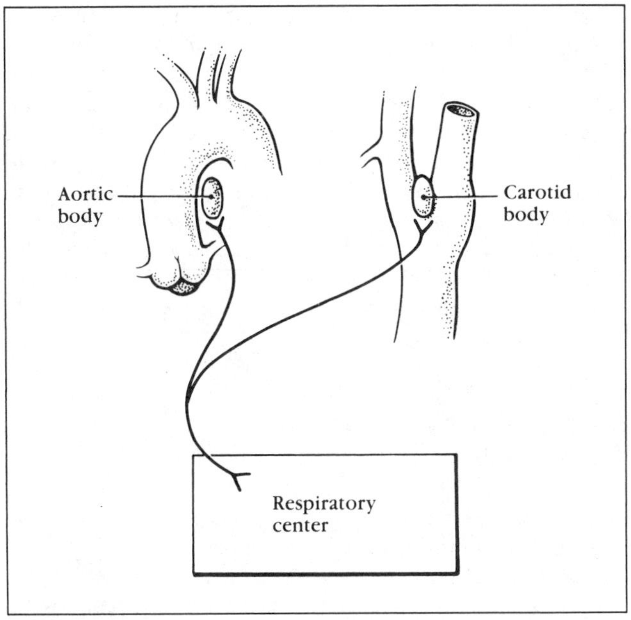

FIGURE 22-10. Decreased oxygen tension causes stimulation of the respiratory center and an increased respiratory rate.

Peripheral Chemoreceptors

Decreased oxygen tension levels in arterial blood are sensed by the peripheral chemoreceptors of the carotid body and aortic arch (Fig. 22-10). The hypoxic stimulus, described as 30 mm Hg oxygen tension less than normal for the person, is transmitted to the respiratory center resulting primarily in the stimulation of inspiratory neurons and effecting an increased respiratory rate through the phrenic nerve. These peripheral chemoreceptors are also sensitive to changes in carbon dioxide and hydrogen, but the direct effect of the central respiratory center overrides the sensitivity from the peripheral receptors [8].

COMPLIANCE AND ELASTANCE

In order to understand pulmonary pathology, it is important to understand the concepts of *compliance* (C) and *elastance* (E), also called *elasticity*. Generally, it can be said that the respiratory system behaves like a pump with a flow-resistive mechanism. The pumping part of the mechanism can be thought of as two separate components: the chest wall with its associated structures and the lungs.

Compliance is a measure of distensibility or how easily a tissue is stretched. In other words, the fewer elastic forces to be overcome in order to stretch a substance, the more compliant it is. Compliance is measured and recorded by the amount of volume change that results from pressure applied. Compare the blowing up of an old balloon with that of a new one. Less pressure is needed to make a large volume change in the old balloon while more pressure is required to make a smaller volume change in the new one. Compliance is thus important because the more compliant a tissue is, the less pressure is needed to stretch it. Using delta (Δ) as a symbol for change, compliance is expressed as follows:

$$C = \frac{\Delta V \text{ (liters) (volume change)}}{\Delta P \text{ (cm water) (pressure change)}}$$

Using the balloon analogy, one can discover which balloon is more compliant if arbitrary numbers are assigned as follows:

Old Balloon	New Balloon
Small pressure needed: 1	Large pressure needed: 10
Large volume change: 10	Small volume change: 3
$C = 10/1$	$C = 3/10$
$C = 10$	$C = 0.33$

From these figures, we find that the old balloon is much more compliant or more easily stretched. It thus has fewer elastic forces to oppose the stretch than the new balloon.

Elastance is the opposite of compliance. Whereas compliance refers to the forces promoting expansion of the lung, elastic forces are those promoting the return to the normal resting position or original shape. Compliance and elastance are closely related in pulmonary dynamics. Compliance refers to the amount of force needed to produce the volume change or stretch. The amount needed depends on the elastic forces at work. A highly compliant rubber band, for example, has few elastic forces, while a less compliant (thicker) rubber band has more elastic forces at work [3]. The thick rubber band takes more work to stretch it and returns much more readily to its original shape than the thin rubber band. Therefore, the thick rubber band is less compliant and more elastant than the thin one. The following formula is used to calculate elastance:

$$E = \frac{\text{pressure change (P)}}{\text{volume change (V)}}$$

The chest wall also has the properties of elastance and compliance, but these properties differ from those of the lungs. To illustrate this difference, imagine that the lungs and chest wall could be separated but remain as living and moving structures retaining all of their unique properties. Each of the two structures could be separated from the pull of the other and could seek its own resting size at an equilibrium between elastance and compliance. In the case of the chest wall, if freed from the lungs, it would seek a much larger resting size than when it was attached to the lungs. Without the inward pull of the lungs, the chest wall size would be abnormally large.

On the other hand, if the lungs could be separated from the chest wall, they would tend to relax to a much smaller size than when they rested against the chest wall. They have more elastic recoil than might be expected from the amount of elastin and fiber contained by them. This is because of a meshlike network arrangement, the structure of which itself increases elastic recoil. This arrangement is termed *nylon stocking elasticity.*

Taking the properties of the lungs and chest wall together, it can be seen that elastance of the lungs prevents overdistention of the thorax while chest wall compliance prevents collapse of the lungs. It was noted on p. 295 that contraction of the diaphragm, an active process, lowered that muscle and increased the size of the thoracic cage. All of this creates a negative intrapleural pressure, causing the movement of air from the atmosphere to the lungs. Relaxation of the diaphragm, a passive process, causes movement of the muscle to its resting position, increased intrapleural pressure, and movement of air from the lungs to the atmosphere. These properties account for the fact that expiration is normally a passive process, while inspiration is an active process.

Many diseases alter the compliance and elastance of either the lung or chest wall, but disease need not affect *both* the elastance and compliance of either structure. In general, bronchopulmonary diseases affect lung compliance, while chest wall compliance is affected by obesity and by diseases of the thoracic skeleton or respiratory nerves. Alveolar edema and atelectasis reduce compliance by reducing the number of inflated alveoli. Compliance of the lung is increased by emphysema and is somewhat increased in the aged person. Usually dynamic measurements of compliance are used rather than estimates of elastance and changes are referred to as *decreased* or *increased* compliance. In the case of pulmonary fibrosis, where there is increased fibrous tissue and stiffening of the lung tissues, compliance is reduced. More pressure than usual is needed to stretch this lung and chest wall system. The total compliance of this lung and chest wall system is then less than the normal. The following is a method for calculating *total compliance:*

$$\text{Normal total compliance} = 0.1\ \text{L (BTPS)/cm}\ H_2O\ \text{(during quiet breathing)}$$

BTPS/cm H_2O refers to the fact that the measurement is calculated at body temperature, at ambient pressure, and with water vapor saturation.

If a person is being mechanically ventilated, measures of compliance provide a useful piece of objective assessment data over a period of time. *Dynamic lung compliance* calculated in this way is not entirely accurate because the true calculation requires static conditions. However, it is accurate enough to be a useful tool for assessing gross changes in total compliance. The following method is used for calculating dynamic compliance:

$$\text{Effective dynamic compliance} = \frac{\text{expired tidal volume (ml)}}{\text{inspiratory pressure (cm } H_2O)}$$

The measure of compliance may be even more useful if related to lung volume. Compliance per lung volume is called *specific compliance.* A decreased specific compliance means that the lung tissues become more rigid and, in severe cases, the pressures needed to expand the lungs adequately over a period of time are more than the person can produce or maintain. This results in hypoventilation. Many disorders, including obstructive disorders, pulmonary edema, and pneumonia may decrease both compliance and lung volume. Specific compliance is also related to lung size and may be reduced by 50 percent in pneumonectomy.

THE MECHANICS OF BREATHING

As has been stated previously, a particular pressure is necessary to cause a change in the volume of the lungs. Volume can be changed by either a high pressure from outside the body forcing air in or a negative pressure from inside the body causing air to move into the lungs. Normally, humans breathe by utilizing negative pressure breathing.

Phases of Ventilation

The phases of ventilation involve the movement of the diaphragm and the other respiratory muscles. As the diaphragm descends, it tends to enlarge the intrapleural space, which causes a negative intrapulmonary pressure; the air then flows into the lungs to equalize the pressure. The subatmospheric or negative pressure, which is necessary for air to flow into the lungs, is accomplished by enlarging the lung and chest cavity. When the chest and lungs enlarge, the pressure inside the thorax is lower than it was before the enlargement. At the end of active effort, the diaphragm relaxes and moves upward, which increases the intrapulmonary pressure to above the atmospheric level. The air moves passively out of the lungs. The elastic recoil of the lung tissue moves the lung to its resting or unstretched state. The phases of ventilation are illustrated in Figure 22-11.

Inspiration, then, is an active process initiated by the contraction of the diaphragm and the outward pull by the intercostals. Air moves from greater to lesser pressure. Expiration is a passive process that occurs when the respiratory muscles relax and the intrapleural pressure increases above the atmospheric level. Even when the system is relaxed, the lung is continually pulling in and attempting to get to its smaller relaxed size. This process creates a negative intrapleural pressure and explains one of the reasons that air is pulled into the chest when the chest wall is punctured.

Airway Size Changes

The size of the airways is also affected by the process of ventilation. The airways are attached to and supported by the lung parenchyma. Since the lungs are expanding to fill a

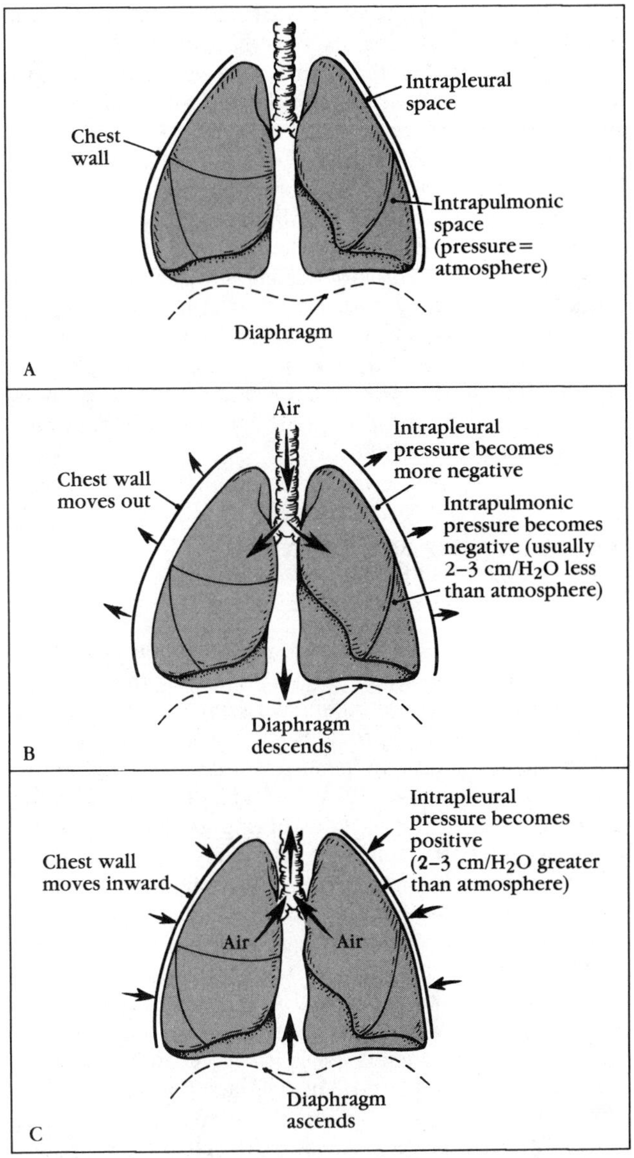

FIGURE 22-11. Phases of ventilation. A. No movement of air. B. Air moves from the environment to the intrapulmonary space. C. Air moves from the intrapulmonary space to the environment.

larger space on inspiration, all of these structures, including the airways and alveolar ducts, are pulled to a larger size. The airway and alveolar duct size is then reduced as lung volume decreases during expiration. During quiet ventilation some of the smaller airways close during the expiration. Because of the effects of gravity airway closure is more pronounced in the supine position.

Airway Resistance

During respiration, the volume of the thorax and consequently of the airways is changing. The airway offers resistance to airflow, the amount of which directly affects the amount of pressure needed to move air into and out of the lungs.

Pressure-flow relationships may be quite complex even in simple straight tubes. Since the respiratory tree is a series of branching tubes of varying sizes, pressure-flow relationships become more complex.

The amount of pressure lost because of friction depends on the flow pattern of the air. The two major air flow patterns are *laminar flow* and *turbulent flow* (Fig. 22-12). In laminar flow, the gas within the airways is like very thin cylinders moving inside each other. The cylinder on the outside moves slowly and each inner cylinder of air moves progressively faster. Gas density has no influence on the velocity of this type of flow. Basically, the gas flow is along a straight line with little friction to the molecules. However, when an airway caliber changes, the laminar pattern is altered. Additional pressure may be needed to reaccelerate the gas and to reestablish a laminar flow pattern.

When flow rates are high or when airways are partially obstructed or collapsed, turbulent air flow occurs. In normal lungs, turbulent flow occurs in the large central airways because of molecular collision and resistance at the sides of the tubes. Laminar flow occurs more readily in the small peripheral airways, which are characterized more by straight, smooth tubes.

Change in airway width greatly alters the resistance present. When airways widen, resistance is greatly diminished and air flows through easily. When airways narrow, resistance is increased and air moves through them with much more difficulty. It takes more pressure to move air through a narrow airway than a wide one. Studies have shown that if airway radius is reduced by one-half, resistance is increased by 16 times [19]. This fact has great importance for individuals whose airways are narrowed by bronchospasm or pressure from tumors or infectious processes around the airways. Increased airway resistance causes an increase in the work of breathing.

Since airways normally widen on inspiration and narrow on expiration, resistance is generally greater on expiration than on inspiration. This process also explains why air trapping occurs with asthma or chronic lung disease.

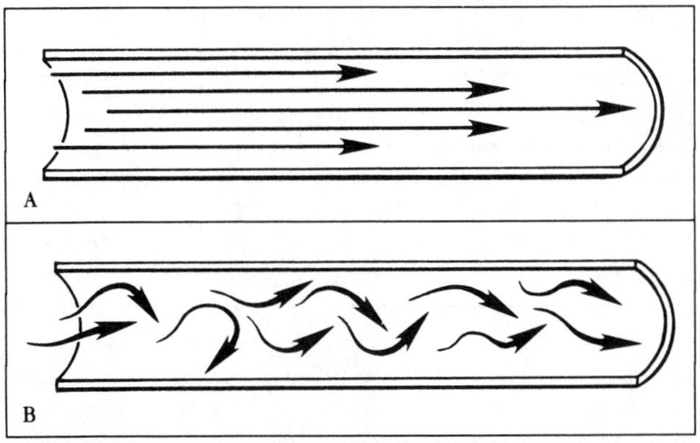

FIGURE 22-12. A. Schematic representation of laminar gas flow. B. Representation of turbulent gas flow.

Although there are many extremely small peripheral airways, they are so tiny that they make little difference in the resistance factors that can be measured. It is postulated that the initial changes of chronic lung disease occur in these airways where they cannot be measured [19]. These airways make up areas called silent zones where diseases can be present without detection.

In normal respiration the bases of the lung tend to ventilate better than the apices in the upright position. This has been demonstrated by having a person inhale radioactive xenon gas and following its diffusion by a radiation camera. During the inspiratory phase the base undergoes a larger change in volume and has a smaller resting volume than the apex. In the supine position this difference disappears and the ventilations become the same. In abnormalities, such as pulmonary edema, the apices tend to ventilate better and the smaller airways in the bases often close [19].

Airway resistance can be altered by many factors. A sigh or deep inspiration usually reduces resistance while forced expiration, even in the normal individual, increases it. Airway compression is the usual cause of increased airway resistance during forced expiration, and this factor is markedly enhanced in persons having diseased or weakened airway walls [13].

Tissue Resistance

In addition to airway resistance, there is also some resistance in the lung and chest wall tissues, called *tissue resistance*. Although the frictional resistance of the tissue movement cannot be measured directly, it can be calculated. In the healthy, young, adult man, tissue resistance is about 20 percent of the total pulmonary resistance. Tissue resistance is rarely increased to the point of being limiting by itself. It is increased in pulmonary sarcoidosis, pulmonary fibrosis, diffuse carcinomatosis, asthma, and kyphoscoliosis. Tissue resistance may be particularly high where there is severe limitation of movement of the thoracic cage as in neurologic disease, musculoskeletal disease, or deformity of the chest structures.

WORK OF BREATHING

The act of breathing requires muscular work to overcome the elastic forces of the lungs and chest wall. Work is also needed to overcome airway and tissue resistance. Initial work is minimal at normal breathing frequency but increases significantly at high breathing frequencies. Resistive work is minimized with a slow, deep respiratory pattern and increases with respiratory frequency. The opposite is true of elastic work. Two-thirds of the work of breathing is against elastic forces prompting the return of the lungs to the resting position. Slow, deep breathing greatly increases the work needed to overcome elastic forces. When the work forces are summarized, respiratory work is the least at a frequency of 14 breaths per minute.

Respiratory pathology usually alters breathing patterns. The pattern finally adopted by the individual will be the one that requires the least work although it will always require more work than the normal pattern. For example, if a flow resistance increase occurs, the breathing may be slow and deep. If compliance is reduced, a rapid, shallow pattern of breathing may be adopted.

The work of breathing, as in other body work, consumes oxygen. Normally, at rest, respiration accounts for about 5 percent of the total metabolic rate. This increases moderately with normal ventilatory changes, but with significant respiratory pathology the work of breathing may increase many times. Ultimately, the ventilatory effort may cost the person more oxygen than it delivers and may produce more carbon dioxide than can be eliminated. This progressive process, without appropriate intervention, continues until respiratory failure ensues.

SUBSTANCES IMPORTANT IN ALVEOLAR EXPANSION

Surfactant

Surfactant, a phospholipid made up of dipalmitoyl-lecithin, is synthesized in the type II or granular pneumocytes lining the alveolus and is secreted to form a film across the alveolar surface. Surfactant provides surface stability and prevents collapse of the alveolar structures.

A deficiency of surfactant will result in an increase in the surface tension in the alveolus during expiration that results in collapse or atelectasis of the alveoli. Amounts of surfactant in the lung vary according to the diameter of the alveoli. As the alveoli inflate, the surfactant spreads out over the surface of the alveolar membrane. As the alveoli empty, the surfactant layer becomes thicker in relation to the decreased space. Smaller alveoli have a thicker layer while larger alveoli have a thinner layer [8].

To be effective it is necessary that the surfactant layer continually be replenished. The half-life of pulmonary lecithin is 14 hours, which suggests that active synthesis must continually take place in the type II cells of the alveoli. Normal ventilation seems to be the most important factor in the replenishment of surfactant, which probably is due to the need for oxygen in the production of this substance. Hypoventilation may lead to atelectasis due to a diminished renewal of surfactant. The underlying problem in this situation is a decreased supply of oxygen with decreased synthesis of surfactant, which leads to a decreased surface tension in the alveoli. The result is widespread collapse of the alveoli.

Surfactant may also function to prevent the transudation of fluid across the alveolar capillary membrane during the respiratory cycle. Fluid exudation from capillary to alveolus has been shown to result from a decrease in the surfactant levels. Therefore, surfactant functions to help keep the alveoli dry.

Without surfactant, the surface tension of the alveoli would be fixed. Greater pressure would be needed to keep

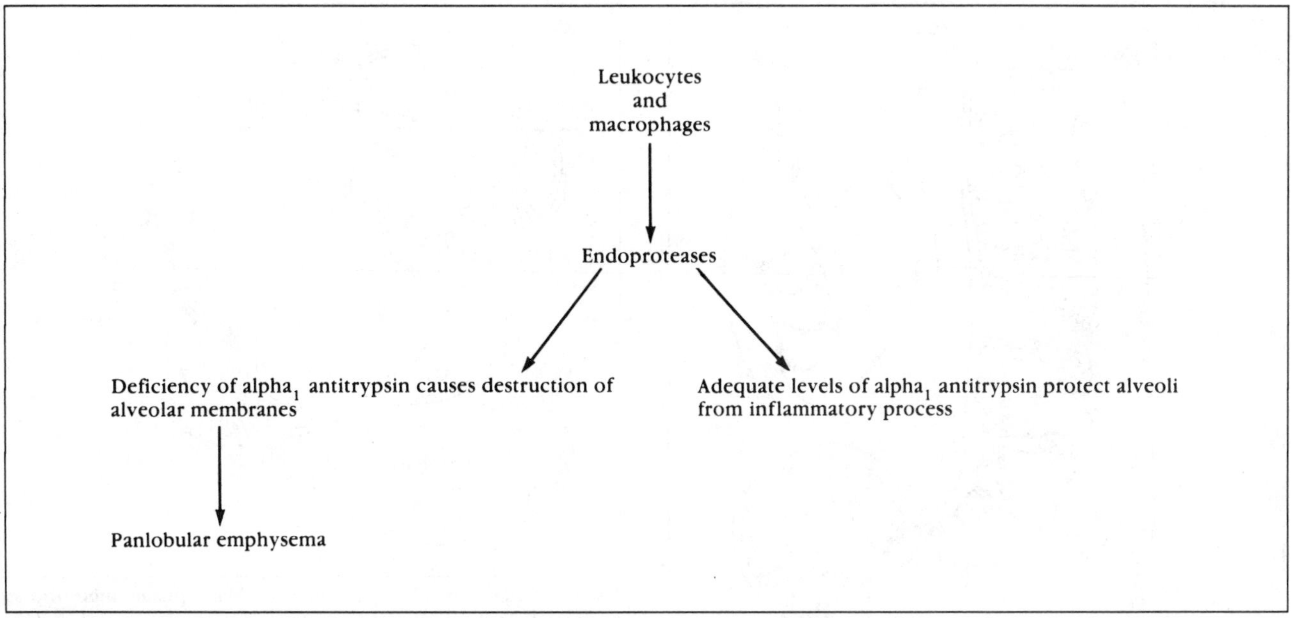

FIGURE 22-13. Postulated mechanism of endoproteases with or without alpha$_1$ antitrypsin.

an alveolus open as its volume and radius would decrease on expiration. Atelectasis would regularly occur at low lung volumes due to collapse of small alveoli. Large inspiratory pressures would be needed to reopen the alveoli. The point of collapse is referred to as the *critical closing pressure*, and the pressure necessary to open a collapsed alveolus must be enough to overcome surface tension.

Disorders that involve destruction, inactivation, or insufficient production of surfactant cause marked changes in pressure-volume relationships, even without changes in the lung or chest wall tissues. Possibly the best known instance of surfactant deficiency is in the infant respiratory distress syndrome (IRDS), also called hyaline membrane disease although the membrane seems to be secondary to the pathology rather than to the cause of the disease. The condition is closely associated with prematurity and appears to be caused by immaturity of the type II cells and a deficiency of surfactant synthesis. Further discussion of the related problem, adult respiratory distress syndrome (ARDS), is found in Chapter 23.

Alpha$_1$ Antitrypsin

In the search for the cause of emphysema, clinicians noted that some families had a high incidence of the disease and that the onset was at an earlier age. The correlation between the absence of alpha$_1$ antitrypsin (a glycoprotein synthesized by the liver) and familial early-onset emphysema was studied by Laurell and Erickson [11]. The level of alpha$_1$ antitrypsin has been found to be genetically controlled. The homozygous state is linked with early onset of panlobular emphysema. The heterozygous or intermediate states may have greater susceptibility to emphysema, particularly in the presence of repeated inflammatory reactions.

Exactly how alpha$_1$ antitrypsin protects the lung is unknown. A widely accepted hypothesis states that leukocytes and macrophages release endoproteases in the inflammatory response (Fig. 22-13). That these proteases are capable of producing emphysema has been well established in animal research [12, 19]. The endoproteases are neutralized by alpha$_1$ antitrypsin. Without this inhibitor these enzymes attack and destroy the alveolar membrane.

Until recently, it was thought that the prevalence of some degree of alpha$_1$ antitrypsin deficiency in persons with emphysema was low, accounting for about 1 percent of this population. Recent studies have shown this percentage to be much greater, on the order of 25 percent. This compares with 5 percent of the healthy population who have some degree of the deficiency [12].

DEFENSE OF THE AIRWAYS AND LUNGS

Mucociliary Transport or the Mucociliary Escalator System

The *mucociliary escalator system* or the *mucous blanket* provides the major defense of the respiratory tract against disease. The components of this system include the goblet cells, which secrete mucus; the ciliated epithelial cells; and the mucus itself. These components are discussed in the following section.

The *ciliated epithelial cells* of the respiratory tract function to clear the airways by moving fluid forward (Fig. 22-14A). These cells line the entire respiratory tract with the exception of the anterior third of the nose, part of the pharynx, and the alveoli. The surface of each ciliated

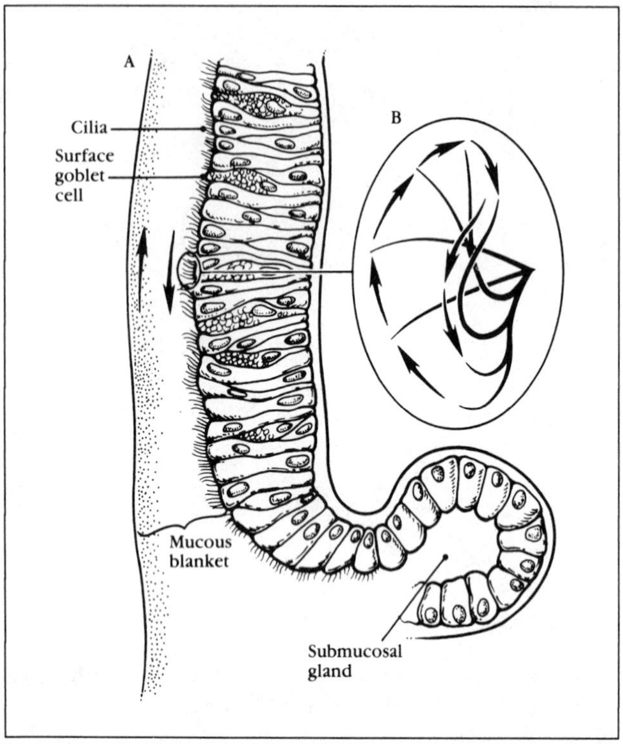

FIGURE 22-14. A. The mucociliary escalator. B. Conceptual scheme of ciliary movement, allowing forward motion to move viscous gel layer and backward motion to take place entirely within more fluid sol layer.

cell contains about 200 cilia. These cilia move in a continuous wave to carry mucus and debris up the airway to the larynx.

From an upright position, the cilia sweep forward about 30 to 35 degrees and then bend to make their recovery (Fig. 22-14B). Comroe likens the cilia to strokes of the oars of a boat:

> Each cilium makes a forceful, fast effector stroke forward, followed by a less forceful, slower stroke backward to get in position again. There is precise timing and coordination of the strokes of a row of cilia so that together they move as a wave [4].

Cilia, beating in sequential waves at 1000 cycles/minute, move the mucus up the airway. Because the ciliary beat is rapid, the mucous layer does not have time to recoil between beats.

A mucous blanket, made up primarily of the secretions of goblet cells that line the airways and mucus-secreting glands located in the larger ciliated bronchi, moves forward on the cilia. Cells in the alveoli may also contribute secretions to the mucous blanket. The rate of secretion of these cells is difficult to estimate because of resorption and expectoration of mucus. The mucous blanket consists of two layers, the sol layer, which surrounds the cilia, and the gel, or surface, layer.

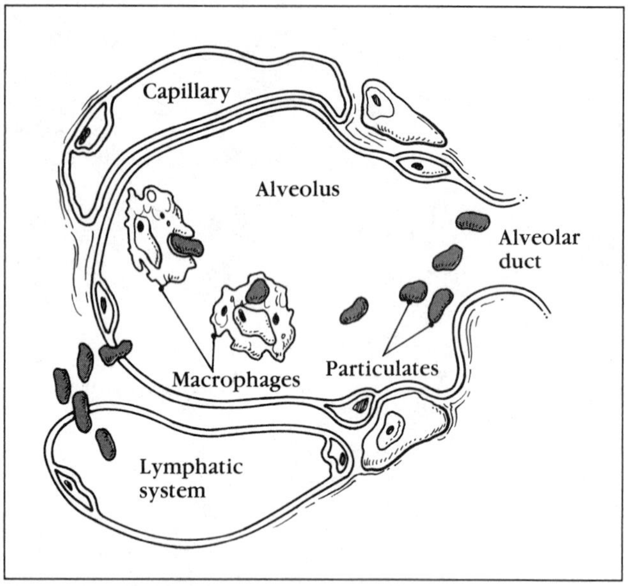

FIGURE 22-15. Alveolar clearance. A. Macrophage ingestion of particulate matter. B. Particles traveling in the alveolar duct. C. Lymphatic clearance of particulate matter. D. Blood flow clearance. E. Carriage of particulates within the macrophages.

The mucous layers retain a constant depth and the rate of transport of mucus increases rapidly as the mucus moves toward the trachea. Some mucus is resorbed in the large airways to maintain a constant depth with little removal by evaporation, because inspired air is virtually 100 percent saturated with moisture by the time it reaches the pharynx. Mucociliary transport is known to be altered by depressed ciliary activity, changes in the property of mucus, and injury to the respiratory epithelium cells.

Mucus is produced primarily by the goblet or mucus-secreting cells that lie along the tracheobronchial tree. These cells produce an estimated 100 ml of mucus per day, continually providing for humidification and protection of the respiratory passages. The mucous covering of the epithelium in the respiratory passages is normally uninterrupted. Adhesive properties of mucus allow for adherence of particles and movement of these particulates out of the respiratory tract. Mucus is normally composed of water, electrolytes, and several types of mucopolysaccharides, which account for the viscosity of the material.

Alveolar Clearance

Mucociliary transport, lymphatic drainage, blood flow, and phagocytosis all contribute to creating a sterile environment within the alveoli. Macrophage activity is the principal *alveolar* defense against particulates. These alveolar macrophages regularly scavenge the surface of the epithelium, digesting foreign material (represented schematically in Fig. 22-15).

Surface tension may play a part in the removal of particu-

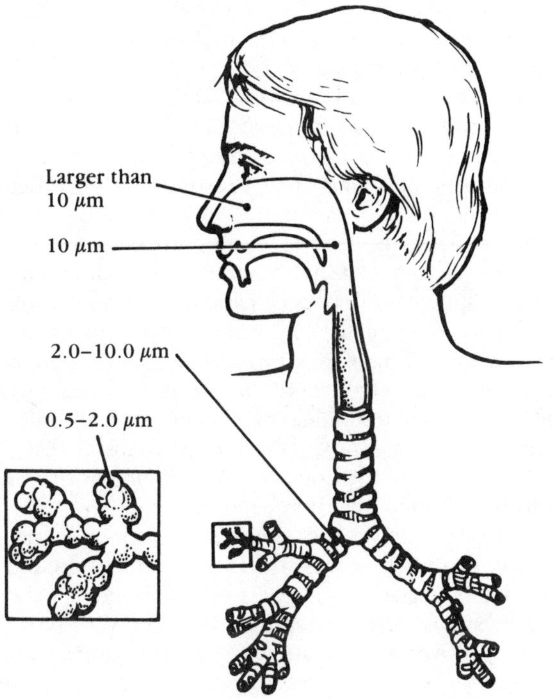

FIGURE 22-16. Deposition of particulates in the airways depends on their size.

lates from the lung. Particulates on a plane move from an area of low surface tension to an area of higher surface tension. Therefore, particulates may move from the environment of alveolar surfactant to the higher surface tension of the respiratory bronchioles and up the mucus escalator to the pharynx [1].

Some particulates are removed to perivascular, peribronchial, and hilar lymph nodes. The lymphatics probably transport the particulates engulfed in macrophages. It is not clear to what extent blood flow is responsible for alveolar clearance. Kilburn hypothesizes that monocytes from the blood enter the air space at the alveolar bronchial junction where they become lung macrophages, engulfing material left there by other mechanisms [10].

Some particulates remain in the lung for protracted periods while others stay for an intermediate period and are cleared. This seems to depend on a number of factors, such as deposition site, nature of the particulate, and host resistance. A small number of particulates remain in the lung indefinitely. Particulates, such as asbestos, silica, and carbon, may stimulate fibroblast proliferation and this can create severe restrictive pulmonary disease.

Deposition of Particulates in the Airways

Under normal conditions, an individual inspires 10,000 to 12,000 liters of air daily. Each liter of urban air may have several million particles suspended in it, the majority of which are deposited along the respiratory tract and are cleansed by the defenses of the lung. Particles smaller than 0.5 μ in diameter usually remain suspended in inhaled air and are expelled from the lung during expiration.

The first site of deposition of particulates in the airway is the nose (Fig. 22-16). Particulates larger than 10 μ in diameter are filtered out in the nares or trapped in the nasal mucosa. It is the inertia of large particles that determines deposition at these sites. Their large mass and high linear velocity force them to rain out in the nose. Along with being filtered, the warming and moistening of air in the nose allows the defense mechanisms of the lower respiratory tract to function more effectively.

As the inhaled air flows over the tonsils and adenoids, particulates are deposited by impaction. These structures are ideally located in the airway to entrap debris that passes over them. In addition to mechanical defense, the tonsils and adenoids may function in the immunologic reaction. Farther along the respiratory tract linear velocities of air decrease as the surface area increases, which allows particulates in the range of 2 to 10 μ to be deposited on the mucociliary blanket by sedimentation.

Particulates smaller than 2 μ reach the alveoli by gravitational forces and, to a lesser extent, by the Brownian movement, which describes the random movement of molecules due to thermal energy. The particulates are removed primarily by mucociliary transport and phagocytosis. Smaller particles may present more of a threat to the lung than larger ones because they penetrate more deeply and stay longer in the lung.

Along with size, the aerodynamic properties of particulates and deposition sites must be considered. Asbestos particles, up to 300 μ in size, have been shown to reach the lung periphery where, because of their aerodynamic properties, rather than their size, they behave as particles of about 1 μ [15]. This explains why asbestos often severely damages the distal portions of the lung.

Reflexes of the Airways

The respiratory tract is equipped with reflexes that rid it of debris and protect it from inhaled foreign substances. As is true of other mechanisms, the hypoactivity or hyperactivity of these reflexes create conditions that are detrimental to the host.

The *sneeze reflex* is one of the defenses against irritant materials. Particulates or irritants stimulate sensory receptors of the trigeminal nerves resulting in the sneeze response. The sneeze is characterized by a deep inspiration followed by a violent expiratory blast through the nose.

The *cough reflex* is important in clearing the trachea and large bronchi of foreign matter by expectoration or swallowing. Irritants cause different impulses to be carried by the vagus nerve to the medulla. Conscious control can also initiate the cough mechanism. The cough reflex initiates a deep inspiration. The glottis then closes, the diaphragm relaxes, and the muscles contract against the closed glottis. Maximum intrathoracic and interairway pressures are produced that create a narrowing of the trachea. When the glottis opens, the combination of the large pressure differential between the airways and the atmosphere coupled with tracheal narrowing create air flow through the trachea at a rate that is nearly the speed of sound [17]. This is very effective in propelling secretions toward the mouth. While the cough is more effective in clearing the major airways, it also may help clear the peripheral airways through a milking action created by the high intrathoracic pressures. This may deliver secretions from the peripheral airways to the main bronchi for expulsion by coughing.

Along with other mechanisms, reflex *bronchoconstriction* protects the upper and lower airways from mechanical and chemical irritants. Both cough and reflex bronchoconstriction are initiated in the subepithelium of the airways by receptors sensitive to irritants. For example, when the receptors are exposed to dust, the reflex narrowing of the airways, along with cough, increases the linear velocity of airflow and assists in the removal of dust from the airways. Reflex bronchoconstriction also protects the alveoli from harmful fumes and prevents gases from entering the pulmonary circulation. The removal of gases from the inspired air depends on their solubility in water. Highly soluble gases, such as sulfur dioxide and acetone, are removed in the upper respiratory tract. Less soluble gases such as nitrous oxide and ozone reach the peripheral lung. This accounts for the observation that sulfur dioxide inhalation results in bronchitis while nitrous oxide inhalation may lead to pulmonary edema. The protection offered by reflex bronchoconstriction is dose- and time-related, which means that if exposure to the toxic fumes is brief or of low concentration, reflex bronchoconstriction may protect the lungs.

DEFENSES AGAINST INFECTION

Defense Against Microbial Agents

The invasion of the lung by microbial agents presents special problems in the defense of the lung. Microorganisms have the ability to replicate themselves and conceivably one organism could multiply and completely permeate the lung tissue. The defenders against infectious agents must act quickly to kill the organisms before they have sufficient opportunity to multiply, which can be in minutes to hours. Current research indicates that the alveolar macrophage system is the primary bactericidal mechanism for the clearance of infectious agents from the lungs [6].

The *alveolar macrophages* ingest bacteria at such a rapid rate that the majority are destroyed in situ. The rate of bacterial killing in the lung exceeds the rate at which the bacteria are transported out of the lung. This has been demonstrated by radioactive-tracer-labeled bacteria. In 24 hours, 30 to 40 percent of the radioactivity is cleared, but nearly all bacteria are killed. This is known as *net bacterial lung clearance.* Three factors contribute to this process: (1) physical transport out of the lung, (2) in situ bacterial killing, and (3) bacterial multiplication [9].

The rate of bactericidal activity by the macrophages is influenced by different bacterial strains. For example, *Staphylococcus aureus* is removed at a faster rate than *Proteus mirabilis.* Some organisms are readily inactivated by phagocytosis while others appear resistant to this process.

Conditions in the metabolic environment such as hypoxia, acidosis, and high levels of cortisol slow net bacterial lung clearance. Ethyl alcohol and tobacco smoke have been shown to depress clearance, but all organisms are not depressed equally. For example, alcohol completely suppresses the killing of *P. mirabilis* but not of *S. aureus* or *S. albus* [9]. This selective action on the alveolar macrophages has important clinical ramifications. In chronic obstructive lung disease, mixed flora are constantly present in the respiratory tract yet one predominant organism will be responsible for lung infection when it occurs.

Acute viral infections predispose the host to bacterial infections in the lung. Viruses appear to interfere with the alveolar macrophages and suppress their bactericidal ability. The greatest susceptibility appears between the sixth and tenth day following the acute viral infection during which time superimposed bacterial pneumonias frequently develop.

The dynamics of differing responses to bacteria, fluctuations in host resistance, and environmental changes may permit one or another organism to multiply at any given time. All of these factors influence the fate of the microorganism, whether it will remain in a localized area or whether it will be disseminated throughout the body.

Immunologic Defense of the Lungs

Closely associated with the macrophage system is the *immunologic defense of the lungs*. The cells involved in the specific immune response have been described in Chapter 9. These cells include the T lymphocytes (thymic-dependent) and the B lymphocytes (bone-marrow derived), which function in a complex, interacting pattern to provide for immunity and for defense of the body against foreign invasion.

Specialized B lymphocytes become immunoglobulin-secreting plasma cells that assist the macrophages in the inactivation of infectious material. This action is called the *humoral response* and involves five classes of immunoglobulins, IgG, IgM, IgA, IgD, and IgE. The first three classes are important in the control of infectious diseases. IgG and IgM provide the primary and secondary antibody response against pathogens, by facilitating opsonization and phagocytosis of bacteria.

Two types of IgA have been identified and are labeled *secretory IgA* and *serum IgA*. Secretory IgA is the major immunoglobulin found at the surfaces of the mucous membranes. On the respiratory mucosa, IgA protects the lung against viral and bacterial invasion. It may function by inhibiting the adherence of the organisms to the mucosal surfaces. Persons with chronic bronchitis frequently have low levels of IgA, which apparently results in a high incidence of recurrent pulmonary infections [5].

The T lymphocytes provide for cell-mediated immunity. They play a major role in the attraction of macrophages to the site of an infection. Tuberculosis is an excellent prototype for the understanding of this response. Inhaled tubercle bacilli travel from the lung to the lymph nodes where the macrophages engulf, process, and concentrate the antigens of the bacilli. A few T lymphocytes bearing receptors for tuberculin antigens react with the bacillus and undergo multiplication. These T cells circulate back to the lungs and release chemical mediators that induce macrophages and other leukocytes to kill the bacteria.

Humoral and cell-mediated immunity function together to protect the body from infection. Both systems are essential for maximum defense of the body.

Interferon

Interferon is a protein that inhibits viral replication. Production and regulation of interferon appears to take place within the cell. Cells react to viruses by producing the interferon that causes unaffected surrounding cells to synthesize another protein that protects the cell by preventing viral replication. It appears that all cells produce interferon when exposed to a virus, but viruses differ in their ability to act as interferon inducers. It is thought that lymphocytes assist the host to counteract viruses and these lymphocytes have the ability to produce interferon. Because of this it has been suggested that interferon may be the mediator of the cellular immune response with certain viruses.

Interferon may also be important in protecting the organism against bacteria and tumors. It has been used experimentally in the treatment of cancer and in viral infections in immunosuppressed individuals.

Alveolar macrophages, immunologic defenses, lymphatic drainage, and blood flow act together to guard the lungs against infection. The respiratory tract receives many pathogens daily requiring an active defense system.

NORMAL GAS EXCHANGE

Oxygen makes up about 21 percent of the atmospheric air while most of the remaining 79 percent is nitrogen. Carbon dioxide in the atmosphere is only a minute percentage (approximately 0.02%) and minuscule amounts of other trace gases, such as argon, neon, and helium, are present.

Oxygen Transport to the Tissues

The oxygen tension or partial pressure of oxygen at sea level is equal to the barometric pressure of 760 mm Hg multiplied by the fraction of oxygen in dry air (20.93%), which equals 159 mm Hg. However, as the inspired air is warmed and humidified in the upper airways, it is diluted by water vapor and this causes the oxygen tension to fall to 149.3 mm Hg [5]. The inspired air is then further diluted by carbon dioxide in the lower airways and alveoli. Factors that lower inspired oxygen concentration or that raise alveolar carbon dioxide levels will lower alveolar oxygen levels and hence lower arterial blood oxygen tension, which may reduce the delivery of oxygen to the tissues. Table 22-1 displays the normal blood gas pattern seen when arterial blood is drawn for analysis.

TABLE 22-1. Arterial blood gas values

Oxygen	
Tension	75–100 mm Hg breathing room air
Saturation	96–100% of capacity
Carbon dioxide	
Tension	35–45 mm Hg
Arterial pH	7.35–7.45
Bicarbonate	22–26 mEq/L
H_2CO_3	1.05–1.35 mEq/L (always 3% of PCO_2)

Oxygen is delivered by a linked chain of transfers from the atmosphere to the alveoli to the blood and then to the tissues and cells of the body. It diffuses from areas of higher partial pressure to areas of lower pressure. It is transported initially from the air of the atmosphere to the larger airways by movements of the diaphragm and chest wall that cyclically lower the intrathoracic pressure. This process results in the movement of air in and out of the lungs (*ventilation*) and then delivers it by the smaller peripheral airways to the alveoli (*distributes it*). It then crosses the alveolar-capillary membrane (*diffusion*) and is carried in the plasma, bound chemically to the hemoglobin. During the process of *perfusion* blood is delivered past the alveoli for the purpose of gas exchange. At the capillary level it diffuses into the tissue fluid surrounding the cells and then to the cells themselves where it is metabolized. Oxygen is essential for cellular metabolism and the cells have no capability to store it. Without constant delivery of oxygen, tissue hypoxia and anaerobic metabolism result. *Tissue hypoxia* is defined as inadequate critical oxygen tension to meet the needs of the cell. *Critical oxygen tension* is that "cellular oxygen tension at which the mitochondrial respiratory rate begins to decrease" [18].

Tissue hypoxia is not synonymous with *arterial hypoxemia*, which refers to a decreased oxygen tension in the arterial blood. Tissue hypoxia and arterial hypoxemia may exist simultaneously or independently of each other. Arterial hypoxemia can be measured by arterial blood gas measurement. Tissue hypoxia cannot be directly measured but is assessed on the basis of clinical signs and symptoms.

The relationship between arterial and tissue oxygenation is explained in large part by the relationship between hemoglobin and oxygen. Oxygen and carbon dioxide diffuse across a membrane along a gradient from higher pressure to lower pressure. Most of the oxygen is transported to the body cells in chemical combination with hemoglobin. *Hemoglobin* is a complex spherical molecule that is made up of four heme groups, each of which is enfolded in a chain

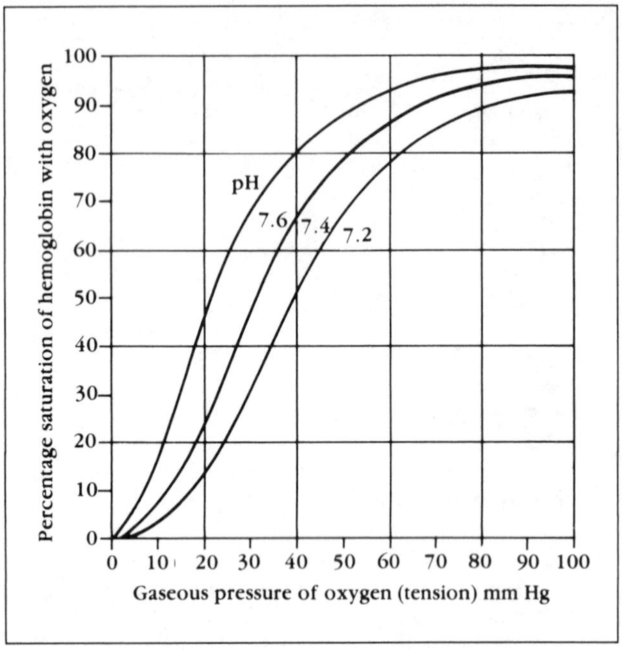

FIGURE 22-17. The oxyhemoglobin dissociation curve.

of amino acids. Each of the heme groups can combine with an oxygen molecule, which gives the hemoglobin the capability of carrying four oxygen molecules per hemoglobin molecule. Hemoglobin combined with oxygen is termed *oxyhemoglobin* (HbO_2) while oxygen-free hemoglobin is called *reduced hemoglobin* (Hb) (see Chap. 14).

In the adult, normal hemoglobin levels range from 12 to 16 gm/dl of blood. It has been found that 1 gm of hemoglobin fully saturated can carry 1.34 ml of oxygen. Each milliliter of blood with an oxygen tension of 100 mm Hg can carry about 0.03 ml of dissolved oxygen. This means that 100 ml of blood with a hemoglobin of 15 gm and 100 percent saturation has an oxygen content of about 20.4 ml of oxygen, which is expressed as *volumes percent*. A very small percentage of oxygen is carried dissolved in the plasma, but hemoglobin is by far the most important method of oxygen transport in the blood.

Oxyhemoglobin Dissociation Curve

The affinity of hemoglobin for oxygen has been plotted on an *oxyhemoglobin dissociation curve* (Fig. 22-17). It is derived by plotting oxyhemoglobin saturation (the percent of hemoglobin that has combined with oxygen) against the oxygen tension (mm Hg) to which it is exposed. Since oxyhemoglobin dissociation is readily reversible, the curve reflects the ease with which hemoglobin gives up oxygen as well as the ease with which it takes up oxygen. This is important because, to a large extent, oxygen delivery to the tissues depends on the ease with which hemoglobin gives up its oxygen once it reaches the tissues.

In studying the oxyhemoglobin dissociation curve, it is readily apparent that the initial portion is very steep and then flattens. The upper portion of the oxyhemoglobin curve is flat showing that when the oxygen tension (PO_2) is 70 mm Hg or above, the hemoglobin becomes nearly fully saturated. When the available oxygen begins to fall below 60 mm Hg, the degree of saturation also falls rapidly. Note in Figure 22-18 that when the PO_2 falls to 40 mm Hg, the saturation of hemoglobin is 75 percent or approximately the level of venous blood. At 20 mm Hg PO_2 the saturation is 35 percent, which is intolerable for any length of time.

Many factors alter the affinity of hemoglobin for oxygen. Some of these are summarized in Figure 22-18. An increase in hemoglobin affinity for oxygen makes the curve shift to the left and oxygen is given up less readily. Alkalemia, hypothermia, and hypocarbia are among factors that can cause a leftward shift. Conversely, acidemia, hypercarbia, and hyperthermia reduce the affinity of hemoglobin for oxygen and cause, by inference, increased oxygen availability to the tissues. Noted on the curve is the *shift to the right*. Figures 22-18B and C show the effects of pH and body temperature on the affinity of hemoglobin for oxygen.

Other factors that affect tissue oxygenation are summarized in Table 22-2. Oxygen content of arterial blood is determined by a combination of alveolar oxygenation, hemoglobin level and quality, and hemoglobin affinity for oxygen. Oxygen delivery to the tissues depends on the status of the cardiovascular system and regional perfusion. At the tissue level, oxygenation depends on vascularity, diffusion characteristics, and intracellular mechanisms.

Carbon Dioxide Transport

Carbon dioxide is produced as the end product of metabolic combustion and travels the opposite pathway along pressure gradients from tissues to blood to alveoli to airways and then out to the atmosphere. Total amounts of oxygen consumed and carbon dioxide produced are *not* determined by the quantity of ventilation, but rather by the actual *metabolic demands* of the cells. The body at rest requires about 250 cc of oxygen per minute and produces about 200 cc of carbon dioxide per minute as a result of its continuing metabolic cellular requirements. Heavy exercise may increase the production of carbon dioxide up to 20 times this volume.

The normal matchup between ventilation and perfusion serves the ultimate purpose of supplying oxygen and eliminating carbon dioxide from the cells and eventually from the body. Alveolar ventilation is about 4 liters of air per minute. Cardiac output and resulting tissue perfusion is about 5 liters of blood per minute.

Because carbon dioxide diffuses about 20 times as easily as oxygen, tissue carbon dioxide diffuses rapidly into the venous end of the capillaries with a gradient of less than 1 mm Hg. Venous blood entering the lungs with a PCO_2 of 46 mm Hg readily transfers carbon dioxide into the alveoli (Fig. 22-19). With normal alveolar ventilation, the alveolar carbon dioxide ($PaCO_2$) of 40 mm Hg is in equilibrium

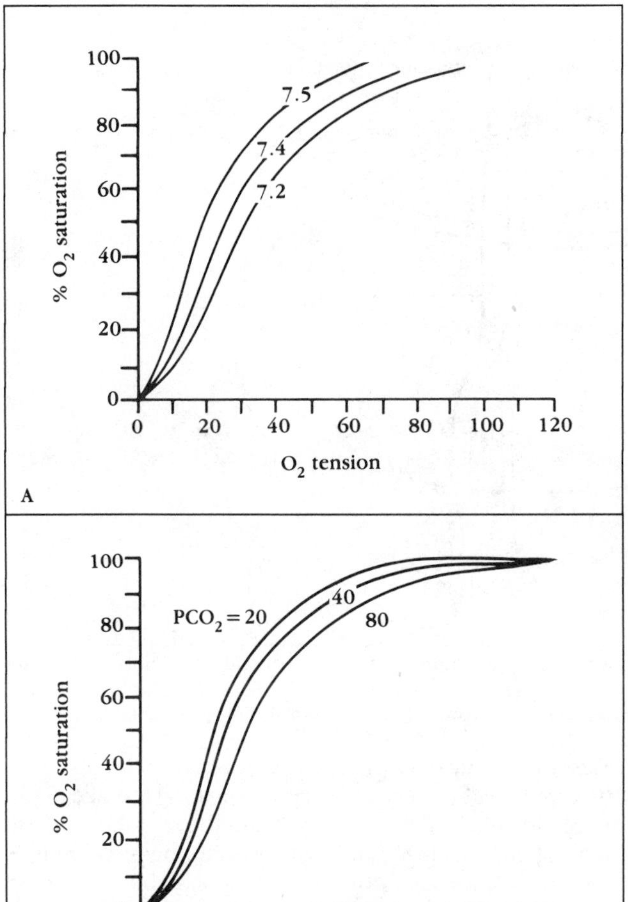

FIGURE 22-18. A. Effects of pH on oxyhemoglobin dissociation curve. B. Effects of PCO_2 on oxyhemoglobin dissociation curve. C. Effects of temperature on oxyhemoglobin dissociation curve.

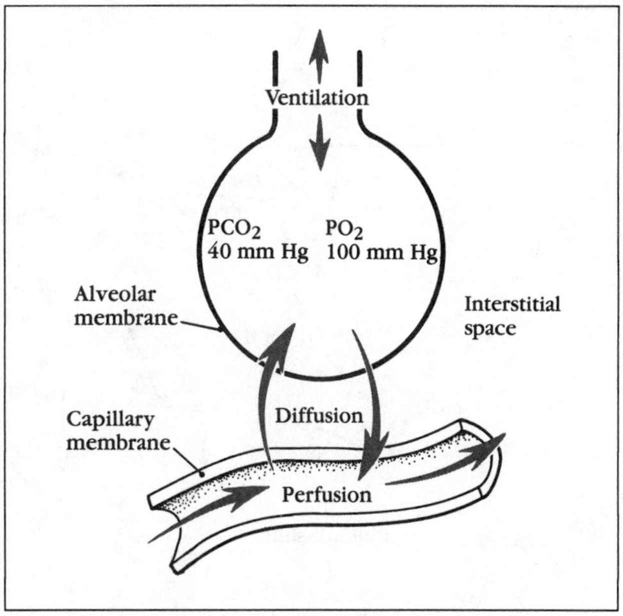

FIGURE 22-19. Movement of gases across the alveolocapillary membrane due to ventilation, diffusion, and perfusion.

TABLE 22-2. Factors that affect tissue oxygenation

Oxygen tension arterial blood
Hemoglobin content
Hemoglobin saturation
Blood flow to tissues
Diffusion of oxygen to tissues
Diffusion of cabon dioxide

with the resulting arterial carbon dioxide ($PaCO_2$) of 40 mm Hg. The level of both alveolar and arterial carbon dioxide is directly and inversely proportional to the volume of alveolar ventilation ($\dot{V}A$). Thus, in alveolar hypoventilation, halving the alveolar ventilation from 4 to 2 liters per minute doubles the $PaCO_2$ from 40 to 80 mm Hg. In hyperventilation doubling the alveolar ventilation from 4 to 8 liters a minute halves the $PaCO_2$ to 20 mm Hg.

Blood carries carbon dioxide in three different forms: (1) Five percent or less of the carbon dioxide is transported to the lungs in the *plasma* as *dissolved carbon dioxide*. (2) Nearly 70 percent of the carbon dioxide diffuses into the red blood cells and is carried in the form of *bicarbonate*. (3) Approximately 25 percent of the carbon dioxide is carried in the red blood cell bound to the hemoglobin.

Figure 22-20 illustrates the reaction of carbon dioxide as it is carried dissolved in the red blood cell. It is important to note that this is a reversible reaction that occurs rapidly at the tissue level where carbon dioxide is picked up and in the lungs where it is released. Most carbon dioxide diffuses into the red blood cells where it is catalyzed in a reaction with carbonic anhydrase and water to form carbonic acid. This carbonic acid immediately dissociates into hydrogen

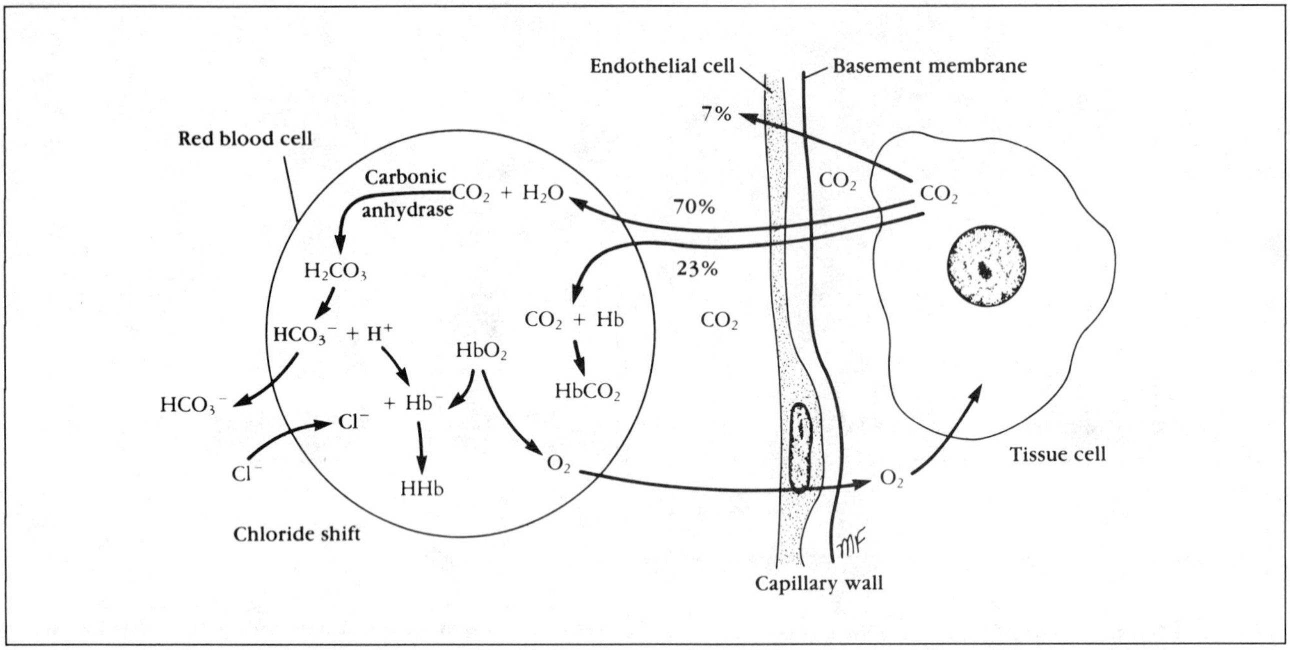

FIGURE 22-20. Methods of carbon dioxide transport in the red blood cell (RBC). (From R. S. Snell, *Clinical Histology for Medical Students.* Boston: Little, Brown, 1984.)

ions (H^+) and bicarbonate ions (HCO_3^-) that can diffuse back into the plasma or may stay in combination with a positive ion in the red blood cell. The excess hydrogen ion formed in this reaction usually binds with the hemoglobin molecule to form hydrogen hemoglobin (HHb). If significant amounts of HCO_3^- diffuse into the plasma, a negative ion is drawn into the red blood cell to equalize the electrochemical gradient. This ion is usually chloride and the process for its movement is called the *chloride shift*. This process can provide bicarbonate to the plasma when the pH is decreased. Normally, in the lungs a reverse process occurs very rapidly. The hydrogen is released from the hemoglobin and recombines with the bicarbonate to form carbonic acid, which dissociates into carbon dioxide and water. The carbon dioxide diffuses out of the red blood cell into the alveolus and is blown off in the exhaled air.

Carbon dioxide may react directly with hemoglobin and be carried in a loose chemical bond directly on the hemoglobin molecule. This is referred to as *carbaminohemoglobin* and accounts for about 25 percent of the carriage of carbon dioxide to the lungs. In the pulmonary capillary bed, the carbon dioxide is simply released to the alveolus and blown off in the exhaled air.

Ventilation-Perfusion Relationships

Arterial oxygenation is affected not only by ventilation but also by the *blood supply to the lung*. Abnormalities in pulmonary blood flow (perfusion) or in relationships between ventilation and perfusion ($\dot{V}a/\dot{Q}$ ratio) will alter arterial oxygen tension and, subsequently, oxygenation of body tissues.

Exchange of oxygen and carbon dioxide occurs as blood circulates through the pulmonary capillary bed. The capillaries are arranged so that each is adjacent to an alveolus. The capillaries are very small, approximating the size of the red blood cell. The capillary wall and the alveolar wall are each only one cell thick so that the diffusing membrane is very thin. Gases, therefore, diffuse across the membrane with little difficulty (Fig. 22-21).

Each red blood cell (RBC) stays in the pulmonary capillary bed about 1 second and exchanges gases with two or three alveoli during this time. Approximately 70 ml of blood is normally exchanging gases at a given moment in the pulmonary capillary bed of an adult, in contrast to the large volume of air that is moved by the alveoli with each breath. This is an important, if temporary, safeguard against oxygen lack. Storing oxygen, even for a few moments, guards against the extra oxygen needs encountered during breath holding [19].

In addition to moving blood to the blood-gas barrier for gas exchange, the pulmonary circulation also functions to provide a reservoir for blood, filter small thrombi from the blood, and trap white blood cells.

Generally, the pulmonary circulation is a low pressure system with pressures much lower than the systemic circulation. The normal mean pulmonary artery pressure (PAP) is 14 mm Hg. Since the mean left atrial pressure of the heart is about 5 mm Hg, the driving pressure across the pulmonary bed is only about 9 mm Hg. Pressure in the pulmonary artery or in the pulmonary capillary bed may be increased by pathology but an increase in one does not necessarily mean a corresponding increase in the other. The pulmonary and systemic circulations are compared in Table 22-3. Table 22-4 gives the normal pressures in the heart and the pulmonary circulation.

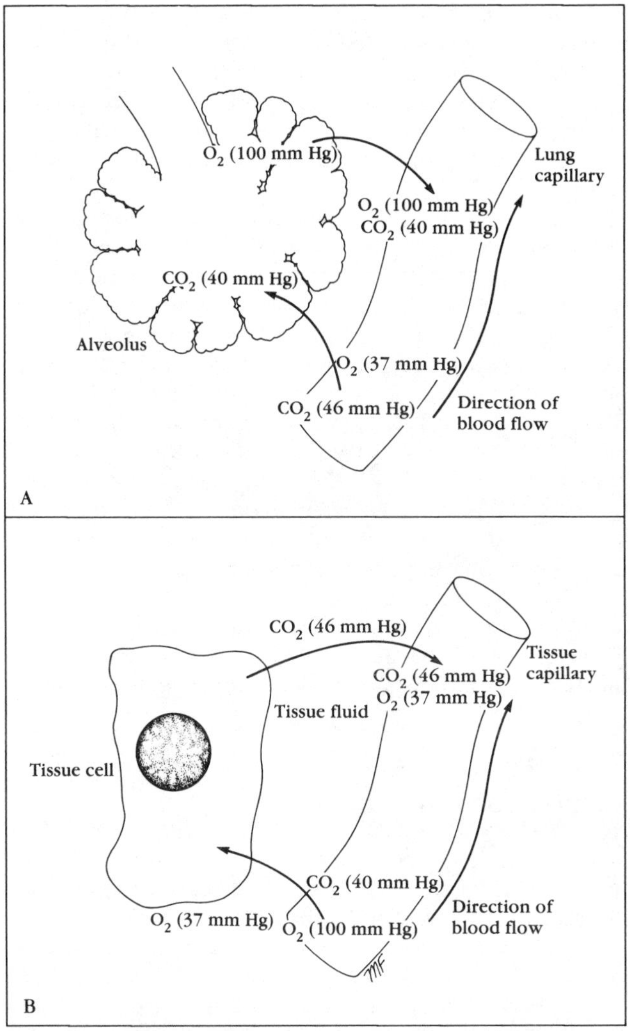

FIGURE 22-21. A. Representation of gas exchange at alveolus. B. Representation of gas exchange at tissue level. (From R. S. Snell, *Clinical Histology for Medical Students.* Boston: Little, Brown, 1984.)

Both acidemia and hypoxemia can stimulate constriction of the pulmonary arteries and thus increase resistance in the pulmonary capillary bed. Either of these conditions causes vasoconstriction alone and together they provide a synergistic effect. Once this vasoconstriction occurs and persists for some time, it may cause an adverse effect on the right ventricle because of increased work needed to pump blood into the constricted pulmonary vasculature. Over a period of time this may lead to right ventricular hypertrophy (RVH) and subsequent right ventricular failure.

Approximately 10 to 20 percent of the total blood volume resides in the pulmonary vascular bed at any given time. The bed is capable of accepting several times this amount, which allows it to accommodate variations in cardiac output or blood volume. The distensibility of the bed is accomplished both by the dilatation of pulmonary vessels and by the opening of closed or unused vessels. This distention of the pulmonary vascular bed reduces pulmonary vascular resistance until its capacity is reached. Then as increases in blood flow cannot be accommodated, pulmonary vascular resistance increases.

Perfusion changes more rapidly from the top to the bottom of the upright lung than does ventilation. Therefore, the ventilation-perfusion ratio decreases down the lung. If the individual is in the upright position, pulmonary blood flow increases linearly from top to bottom due to gravitational forces [13]. At the apex the pulmonary arterial pressure is just sufficient to raise minimal amounts of blood

TABLE 22-3. Differences between pulmonary and systemic circulations

Pulmonary	Systemic
Pressures low: 25/8 mm Hg (mean: 14)	Aortic pressure about 100 mm Hg
Walls very thin with little smooth muscle	Artery walls thick-walled with much smooth muscle
System rarely concerned with directing blood between regions (except in case of localized alveolar hypoxia); keeps work of right heart low	Regulates and distributes blood supply throughout body
Pressure changes within lungs, symmetric and of low magnitude	Asymmetric pressure changes of great magnitude throughout body
Capillaries surrounded by gas have little support; therefore, collapse or distend depending on pressure within and around them	Surrounded by tissue; less easily changes caliber
Pressure may be determined by arteriolar/alveolar gradient or arteriolar/venous gradient	Pressure determined by arteriolar/venous gradient
Pulmonary vascular resistance is $^1/_{10}$ that of systemic circulation; able to reduce resistance as pressure in system rises	Resistance is 10 times that of pulmonary circulation; less able to lower resistance when needed

TABLE 22-4. Approximate normal pressures in the heart and pulmonary circuit

Superior vena cava	6–10 mm Hg
Inferior vena cava	6–10 mm Hg
Right atrium	2–5 mm Hg
Right ventricle	25/0–5 mm Hg
Pulmonary artery	25/10 mm Hg
Pulmonary capillary bed	8–12 mm Hg
Left atrium	5–10 mm Hg
Left ventricle	120/0–10 mm Hg
Aorta	120/80 mm Hg
Systemic arteriole	30 mm Hg

to the top of the lung and perfuse the apices. Capillary pressure is very low. If blood volume is reduced for some reason, such as systemic blood loss or pulmonary capillary destruction, there may be decreased or absent apical perfusion.

The blood flow to the lungs changes with exercise and position. With exercise, all areas of the lung receive increased blood flow. When a person lies down, blood flow from the apex to base becomes uniform.

The concept of regional differences in ventilation has important ramifications for the person with asymmetric lung pathology. An example might be the person whose left lung on x ray appears to be *whited out* by a process such as pneumonia. In order to maximize ventilation, perfusion, and gas exchange, the person should not be positioned on the left side. Instead, the abilities of the unaffected lung should be capitalized on with back- and right-sided turning. Arterial blood gas values can be significantly affected with this type of positioning.

As previously mentioned, the perfusion gradient down the lung exceeds the ventilation gradient. In order to state a $\dot{V}a/\dot{Q}$ ratio, ventilation and perfusion must be expressed in the same units. For example, a blood flow of 6 liters/minute and ventilation of 5 liters/minute in the average adult male results in ventilation-perfusion ($\dot{V}a/\dot{Q}$) ratio of about 0.8:1.0 or 0.8. In the normal person, the deviation from a ratio of 1 is largely due to anatomic dead space. Normally, a portion of the air inspired does not come in contact with the alveoli and does not participate in gas exchange. This *anatomic dead space* usually remains relatively constant, but *alveolar dead space* (where alveolar gas does not participate in blood-gas exchange) may be significantly altered in pathologic states. The $\dot{V}a/\dot{Q}$ ratio is altered in conditions where alveolar dead space ventilation and thus physiologic dead space ventilation is increased. A higher than normal amount of inspired gas is wasted with the result that a lower than normal amount of inspired gas is exchanged with the blood. To compensate for this wasted ventilation and to maintain a normal PaO_2 and $PaCO_2$, total ventilation must increase. This will move more inspired gas per minute to improve exchange with the blood. If the body is incapable of increasing ventilation and blood flow enough to maintain adequate gas exchange, then carbon dioxide retention and hypoxemia may result. In any case the work of breathing is increased. If the body is incapable of altering ventilation and blood flow to meet this need, altered blood gases, decreased cellular oxygenation, and clinical symptoms will occur.

The opposite of *dead space ventilation* is *shunting*. All cardiopulmonary and pulmonary disease leads either to dead space ventilation or shunting or both. Shunting refers to an area that is perfused but not ventilated (Fig. 22-22). A small amount of shunting (less than 2.5% of cardiac output) is normal; it occurs because not all blood is exchanged at the alveolocapillary line. This accounts for the fact that normal oxygen saturation of hemoglobin in arterial blood gases is 96 to 100 percent. Pathologic amounts of shunting may be caused by such problems of nonventilation as atelectasis and pneumonia (see Chap. 23).

In shunting, the $\dot{V}a/\dot{Q}$ is decreased. The blood returning from the affected areas of the lung mixes with the blood returning from the oxygenated areas. This lowers the total level of oxygen in the arterial blood resulting in a lowered PaO_2.

If shunting is not severe, the body can compensate for the amount of carbon dioxide that is not excreted by the shunted areas. Hyperventilation of the unaffected areas can blow off enough carbon dioxide to compensate. Oxygen exchange cannot be compensated for so readily because carbon dioxide is much more readily diffusible than oxygen. If compensation occurs, it will lead to a blood gas pattern of normal $PaCO_2$ with hypoxemia. If the body is unable to compensate adequately for the carbon dioxide, exchange blood gases will show acidemia, hypoxemia, and hypercapnia. A compromised pulmonary or cardiovascular system could lead to loss of ability to compensate for the demands of shunting or other abnormalities.

Both shunt and dead space defects are often referred to as $\dot{V}a/\dot{Q}$ mismatching. All other factors being equal, the lung with a $\dot{V}a/\dot{Q}$ mismatch will not be able to exchange as much oxygen and carbon dioxide as the lung with a normal $\dot{V}a/\dot{Q}$ ratio.

RESPIRATORY REGULATION OF ACID-BASE EQUILIBRIUM

As has been described in Chapter 6, the major buffers are hemoglobin, the plasma proteins, and the carbonic acid-bicarbonate system. Any increase in carbon dioxide concentration in the blood causes a shift in the blood pH toward the acidic side and any decrease in the carbon dioxide level causes it to shift toward the alkaline side. Therefore, the amount of carbon dioxide present in the blood affects the pH significantly. This carbon dioxide, usually in the form of carbonic acid (H_2CO_3), is closely regulated by the physiologic buffer system of the lungs.

If the metabolic rate increases, the rate of carbon dioxide formation increases and, conversely, if the rate of metabolism decreases the formation of carbon dioxide also decreases. Alveolar ventilation also changes according to nervous control of respiration through the *chemoreceptors* in the medulla. These chemoreceptors are extremely sensitive to minute changes in the carbon dioxide level and stimulate an increase or decrease in the respiratory rate. If the blood pH declines to 7.0, the alveolar ventilation may increase up to 5 times above the resting value. Also, an increase in the pH above 7.4 may decrease the alveolar ventilation to one-half the normal value. Thus, the respiratory rate and the depth of respiration, physiologically, can retain or blow off excess carbon dioxide according to the pH of the blood.

The two major alterations in acid-base balance related to pulmonary function are *respiratory acidosis* and *alkalosis*. Respiratory acidosis is always due to some factor that com-

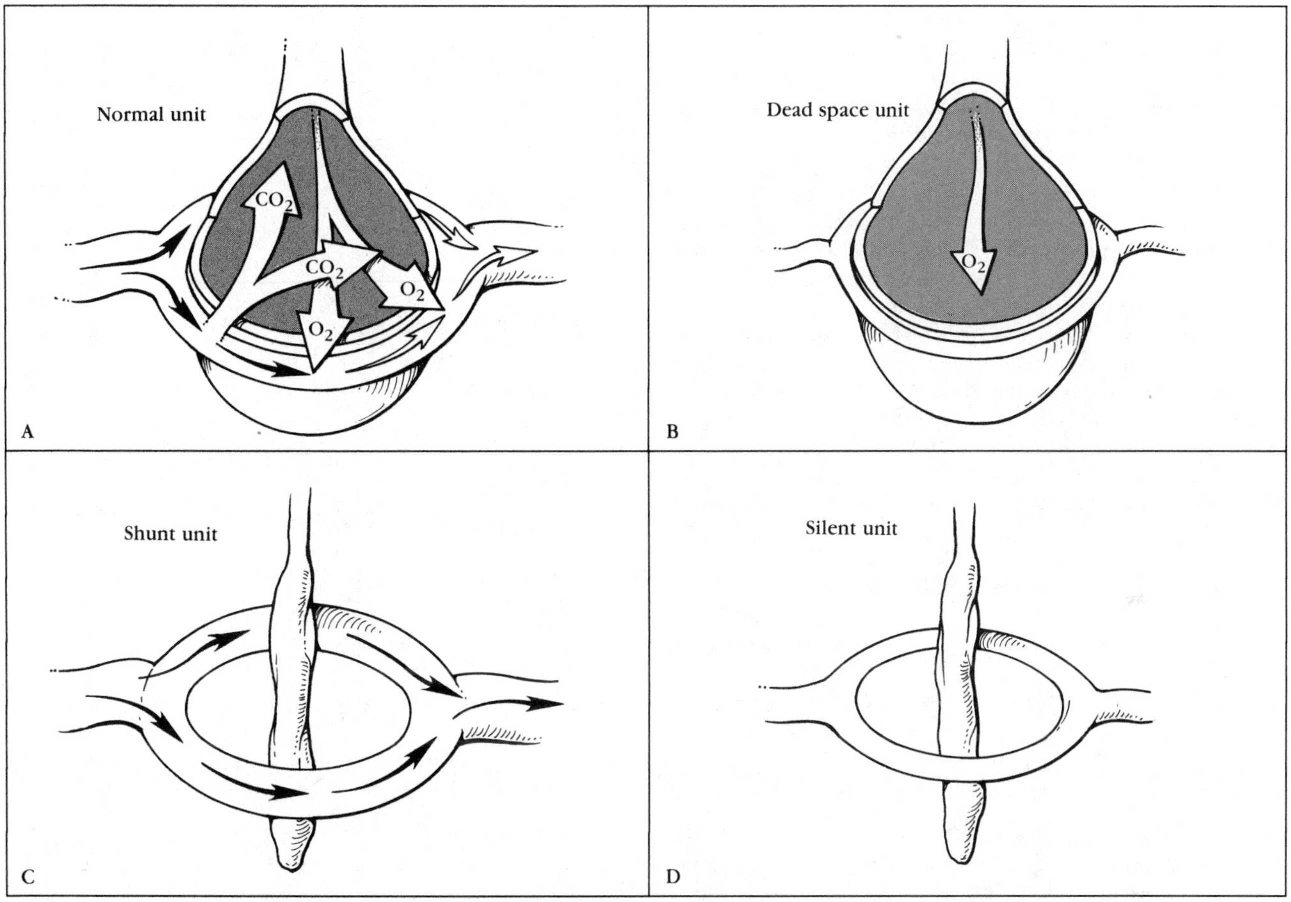

FIGURE 22-22. A. Schematic representation of normal alveolar-capillary unit. B. Representation of ventilation without perfusion. C. Representation of perfusion without ventilation. D. Representation of neither perfusion nor ventilation.

promises ventilation. Thus, hypoventilation leads to retained carbon dioxide, causing an excess of carbonic acid in the blood. The excess carbon dioxide or hydrogen ion is a powerful stimulus for the central chemoreceptor in the medulla oblongata, which initiates a response increasing respiratory rate and depth.

Respiratory alkalosis results from hyperventilation, which blows off carbon dioxide, leading to a decreased carbonic acid and a shift of the pH to the alkaline side.

The Henderson-Hasselbalch equation expresses the relationship of the pH to bicarbonate and PCO_2 showing a direct relationship to bicarbonate and an inverse relationship to PCO_2. In formula it is expressed as follows [2]:

$$pH \propto \frac{HCO_3^-}{PaCO_2}$$

The reader is referred to Chapter 6 for a more detailed discussion of acid-base balance.

PULMONARY FUNCTION TESTING

Pulmonary function testing (PFT) measures many variables including the lung volumes. PFTs are important tools in the diagnosis and evaluation of pulmonary status. The spirometric tests have the limitations of recognizing abnormalities only when they are relatively diffuse. Therefore, spirometric studies may be normal in early disease states or in localized rather than diffuse conditions. When an abnormality of a PFT exists, other clinical data must be collected prior to making an accurate diagnosis. The effectiveness of spirometry also is totally dependent on the ability and cooperation of the persons being tested. Pulmonary function study results are evaluated in relation to predicted normals. Tables of norms based on age, sex, and size are used by physicians to predict normal values for each person. The tables of norms are not totally reliable because of the individual differences between persons. One person, for example, may normally have a greater than predicted vital capacity, which may actually be compromised even though the test results are in the normal range according to the tables.

Pulmonary function testing provides a yardstick in the diagnosis of the amount of disability occurring in the course of pulmonary disease. The tests are used in many settings to diagnose and manage patients with pulmonary or cardiac disability, and in epidemiologic surveys for industrial hazards or community disease risks.

Lung contents can be divided into four lung capacities or compartments, each of which is made up of two or more volumes (Fig. 22-23). The *lung volumes* usually are measured as follows:

1. *Tidal volume* (V_T) is the volume of gas moved into and out of the lungs with each breath. The normal tidal volume is only a small percentage of the amount of air that the lungs are capable of moving.
2. *Expiratory reserve volume* (ERV) is the additional amount of gas or air that can be forcefully exhaled after a normal expiration is complete.
3. *Residual volume* (RV) is the amount of air remaining in the lungs after a forced expiration.
4. *Inspiratory reserve volume* (IRV) is the maximum volume of air that can be inhaled after a normal resting inspiration.

The *lung capacities* are as follows:

1. *Total lung capacity* (TLC) is the maximum volume of gas that the lung can hold. All of this gas is not available for exchange because it includes dead space gas. The total lung capacity equals the inspiratory reserve volume plus the tidal volume plus the expiratory reserve volume plus the residual volume ($TLC = IRV + V_T + ERV + RV$).

2. *Functional residual capacity* (FRC) refers to the volume of gas remaining in the lungs at the end of a spontaneous expiration and includes the expiratory reserve volume and the residual volume ($FRC = ERV + RV$). The functional residual capacity decreases in conditions such as obesity that affect the chest wall mass. With an increased FRC it would take more change in the ventilatory rate or more time to reduce a given high carbon dioxide level than with a normal FRC.

3. *Vital capacity* (VC) can be measured either as expiratory vital capacity or inspiratory vital capacity. *Expiratory vital capacity* is the maximum volume of gas that can be exhaled after the deepest possible inspiration. Usually expiratory VC equals *inspiratory VC*, which is the maximum amount of gas that can be inhaled after the fullest possible expiration. *Total vital capacity* therefore equals inspiratory reserve volume plus tidal volume plus expiratory reserve volume ($VC = IRV + V_T + ERV$). It equals about 5000 cc in men. In severe obstructive pulmonary disease, the inspiratory vital capacity may be much greater than the expiratory vital capacity. The vital capacity increases with height, usually is greater in men, and is roughly proportional to lean body weight in young adults. Vital capacity decreases slightly in the supine position due to the splinting of posterior rib movement and reduced diaphragmatic action. On quiet breathing, the lungs are roughly one-third inflated in the supine position and one-half inflated in the upright position.

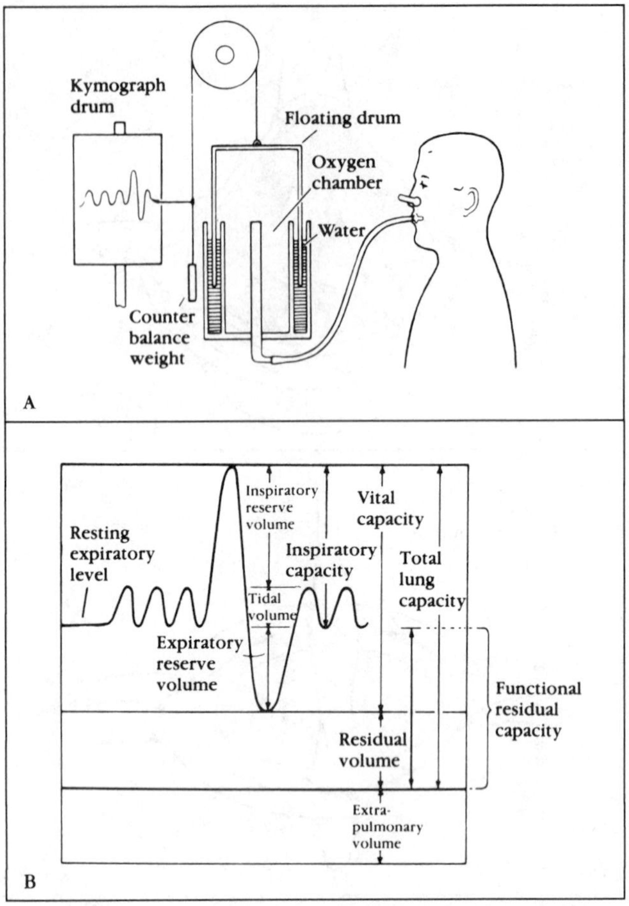

FIGURE 22-23. A. Structure of the spirometer used for direct measurement of lung volumes. B. Components of lung volume. (From E. E. Selkurt, *Basic Physiology for the Health Sciences* [2nd ed.]. Boston: Little, Brown, 1982.)

4. *Inspiratory capacity* (IC) is the maximum volume of air that can be inhaled from a resting position. It equals the tidal volume plus the inspiratory reserve volume ($IC = V_T + IRV$.

The residual volume, total lung capacity, vital capacity, and functional residual capacity are not anatomically fixed, but depend on elastic characteristics and muscle forces. Age changes all lung volumes and capacities by decreasing the elastic recoil as the age increases. The resting position (at the end of quiet expiration) shifts in the direction of inspiration so the residual volume and functional residual capacity increase slightly and the vital capacity decreases with age. This decrease is partially due to the stiffening of the thoracic cage and decrease in the chest mobility.

Besides the lung volumes, the forced *expiratory vital capacity* can yield much information in persons with chronic obstructive disease.

In Figure 22-23 point A is a beginning of the forced expiration and point B is its completion. The shape of the curve

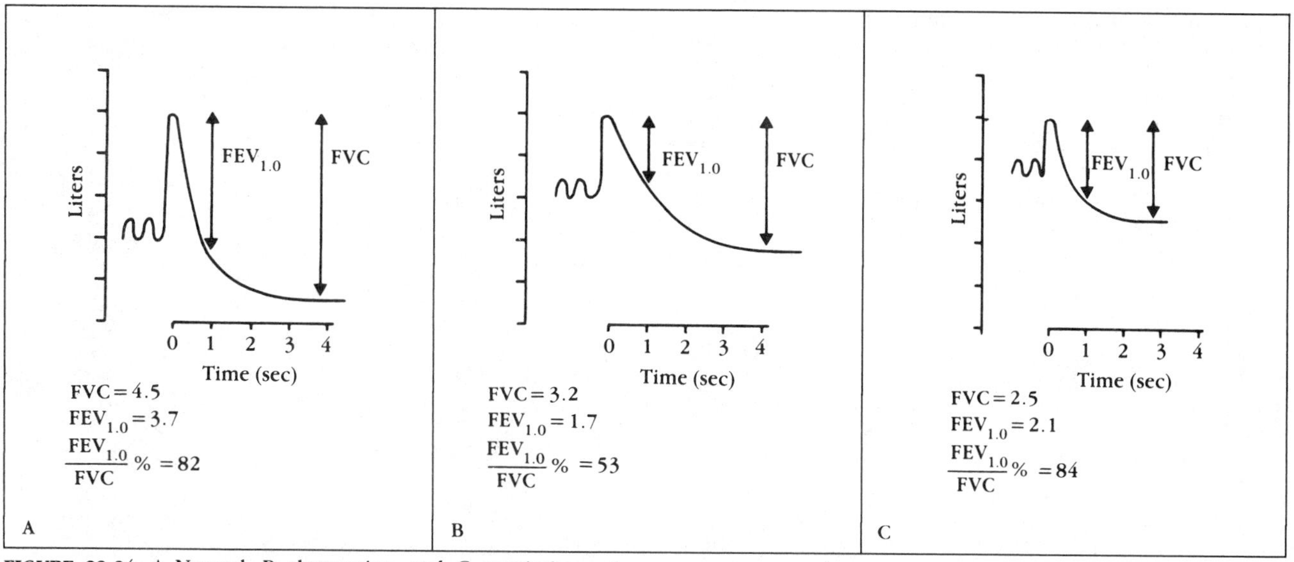

FIGURE 22-24. A. Normal, B. obstructive, and C. restrictive patterns of a forced expiration. (From H. A. Braun, F. W. Cheney, Jr., and C. P. Loehnen, *Introduction to Respiratory Physiology* [2nd ed.]. Boston: Little, Brown, 1980.)

is important in indicating abnormalities. Generally, in obstructive disease, the expiration takes much longer than normal and is less complete because of premature airway closure and subsequent air trapping (Fig. 22-24). In restrictive disease, the shape of the curve may be normal, but compressed due to the smaller chest volume without changes in the actual air flow (Fig. 22-24C). The curve is measured to determine the *FEV*$_{1.0}$. This is the volume of air expired in the first second of the forced expiratory maneuver. The volume obtained by the $FEV_{1.0}$ is placed over the FVC to get a ratio or percentage. Normally, the $FEV_{1.0}$/FVC is 80 percent, which means that 80 percent of the total volume is expired in the first second. Generally, in restrictive lung disease, both FVC and $FEV_{1.0}$ are reduced. In contrast, obstructive disease tends to reduce the $FEV_{1.0}$ much more than the FVC (Fig. 22-24B). Mixed restrictive and obstructive patterns are not uncommon and the $FEV_{1.0}$ may also be affected by changes in airway resistance, elastic recoil, and in lung compliance [13].

Alveolar ventilation, or the amount of gas actually reaching the exchange area, refers to the tidal volume minus the dead space. This is calculated as follows:

$$\dot{V}_A = (V_T - V_D) \times f$$

$\dot{V}_A$ is alveolar ventilation in 1 minute. The dot indicates that it is a timed measurement; f equals respiratory frequency. Most physicians estimate dead space from standard tables; however, an easy approximate value is that it equals an adult's ideal weight in pounds.

Minute ventilation is the total amount of air entering or leaving the body per minute. It is calculated by multiplying the tidal volume times the respiratory rate. It includes the anatomic dead space. The formula for this calculation is as follows:

$$\dot{V}_E = V_T \times R$$

REFERENCES

1. Asmundson, T., and Kilburn, K. Mechanisms of Respiratory Tract Clearance. In M. J. Dulfano (ed.), *Sputum: Fundamentals and Clinical Pathology.* Springfield, Ill.: Thomas, 1973.
2. Braun, H. A., Cheney, F. W., Jr., Loehnen, C. P. *Introduction to Respiratory Physiology* (2nd ed.). Boston: Little, Brown, 1980.
3. Burrows, B., Knudson, R., and Kettel, L. *Respiratory Insufficiency.* Chicago: Year Book, 1975.
4. Comroe, J. H. *Physiology of Respiration* (2nd ed.). Chicago: Year Book, 1974.
5. Fitzgerald, M., Carrington, C., and Gaensler, E. Environmental lung disease. *Med. Clin. North Am.* 57:593, 1973.
6. Green, G. Pulmonary clearance of infectious agents. *Annu. Rev. Med.* 19:315, 1968.
7. Guyton, A. *Textbook of Medical Physiology* (6th ed.). Philadelphia: Saunders, 1981.
8. Jacques, J. A. *Respiratory Physiology.* New York: McGraw-Hill, 1979.
9. Johansen, W., and Gould, K. Lung defense mechanisms. *Basics Respir. Dis.* 6:2, 1977.
10. Kilburn, K. An hypothesis for pulmonary clearance and its implications. *Am. Rev. Resp. Dis.* 98:449, 1968.
11. Laurell, C., and Erickson, S. Electrophorphetic alpha$_1$ antitrypsin deficiency. *Scand. J. Clin. Lab. Invest.* 15:132, 1963.
12. Lieberman, J. Alpha$_1$ antitrypsin deficiency. *Med. Clin. North Am.* 57:691, 1973.
13. MacDonnell, K., and Segal, M. *Current Respiratory Care.* Boston: Little, Brown, 1977.
14. Morrow, P. Dynamics of Dust Removal from Lower Airways. In A. Bouhuys (ed.), *Airway Dynamics.* Springfield, Ill.: Thomas, 1974.
15. Selkurt, E. *Basic Physiology for the Health Sciences* (2nd ed.). Boston: Little, Brown, 1982.

16. Tisi, G., and Brauwald, E. Cough and Hemoptysis. In K.J. Isselbacher, et al. (eds.), *Principles of Internal Medicine* (9th ed.). New York: McGraw-Hill, 1980.
17. Trout, C., et al. Perspectives in Critical Care. Unpublished.
18. Walter, J. B. *An Introduction to the Principles of Disease* (2nd ed.). Philadelphia: Saunders, 1982.
19. West, J. *Respiratory Physiology: The Essentials*. Baltimore, Williams & Wilkins, 1974.

CHAPTER 23
RESTRICTIVE ALTERATIONS IN PULMONARY FUNCTION

LEARNING OBJECTIVES

1. Define *restrictive pulmonary disease.*
2. Describe compression and absorption atelectasis.
3. Discuss the role of surfactant in the production of atelectasis.
4. Discuss ventilation-perfusion abnormalities in atelectasis.
5. List the clinical manifestations of this condition.
6. List organisms and areas that are affected in upper respiratory tract infections.
7. Describe the etiologic factors in bacterial pneumonia.
8. Discuss the pathophysiology of pneumococcal pneumonia.
9. List the cause of tuberculosis and the role of individual susceptibility in disease production.
10. Describe the pathophysiology of primary and reinfection tuberculosis.
11. List two causes of aspiration pneumonia and describe the danger of each.
12. Discuss the cardiac and noncardiac causes of pulmonary edema.
13. Describe, in detail, the pathophysiology of alveolar and interstitial pulmonary edema.
14. Discuss how restrictive pulmonary disease can occur in a person having a simple rib fracture.
15. Describe the hemodynamics of flail chest abnormality.
16. List and describe disease-induced pleural effusion.
17. Outline the clinical manifestations of pleural effusion.
18. Describe tension pneumothorax.
19. Review central nervous system control of respiration.
20. Indicate how a head injury may affect respiration.
21. Define *Guillain-Barré syndrome.*
22. Describe the pulmonary problems that may occur with Guillain-Barré syndrome.
23. Describe the onset of respiratory failure in Duchenne's muscular dystrophy.
24. List at least four substances that may cause pneumoconiosis.
25. Outline the way in which silicosis and asbestosis can cause a restrictive process.
26. Indicate how particulate matter is cleared in coal worker's pneumoconiosis.
27. Relate the development of pulmonary fibrosis to emphysematic changes in the pneumoconioses.
28. Define byssinosis.

29. Indicate two chest deformities that may cause restrictive pulmonary disease.
30. Explain why restrictive pulmonary disease can occur in obese individuals, especially in those afflicted by the Pickwickian syndrome.
31. Define the role of surfactant in the production of the idiopathic respiratory distress syndrome of newborns (IRDS).
32. Describe, in detail, the pathophysiology of the adult respiratory distress syndrome (ARDS).
33. List at least 10 conditions that may lead to ARDS.

Restrictive pulmonary disease is an abnormal condition that causes a decrease in the total lung capacity and the vital capacity. It involves difficulty in the inspiratory phase of respiration. In this chapter a group of conditions are considered, some of which do not precisely fit the above definition but which may lead to significant restriction. The following conditions are described in this chapter: atelectasis, infectious disease of the respiratory tract, aspiration pneumonia, pulmonary edema, pleural effusion, pneumothorax, trauma to the lungs and thorax, neuromuscular disease, central nervous system depression, pneumoconiosis, pulmonary fibrosis, thoracic wall deformity, obesity, and idiopathic respiratory distress syndrome. Table 23-1 classifies these conditions according to the source of the problem.

ATELECTASIS

This very common acute restrictive disease involves the collapse of previously expanded lung tissue or incomplete expansion at birth. It is usually described as a shrunken, airless state of the alveoli.

The two major alterations that occur with atelectasis are compression of the lung tissue from a source outside the alveoli and absorption that involves gas absorption from the alveoli. *Compression atelectasis* may be produced by such conditions as pneumothorax, pleural effusion, or tumors within the thorax. *Absorption atelectasis* occurs when secretions in the bronchi and bronchioles obstruct these airways and prevent the movement of air into the alveoli. The air trapped in the alveoli is absorbed and the alveolar sacs collapse. The stasis of secretions in the larger airways provides an excellent medium for bacterial growth and stasis pneumonia. Figure 23-1 illustrates the two conditions.

Atelectasis is a common postoperative complication due to retained secretions. The surgical patient has a decreased protective cough response due to medications and pain. An ineffective cough reflex, diminishing the tidal volume, and a decreased sigh mechanism lead to inadequate alveolar expansion. Increased viscosity of sputum results, with a tendency for secretions to gravitate to the dependent areas.

Adults are susceptible to atelectasis, particularly in the right middle lobe, which is more vulnerable because of the angle of convergence of its bronchus with the right main bronchus. The right middle lobe also seems to have an increased susceptibility to bacterial pneumonia, which tends to flourish in copious pooled secretions.

As was noted in Chapter 22, the natural tendency of the lungs is to collapse. In other words, the elastic forces are constantly trying to force the lung tissue inward. These forces are opposed by the negative intrapleural forces and chest wall expansion. When airflow into the alveoli is obstructed, alveolar sacs collapse and produce little or no surfactant. Surfactant, due to its short half-life, must be constantly replenished and this requires normal ventilation. To offset the tendency toward collapse, collateral communication often occurs through the pores of Kohn, the amount of

TABLE 23-1. Restrictive diseases

Category	Examples of disease entities	Summary of pathology	Assessment of findings
Respiratory center depression	Narcotics and barbiturate dependence	Direct depression of respiratory center	Respiratory rate: <12/minute; associated signs of hypoventilation
	Central nervous system lesions, head trauma	Injury to or impingement on respiratory centers	Hyper- or hypoventilation; cerebral edema and its signs
Neuromuscular	Guillain-Barré syndrome	Acute toxic polyneuritis; intercostal paralysis leads to diaphragmatic breathing; vagal and SNS paralysis lead to reduced ability of bronchioles to constrict, dilate, react to irritants	Reduced negative inspiratory pressure, V_T, V_C, compliance, breath sounds; hypoxemia, hypercapnia
	Duchenne's muscular dystrophy	Genetic; thoracoscoliosis; paralysis of intercostals, abdominal muscles, diaphragm, accessory muscles	Pulmonary symptoms appear late; reduced IC, ERV, V_C, V_T, FRC, compliance PO_2; elevated PCO_2; abnormal respiratory patterns
Restriction of thoracic excursion			
Thoracic deformity	Kyphoscoliosis, pectus excavatum	Deformity of chest compresses lung tissue and limits thoracic excursion	Reduced breath sounds in affected areas, probably with rales; reduced compliance, TLC, V_C, ERV; signs of hypoventilation, hypoxemia, increased work of breathing
Traumatic chest wall instability	Flail chest	Fracture of a group of ribs leads to unstable chest wall; reduced intrathoracic pressure on inspiration pulls area in and causes pressure on parenchyma; this increases work of breathing and hypoventilation	Obvious flail, unequal chest excursion, bruising, skin injuries, localized pain on inspiration, dyspnea, reduced breath sounds with rales and rhonchi; reduced compliance, ERV, TLC, V_C, PO_2
Obesity	Pickwickian syndrome	Excess abdominal adipose tissue impinges on thoracic space and diaphragmatic excursion; increased weight of chest restricts thoracic excursion	Somnolence, twitching, periodic respirations, polycythemia, right ventricular hypertrophy/failure; reduced compliance, ERV, TLC, V_C, PO_2; elevated PCO_2; distant breath sounds
Pleural disorders	Pleural effusion	Accumulation of fluid in pleural space secondary to altered hydrostatic or oncotic forces	Unequal chest expansion; dullness and reduced breath sounds in affected area; may be constant chest discomfort; dyspnea if amount of fluid large; if over 250 ml, will show on x ray; if large, bulging of intercostal spaces
	Pneumothorax	Accumulation of air in pleural space with proportional lung collapse	Hyperresonance; reduced breath sounds; tracheal deviation away from pneumothorax; tachycardia; unequal chest expansion; breath sounds reduced or absent; shows on x ray
Disorders of lung parenchyma	Pulmonary fibrosis	Many possible causes: occupational sarcoid, etc.	Reduced compliance, hypoxemia, hypercapnia, and their consequences
	Tuberculosis	Bacterial invasion leads to scarring, reduced compliance, and reduced lung function	Visible on x ray; positive skin test, sputum; malaise, weight loss, fatigue, evening fever with night sweats, cough, hemoptysis
	Atelectasis	Obstruction of bronchioles, shrunken airless alveoli; reduced compliance; right-to-left shunting	Dyspnea, tachycardia, cough, fever, decreased chest wall expansion, hypoxemia, x ray evidence

TABLE 23-1. (continued)

Category	Examples of disease entities	Summary of pathology	Assessment of findings
Disorders of lung parenchyma	Adult respiratory distress syndrome (ARDS)	Widespread atelectasis; loss of surfactant; interstitial edema, formation of hyaline membrane	Dyspnea, tachypnea, grunting, labored respirations, hypoxemia, occasional hypercapnia, cyanosis; x ray shows bilateral patchy infiltrates
	Pulmonary edema	Increased pulmonary capillary pressure leads to interstitial and alveolar edema	Hypoxemia, tachypnea; signs of CHF, x ray butterfly infiltrates, rales
	Aspiration pneumonia	Chemical irritant from aspirant leads to bronchoconstriction, necrosis, and fibrosis of airways	Hypoxemia, signs of ARDS, wheezing, tachypnea, tachycardia
	Pneumoconiosis	Inhalation of pollutants, results in scarring, fibrosis, and secondary emphysema	Slow developing pulmonary signs of dyspnea, hypoxemia, hypercapnia, cor pulmonale

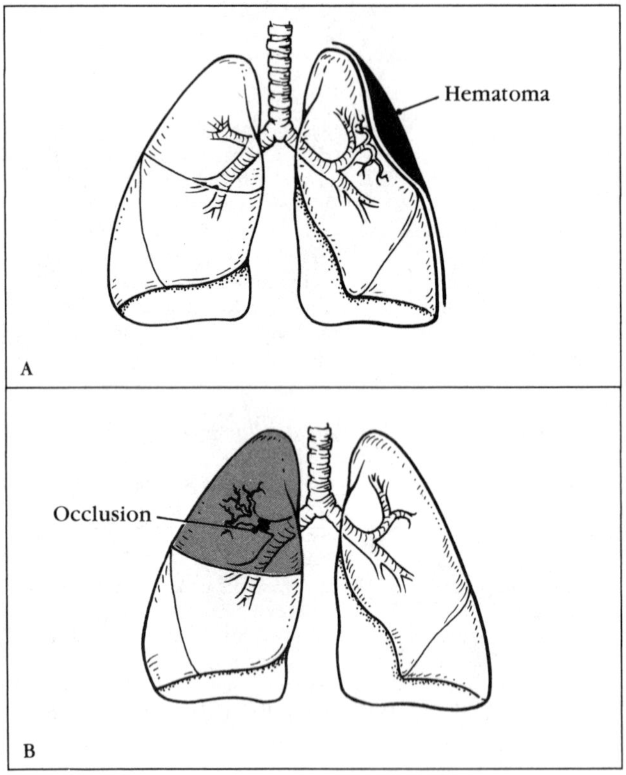

FIGURE 23-1. A. Compression of lung tissue by hematoma. B. Right upper lobe atelectasis caused by broncial occlusion.

which partly depends on the overall degree of inflation of the lungs (Fig. 23-2).

Perfusion to the collapsed airways is not affected so that the blood shunts by the ineffective alveoli and is not oxygenated. This results in a *perfusion without ventilation* shunt or a direct right-to-left shunt across the lungs (Fig. 23-3). Therefore, if significant atelectasis is present, there will also be significant hypoxemia.

One can readily see that the process of atelectasis may occur in many situations. It may also occur alongside obstructive conditions with a portion of lung tissue being hyperinflated and adjacent sections collapsed.

The clinical manifestations of this condition depend on the amount of atelectasis present. Presence of rales in the bases and/or diminished breath sounds are common in postoperative atelectasis. In mild cases there may be no symptoms but as it progresses, or becomes more widespread, dyspnea, tachycardia, cough, fever, and disturbances in chest wall expansion may occur. Blood gas analysis shows hypoxemia when significant atelectasis is present. Hypercapnia and decreased pH may herald a progression toward respiratory failure (see Chap. 25).

INFECTIOUS DISEASE OF THE RESPIRATORY TRACT

Infectious processes can involve either the upper or lower respiratory tract or both. These may be caused by viruses, bacteria, rickettsia or fungi, and be mild, self-limiting, or very debilitating.

Upper Respiratory Tract Infection

The upper respiratory tract functions to warm, humidify, and filter the air; in this process it is exposed to a wide variety of pathogens that may lodge and grow in various areas depending on the susceptibility of the host. Pathogens may lodge in the nose, pharynx (particularly the tonsils), larynx, or trachea and may proliferate if the defenses of the host are depressed. The spread of the infection depends on the resistance mounted by the host to the pathogen and on the virulence of the organism. Figure 23-4 shows the defensive anatomy and physiology of the upper respiratory tract including the mucociliary blanket, which normally provides a very efficient cleansing mechanism for expelling foreign material.

An example of an *upper respiratory tract infection* is the sore throat (nasopharyngitis), which, if caused by the bacteria hemolytic streptococci, leads to suppuration in the nasopharynx and tonsils that may spread to the sinuses.

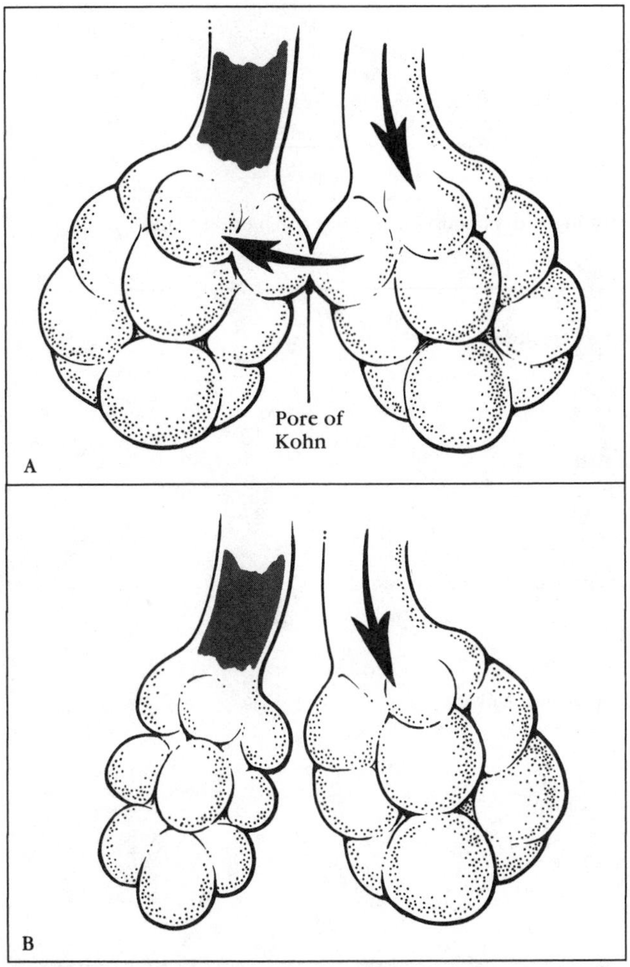

FIGURE 23-2. A. Demonstration of collateral communication between the alveoli through pores of Kohn. B. Atelectasis occurring without this communication.

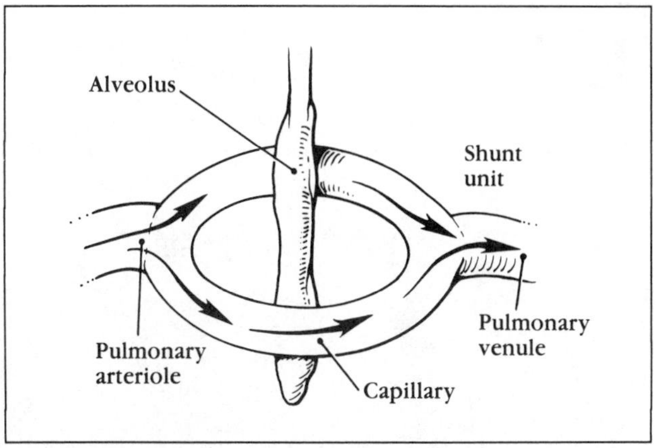

FIGURE 23-3. Shunt unit demonstrating a right-to-left shunt across the pulmonary bed.

Susceptible individuals may later develop a reaction to the organism that is manifested as rheumatic fever (see Chap. 19).

Viruses also can cause pathology of the upper respiratory tract. Influenza, for example, is characterized by an acute inflammation of the nasopharynx, trachea, and bronchioles, leading to edema, congestion, and necrosis of these structures. The common cold is characterized by an acute inflammation of the nasopharynx, pharynx, larynx, and trachea resulting in swelling of the mucous membranes and mucopurulent serous exudate. The purulence is due to secondary bacterial infection.

Lower Respiratory Tract Infection

Infectious processes of the lower respiratory tract can be caused by any of the pathogens that affect the upper respiratory tract. These lead to a variety of pathologic and clinical appearances, depending on host resistance and virulence of the organism.

BACTERIAL PNEUMONIA. Bacterial pneumonia is a common infectious process that presents a threat to life for many of our population, especially the aged and chronically ill. This threat has been drastically reduced by antimicrobial preparations, which have decreased the death rate, shortened the course of the disease, and prevented many serious complications, such as empyema.

In order for bacteria to successfully invade the lung, there must be an alteration in net bacterial lung clearance. This alteration may occur as a result of decreased bacteriocidal ability of the alveolar macrophages or increased susceptibility of the host to infection. Normally, the bacteriocidal activity of macrophages is extremely important in supplementing the mucociliary escalator system in removing pathogens.

Pneumococcal pneumonia (Streptococcus pneumoniae), the most common bacterial pneumonia, follows an orderly sequence in the lung; the severity of the disease depends greatly on host resistance and/or medical intervention. While infection may develop in healthy persons, underlying factors (e.g., malnutrition, alcoholism, aging) seem to increase risk. Pathophysiologically, an initial acute inflammatory response occurs that brings excess water and plasma proteins to the dependent areas of the lower lobes. Red blood cells, fibrin, and polymorphonuclear leukocytes infiltrate the alveoli. The bacteria are contained within segments of pulmonary lobes by this cellular recruitment causing consolidation of the leukocytes and fibrin within the involved area.

The inflammatory exudate is seen progressing through stages including *hyperemia, red* and *gray hepatization,* and finally terminating in *resolution*. Hyperemia, also called the stage of congestion, is characterized by engorgement of the alveolar spaces with fluid and blood. Red hepatization refers to the red appearance of affected lung tissue, which demonstrates the consistency of liver tissue. The stage of gray hepatization occurs when an increasing number of leukocytes infiltrate the alveoli causing a solid, grayish tissue [1]. During resolution, the polymorphonuclear

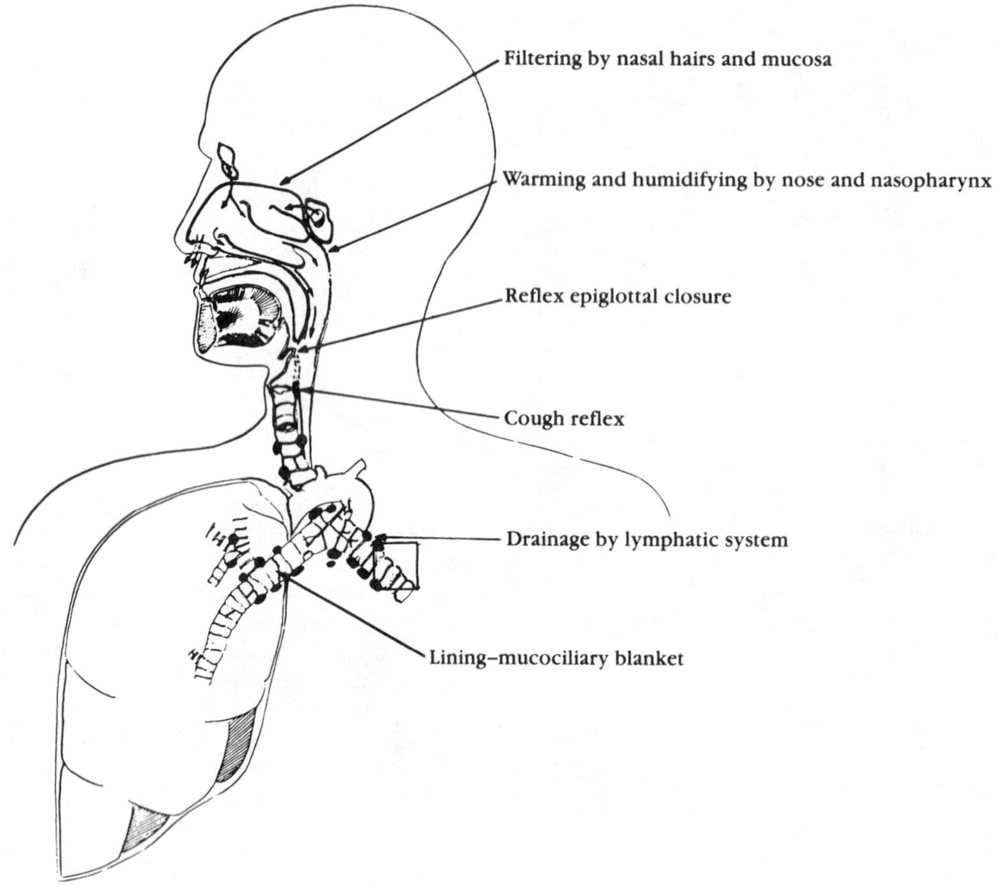

FIGURE 23-4. Defense of the respiratory tract. (Adapted from K. MacDonnell, *Current Respiratory Care.* Boston: Little, Brown, 1977.)

leukocytes are replaced by macrophages that are highly phagocytic and destroy the organisms.

The filling of alveoli with exudate or consolidation causes them to become airless. Sustained perfusion with poor ventilation occurs in the consolidated area, but this rarely is severe enough to cause a true hypoxemic picture. Resolution of the infection takes place as exudate is lysed and resorbed by the neutrophils and macrophages. The lymphatics carry exudate away from the site of infection resulting in the restoration of both structure and function of the lung. The clinical manifestations of pneumococcal pneumonia include fever, cough, pleuritic chest pain, and production of rusty-colored or blood-streaked sputum.

Bacterial pneumonia also may result from other bacteria including the *Staphylococcus, Streptococcus, Klebsiella,* and *Pseudomonas* organisms. At times, these organisms are opportunistic and follow the debilitation of the individual by another infection or disease process. They often are complicated by abscess formation, empyema, and pleural effusion.

VIRAL PNEUMONIA. Viral pneumonias are frequently mild and self-limited in adults but may be rapidly proliferative and fatal in children. A more important problem with virus infection is that the terminal and respiratory bronchioles become damaged and then are susceptible to secondary bacterial invasion that spreads to the surrounding alveoli. The common types of viruses involved are the influenza virus, the adenovirus, and the chicken-pox virus.

TUBERCULOSIS. Tuberculosis is caused by the *Mycobacterium tuberculosis*, which is classified as an acid-fast bacillus because of its staining property. This disease is most commonly seen in malnourished persons and the spread of the disease is closely related to host resistance. Transmission of the disease occurs through droplets from persons with an active tuberculous process. The portal of entry is usually the respiratory system but may also be the skin or gastrointestinal tract. Respiratory transmission begins with the inhalation of the mycobacteria; because of small particulate mass, the organisms are deposited in the lung periphery, usually in the lower part of the upper lobe or the upper part of the lower lobe (Fig. 23-5). In the primary infection, the mycobacteria become surrounded by polymor-

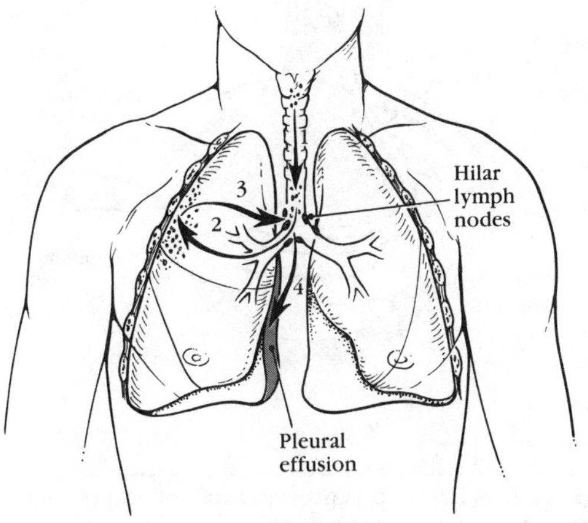

FIGURE 23-5. Tubercular organisms are usually deposited in the lung periphery either in the lower part of the upper lobe or the upper part of the lower lobe. *Arrows* and numbers (*1–4*) indicate entrance deposition spread to hilar lymph nodes and pleural effusion.

phonuclear leukocytes (PMNs) and inflammation results. After a few days, macrophages replace the PMN leukocytes. Some mycobacterial organisms are carried off by the lymphatics to the hilar lymph nodes. The combination of the initial lesion and lymph node involvement is called the *Ghon complex*, but this rarely results in spread to other body organs. Macrophages engulf the mycobacteria and are called *epitheloid cells*. These epitheloid cells join together to form giant cells that ring the foreign cell. Within the giant cell, caseous necrosis develops, probably a result of acquired hypersensitivity to the organism. Caseous necrosis has a characteristic granular, cheesy appearance. The area surrounding the central core of necrosis is ringed with sensitized T lymphocytes. Fibrosis and calcification develop as the lesion ages, resulting finally in a *granuloma*, which is called a *tubercle*. Collagenous scar tissue encapsulates the tubercle, effectively separating the organisms from the body. The organisms may or may not be killed in the process, but sensitized T lymphocytes develop to enhance the bactericidal ability of the macrophages. This development results in a cell-mediated immunity that usually lasts through life and can be demonstrated by administering purified protein derivative of the bacilli (PPD). A positive inflammatory wheal response indicates the presence of memory T cells for the mycobacteria.

Following initial exposure, 5 percent of individuals who inhale the mycobacteria will develop clinical tuberculosis. The clinical manifestations are variable and include night fever, cough, and symptoms of airway obstruction from hilar node involvement. The disease may spread involving the meninges, kidneys, bones, or other structures. In a small number of individuals, the actual disease develops years after the initial exposure. The mycobacterial organisms not destroyed by alveolar defenses lie dormant until a decrease in host resistance allows the original focus to become a source of progressive disease. This *postprimary,* or *reinfection, tuberculosis (secondary tuberculosis)* is most frequently seen in persons who have developed a secondary immunodeficiency, especially from cancer, cirrhosis of the liver, or diabetes mellitus.

ASPIRATION PNEUMONIA

Aspiration usually refers to the inhalation of gastric contents, food, water, or blood into the tracheobronchial system. Aspiration pneumonia results when the material is propelled into the alveolar system and most frequently occurs after vomiting or near-drowning.

Aspiration of gastric contents is relatively common and is especially associated with impaired consciousness, which includes such conditions as: cardiac arrest, seizures, strokes, and general anesthesia. The gastric contents are very acidic having a pH of less than 3. Aspiration of this acidic material results in a chemical irritation and destruction of the mucosa of the tracheobronchial tree. In the lungs, areas of hemorrhage and edema occur especially in the dependent portions. The severity of the response depends on the patient's physiologic status and the quantity and acidity of the aspirant.

Following aspiration, respiratory distress usually begins abruptly with evidence of bronchospasm, dyspnea, tachycardia, and cyanosis. Severe hypoxemia frequently occurs and may precipitate the adult respiratory distress syndrome [4].

Aspirated foodstuffs may be diagnosed by their content or appearance. Lipid-laden macrophages, for example, indicate that fats have been aspirated and have caused an acute or chronic pneumonia [8]. Foodstuffs may cause mechanical obstruction to the airway or chemical irritation to the mucosal lining, especially if they are mixed with the acid gastric secretions.

In *drowning* or *near-drowning*, aspiration of water usually causes intense laryngospasm, which is not enough to protect the alveoli from fluid. The result of near-drowning is severe hypoxemia and acidosis. Sea water aspiration may lead to a secondary pulmonary edema because of the high sodium content of the water [4]. The close relationship between near-drowning and the adult respiratory distress syndrome may, in part, be due to washing out of surfactant from the alveolar linings.

PULMONARY EDEMA

The pulmonary vascular system has a great capacity to accommodate increased amounts of blood up to 3 times its normal volume, but at a critical pressure point fluid moves across the alveolocapillary line and pulmonary edema occurs. *Pulmonary edema* is simply an accumulation of fluid in the tissues (interstitium and alveoli) of the lung.

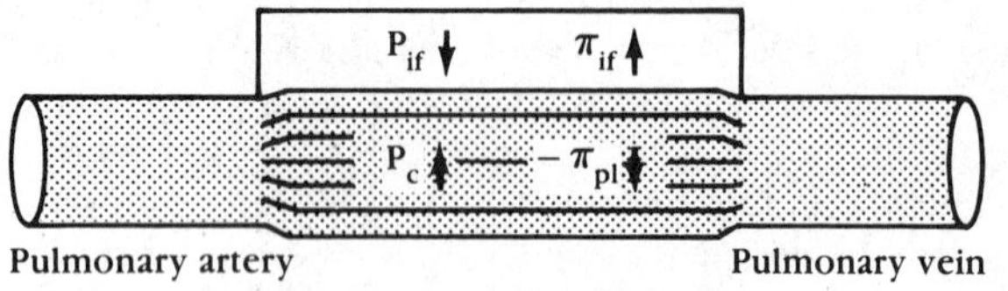

Fluid accumulation = $K[(P_c - P_{if}) - \sigma(\pi_{pl} - \pi_{if})]$
K = filtration coefficient
P_c = capillary hydrostatic pressure
P_{if} = pericapillary hydrostatic pressure
σ = reflection coefficient
π_{pl} = colloid osmotic pressure of plasma
π_{if} = colloid osmotic pressure of pericapillary fluid

FIGURE 23-6. Starling equation for transcapillary exchange. The reflection coefficient (σ) is a correction factor that relates to the effective difference in the osmotic pressure of proteins that operates across the capillary wall. (From A.P. Fishman, *Pulmonary Disease and Disorders.* New York: McGraw-Hill, 1980.)

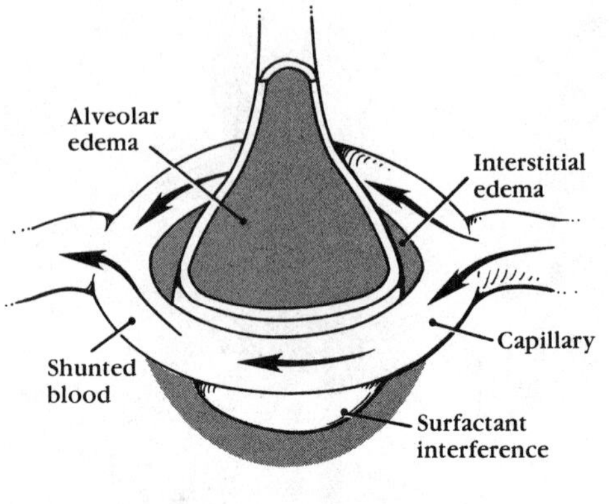

FIGURE 23-7. Schematic representation of interstitial alveolar edema, right-to-left shunting, alveolar edema, and surfactant interference.

Understanding of the mechanism by which pulmonary edema occurs is enhanced by the understanding of *Starling's equation* (Fig. 23-6). Hydrostatic and osmotic pressures are the major forces that affect movement of water across the capillary membrane (see Chap. 5). The normal hydrostatic pressure in the pulmonary capillaries is approximately 7 to 10 mm Hg, which is estimated from the pulmonary wedge pressure. The plasma oncotic pressure is approximately 25 mm Hg. Therefore, the alveoli tend to stay "dry" because the pressures oppose fluid movement into the interstitium and alveoli [5].

Pulmonary edema fluid is distributed positionally. Normally, when a person is in the upright position, the hydrostatic pressures are higher in the lung bases than at the apices [5]. Acute pulmonary edema may show bizarre patterns of distribution because of variations in the transmission of pleural pressures in different areas of the lungs but in chronic pulmonary edema the fluid tends to accumulate at the lung bases.

Hydrostatic pressure in the pulmonary bed must increase to a level of approximately 25 to 30 mm Hg in order for pulmonary edema to occur when there is normal capillary permeability and an intact alveolar system. Lymphatic drainage of a few ml/hour is usually sufficient to drain any excess protein and fluid that does not move back into the capillary. Lymphatics are probably sparse in the alveolar regions and more plentiful in the peribronchial and perivascular spaces, but these can increase lymph-carrying capacity six- to tenfold, so that a chronic increase in the hydrostatic pressure can be compensated for by increased lymphatic drainage [14].

The most common cause of pulmonary edema is left ventricular failure (LVF). This is discussed in more detail in Chapter 18. Left ventricular failure may be due to such pathology as acute myocardial infarction, hypertension, or mitral valve disease. Pulmonary edema may also result from acute inflammation, poisoning with certain gases (especially chlorine and nitrogen peroxide), pulmonary aspiration of gastric juice, excessive volume overload, some cases of cerebral damage, and smoke inhalation. These are summarized in Table 23-2. The mechanisms for producing the edema are different, but all result in increased interstitial or alveolar fluid. Figure 23-7 summarizes these mechanisms. In the case of acute inflammation, the result is alveolar damage, which leads to increased permeability and fluid exudation into the alveoli. In cerebral damage, the reaction of the body is to increase sympathetic nervous system stimulation resulting in diversion of blood to the lungs, which increases the hydrostatic pressure and causes the edema. Fluid overloading rarely occurs with a normal heart but occurs when the fluid volume to be pumped exceeds the ability of the heart to pump all of the fluid. Smoke inhalation may be injurious due to the chemical pneumonitis from the fumes, gases, and particulate matter [13]. Intraal-

TABLE 23-2. Causes of pulmonary edema

Cause	Precipitating event
Increased capillary hydrostatic pressure	Myocardial infarction, mitral stenosis, fluid overload, pulmonary venoocclusive disease
Increased capillary permeability	Inhaled or circulating toxins, radiation, oxygen toxicity
Lymphatic insufficiency	Silicosis, lymphangitis, carcinomatous
Decreased interstitial pressure	Rapid removal of pleural effusion or pneumothorax, hyperinflation
Decreased colloid osmotic pressure	Overtransfusion, hypoproteinemia
Unknown etiology	High altitude, heroin, neurogenic causes

Source: J.B. West, *Pulmonary Pathophysiology: The Essentials.* Baltimore: Williams & Wilkins, 1977. P. 117. (Reprinted with permission.)

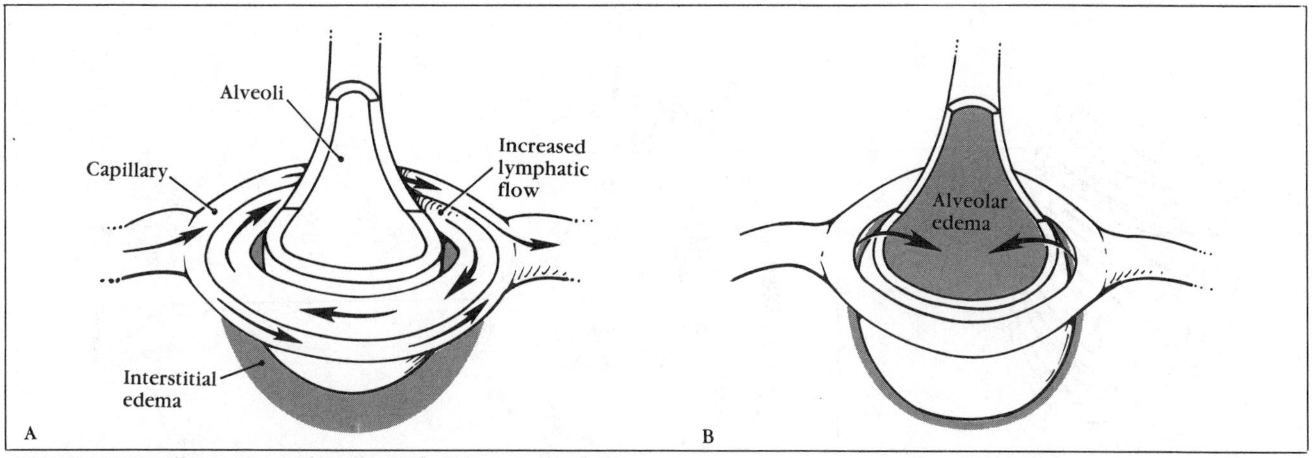

FIGURE 23-8. Illustration of stages of pulmonary edema. A. Interstitial pulmonary edema and increased lymphatic flow. B. Alveolar pulmonary edema.

veolar hemorrhage, congested, edematous alveoli, and interstitial edema may all result from this type of injury.

Pulmonary edema due to heart failure occurs when the left side of the heart is no longer able to accept all of the output sent to it from the right side of the heart. As a result, a small amount of blood is dammed back into the pulmonary circulation with each beat of the heart. Gradually, the blood accumulation exceeds the distensible capacity of the pulmonary vasculature. The excess blood accumulation in the pulmonary tree increases the pulmonary capillary hydrostatic pressure. This pressure increase is most severe in the dependent areas of the lung, accounting for increased fluid buildup in the bases of the lungs.

Pulmonary blood pressure is also raised by reflex vasoconstriction of the pulmonary vessels that occurs in response to hypoxemia, which may result from the decreased cardiac output. As pressure in the pulmonary circulation increases, fluid is forced into the pulmonary interstitial spaces. This phenomenon is known as *transudation*.

Pulmonary edema actually occurs in two stages (Fig. 23-8). The first stage is ***interstitial edema***. In this stage, there is fluid accumulation in the peribronchial and perivascular spaces. The lymphatics attempt to decrease this fluid by widening and increasing the rate of lymphatic flow. Some widening of the alveolar walls may also occur at this stage. Interstitial pulmonary edema widens the distance between the alveoli and pulmonary capillaries but little effect on gaseous exchange occurs in the early stages.

The second stage occurs when interstitial hydrostatic pressure is so high that it pushes fluid into the alveoli resulting in *alveolar edema*. The alveoli fill, one at a time, diluting the surfactant with the incoming fluid. This reduces the surface tension in the alveoli and predisposes the affected alveoli to collapse. Some alveoli may be compressed by surrounding edematous alveoli while others are not aerated because the airways that supply them are filled with fluid. When no oxygen is present in the alveoli, right-to-left shunting occurs and sometimes the shunt may be as large as 50 percent, resulting in severe hypoxemia and later, hypercapnia. This ventilation-perfusion ($\dot{V}/\dot{Q}$) abnormality is called a ***shunt unit*** (see Fig. 23-7).

The symptoms of pulmonary edema are directly attributable to its pathophysiology. The onset of symptoms may be sudden or gradual. If the pulmonary edema is mild and develops slowly, the major symptoms are wheezing, paroxysmal nocturnal dyspnea (PND), and dry cough. When it is fully developed, there is dyspnea, orthopnea, wheezing, and productive cough. The person expectorates profuse amounts of frothy sputum that initially may be white and frothy in appearance, progressing to pink-tinged or bright red expectoration.

In pulmonary edema, the elastic work of breathing is greatly increased because the interstitial fluid accumulation causes lung stiffening and loss of compliance. This, along with the hypoxemia, leads to a pattern of rapid, shallow breathing. The lungs are filling with fluid, which causes moist bubbling, rales, and wheezing. Abnormal heart sounds are common in pulmonary edema due to heart failure. Chest x ray will show cardiomegaly, and the fluid accumulation will appear as confluent patchy opacifications that are concentrated centrally in the lungs having the appearance of a butterfly or bat's wing [15]. Arterial blood gases reflect the degree of hypoxemia and/or hypercapnia.

TRAUMATIC INJURIES OF THE CHEST WALL

Traumatic injuries of the chest wall are common results of automobile accidents or other injuries. These may be simple, such as a rib fracture, or as serious as the flail chest abnormality.

The most common chest wall injury is the ***simple rib fracture***. Because this causes inspiratory pain, there is voluntary splinting, which results in restricted tidal volume and an increased respiratory rate. The victim voluntarily inhibits the urge to cough. The young, previously healthy person usually tolerates a fractured rib well, but a person with underlying pulmonary disease or the aged individual may develop impaired clearance of secretions, atelectasis, pneumonia, or even respiratory failure. The condition is further aggravated if chest strapping and narcotic analgesics are used. Chest strapping limits the ability to take a

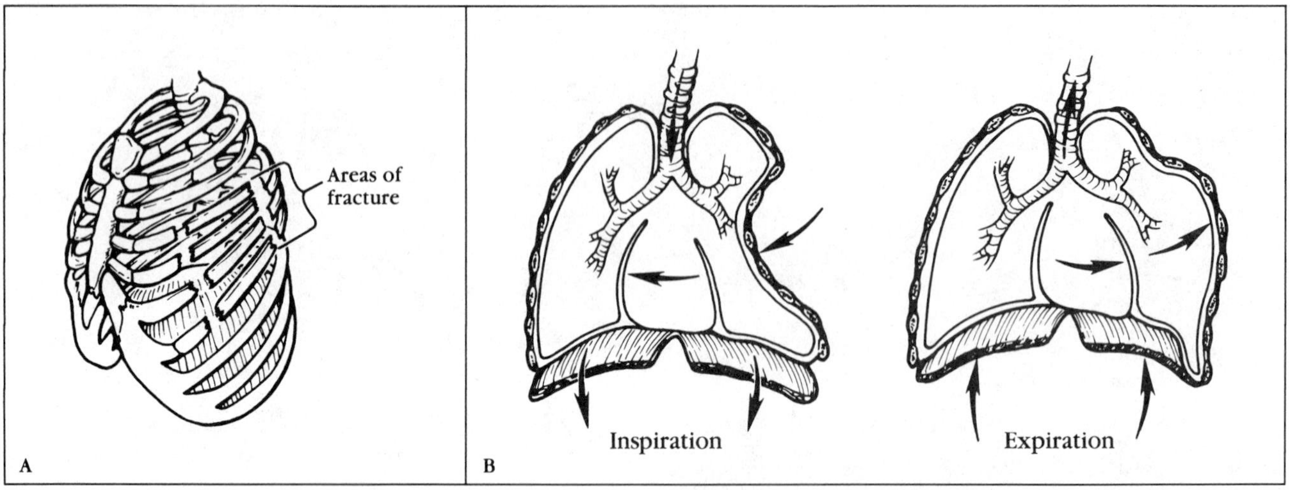

FIGURE 23-9. A. Chest wall injury that can produce the flail chest abnormality. B. Physiology of flail chest abnormality.

deep breath and thus enhances the risk for atelectasis and pneumonia. Compliance and all measures of lung volume are reduced. The respiratory drive and the cough reflex may be depressed by administration of narcotic analgesics.

If several adjacent ribs in an area are fractured, the stability of that area of chest wall may be lost (Fig. 23-9). As a result, when the patient inspires and intrathoracic pressure is lowered, that area of the chest wall is sucked in. The lung tissue underlying does not expand and gas exchange becomes impaired. Compliance is reduced. When the victim exhales, the affected area of the chest is elevated somewhat because of the increased intrathoracic pressure, creating a paradoxical movement during the ventilatory cycle. This injury increases the work of breathing and impairs ventilatory efficiency. The more the affected person works to maintain adequate ventilation, the more paradoxical the respiratory motion. In severe cases, a pendulum movement of the mediastinum may occur with each breath, putting pressure on the otherwise unaffected lung. The paradoxical motion may increase the central venous pressure while decreasing the venous return to the heart, resulting in a decreased blood pressure. Normal breathing is impaired and coughing is impossible, resulting in hypoventilation, hypoxemia, and even respiratory failure. Clinical manifestations of the *flail chest abnormality* include the obvious signs of chest wall trauma, "flail" movement with unequal chest excursion, severe dyspnea, pain especially on inspiration, rales, or reduced breath sounds. Chest x ray will show evidence of fractured ribs and blood gases will indicate the degree of hypoxemia.

PLEURAL EFFUSION

Pleural fluid is normally produced in quantities just sufficient to lubricate the surfaces of the visceral and parietal pleura so as to provide a smooth sliding surface. This small amount of fluid is constantly being replenished and resorbed, maintaining a constant amount in the pleural space.

Pleural fluid accumulation or effusion may result from disease or trauma. Diseases that may lead to accumulation of pleural fluid include neoplasms, infections, thromboemboli, and cardiovascular and immunologic defects. Thoracic trauma may cause bleeding into the pleural space.

Pleural effusions are frequently divided into the categories of transudates and exudates. Generally, inflammatory diseases and those of tissue destruction produce exudates with a specific gravity above 1.017 and a high concentration of protein and lactic acid dehydrogenase (LDH). Transudates, which are produced by diseases such as congestive heart failure, show lower values for these components with protein below 3.5 gm/dl and LDH below 200 units [6].

The accumulation of pleural transudates is sometimes referred to as *hydrothorax*. If the effusion contains purulent material, it is called *empyema*. If the empyema ultimately leads to fibrous fusing of the lung and chest wall, it is called *fibrothorax*. If the pleural fluid contains blood it is called *hemothorax*.

Fluid in the intrapleural space occupies space and displaces lung tissue (Fig. 23-10), by reducing the amount of lung expansion possible by direct pressure on the tissue; it may cause a mediastinal shift, which puts pressure on the opposite lung as well. Compliance decreases, altering the ventilation and perfusion on the affected side. When the fluid is removed from the pleural space, lung tissue reexpands allowing ventilation and perfusion to return to normal.

Clinical manifestations depend on the rate of the effusion. A hemothorax from a ruptured thoracic aneurysm, for example, will cause rapid blood accumulation and dramatic signs and symptoms from blood loss and a mediastinal shift. In a slower process, 2000 ml of fluid in the pleural space may accumulate before dyspnea is noted. The common symptoms relate to the amount of pulmonary embarrassment produced and these include dyspnea, blood gas abnormalities, cyanosis, and jugular venous distention.

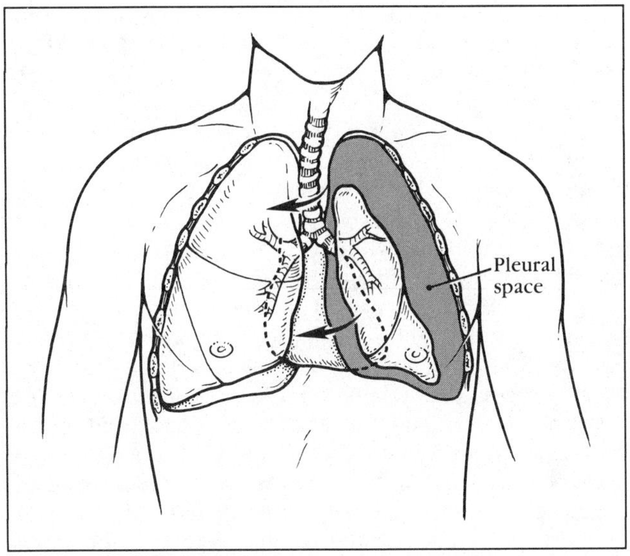

FIGURE 23-10. Pleural effusion. Fluid has collected in the pleural space and displaced lung tissue. Also note shift of fluid into the mediastinum and tortion of the bronchus.

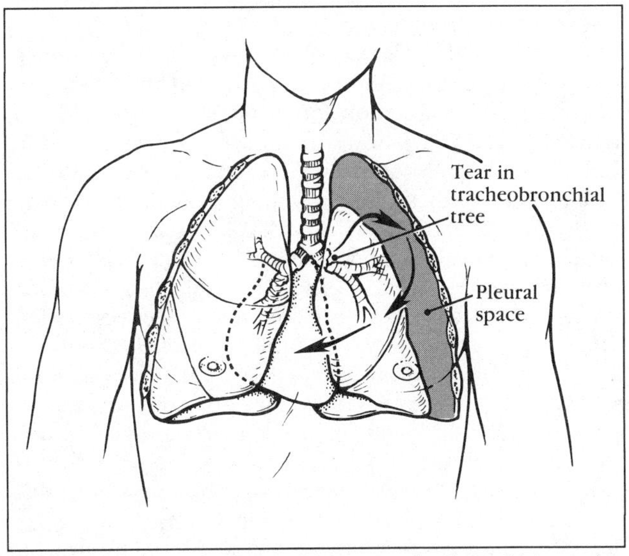

FIGURE 23-11. Pneumothorax. Tear in tracheobronchial tree has caused collapse of the lung and shifting of the mediastinum to the unaffected side.

Pneumothorax

Pneumothorax occurs when air enters the pleural space (Fig. 23-11). Once this occurs, lung tissue is displaced in much the same way as if fluid had entered the space except that the displacement is due to air in the intrapleural space.

Air may enter the pleural space from an opening in the chest wall or from the lungs themselves. Some of the causes of pneumothorax from the lungs include puncture by a fractured rib, spontaneous rupture of a superficial bleb, or rupture of a bleb during vigorous mechanical ventilation. Tracheobronchial rupture due to trauma may also cause pneumothorax. Surgical pneumothorax occurs as a part of every thoracotomy. *Spontaneous pneumothorax* may occur in individuals with emphysema when a bleb on the surface of the lung ruptures and releases air into the pleural spaces.

Pressure in the potential intrapleural space is normally lower or more negative than intraalveolar pressure. Therefore, if there is a break in either the integrity of the lung through the visceral pleura or the chest wall through the parietal pleura, air rushes to the area of lowest pressure, that of the pleural space. This will continue as long as the air leak is present. Sometimes air leaks into the pleural space on inspiration but the tissue seals itself on expiration and outward leakage does not occur. This results in *tension pneumothorax*, which is a life-threatening condition of air build-up in the space with displacement of the structures within the mediastinum. This displacement to the opposite side affects the other lung and may impede the venous return to the heart.

Clinical signs of a significant pneumothorax may include dyspnea and chest pain of sudden onset. Tracheal deviation toward the unaffected side and reduced vesicular or bronchial breath sounds on the affected side may occur. Arterial blood gases may reveal acute hypoxemia at the outset. The degree of all of the clinical signs depends on the extent of the pneumothorax. Symptoms of tension pneumothorax include increasing respiratory distress and cyanosis, bulging sternum, distended neck veins, elevated central venous pressure, and hypotension.

CENTRAL NERVOUS SYSTEM (CNS) DEPRESSION

The respiratory center is made up of groups of nerve cells that are scattered through the reticular formation in the medulla oblongata. This brainstem structure is responsible for the respiratory rhythm. Although this structure is the major respiratory control, the pons functions in the coordination of breathing. The respiratory neural structure in the pons is called the *pneumotaxic center*. Stimulation of this center increases respiratory frequency, while depression of the center slows respirations. The apneustic center also modifies the respiratory pattern. Cranial or cerebral trauma or central nervous system lesions, such as malignancies, brain abscesses, and other conditions may result in injury to or impingement on the mediators of respiration and result in alterations of respiratory patterns.

If head injury affects the pneumotaxic center or the respiratory center in the medulla, it may alter the rate, rhythm, and depth of respiration. Apnea may also occur. If CNS depression has occurred because of trauma or disease, there is frequently a decreased ventilatory drive, decreased responsiveness to ventilatory stimuli, and absence of the sigh mechanism. The result is a restrictive pathology that decreases the total lung capacity [11].

Increasing intracranial pressure may lead to pressure on the respiratory center and change in breathing patterns but more common than this is hypoxemia in obtunded individuals due to the acute restrictive disease. There is also a

TABLE 23-3. Neuromuscular diseases exhibiting respiratory insufficiency

Spinal cord disease
Trauma
Quadriplegia
Paraplegia
Poliomyelitis
Motor nerve disease
Acute idiopathic polyneuritis
Guillain-Barré syndrome
Landry's ascending paralysis
Tick-bite paralysis
Porphyria
Myoneural junction disease
Myasthenia gravis
Myasthenic syndrome
Muscle-wasting disease
Muscular dystrophy
Congenital myotonia
Tetanus

depression of the airway reflexes, which increases the risk of obstruction and aspiration.

NEUROMUSCULAR DISEASES

Many types of neuromuscular disease processes may cause impairment of the respiratory system. The most common ones are summarized in Table 23-3. These can lead to an acute or chronic restrictive pulmonary process. Two of these processes, the Guillain-Barré syndrome and Duchenne's muscular dystrophy are discussed in the following section.

Guillain-Barré Syndrome

Guillain-Barré syndrome, which is named after the two individuals who originally described this condition, is an acute toxic polyneuritis. Typically, in its early stages, it is mistaken for a flu syndrome. As it progresses it is accompanied by varying degrees of muscular weakness and paralysis. It almost always follows a viral upper respiratory tract infection and has been shown to be associated with the virus of mononucleosis. This condition appears to result from an individual hypersensitivity response to a particular type of virus (see Chap. 45). The respiratory muscles typically become involved and death, if it occurs, is most frequently due to respiratory complications.

The pulmonary problems in Guillain-Barré syndrome are threefold. First, there is paralysis of the internal and external intercostal muscles, which reduces functional breathing ability. The breathing then becomes entirely diaphragmatic leading to reduced tidal volume, hypoxemia, and hypercapnia [7]. Second, there is paralysis of the preganglionic fibers of the vagus nerve and of the postganglionic fibers of the sympathetic nervous system. With vagal paralysis there is loss of the normal protective mechanisms that respond to bronchial irritation, foreign bodies, etc. There is also loss of reflex bronchoconstriction. Paralysis of the sympathetic postganglionic fibers causes loss of bronchodilation. Third, the gag reflex is diminished or absent.

Pathologically, segmental loss of myelin sheath in the peripheral nerves may be seen. Other body areas are also affected by the paralysis, but this is not life-threatening. Even though the syndrome may last for a few weeks, complete recovery often occurs if respirations are adequately supported during the acute stage.

Clinical manifestations include the rapid onset of symmetric weakness beginning in the legs and moving upward. The muscles are flaccid and sensory changes may or may not be present. Muscles of the pharynx and larynx may lead to swallowing and gag reflex impairment. Cough reflex is depressed, and superimposed respiratory infection frequently occurs. Functional return is variable and usually progresses in a reverse pattern with respiratory improvement occurring first, followed by functional improvement, beginning with the upper extremities and finally terminating in the lower extremities. Various types of residual impairment have been described.

Duchenne's Muscular Dystrophy

The most common, rapidly progressive type of muscular dystrophy is Duchenne's muscular dystrophy (DMD). Two types of the disease are described according to its progression. One form is rapidly progressive and the other progresses more slowly. Both forms of DMD are hereditary, being X-linked recessive. Women are the carriers, while their sons tend to manifest the disorder (see Chap. 38).

Muscular weakness results leading to difficulty walking in the early years of life. Thoracoscoliosis and respiratory muscle weakness then progresses rapidly. The muscles seem to weaken in this order: intercostals, abdominal muscles, diaphragm, and accessory muscles of respiration. Despite this respiratory impairment, studies show that alveolar hypoventilation occurs only as an acute or terminal event. As the severity of respiratory involvement progresses, many DMD patients are left with the use of only the accessory muscles of respiration. As a result, they may display unusual breathing patterns such as frog breathing, gulping air, head bobbing, and pursed-lip breathing [2]. The final acute respiratory failure is often triggered by an acute respiratory infection.

RESPIRATORY DISEASES CAUSED BY EXPOSURE TO ORGANIC AND INORGANIC DUSTS

Many organic and inorganic dusts have been identified as injurious to the lungs. The group of diseases caused by these dusts are collectively called the *pneumoconioses*. In the following paragraphs, silicosis, coal worker's pneumoconiosis, byssinosis, and asbestosis are discussed briefly.

Silicosis

Silicosis is probably the best known and the most severe of the industrial diseases. It results from the inhalation of silicon dioxide. Workers at occupations with high silica exposure include masons, potters, sand blasters, and foundry workers. Coal workers occasionally develop silicosis if they are exposed to coal dust in the mine.

The main characteristic of silicosis is fibrosis, which is manifested initially as hard nodules of about 1 mm in diameter in lung parenchyma that increase in size and coalesce as the disease progresses. It is believed that the silica particles cause lysis of the macrophages that ingest them [9]. Immune response may then be responsible for the development of the fibrotic lesion. Among the industrial inhalants, silica is particularly dangerous because of its effect on the macrophages allowing the fibrotic lesions to proceed unchecked. All of this causes very severe restrictive pulmonary disease.

Coal Worker's Pneumoconiosis (Black-Lung Disease)

The efficiency of alveolar clearing of coal dust has been demonstrated by Davies [3]. He found that although miners may inhale 100 to 150 gm of dust per year, only 0.5 gm could be recovered by autopsy. Most coal dust is removed by the alveolar macrophages, with the remaining coal dust accumulating in the macrophages. Over time the dust-laden macrophages gather at the perivascular structures and local fibrosis ensues. Early in the disease the process is manifested as a restrictive process with progressive fibrosis. As the disease progresses, dilatation of the respiratory bronchioles occurs as a result of the traction created by the contracting fibrous tissue. Centrilobular emphysema results from the dilatation and destruction of the respiratory bronchioles. The walls of the bronchioles break down, forming single spaces. If exposure to coal dust continues, centrilobular emphysema may occur throughout the lung. Panlobular or primary emphysema characterized by destruction of the alveoli rather than the more central respiratory bronchioles is not observed in relationship to dust inhalation.

A small percentage of those afflicted with simple pneumoconiosis due to silica or coal dust develop a more complicated form of the disease characterized by massive pulmonary fibrosis and chronic restrictive pulmonary disease. While it is generally accepted that simple pneumoconiosis is related to the quantity and composition of dust retained in the lung, the etiology of complicated pneumoconiosis is not as clear. It has been suggested that the process involves an immunologic mechanism and that it results in the development of massive fibrotic lesions. In the past, the recovery of the tuberculin bacillus from the lungs of miners with complicated pneumoconiosis led researchers to conclude that the bacillus was the mediator of the immunologic defense. However, this theory has not been substantiated and the pathogenesis of this condition remains obscure.

Byssinosis (Brown-Lung Disease)

Bronchoconstriction also occurs as a result of hypersensitivity to inorganic and organic dusts. An example is byssinosis, which results from long-term exposure to cotton dust. Cotton dust extracts have been shown to cause bronchoconstriction and it is now believed that exposure to cotton dust causes a discharge of naturally produced histamine leading to bronchospasm. When histamine stores are depleted, reactivity to cotton dust decreases, which explains the dynamics of *Monday fever*. During a short layoff, histamine stores are replenished and exposure to the dust on Monday causes the histamine to be released. Histamine stores are depleted as the work week progresses, resulting in disappearance of symptoms and improved ventilatory capacity [16].

Textile workers experienced chest tightness, low-grade fever, and dyspnea. The symptoms were more pronounced on Monday after a weekend away from the factory. Hence, the syndrome became known as "Monday fever." Later in the week, the symptoms gradually disappeared. Researchers demonstrated that the textile workers had decreased ventilatory capacities and increased airway resistance during the Monday workday.

Asbestosis

Occupational exposure to asbestos has occurred in the mining, manufacturing, and application areas. The main use for asbestos is in asbestos cement products for construction. The most important health-related effects from asbestos exposure are pulmonary fibrosis and tumors. Particles of asbestos may be cleared by the mucociliary escalator system or, if deposited deep within the lung parenchyma, may be partially or completely engulfed by alveolar macrophages [5]. Some of the fibers may be removed through lymphatic circulation.

Diffuse pulmonary fibrosis resulting from asbestos exposure is termed *asbestosis*. The fibrosis initially affects the alveolar walls and gradually involves the interstitium. Prominent symptoms include exertional dyspnea, severe nonproductive cough, clubbing of the fingers, and, ultimately, symptoms of respiratory failure [5]. Rales and restriction of lung inflation are common clinical findings. Pleural changes may be associated and include hyaline plaques that undergo calcification. Recurrent exudative pleural effusions may also be associated.

PULMONARY FIBROSIS

Pulmonary fibrosis refers to a chronic restrictive condition that involves diffuse fibrosis of the lung tissue, and results in severe loss of compliance with lung stiffness. As has been indicated above, fibrosis is frequently due to occupational exposure to substances such as glass dusts, coal dusts, and other substances. In cases where the cause is unknown, the disease may be referred to as the *Hamman-Rich syndrome*, or unusual interstitial pneumonitis [12]. *Sarcoidosis* is another disease that includes among its features a severe diffuse pulmonary fibrosis. Severely decreased compliance and diffusing capacity may lead to hypoxemia and cor pulmonale.

THORACIC DEFORMITY

Many chest deformities are not severe enough to compromise pulmonary status. However, severe deformities will

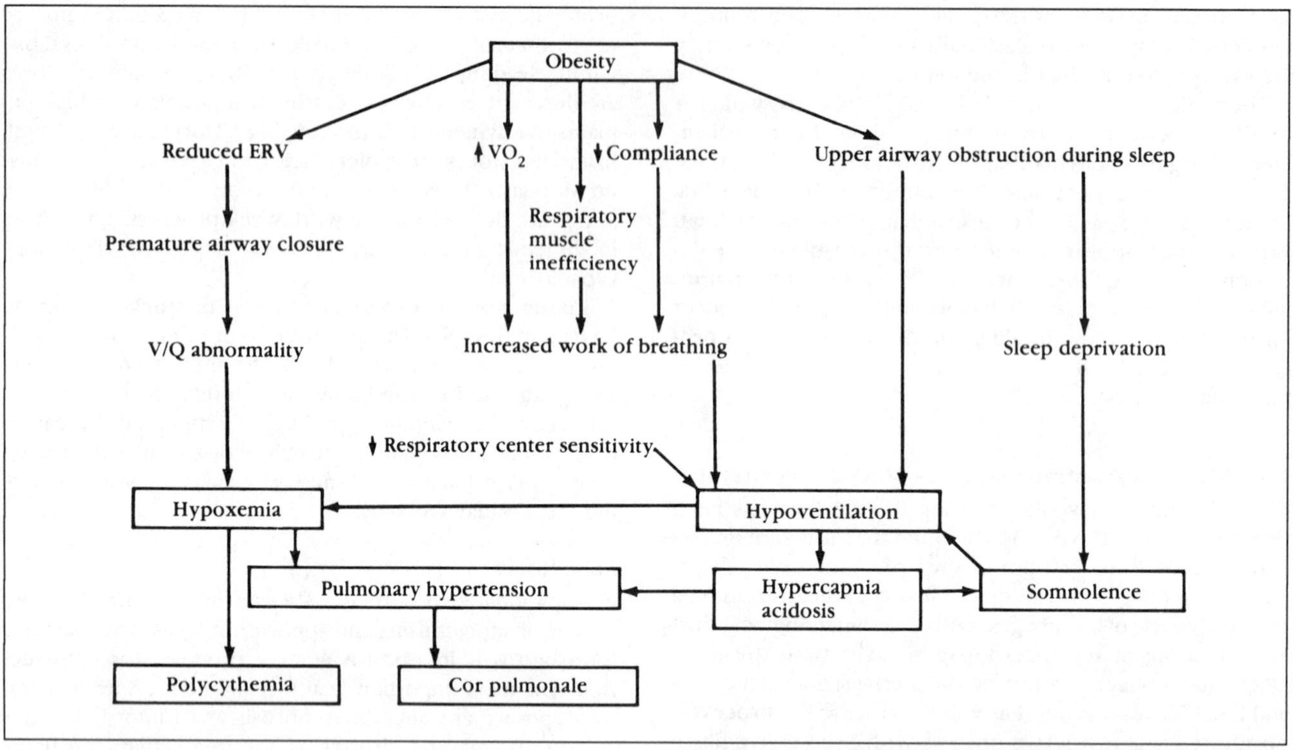

FIGURE 23-12. Pathogenesis and pathophysiology of obesity hypoventilation syndrome. (From S. Farzan, *A Concise Handbook of Respiratory Diseases*. Reston, Va.: Reston Pub., 1978.)

compress lung tissue in one or more areas of the chest and may limit thoracic excursion. Severe *kyphoscoliosis*, in which the body is essentially twisted over to one side, is one example. Another example is *pectus excavatum* or *funnel chest*, in which the lower end of the sternum is caved in because of attachment to the spine by thick fibrous bands. *Pectus carinatum*, or pigeon breast, causes abnormal prominence of the sternum, and the rib structure may limit respiratory movement. Many other deformities also occur that restrict pulmonary status.

In general, severe thoracic deformities compress areas of lung tissue and limit chest expansion, leading to areas of small lung volume and atelectasis. Compliance, total lung capacity, and other volume measurements are reduced. The pulmonary vascular bed in the affected areas is also reduced, resulting in an increased work of breathing, alveolar hypoventilation and the consequences of the hypoxemia.

Because of the wide variety of deformities and their effects on pulmonary status, the pulmonary function of each affected person must be carefully assessed. Generally, the effect of pectus excavatum is not severe, while the effect of kyphoscoliosis varies from mild to very severe.

OBESITY

Severe obesity results in restriction of ventilation, especially in the supine position. The *Pickwickian syndrome*, or the obesity hypoventilation syndrome, is related to morbid obesity and presents a picture of hypoventilation, somnolence, severe hypoxemia, polycythemia, and cor pulmonale [4]. The term, used for a clinical syndrome associated with extreme obesity, comes from Charles Dickens's description of a fat boy.

Severe obesity causes pulmonary restriction by two means: (1) The extreme excess of adipose tissue in the abdomen tends to force the thoracic contents up into the chest and thus restricts diaphragmatic excursion. (2) The weight of the chest wall greatly increases the amount of work required to move the chest for inspiration. This is especially true for the woman with pendulous breasts. Severe obesity, then, results in reduced compliance, expiratory reserve volume, total lung capacity, and vital capacity with all of these reductions due to a great increase in the work of breathing and great susceptibility to respiratory infections. Arterial blood gas studies reveal hypercapnia and hypoxemia.

Severely affected individuals have depression of the ventilatory drive and may have apneic episodes due to upper airway obstruction during sleep. Somnolence is characteristic and may be related to sleep deprivation that occurs as a result of frequent awakenings following the airway-obstructive episodes. Figure 23-12 shows the development of the Pickwickian syndrome.

IDIOPATHIC RESPIRATORY DISTRESS SYNDROME OF THE NEWBORN (IRDS)

This syndrome is the most clearly understood abnormality that involves surfactant deficiency. The development of the surfactant layer occurs late in fetal life, at about the twenty-eighth to the thirty-second week of gestation. Infants born before the twenty-eighth week are at a greater risk for developing acute respiratory distress and this is still a major cause of death in premature infants. The severity of the respiratory distress and the mortality have been shown to be related to the gestational age at birth.

The pathology of IRDS includes inadequate pulmonary expansion and diffuse atelectasis, which is of a primary type because the lungs have never been expanded. Increased pulmonary vascular resistance occurs because of high pulmonary arterial pressures, presumably due to increased pulmonary arteriolar resistance. The resulting increased pressure creates a higher than normal pressure on the right side of the heart. This high pressure perpetuates the fetal circulation by keeping the foramen ovale and the ductus arteriosus patent. The IRDS or hyaline membrane disease is characterized by large right-to-left shunting that accentuates hypoxemia and hypercapnia in later stages and is increased by hypoxemia, which leads to increased right heart pressures. Ischemic injury in the lung fields causes leaking of fluid into interstitial and alveolar spaces and formation of the hyaline membrane. There is vascular engorgement, dilated lymphatics, and cellular debris lining the alveoli, with evidence of degenerating epithelial and endothelial cells in the alveolocapillary membrane. The hyaline membranes are apparently composed of plasma, fibrin, necrotic epithelial cells, and amniotic fluid and contribute to the respiratory distress [1]. Extensive atelectasis occurs with widespread infiltration of the pulmonary tissue [4].

Clinical manifestations include dyspnea from the first moments of life and rapid, shallow respirations. Retraction of the lower ribs on inspiration and an expiratory grunt usually occur. Hypoxemia is characteristic and an elevated PCO_2 with respiratory and/or metabolic acidosis may complicate the picture.

Treatment measures are improving the prognosis in this condition. Continuous positive airway pressure (CPAP) is used with good results to improve oxygenation but the condition still carries about a 50 percent mortality.

ADULT RESPIRATORY DISTRESS SYNDROME (ARDS)

The adult respiratory distress syndrome is a condition characterized by severe hypoxemia and progressive loss of lung compliance. It causes severe restrictive disease. ARDS is known by a number of other names including shock lung, traumatic wet lung, capillary leak syndrome, postperfusion lung, congestive atelectasis, and posttraumatic pulmonary insufficiency.

ARDS is never a primary disease but occurs secondarily to some other insult to the body. General etiologic factors have been identified and classified as to the mechanism of causation. These are summarized in Table 23-4. The categories described are the following: (1) reduced perfusion, (2) increased capillary permeability, (3) direct tissue and capillary insults, and (4) others, with obscure mechanisms.

TABLE 23-4. Underlying causes that can precipitate adult respiratory distress syndrome (ARDS)

Reduced perfusion
Cardiogenic shock
Trauma
Major burns
Fat embolus
Hemorrhage
Severe hypovolemia
Increased capillary permeability
Sepsis
Pneumonia
Noxious fume or smoke inhalation
Reactions to drugs
Venoms or toxins
Immune complex diseases
Overtransfusion of crystalloids
Uremia
Direct tissue and capillary insults
Aspiration of GI contents
Rapid decompression
Near-drowning
Oxygen toxicity
Hypoxemia
Fluid overload
Starvation
Other mechanisms, not well understood
High altitude reactions
Sudden changes in intrathoracic pressure
Central nervous system injuries
Narcotic overdose
Cardiopulmonary bypass

The causes of ARDS are many, but these result in essentially the same pathologic process. One may note an overlap of mechanisms from one category to the next.

The pathologic effects of ARDS are very similar despite the initiating underlying condition. These are summarized in Figure 23-13. The insult leads to capillary congestion and a consequent alteration of capillary permeability. Endothelial cell damage occurs as does malfunction of the type II pneumocytes. The activity of these cells decreases and this results in decreased production of surfactant. Exudation of fluid into the pulmonary interstitium and eventually to the alveoli occurs. This causes lung stiffening (loss of compliance) and dilution of surfactant. The compliance alteration and surfactant dilution work together to lead to widespread atelectasis, which causes hypoxemia. In addition, there may be pulmonary interstitial edema and hemorrhage, the formation of alveolar exudate or hyaline membrane, and a predisposition to pulmonary secondary infection. The widespread atelectasis leads to an increased right-to-left shunt across the pulmonary capillary bed, causing critical hypoxemia.

Oxygen Toxicity

A special pulmonary pathophysiologic process has been described in individuals exposed to high levels of oxygen for more than 24 to 36 hours. The continuous breathing of

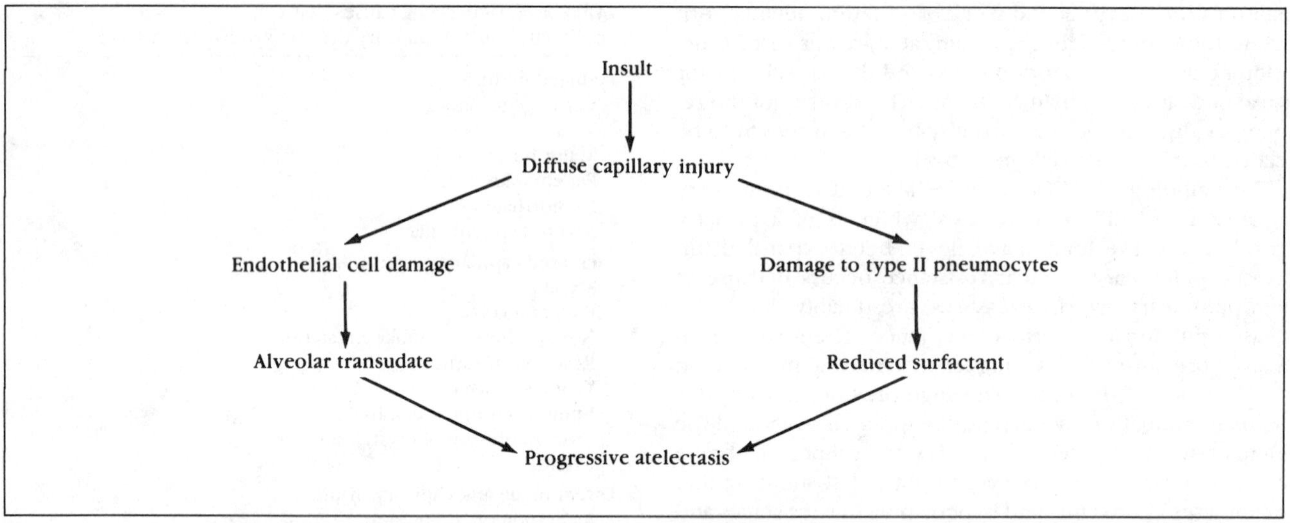

FIGURE 23-13. Simplified pathogenesis of adult respiratory distress syndrome (ARDS).

high concentrations of oxygen leads to diffuse parenchymal damage resulting in interference with the production of surfactant and formation of hemorrhagic exudate with fibrin in the alveoli, alveolar ducts, and the respiratory bronchioles. The earliest changes involve thickening of interstitial spaces with fluid containing fibrin, polymorphonuclear leukocytes, and macrophages. Two special processes explain the resulting dysfunction: (1) Breathing pure oxygen results in absorption of the gas from the alveoli. Nitrogen, normally present in atmospheric gas, is not present under these circumstances and therefore does not exert its function of keeping the alveoli expanded. The result is alveolar collapse. (2) Oxygen has a toxic effect on the surfactant-producing cells so that this vital substance is not being produced in adequate quantities; without adequate surfactant the alveoli tend to collapse and fluid exudes from the capillaries to the alveolar sacs [10].

The results of this process are progressive hypoxemia and reduced lung compliance despite the administration of high levels of oxygen. Any individual whose oxygen tension is decreasing while receiving high concentrations of oxygen should be considered a prime candidate for ARDS.

Those persons at a high risk for ARDS should be observed for onset of the condition throughout the first 96 hours after insult. No previous history of lung disease may be obtained but persons with previous lung pathology are somewhat more susceptible to development of this problem. Obvious observable symptoms include extreme dyspnea, tachypnea and grunting, and labored respirations that occur late in the phenomenon. Therefore, the arterial blood gases of those persons developing the disease indicate decreasing PO_2 despite oxygen therapy. If the arterial PO_2 is not correctable to above 50 when a person is receiving 100% oxygen, there should be a high index of considered suspicion for this condition. Usually, clinical deterioration is rapid and progressive. Hemoptysis and cyanosis may or may not occur. The hypoxemia and increased work of breathing may initially lead to metabolic acidosis. As respiratory muscles tire, a respiratory acidosis will occur. The chest x ray will show progressive, patchy, bilateral infiltrates. Improvement in the prognosis for these persons is occurring with the use of positive end expiratory pressure on volume cycled ventilators but it still remains poor.

REFERENCES

1. Anderson, W. A. D., and Scotti, T. *Synopsis of Pathology* (10th ed.). St. Louis: Mosby, 1980.
2. Beckerman, R. Respiratory Aspects of Progressive Neuromuscular Disorders of Children. University of Arizona at Tucson. Unpublished, 1976.
3. Davies, C. N. A comparison between inhaled dust and the dust recovered from human lungs. *Health Phys.* 10:129, 1964.
4. Farzan, S. *A Concise Handbook of Respiratory Diseases.* Reston, Va.: Reston Pub., 1978. P. 165.
5. Fishman, A. P. *Pulmonary Diseases and Disorders.* New York: McGraw-Hill, 1980.
6. Isselbacher, K. J., et al. (eds.), *Harrisons's Principles of Internal Medicine* (9th ed.). New York: McGraw-Hill, 1980. Pp. 1265–1267.
7. Kealy, S. L. Respiratory care in Guillain-Barré syndrome. *Am. J. Nurs.* 1:59, 1977.
8. MacDonnell, K., and Segal, M. *Current Respiratory Care.* Boston: Little, Brown, 1977. P. 172.
9. Muir, D. *Clinical Aspects of Inhaled Particulates.* Philadelphia: Davis, 1972.
10. Pierce, A. Oxygen toxicity. *Basics Respir. Dis.* 1:5, 1975.
11. Shapiro, B., Harrison, R., and Trout, C. *Clinical Application of Respiratory Care.* Chicago: Year Book, 1975. Pp. 357–358.
12. Sodeman, W., and Sodeman, T. *Pathologic Physiology* (6th ed.). Philadelphia: Saunders, 1979. P. 462.
13. Surveyer, J. Smoke inhalation injuries. *Heart Lung* 9:825, 1980.
14. West, J. *Respiratory Physiology: The Essentials.* Baltimore: Williams & Wilkins, 1974. P. 47.
15. West, J. *Pulmonary Pathophysiology: The Essentials.* Baltimore: Williams & Wilkins, 1977. P. 115.
16. Ziskind, M. Occupational pulmonary disease. *Clin. Symp.* 30:4, 1978.

CHAPTER 24
OBSTRUCTIVE ALTERATIONS IN PULMONARY FUNCTION

LEARNING OBJECTIVES

1. Define the term *obstructive pulmonary disease.*
2. Differentiate between acute and chronic bronchitis.
3. Describe the pathophysiology of an acute asthmatic attack.
4. List two precipitating factors for an asthma attack.
5. List and describe the symptoms that result from bronchoconstriction.
6. Define *pulsus paradoxus.*
7. List the conditions that are classified as chronic obstructive pulmonary disease (COPD).
8. Define the pathology of bronchiectasis.
9. Describe the signs and symptoms seen with bronchiectasis.
10. Discuss the basis for the development of cystic fibrosis.
11. List the pathologic features of cystic fibrosis.
12. List the criteria used in diagnosing cystic fibrosis.
13. List at least two risk factors in the development of chronic bronchitis.
14. Describe the pathophysiology of chronic bronchitis.
15. Differentiate chronic bronchitis from emphysema on the basis of pathologic and clinical features.
16. Relate similarities of chronic bronchitis and emphysema.
17. Describe the interrelationships of all the obstructive pulmonary diseases.
18. Describe the pathology of the different types of emphysema.
19. Discuss the pathophysiologic course of emphysema.
20. Define *hypoxia*, *hypoxemia*, and *hypercapnia.*
21. Explain why polycythemia occurs with chronic obstructive pulmonary disease.
22. Differentiate between compensated and uncompensated respiratory acidosis.

In general, obstructive pulmonary conditions cause obstruction to airflow within the lungs with less resistance to inspiration and more resistance to expiration, resulting in a prolongation of the expiratory phase of respiration. Many conditions can cause obstruction to airflow; the more prominent ones are detailed in this chapter.

ACUTE OBSTRUCTIVE AIRWAY DISEASE

The classification of an acute obstructive airway disease is dependent on an episodic nature of the condition. The two major entities in this classification are acute bronchitis and asthma. In both conditions, the obstructive process is intermittent and reversible.

Acute Bronchitis

Acute bronchitis is a common condition caused by infection and inhalants that results in inflammation of the mucosal lining of the tracheobronchial tree. Increased mucus secretion, bronchial swelling, and dysfunction of the cilia lead to increased resistance to expiratory airflow usually resulting in some air trapping on expiration.

Bronchitis causes cough and production of large amounts of usually purulent mucus with associated wheezing if there is significant air obstruction. Once the stimulus for bronchitis is treated or removed, the bronchial swelling decreases and the airways return to normal.

Asthma

Asthma is an episodic, acute airway obstruction that results from stimuli that would not elicit such a response in normal individuals. It has been defined as a disorder characterized by recurrent paroxysms of wheezing and dyspnea that are not attributable to underlying cardiac disease or other disease. This means that the person who has asthma has a tendency toward bronchospasm as a response to a variety of stimuli. The common characteristic of all asthmatic reactions is hyperreactivity of the airways. Between acute attacks, the lungs of the asthmatic individual are usually normal or relatively normal.

While asthma is characterized by wheezing, not all wheezing is asthma. Unilateral localized wheezing may be caused by the aspiration of foreign bodies or by a tumor. Other causes of wheezing include pulmonary emboli, infections, left ventricular failure, cystic fibrosis, immunologic deficiency, and viral respiratory illnesses.

PATHOPHYSIOLOGIC MECHANISMS OF ASTHMA. The causes of asthma may be divided into two major categories: *extrinsic* and *intrinsic*.

Extrinsic asthma more commonly affects the child or young teenager who frequently relates a personal and/or family history of allergy, hives, rashes, and eczema. Skin tests are usually positive for specific allergens, indicating the probability that extrinsic asthma is allergic in nature.

Childhood asthma attacks are usually self-limited and frequently are precipitated by exposure to specific antigens. It is not uncommon for the person who "outgrows" asthma in childhood to develop other allergic manifestations in adulthood. Commonly, the asthmatic child has a decrease in severity and frequency of attacks as he or she matures.

The pathophysiology of the asthma attacks is related to the release of chemical mediators in an IgE–mast cell interaction (see Chap. 11). This results in constriction of the bronchial smooth muscle, increased bronchial secretion from the goblet cells, and mucosal swelling, all of which lead to significant narrowing of the air passages. It is basically an IgE-associated immune reaction in which the allergen evokes an immediate production of histamine and other chemicals by the target organ, which is the lung [8]. The acute respiratory obstruction, resistance to airflow, and turbulence of the airflow are due to the following three responses: (1) bronchospasm, which involves a rhythmic squeezing of the airways by the muscle bands surrounding them, (2) production of abnormally large amounts of thick mucus, and (3) the inflammatory response, including increased capillary permeability and mucosal edema (see Fig. 24-1).

Allergy alone as a basis for the attacks is rare and many mechanisms may be involved. Whatever the mechanisms, once bronchospasm is induced by one agent the airway response to superimposed stimuli is greatly enhanced. For example, if a person having a subclinical response to pollen becomes emotionally upset, the airway response to the emotions may be greatly magnified because of the pollen sensitivity already established. It is important to note that, without a tendency toward bronchospasm, emotions, pollen, or other substances will not produce asthma.

Intrinsic asthma usually affects adults, including those who did not have asthma or allergy prior to middle adulthood. The family history for allergy, eczema, hives, and rashes is usually negative. Attacks are most often related to infection of the respiratory tract or to exercise; emotion, allergy, and other factors also may play a part.

In either type, respiratory infection may be a major precipitator of a severe asthma attack. Both bacterial and viral infections may precipitate the attack, but viruses seem to be more important in this respect.

CLINICAL MANIFESTATIONS OF ASTHMA. The signs and symptoms of an asthmatic attack are closely related to the status of the airways. Bronchospasm leads to both obstruction of the airways and air trapping. Air trapping is probably due to the acute increase in expiratory flow resistance, which means that the inspired air simply cannot be exhaled in the time available before metabolic demands trigger another inspiration. As a result, a portion of each breath is retained. The hyperinflated alveoli exert a lateral traction on the bronchiolar walls so that inspiratory airway diameter is further increased. This may aid slightly in gas exchange but it requires more inspiratory energy to overcome the tension of the already stretched elastic tissue. The pressure of the

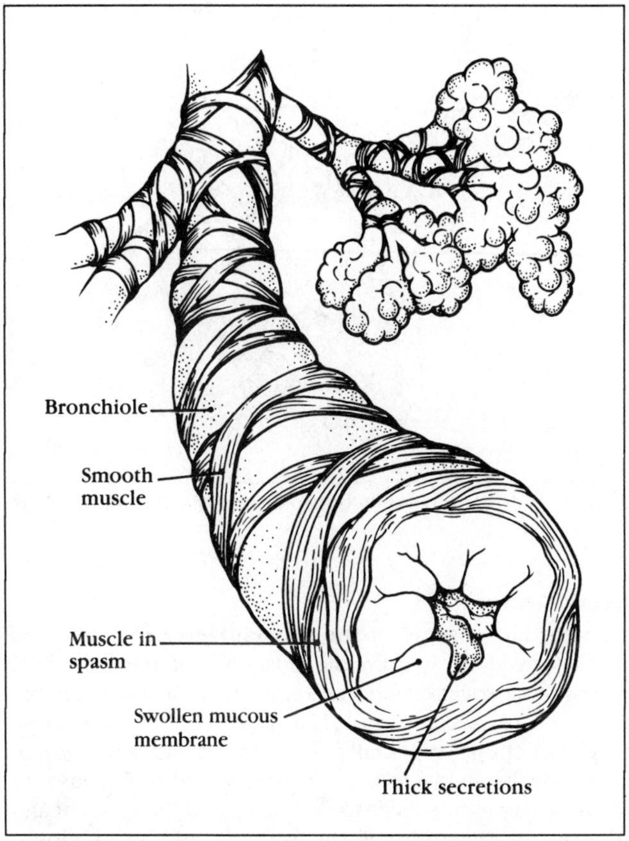

FIGURE 24-1. Bronchial asthma. The bronchiole is obstructed on expiration, particularly by muscle spasm, edema of the mucosa, and thick secretions.

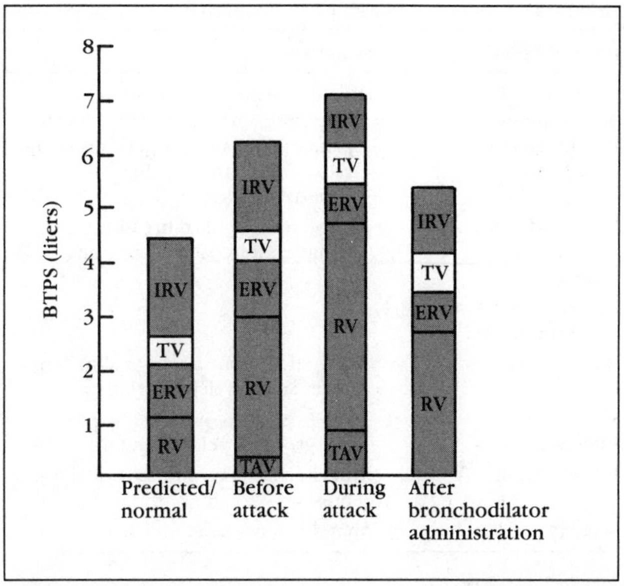

FIGURE 24-2. The normal values are indicated as predicted values: inspiratory reserve volume (*IRV*), tidal volume (*TV*), expiratory reserve volume (*ERV*). Before the attack there is a small trapped air volume (*TAV*) with a larger than usual residual volume (*RV*). During the attack the residual volume increases dramatically. After bronchodilator therapy the trapped air volume and residual volume decrease markedly.

trapped air tends to flatten the diaphragmatic ability to function as the major organ of respiration and may oppose expansion of the lower chest. The costal fibers that are attached to the lower ribs are pulled into a horizontal rather than upright position. They can no longer move up and out so the lower chest cannot expand normally. With the flat, fixed diaphragm, the accessory muscles are called on for chest enlargement with each inspiration. This increases energy cost and also causes increased inflation of the apices rather than the bases. Figure 24-2 shows characteristic pulmonary function studies for an acute asthmatic attack.

Wheezing, a common sign, can be likened to the pulling on the opening of a balloon full of air to make it squeak. The smaller the opening that the air is rushing past, the more squeaking that occurs. In the chest, wheezing results from the squeezing of air past the greatly narrowed airways. Narrowing is caused by bronchospasm plus mucosal edema and obstructive secretions. Since the airways are normally smaller on expiration, expiratory wheezing occurs first. As the attack progresses, there will be both inspiratory and expiratory wheezing.

Pulsus paradoxus, or paradoxical pulse, is an objective measure of bronchospasm. The amplitude of the arterial pulse normally decreases with inspiration and is produced by the pooling of blood in the pulmonary vessels. Due to the respiratory distress in the asthmatic attack, the amount of pooling apparently increases. Pulsus paradoxus is measured by pumping up the blood pressure cuff to above the systolic pressure and lowering the pressure very slowly. With the person breathing quickly and if a paradoxical pulse is present, the Korotkov sounds become audible first during expiration and then during all phases of respiration. The point at which all beats are equally loud is recorded as the bottom of the paradoxical pulse.

Paradoxical pulse is recorded as follows:

Example: $\frac{140 - 120}{60}$

Point at which beats can be heard on expiration = 140
Point at which all beats are equally loud = 120
Diastolic pressure = 60

In this case, the pulsus paradoxus is 20. The normal difference is not more than 8–10 mm Hg.

Fatigue is a major problem in an acute asthma attack. The increased work of breathing leads to increased oxygen consumption until a point is reached at which the individual begins to tire and is no longer able to hyperventilate enough to meet the increased oxygen need. The degree of hypoventilation that results can be accurately assessed by monitoring the arterial carbon dioxide, which may indicate the onset of respiratory failure.

TABLE 24-1. Symptoms of asthma and underlying pathophysiology

Pathophysiology	Symptoms
Bronchospasm Air trapping Diaphragmatic flattening	Dyspnea; orthopnea; coughing; wheezing; chest tightness; elevated paradoxical pulse; tripod position; reduced breath sounds; hyperresonance
Increased work of breathing Fatigue	Tachycardia; labored breathing; air hunger; intercostal retractions
Increased oxygen consumption	
Increased sputum production Dehydration	Thick, sticky sputum; poor skin turgor; other signs of dehydration
Infection	Thick green or yellow sputum
Inflammation	Bronchospasm, eosinophilia if allergy present
Anxiety	Apprehension/panic

A large amount of yellow or green sputum is produced by the bronchial mucosa in an asthma attack. This sputum tends to be thick and obstructive due to its volume, the associated bronchoconstriction, and the associated dehydration. Inflammation is responsible for mucosal edema, which may be due to infection, a common precipitator of the attack (Table 24-1).

Once the attack has subsided and underlying precipitators have cleared, the lungs of the affected individual usually return to normal. There is a significant relationship between asthma and the development of chronic obstructive lung disease later in life.

CHRONIC OBSTRUCTIVE LUNG DISEASE

Chronic obstructive lung diseases are similar to asthma in that there is obstruction to expiratory airflow and that exacerbations and remissions commonly occur. The acute and chronic obstructive diseases differ in that the lung tissues do not return to normal between exacerbations in chronic lung disease. Instead, the pulmonary damage is a slowly progressive process.

The term *chronic obstructive lung disease* (COPD or COLD) refers to a group of conditions associated with chronic obstruction to airflow within the lungs. Usually the term is used to refer to emphysema or chronic bronchitis, but it may also include bronchiectasis and cystic fibrosis. Asthma, considered in this chapter as an acute obstructive condition, is also often grouped with these pulmonary conditions. Of these diseases, the obstruction of chronic bronchitis, bronchiectasis, and cystic fibrosis chiefly results from secretions, while emphysematic obstruction is anatomic in nature. Pneumoconiosis is often classified with chronic obstructive diseases but because of the underlying pathogenesis it is discussed in Chapter 23.

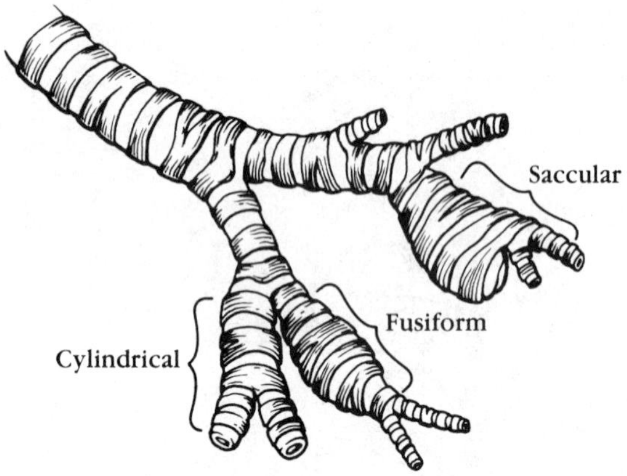

FIGURE 24-3. Various types of bronchiectasis; the morphology varies.

Bronchiectasis

This chronic disease of the bronchi and bronchioles is characterized by irreversible dilatation of the bronchial tree and is associated with chronic infection and inflammation of these passageways. It is usually preceded by respiratory infection, especially bronchopneumonia, which causes the bronchial mucosa to be replaced by fibrous scar tissue. This process leads to destruction of the bronchi and permanent dilatation of the bronchi and bronchioles, which allows the areas affected to be targets for a chronic, smoldering infection (Fig. 24-3).

This disease affects all ages and both sexes, often with onset of the disease in childhood. Usually the initiating event is an infection, such as pneumonia or bronchitis. It is not known whether the condition begins as an infection or if it is due to abnormal structure of the bronchial walls [2]. It frequently exists as an asymptomatic condition but may progress to a disabling or life-threatening condition.

The lower lobes are the most vulnerable and usually are filled with a yellow green infected material that may spread to the pleural cavity. It may or may not be associated with an acute inflammatory exudate with bronchial ulceration or abscess [6].

The common symptoms are cough and symptoms of infection. The person affected raises large amounts of mucopurulent sputum and occasionally hemoptysis occurs.

Cystic Fibrosis (Mucoviscidosis)

This is a hereditary disorder that involves the secretion of large quantities of viscous material. It affects the sweat glands, bronchi, pancreas, and mucus-secreting glands of the small intestine. It may be seen shortly following birth, in young children, and in early adulthood.

The pathologic features include a high concentration of sodium and chloride in the sweat, and abnormal mucus secretion and elimination. Secretion of tenacious mucus throughout the airways produces airway obstruction leading to various combinations of atelectasis, pneumonia, bronchitis, emphysema, and other respiratory conditions. Bacterial secondary infection is common.

Associated pancreatic insufficiency causes abnormal stools, malnutrition, and abdominal distention. Intestinal obstruction is common in the neonate.

The clinical manifestations are variable, with some individuals having mainly gastrointestinal symptoms while others develop severe pulmonary problems. All of the manifestations relate to inability to handle excessive secretions. Pulmonary signs and symptoms are very common and include chronic cough, persistent lung infections, chronic obstructive lung disease, and cor pulmonale.

To diagnose the disease, at least three of the following four criteria are essential [6]:

1. Increase in sodium and chloride in the sweat
2. Deficient pancreatic enzymes in the gastrointestinal secretions
3. Chronic pulmonary infections, especially with *Pseudomonas aeruginosa* and *Staphylococcus aureus*
4. A family history of the problem

The prognosis is variable with survival past the age of 20 increasing, although gastrointestinal and pulmonary problems are continually encountered.

Chronic Bronchitis

Continued bronchial inflammation and progressive increase in productive cough and dyspnea are classic features of *chronic bronchitis*. Usually the bronchial mucosa is responding to chronic irritation.

Pathophysiologically, there is thickening and rigidity of the bronchial mucosa resulting from vasodilatation, congestion, and edema. The mucosal areas may be infiltrated with lymphocytes, macrophages, and polymorphonuclear leukocytes. Excessive secretion plus narrowing of the passageways first causes obstruction to maximal expiration and later to maximal inspiratory airflow [7].

This bronchitis is closely related to emphysema but is usually defined as an abnormality that involves excessive secretion of mucus and bronchial inflammation, while emphysema involves the degeneration of the alveolar parenchyma. Bronchitis is closely related to cigarette smoking and/or other environmental pollutants and may lead to the following: (1) increased airway resistance with or without emphysematic changes, (2) right heart failure (cor pulmonale), and (3) dysplasia of the respiratory epithelial cells that may undergo malignant change [6].

The clinical manifestations for the bronchitic person include cyanosis, copious production of sputum, mild degrees of hyperinflation, marked hypercapnia, and severe hypoxemia. Heart failure with manifestations of right-sided failure occur early in the course of the disease. These manifestations include jugular venous distention, cardiac enlargement, liver engorgement, and peripheral edema. These persons have often been called the "blue bloaters" because of the presence of marked cyanosis and edema. The clinical picture is variable depending on the amount of emphysema present. Table 24-2 compares the clinical and physiologic features of the two conditions. Bronchitis and emphysema rarely occur in isolation from each other, and some mixture of clinical signs and symptoms is usually present.

TABLE 24-2. Features that distinguish bronchial and emphysematous types of chronic obstructive lung disease

	Bronchial	Emphysematous
CLINICAL FEATURES		
History	Often recurrent chest infections	Often only insidious dyspnea
Chest exam	Noisy chest, slight overdistention	Quiet chest, marked overdistention
Sputum	Frequently copious and purulent	Usually scanty and mucoid
Weight loss	Absent or slight	Often marked
Chronic cor pulmonale	Common	Infrequent
Roentgenogram	Often evidence of old inflammatory disease	Often attenuated vessels and radiolucency
General appearance	"Blue bloater"	"Pink puffer"
PHYSIOLOGIC TESTS		
Lung volumes		
TLC	Normal or slightly decreased	Increased
RV	Moderately increased	Markedly increased
RV/TLC	High	High
Lung compliance		
Static	Normal or low	High
Dynamic	Very low	Normal or low
Airways resistance		
Expiratory	Very high	High
Inspiratory	High	Normal
Diffusing capacity	Variable	Low
Chronic hypoxemia	Often severe	Usually mild
Chronic hypercapnia	Common	Unusual
Pulmonary hypertension	Often severe	Usually mild
Cardiac output	Normal	Often low

Source: B. Burrows, R.J. Knudson, and L. J. Kettel, *Respiratory Insufficiency*. Chicago: Yearbook, 1975. P. 141. (Reprinted with permission.)

Pulmonary Emphysema

This is the most common chronic pulmonary disease and is frequently classified with chronic bronchitis because of the association of the two disease conditions. Emphysema in anatomic terms involves the portion of lung distal to a terminal bronchiole (*acinus*) where gas exchange takes place. Emphysema involves permanent, abnormal enlargement of the acinus with associated destructive changes. It may be classified as *vesicular emphysema* when it involves the spaces distal to the terminal bronchioles and *interlob-*

TABLE 24-3. Comparison of lobular and acinar terminology of emphysema

Lobules	Acini
Panlobular All lung affected; diffuse throughout lung	*Panacinar* Whole acinus affected; diffuse throughout lung
Centrilobular Spaces around central bronchioles affected; usually affects apices	*Centriacinar* Area around alveolar ducts affected; usually affects apices
Periseptal Occurs at periphery of lobule; less common than above types	*Perciacinar* Occurs at the periphery of acinus; less common than above types
Irregular Scarring throughout the acinus irregularly	

TABLE 24-4. Terminology related to the classification of emphysema

Diffuse or generalized emphysema Lobules or acini throughout lung affected

Focal emphysema Emphysema associated with focal dust deposition (e.g., coal dust)

Irregular emphysema Emphysema associated with the shrinkage of fibrotic scars, usually from old disease

Obstructive emphysema Emphysema that is accompanied by demonstrable bronchial obstruction

Bulla An emphysematous space of more than 1 cm in an inflated lung; may occur in any type of emphysema

ular, or *interstitial, emphysema* when it affects the tissue between the air spaces [1]. The commonly used term *pulmonary emphysema* is usually used to designate the vesicular type.

PATHOPHYSIOLOGY OF EMPHYSEMA. Emphysema seems to be due to many separate injuries that occur over a long period of time. The elastin and fiber network of the alveoli and airways is broken down. The alveoli enlarge and many of their walls are destroyed. The alveolar destruction leads to the formation of larger than normal air spaces, or pools, which greatly reduces the alveolar diffusing surface. Once the process begins, it progresses slowly and inconsistently. The alveolar destruction also destroys the support structure for the airways, making them more vulnerable to expiratory collapse. There may be associated airway inflammation and consequent increase in mucus production, although many persons with emphysema produce little or no sputum.

The exact mechanism of injury is yet to be determined. Ischemia may cause the alveolar breakdown, although specific vascular lesions have not been found [3]. Repeated injuries from smoking, infection, and air pollution often lead to emphysema but the exact mechanism of injury has not been identified.

Specific types of emphysema have been shown to be related to a deficiency in the enzyme *alpha$_1$ antitrypsin,* which functions to inhibit the proteases of elastase and collagenase. These proteases are normally major contributors to tissue destruction during the inflammatory process. Without the inhibition of alpha$_1$ antitrypsin, the destruction or digestion of pulmonary tissue occurs, more at the bases than at the apices of the lungs. This circumstance leads to the onset of severe obstructive lung disease early in adult life, often before the age of 40 [5]. The onset of hypoxia and cor pulmonale in these persons heralds a poor prognosis.

The types of emphysema have been classified according to the area of the lung affected. Terminology varies in the classification of emphysema (Table 24-3). The classification is anatomic and may describe lobules or acini. Other descriptive terms are found in Table 24-4. It is important to remember that many types of emphysema cannot be classified with certainty, especially during life. Pulmonary interstitial emphysema is an associated condition that involves overdistention of the alveoli and dissection of air into the perivascular spaces. The dissection may continue into the mediastinum, causing *pneumomediastinum,* or into the pleural cavity, causing *pneumothorax.* Figure 24-4 illustrates the appearance of the different types of emphysema.

Emphysema has a major effect on compliance and elasticity. Because of alveolar wall destruction, fibrous and muscle tissues are lost, making the lungs more compliant or more distensible. Even in severe disease inspiratory airway resistance tends to be normal. Air trapping occurs because of loss of elastic recoil, which increases airway size on inspiration and causes collapse of the small airways on expiration. Thus, a minor obstruction on inspiration is a serious obstruction on expiration. If the expiration is a forced expiration, there is a sharp rise in pressure on the airways that leads to compression of the bronchi and bronchioles. The resultant distention eventually leads to disruption in the alveolar walls and surrounding musculoelastic tissue around the small airways. Figure 24-5 illustrates the difference between normal alveoli and distended alveoli of emphysema.

CLINICAL MANIFESTATIONS OF EMPHYSEMA. The clinical manifestations of emphysema may overlap with those of bronchitis. The person with emphysema has often been called the "pink puffer" on the basis of appearance. Dyspnea is characteristic; in the early stages it occurs with exertion and later progresses to dyspnea at rest. Severe hyperinflation of the lungs may result in an increase in the anteroposterior chest diameter resulting in the typical barrel chest appearance. Dorsal kyphosis, prominent anterior chest, and elevated ribs all contribute to this appearance (Fig. 24-6). The accessory muscles are used to raise the thorax on inspiration and the abdominal muscles are developed in order to actively force air out. There is a resultant prolongation of the expiratory cycle. Pulmonary function tests will show a prolonged FEV with a decreased vital capacity, despite an increase in total lung capacity. Respiratory sounds are frequently decreased unless there is a superimposed infection that may account for expiratory wheezing and rales.

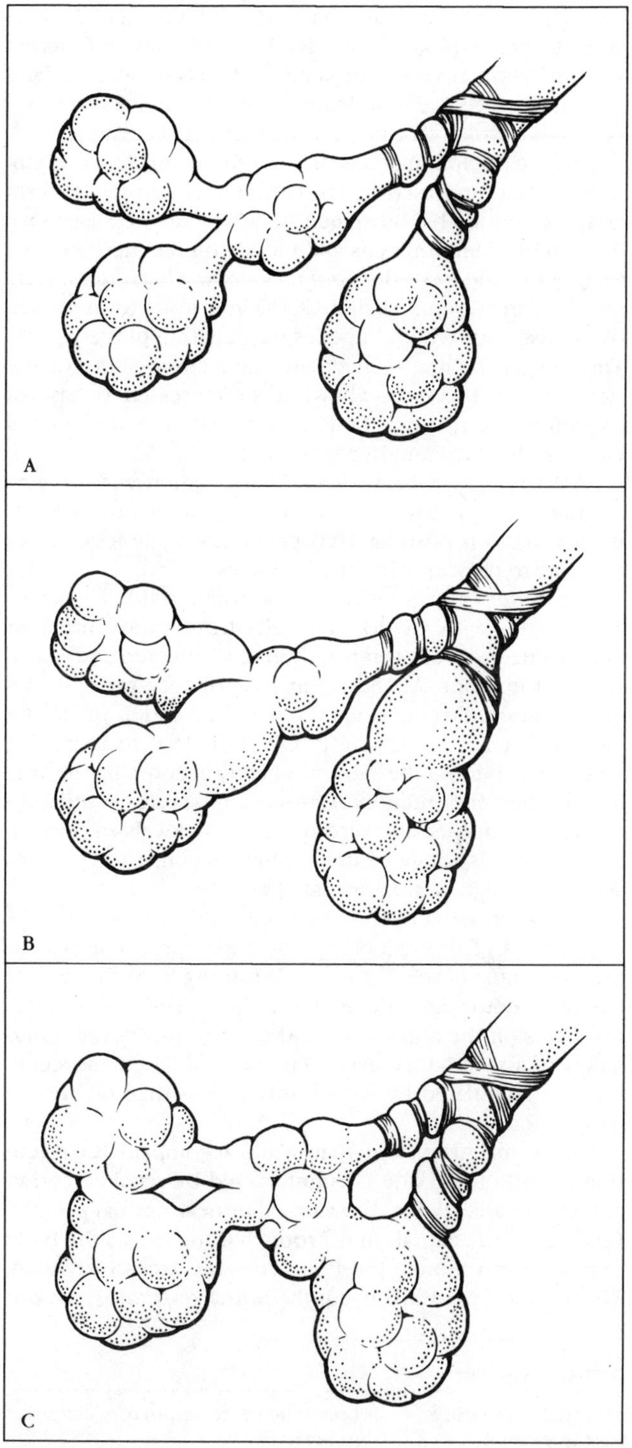

FIGURE 24-4. Alterations in alveolar structure. A. Normal respiratory bronchioles and alveoli. B. Centrilobular emphysema—dilation of the respiratory bronchioles. C. Panlobular emphysema—destruction of the alveolar walls.

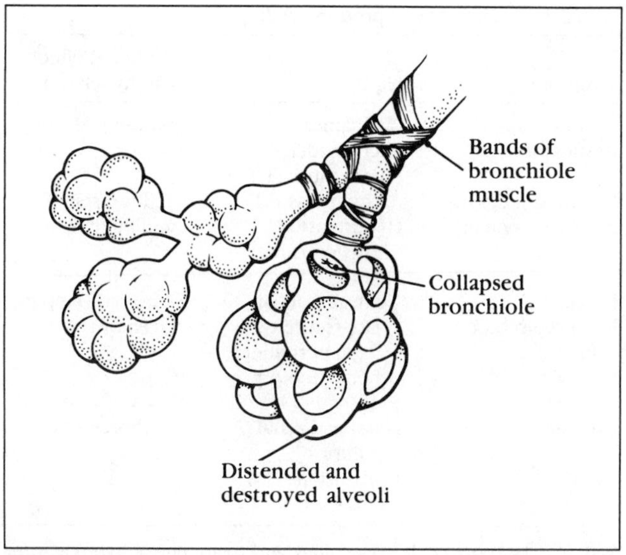

FIGURE 24-5. Compare the distended and destroyed alveoli with normal ones.

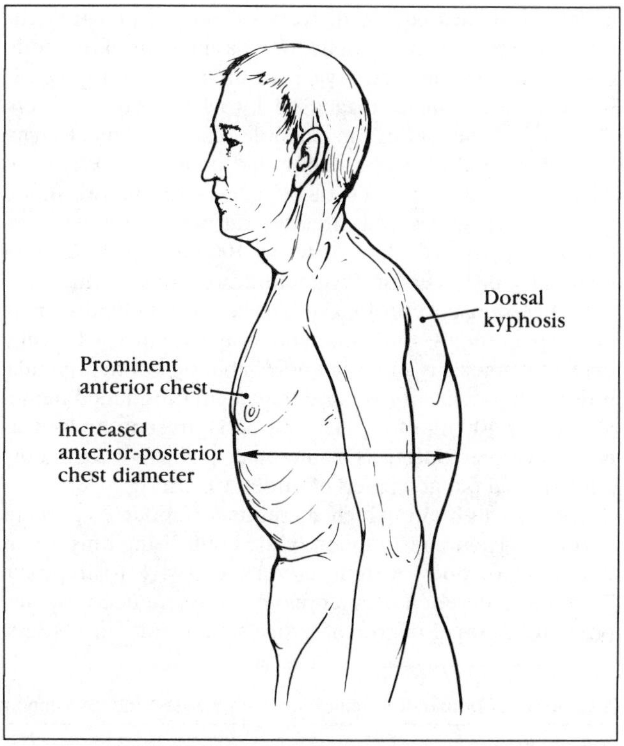

FIGURE 24-6. Barrel chest of emphysema.

TABLE 24-5. Diagnosis of progressive hypoxia

Symptoms	Signs	Additional effects from hypercapnia
Dyspnea	Tachypnea	Severe headache
Restlessness	Tachycardia (bradycardia, late)	Tremor
Impaired judgment	Arrhythmias	Diaphoresis
Personality change	Hypertension (hypotension, late)	Papilledema
Headache	Central cyanosis — late (more than 5 gm of reduced hemoglobin per 100 ml of blood)	Asterixis (flapping tremor)
Impaired motor function		
Confusion	Heart and renal failure	Diaphoresis
Delirium	Convulsions	
Coma	Coma	

Source: J. L. Andrews, Jr., Physiology and treatment of hypoxia. *Clin. Notes Respir. Dis.* 13:4, 1974.

Hypoxia is a very common end result of emphysema. It is defined as inadequate delivery of oxygen to satisfy the metabolic requirements of the organs and cells of the body. Direct measurement of oxygen in the tissue is impossible so hypoxia is usually diagnosed by its end-organ effects. Hypoxia of the brain, for example, causes clinical signs, such as mental changes, stupor, and coma. *Hypoxemia* is defined as reduced levels of oxygen in the blood. Blood gas levels are measured directly and normal oxygen tension in the arterial blood is 80 to 100 mm Hg. A value of 40 mm Hg or lower for oxygen indicates hypoxemia.

As a response to prolonged hypoxia, the individual may develop cyanosis, clubbing, and polycythemia. Clinically evident cyanosis is a late and unreliable sign of hypoxemia. It does not occur unless more than 5 gm of reduced hemoglobin per 100 ml of capillary blood is present. As long as normal cardiac output is maintained, cyanosis occurs only with arterial oxygen levels of under 40 mm Hg.

The human brain, which accounts for about 20 percent of total oxygen consumption while comprising only about 2 percent of body weight, is very sensitive to hypoxia. Therefore, cerebral symptoms may be induced by hypoxemia. A small degree of hypoxemia results in restlessness, change in personality, and impaired judgment. Moderately severe hypoxemia causes impaired motor function and confusion. Severe hypoxemia, at levels between 20 and 30 mm Hg, often causes delirium and coma. Persistent severe hypoxemia can cause permanent cortical damage.

Chronic hypoxemia causes a release of renal erythropoietic factor, which reacts with a plasma protein to form erythropoietin. This substance stimulates an increased production of red blood cells and blood volume increase (see Chap. 14). The resulting *polycythemia* characteristically develops in patients having COPD and leads to increased blood viscosity, which impedes oxygenation of the tissues. The oxygen hemoglobin dissociation curve shifts to the right with hypoxemia, allowing for increased release of oxygen to the tissues. (Table 24-5 summarizes the general effects of hypoxia and hypercapnia.)

Clubbing is commonly seen in association with polycythemia and hypoxemia. The etiology of this disorder is unclear but it is postulated that capillary dilation occurs in an effort to draw oxygen to the tissues.

Hypercapnia (retention of carbon dioxide) is commonly seen with COPD. It results from hypoventilation mostly due to an uneven matchup of ventilation and perfusion in the lungs. At the normal ventilatory rates, inadequate carbon dioxide is excreted and retention of carbon dioxide occurs. Increasing PCO_2 levels lead to increased ventilation due to the central chemoreceptor in the medulla. When the pulmonary disease is severe, ventilation changes do not usually return the PCO_2 levels to normal. In other words, the work of breathing becomes too great to sustain the high ventilatory rate [4].

The hypercapnia becomes chronic and depresses the receptiveness of the medullary chemoreceptor. The person may lose most of the stimuli for breathing from the central chemoreceptor and depend on the peripheral chemoreceptors on the aortic arch and carotid sinuses for stimulation of a ventilatory drive. The peripheral chemoreceptors are stimulated by hypoxemia of less than 60 mm Hg oxygen tension.

The normal pH change that would accompany the retention of carbon dioxide is counteracted by renal retention of bicarbonate, leading to a normal or near normal pH (see Chap. 6). This adaptation is protective and assists the body function even though the PCO_2 remains excessively high. The adjusted pH reflects *compensated respiratory acido-*

TABLE 24-6. Comparative values for compensated and uncompensated respiratory acidosis

Arterial blood gas components	Normal values	Compensated respiratory acidosis (an example)	Uncompensated respiratory acidosis (an example)
pH	7.35–7.45	7.35	7.22
PCO_2	35–45 mm Hg	54 mm Hg	74 mm Hg
PO_2	80–100 mm Hg	62 mm Hg	40 mm Hg
O_2 saturation	95–100%	83%	69%
HCO_3	22–26 mEq/L	32 mEq/L	28 mEq/L
H_2CO_3	1.05–1.35 mEq/L	1.8 mEq/L	2.9 mEq/L

sis. Table 24-6 shows examples of compensated and uncompensated respiratory acidosis. Acid-base balance is described in depth in Chapter 6.

Any of the chronic lung diseases may lead to respiratory failure, which is further discussed in Chapter 25. Further reference material for chronic obstructive lung disease is found in the bibliography at the end of Unit 9.

REFERENCES

1. Anderson, W. A. D., and Scotti, T. *Synopsis of Pathology* (10th ed.). St. Louis: Mosby, 1980.
2. Farzan, S. *A Concise Handbook of Respiratory Diseases.* Reston, Va.: Reston Pub., 1978.
3. Hugh-Jones, P., and Whimster, W. The etiology and management of disabling emphysema. *Am. Rev. Respir. Dis.* 117:2, 1978.
4. Isselbacher, K. J., et al. (eds.). *Harrison's Principles of Internal Medicine* (9th ed.). New York: McGraw-Hill, 1980.
5. Kueppers, F., and Black, L. $Alpha_1$ antitrypsin and its deficiency. *Am. Rev. Respir. Dis.* 110, 1974.
6. Robbins, S., and Cotran, R. *Pathologic Basis of Disease* (2nd ed.). Philadelphia: Saunders, 1979.
7. Sodeman, W., and Sodeman, T. *Pathologic Physiology* (6th ed.). Philadelphia: Saunders, 1979.
8. Weiss, E. Bronchial asthma. *Ciba Clin. Symp.* 27:1, 1975.

CHAPTER 25
OTHER ALTERATIONS AFFECTING THE PULMONARY SYSTEM

LEARNING OBJECTIVES

1. Describe the ventilation-perfusion abnormality occurring with pulmonary embolus.
2. Discuss the underlying risk factors in the causation of pulmonary embolus.
3. List and describe three conditions that favor thrombic formation in the deep veins.
4. Describe the variable clinical manifestations that may be seen with the process of pulmonary embolization.
5. Briefly explain how resolution of emboli occurs.
6. Describe the development of pulmonary hypertension.
7. Define *cor pulmonale.*
8. Define *rhinitis, pharyngitis, sinusitis,* and *laryngitis.*
9. Briefly explain the dangers of laryngeal edema.
10. Classify and briefly describe cancer of the larynx.
11. Define *hamartoma of the lungs.*
12. Discuss some factors predisposing the onset of malignancy in the lung.
13. Describe the pathology, major clinical manifestations, and prognosis of four major types of intrapulmonary malignancy.
14. List the most common sites for metastasis of lung cancer.
15. Differentiate between respiratory insufficiency and respiratory failure.
16. Explain how adaptation can occur in chronic respiratory insufficiency.
17. List the criteria for diagnosing respiratory failure and the other factors that should be taken into account.
18. Describe the clinical manifestations of respiratory failure.
19. Define *carbon dioxide narcosis.*
20. Discuss the prognosis in acute or chronic respiratory failure.

Several of the pulmonary disease processes do not easily lend themselves to strict classification into the restrictive or obstructive patterns. This chapter discusses some of these conditions, including pulmonary embolus, tumors of the lung, and respiratory insufficiency and failure. Respiratory failure may result from many intrapulmonary and extrapulmonary disease conditions, and it is frequently the cause of death in chronic pulmonary disease.

As discussed in Chapter 22, the normal ratio of alveolar ventilation (4 liters/minute) to volume of blood flow in the pulmonary capillaries ($\dot{V}/\dot{Q}$) is about 0.8 because cardiac output averages about 5 liters/minute. A decrease of alveolar ventilation in relation to perfusion occurs in any part of the lung where airways are obstructed by secretions (bronchitis), by expiratory dynamic collapse (emphysema), by muscular spasm (asthma), where alveoli are collapsed (atelectasis), or are filled with fluid (pulmonary edema). These conditions cause increased venous blood flow past nonventilated alveoli with the oxygen-poor mixture being added to the arterial blood and the resultant product being hypoxemia. As has been stated previously, hypoxemia resulting from underventilated alveoli is, in essence, a form of right-to-left shunting of venous blood past the alveoli. The reader is referred to the preceding chapters for a more comprehensive discussion.

Another type of ventilation-perfusion abnormality is the reduction of perfusion in relation to ventilation. This occurs most frequently when pulmonary emboli obliterate arteriolar blood supply, but may occur when cardiac output is reduced because of congestive heart failure. In these examples, ventilated but nonperfused alveoli increase the physiologic dead space because a significant number of alveoli receive inspired air but do not participate in the exchange of oxygen or carbon dioxide.

In conditions in which hypoxemia is the result of a ventilation-perfusion abnormality, the PCO_2 will often be normal or low, since compensatory hyperventilation is able to lower the more easily diffusible PCO_2. Thus, the clinical pattern of ventilation-perfusion inequality is often one of hypoxemia with hyperventilation, a lowered PCO_2, and even respiratory alkalosis. This picture is directly related to the degree of the ventilation-perfusion defect and eventually may result in hypoxemia, hypercapnia, and respiratory acidosis.

PULMONARY EMBOLUS

A pulmonary embolus is defined as an occlusion of one or more pulmonary vessels by matter that has traveled from a source outside the lung. Any foreign material freely traveling in the systemic venous system must finally terminate in the pulmonary vascular bed at some point. For example, if a clot in a small vein dislodges, it travels through progressively larger vessels until it reaches the right ventricle, where it is pumped via the pulmonary artery to the lungs. The usual cause of pulmonary embolus is a thrombus from the deep veins of the legs or pelvis that dislodges and travels with the flow of blood to the lungs. It may also result from a fat embolus; an amniotic fluid embolus; an air embolus; particulate matter injected intravenously; or rarely, gas, parasites, or foreign objects.

Pulmonary embolus is a major cause of death among hospitalized individuals, but the diagnosis is often missed. Estimates vary, but about 50,000 deaths per year in the United States are probably attributable to this condition. It is thought that many persons have thrombi in the venous systems. These may actually embolize but may be diagnosed as a pulmonary infection, as pleurisy, or may not be diagnosed at all. Pulmonary emboli rarely strike the young or healthy but strike a high-risk group that includes bedfast persons, the obese, the elderly, and those with a history of prior emboli or thrombosis. Persons with congestive heart failure, who have abdominal or pelvic surgery, or who have sustained trauma to the legs are also at high risk.

Sequence of Events in Pulmonary Embolization

The right lung is more frequently involved than the left, with the degree of obstruction related to the size of the embolus. It has been shown in some studies that the physiologic consequences of pulmonary embolus are greater than can be explained by the degree of occlusion alone. A large embolus may cause infarction of the lung parenchyma but this is not directly relative to the size of the embolus, because the bronchial arteries continue to supply the lung tissue [3].

As stated before, most pulmonary emboli are the result of thrombi that dislodge from the deep veins of the legs and pelvis. Phlebothrombosis is the most common type of deep vein thrombosis and is frequently seen in immobilized and/or obese persons and in those who have sustained surgical or accidental trauma.

In order for a thrombus of this nature to form, an abnormality must be present, since clotting rarely occurs when there is normal blood flow and vascular integrity. Three conditions have been described that favor clot formation: (1) venostasis, (2) endothelial disruption of the vessel lining, and (3) hypercoagulability.

Local concentration of coagulation factors along with an injury to the venous wall may provide a place for clots to form. As the flow of blood slows or stops over the injured area, the clot begins to form and extends or propagates itself up the vein (Fig. 25-1). It may then retract and pull away from the vessel wall and become a free-floating embolus. Small fragments of the clot may break off and produce multiple areas of embolization to the lungs. Multiple embolization to the pulmonary capillary bed is more common than occlusion of the main pulmonary artery or its branches.

Once the blood clot lodges in the pulmonary capillary bed, it obstructs blood flow beyond the point of the obstruction. Perfusion in the pulmonary capillary bed stops. If large areas are affected there may be infarction of the lung

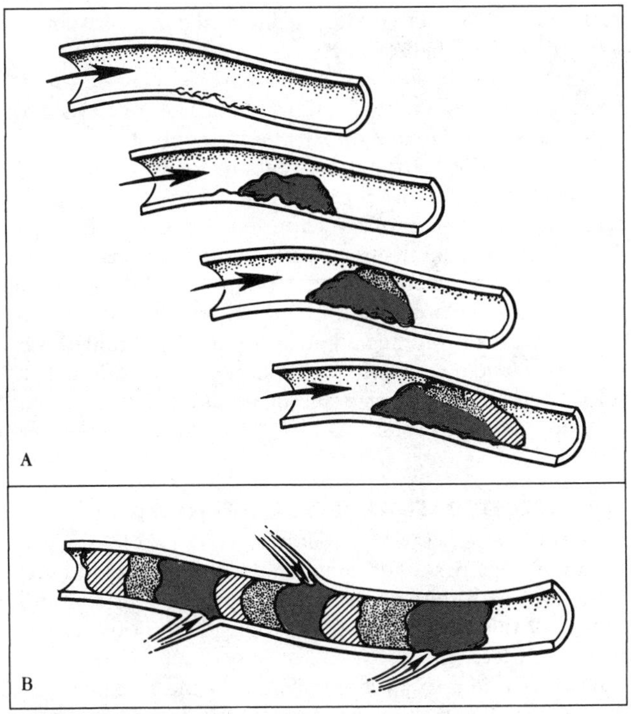

FIGURE 25-1. A. Formation of clot on area of intimal damage, sequence of clot formation. B. Propagation of clot up the length of the vein wall may lead to pulmonary embolus.

tissue, which occurs in perhaps 5 to 10 percent of cases and produces infarcts of varying sizes. The newly formed infarct becomes hemorrhagic but later becomes filled with scar tissue [5].

A wide variety of pathophysiologic responses to a pulmonary embolus occur, depending on the size of the embolus and the ability of the host to compensate. Small obstructions to the blood supply usually create no hemodynamic changes and are called *silent pulmonary emboli.* Larger obstructions may cause increased resistance to pulmonary blood flow, which may lead to right ventricular failure (cor pulmonale). Studies show that more than 50 percent of the pulmonary vasculature must be obstructed to cause significant increase in pressure in the pulmonary artery [6]. Vasoconstriction in the smaller pulmonary arterial vessels is apparently common and may be due to the liberation of vasoactive substances, such as serotonin. This vasoconstriction enhances the risk for pulmonary ischemia and infarction.

As stated earlier, the increase in the pulmonary artery pressure leads to an increased workload for the right side of the heart in pumping blood into the pulmonary circulation. Tachycardia results and progresses to signs of right ventricular failure, including jugular venous distention, hepatomegaly, and peripheral edema. A large saddle embolus obstructing the main pulmonary artery at its bifurcation to the right and left branches leads to acute cor pulmonale, severe shock, and often, sudden death [3].

The process of embolization may be chronic, with small

TABLE 25-1. Signs and symptoms of pulmonary embolus

Initial manifestations
May be clinically silent
Dyspnea of sudden onset
Cough
Fever
Pain: pleuritic or deep and crushing
Hemoptysis
Tachypnea
Anxiety, apprehension, restlessness
Palpitations
Weakness
Diaphoresis
Nausea and vomiting
Shock
Physical examination findings
Splinting of involved side
Cyanosis
Distended neck veins
Area of dullness over involved side
Tachycardia
S3 or S4 gallop
Rales
Localized decreased breath sounds
Localized wheezing
Chest x ray may be normal or may show patchy areas of infiltration
Lung scan and pulmonary arteriogram definitive
Arterial blood gases: frequently show hypoxemia and hypercapnia

emboli being released from a thrombotic focus over months or years. Often undiagnosed, this process may lead to pulmonary embarrassment.

Resolution of the pulmonary embolus occurs by absorption and fibrosis. This may begin as early as a few hours after a small embolic episode. Fibrous replacement converts infarcted lung tissue to scar tissue. Clots are partly or totally dissolved by the fibrinolytic system of the body. Residual material, resistant to fibrinolytic attack, may organize and become small, scarred areas.

Clinical Manifestations

The signs and symptoms of pulmonary embolus vary greatly (Table 25-1). The embolus may be clinically silent with no manifestations at all. The most frequent symptom is the sudden onset of mild, moderate, or severe dyspnea that may occur transiently. Tachypnea that persists is suggestive of pulmonary embolus. Fever and cough, sometimes with associated hemoptysis, often occur. Pain may be absent, mild, or severe and may be manifested as pleural pain or deep, crushing, substernal pain mimicking the pain of myocardial infarction. The pain often occurs with pulmonary infarction and may be oppressive and substernal in nature. Anxiety, apprehension, and restlessness commonly occur in response to hypoxemia. Palpitations and weakness associated with profuse perspiration and nausea and vomiting often are present. If massive embolization has occurred, cardiovascular collapse may result, leading to sudden shock, seizures, or cardiopulmonary arrest.

Clinical signs of pulmonary embolus may include splinting of the involved side, cyanosis, distended neck veins, tachycardia with an increased pulmonic sound, or an S3 or S4 gallop. Rales and decreased breath sounds in the affected areas are frequent findings.

Definitive diagnosis is often difficult. A chest x ray often appears normal and any abnormalities may be of a general nature, such as elevation of the diaphragm, atelectasis, or pleural effusion. The serum enzyme lactic dehydrogenase (LDH), is often elevated. The arterial blood gases may show hypoxemia, hypocapnia, and respiratory alkalosis due to the marked tachypnea. The radioisotope lung scan shows perfusion defects in areas of the lung and provides support for the diagnosis. The pulmonary arteriogram is occasionally performed to provide visualization of the vessels of the pulmonary tree.

Fat Embolization

Fractures of the long bones are the major source of emboli that are composed of fat particles. The origin appears to be from the bone marrow, and the particles enter the bloodstream through the ruptured veins. Fat also may be mobilized from the injured site and may form large globules in the plasma [1]. Alveolar edema often occurs and appears much like the adult respiratory distress syndrome (ARDS). The person affected begins to exhibit marked respiratory distress, fever, and tachycardia [3].

PULMONARY HYPERTENSION

This condition can result from heart and/or lung disease. It refers to an increase in the pulmonary artery pressure, which increases the workload of the right ventricle. Significant pulmonary vascular obliteration must be present in order for the pulmonary arterial pressure to be elevated, because there is normally a large reserve in the pulmonary capillary bed.

The most common picture of pulmonary hypertension involves progressive disease either of the pulmonary vessels or of the lung parenchyma. There is usually hypertrophy of the pulmonary arteries and loss of adaptability of the system to stress factors, such as increased blood flow or hypoxia.

As the process becomes persistent, an elevated, end-diastolic pressure develops in the right ventricle. The right ventricle hypertrophies and further increases its systolic pressure. In the early stages, symptoms of right ventricular failure or *cor pulmonale* (heart failure resulting from lung disease) occur only during periods of increased stress. As it progresses, cor pulmonale is present all of the time, manifested by jugular venous distention, hepatomegaly, and peripheral edema.

The pulmonary artery pressure, which is normally approximately 25/10 mm Hg, is elevated to above approximately 40/15 mm Hg and may be much higher as the disease progresses. At a certain critical point, the right ventricle cannot compensate for the increased pressure and intractable cardiac failure occurs.

Death, from chronic respiratory disease, may be due to heart failure or respiratory failure. Nearly all persons with these diseases exhibit some symptoms of right ventricular failure, also called chronic cor pulmonale.

Other conditions besides chronic obstructive lung disease may cause pulmonary hypertension. Congenital cardiac left-to-right shunts that overload the pulmonary vascular system can eventually cause pulmonary hypertension. Also, some valvular conditions, particularly mitral stenosis, cause increased volume and pressure in the pulmonary vascular bed and eventually pulmonary hypertension. Left-sided heart failure of long-standing duration also may cause pulmonary hypertension.

UPPER RESPIRATORY TRACT ALTERATIONS

Alterations in the upper respiratory tract (URT) are very common, usually self-limiting conditions that include such conditions as rhinitis, pharyngitis, sinusitis, and laryngitis. Cancer of the larynx is a more serious condition that may affect the URT.

Rhinitis refers to an inflammation of the nasal cavities, resulting in a persistent nasal discharge caused by secretory hyperactivity of the submucosal glands of the nasal cavities. The etiology of this condition is commonly either viral, bacterial, or allergic in nature. The viral form is recognized as the common cold. Allergies or exposure to irritants injure the normal cilia of the nasal mucosa. Bacterial growth often follows the initial viral attack.

Pharyngitis usually results from viral or bacterial invasion of the pharynx that causes a sore throat. The appearance of the throat varies depending on the causative agent. Tonsils are often affected and become reddened, swollen, and exude a suppurative discharge. Most pharyngitis is relatively innocuous but untreated streptococcal infections may have systemic effects in some persons. These effects are manifested as scarlet fever, rheumatic fever, rheumatic heart disease, glomerulonephritis, and others. Other organisms, such as the *Corynebacterium diphtheriae* and the *Hemophilus influenzae* may cause grave effects.

Sinusitis is an inflammation of the sinus cavities, often spreading from a rhinitis infection to the sinuses. The most common organisms causing this condition are the group A *Streptococcus pyogenes,* the *Staphylococcus aureus,* and the *H. influenzae.* The infection usually causes localized pain in the frontal, maxillary, ethmoid, or sphenoid sinuses (Fig. 25-2). A purulent exudate indicates bacterial infection that, when severe, is associated with the constitutional symptoms of fever, chills, pain in the sinuses, and nasal obstruction. Chronic cases may be indicated by a postnasal discharge and tenderness over the sinus cavity.

Laryngitis often occurs in persons who overutilize the voice in singing or other vocal activities. It may also be due to any organism that may affect the URT. It affects both vocal cords and is manifested by cough and hoarseness with

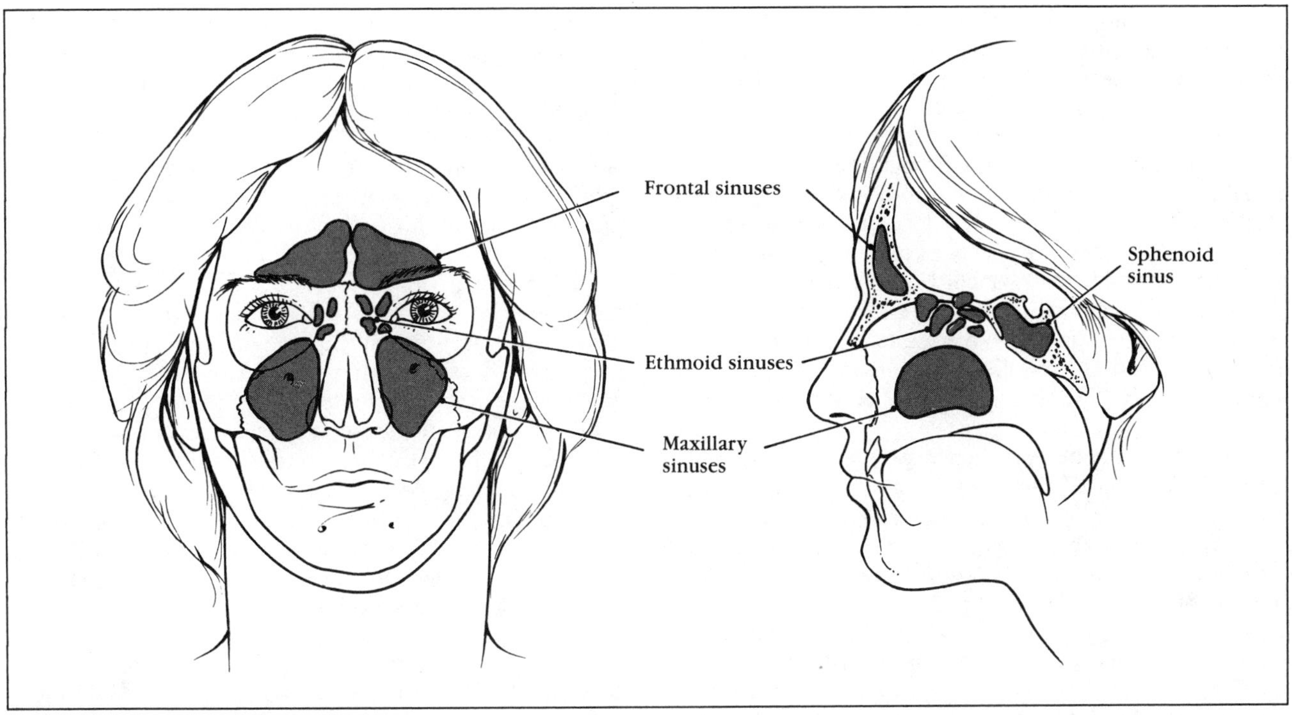

FIGURE 25-2. Location of paranasal sinuses.

loss of the voice. Laryngitis may also be a chronic condition precipitated by overuse of tobacco, straining the voice, or inhalation of toxic gases. Rarely, this condition causes *laryngeal edema* and obstruction to airflow. Complete obstruction causes asphyxia while incomplete obstruction, such as that seen with anaphylaxis, causes laryngeal stridor and respiratory distress.

CARCINOMA OF THE LARYNX

Polyps of the vocal cords are not usually premalignant but the *laryngeal papilloma* is a true neoplasm that has the potential of undergoing malignant transformation. Most persons affected are or have been heavy tobacco smokers.

Most cancers of the larynx arise on the vocal cords and are clinically manifested by hoarseness. This malignancy is closely associated with chronic laryngitis and smoking. It is seen in greater incidence in men after the fourth decade.

Clinical manifestations of cancers of the larynx include pain, a palpable lump, dysphagia, and occasionally respiratory distress. The tumor, being a relatively slow-growing malignancy of the squamous epithelium, is curable in the early stages.

LUNG TUMORS

Tumors of the lung may be benign or malignant. The majority of these tumors are malignant and have an unremitting, progressive course leading ultimately to a poor prognosis. The only benign tumor that is discussed in this section is the hamartoma because it is frequently difficult to differentiate this tumor from a malignancy. The malignant tumors are described according to histologic classification and pathogenesis.

Benign Tumors of the Lung

The *hamartoma* is not a true neoplasm but is a congenital anomaly that frequently leads to tumorlike lesions, containing connective tissue, cartilage, and bronchial epithelium, in the bronchi or lung tissue [1]. The lesions produced are encapsulated, firm, and grayish-white with a rough nodular surface; they appear on chest x ray in the periphery of the lung, in the subpleural area, and endobronchially, making them difficult to distinguish from malignant tumors. These uncommon lung tumors rarely cause any clinical symptoms but must be differentiated from malignancy.

Malignant Tumors of the Lung

FACTORS PREDISPOSING TO MALIGNANCY. Cigarette smoking, air pollution, and industrial chemicals seem to account for the increasing incidence of bronchogenic carcinoma. Statistical evidence supports the relationship between cigarette smoking and certain types of lung cancer. The death rate from lung cancer is twice as high in urban areas as in rural areas, implicating air pollution as an etiologic factor (see Chaps. 12 and 13).

Certain occupations apparently predispose persons to lung cancer. Asbestos workers have about a 10 times greater risk of developing the disease than the general population. More startling, an asbestos worker who smokes has a 90 times greater risk of developing lung cancer than the general population. Other industrial agents that increase risk are uranium, chromate, arsenic, and iron.

Studies performed by Passey suggest a correlation between chronic bronchitis and bronchogenic carcinoma, with the differences in mortality from lung cancer reported in different countries being related to a differing incidence of chronic bronchitis [4]. The excess mucus secretion characteristic of chronic bronchitis may interfere with the bronchial epithelial cells, making them more likely to undergo malignant change [4]. Also, the bronchial mucosa, which is chronically inflamed, exhibits depressed ciliary activity, and airway cleansing is decreased.

GROSS APPEARANCE OF PULMONARY MALIGNANCY. Although variability may occur, the appearance of pulmonary carcinoma may be one of three types: (1) *hilar, infiltrating form*, which causes a large tumor mass that presses on the bronchi; (2) *peripheral* or *nodular form*, which may appear as a single tumor or multiple nodular masses through the lung; or (3) diffuse type, which looks very much like pneumonia and may be difficult to see grossly [1].

MICROSCOPIC APPEARANCE OF PULMONARY MALIGNANCY. The *squamous cell carcinoma* is the most common morphologic type of bronchogenic carcinoma. It causes 45 to 60 percent of lung malignancies. The cell type may be well differentiated but frequently is undifferentiated and quite pleomorphic in appearance. It tends to have large, well-outlined areas of tumor growth arising from the bronchi [5]. These invade surrounding tissue in the early stages of the disease but later metastasize readily to the lymph nodes, brain, bone, adrenal glands, and liver. This tumor type has a very high correlation with heavy cigarette smoking. The 2-year prognosis is poor with less than a 50 percent survival rate.

The *small-cell (oat-cell) carcinoma* consists of small, dark cells located between the cells of the mucosal surfaces. These are characterized by rapid growth and early metastasis through the lymphatic system and the blood. This type is rarely seen in the peripheral areas and frequently exhibits large, obstructive growths in the main bronchi [1]. These small-cell carcinomas often secrete substances normally found in other areas of the body, including ACTH (adrenocorticotrophic hormone) and ADH (antidiuretic hormone). The result of ACTH secretion is Cushing's syndrome leading to obesity, osteoporosis, hypokalemia, alkalosis, and other problems. ADH secretion leads to retention of water, hyponatremia, renal sodium loss, anorexia, nausea, and lethargy [2]. The prognosis in this type of malignancy is very poor with only a 3 to 5 percent survival rate for 2 years.

Large-cell undifferentiated or giant-cell carcinoma is distinct from the previous two in that the cell involved is large and very anaplastic. It is more frequently located in the peripheral areas of the lung. These tumor cells do not secrete hormones and also do not tend to grow at the rate of the small-cell type. The overall prognosis still remains very poor with only about 12 percent survival for 2 years.

Adenocarcinoma is a carcinoma of the lungs that has no particular relationship to smoking and carries an equal incidence in men and women. The location of the tumor cells is more often in the periphery of the lungs with a rapid growth rate and early metastasis to the bloodstream. The overall 2-year prognosis is poor with only a 20 percent survival rate.

The propensity for metastasis, at differing rates, is very common with lung cancer. Over one-half of persons afflicted have metastasis at the time of diagnosis. The spread commonly occurs to the pleura, the mediastinum, the lymph nodes, the liver, bone, brain, and adrenal glands.

The clinical manifestations of carcinoma of the lung are difficult to classify. Most of those affected are asymptomatic for a long period or may develop signs of metastasis. The most common symptoms of the primary tumor are cough and expectoration of bloody sputum. Severe hemoptysis may occur. Lymph node enlargement may cause encroachment on the superior vena cava, obstruction, and dramatic signs and symptoms. Chest pain, dyspnea, and hoarseness may be present. X-ray evidence on a routine chest film is frequently the first sign, but by the time a lung tumor is radiologically evident it has usually invaded surrounding structures. Sputum cytology and bronchoscopy help to confirm the diagnosis.

RESPIRATORY FAILURE

Respiratory Insufficiency

Respiratory insufficiency is said to occur when the lungs are not able to exchange adequate amounts of carbon dioxide and oxygen to carry out the normal activities of daily living. In chronic respiratory insufficiency, there is a gradual adaptation of the body to the pulmonary dysfunction. This process of adaptation includes hyperventilation, use of accessory muscles to breathe, circulatory changes to adjust the oxygen delivery to vital organs, and renal compensation to maintain the blood pH [3]. In *acute respiratory insufficiency,* hypoxemia and hypercapnia become severe and the compensatory mechanisms instituted by the body do not adjust the oxygen and carbon dioxide levels sufficiently to supply the body's needs. Inadequate tissue oxygen and severe respiratory acidosis will occur without immediate treatment.

Respiratory Failure

Respiratory failure is the inability of the lungs to meet the basic demands for tissue oxygenation at rest. Respiratory failure can occur as a result of intrapulmonary disorders or nonpulmonary disorders as noted in Table 25-2. It can be seen that a wide variety of conditions can lead to this problem. Table 25-3 indicates that certain precipitating factors may cause the exacerbation of preexisting respiratory insufficiency.

TABLE 25-2. Important disorders leading to respiratory failure, classified according to major areas of involvement

- Intrinsic lung and airway diseases
  - Large airway obstruction
    - Congenital deformities
    - Acute laryngitis
    - Foreign bodies
    - Intrinsic tumors
    - Extrinsic pressure
    - Traumatic injury
    - Enlarged tonsils and adenoids
  - Bronchial diseases
    - Chronic bronchitis
    - Asthma
    - Acute bronchiolitis
  - Parenchymal diseases
    - Pulmonary emphysema
    - Pulmonary fibrosis of various causes
    - Pulmonary edema, cardiac
    - Severe pneumonia
    - Acute lung injury from various causes
  - Vascular disease
    - Massive or recurrent pulmonary embolism
- Extrapulmonary disorders
  - Diseases of pleura and chest wall
    - Pneumothorax
    - Pleural effusion
    - Fibrothorax
    - Thoracic wall deformity
    - Traumatic injury to the chest wall: flail chest
    - Obesity
  - Disorders of respiratory muscles and neuromuscular junction
    - Myasthenia gravis and myasthenialike disorders
    - Muscular dystrophies
    - Polymyositis
    - Botulism
    - Muscle-paralyzing drugs
    - Severe hypokalemia
  - Disorders of peripheral nerves and spinal cord
    - Poliomyelitis
    - Guillain-Barré syndrome
    - Spinal cord trauma (quadriplegia)
    - Amyotrophic lateral sclerosis
    - Tetanus
    - Multiple sclerosis
  - Disorders of central nervous system
    - Sedative and narcotic drug overdose
    - Head trauma
    - Cerebral hypoxia
    - Cerebrovascular accident
    - Central nervous system infection
    - Epileptic seizure: status epilepticus
    - Metabolic and endocrine disorders
    - Bulbar poliomyelitis
    - Primary alveolar hypoventilation

Source: S. Farzan, *A Concise Handbook of Respiratory Disease.* Reston, Va.: Reston Pub., 1978. Pp. 223–224.

TABLE 25-3. Precipitating or exacerbating factors of respiratory failure

- Changes of tracheobronchial secretions
- Infection: viral or bacterial
- Disturbance of tracheobronchial clearance
- Drugs: sedatives, narcotics, anesthesia, oxygen
- Inhalation or aspiration of irritants, vomitus, foreign body
- Cardiovascular disorders: heart failure, pulmonary embolism, shock
- Mechanical factors: pneumothorax, pleural effusion, abdominal distention
- Trauma, including surgery
- Neuromuscular abnormalities
- Allergic disorders: bronchospasm
- Increased oxygen demand: fever, infection

Source: S. Farzan, *A Concise Handbook of Respiratory Diseases.* Reston, Va.: Reston Pub., 1978. Pp. 224.

The criteria for diagnosing respiratory failure depend on the arterial blood gases. A PO_2 of less than 50 mm Hg, and a PCO_2 of greater than 50 mm Hg often are considered the parameters for determining respiratory failure. These are accepted guidelines for diagnosis and are related also to the patient's age, past history, and overall condition. The disorder may exist with hypoxemia as the predominant problem or with a combination of hypoxemia and hypercapnia.

As respiratory failure ensues, the PCO_2 begins to accumulate and leads to a significant respiratory acidosis indicating the inability of the lungs to eliminate the excess carbon dioxide. The normal chemoreceptors for carbon dioxide may become inoperative and the hypoxic stimulus may be the stimulus for the respiratory effort.

The clinical manifestations are dependent on the underlying cause but especially involve the resulting oxygen–carbon dioxide imbalance. Dyspnea may not occur if there is depression of the respiratory center, so that the respiratory rate may be very rapid or slow. Hypoxemia leads to inadequate tissue perfusion with varying degrees of cyanosis depending on how much right-to-left shunting is present. Hypercapnia refers to increased PCO_2 levels above 45 mm Hg. It indicates inadequate alveolar ventilation and the inability to release carbon dioxide. The symptoms, often associated with hypoxemia, include increased pulse and blood pressure, dizziness, headache, mental clouding and central nervous system depression, muscle twitching, and tremor.

Carbon dioxide narcosis, which occurs as the levels of carbon dioxide progressively increase, leads to loss of consciousness, dilation of cerebral blood vessels, increased blood flow to the brain, and constriction of the pulmonary vessels. Respiratory acidosis is frequent and may develop rapidly or slowly depending on renal compensation.

The prognosis with acute or chronic respiratory failure depends on the underlying causative mechanisms and whether improved lung function can occur. Respiratory failure is frequently the cause of death in many pulmonary conditions.

REFERENCES

1. Anderson, W. A. D., and Scotti, T. *Synopsis of Pathology* (10th ed.). St. Louis: Mosby, 1980.
2. Boyer, M. Treating invasive lung cancer. *Am. J. Nurs.* 77:1916, 1977.
3. Farzan, S. *A Concise Handbook of Respiratory Diseases.* Reston, Va.: Reston Pub., 1978.
4. Passey, R. Some problems of lung cancer. *Lancet* 2:107, 1962.
5. Robbins, S., and Cotran, R. *Pathologic Basis of Disease* (2nd ed.). Philadelphia: Saunders, 1979.
6. Sodeman, W., and Sodeman, T. *Pathologic Physiology* (6th ed.). Philadelphia: Saunders, 1979.

BIBLIOGRAPHY

Anderson, W. A. D., and Scotti, T. *Synopsis of Pathology* (10th ed.). St. Louis: Mosby, 1980.

Andrews, J. L., Jr. Physiology and treatment of hypoxia. *Clin. Notes Respir. Dis.* 13:3, 1974.

Andrews, J. L., Jr. Cor pulmonale: Pathophysiology and management. *Geriatrics* 31:91, 1976.

Andrews, J. L., Jr. The clinical roles of pulmonary function testing. *Med. Clin. North Am.* 63:355, 1979.

Antelman, N. Surface tension in the lung. *Point View* 13:10, 1976.

Asmundson, T., and Kilburn, K. Mechanisms of Respiratory Tract Clearance. In M. J. Dulfano (ed.), *Sputum: Fundamentals and Clinical Pathology.* Springfield, Ill.: Thomas, 1973.

Bohning, D., et al. Tracheobronchial particle deposition and clearance. *Arch. Environ. Health* 30:457, 1975.

Bouhuys, A. *Physiology, Environment and Lung Disease.* New York: Grune & Stratton, 1974.

Boyer, M. Treating invasive lung cancer. *Am. J. Nurs,* 77:1916, 1977.

Burrows, B., Knudson, R. J., and Kettel, L. J. *Respiratory Insufficiency.* Chicago: Year Book, 1975. P. 26.

Camner, P., et al. Human tracheobronchial clearance studies. *Arch. Environ. Health* 22:444, 1971.

Camner, P., Jarstand, C., and Philipson, K. Tracheobronchial clearance in patients with influenza. *Am. Rev. Respir. Dis.* 108:131, 1973.

Camner, P., Mossberg, B., and Afzeluis, B. Evidence for congenitally non-functioning cilia in the tracheobronchial tract of two subjects. *Am. Rev. Respir. Dis.* 112:807, 1975.

Cate, T. The role of nasal secretions and serum antibodies in the rhinovirus common cold. *Am. J. Epidemiol.* 84:352, 1966.

Cate, T. Interferons. In V. Knight (ed.), *Mycoplasmal Infections of the Respiratory Tract.* Philadelphia: Lea & Febiger, 1973.

Cherniack, R., Cherniack, L., and Naimark, A. *Respiration in Health and Disease* (2nd ed.). Philadelphia: Saunders, 1972.

Chodash, S. Examination of sputum cells. *N. Engl. J. Med.* 282:854, 1972.

Clements, J. A. Surface tension in the lung. *Sci. Am.* 207:120, 1962.

Cohen, A. B., and Gold, W. M. Defense mechanisms of the lung. *Annu. Rev. Physiol.* 37:325, 1975.

Comroe, J. *Physiology of Respiration* (2nd ed.). Chicago: Year Book, 1974.

Cunningham, J., Richardson, R., and Smith, J. Interstitial pulmonary edema. *Heart Lung* 6:617, 1977.

Davenport, H. W. *ABC of Acid-Base Chemistry: The Elements of Physiological Blood-Gas Chemistry for Medical Students and Physicians* (6th ed.). Chicago: University of Chicago Press, 1974.

Davies, C. N. A comparison between inhaled dust and the dust recovered from human lungs. *Health Phys.* 10:129, 1964.

Dowell, A. R., et al. Lung defense mechanisms: Their importance in respiratory care. *Respir. Care* 22:50, 1977.

Doyle, J. The intracaval filter: New nursing challenge. *RN* 5:39, 1980.

Drachler, D. H. Adult Respiratory Distress Syndrome. Phoenix, Ariz.: Speech at AACN Respiratory Care Symposium, 1976.

Dulfano, M. J. *Sputum Fundamentals and Clinical Pathology.* Springfield, Ill.: Thomas, 1973.

Dulfano, M. J., Adler, K., and Phillippoff, W. Sputum viscoelasticity in chronic bronchitis. *Am. Rev. Respir. Dis.* 104:88, 1971.

Ellis, E. F., and Farr, R. T. (eds.). *Essays in Medicine: A 70's Look at Asthma.* Morris Plains, N. J.: Medcom, 1972.

Ewertz, M., and Shpritz, D. Your best strategy when 'shock lung' strikes. *RN* 10:43, 1980.

Falk, G. A., Okinaka, A. J., and Siskind, G. W. Immunoglobulins in the bronchial washings of patients with chronic obstructive lung disease. *Am. Rev. Respir. Dis.* 105:14, 1972.

Farzan, S. *A Concise Handbook of Respiratory Diseases.* Reston, Va.: Reston Pub., 1978.

Fitzgerald, M., Carrington, C., and Gaensler, E. Environmental lung disease. *Med. Clin. North Am.* 57:593, 1973.

Gaensler, E. A., and Wright, G. W. Evaluation of respiratory impairment. *Arch. Environ. Health* 12:146, 1966.

Ganong, W. F. *Review of Medical Physiology* (8th ed.). Los Altos, Calif.: Lange, 1977.

Gilbert, E., and Huntington, R. *An Introduction to Pathology.* New York: Oxford University Press, 1978.

Goldstein, E., Lippert, W., and Warshauer, D. Pulmonary alveolar macrophages: Defender against bacterial infection in the lung. *J. Clin. Invest.* 54:519, 1974.

Gosselin, R. I. Physiological regulators of ciliary motion. *Am. Rev. Respir. Dis.* 93:41, 1966.

Green, G. Pulmonary clearance of infectious agents. *Annu. Rev. Med.* 19:315, 1968.

Green, G. The Amberson lecture: In defense of the lung. *Am. Rev. Respir. Dis.* 102:691, 1970.

Grossburg, S. E. The interferons and their inducers: Molecular and therapeutic considerations. *N. Engl. J. Med.* 287:122, 1972.

Guenter, C. A. The Respiratory Environment. In C. A. Guenter and M. H. Welch (eds.), *Pulmonary Medicine.* Philadelphia: Lippincott, 1977.

Guenter, C. A., Welch, M. H., and Hogg, J. C. *Clinical Aspects of Respiratory Physiology.* Philadelphia: Lippincott, 1978. P. 151.

Guyton, A. *Textbook of Medical Physiology* (6th ed.). Philadelphia: Saunders, 1981.

Hanson, R., and Dasik, J. The pneumoconioses. *Heart Lung* 6:646, 1977.

Hedley-Whyte, J., and Winter, P. M. Oxygen therapy. *Clin. Pharmacol. Ther.* 8:696, 1967.

Hilding, A. Ciliary streaming in the bronchial tree and the time element in carcinogenesis. *N. Engl. J. Med.* 256:634, 1957.

Hilding, A. Phagocytosis: Mucus flow and ciliary action. *Arch. Environ. Health* 6:61, 1963.

Hugh-Jones, P., and Whimster, W. The etiology and management of disabling emphysema. *Am. Rev. Respir. Dis.* 117:2, 1978.

Isacson, L. Treating pulmonary edema. *Nurs. 78* 8:42, 1978.

Isselbacher, K. J., et al. *Harrison's Principles of Internal Medicine* (9th ed.). New York: McGraw-Hill, 1980.

Jarstand, C., Camner, P., and Philipson, K. Mycoplasma pneumonia and tracheobronchial clearance. *Am. Rev. Respir. Dis.* 110:415, 1974.

Johansen, W., and Gould, K. Lung defense mechanisms. *Basics Respir. Dis.* 6:2, 1977.

Jones, R., and Weill, H. Occupational lung disease. *Basics Respir. Dis.* 6:3, 1978.

Juers, J., et al. Enhancement of bacteriocidal capacity of alveolar macrophages. *J. Clin. Invest.* 58:271, 1976.

Kass, E., Green, G., and Golstein, E. Mechanisms of antibacterial action in the respiratory system. *Bact. Rev.* 30:488, 1966.

Kealy, S. L. Respiratory care in Guillain-Barré syndrome. *Am. J. Nurs.* 1:59, 1977.

Keim, L., Schuldt, S., and Bedell, G. Tuberculosis in the intensive care unit. *Heart Lung* 6:624, 1977.

Kensler, C., and Battista, S. Chemical and physical factors affecting mammalian ciliary activity. *Am. Rev. Respir. Dis.* 92:102, 1966.

Kilburn, K. Functional morphology of the distal lung. *Int. Rev. Cytol.* 37:153, 1974.

Kueppers, F., and Black, L. F. Alpha$_1$-antitrypsin and its deficiency. *Am. Rev. Respir. Dis.* 110:178, 1974.

Laurenzi, G. The mucociliary stream. *J. Occup. Med.* 15:175, 1973.

Laurenzi, G., Yin, S., and Guarneri, J. Adverse effects of oxygen on tracheal mucus flow. *N. Engl. J. Med.* 279:333, 1968.

Lieberman, J. Alpha$_1$ antitrypsin deficiency. *Med. Clin. North Am.* 59:3, 1973.

Loudan, R., and Shaw, G. Mechanics of cough in normal subjects and patients with obstructive lung disease. *Am. Rev. Respir. Dis.* 96:666, 1967.

Luckmann, J., and Sorensen, K. *Medical-Surgical Nursing* (2nd ed.). Philadelphia: Saunders, 1980.

MacDonnell, K., and Segal, M. *Current Respiratory Care.* Boston: Little, Brown, 1977.

Matsuba, K., and Thrubeck, W. Disease of the small airways in bronchitis. *Am. Rev. Respir. Dis.* 107:552, 1973.

McKerrow, C. Silicosis and Coalworker's Pneumoconiosis. In D. Muir (ed.), *Clinical Aspects of Inhaled Particles.* Philadelphia: Davis, 1972.

McKerrow, C., et al. Respiratory function during the day in cotton workers: A study of byssinosis. *Br. J. Ind. Med.* 15:75, 1958.

Meador, B. Why COPD can end in heart failure. *RN* 5:64, 1980.

Miller, D., and Boudrant, S. Effects of cigarette smoke on the surface characteristic of lung extracts. *Am. Rev. Respir. Dis.* 85:692, 1962.

Morgan, T. Pulmonary surfactant. *N. Engl. J. Med.* 284:1185, 1972.

Morrow, P. Dynamics of Dust Removal from Lower Airways. In A. Bouhays (ed.), *Airway Dynamics.* Springfield, Ill.: Thomas, 1974.

Muir, D. *Clinical Aspects of Inhaled Particulates.* Philadelphia: Davis, 1972.

Nadel, J. Mechanisms of airway response to inhaled substances. *Arch. Environ. Health* 16:171, 1968.

Neff, T. A., and Petty, T. L. Long-term continuous oxygen therapy in chronic airway obstruction: Mortality in relationship to cor pulmonale, hypoxia and hypercapnia. *Ann. Intern. Med.* 72:621, 1970.

Newhouse, M., Sanchis, J., and Bienstack, J. Lung defense mechanisms. *N. Engl. J. Med.* 295:990, 1976.

Newhouse, M., et al. Mucociliary Clearance in Children with Cystic Fibrosis. In J. Mangos (ed.), *Fundamental Problems of Cystic Fibrosis and Related Diseases.* New York: Grune & Stratton, 1973.

Notkins, A. (ed.). *Viral Immunology and Immunopathology.* New York: Academic, 1975.

Nysather, J., Katz, A., and Lenth, J. The immune system: Its development and function. *Am. J. Nurs.* 76:1614, 1976.

Parsons, L. C. Respiratory changes in head injury. *Am. J. Nurs.* 71: 2188, 1971.

Passey, R. Some problems of lung cancer. *Lancet* 2:107, 1962.

Pattle, R., Schoch, C., and Battensby, J. Some effects of anesthesia on lung surfactant. *Br. J. Anaesth.* 99:1119, 1972.

Phipps, W., Long, B., and Woods, N. *Medical-Surgical Nursing.* St. Louis: Mosby, 1979.

Polk, B. V. Cardiopulmonary complications of Guillain-Barré syndrome. *Heart Lung* 5:96, 1976.

Purtillo, D. *A Survey of Human Diseases.* Reading, Mass.: Addison-Wesley, 1978.

Radford, E. P., Jr. The Physics of Gases. In W. O. Fenn and H. Rahn (eds.), *Handbook of Physiology: Respiration* (vol. 1). Washington, D. C.: American Physiological Society, 1964. P. 125.

Reichel, J. Pulmonary embolism. *Med. Clin. North Am.* 61:1310, 1977.

Rifas, E. How you and your patient can manage dyspnea. *Nurs. 80* 6:34, 1980.

Robbins, S., and Cotran, R. *Pathologic Basis of Disease* (2nd ed.). Philadelphia: Saunders, 1979.

Rodarte, J. R., and Hyatt, R. E. Respiratory mechanics. *Basics Respir. Dis.* 4:4, 1976.

Sade, J., et al. The role of mucus in transport by cilia. *Am. Rev. Respir. Dis.* 102:48, 1970.

Santa Cruz, R., et al. Tracheal mucus velocity in normal man and obstructive lung disease: Effects of terbuline. *Am. Rev. Respir. Dis.* 109:458, 1974.

Satir, P. How cilia move. *Sci. Am.* 231:44, 1974.

Sears, D., and Reed, A. ARDS: A true test of nursing skills. *Nurs. 80* 5:51, 1980.

Shapiro, B. A. *Clinical Application of Blood Gases.* Chicago: Year Book, 1973. P. 42.

Shapiro, B. A. Intracranial Pressure Monitoring. Tulsa, Okla.: Speech at Perspectives in Critical Care, 1979.

Shapiro, B. A., Harrison, R. A., and Trout, C. A. *Clinical Application of Respiratory Care.* Chicago: Year Book, 1975. P. 61.

Shrake, K. The ABCs of ABGs. *Nurs. 79* 9:26, 1979.

Slonim, N. B., and Hamilton, L. H. *Respiratory Physiology* (3rd ed.). St. Louis: Mosby, 1976. P. 55.

Smith, C., et al. Protective effect of interferon to parainfluenza type I virus. *N. Engl. J. Med.* 275:1145, 1966.

Sodeman, W., and Sodeman, T. *Pathologic Physiology* (6th ed.). Philadelphia: Saunders, 1979.

Stephens, G. *Pathophysiology for Health Practitioners.* New York: Macmillan, 1980.

Surveyer, J. Smoke inhalation injuries. *Heart Lung* 9:825, 1980.

Sweetwood, H. Cardiac tamponade. *RN* 10:35, 1980.

Thomson, M., and Pavia, D. Long term tobacco smoking and mucociliary clearance. *Arch. Environ. Health* 26:36, 1973.

Tisi, G., and Brauwald, E. Cough and Hemopytosis. In M. Wintrobe (ed.), *Principles of Internal Medicine* (7th ed.). New York: McGraw-Hill, 1974.

Tomasi, T., and Grey, H. Structure and function of immunoglobulins. *Prog. Allergy* 16:31, 1972.

Trout, C. A., et al. Perspectives in Critical Care. Unpublished data.

Wade, J. F. *Respiratory Nursing Care* (2nd ed.). St. Louis: Mosby, 1977.

Walter, J. *An Introduction to the Principles of Disease* (2nd ed.). Philadelphia: Saunders, 1983.

Wanner, A., et al. Tracheal mucus flow in beagles after chronic exposure to cigarette smoke. *Arch. Environ. Health* 27:370, 1973.

Wayne, K. S. Adult Respiratory Distress Syndrome in the Adult. University of Arizona at Tucson, 1975. Unpublished.

Weiss, E. B. Bronchial asthma. *Ciba Clin. Symp.* 27:1, 1975.

West, J. B. *Ventilation: Blood Flow and Gas Exchange* (3rd ed.). Oxford, England: Blackwell, 1977. P. 4.

West, J. G. *Respiratory Physiology: The Essentials.* Baltimore: Williams & Wilkins, 1974. Pp. 2–6.

West, J. G. *Pulmonary Pathophysiology: The Essentials.* Baltimore: Williams & Wilkins, 1977.

Wood, R., Wanner, A., and Hirsch, J. Tracheal mucociliary transport in patients with cystic fibrosis and its stimulation effect by terbutylene. *Am. Rev. Respir. Dis.* 111:633, 1975.

Ziskind, M. Occupational pulmonary disease. *Clin. Symp.* 30:4, 1978.

UNIT 10
URINARY EXCRETION

Cammie Quinn
NORMAL URINARY FUNCTION
OBSTRUCTION OF GENITOURINARY TRACT
RENAL FAILURE

Barbara L. Bullock
IMMUNOLOGIC, INFECTIOUS, AND TOXIC ALTERATIONS IN URINARY FUNCTION

The urinary system functions to maintain the concentration of electrolytes and water in the blood. Chapter 26 explains normal renal function and provides a basis for the subsequent chapters concerning different forms of renal pathology. Chapter 27 details the varied immunologic, infectious, and toxic alterations that can affect renal function. Chapter 28 describes the common causes of genitourinary obstruction with special emphasis on the formation of different types of calculi. Benign prostatic hypertrophy and renal tumors are included. Chapter 29 describes renal failure, its causes, and clinical course.

The reader is encouraged to utilize the learning objectives to provide a systematic method for study. The extensive bibliography provides a current and historical perspective on theories of renal function and dysfunction.

CHAPTER 26
NORMAL RENAL AND URINARY EXCRETORY FUNCTION

ANATOMY OF THE KIDNEYS

Macroscopic Anatomy of the Kidneys

Microscopic Anatomy: The Nephron

Blood Supply to the Kidneys

Innervation of the Kidney

PHYSIOLOGY OF THE KIDNEY

Glomerular Filtration

Resorption: Tubules

Proximal Convoluted Tubules

Active Transport

Passive Transport

Loop of Henle

Counter-Current Multiplier Effect

Counter-Current Exchanger

Distal Convoluted Tubules and Collecting Tubules

Sodium and Potassium Resorption

Water Resorption

Secretion: Tubules and Collecting Ducts

Substances That are Secreted

PAH

Hydrogen Ions

Potassium

ACCESSORY URINARY STRUCTURES AND BLADDER

Ureters

Bladder

Micturation Reflex of the Bladder

Urethra

LEARNING OBJECTIVES

1. Identify the location and size of the kidneys.
2. Describe the external structure of the kidneys.
3. Explain the major portions of the internal structure of the kidneys, including the cortex, medulla, and renal pelvis.
4. Identify Bowman's capsule and the glomerulus.
5. List the main layers of the glomerular membrane, including the epithelial, glomerular basement membrane, and endothelial layer.
6. List the parts of the proximal convoluted tubules, loop of Henle, and the distal convoluted tubules.
7. Describe the renal corpuscles and juxtaglomerular apparatus.
8. Identify the collecting tubules, ducts, and papillary duct.
9. Describe the interstitium of the kidneys.
10. Describe the blood supply to the kidneys.
11. Explain the innervation of the kidneys.
12. Explain autoregulation of the kidneys.
13. Describe, in detail, the mechanisms responsible for urine formation, including glomerular filtration, tubular resorption, and secretion.
14. Define *filtration, filtrate, tubular resorption, transport maximum,* and *secretion.*
15. Describe the pressures that are responsible for filtration.
16. Calculate the effective net filtration pressure.
17. Describe active transport of glucose ions and protein from the proximal convoluted tubules.
18. Explain the passive transport of water and ions from the proximal convoluted tubules.
19. Describe hypotonic and hypertonic urine formation and explain the countercurrent mechanisms in the loop of Henle and collecting duct.
20. Explain renal regulation of the renin-angiotensin-aldosterone system.
21. Discuss the antidiuretic hormone and its relation to water regulation in the distal convoluted tubules and collecting tubules.
22. Discuss the secretion of PAH and potassium.
23. Explain the secretion of hydrogen ions and its relation to acid-base balance.
24. Describe the structure of the ureter and the purpose of this special structure.
25. List the layers of the bladder.
26. Explain the micturation reflex.
27. Differentiate between the female and male urethras.
28. Explain the physical characteristics of urine.

In order for the body to maintain a steady state the renal system must function normally. The renal system not only has important roles in removing waste products from the blood, but it also maintains sufficient amounts of electrolytes in the blood. Urine production occurs in the kidneys and urine is transported to the ureters, which empty into the bladder. Excretion of urine from the body occurs through the urethra.

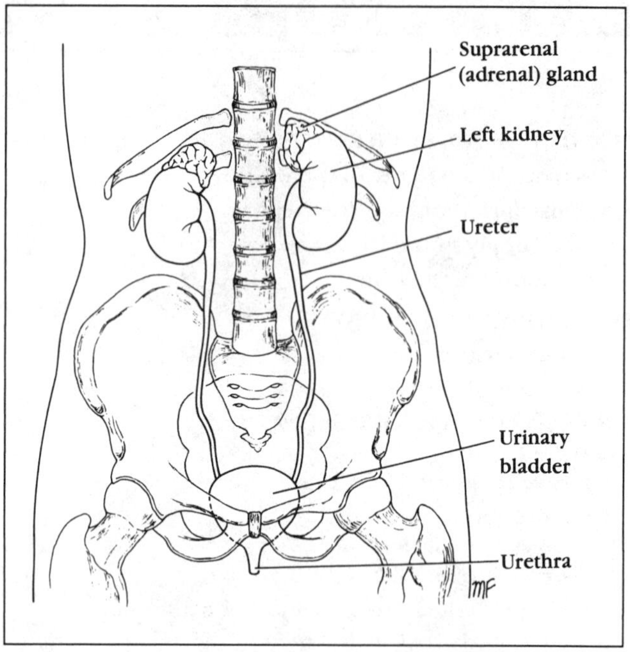

FIGURE 26-1. Posterior abdominal wall, showing kidneys and ureters in situ. *Arrows* indicate three sites where ureter is narrowed. (From R. Snell, *Clinical Histology for Medical Students.* Boston: Little, Brown, 1984.)

ANATOMY OF THE KIDNEYS

Macroscopic Anatomy of the Kidneys

The kidneys are bean-shaped organs, reddish-brown in color, and are located retroperitoneally on either side of the vertebral column extending from the twelfth thoracic vertebra to the third lumbar vertebra. Each kidney is approximately 11.0 cm in length, 5.0 to 7.0 cm in diameter, and 2.5 cm in thickness. The right kidney is slightly lower than the left, because the liver is located above it (Fig. 26-1).

Surrounding the kidneys is a layer of adipose tissue or perirenal fat that aids in protection and support. A fibrous layer of connective tissue called *renal fasciae* encapsulates and anchors the kidneys in place in the abdomen.

Located externally at the concave portion of the kidney is a notch called the *hilus*. The hilus is located in the *renal sinus*, which is a C-shaped cavity in the kidney. Entering the hilus of each kidney are the renal artery and vein, lymphatics, nerves, and the renal pelvis (Fig. 26-2).

The kidneys internally are basically composed of the *cortex* and the *medulla*. The cortex, the outer portion of the kidney, lies under the renal fasciae and is composed of renal columns called *columns of Bertin*. Also originating in the cortex and extending into the medulla are the *uriniferous tubules*, which are made up of the functioning units of the kidneys, the *nephrons*.

The medulla, the inner portion of the kidney, contains an estimated 8 to 18 *renal pyramids*. These are designated "renal pyramids" because they are triangular in shape and striated in appearance due to the collecting ducts, nephrons, and blood vessels of which they are composed. The apex of each pyramid is called the *papilla*.

Below the papillae is a large cavity called the *renal pelvis,* which is interrupted by cuplike extensions called the *minor* and *major calices*. These structures are lined with transitional epithelium. The minor calices, approximately 10 in number, have openings that collect urine from the *collecting ducts* of the pyramids, empty urine into the major calices, approximately three in number, and thus into the renal pelvis where the urine is excreted from the kidney to the ureter (see Fig. 26-2).

Microscopic Anatomy: the Nephron

It is estimated that a pair of kidneys contain 2.5 million nephrons. The nephron is a unique but complex structure; it is composed of Bowman's capsule, the proximal convoluted tubule, the loop of Henle, and the distal convoluted tubule. Many distal tubules empty into one collecting duct.

Bowman's capsule is a cuplike structure that surrounds a capillary network called the *glomerulus;* the two together are called the *renal malpighian corpuscle*. The membrane of the glomerular capillaries is composed of three main layers: *epithelial, glomerular basement membrane (GBM),* and *endothelial* [3]. The main function of the glomerular membrane is the formation of glomerular filtrate or a protein-free solution, which is the initial step in urine formation (Fig. 26-3).

Nephrons are classified as either cortical or juxtamedullary. The glomeruli of the cortical nephrons are found in the outer two-thirds of the cortex. The remaining one-third of the cortical area consists of glomeruli of the juxtamedullary nephrons, which contain a long loop of Henle that extends deep into the medulla (Fig. 26-4) [6].

Lining the inner layer of Bowman's capsule, adjacent to the glomerulus, is a thin layer of *epithelial cells* called *podocytes.* These podocytes have projections called *pedicles* which cover the GBM. Between the pedicles are *slit pores* through which proteins with a molecular weight of less than 50,000 can pass [1]. Since the molecular weight of the plasma proteins is slightly higher, they cannot cross the membrane. Because of the location, numbers, and arrangement of slit pores, there is a large surface area that allows for rapid filtration of fluid and the smaller proteins.

Adjacent to the layer of epithelial cells is the GBM, which consists of a meshwork of fibrillae containing mucopolysaccharides. This meshwork acts to prevent passage of

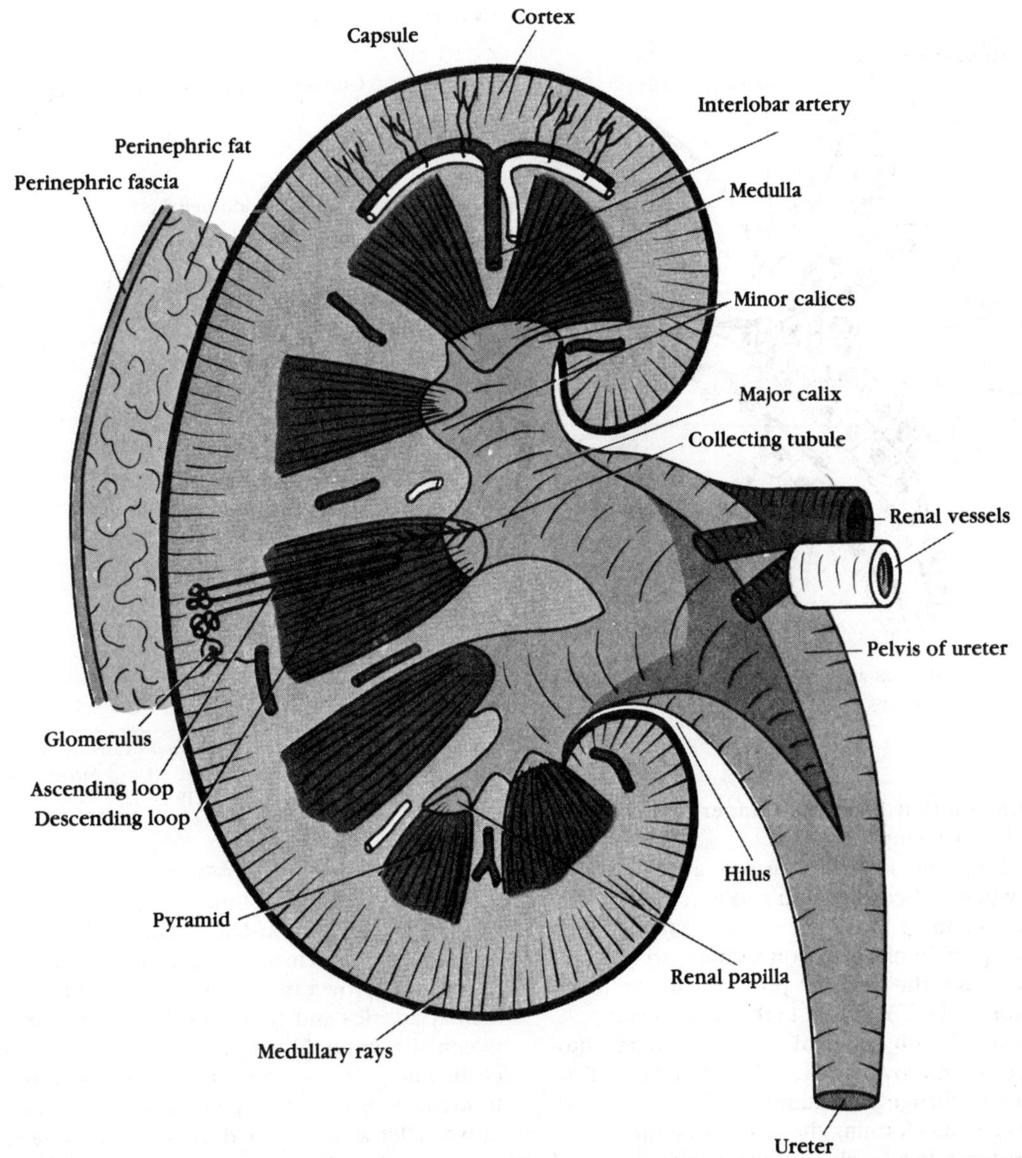

FIGURE 26-2. Longitudinal section through kidney, showing cortex, medulla, pyramids, renal papillae, and calices. Note position of nephron and arrangement of blood vessels within kidney. Note also perinephric fasciae and fat and their relation to renal capsule. (From R. Snell, *Clinical Anatomy for Medical Students* [2nd ed.]. Boston: Little, Brown, 1981.)

large proteins and molecules into Bowman's capsule. The effects of renal disease on the GBM are discussed in Chapters 27 and 29.

The inner layer of the glomerular capillary is composed of *endothelial cells.* This layer consists of thousands of pores or fenestrations that aid in membrane permeability.

Once the glomerular filtrate passes through the glomeruli into Bowman's capsule, it enters the *proximal convoluted tubule* (PCT), which is located in the cortex and is approximately 14 mm in length. Cuboidal epithelial cells line the PCT. On the luminal surface of these cells is a brush border of microvilli that increase the surface area available for secretion and absorption of fluids and solutes. Also located in the PCT cells are mitochondria. The initial portion of the PCT is the *pars convoluta,* which entangles the glomerulus. Leaving the pars convoluta is a straight portion of the PCT called the *pars recta.* More than 65 to 80 percent of the glomerular filtrate is resorbed in the PCT and the remaining 20 to 35 percent proceeds to the loop of Henle.

There are two major portions of the loop of Henle, the *descending limb* and the *ascending limb* (see Fig. 26-4). The thickened descending limb begins in the cortex; as it

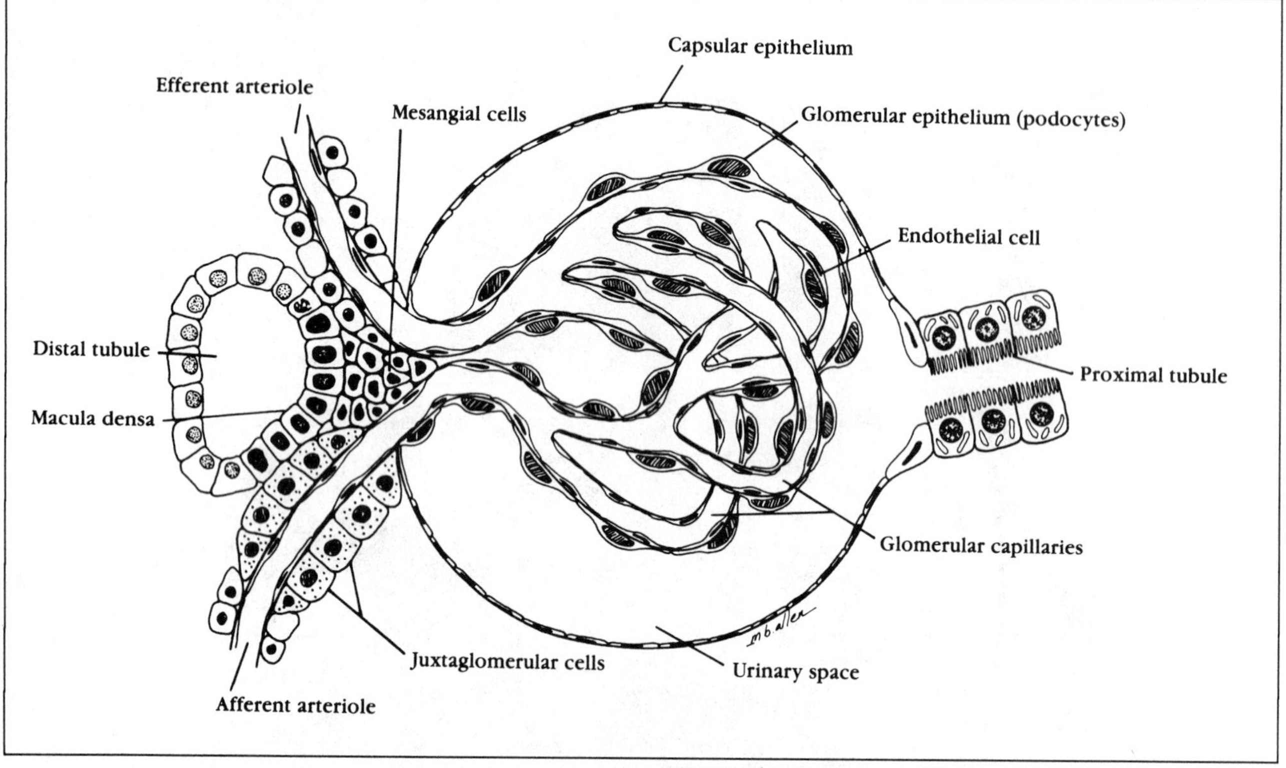

FIGURE 26-3. Appearance of Bowman's capsule with the glomerulus within. (From M. Borysenko, et al., *Functional Histology* [2nd ed.]. Boston: Little, Brown, 1984.)

dips into the medulla it becomes thinner and varies in length from 4.5 to 10.0 mm [2].

The descending limb loops and makes a tight hairpin turn upward, where it becomes thin and is called the thin portion of the ascending limb. The main function of both limbs of the loop of Henle is to concentrate urine. Once urine passes through the limbs, it proceeds to the *distal convoluted tubule* (DCT) located in the renal cortex.

The DCT is lined with cuboidal cells containing mitochondria and fewer microvilli than are found in the PCT. As the cuboidal cells change to columnar cells the area becomes very dense, thus forming the *macula densa*.

The macula densa lies in close contact with the renal corpuscle at the vascular pole or afferent arteriole and forms part of the *juxtaglomerular apparatus* (Fig. 26-5). Located within the apparatus are juxtaglomerular cells that produce an enzyme, *renin*, which functions to transform angiotensinogen to angiotensin I (see p. 362).

The main function of the DCT is to transport electrolytes and water. Two or more DCTs join together to form the *collecting duct*, which conducts the formed urine. The collecting ducts are lined with cuboidal cells, contain few mitochondria, and are located in the renal medulla.

Urine is then transported from the duct to a *papillary duct (of Bellini)*, which opens into the minor calix. Urine is excreted from the minor and major calices into the *renal pelvis, ureters, bladder*, and *urethra*.

Blood Supply to the Kidneys

In a resting state, it is estimated, the kidneys receive 20 to 25 percent of the cardiac output, which is more than 1000 ml/minute. Thus, via the *aorta*, blood enters the hilus of the kidney by a *renal artery*, which branches into segmental arteries and then *interlobar arteries* running between the pyramids of the medulla (Fig. 26-6). At the corticomedullary junction the interlobar arteries convert to *arcuate arteries* that penetrate the cortex and branch into smaller arteries called *interlobular arteries*, thus giving rise to the *afferent arterioles (vas afferens glomeruli)*. The afferent arterioles subdivide into a tuft of capillaries called a *glomerulus*. Blood leaves the glomerulus by the *efferent arteriole (vas efferens glomeruli)* and forms a second network of capillaries called the *peritubular capillary network* that mainly encircles the convoluted tubules (proximal and distal). The special arrangement of capillaries between the arterioles is unique because it allows a higher pressure to be maintained in the glomerulus. Also, the efferent arterioles are smaller in diameter than the afferent arterioles, again causing a higher glomerular pressure due to increased vascular resistance.

The deeper-lying glomeruli or juxtamedullary glomeruli also break up into the peritubular network but have a set of capillaries penetrating the medulla. These thin-walled ves-

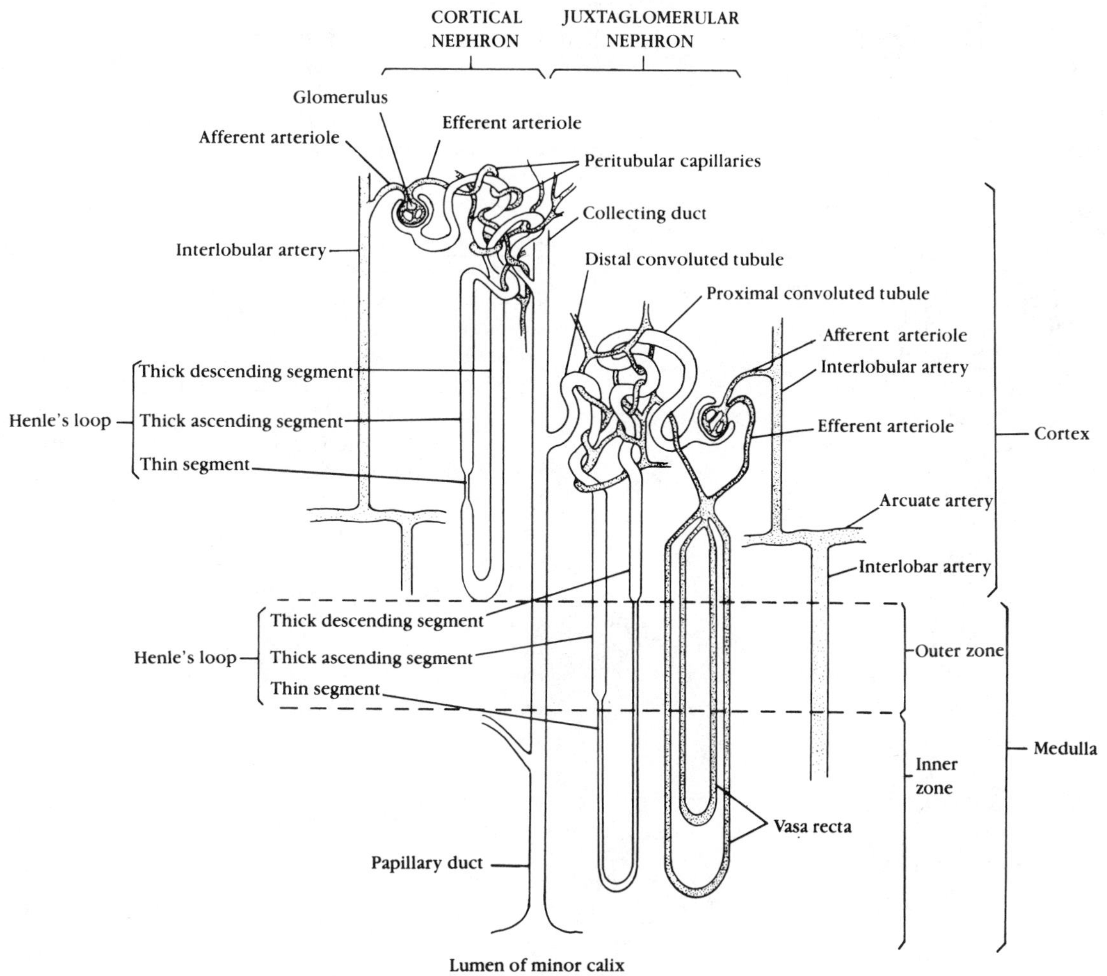

FIGURE 26-4. Structure of cortical and medullary nephrons. Blood supply to the nephron. The vasa recta is shown schematically; this capillary structure normally surrounds Henle's loop. (From M. Borysenko, et al., *Functional Histology* [2nd ed.]. Boston: Little, Brown, 1984.)

sels are in close proximity to the thin ascending and descending loops of Henle and are referred to as the *vasa recta*. The vasa recta aid in the concentration of urine.

The *interlobular veins* are formed from the peritubular capillary network and empty into the *arcuate veins*, into the *interlobar veins*, and converge to form the *renal vein*. Blood from the renal vein leaves the kidney and drains into the *inferior vena cava*.

Innervation of the Kidney

The kidney is innervated mostly by the sympathetic division of the autonomic nervous system. The nerve supply generally follows the distribution of the arterial vessels in the renal parenchyma. The nerve supply to the kidney comes mostly from the celiac plexus and the mesenteric, the upper splanchnic, and the thoracic nerves [5]. The sympathetic nerves, when stimulated, constrict the afferent arteriole and cause an increase in the blood pressure. There has been little research noting the effects of the parasympathetic system on the kidney.

PHYSIOLOGY OF THE KIDNEY

The kidney functions to maintain a constant plasma concentration of nonelectrolytes and water, to maintain the appropriate electrolytes and acid-base balance, and to regulate blood pressure. If the kidneys fail to maintain these steady states and if there are no interventions to relieve this noncompliance, death will result. The composition of urine results from three major mechanisms: glomerular filtration, tubular resorption, and tubular secretion.

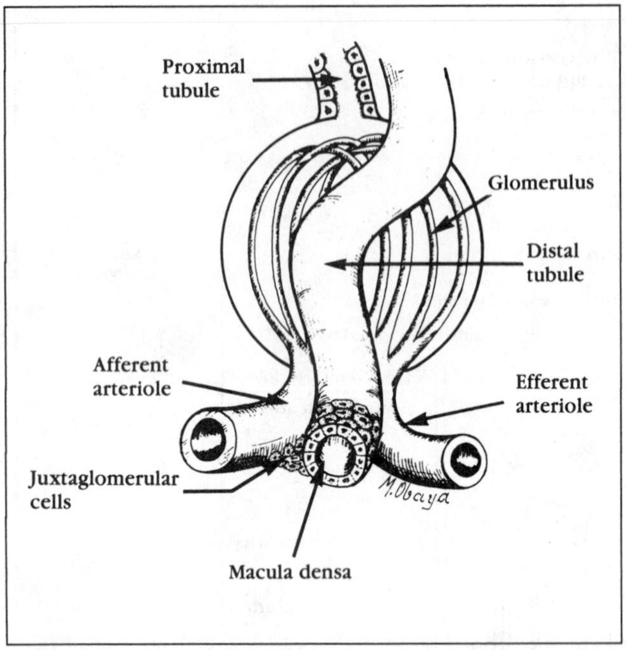

FIGURE 26-5. The relationship of the juxtaglomerular apparatus with the distal convoluted tubule of the nephron. (From S. Papper, *Clinical Nephrology* [2nd ed.]. Boston: Little, Brown, 1978.)

Glomerular Filtration

Filtration, the initial step in urine formation, is the result of pressures that force fluids and solutes through a membrane. The filtration process occurs between the layers of the glomerulus and Bowman's capsule. The fluid resulting from this process is *glomerular filtrate*, a relatively protein-free solution.

Approximately 125 ml/minute or 180 liters/day of glomerular filtrate is produced. Normally, urine output equals approximately 1 to 2 liters/day, which means that the tubules are responsible for resorbing the other 179 liters/day. The measurement of the large quantity of glomerular filtrate each minute is called the *glomerular filtration rate (GFR)*.

The quantity of filtrate and the filtration process are dependent on multiple factors, including the anatomy of the renal corpuscle and the diameter of the arterioles. Various pressures contribute to the outward flow of filtrate into Bowman's capsule and the retention of fluid within the glomerulus. The *hydrostatic pressure* is a simple outward force created by the systemic blood pressure. The *colloid osmotic pressure* is the inward force or pressure that holds fluid within the glomerulus. Figure 26-7 schematically illustrates the relationship of the hydrostatic pressure and the colloid osmotic pressure (see Chap. 5 for further discussion of colloid osmotic pressure).

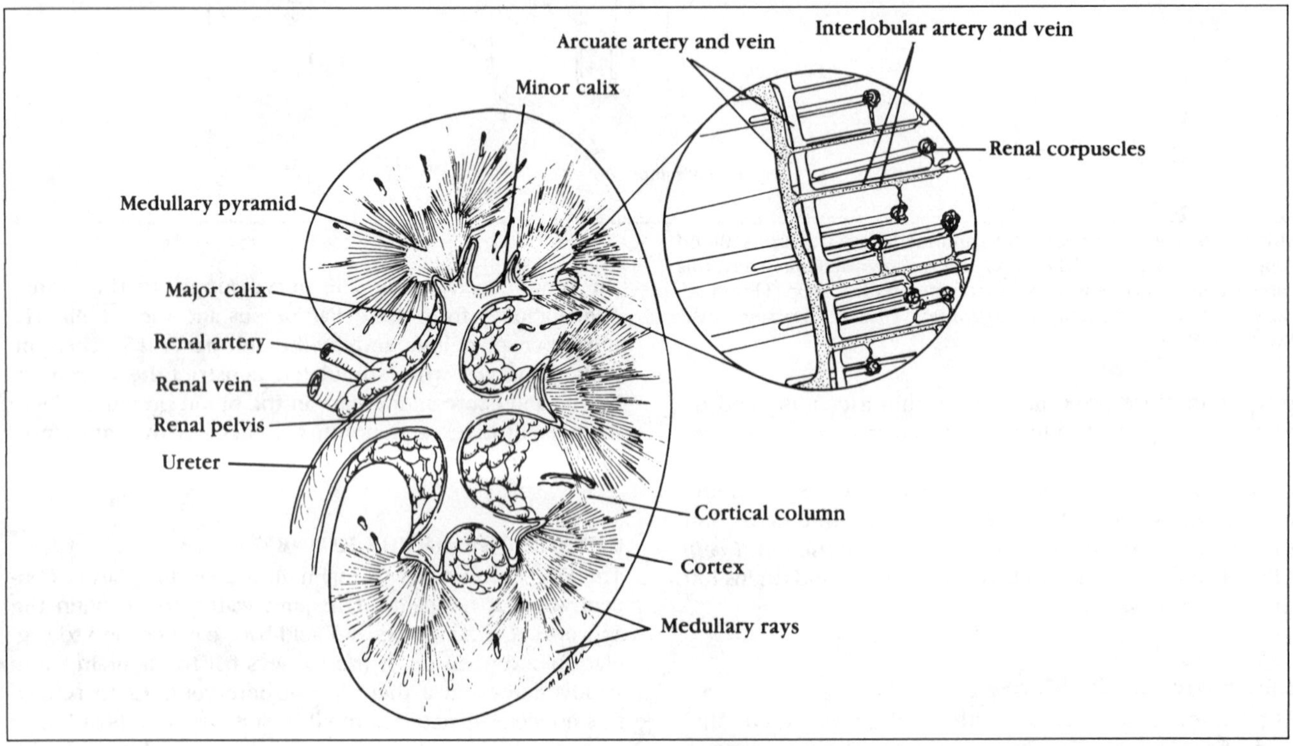

FIGURE 26-6. Hemisected kidney with vascular distribution. (From M. Borysenko, *Functional Histology* [2nd ed.]. Boston: Little, Brown, 1984.)

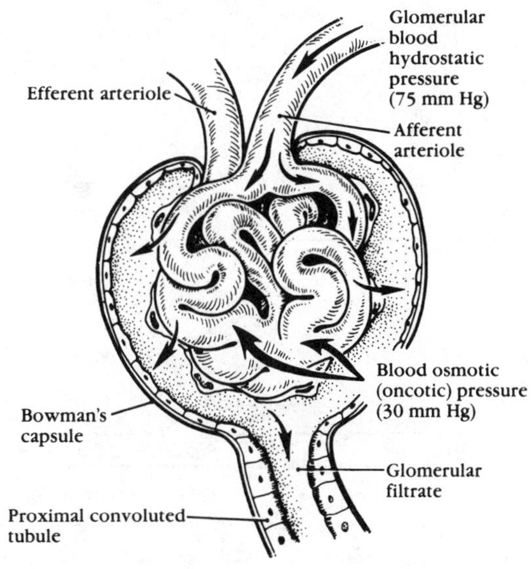

FIGURE 26-7. A schematic representation of the relationship between the hydrostatic pressure and the colloid osmotic pressure.

The pressure that is chiefly responsible for filtration is the *glomerular hydrostatic pressure (GHP).* This pressure forces filtrate out of the glomerulus into Bowman's capsule and normally is approximately 75 mm Hg. It is important to realize that if the GHP decreases to 50 mm Hg, filtration usually will not take place.

Working in opposition to the GHP is the *capsular hydrostatic pressure* within Bowman's capsule, which is normally measured at 20 mm Hg. This pressure is exerted by the walls of Bowman's capsule and the fluid in the renal tubule. Increased capsular pressure causes the GFR to decrease [6].

The other pressure that works in opposition to the GHP is the *blood colloidal osmotic pressure (COP),* normally measured at 30 mm Hg. Since blood contains more protein than filtrate does, the colloidal property constantly exerts an inward force.

The net result of all these pressures — GHP, capsular, and colloidal osmotic — is the *effective filtration pressure (Peff).* To calculate Peff, the following formula can be used:

Peff = GHP −

(capsular pressure + blood colloid osmotic pressure)

For example, if the GHP is 70 mm Hg, the capsular pressure is 28, and the colloid osmotic pressure is 32, then the Peff will be 10 mm Hg (70 − [28 + 32] = 10). If 1 mm Hg effective filtration pressure produces a GFR of 12.5 ml/minute from both kidneys, then 10 mm Hg produces 125 ml/minute, which is a normal rate.

Sympathetic nervous system (SNS) stimulation results in vasoconstriction of the afferent and efferent arterioles, which affects the Peff. Since there is usually greater constriction of the afferent arterioles than the efferent arterioles with sympathetic stimulation, a decrease in the GHP results.

Resorption: Tubules

As described in the previous section, approximately 179 liters of filtrate of the 180 liters filtered per day are resorbed in the tubules. The kidney has the ability to change the composition of urine by excreting different concentrations of substances [3]. This is achieved by resorption and secretion of different substances. For example, when a person ingests a large volume of water, the resulting urine is very dilute; in a dehydrated state the urine output is markedly decreased and the urine becomes very concentrated. *Tubular resorption,* the second step of urine formation, requires movement of solutes between the filtrate and blood of the surrounding vasa recta and peritubular capillaries.

Proximal Convoluted Tubules

In the *proximal convoluted tubules* (PCT), tubular resorption is accomplished by active and passive transport (diffusion or osmosis). Usually the positive ions are transported through the tubules by active transport and negative ions move by passive transport as a result of the electrical differences on the tubular membrane [3].

ACTIVE TRANSPORT. Active transport, the movement of molecules against a concentration gradient requiring an expenditure of energy, causes movement of substances out of the PCT into the plasma. The PCT is able to carry on active transport because of its epithelial cells that contain mitochondria. These cells also have a brush border that increases the surface area for resorption and secretion. Some of the substances that are moved actively include glucose, many electrolytes, amino acids, proteins, and vitamins (Fig. 26-8).

Glucose is actively transported from the tubules into the plasma and normally no glucose appears in the urine. This transport is related to a mechanism called *transport maximum (TM)* in which there is a maximum amount of substance that can be resorbed at any time [4]. If the plasma glucose level exceeds approximately 175 mg/dl, glucose appears in the urine (glycosuria) because the transport mechanism has become saturated with glucose and must return it to the tubules where it is excreted in the urine.

Sodium and *potassium* are actively transported from the tubules into the plasma of the peritubular capillaries by way of the basal channels of the epithelial cells. Since sodium and potassium are positive ions, they set up an electronegative cytoplasm in the epithelial cells; this allows the negative ions to follow the positive ions by passive transport.

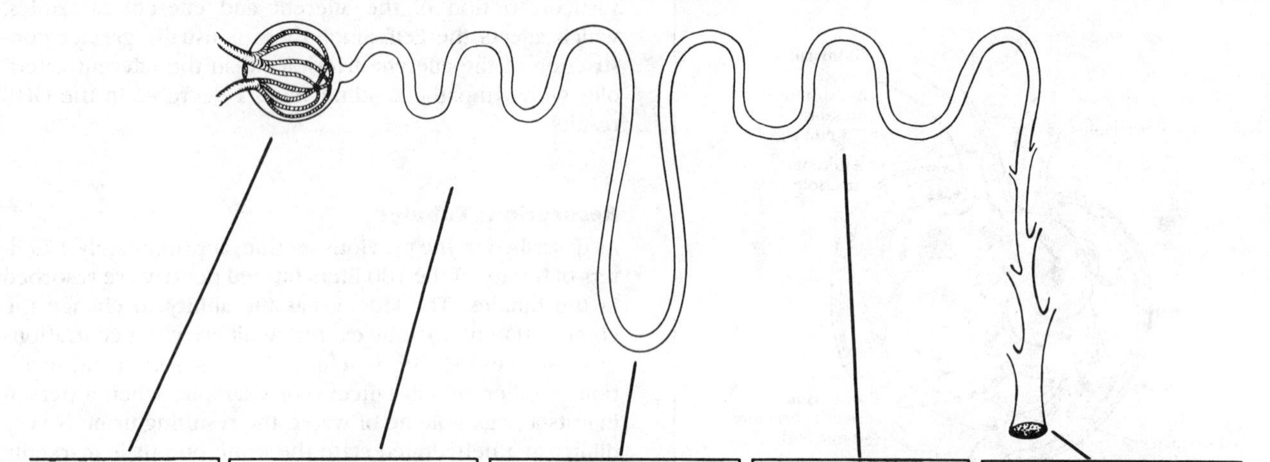

Glomerulus	Proximal tubule	Loop of Henle	Distal tubule	Collecting duct
Filtration	65% Na^+ and H_2O reabsorbed ADH not required All glucose, K^+, urate reabsorbed HCO_3^- reabsorbed H^+ secreted Fluid leaves isotonic	Na^+ transport from ascending limb Countercurrent establishes hypertonic interstitium Fluid leaves hypotonic	Na^+ reabsorbed ADH required for H_2O reabsorption K^+ and urate secreted HCO_3^- reabsorbed H^+ secreted NH_3^+ secreted Leaves hypotonic or isotonic	Water reabsorbed in final concentrating operation ADH required

FIGURE 26-8. Major functions of each portion of the nephron. (From S. Papper, *Clinical Nephrology* [2nd ed.]. Boston: Little, Brown, 1978.)

Proteins are resorbed in the PCT through the process of *pinocytosis*. The proteins attach to the membrane of the brush border of the PCT, are ingested by the tubular cells, and are broken down into amino acids, which are transported into the plasma. If there is increased permeability of the glomerular membrane, large amounts of protein can leak into the filtrate, causing proteinuria.

PASSIVE TRANSPORT. Passive transport, including osmosis and diffusion, involves the movement of substances across a membrane without the expenditure of energy. This transport is accomplished by the established electrical gradient of positive ions, mainly sodium, allowing negative ions and water to diffuse across the tubular membrane.

The removal of *water* from the tubules occurs as the result of the *isosmotic process*, which maintains equal osmotic pressures of fluid inside the tubule and in the plasma. When the solutes are actively resorbed into the plasma, there is a decrease in the concentration of solute in the tubule and an increased concentration in the peritubular capillaries, causing water to move into the peritubular capillary. As much as 65 to 90 percent of water is resorbed by passive transport in the PCT. The role of the kidney in the control of osmolality of the plasma through the transport of water is critical in the maintenance of fluid balance. The excretion of excess water or conservation of water functions to maintain the plasma osmolarity or specific gravity at a fixed 1.010. This regulation is greatly influenced by the antidiuretic hormone (ADH) in the distal convoluted and collecting tubule (see p. 362).

Chloride and *bicarbonate* diffuse across the tubular membrane into the peritubular capillaries by way of the isosmotic process. In the PCT their diffusion occurs because of an electrochemical gradient created by positive ions.

Loop of Henle

The main function of the loop of Henle is to concentrate urine. Hypotonic (dilute) urine is formed by resorption of solutes, leaving water in the water-impermeable ascending loop. In order for the loop of Henle to concentrate or form a hypertonic urine, the *countercurrent mechanism* is utilized.

For this mechanism to be accomplished, there are specific requirements that must be fulfilled: (1) a unique anatomic arrangement of the loops of Henle and the vasa recta (a capillary blood supply), and (2) the inward and outward flows of the countercurrent system. The special anatomic

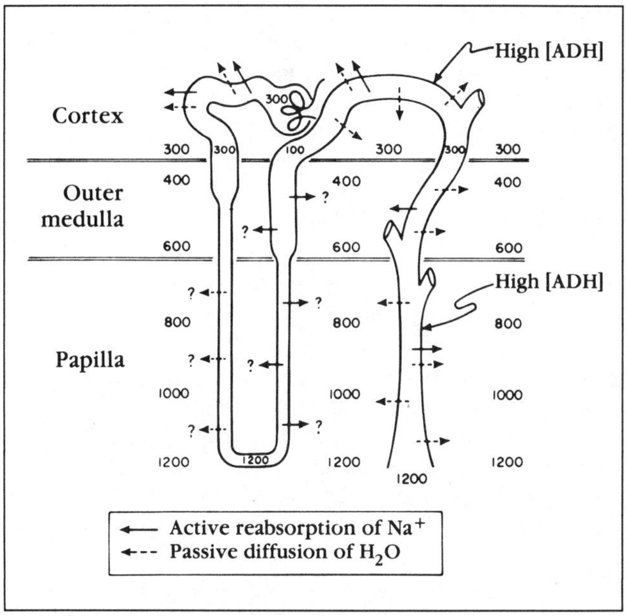

FIGURE 26-9. Operation of the countercurrent mechanism in a normal human during antidiuresis. The numbers refer to the osmolality (mOsm/kg H_2O) of either intratubular or interstitial fluid. Solid arrows denote active resorption of Na^+ (its accompanying anions, mainly Cl^-, being resorbed passively); arrows with a dashed line denote passive resorption of water. The question marks in the loops of Henle indicate that it is not yet known: (1) how much H_2O is resorbed from descending limbs; (2) whether solute transport out of thin ascending limbs is active or passive; and (3) whether Na^+ or Cl^- is actively resorbed from thick ascending limbs. The number of arrows in each nephron segment signifies semiquantitatively the amounts of solute transported relative to water. For example, in ascending limbs of Henle, solute is resorbed to the virtual but not complete exclusion of water, since renal membranes are not absolutely impervious to water. (From H. Valtin, *Renal Function: Mechanisms Preserving Fluid and Solute Balance in Health* [2nd ed.]. Boston: Little, Brown, 1983.)

arrangement of the loop of Henle places the limbs in close proximity not only to themselves, but also to the vasa recta. The limbs go in opposite (descending and ascending) directions. The loops of Henle in 20 to 30 percent of the nephrons extend into the medulla of the kidney and are surrounded by the vasa recta. The resorption through the vessels of the vasa recta is partly responsible for the operation of the concentrating mechanism for urine.

COUNTERCURRENT MULTIPLIER EFFECT. As fluid progresses down the descending limb of the loop of Henle, there can be high concentrations of solute at the loop. The excretion of excess solutes (concentrated urine) requires a hyperosmolality of the medullary interstitial fluid. This hyperosmolality is greater in the long segments of the loop of Henle and may increase to 1200 mOsm/liter at the turn of the loop. Sodium and chloride are transported from the thin segment (descending and loop portion) into the medullary interstitium. Current research indicates that this movement occurs when the interstitial concentration of urea is high, causing osmosis of water into the interstitial area. The sodium and chloride concentration then becomes increased in the thin segment and these ions probably diffuse passively out of this area and into the interstitium [3]. The high concentration of interstitial urea results from increased ADH concentrations. As ADH increases the permeability of the collecting duct to water, it also increases its permeability to urea (see also p. 362). Some sodium is actively transported out of the collecting duct, which is followed by passive chloride movement and this process may also further increase the osmolality of the interstitial fluid. Most of this sodium transport is under the influence of aldosterone.

As sodium, chloride, potassium, and water move up the ascending limb (thick portion), chloride now is actively transported while sodium and other positive ions follow passively [3]. Water is not removed because the ascending limb is impermeable to water. Because this process continuously concentrates the filtrate with sodium chloride in the section of the loop of Henle that is located in the medulla, it is called the *countercurrent multiplier.* As the fluid moves up the ascending loop, the sodium moves out and the filtrate becomes more dilute. As the filtrate passes to the distal and collecting tubules, water is resorbed under the influence of antidiuretic hormone (ADH), resulting in the final regulation of the specific gravity of the urine. Figure 26-9 summarizes the process for countercurrent multiplication.

Urea is also exchanged by this mechanism and excess urea formed is excreted in the urine. Urea is produced through a degradation of amino acids and the amount of this substance formed usually depends on the protein intake in the diet and the ability of the liver to convert ammonia to urea. Normally, the body produces 25 to 30 gm of urea each day but maintains only 8 to 20 mg/dl in the plasma.

COUNTERCURRENT EXCHANGER. As discussed in the previous section, the vasa recta are important in carrying out the countercurrent mechanism. Blood enters the descending limbs of the vasa recta with a solute concentration of 300 mOsm/liter. At this point, sodium, chloride, and urea diffuse from the interstitial fluid into the blood, thus causing a higher osmolality in the blood, which causes water to move back into the blood. At the tip of the U in each of the vasa recta, the osmolality can reach 1200 mOsm/liter for a maximum concentration.

As the blood ascends the vasa recta, water returns to the blood and sodium, chloride, and urea move back by diffusion into the interstitial fluid. When the blood leaves the medulla, the osmolality is slightly higher than that of the blood that enters the vasa recta [7]. This mechanism provides a precise balance between the countercurrent systems and prevents an accumulation of sodium in the interstitium [6]. This entire process by the vasa recta is called the *countercurrent exchange mechanism*.

Distal Convoluted Tubules and Collecting Tubules

SODIUM AND POTASSIUM RESORPTION. The DCT and collecting tubules are responsible for the resorption of sodium but in smaller amounts, depending on the amount of aldosterone in the blood. The release of aldosterone through the *renin-angiotensin aldosterone system* affects sodium resorption at the DCT.

Located in each kidney are special cells called *juxtaglomerular cells*, which make up the juxtaglomerular apparatus. This apparatus produces *renin*, an enzyme, and secretes it into the blood. The stimulus for this secretion is decreased perfusion pressure in the afferent arteriole. Renin then causes splitting of angiotensinogen, a plasma protein, to produce angiotensin I, a polypeptide, which is transformed into *angiotensin II* in the lungs. Angiotensin II causes vasoconstriction throughout the body and stimulates the adrenal cortex to release *aldosterone*. With the release of aldosterone, sodium is transported from the tubules to the blood, passively followed by water; thus, blood volume and the blood pressure are increased. Increasing the blood volume causes the renal cells to receive increased oxygen.

Aldosterone combined with carrier protein enzymes aid in the process of transporting sodium [3]. Potassium is also actively transported in smaller amounts in the DCT and collecting tubules. As the sodium is conserved under the influence of aldosterone, potassium is excreted into the urine.

WATER RESORPTION. Water is regulated in the DCT and collecting tubules by the production of *antidiuretic hormone (ADH)*. This hormone is produced by the hypothalamus and stored and released by the posterior pituitary gland. ADH is secreted by the posterior pituitary when the osmolarity of the plasma increases. ADH directly regulates the permeability of the membranes of the renal epithelial cells.

If there are increased amounts of ADH in the blood, water is osmotically moved from the tubules into the capillaries by increasing the permeability of the tubular membrane. Without ADH, the permeability is decreased, causing water to stay in the tubules and resulting in a very dilute urine.

Secretion: Tubules and Collecting Ducts

Secretion, the final step to urine formation, is the movement of fluid and solute from the blood back into the glomerular filtrate, usually requiring an expenditure of energy to cross the electrochemical gradient. There are active and a few passive secretory mechanisms at various points in the tubules.

Substances That are Secreted

PAH. Organic acids such as para-aminohippurate (PAH) are secreted in the PCT by way of carrier sites. When the plasma PAH concentration is low almost all of it is secreted into the tubules, and very little remains in the blood. The flow of plasma through the kidneys is always slightly greater than the clearance of PAH. Therefore, by knowing the PAH clearance, one can calculate the renal plasma flow (RPF). By knowing the hematocrit and knowing that the average PAH clearance is 630 ml/minute [5], one can calculate the RPF in the following formula:

$$\text{PAH}\,(1-\text{Hct}) = \text{RPF}$$

For example: $630\,(1.0-0.43) = 1158$ ml/minute

HYDROGEN IONS. Hydrogen ions are secreted in the PCT, DCT, and collecting tubules. The number of H^+ ions secreted is dependent on the pH of the extracellular fluid and the amount of buffer in the glomerular filtrate. The normal pH of the urine varies from 4.5 to 8.0 depending on dietary intake and metabolism. If the urine pH decreases to 4.4 secretion becomes inhibited.

When the hydrogen ion concentration is high in the extracellular fluid (plasma), large quantities of hydrogen are secreted. Low hydrogen ion concentrations cause small amounts of H^+ ion secretion.

When ammonia (NH_3^+) is passively secreted by the tubules, it can combine with the actively secreted hydrogen, forming ammonium (NH_4^+). Hence, NH_4 is secreted into the filtrate and sodium (Na^+) is replaced. The exchange of Na^+ and H^+ causes Na^+ to move into the renal capillaries and combine with bicarbonate ion to form sodium bicarbonate. This is one way the renal cells maintain acid-base balance and serve to buffer excess H^+. A special enzyme called carbonic anhydrase, in the renal cells, is necessary in this process and causes the combination of water and carbon dioxide resulting in the formation of carbonic acid (H_2CO_3). When H_2CO_3 dissociates, it forms hydrogen and bicarbonate ions ($H^+ + HCO_3^-$). The hydrogen ions are then exchanged for sodium in the cell.

POTASSIUM. Potassium ions are transported along with sodium from the proximal tubules to the peritubular capillaries and more is resorbed in the distal tubules. This means that less than 10 percent of potassium in the glomerular filtrate actually arrives at the distal tubules. Excretion of excess potassium from the body requires secretion of potassium from the capillaries into the distal tubules and collecting ducts. This is partly under the control of aldosterone. The resorption of sodium leaves a negative electrochemical gradient in the tubules. Electrochemical neutrality must be maintained so the positive potassium takes the place of sodium. Excess potassium is ingested in the normal diet, up to several hundred mEq/day. The secretion method for potassium excretion is an essential process to maintain the normal serum value of 3.5 to 5.0 mEq/liter. Levels of 7 or higher may precipitate cardiac arrhythmias and death (see Chap. 5).

Table 26-1 summarizes some specific characteristics of urine. The variations relate to diet and fluid intake.

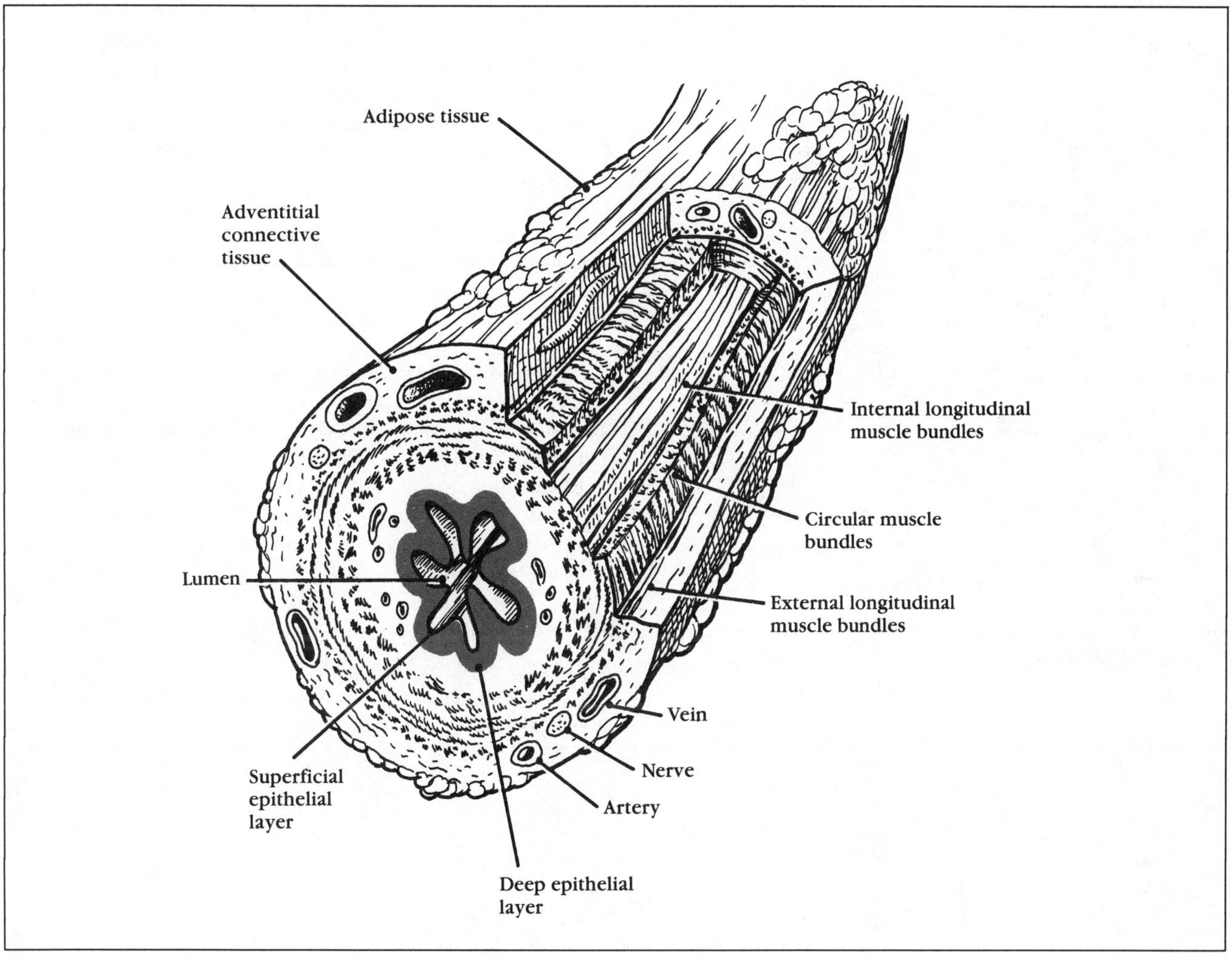

FIGURE 26-10. Structure of the ureter including smooth muscle layers, outer connective tissue, and blood and nerve supply.

ACCESSORY URINARY STRUCTURES AND BLADDER

When urine is excreted from the kidneys, it is transported from the renal pelvis to the ureters by peristaltic wave contractions. The urine is emptied into the bladder, which releases it into the urethra.

Ureters

The ureters vary in length from 25 to 30 cm and are approximately 1.25 cm wide; they enter the bladder at oblique angles. They are composed of three layers of smooth muscle including an inner layer of longitudinal muscle, a middle layer of circular muscle, and an outer layer that is a fibrous coat. There is also a layer lining the ureter that is composed of mucous membrane. This layer, through its mucus secretion, does not allow for permeability by the constituents of urine (Fig. 26-10).

The peristaltic movement of the smooth muscle allows contractions to occur at a rate of 1 to 5 per minute, causing a spurting action by which urine fills the bladder.

TABLE 26-1. Physical characteristics of urine

pH: 4.6–8.0
Amount: 600–2500 ml/24 hours
Color: Amber or straw colored and clear
Specific gravity: 1.003–1.030
Protein: 0–0.1 gm/24 hours
Glucose: 0–0.3 gm/24 hours
RBCs: 1–2/microscopic slide
Urobilinogen: 0–4 mg/24 hours

Source: J. Wallach, *Interpretation of Diagnostic Tests* (3rd ed.). Boston: Little, Brown, 1978.

Bladder

The *bladder,* when empty, is like a deflated balloon; it is located behind the symphysis pubis. When filled with urine it rises into the abdomen and becomes pear-shaped. The bladder is composed of several *layers:* mucosa, submucosa, detrusor muscle, and serous layer. The mucosal layer, containing transitional epithelium, in combination with the *rugae* (multiple folds in the mucosa) allows the bladder to stretch during urinary filling. The submucosa contains connective tissue that connects the mucous layer and the mus-

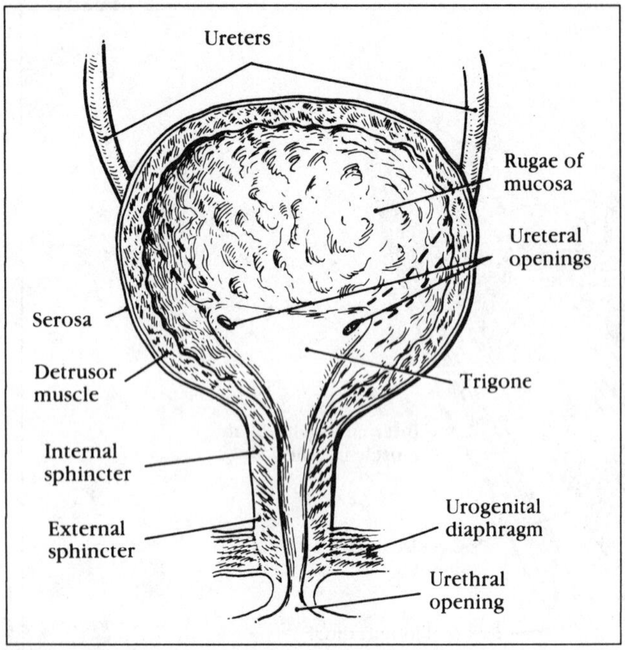

FIGURE 26-11. Structure of the bladder and its internal and external urethral sphincters.

cular layer [5]. The detrusor muscle is composed of longitudinal and circular muscles, allowing for contractility. The serous layer coats the superior portion of the bladder and is formed by the peritoneum.

In the bladder an area called the *trigone* is located at the base of the bladder and is formed by the two ureters and the urethra.

Between the bladder and the urethra there is an *internal urethral sphincter.* Below it is an *external urethral sphincter.* These sphincters are formed by circular muscles and, when stimulated, allow for passage of urine from the bladder into the urethra (Fig. 26-11).

MICTURATION REFLEX OF THE BLADDER. Micturation, or voiding, is the result of a spinal reflex from the sacral portion of the spinal cord. Stretch receptors become stimulated when there is 150 to 300 ml of urine in the bladder. The bladder pressure increases with increased filling and the parasympathetic nerves become stimulated. This causes the *micturation reflex,* which results in contraction of the detrusor muscle and relaxation of the internal sphincter. Urination proceeds unless it is stopped by voluntary contraction of the external sphincter, which is under cerebral control.

FIGURE 26-12. Structure of the female genitourinary anatomy. (From M. A. Miller and D. A. Brooten, *The Childbearing Family: A Nursing Perspective* [2nd ed.]. Boston: Little, Brown, 1983.)

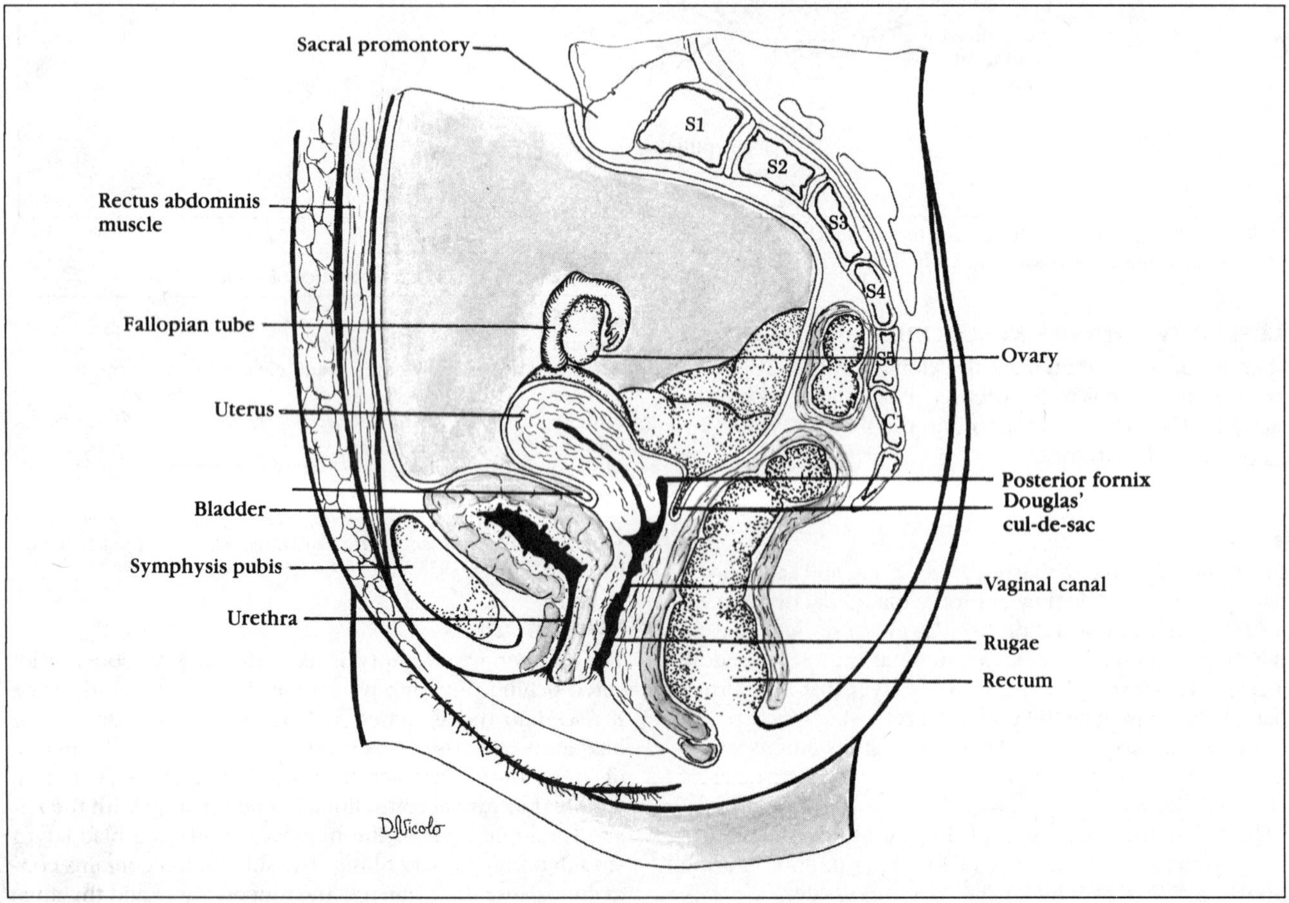

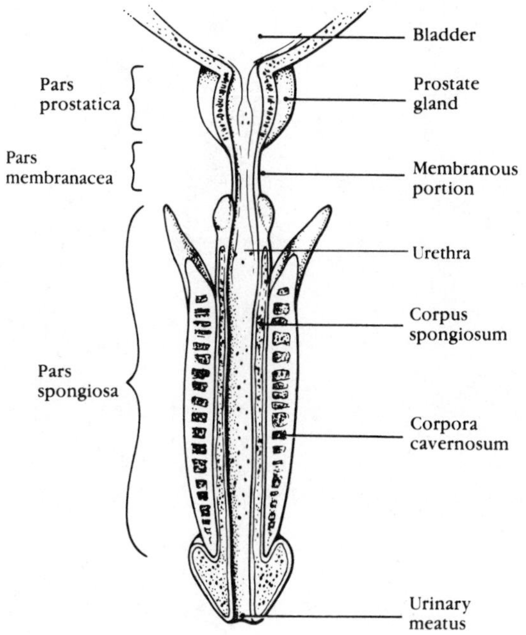

FIGURE 26-13. Structure of the male genitourinary anatomy.

Urethra

The urethra, located at the apex of the bladder, is the final excretory passageway for urine. The urethral opening to the exterior is the urinary meatus.

The female urethra is located posteriorly to the symphysis pubis and anteriorly to the vagina. The urethra is approximately 3.75 cm long and is composed of smooth muscle (Fig. 26-12).

When the male urethra leaves the bladder it passes through the prostate gland (*pars prostatica*), then between a membrane portion (*pars membranacea*) extending from the prostate to the corpus spongiosum of the penis. Finally, the male urethra passes through the corpus spongiosum (*pars spongiosa*) and terminates at the urinary meatus (Fig. 26-13). The male urethra is approximately 20 cm in length and serves the dual purpose of urine transport and semen transport.

REFERENCES

1. Bloom, W., and Fawcett, D. W. *A Textbook of Histology* (10th ed.). Philadelphia: Saunders, 1975.
2. Brenner, B., and Rector, F. C. *The Kidney.* Philadelphia: Saunders, 1976.
3. Guyton, A. *Textbook of Medical Physiology* (6th ed.). Philadelphia: Saunders, 1981.
4. Jensen, D. Functional Anatomy of the Kidney and Related Urinary Structures: Renal Circulation, Blood Flow and Oxygen Consumption. In D. Jensen (ed.), *The Principles of Physiology* (2nd ed.). New York: Appleton-Century-Crofts, 1980.
5. Mitchell, G. A. G. The nerve supply of the kidneys. *Acta Anat.* (Basel) 10:1, 1950.
6. Tortora, G. J., and Evans, R. L. Renal Physiology. In G. J. Tortora, et al. (eds.), *Principles of Human Physiology.* Hagerstown, Md.: Harper & Row, 1982.
7. Valtin, H. *Renal Function: Mechanisms Preserving Fluid and Solute Balance in Health* (2nd ed.). Boston: Little, Brown, 1983.

CHAPTER 27
IMMUNOLOGIC, INFECTIOUS, AND TOXIC ALTERATIONS IN URINARY FUNCTION

LEARNING OBJECTIVES

1. List the major organisms that can cause cystitis.
2. Differentiate between hemorrhagic and suppurative cystitis.
3. Explain the normal protection against infection in the male and female urinary systems.
4. Describe the vesicoureteral reflux.
5. Differentiate between acute and chronic pyelonephritis, pathologically and clinically.
6. State the main cause of end-stage renal disease.
7. Describe antiglomerular basement membrane (anti-GBM) disease using Goodpasture's disease as a model.
8. Explain the significance of crescents in renal pathology.
9. Describe the etiology, pathology, clinical manifestations, and prognosis for poststreptococcal glomerulonephritis.
10. Briefly describe the pathology of rapidly progressive glomerulonephritis.
11. List some etiologic agents of chronic glomerulonephritis.
12. Define *nephrosis*.
13. Explain why persons with nephrotic disease also have hyperlipidemia.
14. Describe the development of edema in nephrotic disease.
15. Describe the relationships between idiopathic nephrotic syndromes, minimal change disease, focal glomerulosclerosis, membranous glomerulopathy, and membrane proliferative glomerulonephritis.
16. Describe how aspirin, phenacetin, codeine, and caffeine can cause nephritis.
17. Outline the mechanisms by which hyperuricemia, hypercalcemia, and hypokalemia can cause tubular or parenchymal alterations.
18. Review the immunologic mechanisms that can cause tubulointerstitial alterations.

Many factors can affect the genitourinary system and can cause relatively innocuous problems or progressive problems leading to renal failure. The most common genitourinary problem is infection of the bladder mucosa that may ascend to the pelvis of the kidney. Immune complexes or antiglomerular basement membrane (anti-GBM) antibody may cause inflammation and increased permeability of the GBM with protein loss into the urine. Nephrosis may follow (see pp. 371–372). Toxic injury to the tubules and interstitium of the kidney may result from exposure of the tubules to a *nephrotoxic* agent. This agent can be *exogenous* (such as pharmaceutical agents) or *endogenous* (such as products of deranged metabolism).

INFECTIONS OF THE GENITOURINARY TRACT

Infections of the genitourinary tract (UTI) are diagnosed by culture of the specific microorganism involved. Active infection is usually considered to be more than 100,000 bacteria/ml of urine in a clean voided specimen. The most common organism causing genitourinary infections is the *Escherichia coli,* an aerobic organism found in large numbers in the lower intestinal area. UTI also may be caused by other organisms, such as *Klebsiella, Proteus,* and *Staphylococcus,* especially in the presence of an indwelling catheter.

Cystitis

Inflammation of the bladder is more common in women than men because of the proximity of the urethral opening and vagina to the anal area. Normally, the urethra contains diphtheroids and *Streptococcus* and *Staphylococcus* organisms. Gram-negative organisms may gain access to the bladder during sexual intercourse, urethral trauma, or as a result of poor hygiene. Normally, these organisms are rapidly expelled by voiding because the urine is acidic and flushes away excess bacteria. In men the prostatic secretions have antibacterial properties.

Risk factors for cystitis include intercourse, pregnancy, neurogenic bladder, other kidney disease, obstructive conditions, and diabetes mellitus. The most dangerous sequel to cystitis is pyelonephritis, which results from organisms in the bladder that have ascended to the renal pelvis. *Vesicoureteral reflux* enhances the risk of pyelonephritis from cystitis (Fig. 27-1). This condition occurs in children who have bladder or urinary tract abnormalities that allow urine to reflux from the bladder to the renal pelvis.

The pathology of cystitis assumes many forms. If there is bloody urine present it is called *hemorrhagic cystitis;* this cystitis is a frequent sequel to chemotherapy or radiation therapy over the bladder area. *Suppurative cystitis* occurs when suppurative exudate accumulates on the endothelial lining of the bladder (Fig. 27-2). The suppurative exudate is composed of polymorphonuclear leukocytes (PMNs) in early stages, but mononuclear infiltrates appear if the condition progresses to chronic cystitis. Ulcerations may be seen in either the acute or chronic stage.

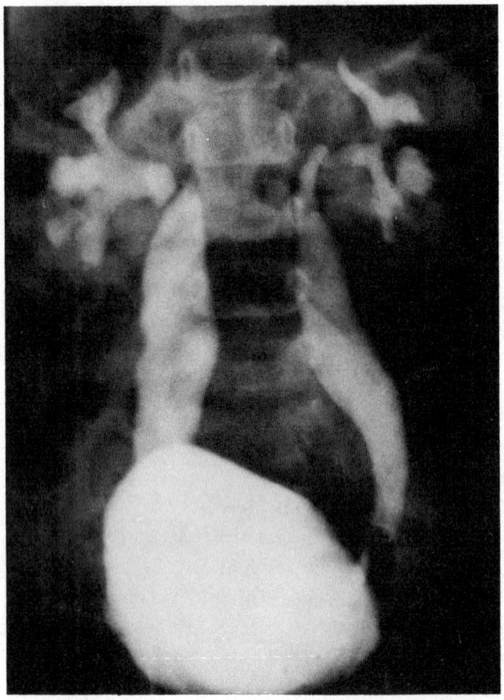

FIGURE 27-1. Grade 4 vesicoureteral reflux in a 2-year-old child. (From S. Papper, *Clinical Nephrology* [2nd ed.]. Boston: Little, Brown, 1978.)

Clinical manifestations include significant bacteriuria in 60 to 70 percent of cases. Some persons may have symptomatic cystitis that cannot be diagnosed by culture [1]. Dysuria, frequency, urgency, and pain over the suprapubic area are classic symptoms. Any individual who has an indwelling catheter for a long period of time has a high risk for developing a cystitis with organisms that become resistant to therapy.

Pyelonephritis

Inflammation of the renal pelvis is called *pyelonephritis.* Because the genitourinary system is continuous, ascending infection from the bladder is the most common cause of pyelonephritis. The infection, as with cystitis, most frequently results from the gram-negative bacteria. Two forms of pyelonephritis have been described. These are the acute and chronic forms.

ACUTE PYELONEPHRITIS (APN). APN usually occurs suddenly with onset of fever, chills, nausea, vomiting, and diarrhea. It may follow a symptomatic or asymptomatic bladder infection or it may result from vesicoureteral reflux. Occasionally, APN is initiated by a bloodborne, virulent organism, but this route of infection almost always signifies the presence of other kidney injury.

Pathologically, APN gives rise to abscesses on the cortical surface of the kidney; these often surround the glomeruli. Glomerular damage is rare but rupture of the tubules may occur. APN also may follow urinary tract obstruction with suppurative exudate filling the renal pelvis. Healing

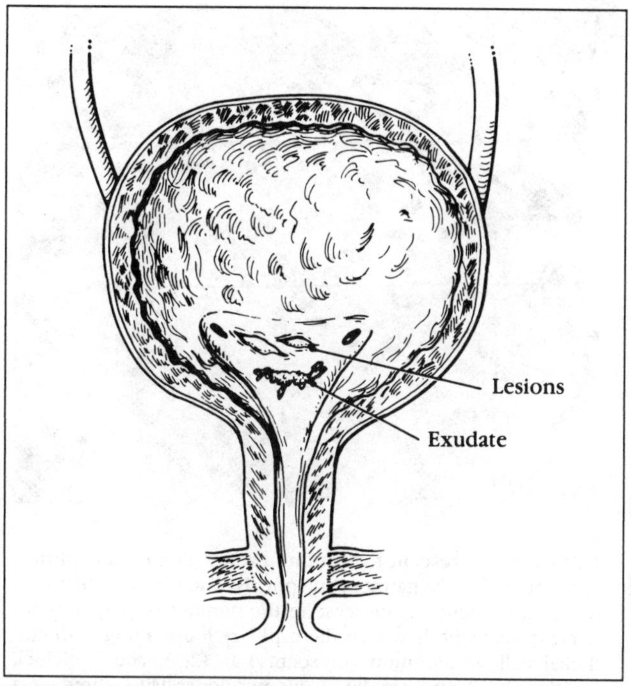

FIGURE 27-2. Suppurative cystitis with ulceration of the bladder mucosa and suppurative exudate on the lining of the bladder.

usually involves scar tissue replacement of affected areas of the cortical surface.

Clinical manifestations of APN include the sudden onset of high fever and chills with the demonstration of marked tenderness on deep pressure on one or both costovertebral areas. Leukocytosis and pyuria with leukocytic casts are common. The identified bacteria are often coated with kidney-produced antibody. In the acute phase some hematuria may be present but it should not persist after the acute manifestations have subsided. The symptoms of APN usually subside with or without treatment, but pyuria may persist for weeks or months.

CHRONIC PYELONEPHRITIS (CPN). CPN is difficult to diagnose except when a history of urinary tract infections, pyuria, and bacteriuria can be elicited. It is a leading cause of chronic renal failure.

Pathologically, scarred, irregular kidneys can be seen with deformity of the calices. Gradual atrophy and destruction of the tubules lead to the impairment of function that results in chronic renal failure. Chronic pyelonephritis has been reported to follow the vascular and hypertensive conditions that affect the glomeruli.

The clinical manifestations are variable with recurrent episodes of APN or the gradual onset of renal insufficiency and failure. Mild proteinuria with lymphocytes and plasma cells is characteristic. While CPN has been linked to bacterial infections, not all affected persons relate a history of UTI. Damage may result from asymptomatic bacterial infection, or other factors besides infection may be involved. [4].

NEPHRITIC GLOMERULAR DISEASE

Glomerular injury is the most common cause of chronic renal failure, with immunologically induced glomerulonephritis causing one-half of the cases of end-stage renal failure [4]. Glomerular injury may result from chemicals, radiation, hypoxemia, and other agents, as well as from immunologically mediated disorders. Two major immunologic mechanisms have been described: (1) antiglomerular basement membrane (anti-GBM) disease, and (2) immune complex glomerular disease.

Antiglomerular Basement Membrane Disease

In this condition, antibodies form that destroy the GBM and cause a rapidly progressive glomerulonephritis (RPGN) (pp. 370–371). It may also involve antibodies that form against the alveolar basement membrane (Goodpasture's disease).

GOODPASTURE'S DISEASE. This rare type II autoimmune disorder affects young men more frequently than women and begins abruptly with no apparent inciting event. It may progress rapidly, causing severe and sometimes fatal hemoptysis, or it may exhibit long remissions. More than 90 percent of individuals affected exhibit anti-GBM antibodies [4]. Pathologically, the glomeruli may show nearly normal configurations or they may exhibit focal or necrotizing proliferations called *crescents.* These characteristic lesions of severe renal disease involve massive proliferation of epithelial cells in crescent-shaped masses within the glomeruli (Fig. 27-3). Deposition of fibrin, complement fragments, and immunoglobins may be found within the crescents. Anti-GBM antibodies may be seen bound to the alveolar basement membrane. These antibodies can cause alveolar damage and pulmonary hemorrhage that may be massive and life-threatening. Rapidly progressive or insidious renal failure may result. Treatment with steroid agents has induced remissions. Renal failure and uremia have been controlled by hemodialysis; a few individuals have received renal transplants.

Immune Complex Glomerular Disease

Many types of glomerular damage are caused by antigen-antibody complexes precipitated in the glomeruli. These complexes have been classified in many ways. Table 27-1 shows exogenous and endogenous systems. Infectious agents are the most frequent causes of immune complex disease, but it also can be associated with many types of autoimmune disease, malignancies, and even thyroiditis. The most common exogenous type is poststreptococcal glomerulonephritis, but nonstreptococcal forms are being identified in increasing numbers [4].

POSTSTREPTOCOCCAL GLOMERULONEPHRITIS (PSGN). The *Streptococcus* organism, of the group A, β-hemolytic type, has been shown to possess nephrotoxic surface proteins. The development of the glomerulonephritis follows an infection by this organism in 1 to 2 weeks. Nasopharyngeal

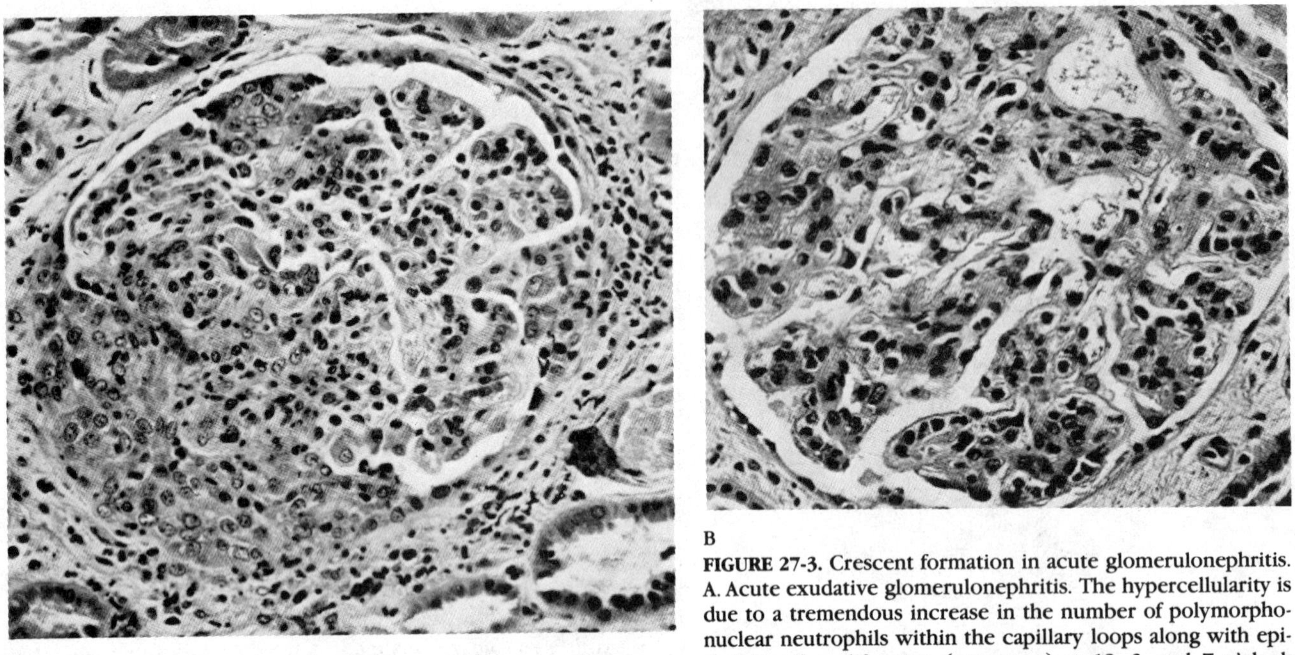

A

B

FIGURE 27-3. Crescent formation in acute glomerulonephritis. A. Acute exudative glomerulonephritis. The hypercellularity is due to a tremendous increase in the number of polymorphonuclear neutrophils within the capillary loops along with epithelial cell proliferation (crescents) at 12, 3, and 7 o'clock positions. B. Acute exudative glomerulonephritis showing a large crescent. (From J. Metcoff, *Acute Glomerulonephritis*. Boston: Little, Brown, 1967.)

infections are the usual source but occasionally a streptococcal skin infection may be the cause. Development of PSGN requires an individual sensitivity to the β-hemolytic *Streptococcus* organism, as is evidenced by the fact that no demonstration of active infection can be seen by blood or urine cultures. Increased ASO (antistreptolysin) titers and depression of the complement factors are common findings.

Pathologically, enlarged hypercellular glomeruli can be demonstrated with proliferation of cells on the epithelial side of the GBM. Infiltration of the area with PMNs and monocytes is followed by interstitial edema and inflammation. "Humps" can be seen on the epithelial side of the GBM and these probably are precipitated antigen-antibody complexes. Increased permeability of the GBM results in loss of red blood cells and protein in the urine. A decrease in the glomerular filtration rate (GFR) leads to sodium and water retention. Hypocomplementemia is frequently associated with and results from large amounts of precipitated complement in the complexes.

The clinical manifestations of PSGN include the acute onset of edema, oliguria, proteinuria, and a characteristic cocoa-colored urine with red blood cell casts. Hypertension is usual and probably results from fluid retention. A markedly elevated ASO titer indicates the presence of circulating antibody to a hemolysin called streptolysin O, which is usually elevated within 2 months after an attack. The erythrocyte sedimentation rate (ESR) is usually increased, indicating inflammation.

PSGN is more frequently seen in children, most of whom totally recover within a week and then exhibit immunity to further infection. Occasionally, PSGN will convert to a type of rapidly progressive glomerulonephritis or a slowly progressive form of glomerulonephritis. In either case, renal failure results. Adults who develop PSGN exhibit a higher incidence of persistant proteinuria, hematuria, and renal failure than do children. A 60 percent total recovery rate is seen in adults [3].

NONSTREPTOCOCCAL GLOMERULONEPHRITIS. Besides the *Streptococcus* organism, other bacteria, viruses, and parasites have been implicated in the etiology of acute glomerulonephritis. These also cause the precipitation of immune complexes and decreased complement levels. As with PSGN, this type of glomerulonephritis occurs following infection and it usually responds well to treatment.

Rapidly Progressive Glomerulonephritis (RPGN)

RPGN leads to the development of renal failure over a period of weeks to months. It may occur as a complication of acute or subacute infectious disease, or from multisystem disease such as systemic lupus erythematosus, or from Goodpasture's disease. It also may occur as an idiopathic or primary condition.

Pathologically, characteristic capillary proliferation with crescents involves more than 70 percent of the glomeruli. Gaps or discontinuities of the GBM also may be associated with the crescents. Anti-GBM antibodies or deposits of immunoglobulins may be demonstrated on the glomerulus. No circulating antibodies are usually detected unless the condition is associated with a specific process for which antibody production can be demonstrated. Table 27-2 lists some of the conditions that may lead to RPGN. The idio-

TABLE 27-1. Exogenous and endogenous antigens that can cause immune complex glomerulonephritis

Antigens	Clinical condition
EXOGENOUS OR FOREIGN ANTIGENS	
Iatrogenic agents	
Drugs, toxoids, foreign serum	Serum sickness, heroin nephropathy (?), gold nephropathy (?), etc.
Infectious agents	
Bacterial: nephritogenic streptococci, *Staphylococcus albus, Corynebacterium bovis,* enterococci, *Streptococcus pneumoniae, Treponema pallidum, Salmonella typhi*	Poststreptococcal glomerulonephritis, infected ventriculoatrial shunts, endocarditis, pneumonia, syphilis, typhoid fever
Parasitic: *Plasmodium malariae, Plasmodium falciparum, Schistosoma mansoni, Toxoplasma gondii, Loa loa*	Malaria, schistosomiasis, toxoplasmosis, filarial loiasis
Viral: hepatitis B, oncornavirus-related antigen, measles, Epstein-Barr virus, cytomegalovirus	Hepatitis, leukemia, subacute sclerosing panencephalitis, Burkitt's lymphoma, cytomegalovirus infection
Perhaps others as yet undetermined	Endocarditis, leprosy, kalaazar, dengue, mumps, varicella, infectious mononucleosis, Guillain-Barré syndrome
ENDOGENOUS OR SELF-ANTIGENS	
Nuclear antigens	Systemic lupus erythematosus
Immunoglobulin	Cryoglobulinemia
Tumor antigens, CEA	Neoplasms
Thyroglobulin	Thyroiditis
Renal tubular antigen	Membranous glomerulonephritis in Japan, sickle cell anemia, renal carcinoma

Source: H. H. Fudenberg, et al. (eds.), *Basic and Clinical Immunology* (3rd ed.). Los Altos, Calif.: Lange, 1980.

pathic form is common and may be identified by enlarged, pale kidneys with cellular proliferation in Bowman's space. The capillary lumens are compressed and distorted with fibrin throughout [5]. The GBM is disrupted; interstitial edema with infiltration of leukocytes leads to degenerative changes of the tubules. When crescent formation is seen it indicates severe glomerular disease. With widespread crescent formation the prognosis for RPGN is bleak, with over 90 percent of affected persons developing chronic renal failure.

The clinical manifestations include a rapid, progressive diminution in renal function; severe oliguria; or anuria with irreversible renal failure in weeks or months [3]. Hypertension, proteinuria, and hematuria are common.

TABLE 27-2. Causes of rapidly progressive glomerulonephritis

Postacute or subacute infections
Streptococcal: beta-hemolytic
Bacteria, viruses, parasites
Idiopathic or primary
Multisystem or autoimmune disease

Chronic Glomerulonephritis (CGN)

CGN is an insidiously developing progressive form of renal dysfunction that usually terminates in end-stage renal failure after years of progressive renal insufficiency. It may result from any form of glomerular disease or it may occur secondarily to pyelonephritis. Pathologically, the glomeruli become scarred and may become totally obliterated. The tubules are atrophic. The glomerulus and renal capsule become infiltrated with lymphocytes and plasma cells. Hyalinization of the glomeruli lead to obliteration of the pathology of the original disease. Vascular sclerosis of arteries and arterioles probably contributes to the arterial hypertension that is almost always associated with this disease.

The progression of the condition is related to the underlying disorder but almost always continues relentlessly to uremia. Proteinuria, hypertension, and azotemia are common, with later manifestations of uremia (see Chap. 29).

NEPHROTIC GLOMERULAR DISEASE

Nephrosis refers to the sequelae of albuminuria that is usually greater than 3.5 gm/day. Hypoalbuminemia of less than 3 gm/dl results in the production of generalized body edema. Hyperlipidemia results from hepatic lipoprotein synthesis, which is stimulated by the decreased serum protein levels. The excess lipids formed are mostly cholesterol in the early stages, but in late stages triglycerides also become elevated.

The loss of protein results from increased permeability of the GBM, which allows the plasma proteins to escape into the urine. The resulting hypoalbuminemia causes a decreased colloid osmotic pressure and systemic edema (anasarca) (Fig. 27-4). Loss of other proteins may lead to decreased levels of immunoglobulins and important hormones.

Nephrosis may result from glomerulonephritis but most nephrosis results from unknown causes. Table 27-3 summarizes some causes of nephrosis. Several of the more common idiopathic syndromes are discussed in this section.

Minimal Change Disease (Lipoid Nephrosis)

This type of nephrosis is the most common type seen in children between the ages of 2 and 8. It results in a decreased GFR and loss or binding together of adjacent glomerular foot processes. This loss and/or binding allows the leakage of albumin and fat particles into the urine. No antibodies have been demonstrated in this condition, but a

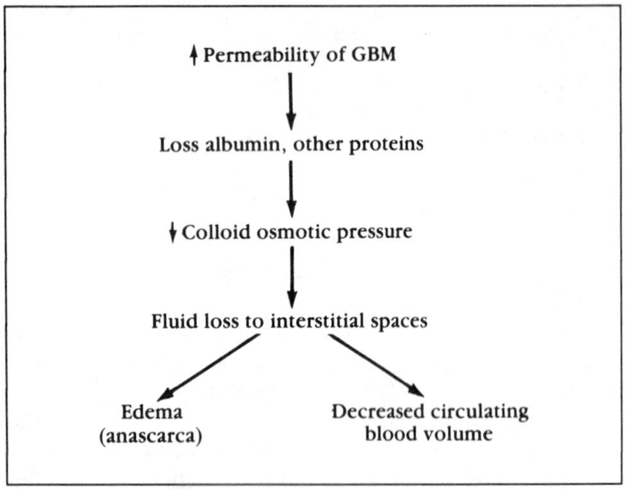

FIGURE 27-4. Production of edema in nephrosis.

relationship with respiratory infections or routine immunization have led to the theory that it is a hypersensitivity reaction. Because it also responds to steroid therapy and is associated with other atopic diseases, it is thought to be T cell related.

The disease is named for its pathologic presentation, which shows few pathologic changes except that the adjacent glomerular foot processes bind together and allow plasma proteins and fats to pass into the urine. The kidney appears edematous and pale.

The clinical course is variable but it is usually characterized by periods of remissions and exacerbations and a 90 percent 10-year survival rate [2]. In a few cases, it progresses to focal glomerulosclerosis and then to renal failure.

Focal Glomerulosclerosis

This condition involves the sclerosis and hyalinization of some of the juxtamedullary glomeruli. Deposits of IgM and C3 fragments are seen by immunofluorescence in the segmental sclerosing lesions [2]. A progressive decline in GFR with increasing albuminuria and hypoalbuminemia occur and renal failure finally results.

Membranous Glomerulopathy

This lesion involves a uniform deposition of protein in the outer glomerular capillary wall with the deposits usually containing IgG. Capillary thickening with basement membrane projections account for the loss of protein in the urine. If the appearance of nephrosis with edema and hypoalbuminemia occurs, the disease generally progresses to renal failure. This disease is usually idiopathic but it may develop in association with systemic lupus erythematosus, exposure to gold or mercury, solid tumors, or some infections. It may progress with increasing renal impairment or it may show a spontaneous and complete remission.

TABLE 27-3. Causes of nephrotic disease

Idiopathic or primary
Minimal change disease or lipoid nephrosis
Focal glomerulosclerosis
Membranous glomerulopathy
Membranoproliferative or mesangiocapillary or lobular glomerulonephritis
Secondary to glomerulonephritis
Poststreptococcal
Autoimmune diseases
Diabetes mellitus
Postinfectious: viral, bacterial, parasitic
Hypersensitivity reaction to drugs or stings

Membranoproliferative Glomerulonephritis (Mesangiocapillary or Tubular GN)

This type of glomerulonephritis involves basement membrane thickening and proliferation of mesangial cells. It apparently does not follow a streptococcal infection but does account for 5 to 10 percent of cases of idiopathic nephrosis in children and adults [3]. Abnormalities of the immune system seem to account for circulating immune complexes, and in some types *hypocomplementemia*, especially of the C3 component, is seen.

The clinical manifestations include any of the manifestations of the nephrotic syndrome. The disease assumes several forms but tends to be slowly progressive and unremitting. About 50 percent of afflicted persons develop chronic renal failure within 10 years [2].

TUBULAR AND INTERSTITIAL DISEASES

Histologic and functional abnormalities of the renal tubules and parenchyma can be caused by many factors. When the etiology is infectious, the term *pyelonephritis* is usually used to describe the process. Nonbacterial factors such as toxins, metabolic imbalances, and immunologic derangements can cause impairment of concentrating ability; metabolic acidosis; and loss of sodium, chloride, potassium, and water. Tables 27-4 and 27-5 list some of the congenital and acquired tubular disorders.

Toxic Mechanisms

The renal tubules and parenchyma sustain damage from nephrotoxic substances because of the large quantities of renal blood flow and the concentration of noxious substances in the tubules. The most common toxic substances are pharmaceutical agents, including phenacetin, aspirin, certain antibiotics, and diuretics. *Chronic analgesia nephritis* is a common cause of renal insufficiency in some countries, such as Australia and New Zealand, and occurs most frequently when mixtures of aspirin, caffeine, phenacetin, and codeine are ingested [3]. The mechanisms may be partly due to the inhibition of prostaglandins' vasodilatory effect by aspirin, which may lead to renal ischemia. Phenac-

TABLE 27-4. Effects of congenital tubular disorders on renal function

Disorder	Altered function
Single tubular defect	
Nephrogenic diabetes insipidus	↓ Reabsorption of water
Renal glycosuria	↓ Reabsorption of glucose Few tubules (normal Tm_G) Most tubules (↓ Tm_G)
Vitamin D–resistant rickets (familial) (? tubular disorder)	↓ Reabsorption of phosphate
Bartter's syndrome	↓ Reabsorption of potassium, ? ↓ reabsorption of sodium
Cystinuria	↓ Reabsorption of selected amino acids (associated jejunal defect)
Hartnup disease	↓ Reabsorption of amino acids other than those in cystinuria or proline or glycine (associated jejunal defect)
Multiple tubular defects	
Idiopathic Fanconi's syndrome	↓ Reabsorption of glucose, amino acids, and phosphate (and potassium and bicarbonate in some)
Renal tubular acidosis	Proximal tubule ↓ Reabsorption of bicarbonate Distal tubule ↓ Excretion of hydrogen ion

Source: S. Papper, *Clinical Nephrology* (2nd ed.). Boston: Little, Brown, 1978.

TABLE 27-5. Selected acquired tubular disorders

Disorder	Primary conditions
Single tubular defect	
Acquired nephrogenic diabetes insipidus	Hypercalcemic nephrocalcinosis Hypokalemic nephropathy Sickle cell disease Interstitial nephritis Medullary cystic disease Medullary sponge kidney Multiple myeloma Postobstructive nephropathy Drugs (lithium, demeclocycline, methoxyflurane, glybenclamide, ? isophosphamide, ? propoxyphene, ? colchicine)
Renal "salt wasting"[a]	Medullary cystic disease Medullary sponge kidney Interstitial nephritis Postobstructive nephropathy
Multiple tubular defects	
Acquired Fanconi syndrome	Cystinosis Galactosemia Glycogen storage disease Lowe's syndrome Luder-Sheldon syndrome Heavy metals: cadmium, copper (Wilson's disease), mercury, lead Multiple myeloma Light-chain nephropathy Outdated tetracycline
Secondary renal tubular acidosis	
Proximal tubule	Fanconi's syndrome (all causes) Hereditary fructose intolerance Hyperglobulinemia Amyloid Renal transplant
Distal tubule	Hypercalciuria Hyperglobulinemia Medullary sponge kidney Amyloid Renal transplant Interstitial nephritis Drugs (amphotericin B, lithium) Toluene "sniffing"

Source: S. Papper, *Clinical Nephrology* (2nd ed.). Boston: Little, Brown, 1978.

etin may have a directly toxic effect on the vasa recta or may cause papillary necrosis. The result is fibrosis, necrosis, and calcification of the papillary areas.

The papilla may be sloughed off and excreted in the urine. The kidneys first lose the ability to concentrate urine; severe renal insufficiency leads to azotemia and electrolyte imbalances. If the drugs are discontinued the renal function tends to improve over a period of time.

Hypersensitivity reactions to antibiotics and furosemide or other thiazide diuretics usually begin about 15 days after exposure to the drug. The reactions are characterized by fever, eosinophilia, hematuria, sterile pyuria, proteinuria, and skin rash [4]. Oliguria and azotemia develop transiently or acute renal failure may develop. When the drug is discontinued complete recovery usually occurs.

Metabolic Imbalances

Abnormal metabolism within the body may lead to the production of metabolites that are toxic to the renal tubules. The three imbalances that most frequently cause problems are: hyperuricemia, hypercalcemia, and hypokalemia.

HYPERURICEMIA. The most common cause of hyperuricemia is gout. Gouty nephropathy results from prolonged elevations of the serum uric acid levels. Crystalline deposits of uric acid are left in the tubules, especially the distal tubules and collecting ducts. The end result is intrarenal obstruction with inflammation and fibrosis of the tubules. Nephropathy is characterized by insidious renal insufficiency with proteinuria and a decreased renal concentrating ability. The precipitated urate bodies induce a *tophus*, which is the urate body surrounded by mononuclear giant cells.

Acute uric acid nephropathy has been reported following the administration of cytotoxic drugs in the therapy of certain leukemias and lymphomas. Uric acid crystals precipitate in the collecting ducts, leading to partial or total tubule obstruction; the obstruction can result in acute renal failure.

HYPERCALCEMIA. Any condition that causes an increase in circulating calcium can result in the increased incidence of calcium stones, obstruction, and nephropathy (see Chap. 28). Deposits of calcium often precipitate in the parenchyma of the kidney. Intracellular accumulation of calcium can disrupt the cell processes, causing cellular death and consequent obstruction of nephrons by cellular debris.

HYPOKALEMIA. When moderate or severe hypokalemia persists for several weeks, a functional decrease in concentrating ability may occur. This ability usually returns to normal when potassium levels are restored.

Immune Mechanisms Affecting the Tubulointerstitial Areas

Allergic drug reactions may cause acute interstitial nephritis. Antibodies to the tubules have been demonstrated by characteristic immunofluorescent studies.

Immune mechanisms may cause a reaction to the renal tubular cells, which is frequently seen in transplant rejections. Also, immune antibodies similar to those causing glomerulonephritis may affect the renal tubules.

REFERENCES

1. Anderson, W. A. D., and Scotti, T. *Synopsis of Pathology* (10th ed.). St. Louis: Mosby, 1980.
2. Glascock, R. J., and Brenner, B. M. The Major Glomerulopathies. In K. J. Isselbacher, et al. (eds.), *Harrison's Principles of Internal Medicine* (9th ed.). New York: McGraw-Hill, 1980.
3. Kincaid-Smith, P. Analgesic nephropathy. *Kidney Int.* 13:1, 1978.
4. Robbins, S., and Cotran, R. *Pathological Basis of Disease* (2nd ed.). Philadelphia: Saunders, 1979.
5. Wilson, C. B., et al. Renal Diseases in Basic and Clinical Immunology. In H. H. Fudenberg, et al. (eds.), *Basic and Clinical Immunology* (3rd ed.). Los Altos, Calif.: Lange, 1980.

CHAPTER 28
OBSTRUCTION OF THE GENITOURINARY TRACT

LEARNING OBJECTIVES

1. Define *benign prostatic hypertrophy (BPH).*
2. Identify the location of the urethra in relation to the prostate gland.
3. Discuss the pathogenesis of BPH, including the hormonal (testosterone, estrogen, dihydrotestosterone) influences.
4. Discuss the pathology of BPH.
5. List the symptoms and complications of BPH.
6. Define *urolithiasis* and *nephrolithiasis.*
7. Describe the composition of renal calculi.
8. Identify the organic matrix and its function in the formation of a stone.
9. List factors that may cause stone formation.
10. Define *staghorn calculi.*
11. Define *hypercalciuria* and *hypercalcemia.*
12. Discuss three classifications of hypercalciuria.
13. Explain the factors that contribute to the production of uric acid stones.
14. Identify the factors causing oxalate stones.
15. Identify the major cause of cystine stones.
16. Discuss the formation of struvite stones.
17. Identify the cause of xanthine stones.
18. List the major benign tumors of the kidney.
19. Define the solid and cystic types of cortical adenomas.
20. Identify the malignant tumors of the kidney.
21. Discuss the pathogenesis of renal cell carcinoma.
22. List the signs and symptoms associated with renal malignancy.
23. Identify the staging mechanism for renal cell carcinoma.
24. Describe the histology of Wilms' tumor.
25. Briefly describe the morphology of tumors of the renal pelvis.

Obstructive renal disorders may cause considerable renal dysfunction, including hemorrhage and renal failure, if they are left untreated. This chapter describes the obstructive conditions of prostatic hypertrophy, renal calculi, and renal tumors.

BENIGN PROSTATIC HYPERTROPHY

Benign prostatic hypertrophy (BPH) is a condition affecting the majority of men over the age of 50. *Hypertrophy* is a misleading term in this condition because the increase in the size of the prostate gland is from hyperplastic proliferation of glandular and cellular tissue (Fig. 28-1).

Normally, the prostate gland weighs 20 gm, surrounds the urethra, and contains four lobes. By the age of 70, the prostate may weigh from 60 gm to as much as 200 gm [28].

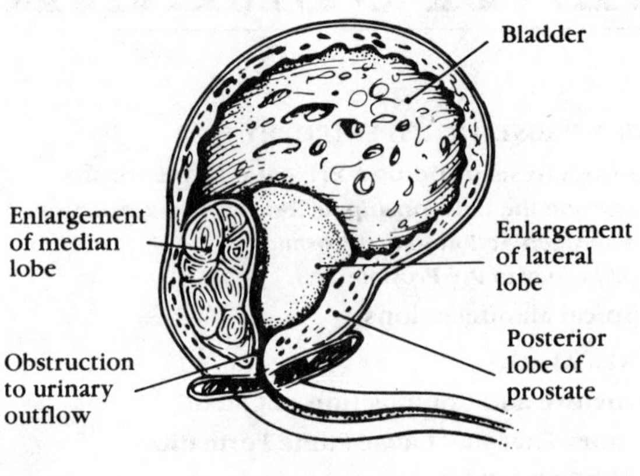

FIGURE 28-1. Enlargement of median and lateral lobes of the prostate gland. Note the obstruction to urinary outflow.

Pathogenesis of Benign Prostatic Hypertrophy

The cause of BPH is unknown but it is believed to result from an imbalance between the male and female sex hormones that occurs with advancing age. Normally, testosterone is the main androgen in the blood and forms two metabolites—dihydrotestosterone and 7 β-estradiol. Dihydrotestosterone metabolizes to 3 α-androstanediol (Fig. 28-2). Dihydrotestosterone is responsible for mediating many of the actions of testosterone. Estradiol is a steroid that possesses estrogenic properties and acts with androgens for many physiologic activities. It can act independently and cause the opposite effect of androgens. Testosterone and its metabolites act together to produce prostatic hyperplasia [38].

AGE AND THE RELATIONSHIP TO TESTOSTERONE AND ESTROGEN. In a person older than 60, the plasma testosterone decreases but BPH can occur 10 to 20 years before demonstrated decreased plasma levels [15]. With aging the estrogen level increases, but this increase does not correlate with the incidence of BPH [1]. The plasma levels of these hormones apparently do not cause BPH, but rather endocrine alterations within the prostate initiate the process [35].

ANDROGEN ACTION IN THE PROSTATE. In the plasma, testosterone binds to two proteins, globulin and albumin. A small percentage of free hormones is in balance with a protein-bound steroid and is able to enter the cells. Within the cell, testosterone is converted by 5 α-reductase enzyme to dihydrotestosterone. It is then bound to a specific androgen receptor protein and the hormone receptor complex changes before entering the nucleus. At this point interaction of steroid-receptor complexes with acceptor sites on the chromosomes results in increased transcription of specific structural genes [17]. These genes cause the formation of new messenger ribonucleic acid (RNA), resulting in the production of new proteins in the cytoplasm [38] (Fig. 28-3).

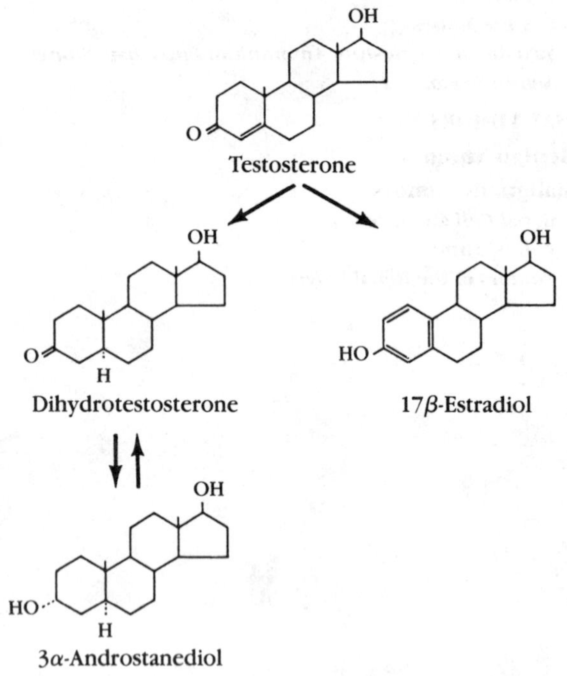

FIGURE 28-2. Plasma testosterone serves as a precursor for two other types of steroid hormones—5α-reduced androgens (dihydrotestosterone and 3α-androstanediol) and 17β-estradiol. (From J. Wilson, The pathogenesis of benign prostatic hyperplasia. *Am. J. Med.* 65:745, 1980.)

The "dihydrotestosterone thesis" indicates a relationship between the dihydrotestosterone concentration and BPH [30]. In human tissues there is not only accumulation of dihydrotestosterone in hyperplastic glands but prostates with earlier periurethral hyperplasia have larger amounts

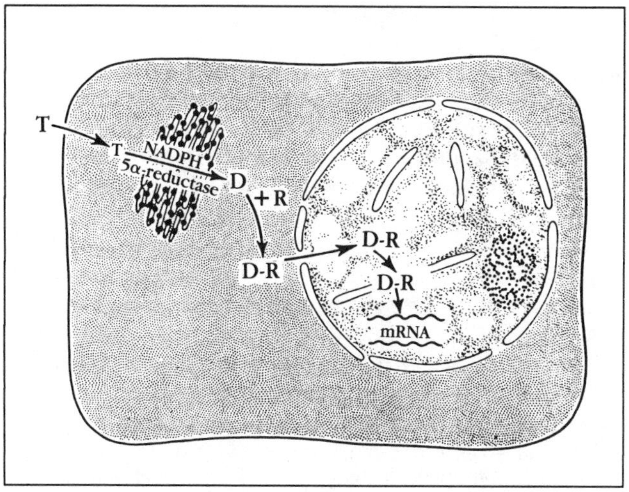

FIGURE 28-3. Current concepts of androgen action in the prostate. (From J. Wilson, The pathogenesis of benign prostatic hyperplasia. *Am. J. Med.* 68:745, 1980.)

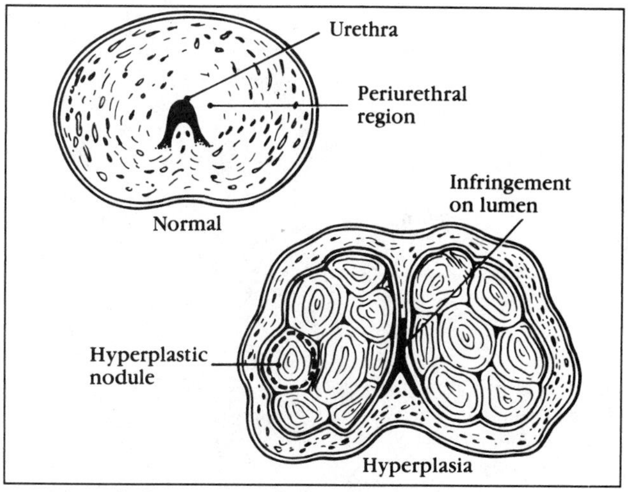

FIGURE 28-4. Comparison of normal prostatic relationship with urethra and hyperplastic infringement on the lumen.

of the hormone in the hyperplastic area than in the normal areas of the same glands. Research has demonstrated the production of BPH in the dog [3, 18, 29].

Estrogen levels increase in the male with aging and act similarly to androgens [15]. Estrogen binds to specific receptors in the cytoplasm and thus goes into the nucleus as a hormone-receptor complex where there is interaction in the chromatin at acceptor sites, resulting in activation of messenger RNA.

Dihydrotestosterone is the hormonal mediator in BPH partly because of decreased catabolism of the molecule and partly because of an increase in intracellular binding of the molecule. Therefore, the process is accelerated because of increased estrogen, which increases the level of the androgen receptor in the gland, thereby resulting in prostatic growth [37].

PATHOLOGY OF THE PROSTATE. Hyperplasia is usually seen in the median and lateral lobes, but the posterior lobe is usually not affected. Seventy-five percent of prostatic carcinomas are found in the posterior lobe [7]. Glands are variable in size and are separated from each other by stroma, including connective tissue and smooth muscle fibers. Enlargement of the lateral lobes compresses the urethra, while enlargement of the medial lobe actually obstructs urine outflow by plugging the urethral orifice (Fig. 28-4) [38].

The hyperplasia, which may be fibromuscular or glandular, results in proliferation of cells, beginning in the periurethral region and causing a smooth and regular appearance of the glands. Located in the adjacent prostatic tissue are areas of ischemia and necrosis encircled by margins of squamous metaplasia. A surgical capsule is formed between the hyperplastic area and the normal tissue. As the periurethral glands enlarge, there is compression of the normal tissue and the urethra.

Clinical Manifestations

When hyperplasia causes significant obstruction, frequency with urination, decrease in force and size of stream, hesitancy, straining to urinate, difficulty in starting and stopping the stream, and inability to empty the bladder will be noted. Complications that may arise from BPH include hydroureter, acute urinary retention of sudden onset, acute renal failure, hematuria, calculi, cystitis, reflux, urinary tract infection, and thickening of the bladder muscles (see Chap. 49).

RENAL CALCULI

Calculi can form in various areas of the renal system. If crystallization occurs in the renal pelvis or calices, it is termed *nephrolithiasis. Urolithiasis* refers to stones anywhere in the urinary tract (Fig. 28-5). The stones may be composed of calcium salts, uric acid, oxalate, cystine, xanthine, and struvite.

When urolithiasis is diagnosed, symptoms may vary from hematuria or oliguria to renal colic. Hematuria results from the damage done by the presence of a stone in the urinary tract, and oliguria may result when the stone obstructs the flow of urine [33, 34]. Renal colic results from spasms as calculi are passed, causing a flank pain that radiates to the abdomen and groin.

Urinary stones or calculi are a common problem. Calculi are present in approximately 0.9 to 5.4 percent of all autopsies [6, 21]. A review of the literature done by Ljunghall and Hedstrand indicated an incidence averaging 7 percent in Scandinavian countries, the United States, and Great Britain [21]. A higher incidence of stones occurs in men, in persons with sedentary life-styles, and in families with a history of stones. The average age for the occurrence of renal stones is 40, but they can occur at any age.

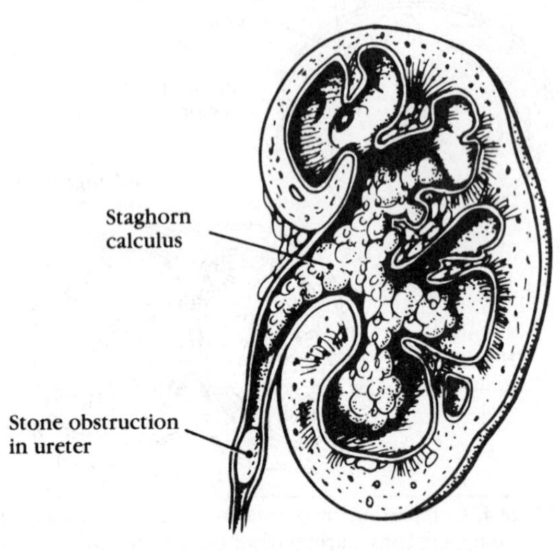

FIGURE 28-5. Staghorn calculus obstructing the entire renal pelvis.

Structure and Composition of Calculi

Calculi vary in shape and size, some being as small as grains of sand while others entirely fill the renal pelvis (staghorn calculi) (Fig. 28-6). They also vary in color, texture, and composition. Stones may occur either unilaterally or bilaterally and may be single or multiple in number.

Stones contain an organic matrix or framework and crystalloids such as calcium, oxalate, phosphate, urate, uric acid, or cystine. The matrix is a mucoprotein that is resorbed by the epithelium of the tubules and then released into the lumen of the tubule, resulting in a site or *nidus* for stone propagation [14].

Factors That May Cause Stone Formation

Stone formation may result from alterations in urine pH, decrease in inhibitors, and supersaturation of urine. All of these factors do not have to be present for urolithiasis to occur. The urine almost always shows an increase in concentration of the stone's constituents [28].

ALTERATIONS IN pH. The solubility of crystalloids is affected by alterations in pH that cause them to leave the urine and attach to the matrix, resulting in crystallization. Stones that form in an acid urine include uric acid, cystine, oxalate, and xanthine stones. In an alkaline urine, a greater incidence of calcium phosphate and struvite stones is seen. Persistent use of medications containing aluminum hydroxide, calcium carbonate, ascorbic acid, and sodium bicarbonate affect the urinary pH and thus increase the risk of stone formation.

DECREASE IN INHIBITORS. A decrease in inhibitors (magnesium, sodium, pyrophosphate, urea, citrate, amino acids, and trace metals) may cause stone formation. The stone must be stable in order to grow to a size that is clinically significant. Urine contains inhibitors for calcium oxalate and calcium phosphate, but not for stones of uric acid, cystine, or struvite [8]. It has been concluded in one study that calculi may result from alterations in several of the urinary components, resulting in abnormal crystal formation or abnormal accumulation of crystals [8].

SUPERSATURATION OF URINE. The main cause of stone formation is a breakdown of the balance between conservation of water and the excretion of materials that are poorly soluble. When the urine becomes saturated with certain materials, crystals may form, aggregating to form a stone [8]. As the insoluble material accumulates the urine reaches a critical point at which it can no longer keep the material in solution. This point is called the *upper limit of metastability* at which time stone growth occurs. Urine pH affects the formation of stones, as some will precipitate in an acid urine while others require an alkaline urine [28].

Types of Stones

Even though many stones are composed of mixtures of substances, stones usually have distinctive characteristics. The majority of renal stones contain calcium, but uric acid, oxalate, cystine, struvite, and xanthine also may predominate.

CALCIUM STONES. Calcium stones are often formed in the presence of hypercalciuria and/or hypercalcemia [24]. Hypercalciuria occurs when there is an increased amount of urinary calcium excretion. Calcium stones are white to grey in color, usually small and soft in texture. Normally, the calcium level in the urine is approximately 75 to 175 mg/24 hours; hypercalciuria occurs when there is a urinary excretion greater than 250 mg/24 hours in women and 300 mg/24 hours in men [31]. Hypercalcemia occurs when the serum calcium exceeds 5 mEq/L in adults [36]. Calcium is excreted in the urine in increased amounts or it may precipitate into the kidney substance (nephrocalcinosis) [12].

There are three major classifications of hypercalciuria: absorptive, resorptive, and renal [26]. Table 28-1 lists the major causes of hypercalcemia and/or hypercalciuria.

Absorptive hypercalciuria results from an exaggerated absorption of calcium from the bowel due to an increased rate of conversion of vitamin D that is often seen with hyperparathyroidism. Absorptive hypercalciuria has also been found with normal levels of serum calcium and phosphorus, normal to low parathyroid hormone levels, and increased filter loads of calcium (Fig. 28-7) [5, 25]. Another explanation for absorptive hypercalciuria is that when there is an increased amount of calcium absorption from the gut, there is an increase in serum calcium, thus causing reduction of parathyroid hormone secretion, which leads to an increased filter load of calcium in the glomerulus.

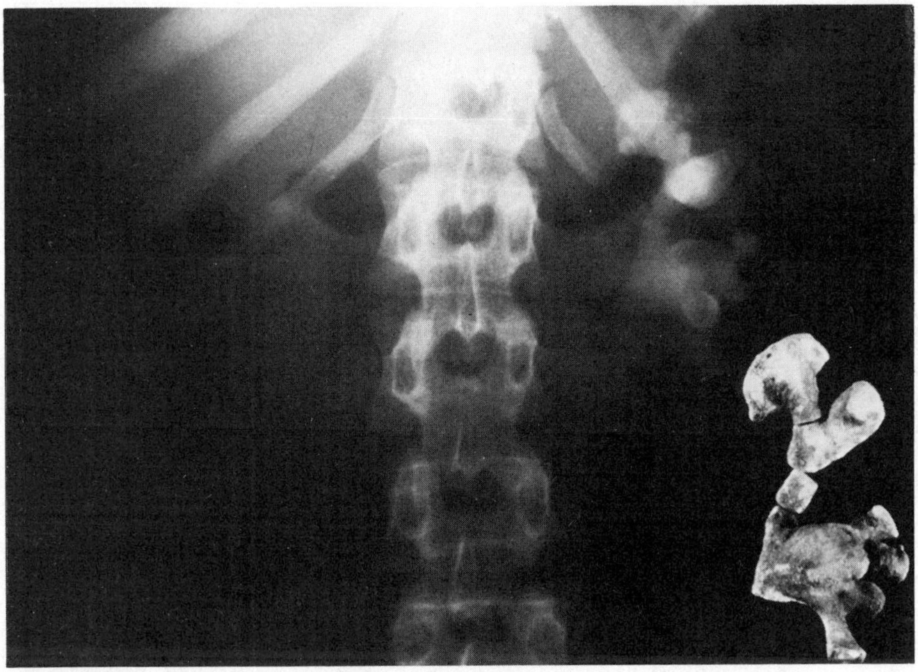

FIGURE 28-6. X-ray appearance of a large staghorn calculus.

TABLE 28-1. Causes of hypercalcemia and hypercalciuria

Increased bone resorption
Hyperparathyroidism—primary and ectopic
Metastatic tumors
Multiple myeloma, lymphoma, leukemia (produce bone-resorbing activity)
Nonmetastatic tumors (produce prostaglandin)
Immobilization osteoporosis
Hyperglucocorticoidism
Hyperthyroidism
Paget's disease
Increased intestinal absorption of calcium
Sarcoidosis
Beryllosis
Absorptive hypercalciuria
Vitamin D excess
Infantile hypercalciuria
Increased calcium intake—milk-alkali syndrome
Renal wasting of calcium
Fanconi syndrome
Renal tubular acidosis
Hypermineralocorticoidism
Renal hypercalciuria

Source: N. A. Knutzman, *Pathophysiology of the Kidney.* Springfield, Ill.: Thomas, 1977.

Resorptive hypercalciuria results when calcium is removed or resorbed from the bone. This can occur in persons who are immobilized, for example, following spinal cord injury. Five to ten percent of persons who are immobilized for prolonged periods of time will develop renal calculi [8]. Stones resulting from resorption abnormality develop over a long period of time (Fig. 28-8).

A renal defect causing hypercalciuria is the result of a tubular defect causing a calcium leak. This defect can be seen in renal tubular acidosis (RTA) in which the distal convoluted tubule and collecting duct are not able to maintain an acid urine. Calcium is not as soluble in an alkaline urine and may precipitate to form stones. In RTA stones may also be the result of a low urinary citrate, an inhibitor of calcium.

Multiple disorders of calcium metabolism result in hypercalcemia including Paget's disease, multiple myeloma, and primary hyperparathyroidism. Sixty to eighty percent of persons with primary hyperparathyroidism at some time develop renal calculi and nephrocalcinosis (the presence of calcium deposits in the renal parenchyma) [16, 26].

URIC ACID STONES. Calculi composed of uric acid cause approximately 10 percent of all kidney stones in persons living in the United States [13]. These stones are yellow to brown in color, smooth and soft in texture, and are formed in an acid urine. Both a urine supersaturated with uric acid and a decreased urinary pH contribute to uric acid stone formation. The more alkaline the urine, the more soluble the sodium urate, but if the urine becomes acid ($pH < 5.5$) and supersaturated, crystallization may occur. In persons with uric acid stones less urinary ammonia is excreted and a more acid urine results.

Hypovolemia, due to dehydration or other causes, contributes to stone formation because of the concentrated uric acid and the low urinary pH that result. Diseases such as the leukemias cause cell necrosis resulting in hyperuricosuria, because purines convert mostly to uric

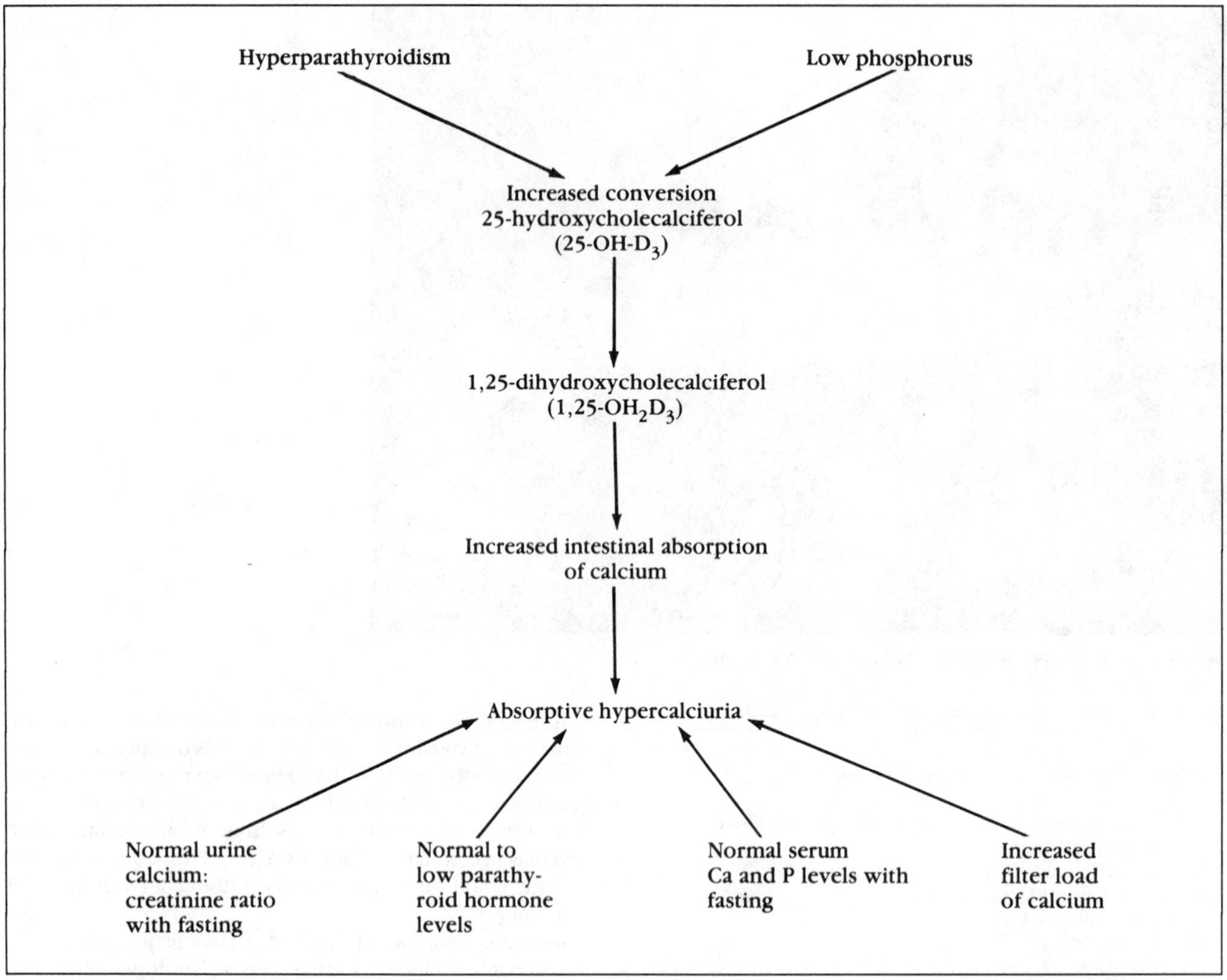

FIGURE 28-7. Absorptive hypercalciuria resulting from hyperparathyroidism or low serum phosphorus.

acids. Massive hyperuricosuria is often seen following chemotherapeutic treatment of certain tumors.

Uric acid stones tend to be staghorn and fill the renal pelvis. They may be reduced in size with medical intervention.

OXALATE STONES. Oxalate stones are hard, gray, and may be smooth or rough in texture. These stones are usually recurrent, and may be formed in a slightly acid or neutral urine. Oxalate, the end product of glycine metabolism, is produced from glyoxylate or glycolate. Oxalate stones can be caused from too much oxalate in a diet, diseases of the intestine, increased amounts of ethylene glycol, and hereditary disorders. Hyperoxaluria may be seen following intestinal bypass surgery and with Crohn's disease.

CYSTINE STONES. Cystine stones are formed in acid urine and are white or yellow in color, small in size, and soft in texture. These stones are characterized by hexagonal crystals that eventually form staghorn calculi. They usually do not occur in adults unless the cystine excretion exceeds 300 mg/day but affected persons often excrete 600 to 1800 mg/day [28]. Cystinuria is due to an inherited renal tubular defect affecting the absorption of the urine amino acids, including cystine, which is the least soluble [20].

STRUVITE OR MAGNESIUM AMMONIUM PHOSPHATE STONES. Struvite stones are the result of urinary tract infection, most commonly with bacteria of the *Proteus* species. These may form following bladder catheterizations and cystoscopies. Chronic antibiotic therapy may predispose the individual to *Proteus* infection. Recurrences of struvite stones have been shown in 27 percent of susceptible persons [8].

The causative bacteria contain the enzyme urease, which functions to split urea into ammonia causing an elevated urinary pH (Fig. 28-9). The organisms are often called "urea-splitters." Staghorn calculi fill the renal pelvis and are

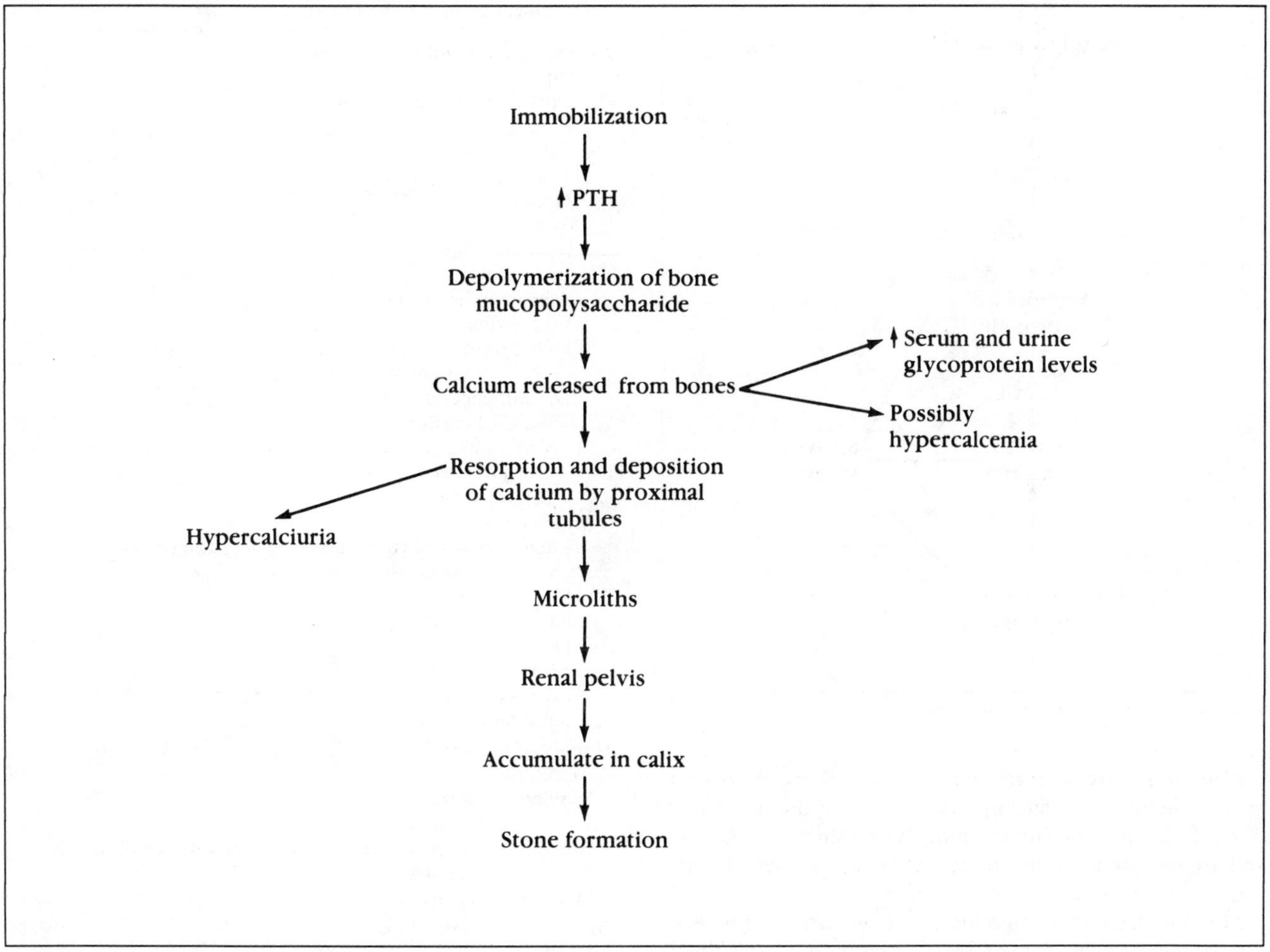

FIGURE 28-8. Resorptive alterations causing stone formation.

difficult to treat. Sometimes a nephrectomy must be performed in order to relieve the obstruction.

XANTHINE STONES. Xanthine stones are rare. They are formed when xanthine is not converted to uric acid, thus causing an increase in excretion of xanthine. This problem is probably the result of a defect in the renal tubules.

RENAL TUMORS

Tumors of the renal system can cause damage to the renal parenchyma whether they are benign or malignant. A renal tumor is usually larger when found by palpation than when it is discovered on a routine radiologic examination. Symptoms are usually late developing and may include complaints of a dull pain in the flank area or hematuria. Renal tumors are classified as benign or malignant and also according to their area of involvement (Table 28-2).

Benign Tumors

Cortical adenomas are usually found during postmortem examinations of elderly people and are the most frequently occurring benign tumors of the kidney. These tumors are usually not larger than 3 cm in diameter and do not produce symptoms unless they enlarge. Two types of cortical adenomas are described [27]:

1. A *solid* type, which can be found in the subcapsular area and the cortex of the kidney and appears yellow, soft, and round
2. A *cystic* type, which is found in the cortex of the kidney and is encapsulated

These adenomas are believed to originate from the tubular epithelium and may be responsible for painless hematuria. They may be difficult to distinguish histologically from small, well-differentiated renal cell carcinomas [28].

Angiomyolysomas are located either in the cortex or in the renal pelvis. These tumors are composed of a combination of blood vessels, fat, and smooth muscle. They usually remain asymptomatic unless they are bilateral when they may cause uremia and death [10]. These tumors may be found in persons with tuberous sclerosis, a familial disease of children characterized by mental retardation, epilepsy, and sebaceous adenomas of the skin.

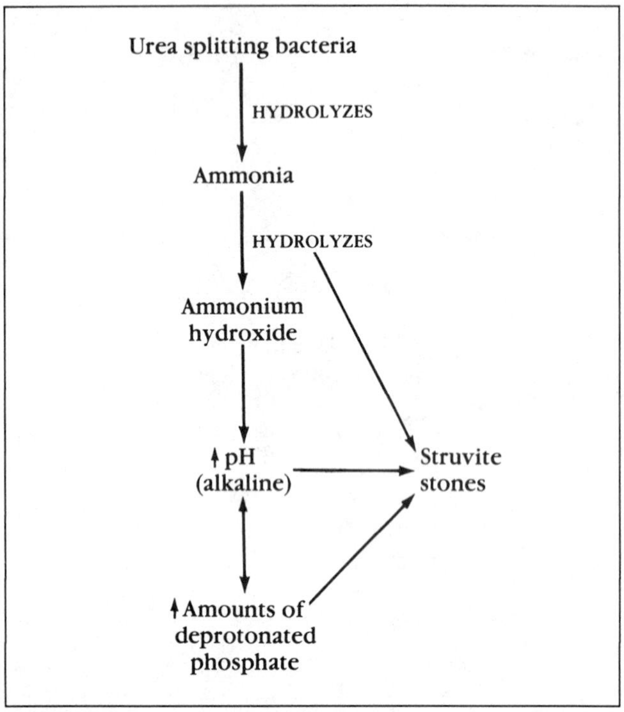

FIGURE 28-9. Formation of struvite stones.

Hemangiomas are rare, benign tumors that can result in massive hematuria, causing renal colic as blood clots pass through the ureters. These tumors have thin-walled sinuses and are usually found in the renal medulla or pelvis. They usually occur singly and are unilateral.

Lipomas are rare, benign tumors originating mainly from the paranephric fat. These tumors, which are usually small in diameter, can be found in the parenchyma, renal capsule, and paranephric tissue.

Juxtaglomerular cell tumors originate from the juxtaglomerular apparatus and are associated with high blood pressure. Histologically, mast cells are frequent with various shapes and sizes of granules in the cytoplasm [28].

TABLE 28-2. Classification of renal tumors

Tumors of the renal parenchyma
- Benign
  - Cortical (tubular) adenoma
    - Solid
    - Cystic
  - Fibroma
  - Lipoma
  - Myxoma
  - Angioma
  - Lymphangioma
  - Hemangiopericytoma
  - Leiomyoma
  - Mixed tumor with combination of above elements (e.g., angiomyolipoma, myxolipoma)
  - Dysontogenetic rests
    - Adrenal cortical rests
    - Chondral and osseous rests
    - Dermoid cysts
    - Endometrioma
- Malignant
  - Adenocarcinoma (tubular) (Grawitz's tumor, hypernephroma)
  - Wilms' tumor
  - Fibrosarcoma
  - Liposarcoma
  - Leiomyosarcoma
  - Angiosarcoma and other compounded sarcomas
  - Metastatic tumors

Tumors of the renal pelvis
- Papilloma
- Papillary transitional cell (epidermoid) or squamous cell carcinoma
- Nonpapillary transitional cell (epidermoid) squamous cell carcinoma
- Mucous adenocarcinoma

Tumors of the renal capsule
- Fibroma
- Lipoma
- Angioma
- Leiomyoma
- Myxoma
- Tumors with combinations of the above elements and their malignant counterpart

Tumors of the paranephric tissue
- Tumors of type found in renal capsule
- Extraosseous osteogenic sarcoma

Source: A. Allen, *The Kidney: Medical and Surgical Diseases* (2nd ed.). New York: Grune & Stratton, 1962.

Malignant Tumors

RENAL CELL CARCINOMAS. Renal carcinomas usually occur between the ages of 50 to 70, are more common in males, and compose 85 to 89 percent of the tumors of the kidney [10]. A higher percentage of renal adenocarcinomas is reported among users of tobacco products. Renal carcinomas or cysts often occur in association with Hippel-Lindau disease, which is a hereditary defect involving angiomas of the retina and cerebellum. Metastasis of renal carcinomas to the lungs, lymph nodes, liver, and other areas is common [19].

Renal carcinomas arise from tubular epithelium and can occur anywhere in the kidney. They vary in size from a few centimeters to multiple centimeters in which the weight may be in kilograms (Fig. 28-10). The tumor may proliferate throughout the kidney to the ureters, invading the hilum, to the renal vein, and the inferior vena cava. The color of these tumors varies from white to yellow to gray [2].

The tumor margins are usually clearly defined, causing pressure on the renal parenchyma. The tumor often spreads or bulges into the renal calices and may extend to the ureter. The tumors characteristically invade the venous system and spread by vascular metastases to the lungs, bone, lymph nodes, liver, and brain. Metastases may occur

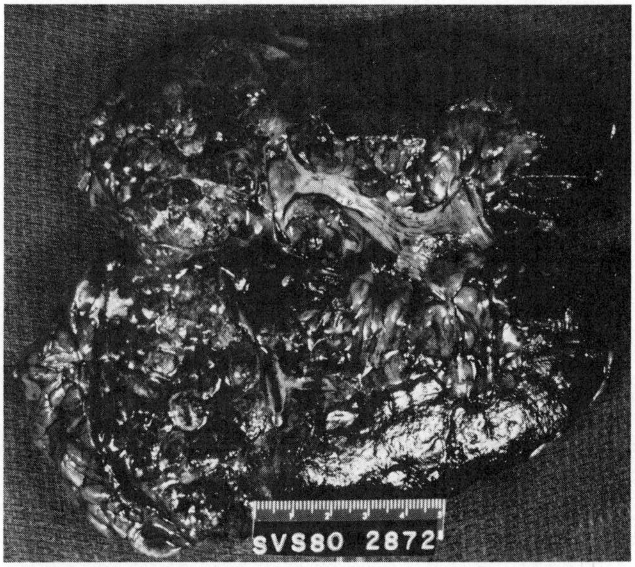

FIGURE 28-10. Renal carcinoma showing enlargement and infiltration of the kidney parenchyma.

TABLE 28-3. Staging of renal carcinomas

TNM staging			
Clinical	Pathologic	Extent of disease	Robson stage
T1	pT1	Tumor within capsule (small)	I
T2	pT2	Tumor within capsule (large)	
T3	pT3	Tumor in perinephric fat	II
T3	V1	Tumor in renal vein	
N1–N3	pN1–pN3	Tumor in regional lymph nodes	III
	V2	Tumor in vena cava	
T4	pT4	Adjacent organ invasion	
M1	pM1	Distant metastases	IV
N4	pN4	Tumor in juxtaregional lymph nodes	

Source: G. Sufrin and G. P. Murphy, Renal adenocarcinoma. *Urol. Surv.* 30:129, 1980.

to almost any organ [19]. Morphologically, the cells may be very anaplastic, giant cells, or clear cells, or they may be more well differentiated.

Another characteristic of renal cell carcinoma is that the abnormal cells produce hormones or hormonelike substances such as erythropoietin, parathyroidlike hormone, renin, gonadotropins, or glucocorticosteroids [28]. The effects of these secretions may lead to diagnosis of the tumor.

The behavior of the tumor is unpredictable, with rapid growth and metastasis being followed by years of slow growth. Metastasis may disappear following nephrectomy.

Symptoms are variable with microscopic or macroscopic hematuria being the most consistent feature. Other symptoms include flank pain, fever, weight loss, and tumor mass that may be palpated.

Regardless of the type and pattern of renal cell carcinoma, there is significant consistency in the staging of tumors (Table 28-3). Prognosis is made from multiple factors that include the staging, the number of the metastases, cellular type, and the size and weight of the tumor [32].

TABLE 28-4. Wilms' tumor study: staging of tumors of the kidney

Stage I	Tumor limited to the kidney and completely resected
Stage II	Tumor extending beyond the kidney but completely resected
Stage III	Residual nonhematogenous tumor confined to abdomen
Stage IV	Hematogenous metastasis
Stage V	Bilateral renal involvement either initially or subsequently

Source: M. Forland, *Nephrology* (2nd ed.). Garden City, N.Y.: Medical Exam., 1983.

WILMS' TUMOR. *Wilms' tumor* is a very malignant tumor that accounts for 6 to 30 percent of abdominal tumors in children, usually occurring between 2 and 5 years of age [23]. By the time the tumor is discovered, a very large abdominal mass is often palpable. Other symptoms that may develop include microscopic hematuria, pain, fever, vomiting, and hypertension due to renal ischemia. Pulmonary metastasis is often present at the time of diagnosis.

Wilms' tumor is grey to yellow, circular in shape with a fibrous capsule, and frequently has solid, cystic, and hemorrhagic areas. Histologically, the tumor contains proliferating embryonic connective tissue with dense nuclei. The glomeruli are primitive with a poorly formed Bowman's capsule, and they lack a basement membrane [23]. At first the tumor is surrounded by a dense capsule and grows by pushing the renal parenchyma out of its path. When the capsule ruptures, metastasis to the lungs, lymphatic system, liver, and brain occurs rapidly.

Multiple factors determine the prognosis for this tumor, but one of the main factors is the stage at the time of diagnosis. The National Wilms' Tumor Study has adopted the staging system seen in Table 28-4 [10]. Long-term survival rates have improved to 90 percent with treatment by chemotherapy, radiotherapy, and surgery [22, 28].

TUMORS OF THE RENAL PELVIS. Of the malignant tumors of the kidneys, the renal pelvic tumors account for 4.5 to 9.0 percent [11]. The papillary tumors have a cauliflower appearance when in the renal pelvis. An RNA virus has been isolated from the papillary tumors, but its importance is not yet understood [9]. Of the renal pelvic tumors, 85 percent are papillary transitional cell carcinomas and when diagnosed, more than one-half of the latter have invaded the pelvic musculature [4, 11].

REFERENCES

1. Bartsch, W., et al. Hormone blood levels and their interrelationships in normal men and men with benign prostatic hyperplasia (BPH). *Acta Endocrinol.* (Copenh.) 90:727, 1979.
2. Bennington, J. L. Histopathology of Renal Adenocarcinoma. In G. Sufrin and S. A. Beckley (eds.), *Renal Adenocarcinoma.* (report No. 10). Geneva: International Union Against Cancer, 1980.
3. Berg, O. A. The normal prostate gland in the dog. *Acta Endocrinol.* (Copenh.) 27:129, 1958.
4. Bloom, N. A., Vidone, R. A., and Lytton, B. Primary carcinoma of the ureter: A report of 102 new cases. *J. Urol.* 103:590, 1970.
5. Bordier, P., et al. On the pathogenesis of so-called idiopathic hypercalciuria. *Am. J. Med.* 63:398, 1977.
6. Brod, J. *The Kidney*. London: Butterworth, 1973.
7. Brosig, W. Conservative Treatment of Benign Prostatic Hypertrophy. In H. Marberger, et al. (eds.), *Prostatic Disease: Proceedings*. New York: Liss, 1976.
8. Coe, F. L. Nephrolithiasis: Causes, classification and management. *Hosp. Pract.* 16:33, 1981.
9. Elliott, A. Y., et al. Isolation of RNA virus from papillary tumors of the human renal pelvis. *Science* 179:393, 1973.
10. Forland, M. (ed.). *Nephrology.* Garden City, N.Y.: Medical Exam., 1977.
11. Frayley, E. E. Cancer of the Renal Pelvis. In D. G. Skinner and J. B. deKernion (eds.), *Genitourinary Cancer.* Philadelphia: Saunders, 1978.
12. Grimes, W. A. Phase contrast study of mechanisms of renal calcification. *J. Urol.* 78:553, 1957.
13. Gutman, A. B., and Yii, T. F. Uric acid nephrolithiasis. *Am. J. Med.* 45:756, 1968.
14. Hallson, P. C., and Rose, G. A. Uromucoids and urinary stone formation. *Lancet* 1:100, 1979.
15. Hammond, G. L., et al. Serum steroids in normal males and patients with prostatic disease. *Clin. Endocinol.* (Oxf.) 9:113, 1978.
16. Hellström, I. Calcification and calculus formation in a series of seventy cases of primary hyperparathyroidism. *Br. J. Urol.* 27:387, 1955.
17. Higgins, S. I., and Gehring, U. Molecular mechanisms of steroid hormone action. *Adv. Cancer Res.* 28:313, 1978.
18. Jacobi, H., Moore, R. J., and Wilson, J. D. Studies on the mechanisms of 32 androstanediol-induced growth of the dog prostate. *Endocrinology* 102:1748, 1978.
19. Karakousis, C. P., and Jennings, E. Renal cell carcinoma metastatic to skeletal muscle mass: A case report. *J. Surg. Oncol.* 17:287, 1982.
20. Kleeman, C. R., et al. Kidney stones: Interdepartmental clinic conference (UCLA School of Medicine). *West. J. Med.* 132:313, 1980.
21. Ljunghall, S., and Hedstrand, H. Epidemiology of renal stones in a middle age population. *Acta Med. Scand.* 197:439, 1975.
22. Margolis, W. S. Chemotherapy in Wilms' tumor. *Cancer* 32:1150, 1973.
23. Marsden, H. B., and Stewart, J. K. *Wilms' Tumors: Recent Results in Cancer Research. Tumors in Children* (vol. 13). New York: Springer-Verlag, 1968.
24. Melick, R. A., and Henneman, P. H. Clinical laboratory studies of 207 consecutive patients in a kidney-stone clinic. *N. Engl. J. Med.* 259:307, 1958.
25. Pak, C. Y., et al. A simple test for the diagnosis of absorptive, resorptive and renal hypercalciurias. *N. Engl. J. Med.*, 292:497, 1975.
26. Pak, C. Y. C., et al. The hypercalciurias: Causes, parathyroid function and diagnostic criteria. *J. Clin. Invest.* 54:387, 1974.
27. Pearse, H. D., and Houghton, D. C. Renal oncocytoma. *Urology* 13:74, 1979.
28. Robbins, S. L., and Cotran, R. *Pathologic Basis of Disease* (2nd ed.). Philadelphia: Saunders, 1979.
29. Schlotthauer, C. F. Observations on the prostate gland of the dog. *Trans. Am. Vet. Med. Assoc.* 81:645, 1932.
30. Siiteri, P. K., and Wilson, J. D. Dihydrotestosterone in prostatic hypertrophy: I. The formation and content of dihydrotestosterone in the hypertrophic prostate of man. *J. Clin. Invest.* 49:1737, 1970.
31. Sudo, M., et al. Renal hemodynamics in uranyl acetate-induced acute renal failure of rabbits. *Kidney Int.* 11:35, 1977.
32. Sufrin, G., and Murphy, G. P. Renal adenocarcinoma (review article). *Urol. Surv.* 30:129, 1980.
33. Summers, W. K., and Jamisan, R. L. The no reflow phenomenon in renal ischemia. *Lab. Invest.* 25:635, 1971.
34. Venkatachalam, M. A., et al. Ischemic damage and repair in the rat proximal tubule: Differences among the S_1, S_2 and S_3 segments. *Kidney Int.* 14:31, 1978.
35. Vermeulen, A., and DeSy, W. Androgens in patients with benign prostatic hyperplasia before and after prostatectomy. *J. Clin. Endocrinol. Metab.* 43:1250, 1976.
36. Wallach, J. *Interpretation of Diagnostic Tests* (3rd ed.). Boston: Little, Brown, 1978.
37. Walsh, P. C., and Wilson, J. D. The induction of prostatic hypertrophy in the dog with androstanodiol. *J. Clin. Invest.* 57:1093, 1976.
38. Wilson, J. D. The pathogenesis of benign prostatic hyperplasia. *Am. J. Med.* 68:745, 1980.

CHAPTER 29
RENAL FAILURE AND UREMIA

LEARNING OBJECTIVES

1. Define *acute renal failure (ARF).*
2. Define *azotemia* and *oliguria.*
3. List three causes of ARF.
4. Describe prerenal, renal, and postrenal causes of ARF.
5. Discuss the two major causes of acute tubular necrosis (ATN).
6. List some of the drugs that can cause nephrotoxic renal failure.
7. Describe the pathologic features of nephrotoxic and ischemic ATN.
8. Discuss the back-leak theory and tubule obstruction in relationship to oliguria.
9. Discuss the theories concerning the pathogenesis of oliguria.
10. Explain arterial occlusion and prostaglandins in relationship to oliguria.
11. Identify four stages of ARF including onset, oliguric, diuretic, and postdiuretic stage.
12. Discuss the pathology of water imbalance, hyponatremia, hyperkalemia, metabolic acidosis, anemia, elevated creatinine, phosphate, and urea during the oliguric stage of ARF.
13. Identify the clinical manifestations characteristic of the diuretic phase of ARF.
14. Define *chronic renal failure (CRF).*
15. List causes and stages of CRF.
16. Discuss the intact nephron theory and its relationship to CRF.
17. Discuss fluid imbalances in CRF.
18. Define *hypothenuria, polyuria,* and *isosthenuria.*
19. Explain how hyponatremia and hypernatremia can occur in CRF.
20. Identify causes of hyperkalemia and hypokalemia in CRF.
21. Discuss three mechanisms that occur in metabolic acidosis in CRF.
22. Explain the relationship of metabolic acidosis and osteodystrophy in CRF.
23. Identify mechanisms that regulate calcium and phosphorus levels.
24. Discuss hyperparathyroidism and vitamin D metabolism in relationship to bone disease.
25. Explain six factors leading to anemia in CRF.
26. Identify the etiology of purpura.
27. Discuss urea metabolism and carbohydrate intolerance.
28. Define *uremia.*

29. List symptoms and causes of the altered neurologic system in relationship to uremia.
30. Identify causes of hypertension in relationship to uremia.
31. List and discuss cardiac abnormalities in relationship to uremia.
32. Discuss the effects of uremia on the respiratory system, including uremic lung, uremic pleuritis, pulmonary edema, and infections.
33. Identify gastrointestinal symptoms in relationship to uremia.
34. Discuss gastrointestinal abnormalities in relationship to uremia, including ulcerations, oral changes, bleeding, and constipation.
35. Define *renal osteodystrophy.*
36. List the causes of renal osteodystrophy.
37. Define *osteomalacia, osteitis fibrosa, soft tissue metastatic calcification,* and *osteosclerosis.*
38. Identify the major hematologic infection in persons with CRF.
39. Discuss dermatologic alterations in relationship to uremia.

Renal failure is the result of failure by the kidneys to remove accumulated metabolites from the blood. The process causes alterations in electrolyte, acid-base, and water balance, as well as the accumulation of substances that are normally totally excreted by the body.

ACUTE RENAL FAILURE

Acute renal failure (ARF) is a clinical syndrome in which the kidneys are unable to excrete the waste products of metabolism, usually because of renal hypoperfusion. This syndrome may lead to *azotemia,* which is the accumulation of nitrogenous waste products in the blood, and to *oliguria,* in which the urinary output is less than 400 ml/24 hours. Approximately 40 percent of ARF cases are non-oliguric.

According to research done by Levinsky and Alexander [23], ARF can result from different causes. The research showed that of 2200 cases of ARF, 43 percent were related to surgery or trauma, 26 percent of individuals had various medical conditions, 13 percent of cases were related to pregnancy, and 9 percent were caused by nephrotoxins. The causes of ARF have been divided into the following three major categories: prerenal, renal, and postrenal.

Causes of ARF

PRERENAL CAUSES. Prerenal acute renal failure results from diminished plasma volume that leads to diminished cardiac output and diminished renal perfusion. Prerenal failure may occur as a result of hypovolemia (e.g., dehydration; hemorrhage; ascites, in which there is pooling of fluid) or from circulatory insufficiency (e.g., shock, congestive heart failure, arrhythmias, prolonged hypotension).

Renal ischemia as a result of central or circulating hypovolemia is a frequent cause of acute tubular necrosis (see p. 387) [9]. The rate and volume of fluid loss determine the degree of circulatory failure. Central hypovolemia may be related to peripheral pooling in septic shock from gram-negative bacteria [9].

RENAL CAUSES. The second major category of ARF results from renal parenchymal changes that damage the nephron [34]. Many factors may cause this condition and the major ones are discussed in this section.

Acute glomerulonephritis may follow streptococcal infection or may result from systemic lupus erythematosus (SLE). These two conditions result from an immunologic reaction causing glomerular abnormalities. The pathologic abnormalities include proliferation of the glomerular cells, necrosis of glomerular capillaries, or exudation of leukocytes into the glomerulus.

Vascular diseases of the kidney may occur following renal occlusion, polyarteritis nodosa, hypersensitivity angiitis, nephrosclerosis, or renal vein thrombosis. The vascular renal diseases are due to abnormalities that may lead to narrowing of the arteries, thickened afferent arterioles, or inflammation and necrosing of the arterial wall.

Severe interstitial nephritis may be seen with acute pyelonephritis, papillary necrosis, sepsis, and certain nephrotoxic drugs. Acute interstitial nephritis often results from hypersensitivity to a pharmacologic agent. This affects the renal interstitium causing edema and infiltration of the area by lymphocytes, eosinophils, and plasma cells.

Acute tubular necrosis (ATN) refers to acute damage to the renal tubular epithelium. Because ATN is the major cause of acute renal failure, it will be discussed in more detail in the following section.

Other causes of ARF include multiple myeloma, hepatorenal syndrome, pregnancy, and acute urate nephropathy.

POSTRENAL CAUSES. The third major category of ARF is postrenal, in which there is obstruction of the urinary tract resulting from urethral obstruction, calculi, benign prostatic hypertrophy, and tumors (see Chap. 28). A unique feature of postrenal failure is that complete cessation of urine flow (anuria) occurs, which does not always happen in renal or prerenal failure.

Acute Tubular Necrosis (ATN)

ETIOLOGY. The two most common causes of ATN are ischemia and nephrotoxic agent exposure (Table 29-1). Ischemia is the most frequent cause, with the duration of renal ischemia determining the extent of damage and the prognosis for return of urinary function. Venkatachalam and associates found that ischemia present for 25 minutes or less caused mild and reversible damage [4]. Studies by Cronin and associates showed that 2 hours of ischemia caused severe and irreversible damage [10].

Nephrotoxic agents cause destruction of tubular cells by direct cellular toxic effects, lysis of RBCs, and intravascular coagulation, precipitation of oxalate and uric acid crystals, and tissue hypoxia [9]. Factors that enhance nephrotoxicity of agents include the hydration status, preexisting renal disease, and the age of the person.

As one ages, the number of nephrons decreases so that drugs become more concentrated in the tubules. Lane and associates found that persons over 75 years of age exposed to nephrotoxic drugs have a much higher incidence of nephrotoxicity than those persons between the ages of 16 and 30 [21].

Antibiotics, including the aminoglycosides, penicillins, cephalosporins, tetracyclines, amphotericin B, and sulfonamides, probably cause the greatest incidence of renal disruption [28].

Radiographic contrast materials containing iodine, solvents, heavy metals, and pigments of hemoglobin and myoglobin also can cause ATN [28].

PATHOLOGY. In the *ischemic type of ATN* a patchy necrosis occurs in the tubules (Fig. 29-1). The main area of necrosis is the straight portion of the proximal tubules, but lesions also occur in the distal tubules.

If severe injury has been sustained, injury to the basement membrane occurs and causes exposure of the tubular lumen to the interstitial space. The mitochondria in the epithelium have been noted to be swollen when viewed with the electron microscope [11]. The areas in which lesions are absent have dilated tubules and flattened epithelium. Damage to the brush border of the proximal tubule cells also results [15, 34].

A characteristic finding of ischemic ATN is the blockage of tubule lumina by casts. Other abnormalities include appearance of leukocytes in the vasa recta, dilation of Bowman's space of the glomerulus, interstitial edema, and inflammatory cells in the interstitium. The glomeruli appear to be normal [11].

In the *nephrotoxic type of ATN* a more uniform appearance is characteristic. Lesions are located in the proximal tubules, but also may occur in the basement membrane and distal tubules when severe injury has been sustained. Usually, less basement membrane disruption occurs with nephrotoxic ATN than ischemic ATN.

Casts, which are debris from cells, obstruct the distal tubules, and necrosis is seen in all nephrons. Interstitial edema, leukocytes in the vasa recta, and inflammatory cells in the interstitium are characteristic.

TABLE 29-1. Nephrotoxic and ischemic mechanisms for the production of acute tubular necrosis

Nephrotoxins
Antibiotics: aminoglycosides (e.g., gentamicin), penicillins, tetracyclines, amphotericin B, sulfonamides
Other drugs and chemicals: phenylbutazone, anesthetic agents, fungicides, pesticides, calcium sodium edetate
Radiographic contrast materials
Organic solvents: carbon tetrachloride, ethylene glycol, phenol, methyl alcohol
Heavy metals: mercury, arsenic, bismuth, cadmium, gold, lead, thallium, uranium
Heme pigments: hemoglobin, myoglobin
Ischemia
Hypovolemia (dehydration, hemorrhage, pooling of fluids in burns or ascites)
Circulatory insufficiency (shock, severe heart failure, arrhythmias, tamponade)

Source: S. Papper, *Clinical Nephrology* (2nd ed.). Boston: Little, Brown, 1978.

PATHOPHYSIOLOGY. *Oliguria* is a cardinal feature of the early stages of ARF with vascular or tubular etiology. However, not all forms of ARF exhibit oliguria, but progressive azotemia occurs due to the impaired renal function. The possible mechanisms for the production of oliguria are shown in Figure 29-2. These are further described below.

Research suggests that *tubular factors* are the primary sources in the pathogenesis of renal insufficiency (Fig. 29-3) [6]. If oliguria is the result of a tubular abnormality, then it is believed to be the result either of *backleakage* or *intratubular obstruction*. Back-leak is one of the oldest theories proposed for the cause of oliguria. It is believed that back-leak is the result of the damaged tubular cells with increased resorption by the renal capillaries [34]. The uranyl nitrate model supports the back-leak proposal.

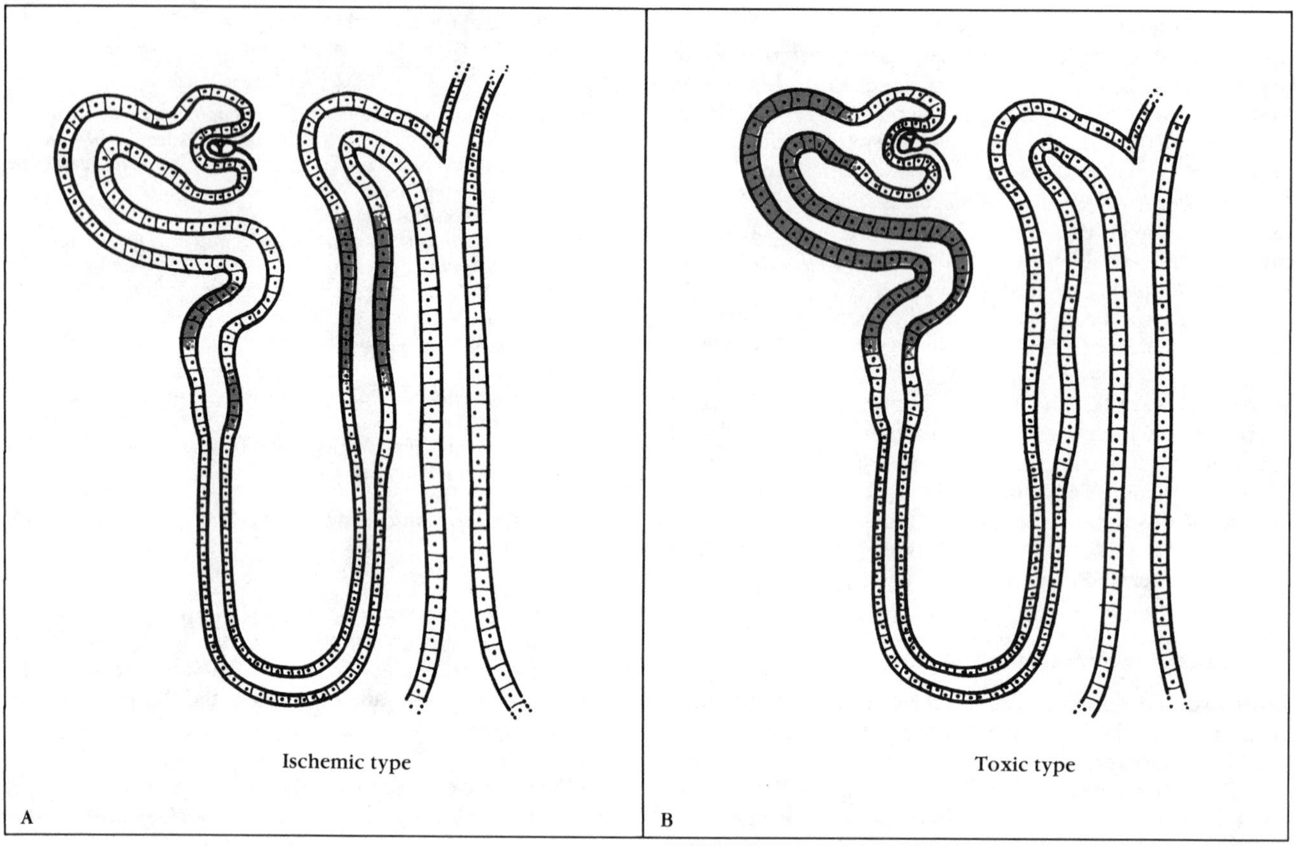

FIGURE 29-1. A. Patchy ischemic necrosis of the proximal tubules. B. Characteristic nephrotoxic injury of large segments of proximal tubule.

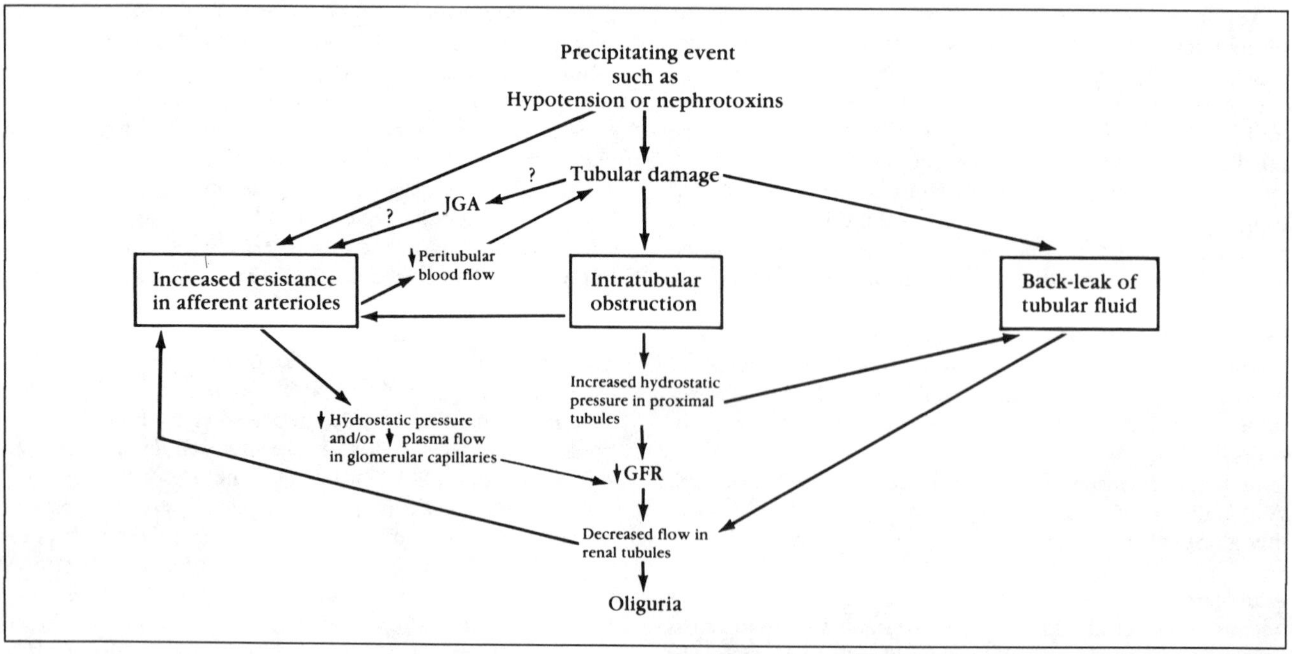

FIGURE 29-2. Possible schema for the causation of oliguria in acute renal failure in which the three major theories of its etiology may be reconciled. The theories are stated in the boxes and the arrows indicate the possible interrelationships among them. (From H. Valtin, *Renal Dysfunction*. Boston: Little, Brown, 1979.)

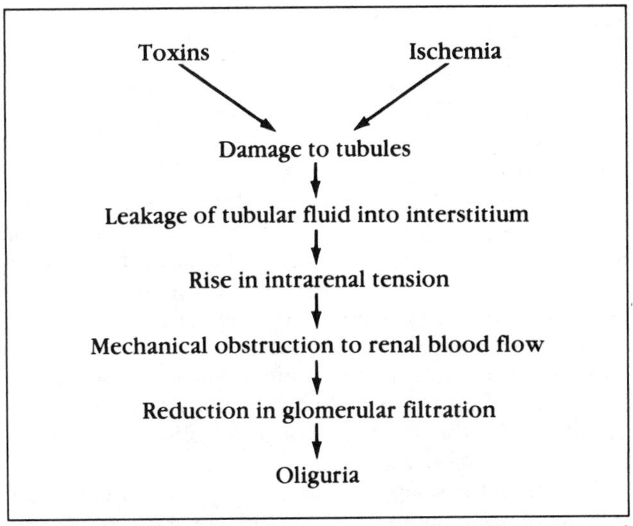

FIGURE 29-3. Chain of events that lead to oliguria in acute renal failure. (From R. Heptinstall, *Pathology of the Kidney* [3rd ed.]. Boston: Little, Brown, 1983.)

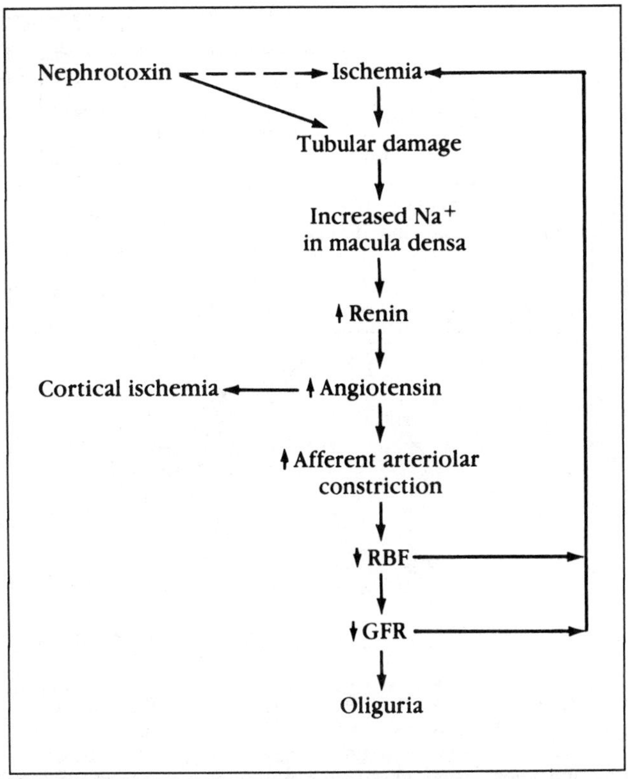

FIGURE 29-4. The possible role of the renin-angiotensin system in the development and maintenance of oliguria (and cortical ischemia) in acute tubular necrosis. (From S. Papper, *Clinical Nephrology* [2nd ed.]. Boston: Little, Brown, 1978.)

When uranyl nitrate is administered to animals there are varying degrees of damage to the pars recta; polyuria occurs in the first 24 to 48 hours with oliguria occurring later [5, 14, 15, 25, 26]. A decrease in the glomerular ultrafiltration coefficient causes a decrease in the GFR. Electron microscopy has shown that there is a reduction in number and size of glomerular capillary endothelial fenestrae between 2 and 17 hours after uranyl nitrate injection [2]. Therefore, tubule leakage appears to be significant in this mode.

Tubular obstruction is believed to be due to casts, debris, and/or interstitial edema. Obstruction may be better understood by examining the *arterial occlusion mode.* If arterial occlusion is induced in rats for 1 hour, oliguria may be present for 1 week or longer and renal blood flow is reduced about one-half [1, 6]. When inulin is administered the clearance test indicates a reduction by 60 to 90 percent [25].

When there is occlusion of the renal arteries, a great number of straight proximal tubules become occluded by swollen blebs of microvilli separated from the brush border of the convoluted segment [14]. Therefore, the arterial occlusion model indicates obstruction, tubular leakage, and vasoconstriction, all of which contribute to the acute renal failure.

If there is no structural damage to the glomeruli, then oliguria may result from *vascular changes,* especially renal artery vasoconstriction. In early stages of ARF, renal vasoconstriction occurs in the renal cortex, resulting in ischemia and a reduction in GFR, and leading to oliguria.

The relationship of the renin-angiotensin-aldosterone (RAA) system to vasoconstriction and oliguria is currently being studied. Renin is released when there is a low plasma volume. In ARF experimental studies have shown increased renin levels (Fig. 29-4) [8, 13, 32].

Thurau and associates have presented a hypothesis regarding vasomotor mechanism (Fig. 29-5). This hypothesis states that initially, when there is renal ischemia, tubular volume is reduced and less sodium chloride is resorbed into the blood. As a result, there is an increase in sodium chloride concentration in the tubular fluid, which is somehow sensed by the juxtaglomerular apparatus (JGA), which then secretes renin. The secretion of renin causes conversion of angiotensinogen to angiotensin, finally leading to vasoconstriction. Thus, constriction of the afferent arteriole results and leads to a decreased GFR, an increased blood urea nitrogen (BUN), and oliguria. The evidence for this hypothesis is conflicting [34].

OTHER THEORIES. Another theory that may explain oliguria in relationship to ARF is that in studies of arterial occlusion in the rat a reduction of renal blood flow occurs, which leads to swelling of the capillary endothelium with the accumulation of sodium and water [17, 22, 32].

Increased vascular resistance due to deficient synthesis of a prostaglandin, a renal vasodilator, is another theory being studied [16, 20]. Further study is necessary to determine the significance of prostaglandin deficiency in ARF.

STAGES OF ARF. The course of ARF can vary tremendously among individuals with different physiologic problems. The four stages of ARF include the (1) onset, (2) oliguric, (3) diuretic, and (4) postdiuretic stages.

Onset is the initial or inciting event that causes necrosis of the convoluted tubules. The course of ARF is related to

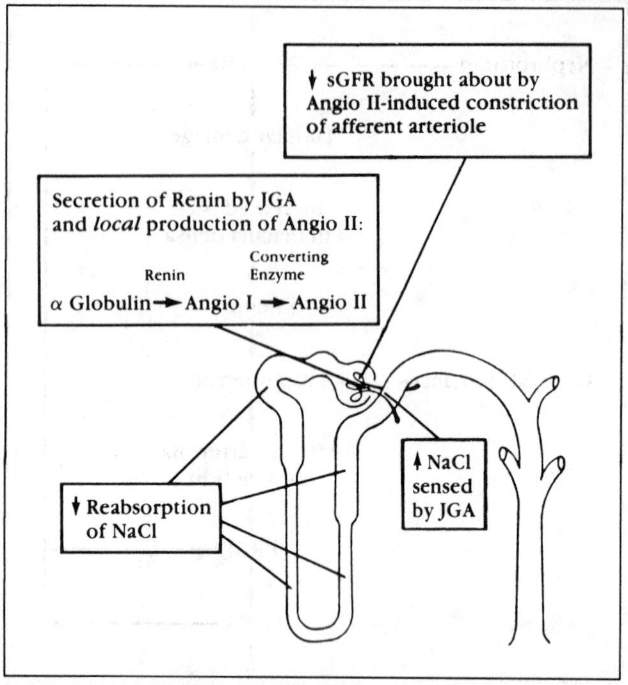

FIGURE 29-5. One theory of the pathogenesis of oliguric acute renal failure. The process is described in the text. JGA = juxtaglomerular apparatus; angio = angiotensin; SGFR = filtration rate of a single glomerulus. (From H. Valtin, *Renal Dysfunction*. Boston: Little, Brown, 1979.)

the magnitude of the inciting insult, the period of hypotension, and the length of time the hemodynamics are altered [9].

In the stage of *oliguria*, about 50 to 100 ml/24 hours of urine is formed. If complete cessation of urine production occurs, a renal obstruction should be investigated. Two major characteristics exhibited during this stage are a urine-specific gravity of approximately 1.010 and spilling of protein in the urine.

Renal blood flow (RBF) is decreased to about one-third of normal, but the GFR falls to less than 1 percent of normal [12]. Because of this, the fluid and electrolyte balance becomes greatly altered.

Water imbalance may occur due to exogenous administration of fluids during the early critical stage. Excess body water may also be related to fat catabolism with a demonstration of mild to moderate hyponatremia. As much as 300 ml of water per day may result from protein and fat catabolism [12]. The hyponatremia that occurs during the oliguric phase is mainly due to the dilution of extracellular fluid, but it also may be due to gastrointestinal disturbances, such as vomiting and diarrhea.

Hyperkalemia often occurs during the oliguric stage. This major electrolyte disturbance is due mostly to decreased renal excretion but also may be related to excessive breakdown of muscle protein. Some other factors that may cause excess potassium to be released from the cells include tissue trauma, acidosis, hypercatabolism, and infection. Potassium levels may rise rapidly and lead to fatal cardiac arrhythmias (see Chaps. 5 and 6).

Metabolic acidosis is sometimes present in the oliguric stage. Because of tubular necrosis, hydrogen is not excreted from the kidneys appropriately and accumulates in the blood.

If ARF persists for 2 to 3 days, nearly all individuals develop a moderate to severe anemia. Anemia is the result of multiple factors, including a mild increase of hemolysis, suppressed erythropoiesis (probably due to lack of erythropoietin and uremic toxins), and increased blood loss from uremic coagulation defects (see p. 396). There are no deficits of iron, B_{12}, or folic acid in the anemia.

Elevations of creatinine, phosphate, and urea result from breakdown of muscle protein and inability to excrete metabolites. With the increase of urea and other nitrogenous wastes in the blood, azotemia progresses.

The *diuretic stage* is characterized by more than 1000 ml of urine output per 24 hours. The diuresis may begin as early as 24 hours after the onset of ARF or it may begin much later. The increased output, as much as 6 liters/day, does not indicate total return of renal function. Tubular function remains altered, which is indicated by the large amounts of sodium and potassium lost in the urine. The serum urea, creatinine, and other accumulated substances act as osmotic diuretics. They also continue to rise during the first days of diuresing. Dehydration may occur due to the inability to conserve water.

Laboratory values indicate a progression toward normal levels and increased production of red blood cells is noted. Wide fluctuations in fluid and electrolyte balance are common during this stage.

The *postdiuretic, or recovery, stage* begins when the urinary output returns to normal. Eventually, sometimes up to a 12-month period, there will be return of GFR, RBF, and tubular function so that the kidneys can again concentrate urine appropriately. Fluid and electrolyte balance improves with alteration in protein intake and prevention of fluid overloading.

PROGNOSIS. The prognosis for individuals with ARF depends on the underlying cause, the onset and severity of the disease, and medical intervention. The mortality varies from 30 to 60 percent with the highest risks being in the traumatized, postoperative, or aged population [1, 9].

CHRONIC RENAL FAILURE

Chronic renal failure (CRF) is an irreversible condition characterized by diminished functioning of the nephrons, which results in decreased GFR, RBF, tubular function, and resorption ability. Progressive stages of renal impairment occur, which have as an end result, end-stage renal disease (Table 29-2).

Multiple conditions that cause CRF primarily affect the renal parenchyma (Table 29-3). Regardless of the cause, the result is damage to the nephrons and glomeruli. This damage may be diffused throughout both kidneys or it may

TABLE 29-2. Stages of chronic renal failure

Stage 1: Decrease renal reserve	Homeostasis is maintained; no symptoms; residual renal reserve 40% of normal
Stage 2: Renal insufficiency	Decreased ability to maintain homeostasis; mild azotemia and anemia; may be unable to concentrate urine and conserve H_2O; residual renal function 15–40% of normal; GFR decreases to 20 ml/minute (normal 100–120 ml/minute)
Stage 3: Renal failure	Azotemia and anemia more severe; nocturia, electrolyte and fluid disorders; difficulty with activities; residual renal function 5–15% of normal
Stage 4: Uremia (end-stage renal disease)	No homeostasis; becomes symptomatic in multiple systems; residual renal function less than 5% of normal

be focal. Progressive loss of nephrons leads to greater dysfunction with more difficulty in maintaining an adequate fluid and electrolyte balance. Systemic effects occur in all of the organs of the body.

The progression toward uremia is usually gradual, being controlled by diet and fluid restrictions for long periods of time. When the kidneys can no longer maintain the fluid and electrolyte balance, dialysis becomes necessary.

Pathophysiology of CRF

The intact nephron theory aids in explaining the pathophysiology of CRF. Experimentation has supported an *orderliness* of impaired renal function in the diseased kidney, which means that total nephron units are lost [7]. This finding lends support to the theory that the manifested net renal function is the result of a decreased number of correctly functioning nephrons, rather than the result of varyingly diseased nephrons [28]. Renal failure eventually affects all of the body systems. These effects are categorized in this section.

Physiologic Problems Caused by CRF

FLUID IMBALANCE. Early in CRF, when the kidneys lose renal function, they are not able to concentrate urine appropriately (*hypothenuria*) and this results in excess water loss (*polyuria*). Hypothenuria is not only related to the diminished number of nephrons, but is also due to the increased solute load per nephron. The increased solute (urea) load results because the intact nephrons carrying the solute and water load for those nephrons are no longer functioning (Fig. 29-6). Osmotic diuresis may result, causing the person to become dehydrated.

As greater numbers of nephrons become dysfunctional, an inability to dilute urine (*isosthenuria*) results [18]. At this stage the glomeruli have hyalinized and plasma cannot be filtered easily through the tubules. Fluid overload with water and sodium retention result.

SODIUM IMBALANCE. Maintaining sodium balance is a serious problem in that the nephrons may excrete as little as 20 to 30 mEq of sodium daily or up to 200 mEq daily. The varying amounts of sodium loss are believed to be related to the intact nephron theory. In other words, the damaged nephrons are unable to exchange sodium, so the intact nephrons receive the excess sodium, causing an excess amount to be excreted in the urine. This excess elimina-

TABLE 29-3. Causes of chronic renal failure[a]

1. Immunologic disorders
   - Glomerulonephritides[b]
   - Lupus erythematosus
   - Polyarteritis nodosa
   - Goodpasture's syndrome
2. Infections
   - Pyelonephritis[b]
   - Tuberculosis
3. Urinary obstruction
   - Prostatic hypertrophy
   - Renal calculi (bilateral or in a single kidney)
   - Urethral constriction
   - Neoplasms
4. Metabolic disorders
   - Diabetes mellitus[b]
   - Amyloidosis
   - Gout
5. Vascular disorders
   - Hypertension (benign and malignant)[b]
   - Infarctions
   - Sickle-cell anemia
6. Hereditary and congenital disorders
   - Alport's syndrome
   - Polycystic disease
   - Renal hypoplasia
7. Nephrotoxins
   - Analgesic nephropathy
   - Other drugs
   - Heavy metal poisoning
   - Industrial solvents
8. Others
   - Radiation nephritis
   - Multiple myeloma
   - Leukemia
   - Hypercalcemia

[a]This list is not exhaustive, and the placement of some diseases into one category rather than another is arbitrary.
[b]These are some of the more common causes of chronic renal failure. Although certain other conditions (e.g., prostatic hypertrophy and renal calculi) have a high incidence, they do not frequently lead to chronic renal falure.
Source: H. Valtin, *Renal Dysfunction*. Boston: Little, Brown, 1979.

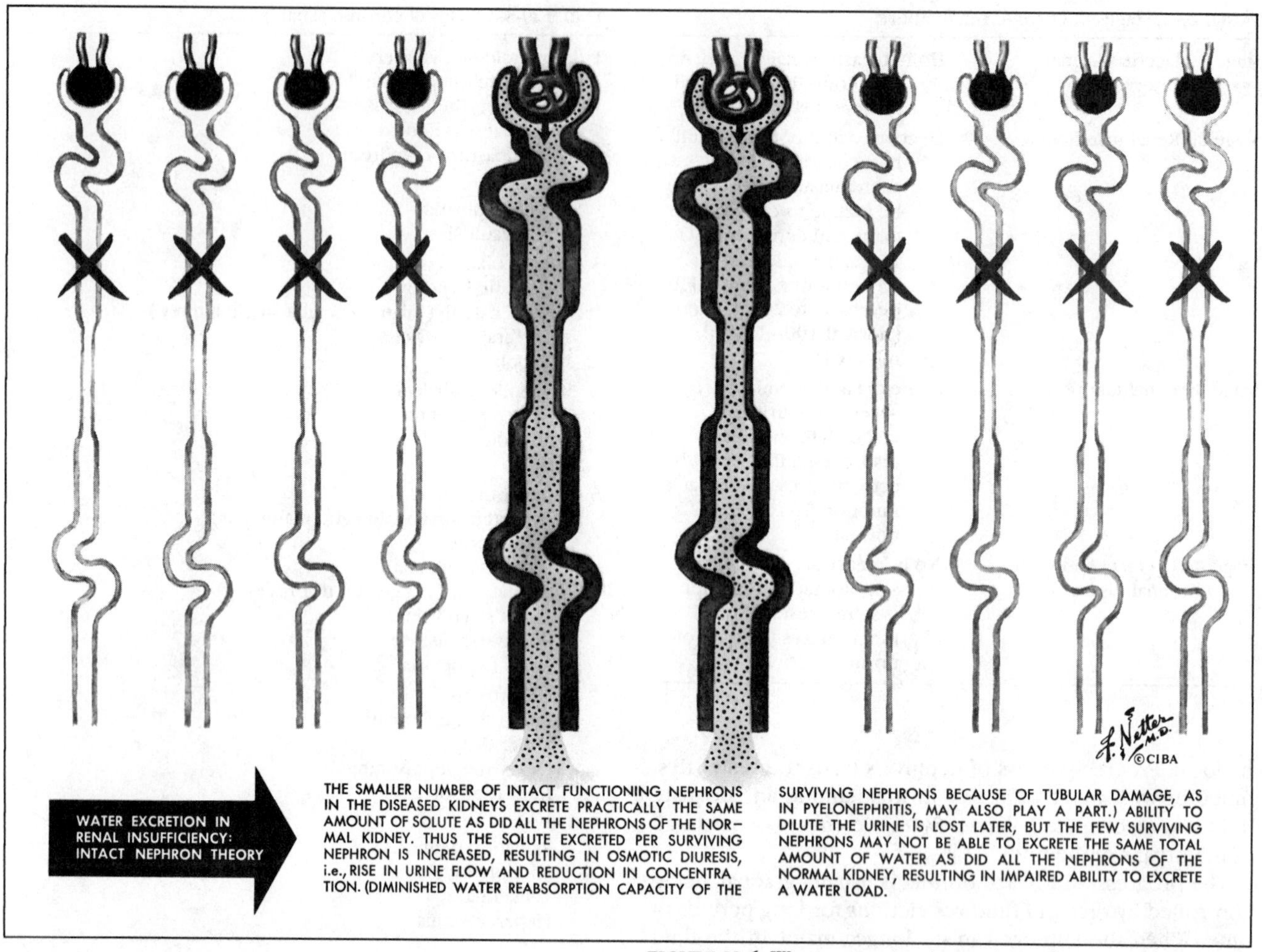

FIGURE 29-6. Water excretion in renal insufficiency. © Copyright 1973, CIBA Pharmaceutical Company, Division of CIBA-GEIGY Corporation. Reprinted with permission from the CIBA COLLECTION OF MEDICAL ILLUSTRATIONS. Illustrated by Frank H. Netter, M.D. All rights reserved.

tion is accompanied by osmotic diuresis, which causes a reduction in GFR and dehydration. Sodium loss may be enhanced by gastrointestinal disturbances, especially vomiting and diarrhea that may aggravate the hyponatremia and the dehydration.

In severe CRF sodium balance can be maintained even though a loss of flexibility in adjusting to sodium levels occurs. A healthy person can reduce urinary excretion of sodium practically to zero or increase excretion to above 500 mEq/day when faced with sodium deficit or excess. If the GFR of a person with CRF has decreased to less than 25 to 30 ml/minute, an obligatory sodium excretion of about 25 mEq /day may occur with a maximum excretion of 150 to 200 mEq [34]. This accounts for the sodium dietary restrictions of 1.0 to 1.5 gm/day in CRF.

POTASSIUM IMBALANCE. Hyperkalemia is rarely a problem in CRF prior to stage 4 if water balance is maintained and metabolic acidosis is controlled. Potassium (K^+) balance is believed to be the result of the adaptations made to the increased potassium presented to each functioning nephron. The mechanism for maintaining K^+ balance is not totally understood, but may be related to enhanced aldosterone secretion. As long as urine output is maintained, the potassium level is usually maintained. Hyperkalemia may result, however, from excessive intake of potassium, certain medications, hypercatabolic illness (infection), or hyponatremia. It also is characteristic in the uremic or end-stage (stage 4) progression.

Hypokalemia also can occur in association with vomiting or excessive diarrhea. In tubular renal disease the nephrons may fail to resorb potassium, leading to increased potassium excretion. If hypokalemia persists, the glomerular filtration rate and concentrating ability decrease and the production of NH_3 increases [7]. HCO_3 decreases and Na^+ is retained. This effect impairs functional ability.

ACID-BASE IMBALANCE. Metabolic acidosis develops because the kidneys are unable to excrete enough hydrogen ion to keep the pH of the blood in a normal range.

Renal tubular dysfunction leads to a progressive inability to excrete H^+ ion. In general, the decreased H^+ excretion is proportional to the decreased GFR [31]. Acids, continually being formed by metabolism in the body, are not filtered as effectively through the GBM; decreased NH_3 is produced; and the tubular cell is dysfunctional. Failure in bicarbonate formation may also contribute to this imbalance.

Part of the excess hydrogen is buffered by the bone salts. As a result, chronic metabolic acidosis increases the possibility of osteodystrophy [33].

MAGNESIUM IMBALANCE. Magnesium level is normal in early CRF, but a progressive reduction in urinary excretion may cause accumulation. A combination of decreased excretion and high intakes of magnesium may result in cardiac or respiratory arrest [12].

PHOSPHORUS AND CALCIUM IMBALANCE. Normally, calcium and phosphorus levels are maintained by the parathyroid hormone, which causes renal resorption of calcium by the kidney, mobilization of calcium from the bone, and depression of tubular resorption of phosphorus.

When the renal function deteriorates to 20 to 25 percent of normal, hyperphosphatemia and hypocalcemia occur, leading to a secondary hyperparathyroidism [19, 33]. This secondary hyperparathyroidism is also associated with altered vitamin D metabolism. Prolonged secondary hyperparathyroidism results in renal osteodystrophy (see Chap. 32).

An activated vitamin D normally is responsible for enhancing calcium absorption in the gastrointestinal tract and increasing resorption of calcium from the bone. When CRF is present, hypocalcemia develops because of decreased absorption of calcium. Figure 29-9 summarizes the development of renal osteodystrophy in chronic renal failure.

ANEMIA. A decreased hemoglobin in persons with CRF is the result of several factors: (1) short life span of red blood cells due to altered plasma; (2) increased loss of red blood cells due to gastrointestinal ulceration, dialysis, and blood taken for laboratory analysis; (3) reduction of erythropoietin due to decreased renal formation and inhibition from uremia; (4) folate deficiency when the person is undergoing dialysis; (5) iron deficiency; and (6) elevated parathyroid hormone, which stimulates fibrous tissue or osteitis fibrosis, taking up bone marrow space and causing the decreased production by the marrow.

The normocytic, normochromic anemia, with hematocrits in the range of 15 to 30 percent, is usually proportionate to the degree of azotemia.

PURPURA. Purpura may develop that is related to platelet impairment from accumulation of nitrogenous wastes. Purpura is characterized by hemorrhage into the skin and is associated with a general increase in bleeding tendencies.

UREA AND CREATININE ALTERATIONS. Urea is a by-product of protein metabolism that accumulates as the uremic stage develops. The blood urea nitrogen (BUN) level is not an adequate indicator of renal disease because the level is elevated with a decrease in GFR and an increased protein intake. Serum creatinine is a better indicator of renal dysfunction because urinary excretion of creatinine equals the amount produced in the body. Therefore, the GFR can be calculated by changes in serum creatinine (Fig. 29-7). With normal renal function, an increase of serum creatinine from 1.0 to 2.0 mg/dl represents a fall of GFR from 120 to

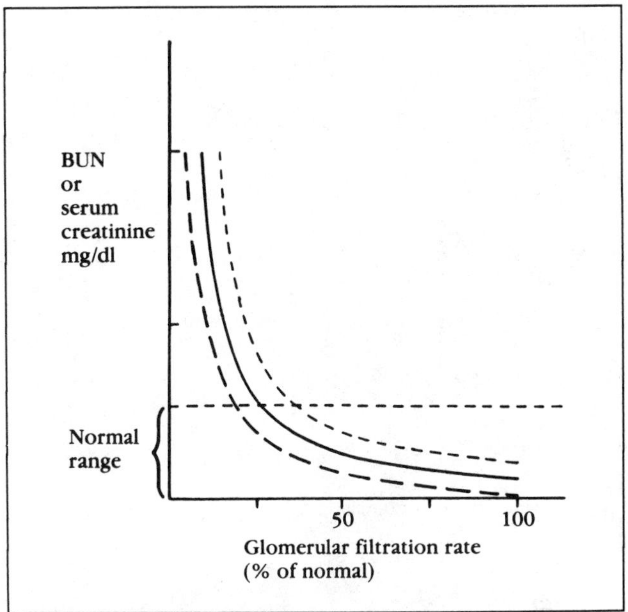

FIGURE 29-7. The relationship of blood urea nitrogen or serum creatinine concentration to glomerular filtration rate. The broken lines indicate that there is a family of curves rather than a single one for all persons. (From S. Papper, *Clinical Nephrology* [2nd ed.]. Boston: Little, Brown, 1978.)

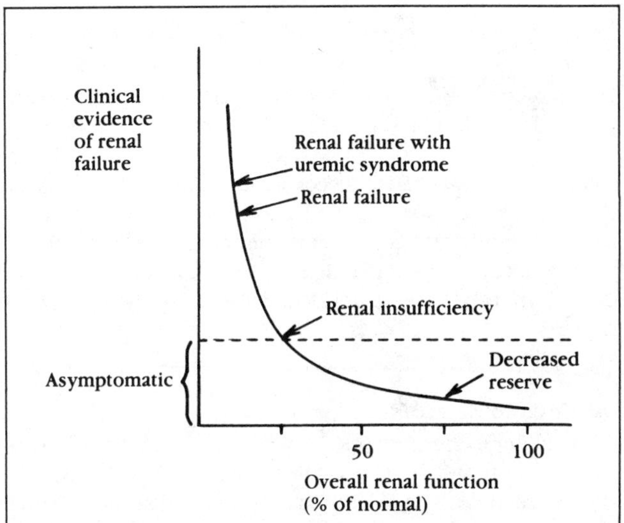

FIGURE 29-8. The relationship of clinical manifestations to renal function. (From S. Papper, *Clinical Nephrology* [2nd ed.]. Boston: Little, Brown, 1978.)

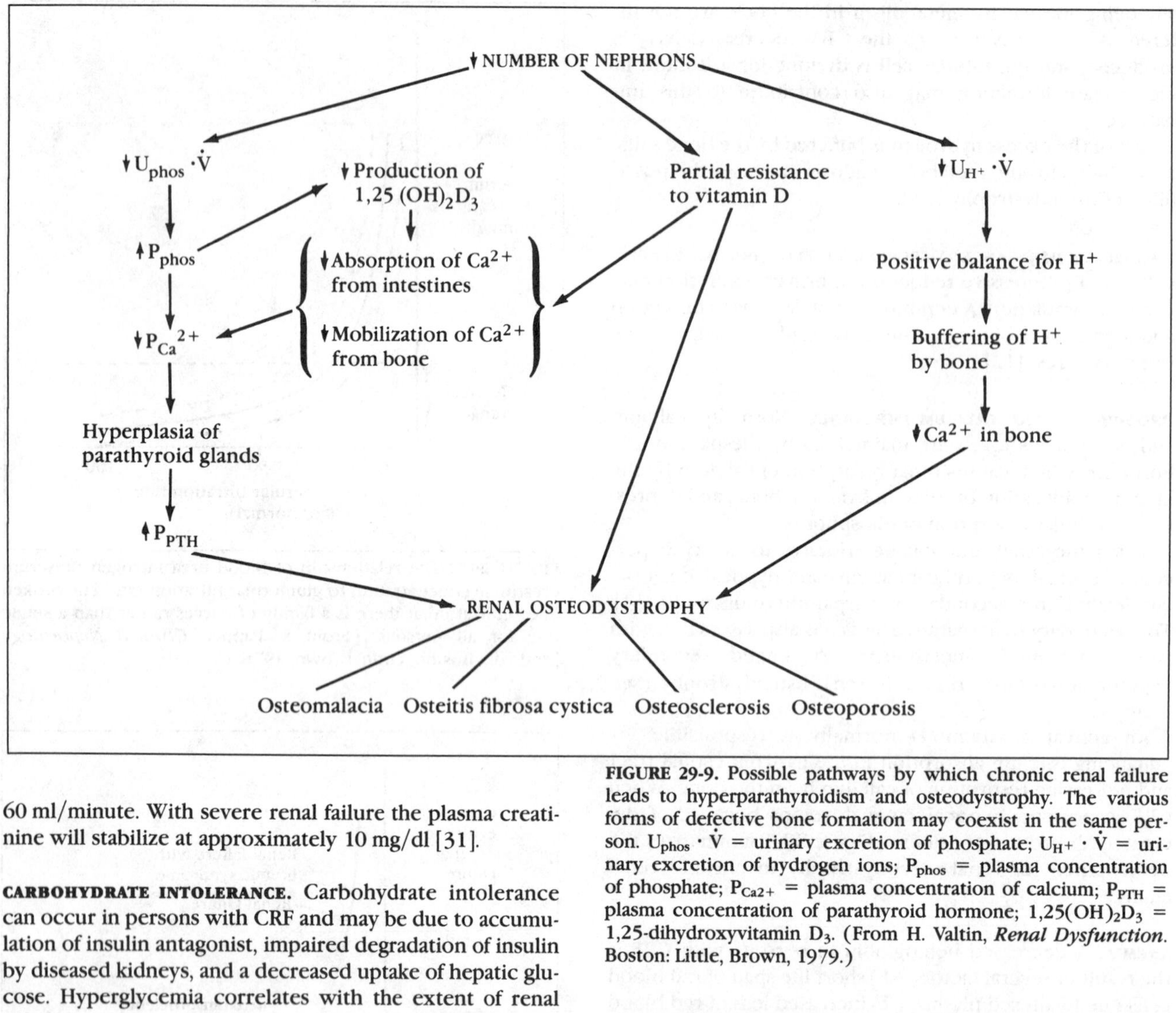

FIGURE 29-9. Possible pathways by which chronic renal failure leads to hyperparathyroidism and osteodystrophy. The various forms of defective bone formation may coexist in the same person. $U_{phos} \cdot \dot{V}$ = urinary excretion of phosphate; $U_{H^+} \cdot \dot{V}$ = urinary excretion of hydrogen ions; P_{phos} = plasma concentration of phosphate; P_{Ca2+} = plasma concentration of calcium; P_{PTH} = plasma concentration of parathyroid hormone; $1{,}25(OH)_2D_3$ = 1,25-dihydroxyvitamin D_3. (From H. Valtin, *Renal Dysfunction*. Boston: Little, Brown, 1979.)

60 ml/minute. With severe renal failure the plasma creatinine will stabilize at approximately 10 mg/dl [31].

CARBOHYDRATE INTOLERANCE. Carbohydrate intolerance can occur in persons with CRF and may be due to accumulation of insulin antagonist, impaired degradation of insulin by diseased kidneys, and a decreased uptake of hepatic glucose. Hyperglycemia correlates with the extent of renal failure.

UREMIC SYNDROME

As renal failure progresses, it eventually becomes symptomatic and the steady state is not maintained. This condition represents stage 4 of CRF or the uremic stage (Table 29-2). The uremic symptoms are described according to the effects that occur on each system (Fig. 29-8).

Neurologic System

As renal failure progresses, central nervous system effects vary and include drowsiness, inability to concentrate, poor memory, hallucinations, seizures, and coma. The alterations are believed to be related to the accumulation of uremic toxins, to deficiency of ionized calcium in spinal fluid with retention of potassium and phosphates, to any hypertensive crises, and to altered fluid loads [24, 30].

Peripheral neuropathy is an early symptom of uremia and begins in the lower extremities. Individuals gradually develop a delayed sensory and motor response, burning sensations, and numbness in the feet and legs.

Cardiovascular System

Hypertension usually results from fluid overloading but may also be related to vascular changes (nephrosclerosis), increased renin secretion, or decreased levels of prostaglandins [24]. Fluid overloading is the result of sodium and water imbalances. Vascular changes include accelerated atherosclerosis and narrowing of the arterioles. *Hyperreninemia* often is noted. The prostaglandins that are secreted by the renal medulla do not function in counteracting the increased peripheral vascular resistance.

Fibrinous pericarditis may develop in end-stage renal disease and may be associated with an excess of pericardial fluid and fibrin formation on the epicardial surface [24].

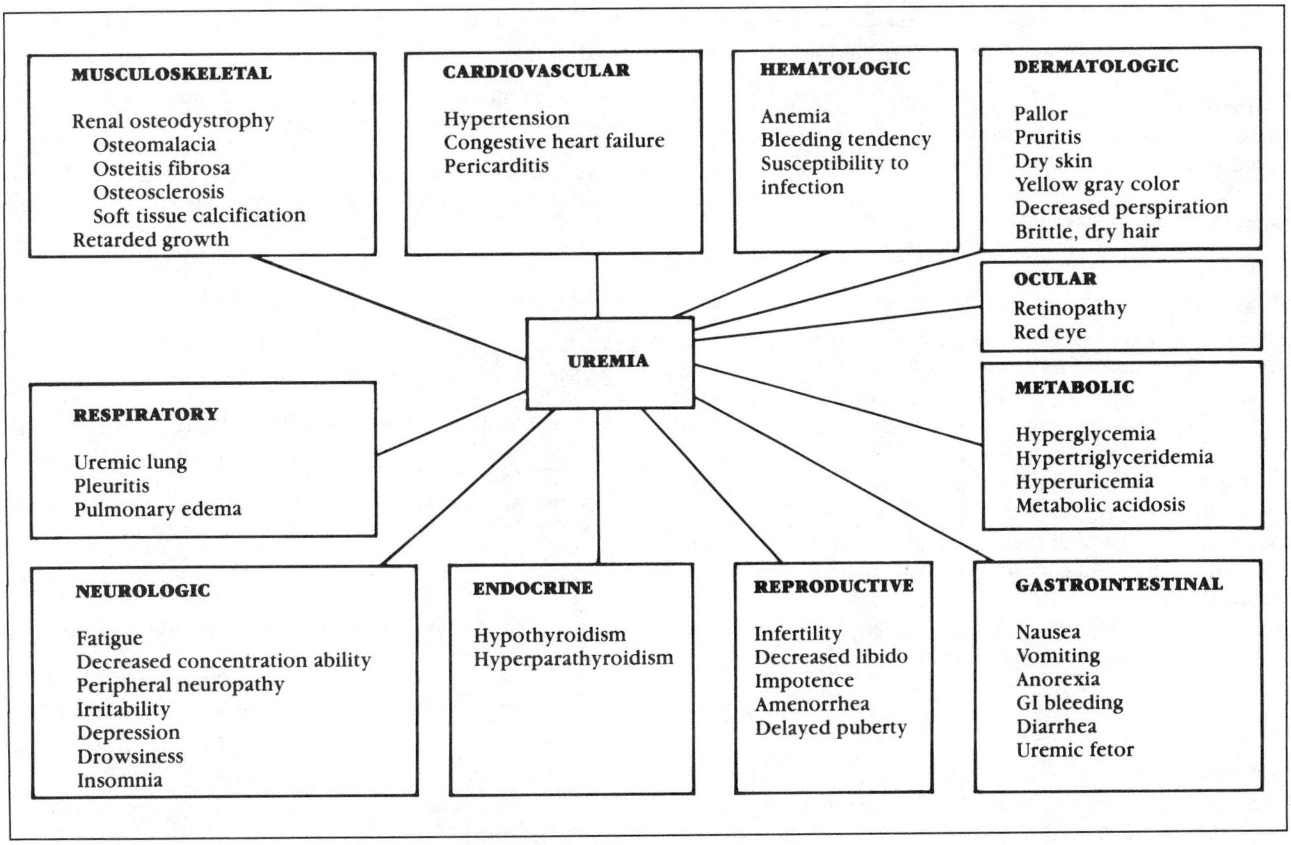

FIGURE 29-10. Systemic effects of uremia. (From S. Lewis, Pathophysiology of chronic renal failure. *Nurs. Clin. North Am.* 16:38, 1981.)

This fluid can cause a cardiac restriction, and even tamponade. Fibrinous pericarditis may be asymptomatic, associated with substernal pain, or symptomatic of cardiac tamponade.

Congestive heart failure results from salt and fluid overloading along with the characteristic hypertension. Pulmonary edema may be manifested by *uremic lung* and respiratory congestion.

Respiratory System

The uremic lung noted on radiologic examination characteristically exhibits "bat wings" and involves perihilar congestion. Pneumonia also is a major threat in CRF because the uremic environment causes a depressed immune response.

Gastrointestinal (GI) System

The most common gastrointestinal symptoms are nausea, vomiting, hiccups, and anorexia. The cause of these symptoms is not well understood, but they are related to the degree of uremia and may improve if hydration is maintained. Ulcers may form anywhere along the gastrointestinal tract. Peptic ulcer disease occurs in up to 25 percent of uremic persons [27]. Gastrointestinal bleeding is a complication that may result from ulcerations and capillary fragility. Uremic fetor, or urine breath, occurs when the salivary urea is broken down to ammonia, causing an unpleasant metallic taste. The oral mucosa is often dry with a yellow brown tongue.

Musculoskeletal System

The effects of altered levels of calcium and phosphorus are illustrated in Fig. 29-9. The resulting faulty bone metabolism, called renal osteodystrophy, is caused by a combination of hyperparathyroidism, calcium and phosphorus alterations, and a decreased synthesis of the active form of vitamin D. Several resulting bone lesions include osteomalacia, osteitis fibrosa, soft tissue calcification, and osteosclerosis (Fig. 29-9).

Osteomalacia is the result of poor tissue utilization of vitamin D that causes accumulation of osteoid material after calcification has ceased. *Osteitis fibrosa* results when fibrous tissue replaces bone tissue. It may be produced from secondary hyperparathyroidism. Soft tissue *metastatic calcification* is the deposition of calcium and phosphate crystals in the synovial tissues and soft tissues, especially the eyes, joints, muscles, and lungs. *Osteosclerosis* is believed to be similar to soft tissue calcification and is due to bone redistribution and remodeling. This lesion causes enhanced bone density mainly affecting the face, skull, and spine.

Renal osteodystrophy causes an enhanced tendency to spontaneous fractures. Many of the complications of this condition can be prevented by using phosphate-binding agents, administering activated vitamin D, and supplementing dietary calcium [3].

Hematologic Alterations

The hematologic effects of uremia include a normocytic, normochromic anemia, and altered hemostasis (see Chaps. 14 and 16). Hemolysis of red blood cells is common; it is related to a decreased survival time of the erythrocytes in the uremic plasma. An increased incidence of hepatitis is associated with the need for blood transfusions and dialysis procedures. Any type of infection may occur because of the depressed immunologic response of afflicted persons [29]. Coagulation defects are caused by platelet defects and are found in most persons with uremia. Abnormal bleeding results, causing a wide range of problems, including epistaxis, purpura, and frank hemorrhage.

Dermatologic Alterations

Skin pallor results from anemia, but there is also a characteristic sallow, yellow pigmentation. Retention of pigmented urochromes results in their deposition in the subcutaneous fat. Dryness of the skin is caused by atrophy of the sweat glands and dehydration. Uremic itching or pruritis is possibly related to excess parathyroid hormone, the skin deposits, or to peripheral neuropathy [24]. Uremic frost may be seen in advanced uremia when the urea deposits are excreted in the sweat and crystallized.

Other organ and system alterations also occur. These are noted in Figure 29-10.

REFERENCES

1. Arendshorst, W. I., Finn, W. F., and Gottschalk, C. W. Pathogenesis of acute renal failure in the rat. *Kidney Int.* 10:5, 1976.
2. Avasthi, P. S., Evan, A. P., and Hay, D. Glomerular endothelial cells in uranyl nitrate–induced acute renal failure in rats. *J. Clin. Invest.* 65:121, 1980.
3. Bennett, W. M., Singer, I., and Coggins, C. H. Guide to drug therapy in adult patients with impaired renal function. *J.A.M.A.* 223:991, 1974.
4. Black, D. (ed.). *Renal Disease* (3rd ed.). Oxford, England: Blackwell, 1972.
5. Blantz, R. C., and Konnen, K. The mechanism of acute renal failure after uranyl nitrate. *J. Clin. Invest.* 55:621, 1975.
6. Brenner, B. M., and Rector, F. C. *The Kidney* (2nd ed.). Philadelphia: Saunders, 1981.
7. Bricker, N. S. On the meaning of the intact nephron hypothesis. *Am. J. Med.* 46:1, 1969.
8. Brown, W. C. B., et al. Renin and acute circulatory renal failure in the rabbit. *Circ. Res.* 30:114, 1972.
9. Chapman, A. (ed.). *Acute Renal Failure.* London: Churchill Livingstone, 1980.
10. Cronin, R. E., et al. Norepinephrine: Induced acute renal failure. *Kidney Int.* 14:187, 1978.
11. Dalgaard, O. Z., and Pedersen, K. J. Ultrastructure of the Kidney in Shock. In G. Ricket (ed.), *Proceedings of the First International Congress of Nephrology.* New York: Karger, 1961. Pp. 165–176.
12. deWardener, H. E. *The Kidney: An Outline of Normal and Abnormal Structure* (4th ed.). London: Churchill Livingstone, 1973.
13. Dibona, G. F., and Saivin, L. L. The renin-angiotensin system in acute renal failure in the rat. *Lab. Invest.* 25:528, 1971.
14. Donohoe, J. F., et al. Tubular leakage and obstruction in acute ischemic renal failure. *Kidney Int.* 13:208, 1978.
15. Dunnell, M. A. A review of the pathology and pathogenesis of acute renal failure due to acute tubular necrosis. *J. Clin. Path.* 27:2, 1974.
16. Fine, L. G. Acquired prostaglandin E_2 (Medullin) deficiency as the cause of oliguria in acute tubular necrosis: A hypothesis. *Isr. J. Med. Sci.* 6:346, 1970.
17. Flores, J., et al. The role of cell swelling in ischemic renal damage and the protective effect of hypertonic solute. *J. Clin. Invest.* 51:118, 1972.
18. Forland, M. (ed.). *Nephrology.* New York: Medical Exam., 1977.
19. Goldman, R., and Bassett, S. H. Phosphorus excretion in renal failure. *J. Clin. Invest.* 33:1623, 1954.
20. Held, E. Protective effects of renomedullary autotransplants upon the course of postischemic acute renal failure in rabbits. *Kidney Int.* 10:5, 1976.
21. Lane, A. Z., Wright, G. E., and Blair, D. C. Ototoxicity and nephrotoxicity of amikacin. *Am. J. Med.* 62:911, 1977.
22. Leaf, A. Regulation of intracellular fluid volume and disease. *Am. J. Med.* 49:291, 1970.
23. Levinsky, N. G., and Alexander, E. A. Acute Renal Failure. In B. M. Brenner and F. C. Rector (eds.), *Renal Failure: The Kidney* (vol. II). Philadelphia: Saunders, 1976. Pp. 806–837.
24. Lewis, S. M. Pathophysiology of chronic renal failure. *Nurs. Clin. North Am.* 16:501, 1981.
25. Mason, J., et al. The early phase of experimental acute renal failure: I. Intratubular pressure and obstruction. *Pfluegers Arch.* 370:155, 1977.
26. Mason, J., et al. The early phase of experimental acute renal failure: III. Tubuloglomerular feedback. *Pfluegers Arch.* 373:69, 1978.
27. Muth, R. *Renal Medicine.* Springfield, Ill.: Thomas, 1978.
28. Papper, S. *Clinical Nephrology* (2nd ed.). Boston: Little, Brown, 1978.
29. Revillard, J. P. Immunologic alterations in chronic renal insufficiency. *Adv. Nephrol.* 8:365, 1979.
30. Robbins, S. L., and Cotran, R. *Pathologic Basis of Disease* (2nd ed.). Philadelphia: Saunders, 1979.
31. Rose, B. D. *Clinical Physiology of Acid-Base and Electrolyte Disorders.* New York: McGraw-Hill, 1977.
32. Semple, P. F., et al. Renin, angiotensin II and III in acute renal failure: Note on the measurement of angiotensin II and III in rat blood. *Kidney Int.* 10:5, 1976.
33. Shalhaub, R. J. The medical management of chronic renal failure. *Med. Times* 107:23, 1979.
34. Valtin, H., *Renal Dysfunction.* Boston: Little, Brown, 1979.

BIBLIOGRAPHY

Allen, A. *The Kidney: Medical and Surgical Disease* (2nd ed.). New York: Grune & Stratton, 1962.

Andreoli, T. E. On the anatomy of amphotericin B–cholesterol pores in lipid bilayer membranes. *Kidney Int.* 4:337, 1973.

Anthony, C. P., and Thibodeau, G. A. *Textbook of Anatomy and Physiology* (10th ed.). St. Louis: Mosby, 1979.

Arendshorst, W. J., Finn, W. F., and Gottschalk, C. W. Pathogenesis of acute renal failure in the rat. *Kidney Int.* 10:5, 1976.

Atkins, G. L., et al. Quantitative aspects of ascorbic acid metabolism in man. *J. Biol. Chem.* 239:2975, 1964.

Avasthi, P. S., Evan, A. P., and Hay, D. Glomerular endothelial cells in uranyl nitrate–induced acute renal failure in rats. *J. Clin. Invest.* 65:121, 1980.

Bartsch, W., et al. Hormone block levels and their interrelationships in normal men and men with benign prostatic hyperplasia (BPH). *Acta Endocrinol.* (Copenh.) 90:727, 1979.

Becker, H., et al. In vivo uptake and metabolism of ^{3}H-testosterone and ^{3}H-5 dihydrotestosterone by human benign prostatic hypertrophy. *Acta Endocrinol.* (Copenh.) 71:589, 1972.

Bennett, W. M., Singer, I., and Coggins, C. H. Guide to drug therapy in adult patients with impaired renal function. *J.A.M.A.* 223:991, 1974.

Bennington, J. L. Histopathology of Renal Adenocarcinoma. In G. Sufrin and S. A. Beckley (eds.), *Renal Adenocarcinoma.* (report no. 10). Geneva: International Union Against Cancer, 1980. P. 61.

Berg, O. A. The normal prostate gland in the dog. *Acta Endocrinol.* (Copenh.) 28:129, 1958.

Black, D. (ed.). *Renal Disease* (3rd ed.). London: Blackwell, 1972.

Blagg, C., and Scribner, B. H. Long term dialysis: Current problems and future prospects. *Am. J. Med.* 68:633, 1980.

Blantz, R. C., and Konnen, K. The mechanism of acute renal failure after uranyl nitrate. *J. Clin. Invest.* 55:621, 1975.

Bloom, N. A., Vidone, R. A., and Lytton, B. Primary carcinoma of the ureter: A report of 102 new cases. *J. Urol.* 103:590, 1970.

Bloom, W., and Fawcett, D. W. *A Textbook of Histology* (10th ed.). Philadelphia: Saunders, 1975.

Bordier, P., et al. On the pathogenesis of so-called idiopathic hypercalciuria. *Am. J. Med.* 63:398, 1977.

Boyce, W. H., et al. Abnormalities of calcium metabolism in patients with "idiopathic" urinary calculi. *J.A.M.A.* 166:1577, 1958.

Brenner, B. M., and Rector, F. C. *The Kidney* (2nd ed.). Philadelphia: Saunders, 1981.

Brenner, B. M., and Stein, J. H. (eds.). *Acute Renal Failure* (vol. 6). London: Churchill Livingstone, 1980.

Bricker, N. S. On the meaning of the intact nephron hypothesis. *Am. J. Med.* 46:1, 1969.

Brod, J. *The Kidney.* London: Butterworth, 1973.

Brosig, W. Conservative Treatment of Benign Prostatic Hypertrophy. In H. Marberger, et al. (ed.), *Prostatic Disease: Proceedings.* New York: Liss, 1976. Pp. 23–29.

Brown, W. C. B., et al. Renin and acute circulatory renal failure in the rabbit. *Circ. Res.* 30:114, 1972.

Chapman, A. (ed.). *Acute Renal Failure.* London: Churchill Livingstone, 1980.

Coe, F. L. Nephrolithiasis: Causes, classification and management. *Hosp. Pract.* 16:33, 1981.

Corea, A. Current trends in diet and drug therapy for the dialysis patient. *Nurs. Clin. North Am.* 10:469, 1975.

Cranston, J. A. Benign enlargement of the prostate gland. *Nurs. Times* 74:789, 1978.

Cronin, R. E., et al. Norepinephrine-induced acute renal failure. *Kidney Int.* 14:187, 1978.

Cummings, K. Nephroureterectomy: Rationale in the management of transitional cell carcinoma of the upper urinary tract. *Urol. Clin. North Am.* 7:569, 1980.

Cummings, N. B. Urolithiasis research: Progress and trends. *Adv. Exp. Med. Biol.* 128:473, 1980.

Dalgaard, O. Z., and Pedersen, K. J. Ultrastructure of the Kidney in Shock. In G. Ricket (ed.), *Proceedings of the First International Congress of Nephrology.* New York: Karger, 1961. Pp. 165–176.

deWardener, H. E. *The Kidney: An Outline of Normal and Abnormal Structure* (4th ed.). London: Churchill Livingstone, 1973.

Dibona, G. F., and Saivin, L. L. The renin-angiotensin system in acute renal failure in the rat. *Lab. Invest.* 25:528, 1971.

Donohoe, J. F., et al. Tubular leakage and obstruction in acute ischemic renal failure. *Kidney Int.* 13:208, 1978.

Droller, M. J. Adenocarcinoma of the prostate: An overview. *Urol. Clin. North Am.* 7:578, 1980.

Droller, M. J. Renal cell carcinoma: An overview. *Urol. Clin. North Am.* 7:675, 1980.

Dunnell, M. A. A review of the pathology and pathogenesis of acute renal failure due to acute tubular necrosis. *J. Clin. Path.* 27:2, 1974.

Elliott, A. Y., et al. Isolation of RNA virus from papillary tumors of the human renal pelvis. *Science* 179:393, 1973.

Fay, F. C. Pulling a patient through acute renal failure. *RN* 11:1978.

Fearing, M. O. Osteodystrophy in patients with chronic renal failure. *Nurs. Clin. North Am.* 10:461, 1975.

Fine, L. G. Acquired prostaglandin E_2 (Medullin) deficiency as the cause of oliguria in acute tubular necrosis: A hypothesis. *Isr. J. Med. Sci.* 6:346, 1970.

Flores, J., et al. The role of cell swelling in ischemic renal damage and the protective effect of hypertonic solute. *J. Clin. Invest.* 51:118, 1972.

Forland, M. (ed.). *Nephrology.* Garden City, N.Y.: Medical Exam., 1977.

Frayley, E. E. Cancer of the Renal Pelvis. In D. G. Skinner and J. B. deKernion (eds.), *Genitourinary Cancer.* Philadelphia: Saunders, 1978.

Geschickter, C. F., and Antonovych, T. T. *The Kidney in Health and Disease.* Philadelphia: Lippincott, 1971.

Goldman, R., and Bassett, S. H. Phosphorus excretion in renal failure. *J. Clin. Invest.* 33:1623, 1954.

Grimes, W. A. Phase contrast study of mechanisms of renal calcification. *J. Urol.* 78:553, 1957.

Gutman, A. B., and Yü, T. F. Uric acid nephrolithiasis. *Am. J. Med.* 45:756, 1968.

Hallson, P. C., and Rose, G. A. Uromucoids and urinary stone formation. *Lancet* 1:1000, 1979.

Hammond, G. L., et al. Serum steroids in normal males and patients with prostatic disease. *Clin. Endocrinol.* 9:113, 1978.

Hautmann, R., Lehmann, A., and Komor, S. Calcium and oxalate concentrations in human renal tissue: The key to the pathogenesis of stone formation? *J. Urol.* 123:317, 1980.

Held, E. Protective effects of renomedullary autotransplants upon the course of postischemic acute renal failure in rabbits. *Kidney Int.* 10:5, 1976.

Hellstrom, J. Calcification and calculus formation in a series of seventy cases of primary hyperparathyroidism. *Br. J. Urol.* 27:387, 1955.

Henkelman, F., and Ostendarp, C. A. Nursing approaches to conservative management of renal disease. *Nurs. Clin. North Am.* 10:431, 1975.

Heptinstall, R. H. Acute Renal Failure. In R. H. Heptinstall, *Pathology of the Kidney* (3rd ed.). Boston: Little, Brown, 1983.

Higgins, S. J., and Gehring, U. Molecular mechanisms of steroid hormone action. *Adv. Cancer Res.* 28:313, 1978.

Horton, R., et al. Altered blood androgens in elderly men with prostatic hyperplasia. *J. Clin. Endocrinol. Metab.* 41:793, 1975.

Jackle, M., and Rasmussen, C. *Renal Problems: A Critical Care Nursing Focus.* Bowie, Md.: Brady, 1980.

Jacob, S. W., and Francone, C. A. *Structure and Function in Man* (2nd ed.). Philadelphia: Saunders, 1970.

Jacobi, H., Moore, R. J., and Wilson, J. D. Studies on the mechanism of 32-androstanediol–induced growth of the dog prostate. *En-*

docrinology 102:1748, 1978.
Jensen, D. *The Principles of Physiology* (2nd ed.). New York: Appleton-Century-Crofts, 1980.
Johnson, H. K., et al. Nursing care of the patient with acute renal failure. *Nurs. Clin. North Am.* 10:421, 1975.
Karakousis, C. P., and Jennings, E. Renal cell carcinoma metastatic to skeletal muscle mass: A case report. *J. Surg. Oncol.* 17:287, 1981.
Kleeman, C. R., et al. Kidney stones: Inter-departmental clinic conference: UCLA School of Medicine. *West. J. Med.* 132:313, 1980.
Klein, M. J., and Valensi, W. J. Proximal tubular adenomas of kidney with so-called oncocytic features: A clinicopathologic study of 13 cases of a rarely reported neoplasm. *Cancer* 38:906, 1976.
Lane, A. Z., Wright, G. E., and Blair, D. C. Ototoxicity and nephrotoxicity of amikacin. *Am. J. Med.* 62:911, 1977.
Leaf, A. Regulation of intracellular fluid volume and disease. *Am. J. Med.* 49:291, 1970.
Leaf, A., and Cotran, R. *Renal Pathophysiology*. New York: Oxford University Press, 1976.
Levinsky, N. G., and Alexander, E. A. Renal Failure. In B. M. Brenner, and F. C. Rector, Jr. (eds.), *The Kidney* (vol. 2). Philadelphia: Saunders. 1976. Pp. 806–837.
Lewis, S. M. Pathophysiology of chronic renal failure. *Nurs. Clin. North Am.* 16:501, 1981.
Ljunghall, S., and Hedstrand, H. Epidemiology of renal stones in a middle age population. *Acta Med. Scand.* 197:439, 1975.
Mancilla-Jimenez, R., Stanley, J., and Blath, R. A. Papillary renal cell carcinoma: A clinical, radiologic and pathologic study of 34 cases. *Cancer* 38:2469, 1976.
Margolis, W. S. Chemotherapy in Wilms' tumor. *Cancer* 32:1150, 1973.
Marsden, H. B., and Stewart, J. K. *Wilms' Tumors. Recent Results in Cancer Research: Tumors in Children* (vol. 13). New York: Springer-Verlag, 1968. P. 225.
Mason, J., et al. The early phase of experimental acute renal failure: I. Intratubular pressure and obstruction. *Pfluegers Arch.* 370:155, 1977.
Mason, J., et al. The early phase of experimental acute renal failure: III. Tubuloglomerular feedback. *Pfluegers Arch.* 373:69, 1978.
Melick, R. A., and Henneman, P. H. Clinical laboratory studies of 207 consecutive patients in a kidney stone clinic. *N. Engl. J. Med.* 259:307, 1958.
Mitchell, G. A. G. The nerve supply of the kidneys. *Acta Anat.* (Basel) 10:1, 1950.
Muth, R. *Renal Medicine.* Springfield, Ill.: Thomas, 1978.
Olsen, S. Renal histopathology in various forms of acute anuria in man. *Kidney Int.* 10:5, 1976.
Pak, C. Y. C., et al. A simple test for the diagnosis of absorptive, resorptive and renal hypercalciurias. *N. Engl. J. Med.* 292:497, 1975.
Pak, C. Y. C., et al. The hypercalciurias: Causes, parathyroid function and diagnostic criteria. *J. Clin. Invest.* 54:387, 1974.
Papper, S. *Clinical Nephrology* (2nd ed.). Boston: Little, Brown, 1978.
Papper, S. The oliguric patient. *Med. Times* 107:70, 1979.
Parks, J., Coe, F., and Favus, M. Hyperparathyroidism in nephrolithiasis. *Arch. Intern. Med.* 140:1479, 1980.
Pearse, H. D., and Houghton, D. C. Renal oncocytoma. *Urology* 13:74, 1979.
Powell, P. H., Smith, P. J. B., and Feneley, R. C. L. The identification of patients at risk from acute retention. *Br. J. Urol.* 6:520, 1980.
Pyrah, L. N., and Raper, F. P. Renal calcification and calculus formation. *Br. J. Urol.* 27:333, 1955.
Revillard, J. P. Immunologic alterations in chronic renal insufficiency. *Adv. Nephrol.* 8:365, 1979.
Roberts, S. L. Renal assessment: A nursing point of view. *Heart Lung* 8:105, 1979.
Rodman, M., and Smith, D. *Pharmacology and Drug Therapy in Nursing* (2nd ed.). Philadelphia: Lippincott, 1979.
Rosenow, E. C. Renal calculi: Study of papillary calcification. *J. Urol.* 44:19, 1940.
Saroff, J., et al. Measurements of prolactin and androgens in patients with prostatic disease. *Surg. Forum* 28:568, 1977.
Schlotthauer, C. F. Observations on the prostate gland of the dog. *Trans. Am. Vet. Med. Assoc.* 81:645, 1932.
Schottelius, B. A., and Schottelius, D. D. *Textbook of Physiology* (18th ed.). St. Louis: Mosby, 1978.
Semple, P. F., et al. Renin, angiotensin II and III in acute renal failure: Note on the measurement of angiotensin II and III in rat blood. *Kidney Int.* 10:5, 1976.
Shalhaub, R. J. The medical management of chronic renal failure. *Med. Times* 107:23, 1979.
Shils, M. E. Renal disease and the metabolic effects of tetracycline. *Ann. Intern. Med.* 58:389, 1963.
Siiteri, P. K., and Wilson, J. D. Dihydrotestosterone in prostatic hypertrophy: I. The formation and content of dihydrotestosterone in the hypertrophic prostate of man. *J. Clin. Invest.* 49:1737, 1970.
Solez, K., Morel-Maroger, L., and Sraer, J. D. The morphology of "acute tubular necrosis" ("ATN") in man. *Kidney Int.* 12:519, 1977.
Sorkin, M. I. Acute renal failure. *Med. Times* 107:33, 1979.
Stein, J. H., et al. Pathophysiology of a nephrotoxic model of acute renal failure. *Kidney Int.* 8:27, 1975.
Steinhausen, M., Eisenbach, G. M., and Helmstädter, V. Concentration of Lissamine green in proximal tubules of antidiuretic and mercury poisoned rats and the permeability of these tubules. *Pfluegers Arch.* 311:1, 1969.
Sudo, M., et al. Renal hemodynamics in uranyl acetate–induced acute renal failure of rabbits. *Kidney Int.* 11:35, 1977.
Sufrin, G., and Murphy, G. P. Renal adenocarcinoma (review of article). *Urol. Surv.* 10:129, 1980.
Summers, W. K., and Jamison, R. L. The no reflow phenomenon in renal ischemia. *Lab. Invest.* 25:635, 1971.
Swyer, G. J. M. Postnatal growth changes in human prostate. *J. Anat.* 78:130, 1944.
Tanner, G. A., Sloan, K. L., and Sophasan, S. Effects of renal artery occlusion on kidney function in the rat. *Kidney Int.* 4:377, 1973.
Thurau, K., and Boylan, J. W. Acute renal success: The unexpected logic of oliguria in acute renal failure. *Am. J. Med.* 61:308, 1976.
Tichy, A., and Marchuk, J. Watch for this renal time bomb. *RN* 11:41, 1978.
Tobiason, S. J. Benign prostatic hypertrophy. *Am. J. Nurs.* 79:286, 1979.
Tortora, G. J., et al. *Principles of Human Physiology*. Hagerstown, Md.: Harper & Row, 1981.
Venkatachalam, M. A., et al. Ischemic damage and repair in the rat proximal tubule: Differences among the S_1, S_2 and S_3 segments. *Kidney Int.* 14:31, 1978.
Vermeulen, A., and DeSy, W. Androgens in patients with benign prostatic hyperplasia before and after prostatectomy. *J. Clin. Endocrinol. Metab.* 43:1250, 1976.
Walsh, P. C., and Wilson, J. D. The induction of prostatic hypertrophy in the dog with androstanediol. *J. Clin. Invest.* 57:1093, 1976.
Weller, J. M. (ed.). *Fundamentals of Nephrology*. Hagerstown, Md.: Harper & Row, 1979.
Whitmore, W. F. Benign prostatic hyperplasia: Widespread and sometimes worrisome. *Geriatrics* 36:119, 1981.
Wilson, J. D. The pathogenesis of benign prostatic hyperplasia. *Am. J. Med.* 68:745, 1980.
Yu, G. S. M., et al. Renal oncocytoma. *Cancer* 45:1010, 1980.

UNIT 11
ENDOCRINE REGULATION

Sue Baldwin
PITUITARY FUNCTION

Camille Stern
FUNCTIONS OF THE ADRENAL, THYROID, AND PARATHYROID GLANDS

Doris Heaman
PANCREATIC FUNCTION

John Marino
DIABETES MELLITUS

Pearl Rosendahl
ENDOCRINE FUNCTION OF THE PANCREAS

The endocrine system is a complex system that coordinates and maintains the steady state through hormone secretion. The secretion of hormones is generally activated by other hormones and/or neural influences and the regulation follows a closely regulated feedback mechanism. Chapter 30 describes pituitary function and explains how alterations in function can affect other body functions. Chapter 31 details the varied functions of the adrenal gland, its role in the stress response, and major alterations in function. Chapter 32 follows normal thyroid activity with discussion of hyperthyroidism, hypothyroidism, and thyroid malignancy. Parathyroid function is also included in this chapter. Chapter 33 includes the normal endocrine secretion activities of the pancreas. Exocrine activities are discussed in Chapter 36. Diabetes mellitus, pancreatitis, carcinoma of the pancreas, and cystic fibrosis are the major pathologies studied in this chapter.

The reader is encouraged to utilize the learning objectives at the beginning of each chapter to organize the study of this unit. The unit bibliography is also helpful in providing direction for further study.

CHAPTER 30
PITUITARY REGULATION AND ALTERATIONS IN FUNCTION

LEARNING OBJECTIVES

1. Recall the normal structure and location of the pituitary gland.
2. Differentiate between the structure and function of the adenohypophysis and the neurohypophysis.
3. Identify the area called the pars intermedia.
4. Define *chromophils* and *chromophobes.*
5. Differentiate morphologically between acidophils and basophils.
6. List and describe the functions of the hormones of the adenohypophysis.
7. List and describe the functions of the two hormones of the neurohypophysis.
8. Describe the feedback method of control between the hypothalamus and pituitary gland.
9. Briefly outline the vascular supply to the pituitary and hypothalamus.
10. List at least four known hypothalamic releasing factors.
11. Clearly differentiate between specific trophic hormones and secretions of the target gland.
12. List and describe the magnitude of effects of growth hormone (GH).
13. Describe the physiologic effects of ADH.
14. Explain the different factors that cause the release of ADH.
15. Briefly describe the effects of oxytocin or uterine contractility, lactation, and fertilization.
16. Explain the mechanical and hormonal effects of pituitary malfunction.
17. Briefly describe conditions and effects of enlargement of the sella turcica.
18. List some causes of deficiency conditions of the anterior pituitary.
19. Define *panhypopituitarism.*
20. Describe the results of deficiencies in single pituitary hormones.
21. Explain how deficiencies in single pituitary hormones affect the metabolism of the entire organism.
22. Specifically describe Sheehan's syndrome.
23. Describe the results of hypersecretion of single pituitary hormones.
24. Differentiate between giantism and acromegaly.
25. Differentiate between Cushing's disease and Cushing's syndrome.
26. Define and explain *ADH deficiency states.*
27. Clearly explain the syndrome of inappropriate ADH secretion (SIADH).
28. List at least six etiologic factors for SIADH.
29. Relate pituitary tumors to hyperpituitarism and hypopituitarism.
30. Describe the morphologic differences in pituitary tumors.
31. List some clinical manifestations of pituitary tumors.

The human organism encompasses complex systems of communication for the purpose of coordinating and maintaining a steady state essential to its bodily functions. Through these communication systems the body monitors the functions and needs of each of its component parts and responds accordingly to maintain normalcy.

Although the nervous system is the dominant controlling influence over the activities and responses of the body, secondary mechanisms exist by which one cell can influence the function of other distantly located cells. The influence is effected through the secretion or inhibition of secretion of a variety of elements into the bloodstream. These elements are referred to as *hormones,* from the Greek root *hormaein,* which means to excite, arouse, or set in motion.

Cells that secrete hormones into the bloodstream may be organized into functional units, as in glands, or may be more diffusely dispersed throughout the tissues. They are called endocrine cells or glands and collectively make up the endocrine system. The cells and glands of the endocrine system each have very specific functions and coordinate with other cells to create an environment conducive to survival of the total organism. Figure 30-1 shows the anatomy and location of the endocrine glands.

Secretion of a given hormone is generally activated by hormonal and/or neural influences on specific target cells by feedback mechanisms. Hormones secreted act selectively on other specific target cells to regulate and maintain normal function.

This chapter is concerned with the pituitary gland. Included are the anatomic structure and physiologic function, the role within the complex communication system for maintaining a steady state, its relationship to the overall endocrine system, and pathologic manifestations of functional imbalance.

MORPHOLOGY OF THE PITUITARY GLAND

Gross Anatomy

The human adult pituitary is approximately 1 cm long, 1.0 to 1.5 cm wide, and 0.5 cm thick. It is a round or ovoid structure and weighs about 0.5 gm. Because of its position beneath the hypothalamus of the diencephalon, it is also called the *hypophysis,* taken from the Greek root *hypon,* meaning under, and *phyeis* meaning to grow. The gland rests in a small depression (hypophyseal fossa) of the sphenoid bone called the sella turcica. It is covered by a tough membrane (diaphragma sellae) through which passes the structure joining the pituitary to the hypothalamus (hypophyseothalamic stalk). This structure is also called the infundibular stalk.

Anatomically and physiologically the pituitary can be divided into three regions, two of which function as distinct and different endocrine organs. The anterior lobe is called the *adenohypophysis,* and may be subdivided into three regions: (1) the pars tuberalis, made up of a small mass of tissue running up along the infundibulum and surrounding

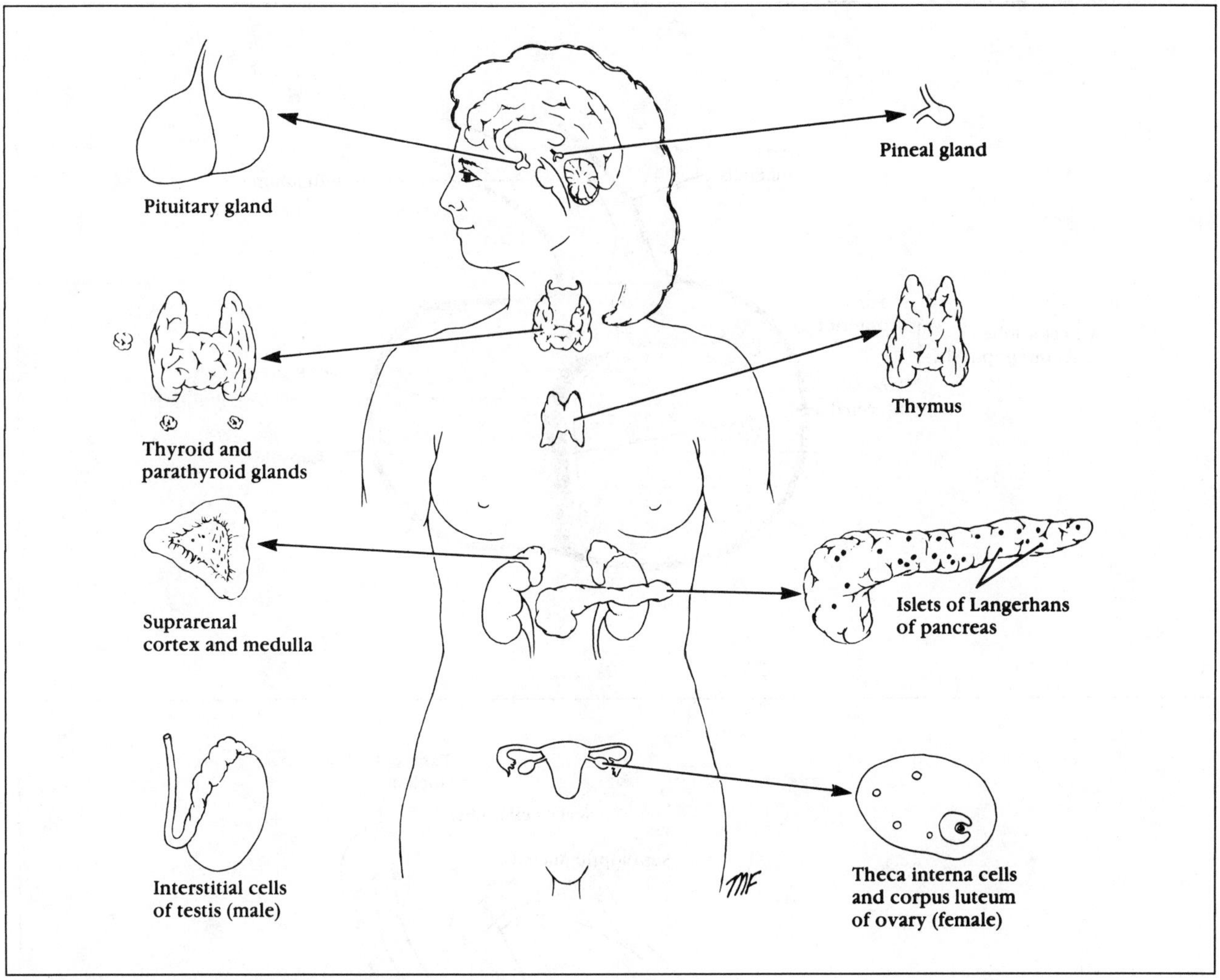

FIGURE 30-1. Location of the endocrine glands.

the stalk; (2) the pars distalis, which forms the bulk of the anterior lobe; and (3) the pars intermedia, or intermediate lobe, made up by the thin layer of cells between the anterior lobe and the neurohypophysis. The posterior lobe is called the neurohypophysis and includes three regions: (1) the neural lobe, (2) the infundibular stalk, and (3) the median eminence of the tuber cincreum, which forms the attachment with the hypothalamus (Fig. 30-2). The intermediate lobe is often considered a separate and distinct lobe. However, since this lobe is poorly developed in the adult human and its function is unknown, it is often categorized as a region of the anterior lobe.

The pituitary develops from a common germ layer, the ectoderm, but originates from two distinctly different embryologic anatomic sources. The adenohypophysis derives from an upward diverticulum of the ectodermal layer of the roof of the mouth or pharyngeal epithelium known as Rathke's pouch. The neurohypophysis originates as a downward ectodermal diverticulum from the hypothalamic portion of the diencephalon. These two lobes come together to form the hypophysis. The junction of the two lobes forms the intermediate lobe. Whereas Rathke's pouch loses its connection with the pharyngeal membrane, the neurohypophysis retains neural tract connections with the hypothalamus. These neural fiber connections play a crucial role in the secretory functions of the neurohypophysis.

The functioning pituitary remains connected to the hypothalamus of the brain through the neural tracts of the infundibular stalk and by an elaborate vascular system. These neural and vascular pathways are essential to the function of the pituitary, which is the bridging of the nervous system with the endocrine system [6].

Histology

ADENOHYPOPHYSIS. Traditionally, anterior pituitary cells have been classified on the basis of their staining properties. Many of these cells contain secretory granules but some are sparsely granulated or considered to be agranular. Cells containing secretory granules (granulae) are called

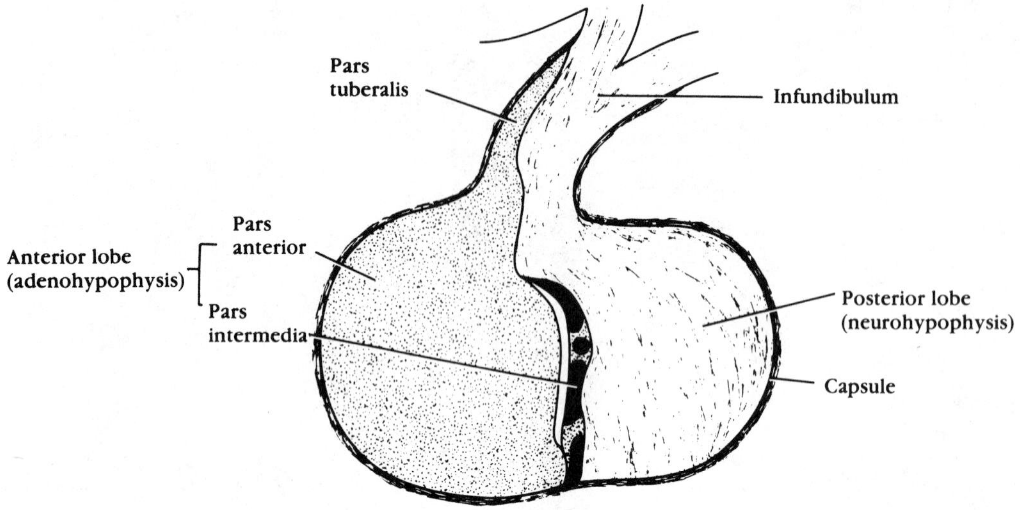
Pars
tuberalis
Infundibulum
Pars
anterior
Anterior lobe
(adenohypophysis)
Pars
intermedia
Posterior lobe
(neurohypophysis)
Capsule

A

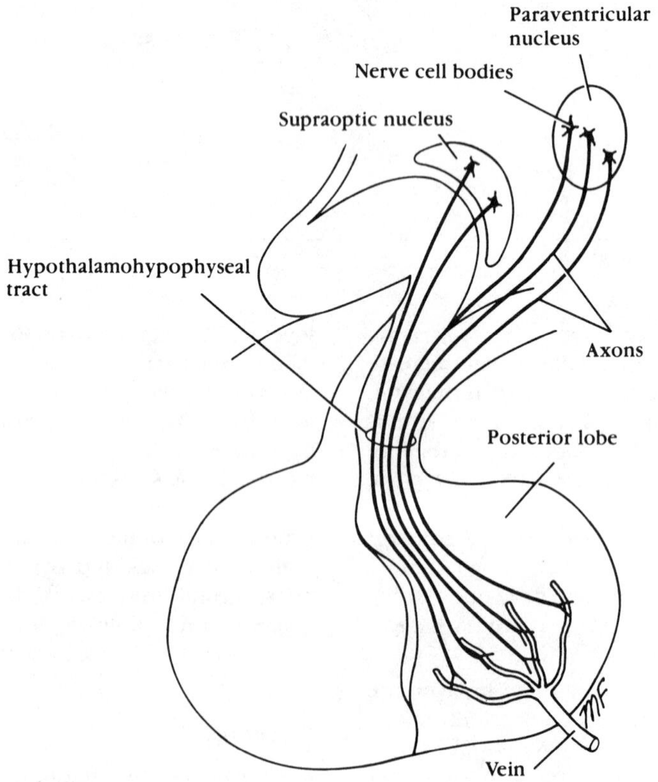
Paraventricular
nucleus
Nerve cell bodies
Supraoptic nucleus
Hypothalamohypophyseal
tract
Axons
Posterior lobe
Vein

B

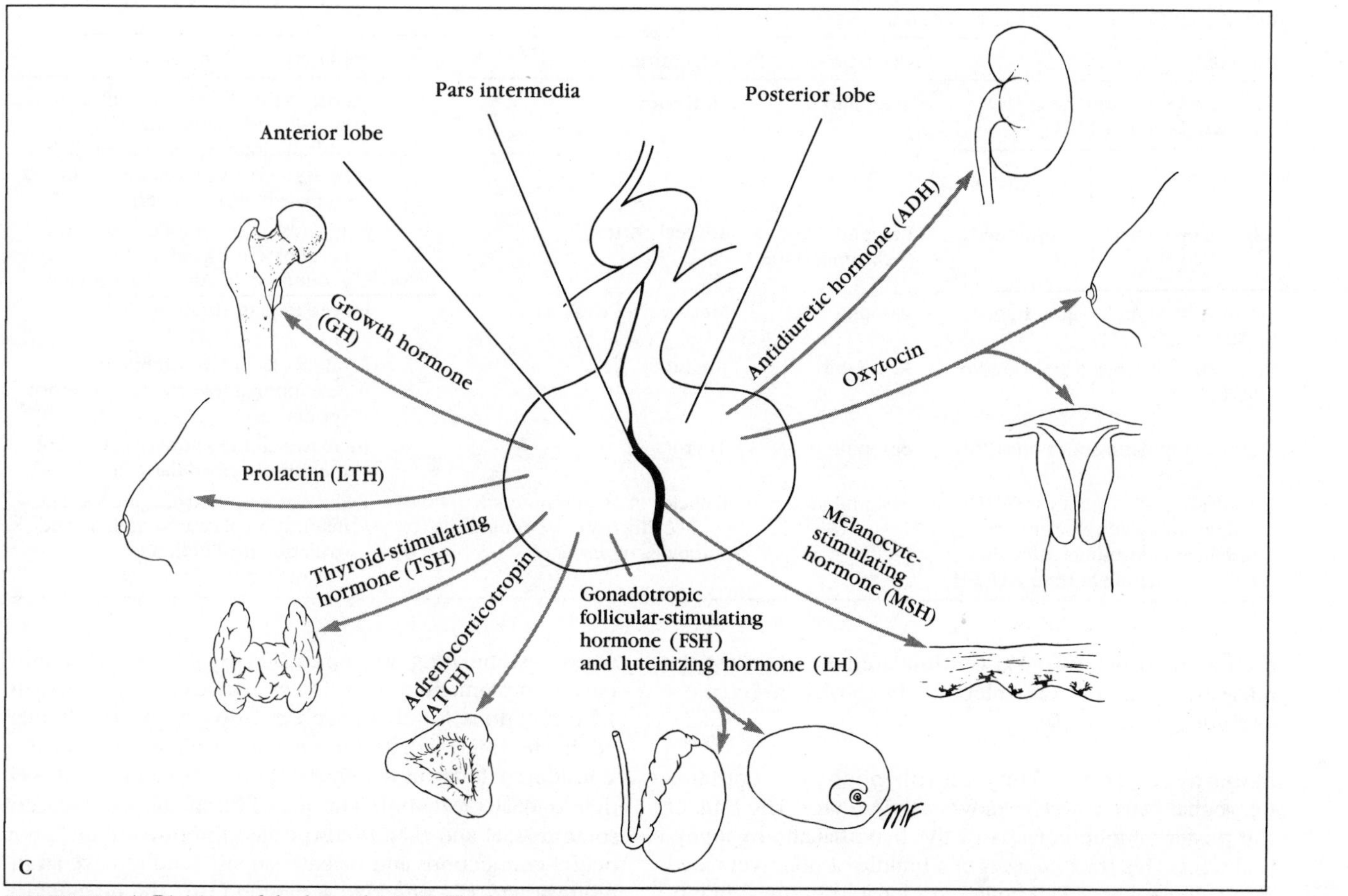

FIGURE 30-2. A. Divisions of the hypophysis. B. The hypothalamo-hypophyseal tract. C. Diagram showing how the pituitary gland controls the body.

chromophils, while those only sparsely granulated or agranular are called *chromophobes* [10].

Chromophobes compose approximately 50 percent of the total cellular populations of the adenohypophysis. These cells stain poorly. They are considered to have no secretory functions and to serve as precursors of secretory cells [6]. This view has been subject to question, however, since tumors containing chromophobe cells exclusively are associated with excessive secretion of various anterior pituitary hormones, and some studies seem to indicate that chromophobe cells do sometimes have secretory function [3].

Chromophilic cells are subdivided on the basis of their staining properties. Secretory granules of these cells take up either acidic or basic stains and are therefore called *acidophilic* or *basophilic* cells.

Acidophils (alpha cells) make up approximately 35 to 40 percent of the cells of the adenohypophysis. They are considered to be responsible for the secretion of growth hormone (GH) and luteotrophic hormone (LTH), also called prolactin.

Basophils (beta cells) make up 10 to 15 percent of the cells of the adenohypophysis. They are believed to secrete thyrotropic hormone, also called thyroid-stimulating hormone (TSH), and luteinizing hormone (LH), also called interstitial cell–stimulating hormone (ICSH). Basophils are thought to be partially responsible for the secretion of adrenocorticotropin (ACTH), also called corticotropin. Recent findings indicate that chromophobic cells, which have previously been considered to be nonsecretory, may also play a role in the secretion of corticotropin.

Acidophils and basophils can be further subdivided on the basis of histochemical reactions, shape, and location. With new immunofluorescent techniques, as many cell types can be identified as there are known anterior pituitary hormones, and a particular cell type can be assigned to each hormone [4]. In addition, the anterior pituitary secretes β-lipoprotein (β-LPH), although its physiologic role is not clearly understood at this time. A summarization of these cell types in relation to hormones secreted is depicted in Table 30-1.

The foregoing discussion represents an attempt to simplify cellular-hormonal relationships; however, it is recognized that, in actual fact, no simple one-to-one interaction exists. A review of Table 30-1 shows that in at least two instances, two hormones are secreted by the same type of cell. In other instances, secretion of a given hormone may be stimulated by a multiplicity of factors. For example, se-

TABLE 30-1. Cell types in relation to hormones secreted

Hormone	Cell type	Target organ	Function
Somatotrophic hormone (STH); growth hormone (GH)	Acidophil	All tissues	Increases rate of protein synthesis in all cells; decreases rate of carbohydrate utilization throughout body; increases mobilization of fats and use of fats for energy
Adrenocorticotrophic hormone (ACTH)	Basophil, large chromophobe	Adrenal cortex	Regulates secretion of cortisol and corticosteroids; enhances production of adrenal androgens
Melanocyte-stimulating hormone (MSH)	Basophil	Melanocytes of skin	Increases pigmentation
Prolactin or luteotrophic hormone (LH)	Acidophil	Breasts	Produces lactation; stimulates development of alveolar secretory system
Thyroid-stimulating hormone (TSH)	Basophil	Thyroid	Increases all the known activities of the thyroid glandular cells
Gonadotrophic hormones (GTH): follicle-stimulating hormone; luteinizing hormone; interstitial cell–stimulating hormone (ICSH)	Basophil	Follicles of ovaries, interstitial cells of Leydig testes, seminiferous tubules of testes	Regulates spermatogenesis; regulates maturation of ovarian follicle and ovulation production of testosterone

cretion of prolactin is also stimulated by thyrotropin releasing hormone and inhibited by prolactin release–inhibiting hormone [9].

NEUROHYPOPHYSIS. The neurohypophysis contains neuroglial cells and cells known as pituicytes. The bulk of the posterior lobe consists of the hypothalamo-hypophyseal tract. This tract consists of a bundle of nonmyelinated nerve fibers whose cell bodies are located in the supraoptic nucleus of the hypothalamus near the optic chiasma, and in the paraventricular nucleus in the wall of the third ventricle. Axons from these cell bodies traverse the hypophyseal stalk to terminate in the posterior lobe in close proximity with the vessels composing the capillary plexus. Pituicytes are found along the nerve terminals of the neurohypophysis and serve no known endocrine function. Neurosecretory material known as Herring bodies is dispersed throughout the axoplasm of the fibers of the hypothalamo-hypophyseal tract and plays a role in hormone secretion. The neurohypophysis stores and releases two hormones. These are *oxytocin* and *antidiuretic hormone* (ADH), also known as vasopressin.

PARS INTERMEDIA. The intermediate lobe separates the adenohypophysis from the neurohypophysis. The neural side is made up of *basophilic* cells organized in multiple layers. Some uncertainty has existed regarding the exact function of this lobe. Ganong discusses the physiologic function within the following framework [3]: Intermediate lobe cells and corticotropes of the anterior lobe both synthesize a precursor protein called proopiocortin. In the cortitrops this precursor is hydrolized to ACTH and β-lipotropin (β-LPH) and these hormones are secreted. It may be further hydrolyzed in intermediate lobe cells to α-melanocyte–stimulating hormone (α-MSH) and β-melanocyte–stimulating hormone (β-MSH). Melanocytes influence skin pigmentation. In lower animals the intermediate lobe functions for this purpose. However, in the human adult, the intermediate lobe is very rudimentary and it is considered doubtful whether it synthesizes and secretes either α-MSH or β-MSH. The pars intermedia may secrete some α-MSH and β-MSH, also called intermedin, but poor neural connections and vascular supply tend to have an inhibitory effect in effective secretion [15]. The pigmentary changes encountered in several endocrine diseases, such as the abnormal pallor seen with hypopituitarism and hypopigmentation seen with adrenal insufficiency, are attributed to changes in circulating ACTH. Since α-MSH has a common 13–amino acid sequence with ACTH, this hormone has melanocyte-stimulating activity.

RELATIONSHIP OF THE PITUITARY TO THE HYPOTHALAMUS

Although the pituitary has been called the "master gland," it is now known that many pituitary functions are controlled by the hypothalamus. Secretion of pituitary trophic hormones is activated by signals from the hypothalamus through a complex humoral and neural communication system.

Hypothalamic Secretion of Release and Inhibiting Factors

Through feedback and other mechanisms of communication, specialized neurons in the hypothalamus are stimulated to synthesize and secrete substances called hypothalamic-releasing and -inhibiting factors. The function of releasing and inhibiting factors is to regulate the secretion of pituitary trophic hormones, which, in turn, control the

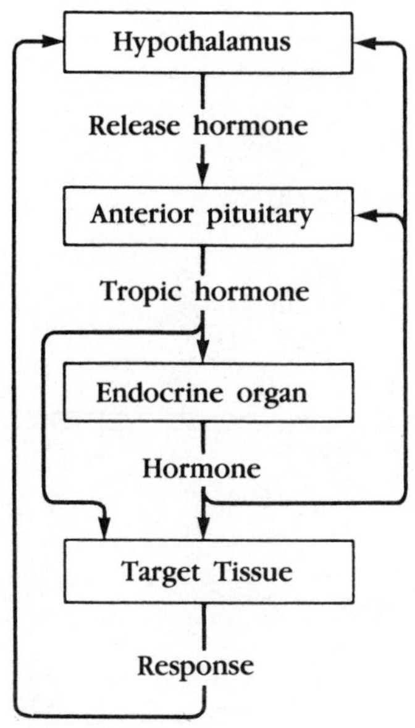

FIGURE 30-3. Negative feedback system for maintaining hormone balance.

secretion of hormones by target glands of the pituitary, for example, the thyroid, adrenals, and gonads.

The hypothalamus has the capacity to secrete a corresponding release factor for each anterior pituitary hormone. For some pituitary hormones, it also secretes a corresponding inhibiting factor. For all hormones except prolactin, the releasing factor is of most importance in regulation. For prolactin, however, the inhibiting factor is thought to exercise the most control. For the growth hormone, both the release and inhibiting factors may control.

An inverse relationship exists between the blood levels of hormones of the various pituitary target organs and synthesis and secretion of the related pituitary trophic hormone. Control of secretion through negative feedback occurs by the following mechanism: When the circulating plasma level of any given target organ hormone is elevated above the level of body need, the hypothalamus, which serves as a collecting center for information, is able to sense this imbalance. It does so by encoding information concerning plasma concentration of the hormone as well as various other stimuli in its humoral and neural environment. The hypothalamus interprets this information and responds by releasing a secretion-inhibiting factor (IF), which signals the pituitary to cease secretion of the specific controlling trophic hormone. Cessation of trophic hormone release in turn acts to halt release of hormones by the target organ and therefore lowers plasma concentrations of the hormone in question until a state of balance is reached. Conversely, when the circulating plasma concentration of a target organ hormone falls below some critical level, the hypothalamus secretes a hormone-releasing factor (RF) to signal for increased secretion of the target organ hormone. Through the same circuit, this information is relayed to the target organ, which acts to increase secretion and restore hormone balance (Fig. 30-3). Although the concept of negative feedback is a valid one, it does not explain all of the complex interrelationships of hypothalamic-pituitary functioning. It does not explain all changes in the plasma levels of hormones resulting from a multiplicity of influences in the body's internal and external environment. Emotion, trauma, and diurnal changes create hormonal variations and other influences.

Hypothalamic-Pituitary Neural and Circulatory Structures

In order to understand clearly the influence of the hypothalamus on the pituitary, it is necessary to understand the neural and circulatory structure essential to their interrelationship. It will be remembered from previous discussion that the lobes of the pituitary each function as a distinct and different endocrine gland. Therefore, the structural relationship of each with the hypothalamus is different. The mode of transmission of signals from the hypothalamus is through neural connections for the neurohypophysis and through a complex vascular portal system for the adenohypophysis.

ADENOHYPOPHYSIS. The adenohypophysis secretes or fails to secrete its hormones into the circulation as a result of signals from the hypothalamus that arrive by the hypothalamic-hypophyseal portal system. The communication system between the hypothalamus and the adenohypophysis utilizes two capillary plexuses organized in series within the structures. Branches of the internal carotid and posterior communicating arteries of the circle of Willis give origin to the superior hypophyseal arteries. These arteries immediately branch to form a network of fenestrated capillaries called the primary plexus located on the ventral side of the hypothalamus (Fig. 30-4). Some capillary loops also penetrate into the median eminence and serve the dual functions of supplying nerve cells around the base of the hypothalamus and of receiving regulating factors secreted by hypothalamic cells.

The primary plexus drains into the sinusoidal hypophyseal portal vessels that carry blood down the infundibular stalk to the anterior pituitary. After reaching the adenohypophysis, the vessels again form a capillary network called the secondary plexus. These vessels serve the purpose of maintaining the cells of the anterior pituitary and delivering the regulatory factors from the hypothalamus to each cell. Vessels of the secondary plexus drain

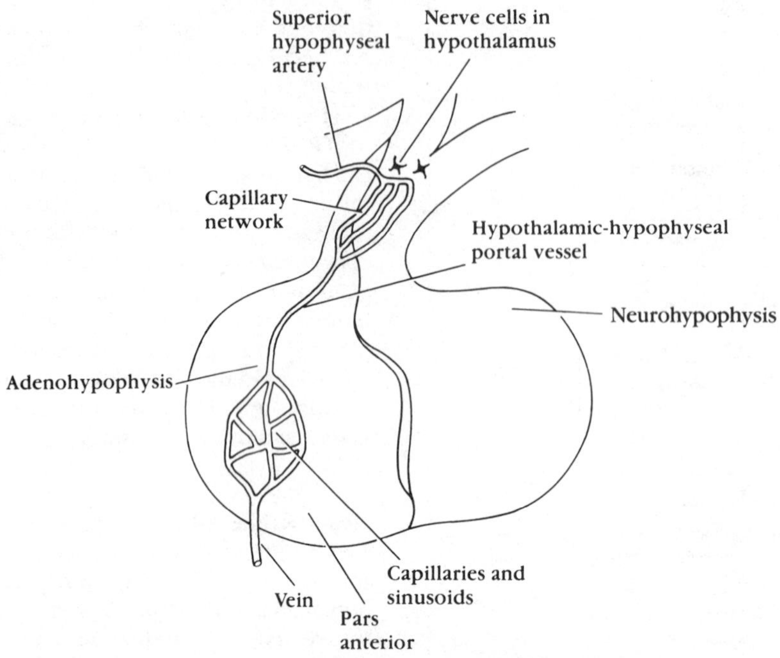

FIGURE 30-4. The hypothalamic-hypophyseal portal system.

into the anterior hypophyseal veins. From here, hormones are ultimately transported to their target glands. The system begins and ends in capillaries and is called the *hypothalamic-hypophyseal portal system* [5].

A number of studies lend support to the hypothesis that anterior pituitary function is achieved through neural as well as vascular communication input. The anterior pituitary, however, is poorly supplied with neural tracts from the hypothalamus. Studies have shown that there are no secretomotor nerve fibers in the anterior pituitary and only a sparsity of vasomotor fibers [4]. The following is a summation of the probable mechanism through which neural transmissions take place. The unusual vascular system of the pituitary functions to facilitate transmission of signals from the CNS to the adenohypophysis. As discussed previously, before reaching secretory cells of the gland, arterial blood passes through the primary plexus, which extends into the median eminence. A significant number of nerve fibers terminate in the vicinity of these capillaries. These nerve fibers release neurosecretory products that are carried through the capillary sinusoids of the anterior lobe through hypophyseal portal vessels to effect release of anterior pituitary hormones [3].

Neural signals may arise from external stimuli such as heat or cold or from internal stimuli such as emotion. Other neural stimuli that exert an influence but are as yet poorly understood include sleep-related and diurnal or circadian rhythms.

NEUROHYPOPHYSIS. The neurohypophysis, unlike the adenohypophysis, contains no cells with secretory granules. It will be remembered that embryologically, the posterior pituitary arises essentially as an invagination from the hypothalamus and retains neural tract connections from this area.

Cell bodies located in the supraoptic nucleus of the hypothalamus synthesize the antidiuretic hormone (ADH). Synthesis of oxytocin, the second hormone secreted by the posterior lobe, takes place in the paraventricular nucleus.

The neurosecretory process occurs in the following sequence. Hormone biosynthesis takes place within the cell bodies of the supraoptic or paraventricular regions of the hypothalamus in the form of hormonally inactive precursors. The active hormone is thought to be cleaved from the precursors during the 1- to 2-hour period in which they are transported down the axons of the neuron fibers to the posterior pituitary gland. A by-product of this cleavage is the protein *neurophysin*. The posterior pituitary contains two distinct neurophysins [3]. One is associated with antidiuretic hormone (ADH) and another with oxytocin. Hormones are stored in the posterior pituitary until release is triggered by the hypothalamus. Since neurosecretory cells retain their capacity to conduct electrical impulses, stimulation from the cell bodies in the hypothalamus are conducted down the axons of the neurosecretory fibers to trigger hormone release.

FUNCTIONS OF THE ANTERIOR PITUITARY

It is known that the adenohypophysis secretes at least six hormones, four of which directly control the functioning

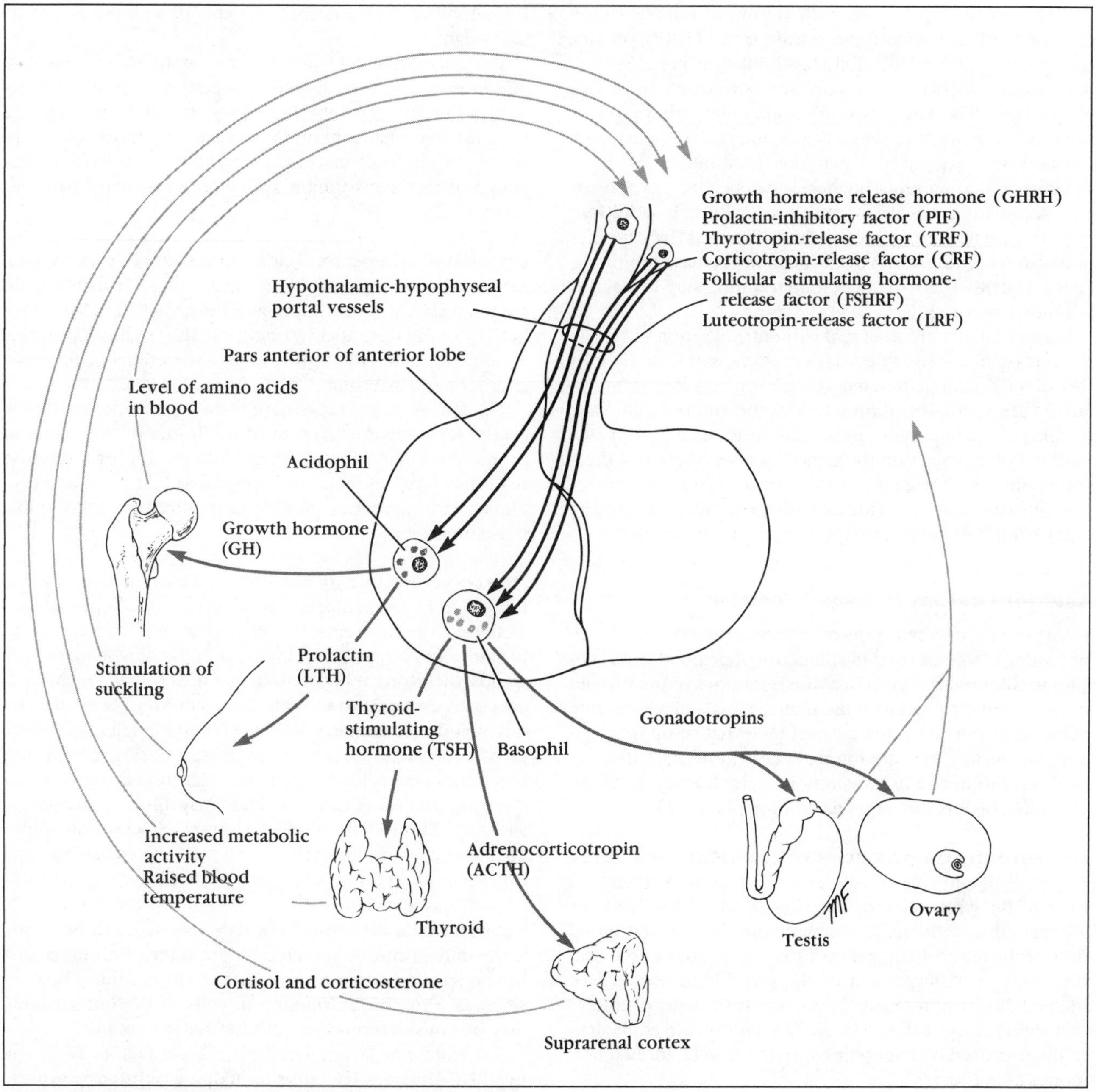

FIGURE 30-5. The mechanisms involved in controlling the activities of the pars anterior of the anterior lobe of the pituitary gland. Note the important feedback mechanisms.

of specific target glands—the thyroid, the adrenals, and the gonads. Hormones that control the functioning of target glands are called *trophic* from the Greek *trophos,* meaning to nourish, or *tropos,* meaning to turn toward. The six peptide hormones secreted by the anterior pituitary are (1) growth hormone, also called somatotropin (STH or GH); (2) adrenocorticotrophic hormone, also called corticotropin (ACTH); (3) thyroid-stimulating hormone, also called thyrotropin (TSH); (4) follicle-stimulating hormone (FSH); (5) luteinizing hormone (LH); and (6) prolactin (Fig. 30-5; see Table 30-1).

All, except growth hormone and prolactin, regulate the functions of other endocrine glands and are, therefore, trophic hormones. Growth hormone, ACTH, and prolactin are polypeptides, while TSH, LH, and FSH are glycoproteins. Growth hormone stimulates the secretion of somatomedin from the liver, which acts as an intermediary in the action of GH itself.

As discussed earlier, secretion of pituitary hormones is regulated by hypothalamic release or release-inhibiting factors. Release factors include thyrotropin release hormone

(TRH), somatotropin or growth hormone release factor (SRF or GHRF), corticotropin release factor (CRF), prolactin release factor (PRF), follicle-stimulating hormone release factor (FSHRF), and luteinizing hormone release factor (LHRF). The latter two are sometimes grouped into the single classification of gonadotropins since their target organs are the gonads. When this terminology is used, the corresponding releasing hormone is called gonadotrophic-stimulating release hormone (GnsRH). In addition, two release-inhibiting factors are liberated by the hypothalamus. These are growth hormone release-inhibiting factor (GHRIF), also called somatostatin, and prolactin-inhibiting factor (PIF).

Release factors are liberated by neurosecretion, which is the release of a substance from nerve endings directly into the bloodstream. Liberated release or release-inhibiting factors are carried to the sinuses of the anterior pituitary. Within the adenohypophysis, the release and release-inhibiting factors act on the glandular cells to control their secretions. The mechanisms that trigger synthesis and release of the factors include feedback as well as various other stimuli in the internal and external environment.

Anterior Pituitary Hormonal Function

THYROID-STIMULATING HORMONE (THYROTROPIN, TSH). The physiologic role of thyroid-stimulating hormone is to activate synthesis and secretion of the hormones of the thyroid gland in order to maintain the size of the gland and its rate of blood flow. The pathologic problems that result from derangements in TSH secretion are synonymous with those of hypersecretion and hyposecretion of the hormones of the thyroid, which is the target gland (see Chap. 32).

ADRENOCORTICOTROPHIC HORMONE (CORTICOTROPIN, ACTH). The physiologic role of adrenocorticotrophic hormone is to regulate synthesis and secretion of adrenal steroids by adrenal cortical tissue. It also maintains the size and blood flow of the adrenal cortex. Excessive secretions of the cortex result in enlargement of the gland, and absence or marked diminution results in atrophy. Pathologic problems that stem from imbalance in ACTH secretion are equivalent to those caused by hyper- or hyposecretion of adrenal hormones (see Chap. 31).

FOLLICLE-STIMULATING HORMONE (FSH). In men, the target organs for FSH are the testes where the hormone directly stimulates the germinal epithelium of the seminiferous tubules to activate and facilitate the rate of spermatogenesis. For optimal effects it appears to require the concomitant presence of LH in both men and women. These hormones are sometimes used in the treatment of infertility in both men and women.

In women, the target organs for FSH are the ovaries; FSH is essential for the normal cyclic growth of the ovarian follicle. It is responsible for the development and growth of a large number of graafian follicles and for an increased ovarian weight.

The gonadotropins stimulate the synthesis of testosterone in men and estradiol and progesterone in women. As with other anterior lobe hormones, secretion is triggered from the hypothalamus and is mediated by feedback mechanisms. Therefore, increased circulation levels of androgens and estrogens inhibit FSH secretions (see Chaps. 48 and 50) [2].

LUTEINIZING HORMONE (LH)—INTERSTITIAL CELL STIMULATING HORMONE (ICSH). Target organs for LH in the male are the testes, where it stimulates the growth and secretory activity of the testicular interstitial cells (Leydig cells). This action stimulates the synthesis and secretions of the male androgen testosterone.

The female target organs are the ovaries, where LH is essential for ovulation. Action of the hormone functions to promote readying of the ovaries follicle and for formation of corpus luteums from the ruptured follicle. As noted previously, the presence of FSH is required to accomplish these functions [7].

PROLACTIN (LACTOGENIC HORMONE). The predominant physiologic roles for prolactin are in breast development and lactation. The hormone acts in synergism with estrogen to promote growth and development of the female mammary glands; therefore, it is said to have a dual role in lactation. It acts with estrogen to prepare the mammary glands for lactation and then initiates secretion of the nutrients of these glands. Prolactin secretion increases during pregnancy, reaching a peak with delivery. The secretion is regulated by a release-inhibiting factor. Release may also be initiated by suckling. The initiation and adequacy of secretion shows physiologic variations associated with sleep, stress, and other stimuli as do other pituitary hormones.

GROWTH HORMONE (SOMATOTROPIN, GH). Growth hormone is the only hormone secreted by the anterior pituitary that has no specific target organ and, therefore, cannot be classified as a trophic hormone. All cells of the human body may be considered target cells for this hormone.

Somatotropin is regulated by release factors from the hypothalamus and by somatomedin, a substance synthesized in the liver. Since growth is a complex phenomenon, many other factors play a role in the rate and mode of growth. Action of GH is influenced by other hormones such as thyroid hormone, insulin, the steriods, and androgens. It is also influenced by nutritional status, exercise, stress, diurnal variations, and sleep. Secretion of GH is suppressed by an inhibiting factor (somatostatin). The growth hormone varies from other hormones in that it is species specific. In the presence of imbalance, only growth hormones synthesized from a human organism source (usually cadaveric) are effective for treatment. Effects of growth hormone may be summarized as follows:

1. *Effects on growth of bone and cartilage.* Growth hormone exerts an indirect rather than direct effect on the growth of bone and cartilage. It stimulates growth of these structures by promoting the synthesis of a number of proteins that are collectively called somatomedin. These proteins are known to be formed in the liver and probably in the muscle and kidneys also. Somatomedin acts directly on the bone and cartilage to promote growth. It is essential to the depositing of chondroid sulfate and collagen [5]. Because the formation of cartilage is accelerated and the epiphyseal plates widen, additional matrix is formed at the ends of long bones. Through this mechanism, linear structure is increased. After the period of development at which the epiphyses are closed, linear growth is no longer possible. Therefore, excessive growth hormone after adolescence results in thickening of bones and tissues.

2. *Effects on protein metabolism.* Growth hormone facilitates the transport of amino acids through the cell membrane. This increase in amino acid concentrations in the cells is thought to be partially responsible for increased protein synthesis. It is also believed to exert a direct effect on ribosomes to make them produce greater numbers of protein molecules [5]. As a result of these mechanisms, it creates a positive nitrogen and phosphorous balance and is therefore a protein anabolic hormone.

3. *Effects on RNA formation.* Growth hormone stimulates the transcription process in the nucleus, causing increased formation of RNA. This, in turn, promotes growth by promoting protein synthesis.

4. *Decreased catabolism of protein.* In addition to an increase in protein synthesis, a decrease in the breakdown of cell proteins occurs. The reduction is believed to result from growth hormone's ability to mobilize free fatty acids from adipose tissue to supply energy. This response acts as a protein sparer as well as a carbohydrate sparer [5].

5. *Effects on electrolyte balance.* Growth hormone increases gastrointestinal absorption of calcium and reduces Na^+ and K^+ excretion [3].

6. *Effects on fat and glucose metabolism.* Growth hormone exerts a strong influence in stimulating fat catabolism in adipose tissue. This action results in the production of large amounts of acetyl coenzyme A, which acts as a ready source of energy and has the effect of reducing the utilization of glucose for energy (glucose sparing). In the presence of excessive quantities of GH, several potential problems may develop from this action. The response may result in increased ketone levels in the blood (ketogenic effect) or it may increase concentration of liver lipids (fatty liver). The glucose-sparing effect of fat catabolism results in storage of increased amounts of glucose in the cells as glycogen. When cellular capacity becomes saturated, an increase in circulating blood levels of glucose occurs (diabetogenic effect), resulting in increased demand for insulin. If this effect persists long enough, exhaustion of the beta cells of the islets of Langerhans occurs and diabetes mellitus results. Growth hormone is not the only anterior pituitary hormone that increases blood glucose levels, however. ACTH, TSH, and prolactin all have this capacity.

7. Two additional facts seem important to the understanding of all growth hormone ramifications. First, GH fails to cause growth if carbohydrate is lacking. Second, growth hormone secretion is increased during episodes of hypoglycemia. Failure of GH secretion during periods of hypoglycemia is seen in adult hypopituitarism.

As these effects indicate in normal functions, growth hormone has many functions other than those of stimulating and supporting growth in the developing child. Although secretion and the subsequent physiologic effects are most pronounced during the early developing years, secretion and release are essential to many bodily functions throughout life.

FUNCTIONS OF THE NEUROHYPOPHYSIS

Unlike the adenohypophysis, the neurohypophysis does not function as an endocrine gland. Posterior pituitary hormones are synthesized in the hypothalamus and are stored in the posterior lobe to await the signal from the hypothalamus for release.

Cell bodies located in the supraoptic nuclei of the hypothalamus are considered to be largely responsible for synthesis of antidiuretic hormone (ADH) while cell bodies located in the paraventricular nuclei synthesize oxytocin. It is recognized, however, that both supraoptic and paraventricular nuclei cell bodies synthesize some amount of each of the two hormones secreted by the neurohypophysis (Fig 30-6).

Synthesis and secretion of posterior lobe hormones takes place in a two-step process [4]. In the first step, a hormonally inactive precursor is synthesized in the specified cells of the hypothalamus. This precursor is transported via secretory granules, down the neuron fibers of the hypothalamic-hypophyseal tract. The actual hormone is believed to be separated from the precursor during the period in which the granules traverse the axons of this tract to reach the posterior lobe. Hormones are then stored in the posterior pituitary until appropriate stimulus for secretion is initiated by the hypothalamus. Since neurosecretory cells and fibers also have the capacity to conduct electrical impulses, action potentials initiated by appropriate stimulus to cell bodies of the hypothalamus are conducted down the axons of the neuron fibers to stimulate release of the hormones.

Physiologic Action of Antidiuretic Hormone (ADH)

The kidneys are the specific target organs of ADH. In the presence of ADH, the distal tubules and collecting ducts of the nephrons become more permeable to water causing an increased water resorption. This results in decreased con-

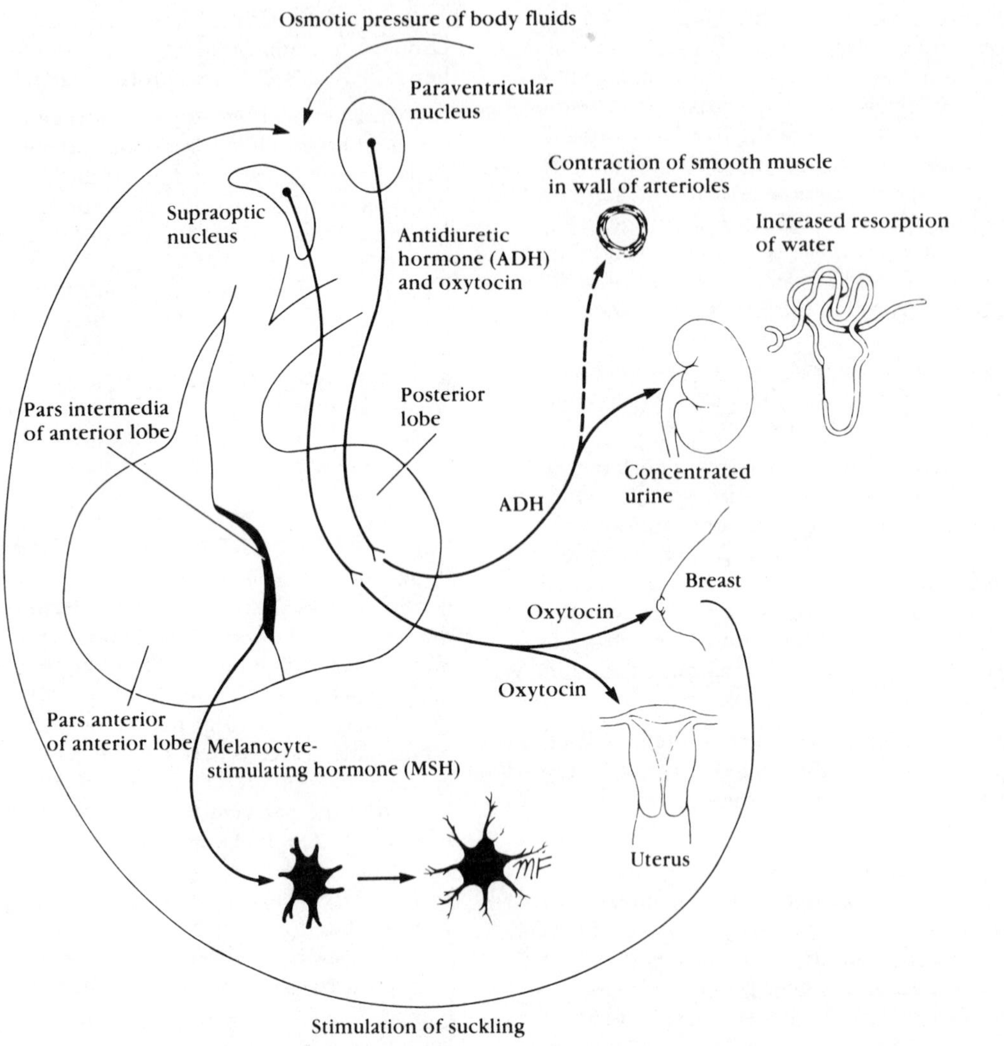

FIGURE 30-6. The mechanisms involved in controlling the activities of the posterior lobe of the pituitary gland. Note that the pars intermedia controls the melanocytes of the skin, but it is not under the control of the hypothalamus.

centration (osmotic pressure) of the extracellular fluid (plasma). It is known that in the absence of ADH, tubules and collecting ducts of the nephron are almost completely impermeable and little or no water is resorbed [5].

ADH also has a vasopressor effect when administered in large doses and may cause hypertension. The effect is caused by direct action of ADH on smooth muscles in the vascular wall. The effect may act to improve systemic fluid volume by reducing the size of the vascular bed.

REGULATION OF ADH BY THE HYPOTHALAMUS. Increased osmolarity of plasma and decreased circulating vascular volume are recognized as the major physiologic stimuli for initiating ADH secretion. Both osmoreceptors and volume receptors influence the hypothalamus to initiate the signal for release of ADH [4].

Osmoreceptors located in the hypothalamus consist of small vesicles surrounded by a semipermeable membrane in which nerve endings are embedded. Increased osmolarity of plasma in the vicinity of the hypothalamus causes water to move out of these osmoreceptors, decreases their volume, and reduces the degree of stretch sensed by neurons. This response presumably stimulates the hypothalamus and initiates the electrical impulse that signals for pituitary release of ADH.

Although the exact location of volume receptors is not known, they are generally thought to be located outside the CNS, probably predominantly in the thoracic cavity. Apparently the circulating vascular volume sensed in the thoracic region, rather than the vascular volume of the total body, is the crucial factor in ADH release. For example, a shift in blood volume, caused by pooling of blood in the periphery, is accompanied by ADH release as is change from a supine to a sitting or standing position. Exposure to high temperatures, which shifts blood from deeper to superficial regions, increases ADH secretion, while exposure to cold temperatures, which shifts blood from superficial to deeper regions, reduces its secretions. Positive pressure respiration, which decreases blood volume in the great veins of the thorax, results in ADH release.

OTHER FACTORS REGULATING ADH SECRETION AND RELEASE. As previously noted, feedback mechanisms protect blood osmolarity and volume balance through influence on ADH secretion. When all factors are in balance, uniform secretion of ADH maintains the fluid balance. When body fluids are depleted or osmotic pressure rises, appropriate mechanisms are activated and ADH is released. This stimulates the kidneys to resorb more water, which restores blood volume or reduces osmotic pressure, and balance is achieved. The state of balance inhibits release of ADH until further need arises (see Fig. 30-6).

Other factors also may influence ADH secretion. These include trauma, pain, anxiety, and drugs such as nicotine, morphine, and tranquilizers. Alcohol inhibits secretion, which partially accounts for the diuresis associated with excess intake of alcohol.

Oxytocin

UTERINE EFFECTS. Oxytocin has the capacity to stimulate the contraction of smooth muscle in a number of organs in the human body. A major physiologic role of this hormone is stimulation of smooth muscle cells in the pregnant uterus. It is released in large quantities during the expulsive phase of parturition. The mechanism by which oxytocin release is triggered has been described as follows: When labor begins, the tissues of the uterine cervix and vagina distend and become stretched. This stretch reflex initiates afferent impulses to the hypothalamus and stimulates the synthesis of oxytocin in cell bodies of the paraventricular nucleus. Oxytocin then migrates down the nerve fibers of the hypothalamic-hypophyseal stalk to the neurohypophysis. From here it is released into the circulation and is carried by the blood to the uterus, where it acts on smooth muscle cells to reinforce uterine contraction. Since greater amounts of this hormone are found in the blood during the expulsive stage of labor, it appears that the quantity of oxytocin released depends on the forcefulness of uterine contractions and the degree of stretch of cervical and vaginal tissues. It is recognized that oxytocin may be one of the factors that precipitate labor [4].

LACTATION EFFECTS. A second major role of oxytocin is in the ejection of milk from the lactating breast. Milk formed by cells of the breast is stored until suckling begins. For approximately 30 seconds to 1 minute after suckling is initiated, no milk is ejected. This is called the latent period. During this period suckling stimuli to the nipple of the breast initiates signals that are transmitted to neuron cell bodies in the paraventricular and supraoptic nuclei to initiate posterior pituitary release of oxytocin. Circulating blood transports oxytocin to the breasts where it initiates contraction of myoepithelial cells to force milk out of the alveoli into the ducts and lacteal sinuses opening to the nipple for milk ejection [4]. Since epinephrine inhibits oxytocin secretion, emotion, anxiety, and pain can inhibit oxytocin release.

EFFECTS ON FERTILIZATION. Distention and stretch of vaginal and cervical tissues during intercourse increases the secretion of oxytocin. Uterine contractions experienced during orgasm have been attributed in part to this increased secretion. It has also been postulated that oxytocin facilitates fertilization by causing uterine propulsion of semen upward through the fallopian tube [5].

INTRODUCTION TO PITUITARY PATHOLOGY

Malfunctions of the pituitary gland result from one or more of the following: (1) invasive or impinging tumors of the pituitary or hypothalamus, (2) vascular infarction within the gland, (3) mechanical damage from trauma or surgery, (4) inflammatory processes, (5) genetic or familiar predisposition, (6) developmental and structural anomalies of the gland itself, (7) feedback from prolonged malfunction of one or more of its trophic glands, (8) autoimmune responses, or (9) idiopathic origin [7, 8].

Symptoms of pituitary malfunction may be precipitated by changes in hormonal balance or by purely mechanical forces. For example, tumors of the pituitary effect malfunction by pressure from their space-occupying properties, by destruction of tissue, and by contributing to hypersecretion as a result of tumor cell secretory capacity. More advanced or larger lesions may impinge on surrounding tissues, such as the optic chiasma or the area of the third ventricle, producing visual disorders, headaches, or other neurologic changes [9]. Vascular and tumor infarctions, structural and developmental anomalies or inflammatory processes, and autoimmune responses influence functioning by compromising or destroying tissue. Feedback from malfunction of a target gland can result in hyperplasia of the pituitary.

Since the pituitary is a crucial link in the production of a variety of hormones, abnormalities of the gland often alter normal hormone secretion. Pressure or tissue destruction may compromise function and result in problems associated with hyposecretion of the gland. Conversely, since many tumors of the pituitary are hormone-secreting, the presence of tumorous lesions may result in problems stemming from hypersecretion of the gland.

Factors that influence hormone secretions of the pituitary inevitably influence functions of the specific endocrine gland(s) dependent on the hormone(s). For example, conditions that stimulate hyperfunctioning properties of the pituitary initiate excessive activation of the target organ(s), while suppression or destruction of pituitary tissue with loss of trophic hormone secretions results in target organ hypofunctions.

For convenience, discussion of pituitary pathologies may be categorized as disorders of the adenohypophysis or of the neurohypophysis. They may be further subdivided as disorders of hyperfunctioning or of hypofunctioning. Since the anterior and posterior lobes of the pituitary operate in general as distinct and separate functional units, malfunctions of each of the glands differ characteristically.

PATHOLOGY OF THE ANTERIOR PITUITARY

Four types of anterior pituitary disorders are usually described: (1) enlargement of the sella turcica with or without evidence of a space-occupying lesion, (2) visual disorders, (3) symptoms of hypopituitary hormone secretion, and (4) symptoms of hyperpituitary hormone secretion [7]. Hormone deficiencies resulting in malfunction may be classified as primary, secondary, or tertiary. Primary deficiencies occur as a result of disease of the target gland. Secondary deficiencies result from pituitary lesions or disorders. Tertiary deficiencies result from hypothalamic disorders.

Evaluation of persons with pituitary diseases may include radiologic, neuroophthalmic, and/or endocrine diagnostic studies. The type of test used and the extent of testing is dependent on the symptoms described. Radiologic studies include plain skull x rays, computerized axial tomography (CAT) scanning, pneumoencephalography, and arteriography. Neuroophthalmic evaluation is done by formal visual field examination using tangent screening. Endocrine studies include plasma levels and urinary excretion levels of each of the pituitary and target gland hormones.

Enlargement of the Sella Turcica

An increase in the size of the sella turcica often results from erosion of this structure caused by pressure from lesions in the pituitary region. Enlargement may be caused by pituitary adenomas, craniopharyngiomas, meningiomas, epithelial cysts, granulomas, malignant tumors of primary origin, or metastasis from carcinoma of the breast. Enlargement may result from nontumorous enlargement of the sella called empty sella syndrome. Sella enlargement may also result from primary hypothyroidism or hypogonadism, which may be attributed to hyperplasia of the thyrotrophs or gonadotrophs since it is accompanied by elevated thyrotropin or gonadotropin levels [7].

Endocrine evaluation for an enlarged sella turcica should include assessment of thyroid and adrenal hormone levels along with basal gonadotropin levels. Basal prolactin levels are important since more than one-half of pituitary tumors secrete prolactin.

EMPTY SELLA SYNDROME. This condition is classified as primary or secondary according to its underlying cause. Primary, or idiopathic, sella syndrome results from an abnormally large opening through which the hypophyseal stalk passes. This is often a developmental defect. With increased intracranial pressure, the arachnoid membrane tends to herniate through the opening, creating a sac filled with cerebrospinal fluid. This compresses the pituitary gland against the wall of the sella turcica, creating the appearance of an empty sella (Fig. 30-7). The condition may also occur as a consequence of necrosis of a pituitary adenoma or of Sheehan's syndrome, both of which are discussed later in this unit. Empty sella can develop secondary to spontaneous infarctions or regression of a tumor. The secondary variant of empty sella syndrome results from ablation of the gland by irradiation or surgery.

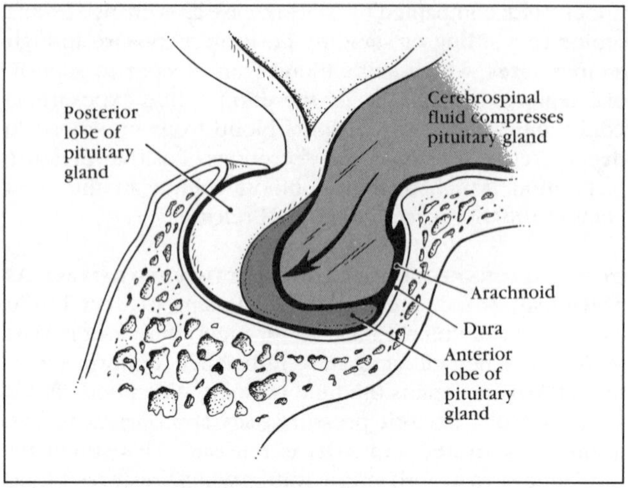

FIGURE 30-7. Empty sella syndrome.

On x-ray, the sella may appear enlarged or normal in size. The clinical picture for primary disease is rarely manifested as pituitary hypofunction. When hypofunction occurs, it is usually evidenced by impaired growth hormone and gonadotropin secretion.

Approximately 90 percent of persons with primary sella syndrome are female. It is evidenced most often in obese, hypertensive, middle-aged women who have borne many children. The tendency for the pituitary to enlarge during pregnancy and regress afterward may be the basis of pathogenesis. Headache is a common symptom. Visual field defects are rare but do occur in persons who have infarction of a pituitary tumor with subsequent development of empty sella or when the optic chiasma becomes prolapsed into the sella.

Hypopituitarism (Panhypopituitarism)

This syndrome may be initiated by any destructive process or by lesion of the pituitary gland. The most common processes are Sheehan's pituitary necrosis, nonsecreting adenomas, and craniopharyngioma [9]. Other causes include cysts, inflammation of the pituitary as a result of diabetes, meningitis, sarcoidosis, tuberculosis, syphilis, metastatic malignancy, and granulomas that may be nonspecific. Anterior pituitary hormone deficit may occur singly or in various combinations of multiple pituitary hormone secretion deficits. The speed of onset and extent of hormone deficiency depend on the nature and size of the precipitating cause. Onset may be acute and life-threatening as in acute adrenocortical insufficiency. More often, however, onset is slow and may occur over a period of months or years.

Clinical manifestations in adults suffering from panhypopituitarism may include absence of axillary and pubic hair, genital and breast atrophy, skin pallor, pallor of nipples, fine skin wrinkling (especially of the face), intolerance to cold, premature aging, poor muscle development, amenorrhea in premenopausal women, loss of previously normal libido and potency in men, and multiple endocrine deficiencies. General physical deterioration occurs and includes weakness, easy fatiguability, slothfulness, and indifference to surroundings. Shortness of stature may be evident if onset occurs before puberty. If hypothyroidism is marked, overweight is common. Reduced visual acuity, optic atrophy, and hemianopsia may occur if there is suprasellar expansion of the lesion or mass.

Diagnosis is made on the basis of history and physical examinations, neuroophthalmic examinations, and plasma immunoassay of TSH. Treatment consists of replacement of function through replacement of hormones. Thyroid replacement, cortisone, or hydrocortisone may be used as indicated. In women, diethylstilbestrol or premarin provides maintenance of secondary sex characteristics, while androgens or testosterone can restore libido and potency in men [2, 9].

Deficiency of Single Anterior Pituitary Hormones

PROLACTIN DEFICIENCY. Postpartum failure to lactate is the only symptom of clinical significance in prolactin secretion deficit. This specific hormone deficiency has classically been associated with the postpartum pituitary necrosis that results from hemorrhage and shock during delivery (Sheehan's syndrome).

GONADOTROPIN DEFICIENCY (ADIPOSOGENITAL DYSTROPHY OR FRÖHLICH'S SYNDROME). As previously stated, hypogonadism is the most common pituitary deficiency among adults. Deficiency in the premenopausal adult woman is manifested by amenorrhea, breast and uterine atrophy, and cornification of the vaginal orifice. The adult man experiences testicular atrophy and decreased libido, potency, beard growth, and muscle tone. When onset of the deficiency occurs prior to puberty the manifestations exhibited include an eunuchoid appearance, lack of development of secondary sexual characteristics, and infertility. Men fail to develop facial hair, an adult male voice, or normal genitalia. Women fail to manifest normal breast development or onset of menses. Both sexes may exhibit absence of axillary and pubic hair. The most common tumors responsible for the syndrome are the craniopharyngioma and chromophobe adenoma [1, 7].

THYROTROPIN DEFICIENCY. Hypothalamic or pituitary hypothyroidism exhibits some symptoms in common with primary hypothyroidism but is usually less severe. Isolated TSH deficiency is rare, however, and symptoms of other anterior lobe hormone deficiency are usually exhibited concomitantly. This factor usually distinguishes pituitary from primary hypothyroidism. In pituitary hypothyroidism, fine wrinkling of the skin and loss of secondary sex characteristics, which are related to gonadal insufficiency, are distinguishing characteristics. The hair is dry but not coarse as in the primary form and tongue enlargement is usually not present. Menstrual history is significant since menorrhagia is common in primary hypothyroidism while amenorrhea is expected in the pituitary form [7].

ACTH DEFICIENCY. ACTH deficiency is the most serious of the endocrine deficiencies in patients with pituitary disease [7]. Like pituitary hypothyroidism, ACTH deficiency is usually associated with other pituitary hormone deficiencies; this can be a characteristic, distinguishing pituitary origin from adrenal origin of disease. Symptomatology includes poor response to stress, nausea, vomiting, hyperthermia, and collapse. Decreased skin and nipple pigmentation is exhibited, which also distinguishes pituitary hypoadrenalism from primary adrenal disease (see Chap. 31).

GROWTH HORMONE DEFICIENCY (LORAIN-LÉVI SYNDROME). This condition results from pituitary insufficiency of growth hormone that affects children in the formative years. It is usually caused by a suprasellar cyst or craniopharyngioma, resulting in hypothalamic or pituitary hypofunction. It is often associated with evidence of sella turcica destruction seen on x ray. It can also be caused by ischemic necrosis and inflammatory changes. Dwarfism is not always exhibited but the physical characteristics are sometimes those of the symmetric dwarf with retention of infantile proportions (see Fig. 30-8). Other characteristics include lack of sexual development associated with bright rather than dull mentality. Persons suffering from this disease who reach adulthood have been described as graceful and attractive children, Peter Pans who refuse to grow up [3]. In these cases the growth and gonadotrophic hormones are deficient, while thyrotropic hormone and ACTH are unimpaired. In some cases an appearance of premature senility is evident with dry, wrinkled skin.

The characteristics of anatomic symmetry without gross deformity and normal mentality distinguish the person with Lorain-Lévi syndrome from genetic dwarfism and cretinism [8].

SHEEHAN'S SYNDROME. This manifestation of depressed pituitary function was first associated with pituitary necrosis occurring after a delivery complicated by hemorrhage and shock. In the course of pregnancy, the pituitary gland enlarges and develops increased circulation. In the event of acute blood loss, which sometimes accompanies labor and delivery, thrombi formation occurs from the slowed and

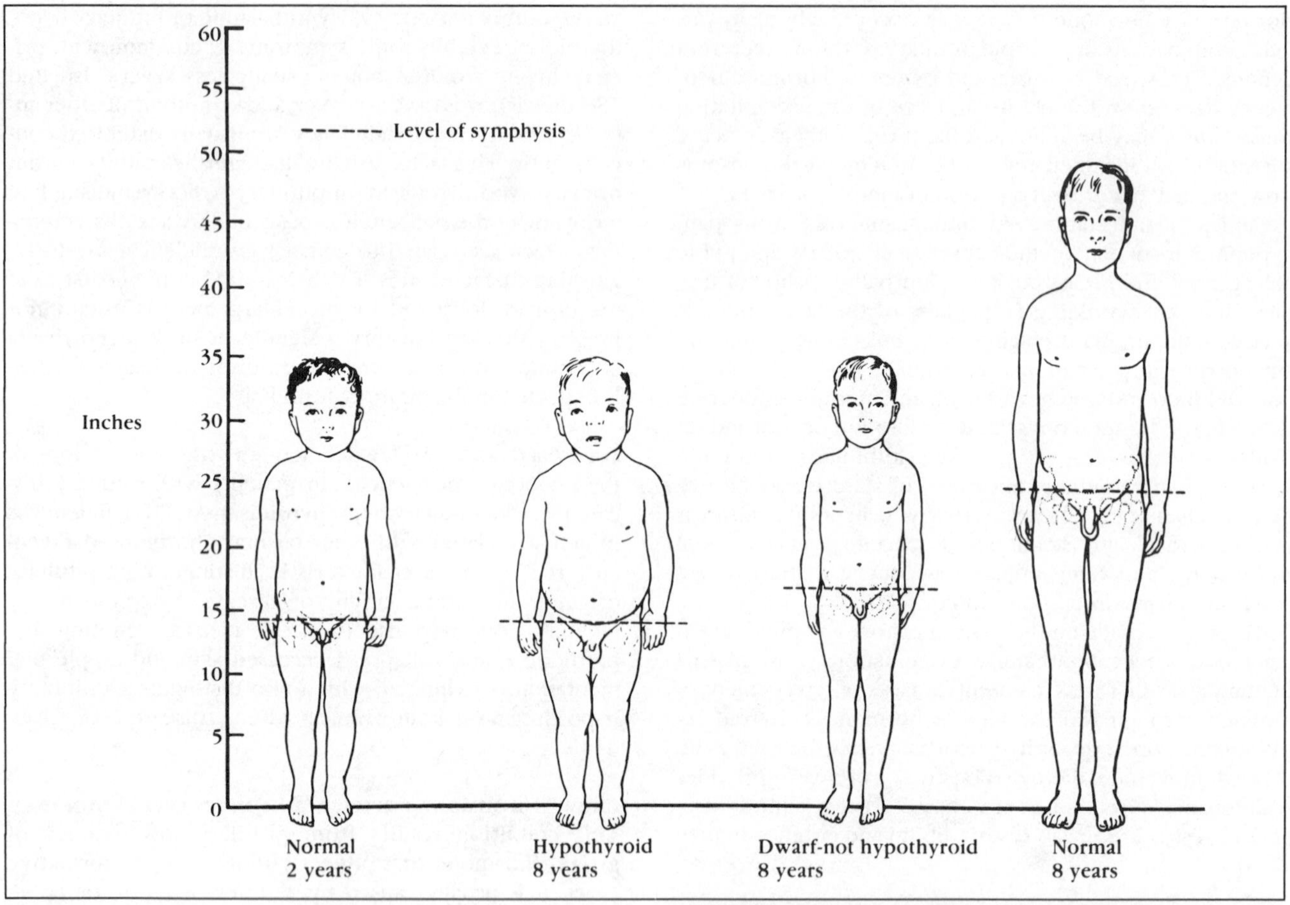

FIGURE 30-8. Normal and abnormal growth. Hypothyroid dwarfs retain their infantile proportions, whereas dwarfs of the constitutional type and, to a lesser extent, of the hypopituitary type have proportions characteristic of their chronologic age. (From L. Wilkins, *The Diagnosis and Treatment of Endocrine Disorders in Childhood and Adolescence* [3rd ed.]. Springfield, Ill.: Thomas, 1966.)

reduced circulation. The end result is infarction and necrotic destruction of glandular tissue, which becomes the basis of hypofunction of the gland. There may sometimes be a lag of months between the intrapartum incident and full development of symptoms. Symptoms that characterize the syndrome, however, are common to a variety of pathologic processes that destroy a significant proportion of pituitary function. Therefore, the syndrome may be produced by any destructive lesion of the pituitary.

Symptoms of the syndrome depend on the degree of impairment of pituitary function relative to the extent of tissue destruction. They may include (1) gonadal atrophy, (2) amenorrhea, (3) impotence and loss of libido, (4) loss of pubic and axillary hair, (5) loss of skin pigmentation, especially around the nipples, (6) flabby facies with thinning of eyebrows, (7) increased sensitivity to cold, (8) sluggish mentality, with slow, soft speech, (9) impalpable thyroid, and (10) hypotension. Hypoglycemia and achlorhydria are frequently present. Characteristic facial appearance similar to that of myxedema is apparent and the condition is sometimes called pituitary myxedema [7].

HYPOPHYSEAL CACHEXIA OR SIMMONDS' DISEASE. This condition may occur at any age, but is more prevalent in the postpubertal period. It occurs twice as frequently in women as in men. Profound cachexia is sometimes evident as is premature senility (progeria). Growth is arrested if the onset occurs before puberty. The clinical syndrome represents that of hyposecretion of gonadotropin, thyrotropin, and ACTH. Perhaps the most common picture is that of pituitary hypothyroidism and hypoadrenalism [9].

Table 30-2 depicts the etiologies of pituitary disease. Evaluation and diagnosis are by physical examination, neuroophthalmic evaluation, and baseline hormone levels.

Hyperpituitarism

Pathologic problems arising from pituitary hormone hypersecretions result from the presence of functioning adenomas of the gland itself. Those adenomas produce an excess secretion of either prolactin, growth hormone, or ACTH [7].

HYPERPROLACTINEMIA. Women with prolactin-secreting adenomas may exhibit galactorrhea, amenorrhea, or de-

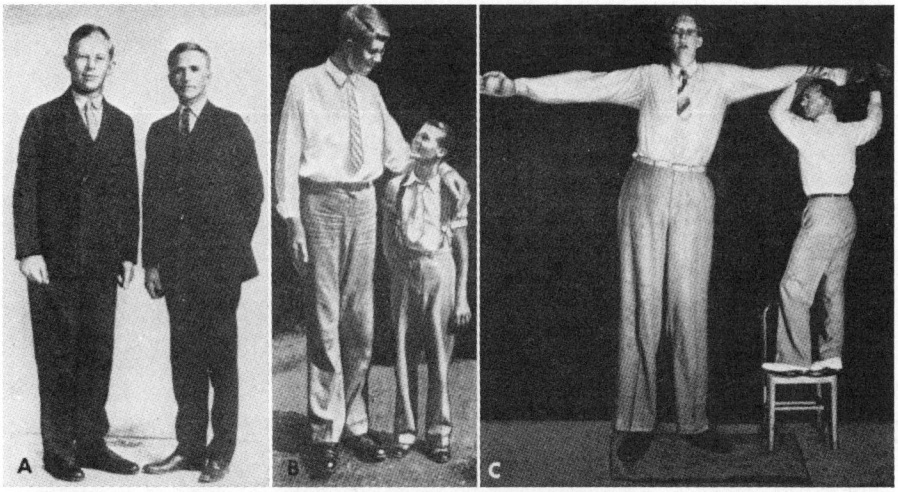

FIGURE 30-9. One of the most notable examples of growth hormone excess in the human was Robert Wadlow, later known as the "Alton giant." Although weighing only 9 pounds at birth, he soon began to grow excessively and by 6 months of age weighed 30 pounds. At 1 year he had reached a weight of 62 pounds. Growth continued throughout his life. Shortly before his death, which occurred at age 22 from cellulitis of the feet, he was found to be 8 feet, 11 in., in height and 475 pounds in weight by the careful measurements of Dr. C. M. Charles. A. Age: 9 years; height: 6 ft, 1 in. (shown with his father). B. Age: 13 years; height: 7 ft, 2 in. (shown with a friend of the same age). C. Age: 20 years; height: 8 ft, 6 in.; weight: 430 lb. (A and B from F. Fadner, *Biography of Robert Wadlow.* 1944. Courtesy of Bruce Humphries, Publishers. C is courtesy of Drs. C. M. Charles and C. M. MacBryde.)

TABLE 30-2. Etiology of pituitary disease

Congenital or hereditary conditions
Single hormone deficiency
Multiple hormone deficiency
Hypothalamic deficiency
Neoplasms
Pituitary tumors
Hypothalamic disorders: metastatic or other neoplasms
Vascular malformations
Postpartum necrosis (Sheehan's syndrome)
Intracranial aneurysm or arteriovenous malformation
Pituitary infarction
Vasculitis
Infections
Tuberculosis
Meningitis
Syphilis
Trauma: head injury
Radiation
Miscellaneous
Emotional deprivation in children
Tay-Sachs disease
Drugs
Sarcoidosis
Other

Source: K. J. Isselbacher, et al. (eds.), *Harrison's Principles of Internal Medicine* (9th ed.). New York: McGraw-Hill, 1980.

pressed libido. Some exhibit evidence of decreased estrogens and hirsutism (excessive hair growth in inappropriate places). These occurrences are believed to be the result of depression of ovarian function or stimulation of adrenal androgen function. Men with prolactin-secreting adenomas do not exhibit galactorrhea because of lack of development of acini in the male breast. These lesions in men usually present only as space-occupying lesions with hypogonadism. Diagnosis and evaluation are through radiologic studies and basal prolactin level studies.

ACTH HYPERSECRETION. Excess secretion of ACTH by the pituitary gland results in Cushing's disease. Manifestations of Cushing's syndrome are detailed in Chapter 31. Cushing's disease of pituitary origin is most frequently due to a basophil ACTH-secreting adenoma of the gland, although rarely it is due to basophil carcinoma. Excess ACTH causes hyperplasia and hyperfunction of the adrenal cortex.

HYPERSECRETION OF GROWTH HORMONE. Hypersecretion of GH occurring before the age of puberty results in giantism. This pituitary abnormality has been defined as height exceeding 80 in. in adults or a height exceeding three standard deviations above the mean for age in children. The disorder occurs as a result of oversecretion of growth hormone by a pituitary adenoma in a growing child before closure of the epiphysis. Before epiphyseal closure, growth is linear and symmetric.

Clinical features of giantism include symmetric growth of stature to enormous proportions, sometimes reaching 8 to 9 feet in height (Fig. 30-9). Symmetry occurs because both epiphyseal and oppositional bone growth occur concurrently. Affected persons do not develop the distortions that are characteristic of acromegaly. Persons with giantism experience many of the symptoms common with acromegaly. They suffer with osteoporosis and muscle weakness. Cardiac hypertrophy is also common and many patients with this problem ultimately die of cardiac failure. Thyroid enlargement and adrenal cortical hyperplasia occasionally occur. Early in the course of the disease persons with giantism may be unusually strong. Later, as the disease progresses, they may develop pituitary insufficiency with weakness and hypogonadism [7].

By definition, acromegaly means "enlargement of the acral parts or the extremities." It occurs when growth hormone–secreting tumors of the pituitary develop after the age of puberty and after fusion of the epiphysis has occurred. After epiphyseal closure, linear growth of bones is no longer possible. A thickening of tissues occurs and growth takes place in the acral areas.

Acidophilic or mixed acidophilic and chromophobic adenomas are predominantly responsible for these tumors. Growth of the tumor may ultimately destroy normal cells. As a consequence, hypopituitarism may develop as the disease progresses. Both sexes are affected equally and the problem is most often detected in the third or fourth decade of life. The disease is slow and insidious in progression and often goes undetected for years. Persons with the disease may first notice progressive increase in ring, shoe, hat, and glove sizes. The skull and head increase in size and the fingers and hands become broad and spadelike. Increased growth of subcutaneous connective tissue of the face produces coarsening of the features (Fig. 30-10). The face assumes a thick, fleshy appearance. There is thickening and enlargement of the lips with accentuated skin folds. The ears and nose become enlarged because of hypertrophy of the cartilages. There is overgrowth of the supraorbital ridge and the cheeks become prominent. Overgrowth of the maxilla produces lengthening of the face and alveolar bone growth results in separations of the teeth. Overgrowth of the mandible results in prognathism (jaw projection). Hypertrophy of the costal cartilage results in increased circumference of the chest. Absorption of bone is rapid and osteoporosis occurs. Acromegalic arthritis develops from proliferation of joint cartilage and effects joints of the long bones and spine. Long bones thicken and become massive in size. There is often bowing of the legs. The skin becomes thickened and hirsutism occurs in females. The tongue enlarges and may protrude from the mouth. The lungs, liver, spleen, kidneys, and intestines enlarge two- to fivefold. There is hypertension, coronary artery atherosclerosis, and marked cardiomegaly. Congestive heart failure often develops. The gonads enlarge but their function is subnormal. The adrenals, thyroid, and parathyroid become enlarged.

The typical physical picture is one of a big, burly person with forward carriage of the head, prognathism, kyphosis, bowlegs, prominent forehead, thickened chest, and husky, cavernous voice. Many men develop impotence and women develop amenorrhea. Apparently, growth of the adenoma impinges on the normal cells and induces other hormone insufficiency.

Diagnosis is by assessment of physical characteristics, serial photography, and laboratory immunoassay of plasma growth hormone levels.

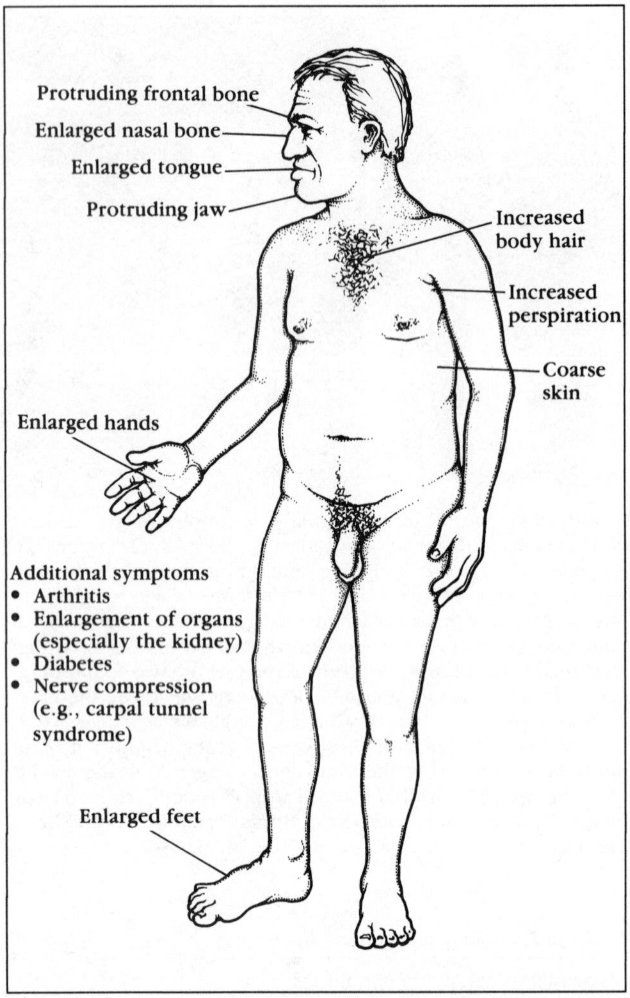

FIGURE 30-10. Composite of all symptoms of acromegaly. (From M. Beyers and S. Dudas [eds.], *The Clinical Practice of Medical-Surgical Nursing* [2nd ed.]. Boston: Little, Brown, 1984.)

PATHOLOGY OF THE POSTERIOR PITUITARY

Pathologic problems stemming from lesions of the neurohypothesis are rare. Posterior lobe pathology is almost always related to primary disease or other processes outside the gland itself. The posterior lobe releases two hormones, ADH and oxytocin, which are synthesized and secreted by the hypothalamus (see p. 408).

Antidiuretic Hormone Deficiency

A deficiency in ADH release results in diabetes insipidus. The underlying causes of development of ADH deficiency have been categorized as follows: (1) neoplastic or inflammatory processes impinging on the hypothalamoneural-hypophyseal axis, such as metastatic carcinoma, abscesses, meningitis, tuberculosis, or sarcoidosis; (2) surgical or radiation injury to the hypothalamoneural-hypophyseal axis, such as hypophysectomy; (3) severe head injuries; and

(4) idiopathic influences. Rarely, the syndrome is familial and inherited as a Mendelian dominant.

The clinical features of diabetes insipidus include polyuria, excessive thirst, and polydipsia. These characteristics are sudden in onset and are pronounced, with urine output reaching 10 or more liters in a 24-hour period. Untreated persons suffering from the disease may have to take in and excrete fluids on an hourly basis or less. Urine is pale in color and concentration is well below that of serum levels.

Diagnosis is on the basis of clinical manifestations, dehydration tests, and response to vasopressin administration. Treatment is through use of vasopressin, usually by nasal spray.

Inappropriate ADH Secretion (SIADH)

Inappropriate ADH release is defined as persistent release of ADH unrelated to plasma osmolarity or volume deficit. The result is excessive resorption of water in the renal system and excessive retention of water with expansion of fluid volume. Fluid overload, hyponatremia, and hemodilution result.

SIADH may occur from a stimulus inside the hypothalamic-hypophyseal system or one from an outside source (Table 30-3). It may occur as a result of a tumor of the hypothalamus or hypophysis that impinges on tissues that control secretions. More often, however, it is the result of secretions of ADH by nonendocrine tumors. Oat-cell bronchogenic carcinoma is the most common ADH-secreting lesion causing SIADH. Other conditions capable of this ectopic secretion include carcinoma of the pancreas, lymphoma, bronchogenic tuberculosis, Hodgkin's disease, and thymoma. Less frequently, disorders of the CNS such as subdural hematoma and CNS infections are the basis of malfunction.

Treatment includes fluid restriction, diuretics, assessment and supplementation of electrolyte balance, assessment for evidence of CHF, and treatment for the underlying cause of the syndrome.

TABLE 30-3. Causes of SIADH

Malignancy
Oat-cell carcinoma of lung
Carcinoma of pancreas
Lymphosarcoma, reticulum-cell sarcoma, Hodgkin's disease
Carcinoma of duodenum
Thymoma
Nonmalignant pulmonary disease
Tuberculosis
Lung abscess
Pneumonia
Central nervous system disorders
Skull fracture
Subdural hematoma
Subarachnoid hemorrhage
Cerebral vascular thrombosis
Cerebral atrophy
Acute encephalitis
Tuberculous meningitis
Purulent meningitis
Guillain-Barré syndrome
Lupus erythematosus
Acute intermittent porphyria
Physical or emotional stress
Pain
Drugs
Chlorpropamide
Vincristine
Cyclophosphamide
Carbamazepine
Oxytocin
General anesthesia
Narcotics
Barbiturates
Thiazide antidepressants
Tricyclic antidepressants
Miscellaneous
Hypothyroidism
Positive pressure respiration

Source: K. J. Isselbacher, et al. (eds.), *Harrison's Principles of Internal Medicine* (9th ed.). New York: McGraw-Hill, 1980. P. 1692.

TUMORS OF THE PITUITARY

Adenomas

Except in children, the most common neoplasms of the pituitary are the adenomas. Pituitary adenomas may be classified according to the type of cell predominantly involved. For example, they may be acidophilic or basophilic. They may also be classified according to their secretory qualities. They may interfere with pituitary functions by virtue of their space-occupying properties or by secretions of various hormones. In general, problems stemming from the space-occupying factor are the result of destruction or suppression of tissue. Those stemming from secretory properties result in hypersecretion or hyperfunction. All lesions may produce CNS symptoms or visual problems because of their space-occupying properties, depending on the size and locations of the lesion.

CHROMOPHOBIC ADENOMAS. These adenomas are the most commonly occurring lesions and are usually without hormonal function. They usually become apparent clinically because of their compressive effect or because of impingement on adjoining structures. The tumor interferes with acidophilic cells, so that growth may be retarded and sexual infantilism may be evident. Pressure on the posterior pituitary may occur and, if the tumor breaks through the roof of the sella, Fröhlich's syndrome may result. The tumor has a poor blood supply so that foci of necrosis and hemorrhage may occur. Rarely, ACTH is synthesized by this type of adenoma.

The chromophobe adenomas occur equally in both sexes and are often large in size, expanding and eroding the sella turcica. Sometimes they compress the optic chiasma and are exhibited by visual symptoms.

ADENOMAS INFLUENCING GROWTH. These lesions are formed almost entirely of acidophils and contain a high content of growth hormone. They tend to be smaller in size than nonsecreting chromophobe adenomas and have a lesser hemorrhagic quality. They are usually confined to the sella turcica, which shows evidence of expansion on x ray. They are usually manifested by acromegaly or giantism [9].

PROLACTIN-SECRETING ADENOMAS. These adenomas range in cellular composition from those consisting predominantly of acidophils to ones containing sparsely granulated chromophobes. They vary in size from microscopic to the size of large nonsecretory chromophobe adenomas. The presenting clinical picture is one of inappropriate lactation and amenorrhea [9].

ACTH-SECRETING TUMORS. ACTH-secreting adenomas are usually composed largely of basophils, although some have chromophobe cells, and range in size from microscopic to being large enough to expand the sella turcica. The larger adenomas may exhibit malignant features. They not only invade surrounding tissues but exhibit bloodborne metastasis.

THYROTROPIN-SECRETING ADENOMAS. These are extremely rare lesions that generally show chromophobe but occasionally show basophilic characteristics [9].

CRANIOPHARYNGIOMA (RATHKE'S POUCH TUMOR). Derived from remnants of Rathke's pouch these lesions commonly occur in young children and are generally cystic, although some are solid. They are usually well encapsulated and are generally benign, although some develop malignancy. Many contain sufficient calcification to be visualized by x ray. They may reach considerable size (8–10 cm in diameter). Because of location, they frequently compress the optic chiasma and pituitary, leading to visual impairment [9].

Malignant Tumors

PRIMARY LESIONS. Although they are rare, primary malignant lesions do occur in the anterior lobe of the pituitary. They occasionally arise in preexisting benign adenomas or craniopharyngiomas. Characteristically, they are fast-growing and rapidly exhibit clinical manifestations. They are also massive and exhibit extensive invasion of nearby structures; distant metastasis may occur, especially to the liver. The distinction between a rapidly growing adenoma and a carcinoma is often difficult to make [8].

SECONDARY LESIONS. Metastases to the pituitary are rare. They occur most often with carcinoma of the breast, lung, and thyroid in that order.

REFERENCES

1. Boyd, W., and Sheldon, H. *Introduction to the Study of Disease* (8th ed.). Philadelphia: Lea & Febiger, 1980.
2. Christy, N. The Anterior Pituitary. In P. B. Beeson, et al. (eds.), *Cecil Textbook of Medicine* (15th ed.). Philadelphia: Saunders, 1979.
3. Ganong, W. F. *Review of Medical Physiology* (10th ed.). Los Altos, Calif.: Lange, 1981.
4. Goodman, H. M. The Pituitary Gland. In V. B. Mountcastle (ed.), *Medical Physiology* (14th ed.). St. Louis: Mosby, 1980.
5. Guyton, A. C. *Textbook of Medical Physiology* (6th ed.). Philadelphia: Saunders, 1981.
6. Jenson, D. *The Principles of Physiology* (2nd ed.). New York: Appleton-Century-Crofts, 1980.
7. Kohler, P. O. Diseases of the Hypothalamus and Anterior Pituitary. In K. J. Isselbacher, et al. (eds.), *Harrison's Principles of Internal Medicine* (9th ed.). New York: McGraw-Hill, 1980.
8. Robbins, S. L., and Angell, M. *Basic Pathology* (3rd ed.). Philadelphia: Saunders, 1981.
9. Robbins, S. L., and Cotran, R. S. *Pathologic Basis of Disease* (2nd ed.). Philadelphia: Saunders, 1979.
10. Tortora, G., et al. *Principles of Human Physiology*. Hagerstown, Md.: Harper & Row, 1981.

CHAPTER 31
ADRENAL MECHANISMS AND ALTERATIONS

LEARNING OBJECTIVES

1. Discuss the normal anatomy of the adrenal gland.
2. Describe the mechanisms of regulating adrenocortical hormone secretions.
3. Identify the pattern of synthesis of each of the major hormones of the adrenal cortex.
4. Outline the physiologic effects of mineralocorticoids, glucocorticoids, and androgen hormones.
5. Identify the process that results in Cushing's syndrome.
6. Define *Cushing's syndrome* and its major clinical manifestations.
7. Differentiate between primary and secondary aldosteronism.
8. Describe the pathologic process and resulting physical changes of the adrenogenital syndromes.
9. Outline the clinical manifestations of primary adrenocortical insufficiency.
10. Compare primary and secondary adrenocortical insufficiency.
11. Discuss the clinical presentation of adrenal crisis.
12. Describe catecholamine biosynthesis and storage.
13. Describe the etiology of pheochromocytoma.
14. Outline the major clinical features of pheochromocytoma.

The adrenal cortex and the adrenal medulla share adjacent housing but have no similar function. The hormonal anatomy and physiology of both of these structures is discussed in this chapter. Altered states of function are also included.

ANATOMY OF THE ADRENAL GLANDS

The adrenal, or suprarenal, glands are located retroperitoneally at the superior pole of each kidney. Although structurally housed together, the adrenal cortex and adrenal medulla are separate organs, in both tissue origin and physiologic function.

The adrenal glands are rather flat in shape, with the right gland having a pyramidal appearance and the left having a curved and semilunar shape (see Fig. 31-1). A thick, fibrous capsule surrounds the glands, and peritoneal fasciae, independent of the kidneys, provide the support. The usual weight of each gland in a normal adult is between 3 and 6 gm and in general, the glands tend to be slightly heavier in males [3].

Arterial blood supply is from the renal, or inferior, phrenic arteries or directly from the abdominal aorta. Once inside the gland, the vessels break up into sinusoids and drain medially into the glands. Venous drainage is different for the right and left glands. The right adrenal gland empties venous blood directly into the vena cava, while the left gland empties into the left renal vein (Fig. 31-1). Nervous innervation is both sympathetic and parasympathetic. Nerves enter through the cortex and progress to the medulla.

The adrenal cortex, golden yellow in color, encompasses the medulla, which is more medially located. Three distinct layers compose the cortex. The first is the *zona*

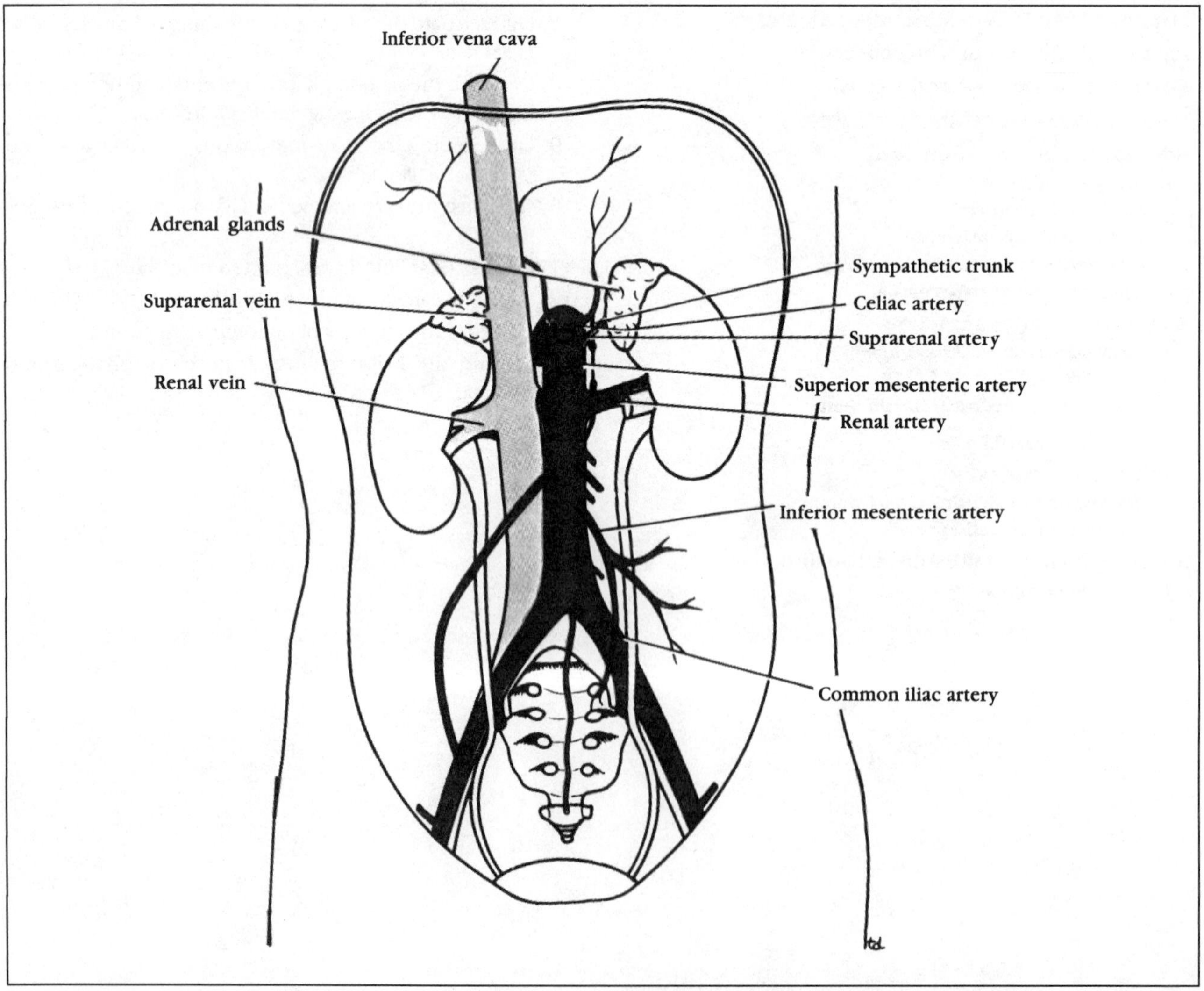

FIGURE 31-1. Position of the adrenal glands on the kidneys. (From R. Snell, *Clinical Anatomy for Medical Students* [2nd ed.]. Boston: Little, Brown, 1981.)

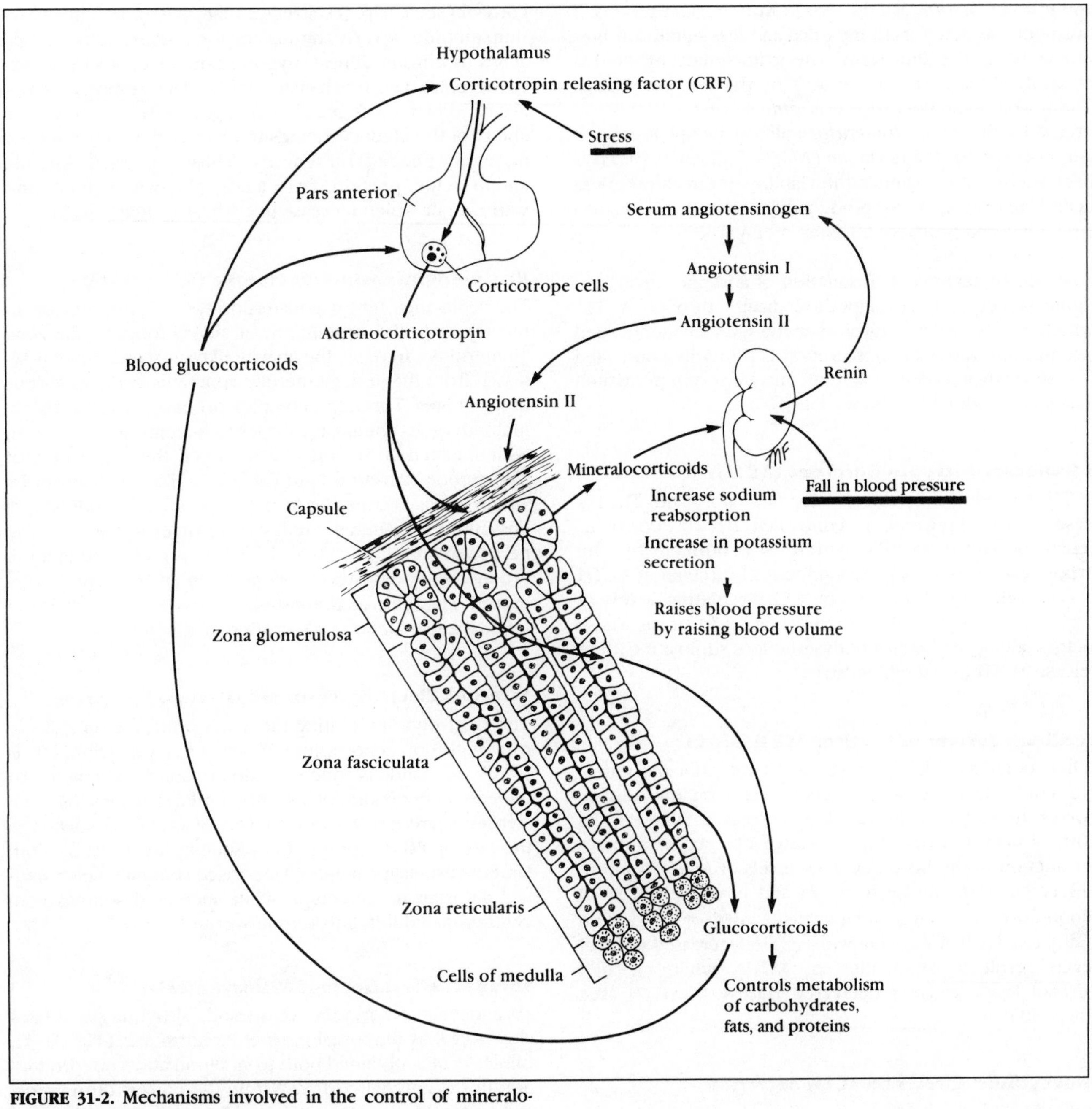

FIGURE 31-2. Mechanisms involved in the control of mineralocorticoid secretion and the glucocorticoid secretion of the suprarenal (adrenal) cortex.

glomerulosa, composed of a thin layer of irregularly shaped cuboidal cells. Immediately beneath is the second layer, the *zona fasciculata*. Cuboidal cells of this layer run in long strands and are separated by the sinusoidal spaces. During periods of inactive glandular function the cells of this layer become filled with vacuoles, but during periods of active function the cells become very compact. The third layer of the cortex, the *zona reticularis*, is composed of groups of cells of very irregular shape (Fig. 31-2).

The adrenal medulla lies central to, and is surrounded by, the adrenal cortex. Its appearance is flat and gray [3] and it is composed of sheets of irregularly shaped masses of cells with small nuclei apparent. The cells are surrounded by sinusoidal blood vessels.

THE ADRENAL CORTEX

Adrenocortical Hormones

The adrenal cortex is responsible for secretion of three major groups of steroid hormones. The *mineralocorticoids* and *glucocorticoids* are the two most important groups of hormones secreted, with the third and less significant hormones being the androgens. The major glucocorticoid is *cortisol*, which is secreted mostly by the zona fasciculata. The major mineralocorticoid is *aldosterone*, which is secreted by the *zona glomerulosa* almost independently of adrenocorticotropic hormone (ACTH) influence. ACTH is necessary to only maintain the viability of the glomerulosa cells. The androgens are produced by the cells of the zona fasciculata and probably the zona reticularis.

CONTROL OF SECRETION. Regulation of adrenocortical hormone secretion is accomplished mainly through ACTH, which exerts direct control over the glucocorticoids and sex steroids. Aldosterone secretion is primarily controlled by the renin-angiotensin system, and by serum potassium and serum sodium levels (see Fig. 31-2).

Adrenocorticotropin Hormone (ACTH)

ACTH is produced by the anterior pituitary gland. The release of this hormone is controlled by corticotropin-releasing factor (CRF), which is produced by the hypothalamus. Normally, the amount of circulating ACTH is controlled by three factors: (1) circulating levels of cortisol, (2) individual biorhythms, and (3) stress. These factors, along with states of dysfunction, stimulate CRF to release ACTH into the bloodstream.

Feedback System of Cortisol-ACTH Levels

When circulating levels of cortisol (the principal glucocorticoid) decrease, ACTH acts directly on the adrenal cortex to stimulate production. Increased secretion of cortisol occurs within a few minutes after ACTH initiates production of the hormone. Low levels of ACTH result in decreased hormone biosynthesis and in decreased renal blood flow. Thus, circulating levels of cortisol respond directly to a feedback system with ACTH. Decreased cortisol levels result in stimulation of ACTH, while elevated cortisol levels cause a decreased release of ACTH (see Chap. 30).

Biorhythms: Effects on ACTH Secretion

Individual biorhythms, or *circadian rhythms*, affect the normal circulating levels of ACTH. The pattern is related to sleep periods and may be altered by changes in daily activity [2]. In the hours prior to and just after waking, ACTH levels reach the highest peak of the 24-hour day. The levels will decrease continually during the remainder of the day. In relation to this, cortisol levels rise at approximately the same times as the ACTH levels and will also decline as the day progresses.

Stress Effects on ACTH Secretion

Any physical or emotional stress increases the secretion of ACTH, resulting in increased production and secretion of cortisol (see Chap. 3). Stresses that may initiate this reaction include severe trauma, major surgery, any severe acute or chronic illness, hypotension, or exposure to extreme cold. The mechanism behind this response is not clearly understood, but it is thought to be related to the ability of the glucocorticoids to provide the body with the materials needed for energy. These materials include amino acids, protein, fatty acids, glucose, sodium, and water, all of which increase in a stressful situation [1].

Renin-Angiotensin-Aldosterone (RAA) System

The renin-angiotensin-aldosterone system is the major influence over the production of aldosterone by the zona glomerulosa. Initially, the enzymelike substance renin is released from the juxtaglomerular apparatus in the nephrons of the kidney. Through a complex process of hydrolysis, renin undergoes chemical changes to become angiotensin II, which exerts a strong control over the regulation of aldosterone secretion (see Fig. 31-2). The mechanism by which this is accomplished is not completely understood. Possibly, it is related to cholesterol conversion by the adrenal cortex. It is known that the action is rapid, and that the production of aldosterone stops when angiotensin II is removed. The renin-angiotensin-aldosterone system does not influence production or secretion of cortisol.

Effect of Electrolytes on Aldosterone Secretion

The electrolyte exhibiting the major influence on aldosterone secretion is potassium. When serum potassium levels are elevated aldosterone secretion becomes increased. An increase in potassium of less than 1 mEq/L triples the aldosterone secretion. Lowered levels of potassium decrease the rate of aldosterone release. Sodium functions by similar, but reverse, principles. Decreased sodium levels stimulate aldosterone secretion, while increased sodium concentrations inhibit aldosterone secretion.

Adrenocortical Hormone Biosynthesis

Adrenocortical hormone, or steroid, biosynthesis utilizes cholesterol as the initial basis of its hormones (Fig. 31-3). Cholesterol is obtained both from blood and from production in the adrenal cortex. Within the cortex, during normal states of activity, cholesterol is stored within lipid droplets in the cytoplasm of the cells. Although the adrenal cortex is capable of synthesizing cholesterol for steroid production, approximately 80 percent is taken from the cholesterol stores within the cortex that were obtained from cholesterol circulating in the bloodstream [5]. During periods when the cortex is not being stimulated by one of the regulating mechanisms, available cholesterol remains in storage, and the production of steroid hormones is minimal [13].

Stimulation from any of the adrenal regulators begins the process of steroid biosynthesis. Cholesterol undergoes many chemical and enzymatic conversions in the process of manufacturing steroids. In this series of changes, the one

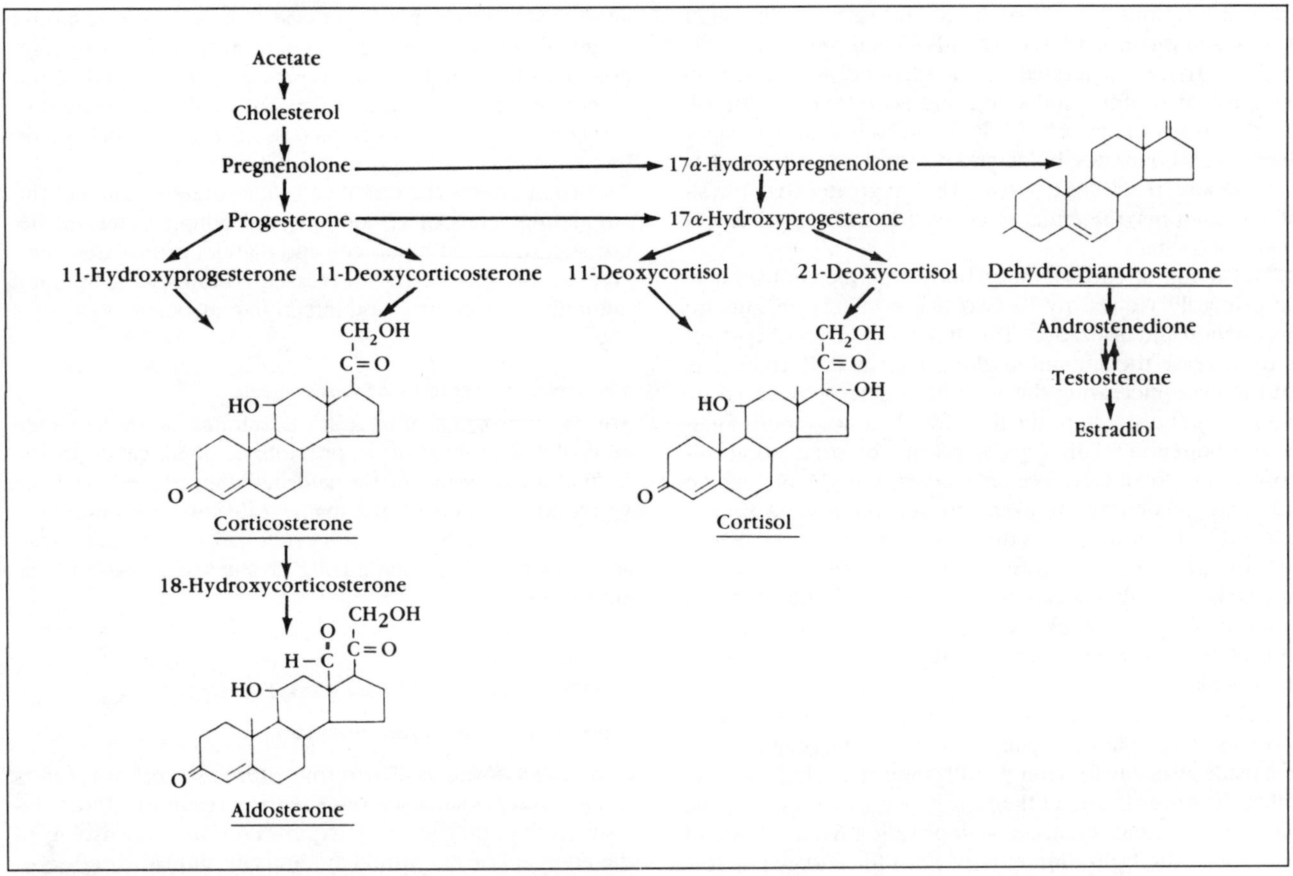

FIGURE 31-3. Formation of adrenocortical hormones. (From D. Jensen, *The Principles of Physiology* [2nd ed.]. Appleton-Century-Crofts, 1980.)

step through which all steroids must pass is the conversion of cholesterol to pregnolone. At this point, the production of the major hormones occurs by different and individual mechanisms.

Transport of Steroid Hormones

After steroid biosynthesis, the steroid hormones are released into the bloodstream to be carried to the tissue cells. In the blood they bind to specific proteins known as *transcortins*, or *corticosteroid-binding globulins* (CBG), which have an affinity for all major steroids. Binding causes inactivation of the steroid hormones, excretion of the steroid by the kidneys, and prevention of excess tissue uptake. At the target site the steroids are released to exert their physiologic action.

Physiologic Actions of Mineralocorticoids

The principal mineralocorticoid that exerts a physiologic action is aldosterone. Almost all mineralocorticoid activity is produced by this steroid, but cortisol also contributes slightly. The single most important action of aldosterone is sodium retention. Because of this action and its resultant effect on intracellular and extracellular fluid volume, aldosterone has a profound effect on fluid balance.

The retention of sodium results in a simultaneous loss of potassium by excretion in the urine. This exchange of ions takes place in the distal renal tubules. Along with the sodium retained, water retention also occurs [8]. Any excess or deficit in normal circulating aldosterone can lead to a variety of basic electrolyte disturbances with resultant effects on body functions.

In addition to the tubules, aldosterone acts on other tissues to achieve sodium retention. Salivary and sweat glands are influenced to conserve sodium in extreme heat. The absorption of sodium by the intestinal mucosa prevents excess sodium loss in fecal waste. Aldosterone also acts to conserve sodium by influencing the exchange of intracellular and extracellular water.

Physiologic Actions of Glucocorticoids

Glucocorticoids are named for their ability to regulate serum glucose levels by a variety of mechanisms. Their effect, however, is not as pronounced or prolonged as that of the regulating ability of insulin. In looking at the total picture of the effects of glucocorticoid activity, the primary action in the tissues is catabolic, with increased breakdown of proteins and increased nitrogen excretion. But in the liver anabolic actions occur, such as increased amino acid uptake and increased synthesis of RNA and protein.

The activities generated by the glucocorticoids are accomplished by the production and secretion of cortisol. Cortisol plays an important role in the control and metabolism of carbohydrates, lipids, and proteins; as well, it assists in metabolic reactions to stress. Also, in greater than physiologic amounts, the effect of cortisol in inflammation and allergies is vital.

The action of cortisol on carbohydrate metabolism may be primarily viewed by its two major effects on glucose production and utilization. The first major effect of cortisol is to increase the amount of glucose formed. Cortisol acts on the liver, increasing the amount of glucose released by enhancing the ability of the liver for gluconeogenesis (glucose production). This is accomplished by stimulating adipose tissue to release free fatty acids, the gluconeogenic substrate needed by the liver. The second major action of cortisol is that it decreases the utilization of glucose by the tissues. In muscle, adipose, and lymphatic tissues, the uptake and metabolism are reduced. Through these actions —increased gluconeogenesis and the inhibition of glucose utilization by tissues—serum glucose concentrations are increased.

By stimulating the release of fatty acids from tissue stores into the plasma, lipids in the form of free fatty acids are made available for energy utilization. This ability to mobilize fat stores is one of the factors that cause a metabolic alteration in times of stress or deprivation from the use of glucose to the utilization of fatty acids for energy [7]. It is not understood how cortisol acts to initiate the mobilization of fatty acids nor is it known why fat deposits are removed from one area of the body and deposited in another, as may easily be seen in adrenocortical dysfunction (see p. 427).

The effects of cortisol on protein are twofold. First, it decreases protein stores in all tissues of the body except the liver. This is carried out by preventing the synthesis of protein and by breaking down protein stores in the cells into amino acids. Second, protein synthesis in the liver is stimulated. Amino acids are released into the liver from the cellular protein catabolism, thereby increasing the amount of amino acids available to the liver for protein synthesis.

The exact mechanism by which cortisol responds to stress is not completely understood, yet it is recognized as being almost essential for survival of the human organism. Any extreme physical or emotional stress may initiate the response, including severe trauma, emotional upset, chronic or debilitating diseases, infection, or extreme temperatures (Fig. 31-4).

Administration of glucocorticoids, specifically cortisol, in larger than normal amounts decreases the inflammatory response to infection or injury. Each step of the process of inflammation is blocked by steroids. Cortisol reduces the passage of water into and out of the cell and decreases the amount of fibrous tissue formation [8]. Also, allergic processes are stopped with the administration of cortisol by altering the inflammatory process that occurs in response to any allergen. The exact mechanism by which the components of the inflammatory process are blocked is not completely understood, but it is believed to be related to the ability of the glucocorticoids to stabilize cell membranes and prevent rupture of the lysosomes [3].

Cortisol affects the blood cells in a variable manner. The circulating levels of eosinophils and lymphocytes are decreased, while red blood cell and platelet production is increased. Because of the decreased lymphocytes, humoral immunity is decreased and infection may occur [7].

Physiologic Actions of Androgens

Adrenal androgens, or male sex hormones, produced in the adrenal cortex have little physiologic significance in the normal adult. Some of the androgens produced are converted to testosterone, the major male sex hormone. However, hypersecretion of the cortex can cause the appearance of dramatic masculinizing changes as a result of the androgens.

ALTERED ADRENOCORTICAL FUNCTION

Adrenocortical Hyperfunction

CUSHING'S SYNDROME. The term *Cushing's syndrome* refers to the clinical manifestations seen as a result of excess glucose production caused by hypersecretion of cortisol from the adrenal cortex. Although clinically similar, three separate factors may cause Cushing's syndrome: (1) adrenal neoplasms, (2) hypersecretion of ACTH by the anterior pituitary, and (3) ectopic ACTH syndrome [13].

The growth of adrenocortical cells into a tumor that secretes cortisol causes cellular growth and further secretion of cortisol. As cortisol secretion increases, it is no longer controlled by ACTH. Eventually, cortisol secretion by the neoplasm will exceed that of normal adrenocortical cells, at which point the normal cells may cease production of cortisol altogether. Cortisol-secreting tumors of the adrenal glands rarely secrete excessive androgenic hormones.

The disorder that is considered to be true Cushing's disease results from cortisol oversecretion caused by excessive release of ACTH from the anterior pituitary gland. This causes increased secretion and release of both cortisol and androgenic hormones.

The third form of Cushing's syndrome occurs from excess production of ACTH by a neoplasm not located in the adrenal gland. This particular form is often found in persons with oat-cell carcinoma of the lung [5]. Other malignant neoplasms may secrete ACTH, causing this peculiar paraneoplastic syndrome.

In addition to hypersecretion of cortisol, two other factors are apparent in Cushing's syndrome, regardless of etiology. These are the absence of circadian rhythm changes in the release of ACTH and cortisol, and the lack of in-

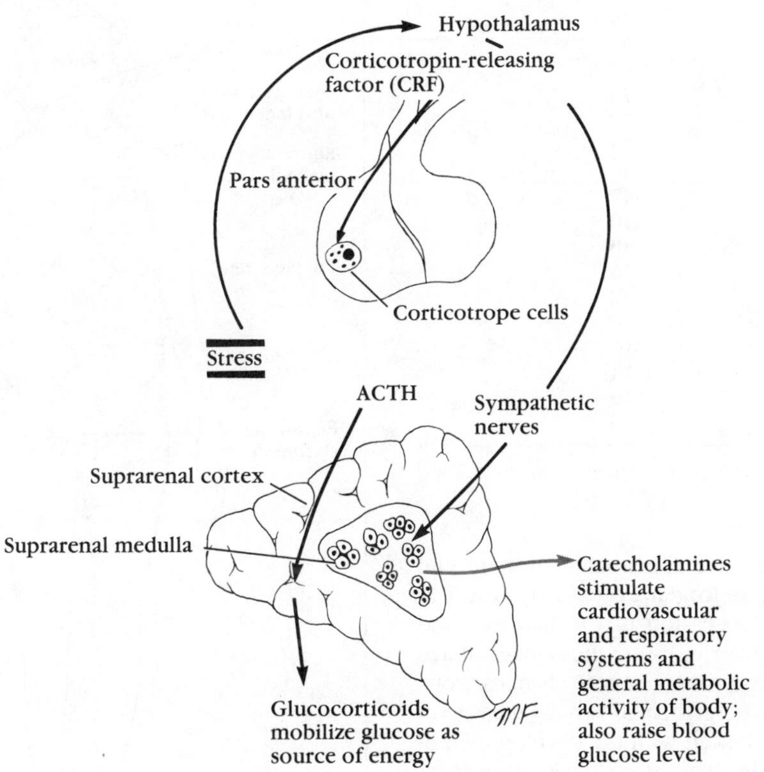

FIGURE 31-4. The effect of stress on the activities of the suprarenal gland.

creased ACTH and cortisol secretion in response to stress [6].

With increased cortisol secretion there is an increased rate of gluconeogenesis resulting in elevated serum glucose levels. Eventually, the islet cells of the pancreas are no longer able to produce sufficient amounts of insulin, and diabetes mellitus results [7]. Loss of protein occurs almost everywhere in the body with the exception of the liver. In the muscular system, the loss of protein results in decreased strength and muscle wasting. Humoral immunity is reduced, decreasing the threshold to infection. Skin tissues lose collagen and become very thin, tearing and bruising easily. In the bones, osteoporosis can cause weakness and actual bone fractures. Hyperpigmentation may be seen and is due to the melanostimulating properties of ACTH. (ACTH has approximately one-thirtieth the stimulating properties of melanostimulating hormone.)

In general, the clinical signs and symptoms vary only slightly with the etiology of the disease. Although scattered in the population, Cushing's syndrome is 4 times more frequent in women than in men; the peak ages affected are 35 to 50 years [8]. Androgens are responsible for a few of the bodily changes, but most of the abnormalities seen are a direct result of hypercortisolism. The three most classic manifestations seen are truncal obesity, purple striae, and round facial features. The frequency of different clinical effects is noted in Table 31-1.

Truncal obesity results from the mobilization of fat in the lower parts of the body to the trunk, causing the abdomen to be greatly protuberant, even as the extremities become thin and wasted. Often, persons affected with Cushing's syndrome are unable to rise from a squatting position without assistance. The enlarged abdomen is characteristic and may be an extension of thoracic accumulation of fat, the "buffalo torso." Fat accumulation around the neck and cervical area is termed the *buffalo hump*. Purple striae appear on the abdomen as a result of the stretching of the abdominal skin when the fat cells are being deposited. Their appearance is purple as a result of the collagen deficit in the skin tissues. Round and full facial features, often called a "moonface," also result from the hypercortisolism (Fig. 31-5).

Other manifestations also often occur. Excessive androgen secretion results in excess hair growth, which is especially prominent in women, often on the face. Androgen

TABLE 31-1. Clinical effects of Cushing's syndrome

Effects	Percent
Obesity	94
Facial plethora	84
Hirsutism	82
Menstrual disorders	76
Hypertension	72
Muscular weakness	58
Back pain	58
Striae	52
Acne	40
Psychologic symptoms	40
Bruising	36
Congestive heart failure	22
Edema	18
Renal calculi	16
Headache	14
Polyuria/polydipsia	10
Hyperpigmentation	6

Source: P. Felig, et al. *Endocrinology and Metabolism.* New York: McGraw-Hill, 1981. P. 472.

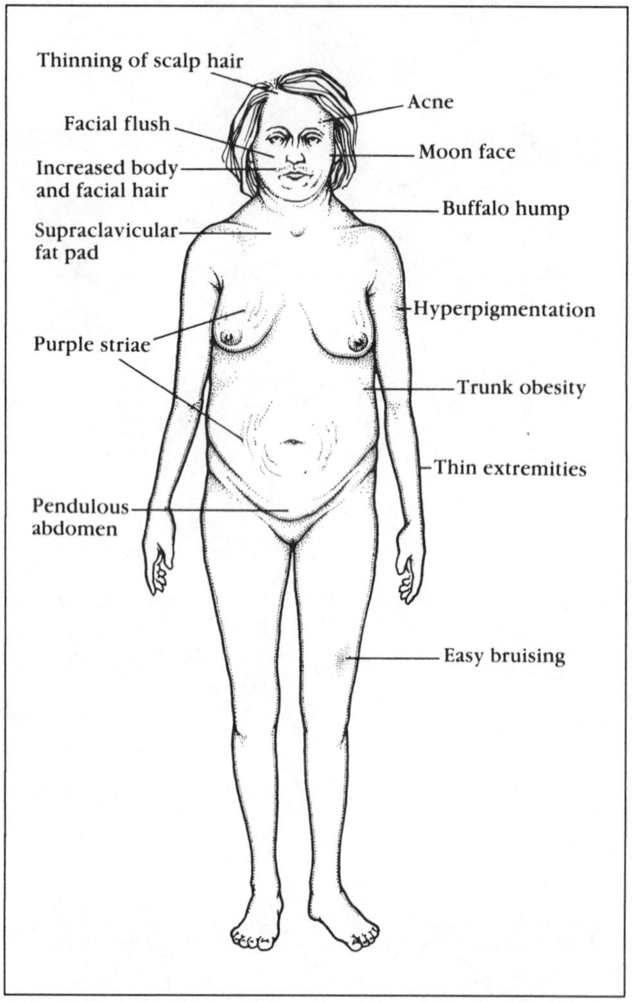

FIGURE 31-5. A composite of symptoms in Cushing's disease. (From M. Beyers and S. Dudas [eds.], *The Clinical Practice of Medical-Surgical Nursing* [2nd ed.]. Boston: Little, Brown, 1984.)

hormones may also cause the appearance of acne and oligomenorrhea. Extreme androgen excess may result in coarsening of the voice, recession of the hairline, and clitoral hypertrophy. Psychiatric disturbances may surface with personality alterations or more severe changes. Polyuria may result from the hyperglycemia. Varying degrees of hypertension are exhibited often with the development of left ventricular hypertrophy. The mortality is 50 percent or greater with Cushing's syndrome unless treatment is received. Death usually results from a severe infection.

When Cushing's syndrome appears in children, growth ceases. If treatment is not begun before the epiphyses of the bones have sealed, the short stature of the child will be permanent [13].

PRIMARY ALDOSTERONISM. Primary aldosteronism, also known as *Conn's syndrome*, is the result of excessive and uncontrolled secretion of the mineralocorticoid aldosterone. The usual cause is the appearance of an adrenocorticol adenoma. Rarely, it results from adrenal hyperplasia. Since it is the function of aldosterone to conserve sodium and waste potassium, the clinical features of this disorder are a direct result of that function.

The principal features of primary aldosteronism are hypernatremia and hypokalemia. Therefore, this condition may be suspected in any hypertensive patient who concurrently exhibits hypokalemia (less than 3.5 mEq/L). The conservation of sodium leads to retention of water, resulting in increased volume in the extracellular and vascular compartments, which in turn results in arterial hypertension. This condition may resemble hypertension of cardiovascular disease origin.

Loss of potassium may result in a variety of manifestations, depending on the severity of the depletion. The most common result is muscle cramps and weakness. Occasionally, it may progress to tetany, and even muscle paralysis as a result of the hypokalemia. Changes in the pattern of cardiac conduction may develop.

Alterations in renal function are apparent since this is the primary site of sodium conservation. Polydipsia, polyuria, and nocturia develop in response to the sodium-induced increased fluid volume and volume-dependent hypertension.

SECONDARY ALDOSTERONISM. The occurrence of secondary aldosteronism results from stimulation of aldosterone secretion from outside the adrenal cortex. Usually, this is stimulated by the renin-angiotensin system. Almost any factor decreasing the blood supply to the kidney will result in an increase in plasma renin levels. Thus, the mechanism is somewhat compensatory: increased renin leads to increased aldosterone secretion and sodium conservation. Water retention results from sodium conservation, leading to increased blood flow to vital organs. Edema, however, will only occur in the presence of preexisting or underly-

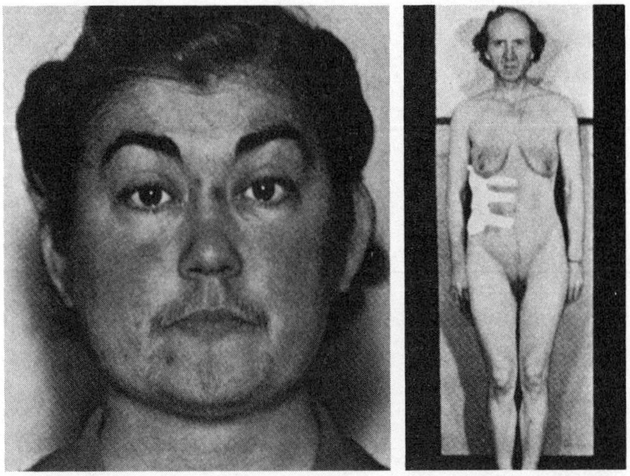

FIGURE 31-6. Adrenogenital syndromes of the female. (From R. Williams, *Textbook of Endocrinology* [6th ed.]. Philadelphia: Saunders, 1981.)

ing cardiovascular disease. Secondary aldosteronism will exhibit a combination of elevated plasma renin levels and aldosterone levels [13].

ADRENOGENITAL SYNDROMES. The adrenogenital syndromes are the result of adrenocortical overproduction of androgens, caused by tumor, or adrenocortical hyperplasia. In all of the adrenogenital syndromes, the ultimate result is the same—virilization and masculinization. The age and sex of the affected person will determine the nature and severity of the disorder.

Androgens are ultimately converted to the male hormone, testosterone. Testosterone is extremely potent and only small amounts are required to produce bodily changes. In the adult male, the masculinizing effects are masked by the production of testosterone from the testes. It is in children and in adult females that the virilization becomes most apparent.

Young boys begin to develop secondary sex characteristics, regardless of their age at the time of onset. Females respond to androgen stimulation with hirsutism, clitoral hypertrophy, and other masculinizing effects (Fig. 31-6).

CONGENITAL ADRENAL HYPERPLASIA. This is one of the most common adrenogenital syndromes and results from a congenital deficiency in the enzymes causing adrenocortical biosynthesis. It is estimated to be found in 1 of 50,000 births in the United States [4]. There is not an absence of the enzymes but an error in metabolism pathways of steroid production. The appearance of clinical manifestations is dependent on the point at which synthesis of cortisol, aldosterone, and androgens is blocked. There may be clinical signs and symptoms either of glucocorticoid or mineralocorticoid deficiency or excess. Also, androgen excess and virilization, or sexual ambiguity, and infantism may be seen. For example, in the most frequently encountered enzyme defect, excessive androgen production in the female fetus may cause modification of the external genitalia to resemble that of a male, while internal structures — uterus, ovaries, and fallopian tubes—are normal and functional.

Adrenocortical Hypofunction

PRIMARY ADRENOCORTICAL INSUFFICIENCY. Also known as Addison's disease, primary adrenocortical hypofunction results from insufficient secretion of the adrenocortical hormones. It is not a common disorder and appears only if 90 percent of the functioning adrenocortical cells have been destroyed [9]. The two major causes of adrenal destruction resulting in this primary form of hypofunction are idiopathic atrophy (80%) and tuberculosis (20%) [6]. Idiopathic atrophy has been attributed to an autoimmune disorder, with adrenal autoantibodies present in many affected persons [5]. In areas where tuberculosis is poorly controlled, the incidence of Addison's disease is much higher. It is interesting to note that in disease of tubercular origin men are usually affected, whereas in idiopathic atrophy women are affected with greater incidence [6].

Clinical manifestations depend on the degree of hormonal deficiency present. Changes in the skin are usually the most dramatic; they occur in about 98 percent of affected persons and help to diagnose the primary (adrenocortical) insufficiency [9]. Skin color changes result from increased ACTH from the anterior pituitary, which is uninhibited by steroid response from the adrenal cortex. Because ACTH has melanostimulating properties, areas of hyperpigmentation become visible especially in the most exposed body areas. Areas of *vitiligo* (pale patches surrounded by excess pigmentation) are also apparent. Muscular weakness and fatigue occur commonly. Many individuals experience hypotension as a result of volume depletion. Nausea, vomiting, weight loss, and diarrhea are the most common gastrointestinal disturbances. Other body changes include loss of hair, mental disturbances, hypoglycemia, and decreased sexual function.

It has been reported with increasing frequency that other physiologic disorders may be associated with primary adrenocortical insufficiency. This association has been referred to as *Schmidt's syndrome*, which refers to an autoimmune endocrine failure along with polyglandular failure [6, 12]. Disorders that may be associated include gonadal failure, thyroid dysfunction, diabetes mellitus, hypoparathyroidism, and pernicious anemia.

ADRENAL CRISIS. Adrenal crisis (Addisonian crisis, acute adrenal insufficiency) usually occurs because of a sudden decrease or absence of adrenocortical hormones. It may be seen in both treated and undiagnosed cases of Addison's disease in which the person is exposed to major stresses, such as trauma, infection, surgery, or major illness. The affected person may develop severe dehydration due to nausea and vomiting. Weakness, confusion, and hypovolemic shock are also associated [12]. Immediate intervention is

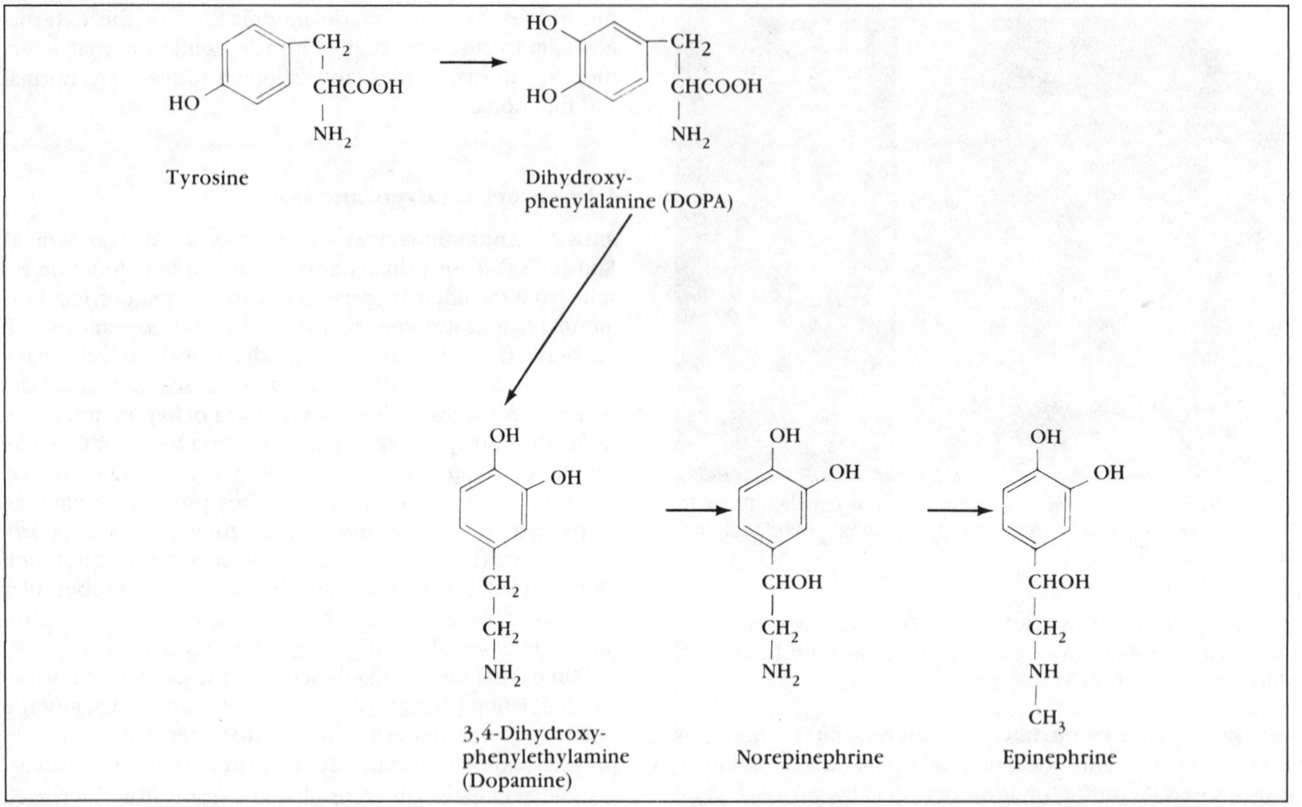

FIGURE 31-7. Steps in the synthesis of norepinephrine and epinephrine from tyrosine. (From I. Danishefsky, *Biochemistry for Medical Sciences*. Boston: Little, Brown, 1980.)

necessary or death will rapidly ensue. The cause of the crisis is not completely understood but it may be due to primary disease within the adrenal gland itself, such as hemorrhage, infection, or infarction [5].

SECONDARY ADRENOCORTICAL INSUFFICIENCY. Secondary adrenocortical insufficiency results from decreased cortisol secretion due to atrophy of the adrenal cortex. Mineralocorticoid secretion is usually not affected. The disorder is a result of decreased ACTH secretion, caused by pituitary or hypothalamic disease, or by therapeutic pharmacologic doses of glucocorticoids. Clinically, the picture may resemble primary insufficiency, except for the absence of hyperpigmentation. When a person is receiving steroid therapy, slow tapering off is required to allow the adrenal gland to return to active production of its own corticosteroids.

THE ADRENAL MEDULLA

The Catecholamines

The most important human catecholamines are epinephrine, norepinephrine, and dopamine, which are synthesized in the brain, sympathetic nerve endings, and chromaffin tissues. It is the function of the adrenal medulla to produce and secrete the catecholamines—epinephrine (adrenalin) and norepinephrine (noradrenalin)—from the chromaffin cells of the medulla. These cells stain readily with chromium salts and function to secrete adrenalin. Adrenal medullary secretion is approximately 80 percent epinephrine and 20 percent norepinephrine [7]. Epinephrine, exerts its greatest effect on the heart, increasing both rate and contractility. It is a potent mediator of the metabolic rate of the body. Norepinephrine, on the other hand, is secreted both by the adrenal medulla and the sympathetic nerve terminals. It exerts its greatest influence on the arterioles, causing vasoconstriction leading to increased blood pressure. Stimulation of the sympathetic nervous system (SNS) causes both direct SNS effects and release of the adrenal medullary hormones.

CATECHOLAMINE BIOSYNTHESIS AND STORAGE. The precursor for catecholamine biosynthesis is tyrosine. Through the processes of hydroxylation, decarboxylation, and methylation, tyrosine will yield norepinephrine and, ultimately, epinephrine (Fig. 31-7). The sequence of the process is as follows [6, 11]:

Tyrosine → dihydroxyphenylaline (dopa) → dopamine (DA)
→ norepinephrine (NE) → epinephrine (E)

It is thought that the tyrosine hydroxylase reaction is the slowest enzymatic conversion, and that this is probably the factor controlling the catecholamine production rate [5].

Catecholamine storage is accomplished by subcellular particles, called granules, which are present in most adrenomedullary cells in the chromaffin granules.

CATECHOLAMINE SECRETION. Release of the catecholamines may occur with acetylcholine stimulation of calcium passage into the chromaffin granules and subsequent liberation into the extracellular fluid [5, 6]. As the adrenal medulla produces the major portion of circulating epinephrine, a small release into the bloodstream occurs almost continuously. Norepinephrine is primarily produced by the sympathetic ganglion cells. Release of large amounts of catecholamines occurs after SNS stimulation.

Extremely stressful situations cause a massive release of epinephrine and norepinephrine, which result in the "fight or flight" syndrome. This enables the body to react effectively to any severe hazard or threat to survival. Physiologic response to this massive release of epinephrine includes increased blood pressure and heart rate, pupil dilatation, decreased peristalsis, and circulatory constriction in all major organ systems except the muscular and cardiovascular. The response to norepinephrine stimulation is similar, but with the major action being increased arterial blood pressure, a result of vigorous vasoconstriction. These responses are apparently normal catecholamine actions that are accelerated to meet the unusual and immediate cellular demands [11].

Altered Function of the Adrenal Medulla

There are no clinically recognized states of altered function of the adrenal medulla. The gland itself is not considered necessary for life, since there are other catecholamine sources in the body. However, the presence of a *pheochromocytoma* in the adrenal medulla will produce apparent states of hyperfunction of the adrenomedullary catecholamines.

PHEOCHROMOCYTOMA. Pheochromocytomas are rare adrenal medullary tumors whose primary clinical manifestation is that of hypertension. Pheochromocytomas originate in the chromaffin cells of the medulla.

During fetal life, the chromaffin cells are widespread in the developing body, and their function is associated with the sympathetic ganglia. After birth, most of the chromaffin cells disappear. Those remaining cluster in the adrenal medulla. While 95 percent of all functioning chromaffin tumors are located in the adrenal medulla, others have been found in chromaffin cells in the chest, neck, and abdomen [5].

Pheochromocytomas occur in either sex, usually between the ages of 25 and 50 years. Children are rarely affected. It is not uncommon for this disorder to affect more than one member of the same family. The tumors are usually benign and are bilateral but a small percentage of malignancy with metastasis occurs. Tumors are well encapsulated and extremely vascular. In a few afflicted persons, the actual tumor may be palpable.

The pheochromocytoma functions to produce and secrete excessive quantities of epinephrine and norepinephrine into the bloodstream, resulting in clinical manifestations of catecholamine excess. Therefore, the individual remains in an accelerated state of response similar to the "fight or flight" response [10].

The primary finding is systemic arterial hypertension. Elevated blood pressures may be sustained or intermittent, mild or malignant, depending on the rate and amount of catecholamine secretion. Sustained elevation can lead to cardiomegaly, left ventricular failure, cardiomyopathy, and ultimately, congestive heart failure. Other metabolic effects include excessive perspiration, palpitations, headaches, hyperventilation, and flushing. Increased incidence of neurofibromatosis, a familial disorder, has been associated with the occurrence of pheochromocytoma.

REFERENCES

1. Brooks, S.M. *Integrated Basic Science* (4th ed.). St. Louis: Mosby, 1979.
2. Catt, K.J. *An ABC of Endocrinology*. Boston: Little, Brown, 1971.
3. Chaffee, E.E., and Lytle, I.M. *Basic Physiology and Anatomy* (4th ed.). Philadelphia: Lippincott, 1980.
4. Dillon, R.S. *Handbook of Endocrinology* (2nd ed.). Philadelphia: Lea & Febiger, 1980.
5. Ezrin, C., Godden, J.O., and Volpe, R. *Systematic Endocrinology* (2nd ed.). Hagerstown, Md.: Harper & Row, 1979.
6. Felig, P., et al. *Endocrinology and Metabolism*. New York: McGraw-Hill, 1981.
7. Guyton, A.C. *Textbook of Medical Physiology* (6th ed.). Philadelphia: Saunders, 1981.
8. Hall, R., Anderson, J., and Besser, M. *Fundamentals of Clinical Endocrinology*. Chicago: Year Book, 1980.
9. Robbins, S., and Cotran, R. *Pathologic Basis of Disease* (2nd ed.). Philadelphia: Saunders, 1979.
10. Sanford, S.J. Dysfunction of the adrenal gland: Physiologic considerations and nursing problems. *Nurs. Clin. North Am.* 15:481, 1980.
11. Sodeman, W.A., and Sodeman, T.M. *Pathologic Physiology: Mechanisms of Disease* (6th ed.). Philadelphia: Saunders, 1979.
12. Tsagournis, M. Acute adrenal insufficiency. *Heart Lung* 7:603, 1978.
13. Williams, R.H. *Textbook of Endocrinology* (5th ed.). Philadelphia: Saunders, 1974.

CHAPTER 32
THYROID AND PARATHYROID FUNCTIONS AND ALTERATIONS

LEARNING OBJECTIVES

1. Describe the normal anatomy of the thyroid gland.
2. Explain the process by which the thyroid hormones are formed.
3. Identify the function of the iodide pump.
4. Describe the mechanism for release and transport of the thyroid hormones.
5. Describe the function of thyrocalcitonin.
6. Describe the effects of the thyroid hormones on metabolic processes, carbohydrate metabolism, and vitamin metabolism.
7. Define *goiter*.
8. Identify the clinical manifestations of hyperthyroidism.
9. Outline the autoimmune component of Graves' disease.
10. Relate the signs and symptoms of Graves' disease to underlying pathophysiology.
11. Differentiate between toxic multinodular goiter and toxic adenoma.
12. Identify the clinical manifestations of hypothyroidism.
13. Identify the cause of cretinism.
14. Describe the physical changes and underlying causes of adult hypothyroidism.
15. Compare thyrotoxic crisis and myxedema coma.
16. Identify the common element in chronic autoimmune thyroiditis.
17. Differentiate the etiology and symptoms of each of the thyroid carcinomas.
18. Describe the normal anatomy of the parathyroid gland.
19. List the effects of parathyroid hormone.
20. Explain the importance of thyrocalcitonin to the parathyroid gland.
21. Describe hypoparathyroidism.
22. Identify the two major causes of hyperparathyroidism.
23. Differentiate between pseudohypoparathyroidism and pseudopseudohypoparathyroidism.
24. Compare the effects of primary, secondary, and tertiary hyperparathyroidism.

The thyroid gland is primarily responsible for controlling the rate of metabolic processes in the body. The parathyroid gland functions to control calcium levels and bone resorption. These two glands are related by proximity and, as recently discovered, by function. In this chapter, normal structure and physiology are explored, with an examination of the major disorders of both glands.

ANATOMY OF THE THYROID GLAND

The thyroid gland is one of the largest endocrine glands in the human body and functions primarily to regulate and control the rate of metabolism. The thyroid is located in the anterior neck, just between the larynx and the trachea (Fig. 32-1). In the normal thyroid, there are two lobes that lie slightly lateral to the trachea, one on either side, and are connected by a thin band of tissue known as an isthmus. Generally, the isthmus lies just below the cricoid cartilage of the trachea. Characteristically, the superior portion of each lobe is somewhat pointed, while the inferior portion is rounded and blunt.

The thyroid is reddish and beefy in appearance, and has a rubbery texture on palpation. In the average adult, the gland weighs 20 to 30 gm. It is enclosed in two layers of connective tissue, with the outer layer being continuous with the cervical fascia of the neck, while the inner layer of connective tissue is closely adhered to the gland itself [11].

Thyroid gland tissue originally develops from the oral epithelium. In an adult, the foreamen cecum, a depression on the dorsum of the tongue, points to the location from which thyroid tissue developed. Rarely, there may be a connecting duct remaining that connects the thyroid gland and the foreamen cecum. This is known as the *thyroglossal duct.*

Blood supply to the thyroid arises from two main pairs of arterial vessels. Branching from the external carotid arteries, the superior thyroid arteries enter and supply the upper portions of the lobes. The inferior thyroid arteries, arising from the subclavian arteries, supply the lower portion of the lobes. It is estimated that 4 to 6 liters of blood per hour circulate through the thyroid gland.

Nervous system control is accomplished primarily from the second to fifth thoracic spinal nerves and through the superior and middle ganglia of the thoracolumbar nervous system controls. Cervical ganglia provide the thyroid with adrenergic stimulation, while the vagus nerve provides cholenergic stimulation.

The body of the thyroid is composed of a mass of tiny follicles that are all approximately equal in size. These follicles, or sacs, are each, in effect, a separately functioning gland the size of a pinhead. It should be noted that the iodine-accumulating function of each follicle is directly proportional to its individual surface area [18]. Although the sacs do not have outside openings, there are rich vascular, lymph, and nervous networks that surround them, exchanging iodine for hormones. The follicles have a single-layer epithelial lining, and an amorphous, secretory fluid—colloid—fills each sac. The primary component of colloid is a large protein molecule called *thyroglobulin,* from which the thyroid hormones are released (Fig. 32-2).

Another distinct cell type, within the thyroid gland, is the *parafollicular* cell. This cell has an ovoid and irregular shape and may be found scattered among the other more numerous thyroid cells.

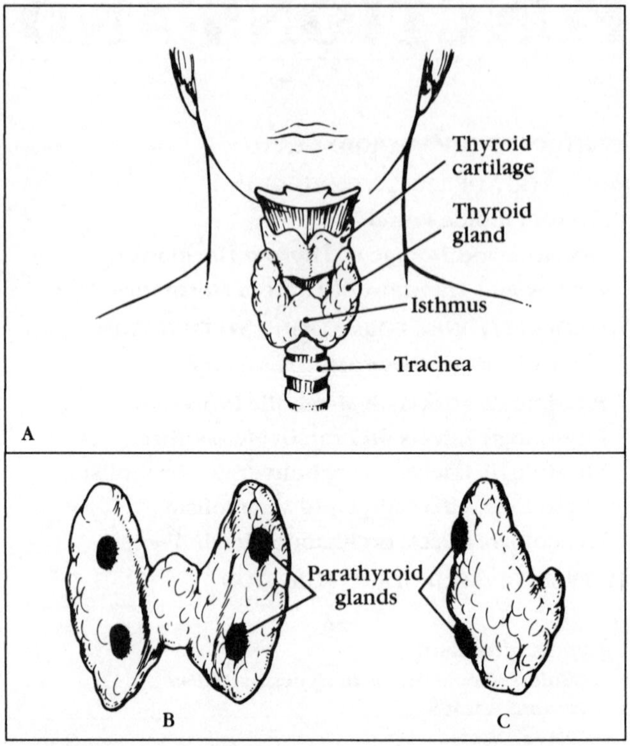

FIGURE 32-1. The thyroid gland. A. Anterior view of thyroid. B. Posterior view showing parathyroid glands. C. Lateral view.

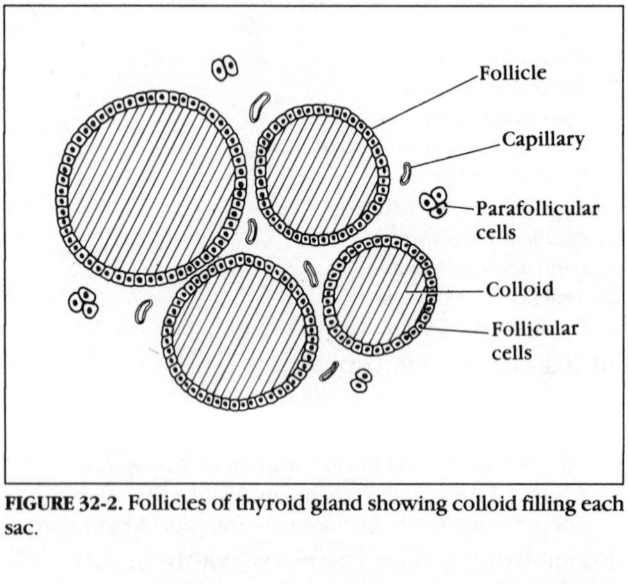

FIGURE 32-2. Follicles of thyroid gland showing colloid filling each sac.

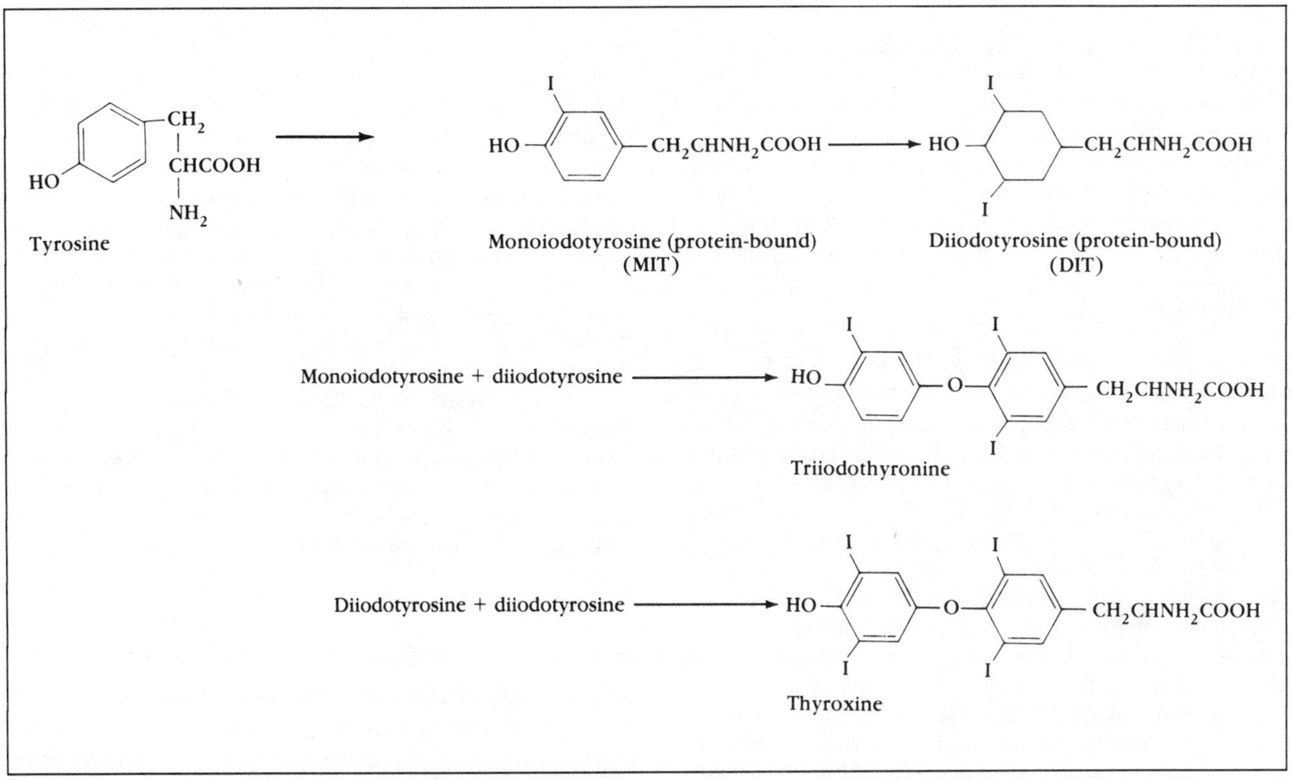

FIGURE 32-3. Tyrosine and compounds formed by its iodination in the thyroid gland; including the thyroid hormones T3 and thyroxine.

PHYSIOLOGY OF THE THYROID GLAND

Thyroid Iodide Pump

Iodide is essential to the normal functioning of the thyroid gland. When iodide enters the body through eating or drinking, it is rapidly absorbed into the bloodstream from the gastrointestinal tract within about an hour. Circulating in the blood, iodide is competed for by the thyroid gland and the kidneys. Approximately two-thirds of the iodide circulating in the bloodstream is excreted in the urine, and the remaining one-third is selectively removed from the blood by the thyroid gland.

Removal of iodide from the circulation is accomplished by means of an "iodide pump" or "trap." Normally, the iodide pump has the ability to concentrate the iodide to about 25 times greater than the concentration in the blood, but at those times when the thyroid gland becomes maximally active, iodide concentration can increase to as high as 350 times greater than blood iodide concentration [8]. Once the iodide is taken into the thyroid cell it is oxidized to the form of iodine [16].

To prevent a basic iodine deficiency, sufficient intake of iodine is necessary. Ordinary table salt contains 1 part sodium iodide to 100,000 parts of sodium chloride in order to provide sufficient quantities of iodine. However, ingested quantities of iodine will still vary, depending on the natural content of iodine in the soil and water in any given environment and on the intake of iodine-enriched salt and foods.

Structure and Storage of Thyroid Hormones

The thyroid iodide trap is an active, energy-requiring mechanism. At the beginning of this process, iodine is removed from the circulation in the form of sodium or potassium iodide. It then passes through the follicular cells and into the colloid. The thyroglobulin molecules in the colloid contain an active amino acid, tyrosine, which will combine with the iodine in the process of forming the thyroid hormones.

The iodine ions must first undergo a change to an active, elemental form of iodine. This occurs under the influence of the enzyme *perioxidase.* Once the iodine is in a simple form, it is able to combine with the tyrosine ring. The active iodine will attach itself to the 3-position of the tyrosine ring to form the molecule *monoiodotyrosine* (MIT). After the formation of MIT, the 5-position of the tyrosine ring becomes iodized. This structure becomes diiodotyrosine (DIT) (Fig. 32-3).

Two separate combinations of these molecules form the two main thyroid hormones. When two DIT molecules fuse in a coupling reaction, thyroxine (T4) is formed. The fusion of molecules of MIT and DIT form triiodothyronine (T3). Nearly 10 times more thyroxine than triiodothyronine is secreted from the thyroid gland but, as it circulates, some of the thyroxine will deiodinate, making only 2 to 3 times as much available to the tissues. Triiodothyronine is 3 to 5 times more active than thyroxine, but the duration of thyroxine is 3 to 5 times longer. Thus, the overall effect of both hormones is similar, and the functions appear to be identical [11].

These thyroid hormones are stored in the follicular colloid as a part of the thyroglobulin molecule. The thyroid gland is unique in its ability to maintain a storage of hormones in the thyroglobulin molecule. In effect, this is a storage mechanism, which functions if synthesis of the thyroid hormones should cease.

Release and Transport of Thyroid Hormones

Although there are other factors that may regulate the release of thyroid hormones, such as iodide concentration, the major regulator is the *thyroid-stimulating hormone* (*TSH, or thyrotropin*) [7]. TSH is a glycoprotein hormone secreted by the anterior pituitary gland. The relationship of TSH and the thyroid hormones exists as a feedback system (see Chap. 30). At any point when T3 and T4 levels become too low in the circulating bloodstream, TSH serves to increase the secretion of T3 and T4. It accomplishes this task by increasing all of the known activities of the thyroid glandular cells [8]. As the blood levels of T3 and T4 begin to rise, the anterior pituitary will decrease secretion of TSH, thereby decreasing the rate of thyroid hormone production. TSH stimulates an increase in the size and number of the follicular cells, thereby increasing their ability to absorb iodide [3]. It also increases the breakdown of thyroglobulin, releasing thyroxine and triiodothyronine hormones from the thyroid gland. Through these mechanisms, adequate levels of hormones are maintained in the bloodstream at all times.

When the hormones are needed, an enzymatic reaction splits the thyroglobulin molecule and frees the hormones for entry into the bloodstream. In the blood, thyroxine and triiodothyronine immediately combine with circulating plasma proteins. The affinity of circulating hormones and proteins is so great that the hormones are released to the tissue cells on a very slow basis. As the hormones enter the cells, both thyroxine and triiodothyronine bind with intracellular proteins where they are again stored. However, they are now inside tissue cells and are available for the nutrition of tissue cells. The hormones have a direct effect on the mitochondria of the cells, resulting in an increased total number, and an increased concentration of oxidative enzymes [2]. Through these actions, the hormones directly influence cell metabolism and metabolic rate. In a period of several days to several weeks, the thyroid hormones will be used.

THYROCALCITONIN: FORMATION AND FUNCTION

In the 1960s another thyroid hormone, *thyrocalcitonin*, was discovered. Its formation and mechanism of action are so different that it must be considered separately from thyroxine and triiodothyronine. Thyrocalcitonin is a large polypeptide containing 32 amino acids. It is synthesized in the parafollicular or "C" cells of the interstitial tissue between the follicular cells of the thyroid [8].

Thyrocalcitonin has a direct effect on bone tissue by counteracting the occurrence of hypercalcemia. An increased serum calcium stimulates the release of this hormone from the thyroid gland. Once released, it inhibits bone resorption, thus inhibiting the rate of release of calcium from the bone tissue to the plasma. This process causes a reduction in blood calcium levels. The action of thyrocalcitonin is essentially the reverse action of the parathyroid hormone (see p. 443). Whereas the action of parathyroid hormone is long-acting and functions constantly to maintain constant levels of circulating calcium, calcitonin only begins to act when there is excess calcium in the blood. It does not serve to block parathyroid hormone, or prevent its release. Calcitonin merely exerts an opposite action on both bone and kidneys. Bone resorption by osteoclasts is inhibited, and in response to calcitonin, the loop of Henle allows calcium to be filtered out and excreted in the urine.

FUNCTION OF THE THYROID HORMONES

Physiologic Effects on Metabolic Processes

Since the thyroid hormones are carried to all parts of the body tissues, their effects are widespread and varied. They exert influence over all major body systems, as well as the most intricate of cell functions. Their major influence in the physiologic body processes is that of increasing basal metabolic rate (BMR), which is simply heat production and energy expenditure in the body. A test to measure BMR is actually a measurement of oxygen consumption. A variety of nonthyroid factors can affect the usefulness of this test.

The basal metabolic rate rises during periods of increased hormone production and secretion, thus increasing energy expenditure and heat production. When this occurs the effect of *calorigenesis,* the utilization of food for energy, is also increased.

Physiologic Effects on Protein Metabolism

Protein synthesis activities are increased by the thyroid hormones. Because of this, the thyroid hormones are essential for normal growth and development in children and young adults. However, when available fat and carbohydrate stores have been depleted, available proteins may be utilized for energy. This protein depletion results in a negative nitrogen balance. It is not clear whether this is a direct result of the thyroid hormone or due to a negative caloric balance [18]. Releasing proteins also releases amino acids, making them available for energy purposes and increases the rate of gluconeogenesis.

Physiologic Effects on Carbohydrate Metabolism

Thyroid hormones affect virtually every function of carbohydrate metabolism. They are responsible for increasing the rate of gluconeogenesis, rapid cellular uptake of glu-

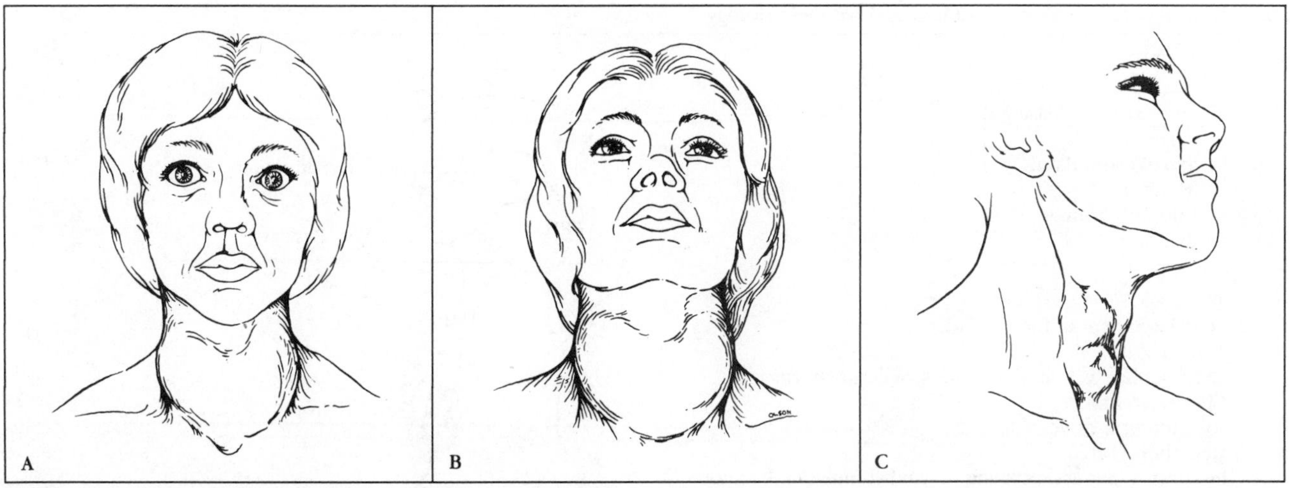

FIGURE 32-4. Thyroid abnormalities. A. Diffuse toxic goiter (Graves' disease). B. Diffuse nontoxic goiter. C. Nodular goiter. (From R. Judge, G. Zuidema, and F. Fitzgerald [eds.], *Clinical Diagnosis* [4th ed.]. Boston: Little, Brown, 1982.)

cose, increasing intestinal absorption of glucose and galactose, and increasing the rate of glucose uptake by adipose tissue.

Especially in carbohydrate metabolism, thyroid hormones are interactive with, or dependent on, other hormones. Insulin secretion is increased, which also enhances carbohydrate metabolism.

Physiologic Effects on Lipid Metabolism

Thyroid hormones essentially stimulate all aspects of lipid or fatty metabolism. The major result of thyroid hormone influence is that of fat storage depletion, especially in the storage of lipids. This leads to increased plasma concentration levels of free fatty acids. Serum cholesterol, however, is lowered by the action of thyroid hormones, probably due to increased intestinal excretion and conversion of cholesterol into bile acids.

Physiologic Effects on Vitamin Metabolism

Because thyroid hormones increase the rate of metabolic processes, they increase the physiologic need for vitamins. Since many vitamins contain enzymes or coenzymes, increased secretion of thyroid hormones causes depletion of vitamins due to the liberation of enzymes unless the intake of vitamins by ingestion is increased.

ALTERED THYROID GLAND FUNCTION

Goiter

The presence of a *goiter,* or enlarged thyroid gland, is not necessarily indicative of thyroid dysfunction, but may demonstrate an insufficient iodine intake [3]. The gland enlarges in an attempt to produce sufficient amounts of thyroid hormones. Various types of disorders can alter the size and state of the thyroid gland. Goiters may appear in states of hypofunction, as well as in states of hyperfunction (Fig. 32-4) [15]. Without the presence of identifiable clinical manifestations, an enlarged thyroid gland is referred to as a *nontoxic goiter.*

Hyperthyroidism

Hyperthyroidism, also known as *thyrotoxicosis,* is characterized by increased T3 and T4 production, often 5 to 15 times normal, resulting in an excess amount of thyroid hormones that are circulated and presented to the tissues. Hyperthyroidism may be related entirely to disease of the thyroid, or the disease may originate from outside the thyroid. It may be permanent or temporary, mild or severe. The severity of the disease may be affected by the patient's age, the duration of hyperthyroid function, and the presence of other disease processes in any other organ systems.

Because of the increased amount of thyroid hormones reaching the cells, all metabolic activities are accelerated. Thus, basal metabolic rate rises, energy expenditure is increased, and heat production also rises.

CLINICAL MANIFESTATIONS OF HYPERTHYROIDISM. The clinical manifestations of hyperthyroidism are varied, and may be manifested in any major organ system (see Table 32-1). One of the primary manifestations is the recognition of a palpable goiter or the growth of a preexisting goiter. In the integumentary system, the skin becomes flushed, warm, and moist. Hair will tend to be very fine and break easily; in some instances there is hair loss. Nails of the fingers and toes also break easily and often separate from the beds.

Hyperthyroid patients are often noted to have a "stare." This is due to upper eyelid retraction and is frequently seen with thyrotoxicosis. Movements of the eyelid are jerky and irregular. Most persons with hyperthyroidism develop some *exophthalmos.* This protrusion of the eyeball may cause difficulty in eyelid closure. The cause of exophthalmos is "edematous swelling of the retro-orbital tissues and deposition of large quantities of mucopolysaccharides in the extracellular spaces . . . ." [8].

TABLE 32-1. Hyperthyroidism: physiology and pathophysiology

PHYSIOLOGY

TRH	=	thyrotropin-releasing hormone
TSH	=	thyroid-stimulating hormone
T3	=	triiodothyronine
T4	=	thyroxine

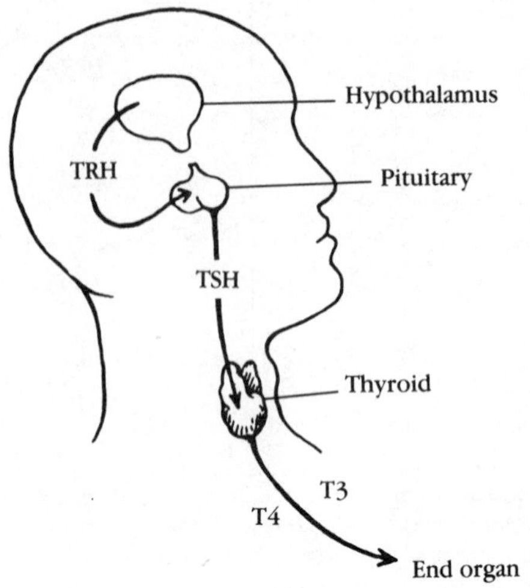

PATHOPHYSIOLOGY

- Diffuse enlargement of the thyroid
  - Graves' disease
  - Activity similar to that of thyroid-stimulating hormone
    - Choriocarcinoma
    - Hydatidiform mole
    - Hepatoma (rare)
    - Pituitary adenoma secreting thyroid-stimulating hormone
- Nodular, enlarged thyroid
  - Graves' disease
  - Toxic multinodular goiter (Plummer's disease)
  - Toxic uninodular goiter (functional thyroid adenoma)
- Tender, enlarged thyroid
  - Subacute thyroiditis
  - Hashimoto's thyroiditis (occasionally tender)
  - Irradiation thyroiditis
  - Iodine thyroiditis (Jodbasedow) (occasionally tender)
- Nonpalpable thyroid
  - Factitious hyperthyroidism — excessive ingestion of thyroid hormone
- Struma ovarii
- Metastatic thyroid carcinoma
- Normal gland (may be nonpalpable)

Source: R. D. Judge, G. D. Zuidema, and F. T. Fitzgerald (eds.), *Clinical Diagnosis* (4th ed.). Boston: Little, Brown, 1982.

Cardiovascular system changes are the most pronounced, due to the increased metabolic demands on the heart. Pronounced tachycardia is always present, even during periods of sleep. Often, systolic blood pressure rises [10]. Palpitations occur due to the increased force of the cardiac contraction. Atrial or supraventricular dysrhythmias are not uncommon. Generally, persons who have no underlying or preexisting cardiac failure are able to maintain the increased rate of cardiovascular function required. However, hyperthyroidism may eventually precipitate congestive heart failure.

Changes in nervous system function are indicated by increasing restlessness and nervousness, a decreased attention span, and a need to be almost constantly in motion, even though fatigue occurs rapidly. Afflicted persons also become emotionally labile, having bursts of temper and rapid mood changes.

In the gastrointestinal system an increased appetite is apparent, but there is usually associated weight loss. Increased food intake is generally insufficient to meet the increased metabolic demands, and there may also be complaints of nausea, vomiting, or diarrhea. The affected person is usually very thin, even emaciated.

Other systemic changes may become apparent. Dyspnea occurs during any periods of increased physical activities. Mild polyuria, heat intolerance, excessive perspiration, and an increased susceptibility to infection may be manifested.

THYROID STORM. Thyrotoxic crisis, or thyroid storm, is an uncommon, but life-threatening, complication of hyperthyroidism. It most frequently occurs after partial or complete surgical removal of a large thyroid gland, in persons poorly prepared (with antithyroid drugs) for thyroid surgery. It may also occur after any extreme stress, such as trauma or infection. Thyroid storm results from a sudden increase in thyroid hormone levels in the bloodstream, resulting in a marked increase in all of the clinical manifestations of hyperthyroidism. Generally, the person develops high fever, profuse diaphoresis, shock, vomiting, and dehydration. The physiologic effects of the hypermetabolic processes are so devastating to the body tissues that those persons in crisis must receive immediate intervention, or death will rapidly ensue.

GRAVES' DISEASE. The most common and well-known form of hyperthyroidism is Graves' disease, also known as exophthalmic goiter, diffuse toxic goiter, Basedow's disease, and primary hyperthyroidism. It is not simply a disease of the thyroid, but a multisystem syndrome that may include major manifestations of hyperthyroidism, diffuse thyroid enlargement, infiltrative ophthalmopathy, infiltrative dermopathy, and generalized lymphoid hyperplasia. These features may occur individually, or in any combination.

Graves' disease may occur at any age but primarily strikes those between the ages of 30 and 50. Generally, women are affected more frequently than men, and it is often seen in more than one member of the same family.

It is now accepted that there is an autoimmune component to this disease. In the 1950s, a specific substance was discovered in the serum of many individuals with Graves' disease. The substance found was an immunoglobulin G1 later termed *long-acting thyroid stimulator (LATS).* LATS has been found to have all of the functions of TSH but the effects are longer lasting, and are not subject to the control of rising levels of thyroid hormones in the blood. In untreated cases of Graves' disease, LATS is found in nearly every case [7].

Heredity and genetic factors are also accepted contributors to the development of Graves' disease. This form of hyperthyroidism is frequently seen in more than one family member and may occur in several generations of the same family. Thus, genetic and autoimmune components are major contributors to the formation of Graves' disease.

It has also been suggested that severe emotional stress may contribute to Graves' disease [3]. Frequently, the appearance of the disease follows a severe emotional or physical trauma.

The outstanding clinical features in a patient with Graves' disease are diffuse and palpable goiter, unilateral or bilateral exophthalmos, pretibial myxedema, and signs of hypermetabolism, or thyrotoxicosis [14, 18]. The onset of symptoms is usually gradual. Complaints of nervousness, irritability, fatigue, heat intolerance, and weight loss are common. These symptoms are a result of the increased metabolic rate.

The thyroid gland is enlarged to 2 to 3 times the normal size, in most cases. It may, however, be massively enlarged, or remain near normal size. Enlargement of the gland is usually symmetric, and the surface is smooth.

Exophthalmos, the most common ocular change, is usually accompanied by periorbital edema. The affected individual will have a characteristic bulging, wide-eyed stare. Often, the eye musculature is so affected that damage to the cornea and sclera occur due to an inability to close the eyes. Exophthalmos usually gradually disappears with treatment of the hyperthyroidism. Infiltrative ophthalmopathy is a more serious and extensive involvement and may cause permanent changes in eye function. It also may cause especially difficult problems in treatment.

Infiltrative dermopathy, commonly termed *pretibial myxedema*, is a dramatic manifestation, generally affecting the pretibial area of one or both legs, causing a barklike appearance of the skin. Localized edema and swelling of the skin and subcutaneous tissues occur. Hyaluronic acid accumulates in the interstitial spaces, and, combining with water, forms edema that is boggy and nonpitting. Individuals exhibiting pretibial myxedema have been found to have a profound immunologic disruption, and it is thought that these dermatologic changes are a direct result of that immunologic reaction [5].

TOXIC MULTINODULAR GOITER. In some persons with a longstanding history of nontoxic goiter, hyperthyroidism may insidiously appear. This disorder is known as toxic multinodular goiter, or *Plummer's disease.* Women are most frequently affected after the age of 50. The origin and etiology of the mechanism that causes nontoxic goiter to become toxic is not known.

The clinical manifestations are mild in comparison to Graves' disease. Thyrotoxicosis signs are less prominent, and serum thyroxine levels are only marginally elevated. Cardiovascular symptoms are the most pronounced. The affected individuals may develop atrial fibrillation, tachycardia, and congestive heart failure; also apparent are muscle weakening and fatigue. It is often difficult to diagnose toxic multinodular goiter because of the slow onset of the disease. The signs and symptoms may be attributed to lethargy and aging.

TOXIC ADENOMA. Toxic adenoma is a less common form of hyperthyroidism. It usually results from the development of a follicular adenoma. These adenomas are subdivided, according to the size of the follicles, into macrofollicular, microfollicular, and embryonal varieties [18]. It may occur in pairs or triplets. The function of the adenoma may be more or less than that of normal thyroid gland tissue, but it is capable of functioning without the stimulation of LATS or TSH.

As the adenoma grows, it begins to take over the function of normal thyroid tissue. Eventually, without intervention, complete atrophy and suppression of the remainder of the thyroid gland occurs [18]. The adenoma must reach the size of 2 to 3 cm before it is capable of producing a state of hyperthyroidism. The lesion may undergo necrosis and hemorrhage of its center. If this occurs, symptoms of thyrotoxicosis will recede, and the remainder of the thyroid gland tissue will resume normal functioning.

Individuals usually affected with toxic adenoma are in the 30- to 40-year age range and generally have a history of a lump in the neck, which has been growing slowly for many years. Clinical features are not pronounced; cardiovascular symptoms are likely to be the most prominent.

Hypothyroidism

Hypothyroidism results when a deficiency of thyroid hormone exists, resulting in a decreased rate of body metabolism and a general slowing down of body processes. The degree of dysfunction is related to the relative amount of hormone deficiency in the tissues.

CLINICAL MANIFESTATIONS OF HYPOTHYROIDISM. Changes in the skin that occur with hypothyroidism result when hyaluronic acid binds with water. The combination produces the baggy, full, edematous skin characteristic in hypothyroidism. Edema is most apparent in the face, hands, and feet. The skin is pale, cool, and very dry. Wounds or breaks in the skin heal very slowly.

Cardiovascular symptoms may closely resemble congestive heart failure. Cardiac output is decreased, as are heart rate and circulating blood volume. Peripheral vascular resistance is increased, ultimately resulting in a decreased flow of blood to the tissues. The term *myxedema heart* refers to the clinical picture of an enlarged heart, with ECG and serum enzyme changes seen with thyroid hypofunction.

The gastrointestinal tract, along with other body functions, slows down under the influence of a hypothyroid state. Most persons have a decreased appetite and, contrary to popular belief, only a slight increase in weight. Decreased peristalsis leads to an accumulation of gas and complaints of constipation.

Hypothyroid effect on the nervous system also decreases function. Thinking and movement begin to slow down. Mental dullness is often apparent. Personality changes may occur, resulting in severe depression or extreme agitation and anxiety. Movements are slow and disorganized, causing the appearance of clumsiness.

Other body system changes also result from hypothyroidism. Muscular pains are common and decreased strength occurs. Decreased renal blood flow and glomerular filtration contribute to the cardiovascular changes. Anemia and changes in the clotting factors occur. And, in both sexes, hypothyroidism decreases sexual drive.

Exactly the opposite of hyperthyroidism, hypothyroidism causes decreased thyroid function and reduced energy metabolism, resulting in a lower metabolic rate. Protein synthesis and degradation are reduced, resulting in growth retardation of bone and muscle tissue. Glucose absorption from the stomach and intestines is delayed, resulting in delayed insulin time. As with protein, the synthesis and degradation of lipids are decreased. The net result is a decreased rate of energy metabolism.

CRETINISM. Thyroid hormone deficiency during embryonic and neonatal life results in a state known as cretinism in infants and young children. It is not readily apparent at birth and it may take several weeks to several months before the hypothyroid state is discovered. The infant becomes sluggish and falls behind the normal rate of growth and development. Mental retardation and delayed growth patterns are characteristic of a cretin.

In appearance, cretins are dwarflike in stature. Their arms and legs are short in relationship to the trunk of the body (Fig. 32-5). The face of a cretin is broad and puffy, and the teeth are usually malformed; the skin is coarse and dry with sparse hair. The abdomen is protuberant, which often results in umbilical hernias. Early recognition and treatment reverse the effects of hypothyroidism in an infant, preventing the onset and development of cretinism.

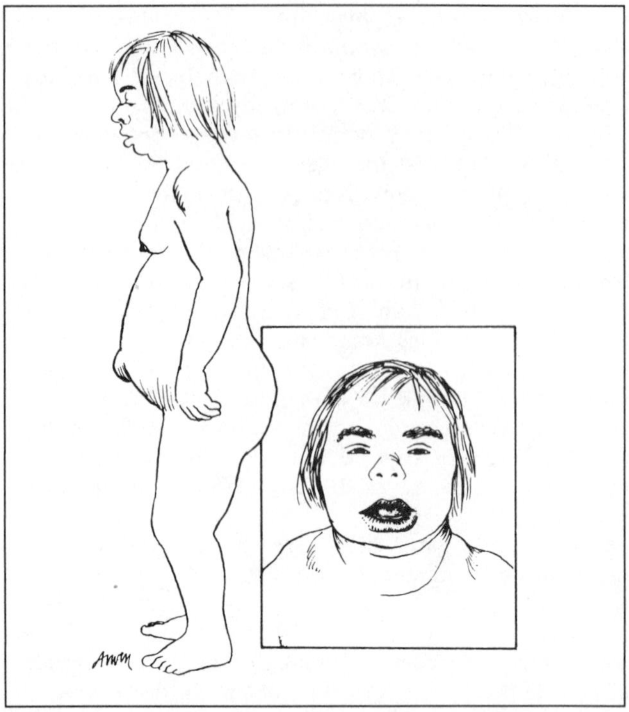

FIGURE 32-5. Hypothyroidism. (From R. Judge, G. Zuidema, and F. Fitzgerald [eds.], *Clinical Diagnosis* [4th ed.]. Boston: Little, Brown, 1982.)

ENDEMIC GOITER. In some areas of the world, an iodine deficiency exists in the environment to the degree that goiters may be common among the people dwelling in that region. The term *endemic goiter* refers to such an area and population. The Great Lakes region of the United States and mountainous areas of other countries, such as the Swiss Alps, are noted for their soil and water iodine deficiency (Fig. 32-6).

Because of the lack of iodine, the thyroid gland is unable to synthesize thyroxine and triiodothyronine, resulting in decreased serum levels of thyroid hormones. Secretion of TSH is increased, and the thyroid gland becomes very hyperplastic, leading to the formation of a goiter that is the attempt by the gland to produce thyroid hormones.

ADULT HYPOTHYROIDISM. Severe hypothyroidism in the adult is often termed *myxedema*. Its onset is slow and may not be recognized for many years. Primary adult hypothyroidism results from the loss or destruction of thyroid gland tissue. This may be caused by an autoimmune or disease process within the thyroid tissue, removal of the thyroid gland, or it may occur following treatment for Graves' disease. Secondary hypothyroidism results from pituitary TSH insufficiency, usually due to a lesion within the pituitary gland.

Early symptoms of adult hypothyroidism are fatigue and lethargy. A goiter may be present, which indicates an attempt to compensate for the deficiency [1]. Also, a marked sensitivity to cold temperatures occurs. A gradual

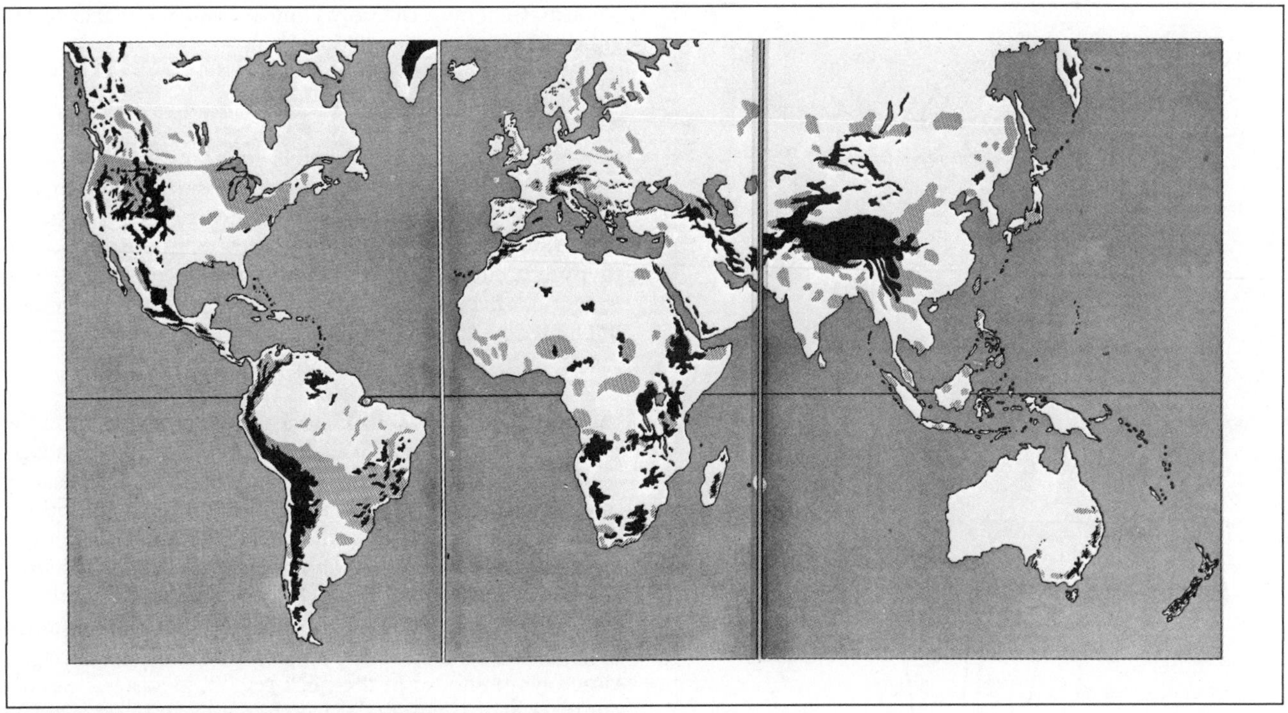

FIGURE 32-6. Regions of endemic goiter and the mountainous terrain with which it is often associated were mapped by the World Health Organization. Areas where iodine-deficiency goiter is endemic are indicated by the gray areas. Populations near seacoasts are seldom affected due to the iodine content of seafood. Not all inland areas are equally affected; the geology and remoteness of mountainous regions (solid black) make them most susceptible. (From W.H. Freeman, Human nutrition. *Sci. Am.* 214, 1978.)

slowing of mental and physical function begins and will progress through the course of the disease. The skin, hair, and nails become very dry, with the hair and nails becoming brittle and breaking very easily. Stiffness and aching in the muscles and joints develop, especially in the morning after waking. A slight weight gain is often noted despite decreased appetite.

As the clinical signs and symptoms continue to develop, the full picture of myxedema may be seen. Thick features, especially in the face, hands, and feet, become apparent, caused by the same process that results in pretibial myxedema in the patient with Graves' disease. Hoarseness of voice and a thick tongue develop. The body temperature is lower than normal, resulting in mild hypothermia. And, finally, mental and physical lethargy progress to an extreme. If untreated this process will continue for many years (Fig. 32-7).

MYXEDEMA COMA. The development of myxedema coma is a medical emergency in persons with hypothyroidism. The comatose state is the most severe expression of profound hypothyroid function [17]. It is usually seen during the winter months and affects mostly elderly myxedematous persons. Any stress, such as extreme cold, trauma, infection, CNS depressants, or physical stress, may precipitate this crisis. Lethargy progresses to coma, with hypotension and hypothermia on examination. The coma results from a continuous slowing of the vital centers; the respiratory center becomes more depressed, cardiac output continues to drop, and cerebral hypoxia increases as a result. Without intervention the mortality is as much as 50 percent [4].

CHRONIC AUTOIMMUNE THYROIDITIS. This form of thyroiditis, also known as *Hashimoto's disease,* is primarily found in women in the 30- to 50-year age range, but it may occur at any age and is thought to be a major cause of hypothyroidism in children [18]. The two most characteristic findings are a large, palpable goiter and a high level of circulating autoantibodies.

The goiter results from hormone biosynthesis defects within the thyroid gland. Because of the failure to produce adequate hormone levels, the pituitary produces TSH abundantly. The result is a goiter without clinical evidence of thyrotoxicosis. Chronic autoimmune thyroiditis may lead to a state of hyperthyroidism but will usually lead to thyroid hypofunction.

Enlargement of the thyroid gland occurs very gradually. The goiter becomes firm and rubbery; usually there is minimal tenderness, although extreme pain can occur. When left untreated, the gland will continue to enlarge over the years.

There is often a family history of chronic autoimmune thyroiditis, or a history of family members with Graves' disease, nontoxic goiter, or primary hypothyroidism. Also,

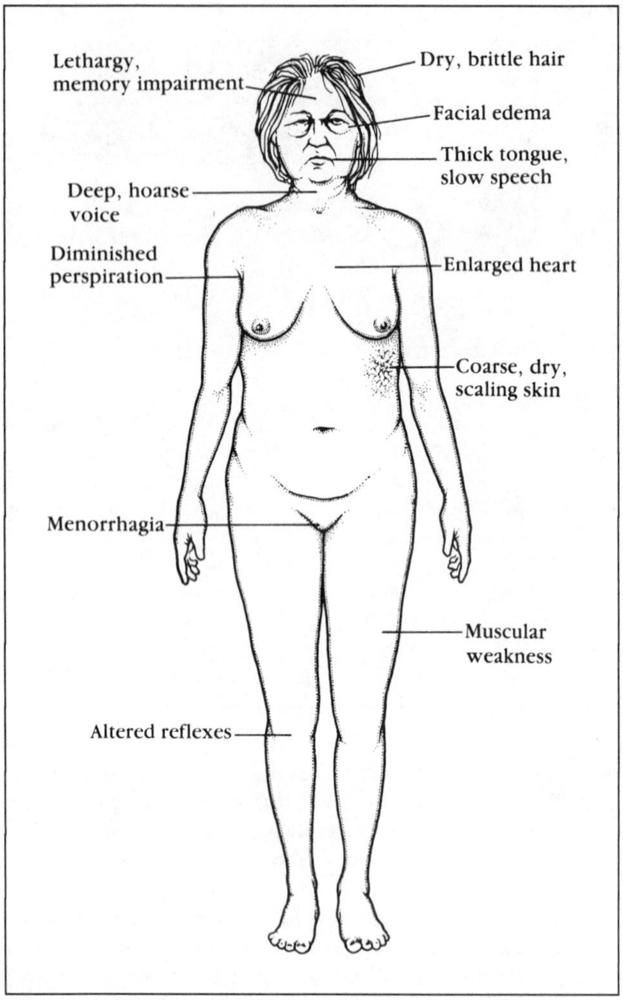

FIGURE 32-7. A composite of the symptoms of myxedema. (From M. Beyers and S. Dudas, *The Clinical Practice of Medical-Surgical Nursing* [2nd ed.]. Boston: Little, Brown, 1984.)

families may show an increased incidence of other autoimmune disorders, such as rheumatoid arthritis, or pernicious anemia.

NONTOXIC GOITER. Sometimes enlargement of the thyroid gland occurs without evidence of alterations in rate of body metabolism. This enlargement is termed a *nontoxic*, or simple, goiter. It commonly occurs at puberty, during adolescence, or during pregnancy. This common disorder occurs in 10 percent of all North American women [5].

A variety of causes may be responsible for the goiter, such as iodine deficiency or genetic enzymatic defects. Any of these causes will result in a decreased rate of production of thyroid hormones, which in turn results in increased secretion of TSH from the pituitary. Hyperplasia of thyroid tissue occurs in compensation and, in mild cases, there is usually no clinical evidence of alteration in function. If thyroid hypertrophy is severe, there may be signs of hyperthyroidism. Generally, the only clinical evidence is that of the enlarged, palpable thyroid gland.

Malignant Thyroid Tumors

Carcinoma of the thyroid gland is not very common and accounts for only a small percentage of the total number of persons diagnosed with cancer. There is no existing evidence supporting a familial tendency or predisposition to thyroid carcinoma, other than the parafollicular type. However, it has been shown that exposure to radiation therapy in childhood dramatically increases the risk of at least two forms of thyroid carcinoma [9].

PAPILLARY CARCINOMA. Papillary carcinoma originates in the papillary cells of the thyroid and is the most common type of thyroid gland cancers, accounting for approximately one-half of all thyroid cancers. It is seen more frequently in children and young adults and more frequently in women. Radiation exposure in childhood contributes to the causation of this malignancy. It is a slow-growing cancer and may remain in the gland for many years. The first appearance may be as a palpable node in the thyroid gland or as enlarged lymph nodes in the neck region. Metastasis can occur through the lymphatics to other areas of the thyroid or, in some cases, to the lungs.

FOLLICULAR CARCINOMA. Follicular carcinoma, as the name implies, originates in the follicular cells and accounts for 20 to 25 percent of thyroid carcinomas. It affects an older population, usually over 40 years of age; it also affects women 2 to 3 times more frequently than men. Childhood exposure to radiation therapy increases the risk in this type of malignancy. There may be invasion of area blood vessels and other areas of thyroid tissue, as this type is more invasive than the papillary type.

ANAPLASTIC CARCINOMA. Anaplastic carcinoma is a highly malignant form of thyroid cancer and accounts for about 10 percent of the thyroid cancers. It is slightly more common in women than in men. Metastasis occurs rapidly, spreading first to the surrounding areas and then to all parts of the body. Initially, the afflicted person may complain of a mass in the region of the thyroid. As the cancer involves structures adjacent to the thyroid, hoarseness, stridor, and a difficulty in swallowing may occur. Life expectancy after diagnosis usually is only several months.

PARAFOLLICULAR CARCINOMA. Parafollicular, or medullary, carcinoma is unique among the thyroid cancers. Only a small number of cases that occur are related to this specific type. It generally affects women more than men and most often patients are past 50 years of age. Parafollicular carcinoma also metastasizes quickly, often to distant sites of the body, such as the lungs, bones, and liver. Its distinctive feature is that it has the ability to secrete calcitonin because of

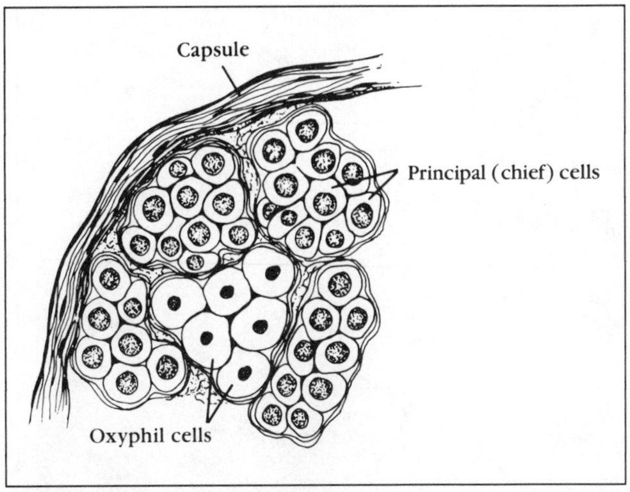

FIGURE 32-8. Parathyroid gland. The cells are arranged in cords by loose connective tissue. The principal cells are predominant in number. Oxyphil cells are recognized by their smaller, more condensed nuclei and larger relative cytoplasmic volume. (From M. Borysenko, et al., *Functional Histology* [2nd ed.]. Boston: Little, Brown, 1984.)

its origin in the parafollicular cells. This particular carcinoma is frequently noted to have familial tendencies.

THE PARATHYROID GLAND

Anatomy of the Parathyroid Gland

The parathyroid glands, four in number, lie posterior and adjacent to the thyroid gland. There is one parathyroid gland in each superior and inferior lateral area of the thyroid. Each gland is small, about the size of a pea, and the combined total weight is approximately 120 mg. The glands are reddish-brown or yellowish-brown and each is enclosed in a small fibrous capsule (see Fig. 32-1).

The parathyroid glands secrete *parathyroid hormone* (parathormone, or PTH). Secretion of this hormone is not under the control of the pituitary gland but is directly regulated by a negative feedback system of the circulating blood levels of calcium. Stated simply, as calcium levels fall, more parathyroid hormone is secreted; as calcium levels rise, hormone secretion is reduced. Almost any factor reducing serum calcium levels will stimulate the release of parathyroid hormone [1].

There are two cell types in the parathyroid gland—the oxyphil cell and the chief (or principal) cell. Oxyphil cells are slightly larger but are not actually engaged in the secretion of hormones and do not have a known function [11]. Chief cells are responsible for production and secretion of the parathyroid hormone.(Fig. 32-8).

Function of the Parathyroid Gland

The parathyroid gland regulates the serum levels of calcium in the body and serves to control the rate of bone metabolism. Vitamin D and calcitonin also affect calcium metabolism. Vitamin D is obtained through dietary ingestion of foods with a high content of vitamin D and through synthesis in the skin. Foods containing vitamin D include milk products and fish-liver oils. Many vitamin D–enriched foods are also available. Vitamin D synthesized in the skin is known as calciferol and is activated on direct exposure to sunlight.

Vitamin D is essential in calcium absorption from the intestinal tract into the bloodstream. It also increases retention of calcium and phosphorus, and serves to control the mineralization of bone matrix. Thus, it plays a major role in relation to controlling and maintaining circulating levels of calcium [14].

Calcitonin, or thyrocalcitonin, which is produced and secreted by the parafollicular cells of the thyroid gland, serves to oppose the action of the parathyroid gland and to lower blood calcium levels. Decreased serum calcium levels are accomplished by transferring calcium circulating in the blood back to the bones (Fig. 32-9).

In order to maintain calcium levels, parathyroid hormone acts on bones, the kidneys, and the intestines to resorb calcium. Some of its most important effects are (1) to increase plasma calcium concentration and decrease plasma phosphate concentration, (2) to increase urinary excretion of phosphate but decrease urinary excretion of calcium, (3) to increase the rate of skeletal remodeling and the net rate of bone resorption, (4) to increase the number of osteoblasts and osteoclasts on bone surfaces, (5) to cause an initial increase in calcium entry into the cells of its target tissues, (6) to alter the acid-base balance of the body, and (7) to increase the gastrointestinal absorption of calcium [18].

EFFECT OF PARATHYROID HORMONE ON BONE RESORPTION.

Since the greatest storage of calcium in the body is in bone, it is here that parathyroid hormone has its greatest effect on increasing the rate of metabolic breakdown of bone tissue. Primarily, this action is exerted on osteoclasts, which are large cells with multiple nuclei that participate in the resorption of bone [8]. After the release of parathyroid hormone, osteoclasts will resorb an area of mineralized bone to release calcium. Parathyroid hormone also stimulates the formation of new osteoclasts and delays the conversion of osteoclasts into osteoblasts, which are the principal cells of bone formation. The overall strength of bone is not substantially altered by this process in a healthy person with a normally functioning parathyroid.

EFFECT OF PARATHYROID HORMONE ON KIDNEY RESORPTION.

The action of parathyroid hormone on the kidneys involves increased resorption of calcium ions and decreased resorption of phosphate ions. These actions occur at different sites in the kidney and by different mechanisms. Decreased resorption of phosphate is due to the effect of parathyroid hormone directly on tubular absorption, and the increase

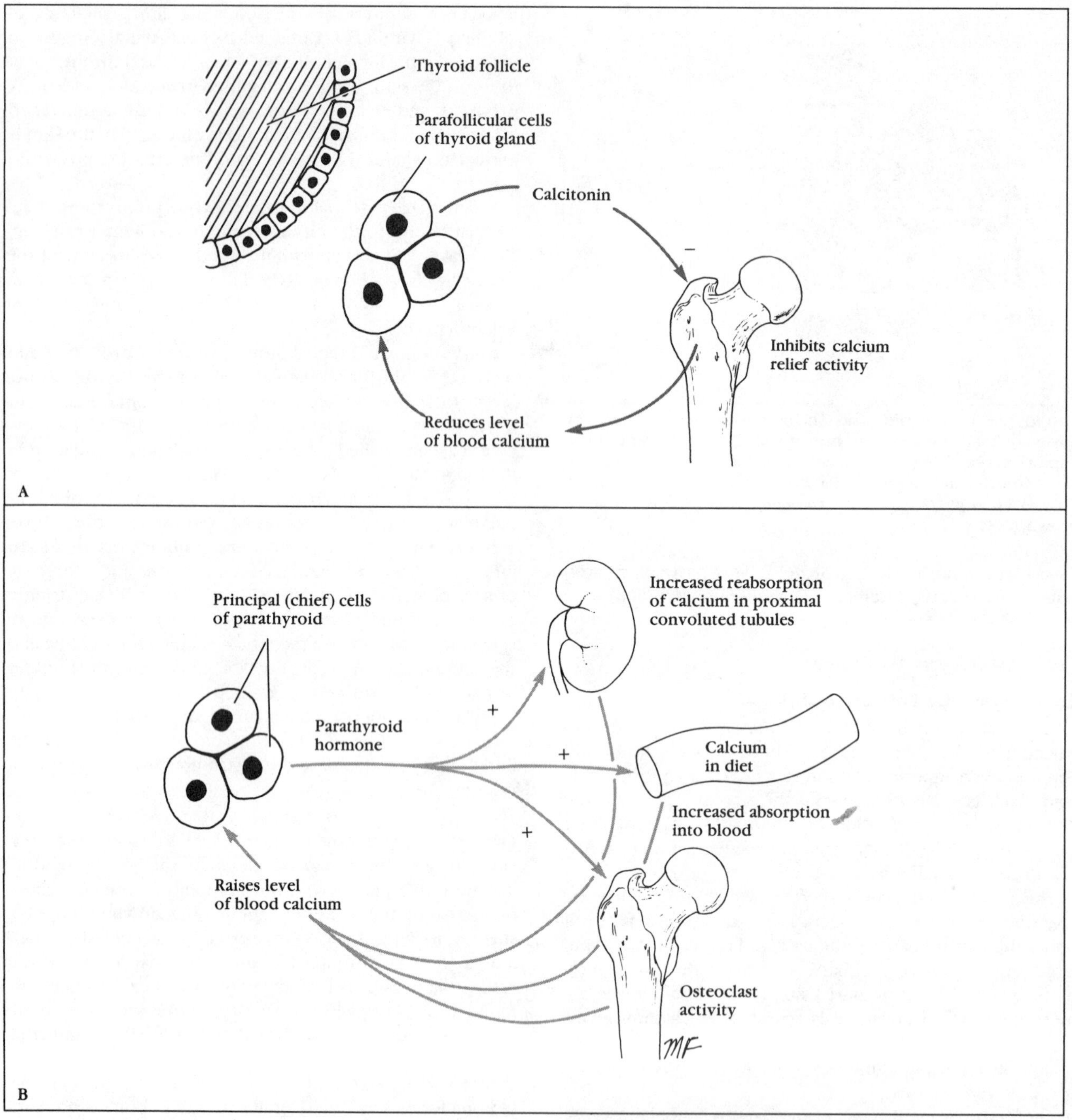

FIGURE 32-9. A. Regulation of calcitonin secretion by the parafollicular cells of the thyroid gland. B. Regulation of the parathyroid gland.

in calcium resorption is due to a direct effect on the distal convoluted tubule. In early research, the effect of parathyroid hormone on the tubular absorption of phosphate was considered to be the primary and most important role. Now, however, it is recognized that this action is secondary to the role of the parathyroid hormone on bone resorption of calcium.

EFFECT OF PARATHYROID HORMONE ON INTESTINAL RESORPTION. Parathyroid hormone also influences the resorption of calcium from the small intestine. It is necessary, however, for activated vitamin D to be present for this process to occur. Resorption of calcium from the intestines also increases absorption of calcium phosphate, thus decreasing the amount of phosphate elimination.

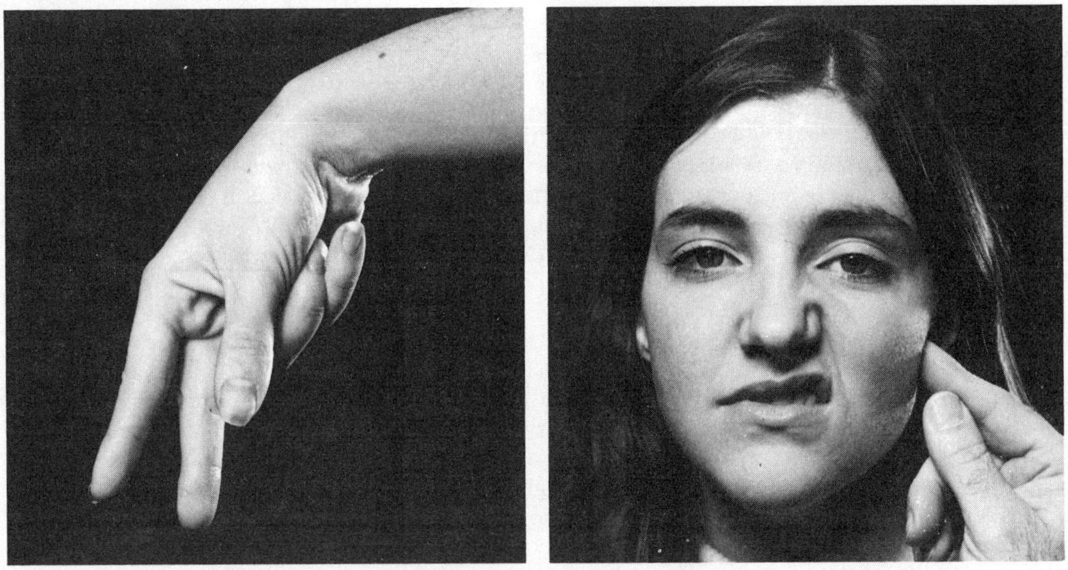

A B

FIGURE 32-10. Diagnostic signs of hypoparathyroidism. A. Carpopedal spasm in Trousseau's sign. B. Facial muscle contraction in Chvostek's sign. (From M. Beyers and S. Dudas, *The Clinical Practice of Medical-Surgical Nursing* [2nd ed.]. Boston: Little, Brown, 1984.)

ALTERED FUNCTION OF THE PARATHYROID GLAND

Hypoparathyroidism

Hypoparathyroidism results when there is insufficient parathyroid hormone secreted, or when the hormone fails to act at the tissue level. Without circulating parathyroid hormone, calcium is not resorbed from bone, kidneys, or the intestines. The resulting effect is a decreased serum concentration of calcium. This in turn causes increased neuromuscular excitability and the symptoms of tetany. Therefore, all of the clinical manifestations result from decreased levels of serum calcium concentration.

CLINICAL MANIFESTATIONS. In 70 percent of cases of hypoparathyroidism, tetany becomes the major clinical manifestation [18]. It begins with a numbness and tingling of the extremities and progresses to stiffness, cramps, and spasms. Carpalspasms are common and are the most prominent symptoms. If serum calcium levels continue to fall, the neuromuscular manifestations will become more severe and pronounced [11]. Laryngeal muscles are very susceptible to spasms, and death by asphyxiation can result if intervention is not accomplished immediately. At the very least, wheezing due to bronchospasm will occur.

When hypoparathyroidism exists for several months to several years, other physical changes may become apparent. Nails become brittle and may atrophy, and horizontal ridges are apparent on the surface. Afflicted persons often experience alopecia in patches on the head and almost complete loss of eyebrows. The skin becomes coarse and dry with patches of brownish pigment visible. Papilledema is often present and may occur with increased intracranial pressure. ECG changes of hypocalcemia show an increased duration of the Q–T interval. Serum calcium levels fall and remain subnormal. Sometimes, personality changes and psychiatric symptoms occur, such as emotional lability, extreme irritability and anxiety, depression, and delirium. Convulsions and grand mal seizures may occur.

There are three clinical signs used to definitively diagnose tetany and hypoparathyroidism. (1) The first test is for a positive Chvostek's sign. A quick tap or light blow over the parotid gland near the ear will produce twitching of the facial muscles especially the upper lip, nose, and eye. (2) Trousseau's sign is elicited by occluding blood supply to the arm for 3 minutes. The result is positive when carpopedal spasms occur (Fig. 32-10). (3) Erb's sign is considered positive when a 6-mV current produces a motor response. Specific positive responses to any of these clinical signs is usually considered diagnostic.

IDIOPATHIC HYPOPARATHYROIDISM. Idiopathic hypoparathyroidism is relatively uncommon. The course of dysfunction is variable. It may be congenital or acquired, mild or severe, transient or lifelong. Generally, the congenital form is related to defective or absent parathyroid glands. Children are most commonly diagnosed, with females being affected twice as often as males. It is widely suspected that an autoimmune state may be related to the idiopathic form. The symptoms produced, including tetany, are usually quite severe.

POSTOPERATIVE HYPOPARATHYROIDISM. More common than the idiopathic form, hypoparathyroidism may be related to damage or removal of the parathyroid glands during thyroid surgery. Removing the thyroid gland without detaching the parathyroids is the most frequent cause. However, any surgery, such as a radical neck dissection, that involves manipulation of the structures of the throat can result in clinical features of hypoparathyroidism.

When damage or partial removal occurs, the remaining parathyroid tissue is usually able to compensate for the loss. Thus, a transient loss of parathyroid hormone occurs. Complete removal of the glands would result in a total loss of parathyroid function, and a severe state of hypocalcemia would rapidly follow.

PSEUDOHYPOPARATHYROIDISM. Pseudohypoparathyroidism, also known as *Albright's hereditary osteodystrophy,* is a form of hypoactive functioning that is familial in origin. It is widely believed to be transmitted by an X-linked dominant gene. Serum hypocalcemia and hypophosphatemia are characteristic of this disorder. The parathyroid glands are normal in size, or slightly enlarged, and there is no deficit in circulating levels of parathyroid hormone. Women are affected twice as frequently as men.

These persons have developmental skeletal abnormalities, and usually exhibit a mild to moderate degree of mental retardation. They are short and stocky in stature, often less than 5 feet tall, and are often obese. The face is very round, due to structural abnormalities in the development of the facial and cranial bones. The metacarpal bones are short and stubby. Usually, there is some degree of subcutaneous soft tissue ossification and calcification that is widespread.

Pseudopseudohypoparathyroidism is a condition very similar to the one described above. The major difference is that the levels of serum calcium and phosphates are normal. Familial tendencies also exist with this disorder.

Hyperparathyroidism

Much more common than hypoparathyroidism, the incidence of this disorder appears to be continually on the increase. The specific etiology of any form of hyperparathyroid function is not well understood. In most cases a single benign adenoma is found to be the cause. It is also thought that a history of long-standing states of hypocalcemia may contribute to the predisposition of hyperparathyroidism. There are three forms of hyperfunction of the parathyroid glands. They are usually recognized as primary, secondary, and tertiary.

PRIMARY HYPERPARATHYROIDISM. Primary hyperparathyroidism is usually characterized by hypercalcemia, resulting from failure of the normal feedback mechanism to decrease secretion of parathyroid hormone. As the serum calcium concentrations rise, parathyroid secretion is no longer reduced and calcium levels continue to increase. The clinical manifestations produced are variable and nonspecific. Some persons experience mild symptoms, while others have severe symptoms. The most common manifestation is in the genitourinary system; renal calculi probably result from precipitation of calcium and phosphate in the kidneys [9].

Other variable symptoms include renal symptoms, skeletal changes, and hypercalcemia. In addition to the formation of renal stones, hematuria may be noted. Gastrointestinal complaints include anorexia, nausea, vomiting, and constipation, as well as generalized abdominal pain [13]. Changes within the skeletal system are diverse. Sometimes, new bone is laid as quickly as calcium is resorbed, and the person will have only mild complaints of vague skeletal pains. At other times, various bone diseases such as osteoporosis or osteomalacia may result.

SECONDARY HYPERPARATHYROIDISM. Secondary hyperparathyroidism may be initiated by a variety of causes that result in a low serum calcium concentration. These causes may include low-calcium diet, pregnancy or lactation, rickets, or osteomalacia. However, in the Western world the usual cause is renal failure. The low calcium levels cause the parathyroid glands to become hyperplastic in order to compensate for the condition that initially caused the low calcium levels. After compensation attempts, calcium may remain low or may attain normal levels (see Chap. 29).

TERTIARY HYPERPARATHYROIDISM. Tertiary hyperparathyroidism results from the same causes as the secondary form, except that hypercalcemia develops from hyperplasia of the parathyroid glands. In some instances, adenomas develop after the onset of secondary hyperparathyroidism. This condition is accompanied by abnormally high calcium levels. Tertiary hyperparathyroidism is often described in persons with renal failure who develop hypercalcemia.

Renal osteodystrophy, which may occur with tertiary hyperparathyroidism, is seen in patients with chronic renal failure who develop hyperphosphatemia [9]. Parathyroid hyperfunction is then necessary to increase serum calcium concentrations (see Chap. 29). Metastatic calcifications in the soft tissues, such as the eyes, lungs, or joints, may occur [6, 12].

REFERENCES

1. Brooks, S.M. *Integrated Basic Science* (4th ed.). St. Louis: Mosby, 1979.
2. Catt, K.J. *An ABC of Endocrinology*. Boston: Little, Brown, 1971.
3. Chaffee, E.E., and Lytle, I.M. *Basic Physiology and Anatomy* (4th ed.). Philadelphia: Lippincott, 1980.
4. Dillon, R.S. *Handbook of Endocrinology* (2nd ed.). Philadelphia: Lea & Febiger, 1980.
5. Ezrin, C., Godden, J.O., and Volpe, R. *Systematic Endocrinology* (2nd ed.). Hagerstown, Md.: Harper & Row, 1979.
6. Fearing, M.O. Osteodystrophy in patients with chronic renal failure. *Nurs. Clin. North Am.* 10:461, 1975.
7. Felig, P., et al. *Endocrinology and Metabolism.* New York: McGraw-Hill, 1981.
8. Guyton, A.C. *Textbook of Medical Physiology* (6th ed.). Philadelphia: Saunders, 1981.
9. Hall, R., Anderson, J., and Besser, M. *Fundamentals of Clinical Endocrinology*. Chicago: Year Book, 1980.
10. Hallal, J.C. Thyroid disorders. *Am. J. Nurs.* 77:417, 1977.

11. Jacob, S.W., et al. *Structure and Function in Man*. Philadelphia: Saunders, 1981.
12. Lewis, S.M. Pathophysiology of chronic renal failure. *Nurs. Clin. North Am.* 16:501, 1981.
13. O'Dorisio, T.M. Hypercalcemic crisis. *Heart Lung* 17:425, 1978.
14. Shaw, K. The nature of the endocrine system: Part 6. The parathyroid glands and calcium metabolism. *Nurs. Mirror* 144:28, 1977.
15. Shaw, K. The nature of the endocrine system: Part 3. The thyroid gland. *Nurs. Mirror* 144:26, 1977.
16. Tortora, G., Evans, R., and Anagnostakos, N. *Principles of Human Physiology*. Hagerstown, Md.: Harper & Row, 1982.
17. Urbanic, R.C., and Mazzafferi, E.L. Thyrotoxic crisis and myxedema. *Heart Lung* 7:435, 1978.
18. Williams, R.H. *Textbook of Endocrinology* (5th ed.). Philadelphia: Saunders, 1974.

CHAPTER 33
NORMAL AND ALTERED FUNCTIONS OF THE PANCREAS

LEARNING OBJECTIVES

1. Describe the anatomy of the pancreas: size, shape, parts, ducts, and cells.
2. Relate the histology of the pancreas to its function.
3. Explain the physiologic regulation of insulin secretion.
4. Describe the metabolic effects of insulin.
5. Explain the actions of glucagon and somatostatin and their effects on metabolism.
6. Discuss the incidence and etiology of diabetes mellitus.
7. Differentiate between the types of diabetes.
8. Relate the stages or degrees of abnormality of diabetes.
9. Explain the pathophysiology of diabetes.
10. Relate the clinical manifestations of diabetes to the pathophysiologic changes.
11. Explain the pathophysiology of complications of diabetes mellitus.
12. Differentiate between ketoacidosis, hyperglycemic hyperosmolar nonketotic coma, and lactic acidosis.
13. Outline the physiologic responses to hypoglycemia.
14. Identify tests used in the diagnosis and evaluation of diabetes mellitus.
15. Explain the pathophysiology of pancreatic islet-cell diseases: hyperinsulinism, Zollinger-Ellison syndrome (gastrinoma), multiple endocrine neoplasia (Werner's syndrome).
16. Discuss the incidence and etiology of acute pancreatitis.
17. Describe the chemical and pathologic changes characteristic of pancreatitis.
18. Relate the clinical manifestations of acute pancreatitis to the histologic alterations.
19. Discuss the complications of acute pancreatitis.
20. Relate laboratory findings of acute pancreatitis.
21. Compare clinical manifestations and complications of acute pancreatitis with chronic pancreatitis.
22. Discuss the incidence, etiology, types, and clinical course of carcinoma of the pancreas.
23. Discuss the incidence and genetics of cystic fibrosis.
24. Describe the pathophysiologic changes that occur in various body systems in cystic fibrosis: gastrointestinal, pancreatic, respiratory, reproductive.
25. Relate the clinical manifestations of cystic fibrosis to the pathophysiologic changes.
26. Discuss laboratory and diagnostic findings related to cystic fibrosis.

The purpose of this chapter is to describe the anatomy, physiology, pathology, and alterations in function of the pancreas. The pancreas plays an important part in the digestion and metabolism of food. Much of its anatomic structure serves gastrointestinal function, but special cells in the islets of Langerhans influence metabolism through the secretion of insulin and glucagon. An excess of insulin causes hypoglycemia and too little causes diabetes. Conversely, an excess of glucagon causes diabetes and too little leads to hypoglycemia. Diabetes mellitus is the most common disease associated with pancreatic islet dysfunction and is a leading cause of death in the United States.

Other disorders discussed in this chapter include inflammation, tumors, and fibrocystic disease (cystic fibrosis). Physiology of digestion and alterations in function are discussed in Unit 12.

ANATOMY AND PHYSIOLOGY

The pancreas is an elongated retroperitoneal gland that lies in the upper portion of the posterior abdominal wall. It resembles a fish with its head and neck lying in the C-shaped curve of the duodenum, its body extending horizontally behind the stomach, and its tail touching the spleen (Fig. 33-1). The head is at the level of the second lumbar vertebra, makes up about 30 percent of the gland, and lies within the concavity of the duodenum. The ***neck***, the narrowed portion between the head and body, joins to the *body*, which accounts for the larger portion of the gland. The tail tapers off from the body. The pancreas is of firm consistency and has a characteristic lobular appearance with a light yellow and slightly pink coloration.

In the adult, the total length of the pancreas varies between 12 and 20 cm, with a width of 3 to 5 cm, and maximal thickness of 2 to 3 cm. The weight is between 70 and 120 gm.

The pancreas is composed of both exocrine and endocrine tissue. The exocrine portion forms the largest mass of the gland and is composed of small groups of *acini* (grapelike formations) where digestive enzymes and large volumes of sodium bicarbonate are synthesized and transported. The acini form a network of larger ducts that eventually drain into the major secretory ducts of Wirsung and Santorini. The duct of Wirsung extends from the surface of the tail of the pancreas to the duodenum at the ampulla of Vater, usually alongside the common bile duct. It empties into the duodenum at the same place as the common bile duct, at the duodenal papilla. In most cases, the sphincter of Oddi surrounds both ducts. In one-third of cases, the duct of Wirsung and the common bile duct form a common channel before terminating at the ampulla of Vater. The accessory duct of Santorini exits from the main duct near the neck of the pancreas and enters the duodenum approximately 2 cm above the main duct.

The endocrine portion of the pancreas, the islets of Langerhans, are embedded between the exocrine units of the pancreas, like small islands. The islets contain four

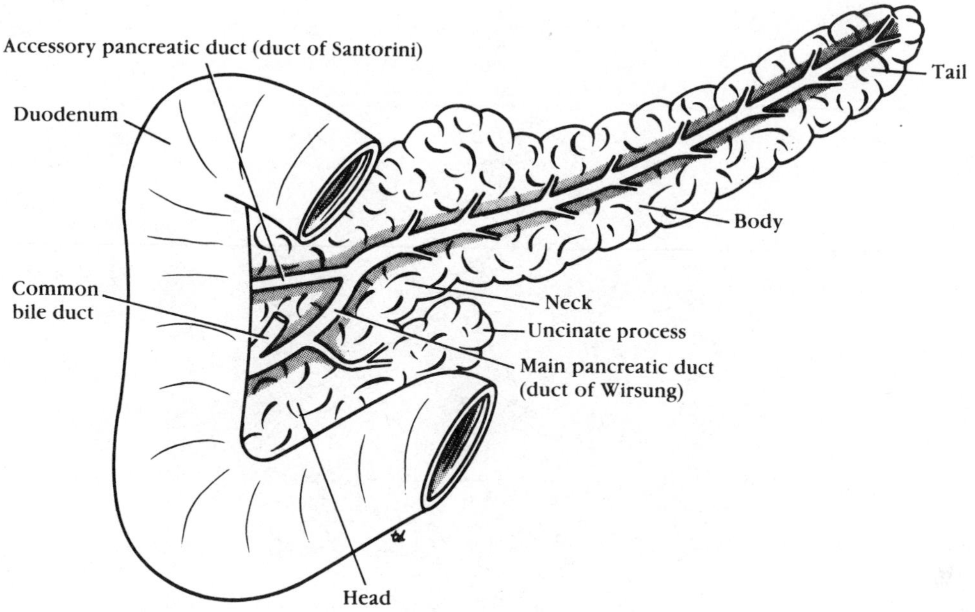

FIGURE 33-1. Parts of the pancreas dissected. (From R. Snell, *Clinical Anatomy for Medical Students* [2nd ed.]. Boston: Little, Brown, 1981.)

types of cells, the *alpha*, *beta*, *delta*, and a recently described *PP* (*pancreatic polypeptide*) cell (Fig. 33-2). These types comprise 20, 70, 5 to 10, and 1 to 2 percent of islet cell population respectively. All of these cells empty their secretions into the bloodstream. Alpha cells secrete *glucagon*, beta cells secrete *insulin*, and delta cells contain secretory granules that secrete *somatostatin*. PP cells have small dark granules and are present not only on the islets, but also on the exocrine pancreas. The PP cells secrete a unique *pancreatic polypeptide* that causes gastrointestinal effects of diarrhea and hypermotility in experimental animals. The physiologic effects in humans are still unknown [16]. Although there are as many as 2 million islets, 20 to 300 μ in diameter, the endocrine portion composes only about 1 percent of the weight of the pancreas.

Physiologic Regulation of Insulin Secretion

The main function of the endocrine portion of the pancreas is the secretion of *insulin*, a hormone essential for normal carbohydrate metabolism. Insulin also influences the metabolism of fats and proteins. Therefore, it functions as a prime hormone for integrating the major metabolic fuels (Fig. 33-3).

Insulin consists of two amino acid chains and is synthesized from a biologically inactive precursor, *proinsulin*, by the beta cells. Recent study indicates that proinsulin itself is derived from an even larger polypeptide, *preproinsulin* [11]. The average adult pancreas secretes an estimated 35 to 50 units of insulin daily.

Insulin is the only known hormone that reduces the circulating glucose levels. Although numerous physiologic factors may alter insulin secretion, output is regulated mainly by blood glucose level through a negative feedback mechanism (Fig. 33-4). When the glucose in the blood that is perfusing the pancreas exceeds approximately 100 mg/dl, there is an immediate beta cell response involving extrusion of the granule's contents from the beta cell. When blood glucose levels fall, the rate of insulin secretion also decreases. The release of insulin is biphasic. Glucose prompts both an immediate and a sustained release as more insulin is synthesized. The feedback mechanism is very rapid-acting with insulin levels reaching 10 to 20 times the basal rate with blood glucose levels of 300 to 400 mg/dl. The cessation of secretion is equally rapid, occurring within minutes after restoration of blood glucose to fasting level [7].

In addition to glucose, amino acids can also stimulate insulin secretion in varying degrees. The most potent stimulants are arginine, lysine, and phenylalanine. Insulin, in turn, promotes transport of the amino acids into the tissue cells.

While insulin secretion is mostly considered in terms of secretion in response to nutrients, measurable amounts of insulin are secreted at a low basal rate between meals and during prolonged fasting. Certain gastrointestinal hormones, secretin, pancreozymin, gastrin, and gastric-inhibiting peptide (GIP), which are released by the gastrointestinal tract after a meal, play a role in stimulating

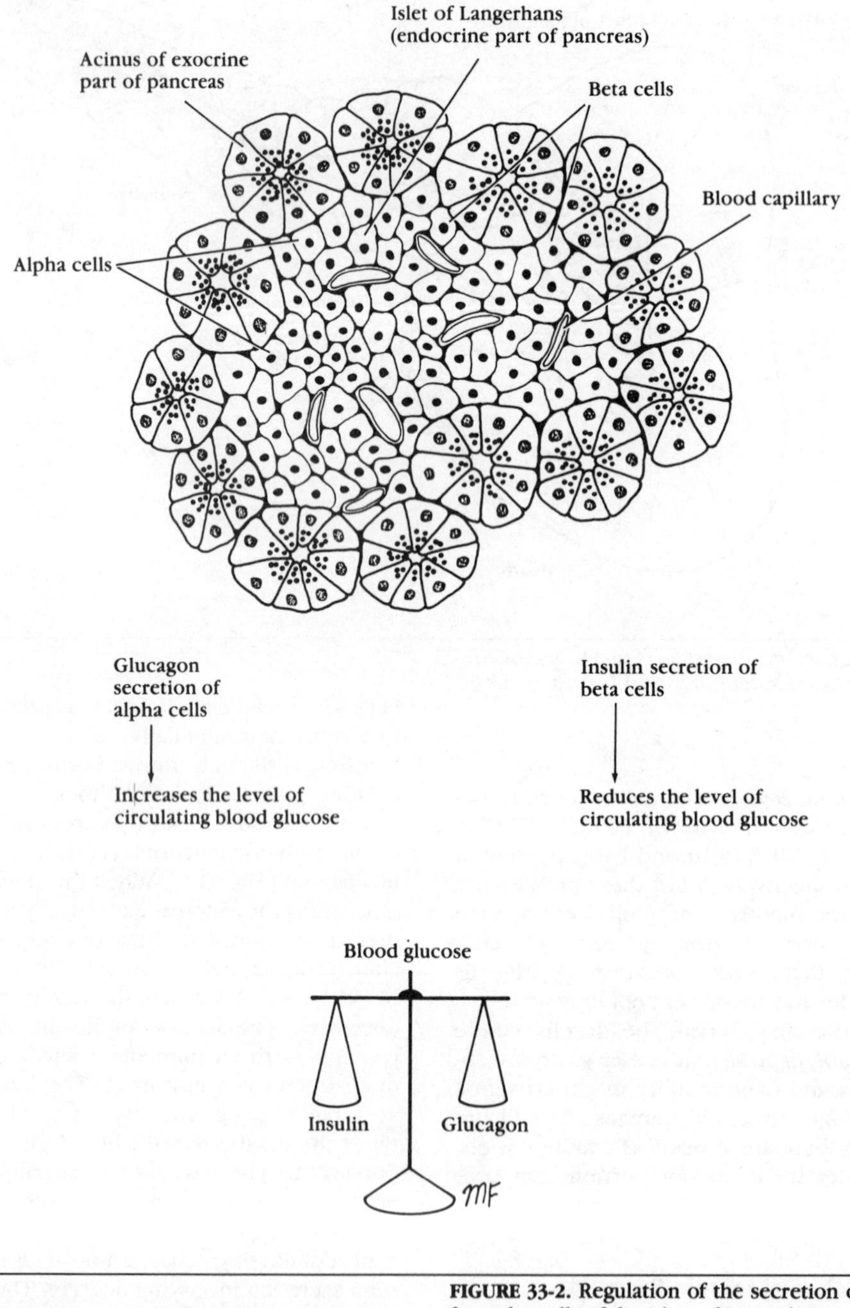

FIGURE 33-2. Regulation of the secretion of insulin and glucagon from the cells of the islets of Langerhans.

pancreatic insulin release [7, 16]. These hormones, released during digestion, cause an "anticipatory" increase in blood insulin preparatory for the glucose and amino acids absorbed from the meal.

Other hormones that either directly increase the secretion of insulin or potentiate glucose stimulation of insulin are glucagon, cortisol, growth hormones, progesterone, and estrogen. Prolonged increased amounts of these hormones can lead to exhaustion of the beta cells and diabetes. High pharmacologic doses of the hormones may also induce diabetes.

The autonomic nervous system also functions in the control of insulin secretion. The alpha-adrenergic activities of the sympathomimetic amines (epinephrine and norepinephrine) inhibit insulin secretion. Although catecholamine stimulation of beta-adrenergic sites increases insulin secretion, the alpha-adrenergic action of epinephrine predominates. Other factors, primarily pharmacologic, that stimulate insulin secretion include sulfonylurea drugs and

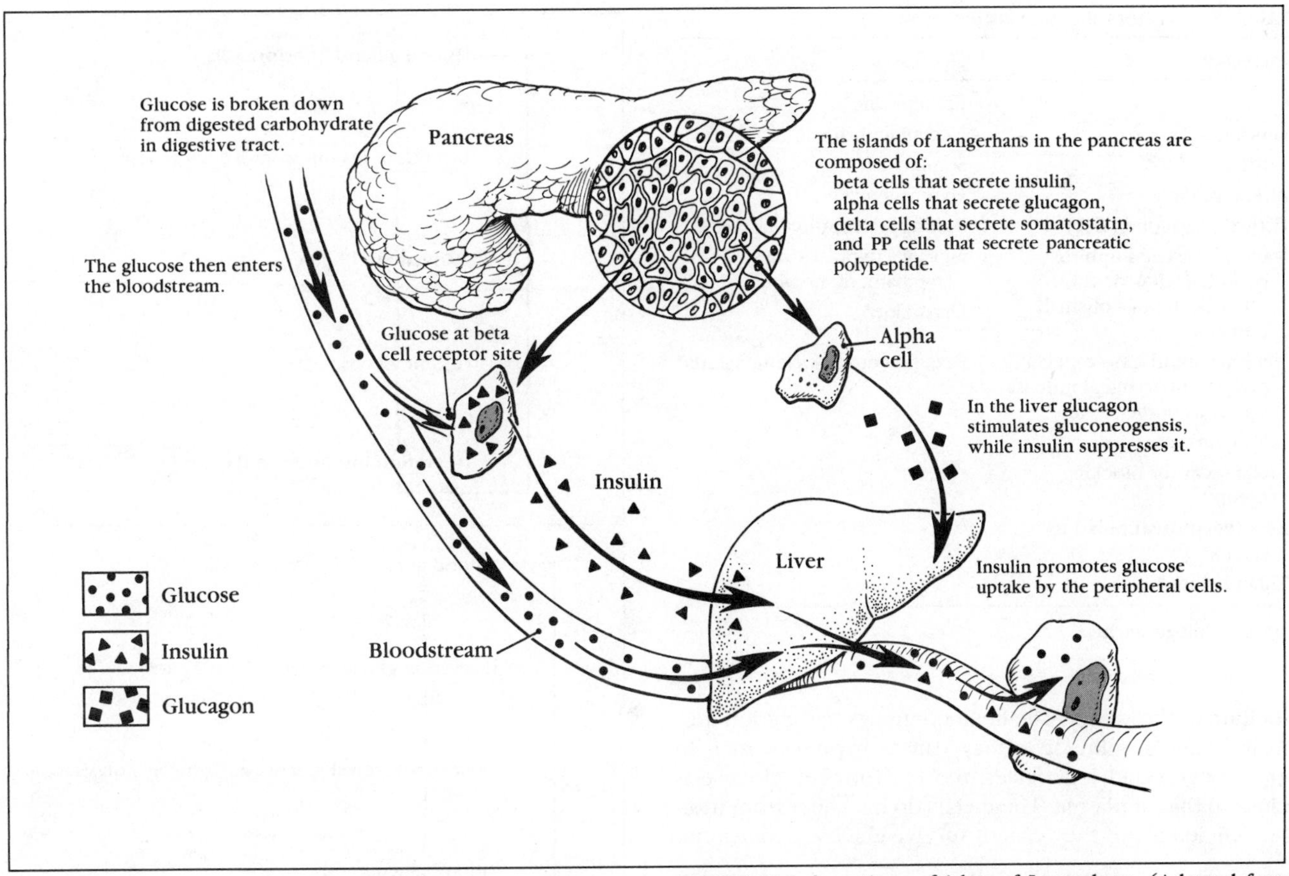

FIGURE 33-3. Secretions of islets of Langerhans. (Adapted from B. Lippe, Diabetology. *Patient Care* 3:17, 1982.)

theophylline. In contrast, beta-receptor blocking agents and diazoxide inhibit secretion (Table 33-1).

Effect of Insulin on Facilitated Diffusion

Insulin is an influential hormone that affects the biochemical function of every organ in the body. Its most important action is to accelerate the transport of glucose across most cell membranes in the body. In the absence of insulin, the rate of transport of glucose into body cells is about one-fourth the normal; when an excess is secreted the rate may be 5 times the normal. Figure 33-5 illustrates the carrier mediated transport of the inside of the membrane and its release transport, by means of a carrier mechanism, called *facilitated diffusion* or carrier transport. *Insulin influences* this transport of glucose into the cell by combining with a receptor protein in the cell membrane. A direct action on the cell membrane is implied since glucose transport occurs within seconds or minutes. Once the glucose concentration inside the cell is equal to the glucose concentration on the outside, additional glucose will not be transferred into the cell. Insulin is especially effective in facilitating transport of glucose in skeletal and adipose tissue, the liver, and the heart. The adipose tissue and skeletal tissue alone make up 65 percent of body weight.

Insulin does not enhance glucose transport into the brain, erythrocytes, leukocytes, intestinal mucosa, or epi-

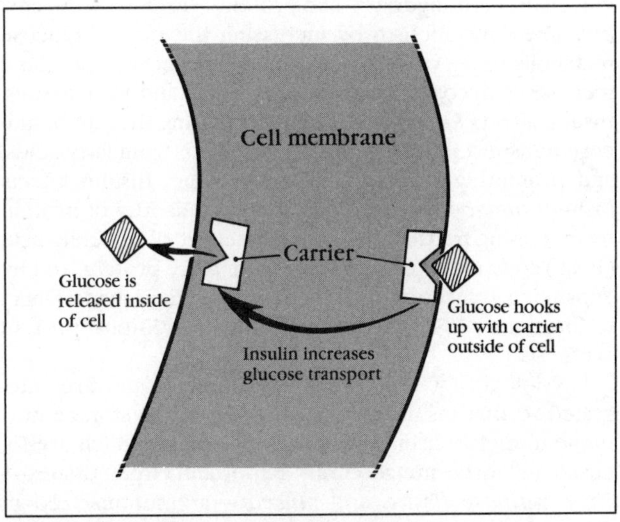

FIGURE 33-4. Insulin increases glucose transport.

TABLE 33-1. Factors affecting insulin secretion

Increases	Decreases
Glucose	Epinephrine
Glucagon	Norepinephrine
Cortisol	Somatostatin
Amino acids	Hypokalemia
Growth hormone (GH)	Fasting (except in diabetes)
Secretin, gastric inhibitory peptide (GIP), possibly other hormones of small intestine	Nervous impulses via sympathetic nervous system Diazoxide*
Nervous impulses—especially oral and pharyngeal mucosa via vagus nerve	Beta-receptor blocking agents*
Sulfonylureas*	
Alpha-receptor blocking agents*	
Beta-receptor stimulating agents*	
Theophylline*	

*Pharmacologic agents

thelium of the kidney. The brain continues to function normally when insulin deficiency causes hyperglycemia. In erythrocytes and leukocytes, the level of free glucose is close to that of plasma. These cells do not suffer from insulin deficiency but they cannot survive glucose deficiency.

Metabolic Effects of Insulin

Insulin functions to stimulate anabolic reactions that involve fats, carbohydrates, and proteins. Insulin affects *carbohydrate* metabolism by increasing the rate of glucose metabolism, decreasing blood glucose concentration, and increasing glycogen stores in the muscle and liver tissues. Insulin affects *fat metabolism* by increasing the rate of glucose transport into fat cells, forming lipids from fatty acids, and promoting storage in adipose tissue. Insulin affects *protein metabolism* and increases the quantity of protein by increasing translation of the messenger ribonucleic acid (RNA) code in the ribosomes to form more protein, and by enhancing transcription of deoxyribonucleic acid (DNA) to form more RNA, thereby resulting in additional protein synthesis.

Physiologically, the diverse effects of insulin are integrated so that insulin functions as the prime storage hormone in metabolism. The actions of insulin, which are focused on three metabolically important target tissues—*liver, adipose tissue,* and *muscle*—are summarized in Table 33-2 and in the following discussion.

LIVER. The role of the liver with respect to insulin and carbohydrate homeostasis is unique because of the following aspects:

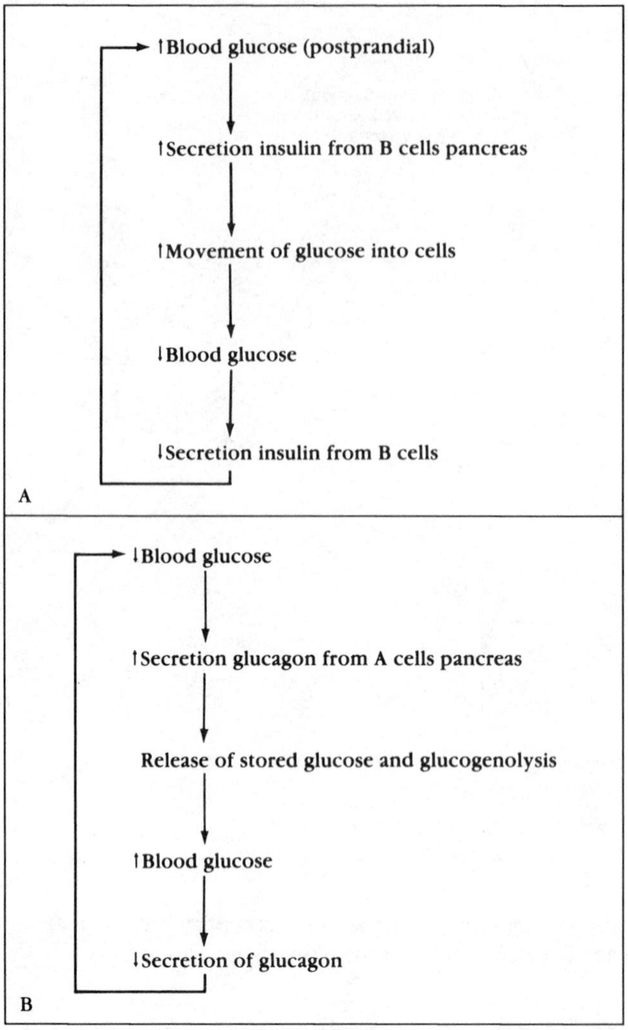

FIGURE 33-5. Negative feedback system of (A) insulin and (B) glucagon.

TABLE 33-2. Target sites and metabolic actions of insulin

	Liver	Adipose cell	Muscle
Carbohydrate	Glycogen synthesis Gluconeogenesis Glycogenolysis	Glucose transport Glycerol synthesis	Glucose transport Glycolysis Glycogen synthesis
Fat	Lipogenesis	Triglycerides Fatty acid synthesis Promotes storage	
Protein	Proteolysis for gluconeogenesis		Amino acid uptake Protein synthesis Protein anabolism

1. Insulin is not necessary for transport of glucose into the liver, since the liver cell is freely permeable to glucose. The uptake is increased by an enzyme, glucokinase, which is responsible for "trapping" of glucose inside liver cells so that intracellular glucose concentration is roughly equal to plasma concentration [1].

2. In the basal state, glucose is continuously released from the liver at a rate of 2.0 to 3.5 mg/kg/minute (200–350 gm/day) [17]. The ability of the liver to release free glucose derives from its capability for glycogenolysis and gluconeogenesis, and its possession of an enzyme, glucose-6-phosphatase, that promotes further breakdown of glycogen into glucose. This process is critical during prolonged fasting when glucose oxidation is minimal in most tissues and glucose is used almost exclusively by the brain. Once the glucose is in the free form, it readily diffuses into the circulating blood and the liver cell membrane.

3. The concentration of insulin in portal blood is two- to tenfold greater than that in peripheral blood. This concentration is due to the secretion of insulin directly into the portal system and the capacity of the liver to remove 50 to 80 percent of insulin reaching it [12].

4. Absorbed hexoses have direct access to the liver via the portal vein prior to circulating to peripheral tissues. Because of the previously mentioned characteristics, the liver plays an important role in the buffering of blood glucose. When there is an excess of insulin and/or glucose, the hepatic cells take up large quantities of glucose, which are deposited as glycogen as well as being converted to fat. When there is an absence of insulin or the blood glucose concentration falls too low, the hepatic cells release quantities of glucose into the blood by breaking down stored glycogen (glycogenolysis) and forming new glucose (gluconeogenesis). Thus, insulin enables the organism to maintain a stable blood glucose balance [3].

ADIPOSE TISSUE. Maintenance of energy balance is a major role of adipose tissue. It is the only tissue that can store a variable amount of "fuel" in the form of fat. The oxidation of 1 gm of fat yields 9 calories. Unlike the liver cell, the fat cell (adipocyte) membrane is capable of excluding glucose. Insulin greatly enhances the transport of glucose into fat cells and promotes fat storage in the adipose tissue.

The metabolism of glucose within fat cells occurs in several steps:

1. Glucose is rapidly phosphorylated with the fat cell.
2. Glucose is further metabolized to 2-carbon fragments (acetyl-coenzyme A), which are converted to fatty acids.
3. A larger portion is degraded by process of glycolysis into alpha-glycero-phosphate. The latter readily combines with free fatty acids to form triglycerides, the primary storage form of fat within the adipose cell.

Through its action on glucose metabolism insulin affects fat storage: It provides 2-carbon fragment precursors for fatty acid synthesis and glycerol for combining and storing these fatty acids as triglycerides. Insulin also enhances fat accumulation through actions unrelated to its effects on glucose metabolism. It inhibits an enzyme within the fat cell, resulting in an inhibition on lipolysis or fat metabolism, and also induces the enzyme necessary for the disposal of plasma triglycerides.

Fatty acids and all of the lipid components of plasma greatly increase in the absence of insulin. High lipid concentrations in the plasma, especially cholesterol, increase the risk of development of atherosclerosis.

MUSCLE. As in adipose tissue, insulin increases transport of glucose across the membrane into muscle cells. Once in the cell, the glucose is metabolized completely to carbon dioxide, or, if oxygen is limited, to lactic acid. After the glucose molecule that enters the cell is phosphorylated, it is used for energy or stored as glycogen. Unlike the liver, glucose cannot be released from stored muscle glycogen into the body fluids because muscle lacks the necessary enzyme, glucose phosphatase, for the conversion [7].

Quantitatively, muscle cell consumption of glucose is small during a resting state. Muscle tissue uses mostly fatty acids for energy because the normal resting muscle membrane is almost impermeable to glucose except in the presence of insulin. However, during exercise, glucose utilization increases greatly. This usage of glucose is not insulin-dependent, for exercising muscle fibers are permeable to glucose in the absence of insulin, because of the contraction process itself [7]. Muscles also use large amounts of glucose in the first few hours after a meal, at which time the blood glucose level stimulates the secretion of large amounts of insulin that increase the transport of glucose into muscle cells.

In summary, insulin functions primarily as a storage hormone. The diverse metabolic effects of insulin at various target tissues demonstrate the integrated and synergistic effect it has on the metabolism of fats, carbohydrates, and protein. Each molecule of glucose that enters a cell is immediately phosphorylated. Adipose tissue and muscles take up glucose only under the influence of insulin, phosphorylate it, and either store it in the form of glycogen or convert it to triglycerides (fatty acids). At the same time, presence of free fatty acids impedes glucose oxidation by insulin muscle and decreases the release of amino acids from muscle for hepatic gluconeogenesis. Glucose uptake by muscle is also stimulated, providing fuel to replace fatty acids whose release from adipose tissue is inhibited by insulin. Fat accumulation is also increased by release of fatty acids at the adipose cell from lipoproteins that arrive via the circulation from the liver and gastrointestinal tract. The antilipolytic action of insulin on the adipose cell increases fat storage, and thereby inhibits gluconeogenesis in the liver by depriving the liver of fatty acids and cofactors used in the gluconeogenesis process.

Physiology of Glucagon

Glucagon, a small protein, is a hormone secreted by the alpha cells of the islets of Langerhans. Its actions are opposite to those of insulin and secretion results in an increase in blood glucose concentration. The major effects of glucagon are stimulation of *glycogenolysis* and *gluconeogenesis* (Fig. 33-3).

Glucagon is very potent and causes glycogenolysis in the liver, which quickly increases blood glucose. Only 1 μg/kg of glucagon can elevate the blood sugar 50 percent within minutes. The hormone can continue to increase blood glucose levels even after the glycogen level in cells has been exhausted by increasing gluconeogenesis in liver cells.

Glucagon secretion is regulated by blood glucose concentration. Changes in blood glucose levels have the opposite effect on glucagon secretion from that on insulin secretion. A decrease in the level of blood glucose increases glucagon secretion. In almost every instance, glucagon has a metabolic effect directly opposite to that of insulin. Insulin promotes storage of glycogen in liver and muscle; glucagon inhibits it. Insulin inhibits glycogenolysis and glucagon promotes it. Insulin inhibits lipolysis and glucagon stimulates it. Thus, a negative feedback system with opposing action of insulin and glucagon maintains blood glucose levels (Fig. 33-5). Glucagon secretion is increased by exercise, starvation, insulin lack, and amino acid ingestion.

Somatostatin (Somatotropin Release Inhibiting Factor [SRIF])

The delta (D) cells of the pancreas and the upper gastrointestinal tract secrete a peptide, somatostatin, that inhibits release of growth hormone, thyrothropin, glucagon, insulin, and gastrin [7, 16, 17]. Somatostatin causes a marked decrease in gastric secretion by the decrease of the antral response to food. The precise role of somatostatin in metabolic processes is not clearly defined, although it has the capability to inhibit both insulin and glucagon secretion [17]. It has been postulated that somatostatin may act as a local regulator of endocrine and exocrine secretion and as a peptidergic neurotransmitter, rather than as a circulating hormone [15].

Regulation of Blood Glucose Concentration

In the normal person, the blood glucose ranges between 80 and 90 mg/dl in the fasting state. This concentration rises to 120 to 140 mg/dl following a meal. The feedback system returns the concentration to normal within about 2 hours following the last absorption of carbohydrates.

Blood glucose level is vital in maintaining nutritional balance in certain tissues, the brain, retina, and germinal epithelium of the gonads, because glucose is the only nutrient that can be used to supply adequate energy. More than one-half of all glucose formed by gluconeogenesis during the interdigestive period is used by the brain.

The liver acts as a reservoir and important blood glucose buffer system for glucose. The liver stores sufficient glycogen to maintain a normal blood sugar for 12 to 24 hours. When blood glucose levels are high, almost two-thirds of the glucose is stored, and when blood glucose concentration falls below normal, the stored glucose is released to maintain the blood glucose. When blood glucose rises to a high level (e.g., following meals), insulin secretion is increased to return blood glucose concentrations to normal.

The glucagon feedback system is stimulated by a decrease in the serum blood sugar, while an increase in blood sugar stimulates the pancreas to secrete insulin. Under normal circumstances, the insulin feedback mechanism is the most important, but in starvation states or excessive utilization of glucose during stress and exercise, the glucagon system becomes very important.

Stimulation of the sympathetic nervous system causes a rise in blood glucose. The release of catecholamines, epinephrine, and norepinephrine stimulates glycogenolysis in the liver, resulting in rapid release of glucose into the circulation.

Growth hormone and cortisol increase blood glucose levels less rapidly than the insulin-glucagon system. Both hormones decrease use of glucose in peripheral cells. Cortisol also stimulates gluconeogenesis, thereby resulting in an increased blood glucose level. Growth hormones and glucocorticoids are secreted during periods of hypoglycemia and decrease the rate of glucose use by most cells of the body. These hormones are less powerful in regulating blood glucose than insulin and glucagon, and require hours rather than minutes to effect a change in the serum glucose.

DIABETES MELLITUS

Diabetes is a metabolic disorder characterized by a relative or absolute lack of the hormone insulin, which results in impaired utilization of carbohydrates and altered metabolism of fats and protein. The term ***diabetes,*** from the Greek word meaning "a siphon," suggests excessive urine formation; the term ***mellitus,*** from the Greek word meaning "*honey*," suggests sweetness.

History

Writings about diabetes can be traced to the Ebers Papyrus, more than 3000 years ago, wherein afflicted persons were described as passing frequent and large amounts of urine. Ayur Veda described the sweetness of the urine and noted that ants were attracted to it. He described weakness, emaciation, polyuria, and carbuncles. Aretaeus, a first-century Greek physician, is credited with naming the disorder. He described the disease as a "melting down of the flesh and limbs into urine." Lipemia of the diabetic blood was noted by Helmunt about 1573 to 1644 A.D. The first diagnostic sign of the disease was established by Thomas Willis in the seventeenth century, when he tasted the urine of his patients and noted its sweet taste. A Paris physician, Michel

Chevreul, discovered that the sweetness was caused by sugar. In 1869 Langerhans, while a medical student, described the group of cells in the pancreas that produce insulin. Elliot Joslin was prescribing dietary restrictions long before the discovery of insulin. In 1921, Banting and Best were able to purify islet cell tissues from dogs and obtained a drop in blood sugar when the tissue was injected into diabetic animals. Within 6 months, insulin was administered to humans and the "rapid melting" and "speedy death" described by Aretaeus were alleviated.

In 1936, long-acting insulins were introduced, protamine being added to prolong the action and zinc being added for stability. In 1942, Hagedorn modified the PZI (protamine zinc insulin) and produced the first intermediate-acting insulin, NPH (neutral protamine Hagedorn). Globin and Lente insulins soon followed. In 1955, oral hypoglycemic agents were introduced. Insulin has been further purified and biosynthetic human insulin has been developed through recombinant DNA techniques.

Classification of Diabetes

Two major clinical types of variants of diabetes have been recognized. *Ketosis-prone, insulin-dependent diabetes or juvenile-onset diabetes (IDDM or JOD)* (Type I) has an onset generally before age 30 in persons who are not obese. Plasma insulin levels are low and respond very little or not at all to insulin stimulators such as glucose or oral hypoglycemics. These persons are ketosis-prone and require exogenous insulin, for the pancreas contains little or no extractable insulin and there is an overall reduction in beta cell mass. At birth, they synthesize insulin, but the level falls with time. About one-third experience a "honeymoon" period, a remission characterized by a temporary restoration of insulin secretion, which is reflected in C-peptide release (measure of residual beta cell secretory capacity), but is followed by a relapse. *Non-insulin-dependent* diabetes of middle and older age (*NIDDM or MOD*) (Type II) usually occurs after age 40, and about 30 percent of affected persons are obese. At birth these persons synthesize insulin, but the level falls as they age and beta cell function deteriorates. These persons are not ketosis-prone. In recent years, a third type, *maturity-onset-diabetes in young people (MODY),* has been more clearly defined. In these persons, diabetes is mild, ketosis-resistant, non-insulin-dependent, and occurs before 25 years of age. Although it is of a type of maturity-onset diabetes, it is seen in children as young as 10. There may be a pattern of inheritance.

Type I (IDDM) and Type II (NIDDM) comprise the majority of diabetic persons. *Secondary diabetes* can also occur in association with other conditions and syndromes, such as pancreatic disease, Cushing's syndrome, insulin-receptor abnormalities, and hormonal or drug-induced disorders. *Gestational diabetes* occurs only during pregnancy. Persons may display varying degrees of glucose intolerance related to metabolic effects of hormones secreted during pregnancy. Clinical manifestations of diabetes may be evident in persons with a predisposition for diabetes; pregnancy is a diabetogenic condition. *Impaired glucose tolerance (IGT)* is a clinical class that includes persons whose glucose tolerance tests are abnormal. These persons are asymptomatic but are recognized at higher risk than the general population for the development of diabetes.

TABLE 33-3. Comparison juvenile-onset (type I) and adult-onset (type II) diabetes

	Juvenile (insulin-dependent)	Adult (non-insulin-dependent)
Age of onset	Frequently before 20; most commonly preadolescence; can occur after 20	Usually after 30; can occur before 30
Onset	Abrupt	Insidious
Body weight	Thin	Usually obese (80%)
Symptoms	Polyuria, polydipsia, polyphagia, weight loss, weakness, fatigue	Polyuria, polydipsia, polyphagia, vulvovaginitis, often asymptomatic
Control	Wide fluctuations of blood sugar in relation to growth, diet, insulin, and exercise	Stable, usually easily controlled
Exogenous insulin	Needed by all	Needed by only 25–30%
Oral hypoglycemics	Not useful	May be useful in 35–40% of cases
Beta cells of pancreas	Destruction or inability of cells to secrete insulin	Secrete inadequate amounts of insulin
Ketoacidosis	Most prevalent first 5 years of known diabetes and in teenage years	Uncommon except with stress, infection
Insulin reactions	Frequent	Uncommon

There are cases that do not fit into any of the types described and there are others that are a combination of types. Therefore, it may be most appropriate to consider diabetes as *insulin-dependent* or *non-insulin-dependent* (Table 33-3).

Stages of Diabetes

Diabetes can also be classified by degree or stage of abnormality based on measurable carbohydrate tolerance and presence or absence of hyperglycemia. Classifications are outlined in Table 33-4 using the American Diabetes Association terminology. The separation between stages is arbitrary. An individual may remain in one stage, progress to

TABLE 33-4. Stages of diabetes

	Prediabetes	Subclinical diabetes	Latent	Overt
Fasting blood sugar	Normal	Normal	Normal or abnormal	Abnormal
Glucose tolerance test	Normal	Normal; abnormal during pregnancy stress	Abnormal	Abnormal
Delayed and/or decreased response to glucose	+	++	+++	++++
Symptoms	None	None	None	Present
Terminology employed by American Diabetes Association	Prediabetes	Suspected diabetes	Chemical or latent diabetes	Overt diabetes

another, or revert to a prior place. Progression or regression of carbohydrate intolerance may occur slowly, never occur, or occur rapidly.

Incidence and Etiology

Diabetes is a common disorder of the endocrine system with about 4.5 to 5.0 million affected individuals in the United States alone. Various theories have been offered to explain the genesis of diabetes. Multifactorial causes such as genetic, metabolic, microbiologic, and immunologic grounds have been cited for the variants of the disease.

Insulin-Dependent Juvenile-Onset Ketosis-Prone Diabetes (IDDM, Type I)

Current thinking leans toward beta cell destruction and lack of insulin in the causation of the *insulin-dependent juvenile-onset ketosis-prone* form of diabetes mellitus (IDDM). Genetic predisposition to beta cell destruction, infection, and autoimmunity have been postulated as mechanisms in the beta cell damage of IDDM.

INFECTION AND AUTOIMMUNITY. Many types of infections have been reported to precede the onset of diabetes mellitus. These include mumps, rubella, varicella, measles, influenza, coxsackievirus B infections, and viral and bacterial pneumonias [10]. Much interest has arisen because of the temporal relationship between the two events, especially in the close time proximity of an infection and the onset of IDDM. In addition, there is a higher incidence of diabetic cases diagnosed during autumn and winter when viral infections are more frequent [8].

Two specific antigen types, HLA-A-B8 and HLA-Bw15, have recently been found to be more common in IDDM, especially in children. These children tend to have high levels of neutralizing antibody titers to certain coxsackievirus types [4]. Islet cell antibodies (ICAs), lymphocytes, monocytes, and eosinophils have been found in the islets of recent-onset IDDM. This finding is strengthened by the association of other autoimmune disorders (e.g., Addison's disease, pernicious anemia, and thyroid disease) with IDDM of juvenile-onset. The NIDDM person lacks this antigenic tendency.

Non-Insulin-Dependent Diabetes Mellitus (NIDDM, Type II)

The causation of *maturity-onset, non-insulin-dependent ketosis-resistant diabetes mellitus* (NIDDM) has been explained as a consequence of a variety of etiologic factors. The following is a summary of several theories that have been offered.

ALTERATION OF INSULIN SECRETION. This theory postulates that NIDDM is not due to a reduction in beta cell mass and insulin production but is due to either inadequate or delayed response to the glucose load. This alteration is demonstrated in NIDDM when the rise in plasma insulin is delayed following oral glucose intake, when peak insulin level is reached after the glucose peak, and when diabetic blood glucose curves in normal, nondiabetic persons (simulated by computer-programmed glucose infusions) are compared with those of NIDDM. The latter secrete less insulin than age-, sex-, and weight-matched normal subjects. Similar findings of impaired insulin secretion have been found in prediabetics [16].

BIHORMONAL THEORY. Normally, a rise in blood glucose level depresses glucagon secretion and a fall in glucose is followed by a rise in glucagon. A relative or absolute hyperglucagonemia has been demonstrated in both forms of diabetes following the ingestion of food or with infusion of an amino acid secretagogue. It is postulated that there is inappropriate control not only of the beta cell but also of the alpha cell, the source of glucagon, as a causative factor in the disease [16].

RESISTANCE TO INSULIN IN PERIPHERAL TISSUES. Insulin resistance exists when a specific quantity of insulin produces less than the normal anticipated biologic effect at target sites. Insulin resistance can be attributed to three principle causes: (1) an *abnormal beta cell secretory product*, such as abnormal insulin molecule or incomplete conversion of proinsulin to insulin; (2) *circulating insulin antagonists* such as anti-insulin antibodies, anti-insulin receptor antibodies, or elevated levels of opposing regulatory hormones (e.g., growth hormone, cortisol, glucagon, or catecholamines); and (3) *receptor defects in target tissues* (e.g., during pregnancy or obesity) [11]. Alterations are demonstrated when the insulin requirements are increased during infection, stress, or endocrine disorders. Reaven proposes that insulin resistance is seen early in NIDDM, but that after a period of prolonged hyperglycemic stress on the islets, beta cell injury and insulin deficiency are secondary [14].

HEREDITY. For centuries it has been noted that diabetes "runs in families," because approximately 40 percent of persons who develop diabetes have a family history of diabetes. In general, it is accepted that there is a genetic component in the etiology of diabetes. Family histories, twin studies, and studies of histocompatibility of antigens confirm this view [13]. One theory, *recessive gene*, holds that diabetes is transmitted as a recessive genetic characteristic that is present in about 20 percent of the population. A second theory, *multifactorial inheritance*, holds that diabetes results from an interaction between several different genes and environmental factors [13]. The finding that IDDM may be of nongenetic origin has stimulated research in the area of nongenetic or environmental causes. Although heredity plays a role in the etiology of diabetes, the mode of inheritance is still uncertain. Insulin-dependent diabetes and non-insulin-dependent diabetes mellitus exhibit genetic differences. Studies of identical twins and first-generation relatives of diabetics reflect a concordance rate (both twins affected) of juvenile-onset, insulin-dependent diabetes mellitus (IDDM) of less than 50 percent, but a concordance rate approaching 100 percent for twins of NIDDM [6]. Therefore, genetic factors seem to play a greater role in the incidence of NIDDM than of IDDM.

AGE. Except for IDDM, increasing age is related to an increased incidence of diabetes. The incidence rises sharply after age 40, probably reflecting a general change in glucose tolerance. The blood glucose is low in childhood, rises progressively, and after age 70 about 15 percent of the population may show a "mild abnormal" glucose tolerance. The separation between diabetes and nondiabetes may present a problem, if the tolerance is not adjusted for age. This increasing incidence of diabetes has been explained as a decrease in body function occurring in all body cells with senescence.

BODY WEIGHT. About 80 percent of NIDDM individuals are obese, and the incidence of diabetes in obese individuals is greater than in the general population. Diabetes and obesity are interrelated in that obesity is associated with insulin insensitivity in target tissues (muscle, liver, and adipose cells). It is well known that blood levels of insulin are higher in the obese individual and take longer to return to the fasting state. Obesity acts as a diabetogenic factor because the accompanying insulin resistance increases the need for insulin. Since the obese are resistant to the effects of insulin, in practice, the obese diabetic responds poorly to treatment with insulin.

SEX. Diabetes is seen more frequently in women. Between the ages of 40 and 60, women diabetics outnumber men almost 2:1. The prevalence rate in females overall is 24.1/1000. This prevalence increases with age. In Japan, Malaya, and India, diabetes is 50 to 100 percent more common in men. In the West Indies, the sex incidence is equal but black women with diabetes outnumber men. The reason for this increased incidence may be related to the late effects of high parity, which may not be manifested until after age 45.

DIET. Certain factors implicate diet as a possible causative factor in the onset of diabetes. The incidence of diabetes is increased in wealthier communities in the United States. The effects of high carbohydrate and high fat diets in the causation of NIDDM have been extensively studied. Modification of dietary intake of carbohydrates minimizes hyperglycemia in these individuals and limitation of saturated fat intake may delay the onset of atherosclerosis.

There are multiple theories, none mutually exclusive, that explain the variants of diabetes. In many cases, there is no single biochemical cause of the disorder, and it can be described only in terms of impairment of carbohydrate intolerance due to multifactorial causes. Likewise, it is difficult to separate those factors that are the result of disease and those that cause disease.

Pathology of Diabetes

The diagnosis of diabetes can only be made on the basis of morphology because in some cases no distinctive lesions are found. Few diseases have as many widespread and systemic lesions as diabetes with major changes occurring in the pancreas, blood vessels, kidneys, and eyes. In classic juvenile diabetes, the number of islets is reduced, degranulation of beta cells and fibrosis of the islets may occur, and there may be lymphocytic infiltration. In maturity-onset diabetes, the number of islets is usually normal, the degree of beta cell granulation is somewhat reduced or may be normal, and hyaline deposits may be observed.

Pathology of the Pancreas

HYALINE DEPOSITS (AMYLOIDOSIS). The most frequently found pancreatic lesion is hyalinization of the islets, a finding present in 30 percent of the pancreatic tissue of diabetics at autopsy [9]. Hyaline, an eosinophilic material, may infiltrate small areas or the entire islet. Progressive accumulation of the deposits may reduce beta cell mass. Hyalinization is more common in older diabetics, is less frequent in the juvenile-onset type, correlates with the duration of the disease, and may occur in nondiabetics.

FIBROSIS. The thickening of the capsule and islets by fibrous connective tissue is a common change, and complete replacement of the islet cells by collagen tissue may occur. This change is correlated with the duration of diabetes, but it also occurs in nondiabetics who have pronounced atherosclerotic changes, and in persons having other types of pancreatic lesions [9].

DEGRANULATION OF BETA CELLS. A reduction in beta cells is a consistent finding and is found more frequently in the younger diabetic. The amount of beta cell granulation correlates with the amount of extractable pancreatic insulin. In most cases of diabetes, total pancreatic beta cell degranulation occurs [9].

VACUOLIZATION (GLYCOGENESIS). Beta granules are replaced by distended foamy vacuolated beta cells. Glycogen accumulation is related to the level and duration of hyperglycemia and is rarely seen in individuals treated with insulin [9].

LEUKOCYTIC INFILTRATIONS. Eosinophils and lymphocytes infiltrate the islets in an inflammatory type of reaction that is referred to as "insulitis." The inflammatory infiltrates are considered a type of immunologic reaction.

HYPERTROPHY AND HYPERPLASIA OF ISLETS. This process occurs infrequently except in the children of diabetic mothers and mothers with a latent diabetic tendency. The hyperglycemia of the mother causes a fetal hyperglycemia and compensatory fetal islet hyperplasia. Hyperplasia of islets has also been reported in diabetics who received tolbutamide therapy [9].

Vascular System Pathology

Vascular lesions are a hallmark of diabetes and are probably related to hyperlipidemia. Electron microscopic studies have revealed microangiopathy—thickening of the walls of the arterioles, capillaries, and venules—in the kidneys, retina, and neural and epidermal vascular beds. It is absent from capillaries of adipose tissue. Atherosclerosis appears mostly in the large vessels in which lipid deposits called *atheromas* or *plaque* are laid down on the intimal surfaces. Fibroblasts and calcium may be deposited and calcified plaques develop. The hyperlipidemia and hypercholesterolemia characteristic of diabetes relates in some way to the high incidence of hypertension in diabetes.

The atherosclerosis is the major factor in the high incidence of myocardial infarction, cerebral vascular accidents, and gangrene of the extremities in diabetes. Coronary atherosclerosis is up to 5 times more prevalent than in the normal population, and myocardial infarction is the most common cause of death. Atherosclerosis develops within a few years of the onset of the disease. Diabetics who have had diabetes for 10 years, whatever the age of onset, usually have significant atherosclerosis [16]. The principal clinical manifestations of peripheral arterial disease are ischemic lesions of the feet and of the lower extremities. In addition, neurotrophic changes cause loss of sensation, which may decrease attention to small injuries that become infected. A small break may lead to cellulitis, lymphangitis, infection, and necrosis of tissue (Figures 33-6 and 33-7). The arterioles also become thickened and microcirculation is impaired.

Pathology of the Kidney

The most characteristic renal changes in diabetes are the glomeruli with three predominant lesions: *nodular glomerulosclerosis, diffuse glomerulosclerosis,* and *exudative lesions.* Approximately 40 percent of deaths in diabetes can be related to kidney failure after 20 to 30 years of the disease [18].

NODULAR GLOMERULOSCLEROSIS. Nodular glomerulosclerosis (Kimmelstiel-Wilson lesion, a specific lesion of diabetes) appears as a round hyaline mass in the glomerulus, resulting in focal thickening of the basement membrane. It is seen in 25 percent of diabetics at autopsy, most frequently in the juvenile type [16].

DIFFUSE GLOMERULOSCLEROSIS. Diffuse glomerulosclerosis involves overall thickening of the basement membrane of the glomerular capillaries, along with increased deposits of matrix in the mesangial portion. This condition is the most common form of nephropathy; and leads to proteinuria, which is initially intermittent, then persistent. Eventually the sclerosis may involve the entire glomerular bed and cause renal failure [16].

EXUDATIVE LESIONS. Exudative lesions in the kidney take two forms. Glassy, brightly eosinophilic, crescentic deposits that hang into the uriniferous space are called "capsular drops." Similar deposits are called "fibrin caps" when they occur on the outer surface of the glomerular capillaries. The capsular drops are diagnostic of diabetes.

OTHER LESIONS. Other common renal lesions affect the vascular supply, the renal pelvis, and medulla. Atherosclerosis and arteriolosclerosis of the renal artery or arterioles are common and may be related to hypertension. The pyelonephritis is usually a bacterial ascending infection of the kidneys, which occurs more frequently in diabetics. *Necrotizing renal papillitis* or renal medullary necrosis involves unilateral or bilateral necrosis of the renal pyramids, which may result in sloughing of necrotic papillae in urine.

Pathology of the Eye

RETINOPATHY. Diabetic retinopathy, the inclusive term for a variety of retinal changes related to diabetes, is the second leading cause of blindness in the United States. This condition is rarely found before the growth-spurt years and develops slowly, corresponding to the duration of the disease. Retinopathy follows alterations in blood flow through the retina and has various manifestations: thickening of retinal capillaries, microangiopathies, and microaneurysms, which

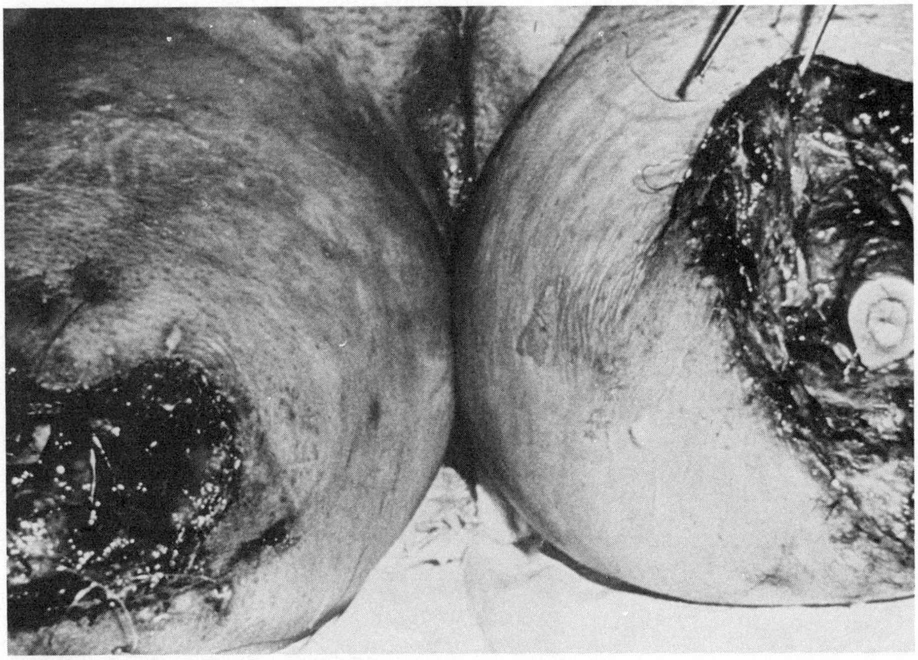

FIGURE 33-6. Necrosis and gangrene of stumps. (Courtesy of Dr. Walter C. Grundy, pathologist.)

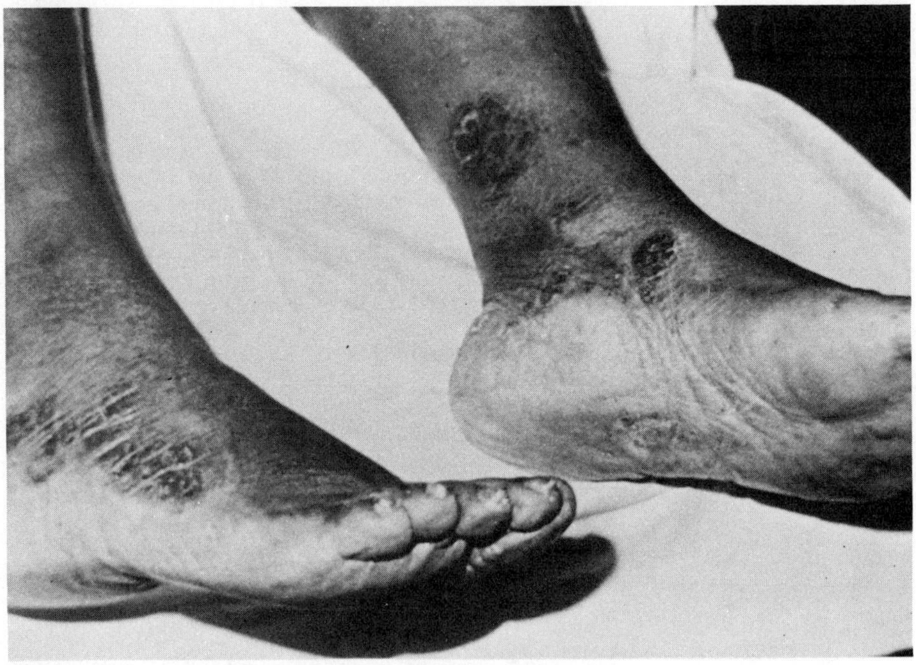

FIGURE 33-7. Atherosclerosis and stasis of lower legs. (Courtesy of Dr. Walter G. Grundy, pathologist.)

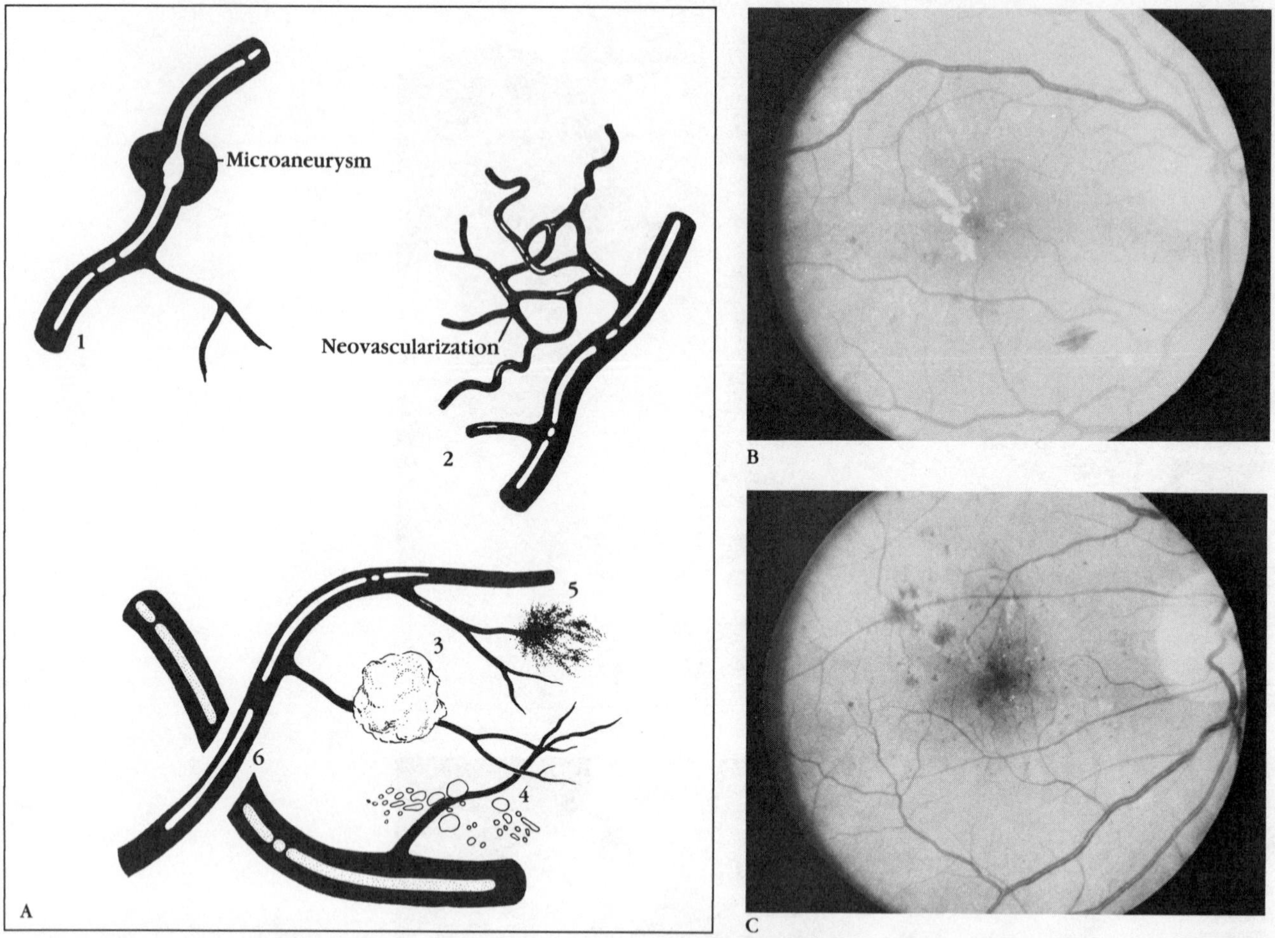

FIGURE 33-8. Characteristic diabetic changes in the retina. A. Blood vessels of the fundus shown with (1) microaneurysms, (2) new vessel formation (neovascularization), (3) soft exudates, (4) hard exudates, (5) hemorrhages, and (6) arteriovenous nicking. B. Diabetic retinopathy with hard exudates. C. Deep retinal hemorrhage. (From R. Judge, G. Zuidema, and F. Fitzgerald [eds.], *Clinical Diagnosis* [4th ed.]. Boston: Little, Brown, 1982.)

are discrete saccular dilatations or outpouchings of vessels (Fig. 33-8). The microaneurysms are asymptomatic; they are seen as discrete, dark-red circular spots near retinal vessels and are diagnostic of diabetes mellitus.

Hemorrhages are usually seen in the macular area between the superior and inferior temporal vessels and resemble red blotches. If located in the area of the fovea they can give rise to destruction of central vision. Exudates occur due to abnormal porosity of the retinal vessels and seepage of fluid into the retina. Soft exudates, called "cotton wool spots," are large, fluffy, and gray-white, and may resolve in several weeks. More commonly seen, hard exudates are yellow in color with discrete sharp edges that may coalesce, take longer to develop, and produce retinal degeneration. Venous changes include enlarged, irregular veins, sometimes resembling a string of sausages.

LESIONS OF THE VITREOUS. Lesions of the vitreous are a most serious complication and include neovascularization or formation of new vessels and fibrous tissue in the fundus. In time, atrophy of new vessels and contraction of fibrous tissue affect central and peripheral vision. Changes between fibrovascular tissue and the vitreous may lead to hemorrhage and retinal detachment.

CATARACTS. Accumulation of sorbital (polyhydroxy alcohol formed from glucose) causes cataracts by accumulating in the lens. Opacities of the lens are common in diabetics, are usually of gradual onset, and are similar to senile cataracts. Transitory lens changes due to dehydration are also seen in diabetics.

Nervous System Pathology

Neurons are vulnerable to the ketoacidosis of uncontrolled diabetes and the hypoglycemia of insulin reactions. Neuropathy may involve the peripheral nerves, brain, spinal cord, cranial nerves, or the autonomic nervous system, but the mechanism of damage is not entirely understood. Two types of neuropathy are seen in the diabetic — polyneuropathy and mononeuropathy.

Polyneuropathy, characterized by myelin degeneration and eventual irreversible injury to axons, is caused by an accumulation of abnormal metabolites and by depletion of substances necessary for nerve cell conduction. The associated sensory loss and motor weakness usually occur first and most severely in the feet.

Mononeuropathy is probably related to ischemia and infarction of the vessels that supply the nerves. Manifestations of nervous system involvement include pain, paresthesia, decreased proprioceptive sensations, motor impairment, and muscle weakness and atrophy. Alterations in the autonomic nervous system may lead to nocturnal diarrhea, atony of the bladder, postural hypotension, and delayed gastric emptying. Disturbances in neural innervation of the pelvic organs lead to sexual impotence in men and orgasmic difficulties in women.

Because of peripheral arterial ischemic disease and neurotrophic changes, the diabetic foot is more susceptible to infection because of loss of sensation. A pathologic condition may not be noticed and may progress rapidly.

Charcot's joints, or neuropathic joint disease, develops because of the trauma and stress of joint motion. Relaxation of supporting structures of the joint leads to cartilage degeneration, recurrent fractures, and collapse of bones. Neuropathic joint disease usually involves the bones and joints of the feet.

Skin Changes

Dry skin is due to dehydration and is seen in poorly controlled diabetes. Poor skin turgor may be related to protein washing and dehydration.

NECROBIOSIS LIPOIDICA EPIDERMIS. This lesion is most frequently found on the shin and usually develops after diabetes has been present for years. In 15 percent of cases, it has been shown to precede clinical diabetes by 2 years. The skin lesion begins as a papule, which progresses to a soft, yellow, ulcerated plaque. Histologically the lesion consists of collagen, surrounded by an inflammatory infiltrate composed of lipid-laden macrophages [18].

DIABETIC DERMOPATHY (SHIN SPOTS). Dermopathy is believed to be due to iron-containing substances that come from small hemorrhages into the skin. These areas appear as hyperpigmented, scaly, atrophic patches and look as though the diabetic has been struck time and time again in the shins. There is no associated pain.

MONILIA INFECTIONS. Monilia infections occur in the diabetic, often in the groin and under the breasts. The high moisture, the glucose content of the skin, and chafing support the growth of *Candida albicans*, especially in the obese person.

LIPOHYPERTROPHY AND LIPOATROPHY. These are specific skin lesions that are caused by insulin injections. Fatty accumulation beneath the skin, similar to a lipoma, may form large bumps with repeated injection of insulin. These sites tend to become fibrous and insensitive to injections, but insulin is absorbed poorly from these areas. Chronic administration of insulin can also cause disappearance of adipose tissue at the site of injections. The use of single peak insulin, a chemically purer form of insulin, around the periphery of the lipoatrophic areas may stimulate some reaccumulation of fat. The atrophic areas can be prevented by rotating injection sites.

XANTHOMAS. Firm, yellowish-pink nodules are found under the epidermis of knees, elbows, periorbital areas, and buttocks as a result of the hyperlipemia of diabetes. Although these nodules are not limited to diabetes, they signify high serum triglyceride levels and disappear with return of triglycerides to normal.

Hepatic Fatty Changes

In long-standing diabetes, fatty changes develop and the size of the liver increases. Infiltration of fat causes it to appear yellowish, and glycogen vacuoles may be found in nuclei of the cells. These liver changes are related to elevated serum lipid levels.

Muscle Changes

Degenerative changes occur in striated muscle of long-standing, poorly controlled diabetes. The pathology is probably related to microangiopathy and neuronal degeneration.

Clinical Manifestations and Complications

Persons with diabetes generally have polydipsia, polyuria, polyphagia, weight loss, and weakness. Many also have infections, particularly *Staphylococcus aureus* and moniliasis.

The predominant pathophysiology of diabetes is due to (1) impaired utilization of glucose by cells; (2) increased mobilization, abnormal metabolism, and deposition of fats; and (3) depletion of protein in body tissues. The manifestations of the disorder occur from insulin deprivation, which results in *hyperglycemia* (blood glucose as high as 200–1000 mg/dl) due to the impaired uptake of glucose, especially into muscle and adipose tissue, and decreased synthesis of glucose by the liver. These two factors, along with an increased dietary intake of carbohydrate, result in an increased blood sugar level. With hyperglycemia, there is an increase in osmotic pressure of the plasma, a shift of fluid to the intravascular compartment, and cellular dehydration. When the blood glucose level reaches approximately 160 to 180 mg/ml, the renal tubules are unable to resorb all of the glucose filtered by the glomeruli and glycosuria occurs. When the blood glucose level reaches 300 to 400 mg/ml, a common occurrence in untreated diabetes, the person may lose as much as 100 gm of glucose into the urine each day. The renal excretion of glucose requires accompanying water and produces an osmotic diuresis, ***polyuria***. The excessive urination also increases loss of water, potassium, sodium, and chloride, resulting in extracellular fluid depletion and compensatory intracellular dehydration. As sodium and potassium are lost, there is electrolyte imbalance, weakness, fatigue, and malaise. Loss of water causes an increase in serum osmolality, which stimulates the thirst center in the hypothalmus and the body's response of *polydipsia*. Because of the loss of large quantities of glucose and semistarvation of the cells, there is a compensatory increase in hunger, *polyphagia*. With the decrease in insulin, an anabolic hormone, there is increased protein and fat catabolism resulting in the release of ketones, nitrogen, and potassium into the circulation. Weight loss, especially in IDDM, is common.

DIABETIC KETOACIDOSIS. The signs and symptoms of diabetic ketoacidosis are pronounced manifestations of uncontrolled diabetes. Polyuria, polydipsia, polyphagia, weakness, and anorexia (plus nausea, vomiting, and abdominal pain) occur in increasing severity. The gastrointestinal symptoms and surgical abdomen may mimic a surgical emergency.

The most important pathogenic element in the causation of ketoacidosis is a marked decrease in insulin production, which leads to hyperglycemia, glycosuria, and progressive metabolic acidosis. Without insulin, the body enters a catabolic state and there is a shift from carbohydrate to fat metabolism. Fats are broken down (lipolysis) for energy faster than they can be metabolized. The ketone acids (acetoacetic and β-hydroxybutyric) and acetone accumulate in the circulation and interstitial fluids. Both acetoacetic and β-hydroxybutyric acids are strong and dissociate to yield hydrogen ions, consequently causing a drop in pH. At a plasma pH of 7.2, the individual's respiratory center is stimulated to prevent further decline in pH, and breathing becomes deep and rapid (Kussmaul breathing). The acetone formed during ketosis is volatile and is blown off during expiration giving the breath a sweet or "fruity" odor. When acidosis depresses their action, ketones are not well metabolized so that acidosis and catabolism are enhanced.

When the lungs are no longer able to maintain the pH by blowing off carbon dioxide, plasma carbonic acid levels rise and acidosis progresses. Further decrease in pH, accompanied by hyperosmolality, dehydration, hypotension, and tissue breakdown contribute to depression of cerebral function and, eventually, lead to coma and death (Fig. 33-9).

HYPERGLYCEMIC HYPEROSMOLAR NONKETOTIC COMA (HHNK COMA). This variation in hyperglycemic diabetic coma has been recognized with increasing frequency. It is characterized by extreme hyperglycemia (800–2000 mg/dl), mild or undetectable ketonuria, and absence of acidosis. The syndrome is seen almost exclusively in the older age group and in individuals with mild diabetes that does not require insulin. The mechanism of HHNK is best understood by considering the principles of osmolality. Without insulin to lower blood glucose, the patient's blood becomes more concentrated, for glucose is a large molecule that cannot pass cell walls easily and draws large amounts of water. The profound hyperglycemia is largely responsible for the increased plasma osmolality that causes an osmotic diuresis. The intracellular fluid is drawn out to help equalize the increasing osmotic pressure of blood hypertonic with sugar. Water in the intracellular fluid moves from cells into the bloodstream, leaving cells dehydrated and shrunken.

Initially, the person's fluid intake can balance the fluid lost to glycosuria. Later, however, intake is not sufficient and dehydration ensues. Gradually, the person becomes more obtunded and unable to respond to thirst. Without treatment with insulin and fluids, the process becomes self-perpetuating [5].

There are similarities between HHNK and ketotic coma. In both there is a shortage of insulin and a defect in utilization of glucose, which result in hyperglycemia, osmotic diuresis, and dehydration. Elevations of urea nitrogen usually occur in both types, although the causes may be different. Metabolic acidosis occurs in both, but less frequently in the hyperosmolar disorder.

The major difference is that large quantities of ketone bodies are produced in ketotic coma but not in hyperosmolar coma. No insulin is secreted in ketotic coma, but some residual ability to secrete insulin remains in hyperosmolar coma. The small quantities of circulating insulin probably prevent the mobilization of fat from tissues and release of ketone bodies. The lesser elevation of plasma growth hormones and cortisol in hyperosmolar coma also account for decreased ketone bodies.

The signs and symptoms of HHNK are polyphagia, polydipsia, polyuria, glycosuria, dehydration, abdominal discomfort, hyperpyrexia, hyperventilation, CNS dysfunction, postural hypotension, and shock. The skin has decreased turgor, mucous membranes are dry, and the eyes are sunken and soft. Some degree of renal impairment is found in many affected persons.

An acute illness or surgery may trigger the onset of HHNK as well as stressful events, for example, diabetes, pancreatic disease, myocardial infarction, hemodialysis, severe myocardial infarction, renal dialysis, severe burns, or hyperalimentation. A number of drugs (corticosteroids, diuretics, diphenylhydantoin, and immunosuppressive agents) may also trigger the syndrome.

The laboratory results are similar to those of ketoacidosis except that the glucose levels are usually higher (often greater than 1000 mg/dl), and serum osmolalities are also more elevated (greater than 350 mOsm/kg H_2O). Bicarbonate concentrations and pH are often normal but may decrease as the syndrome progresses. There is usually no ketoacidosis in the classic cases, but lactic acidosis may result from hypovolemic shock. Plasma acetone is absent or slightly elevated; creatinine and BUN become elevated with renal impairment. Compared with ketoacidosis, there is less elevation of the plasma free fatty acids (FFA), growth hormone (GH), and cortisol. The prognosis in hyperosmo-

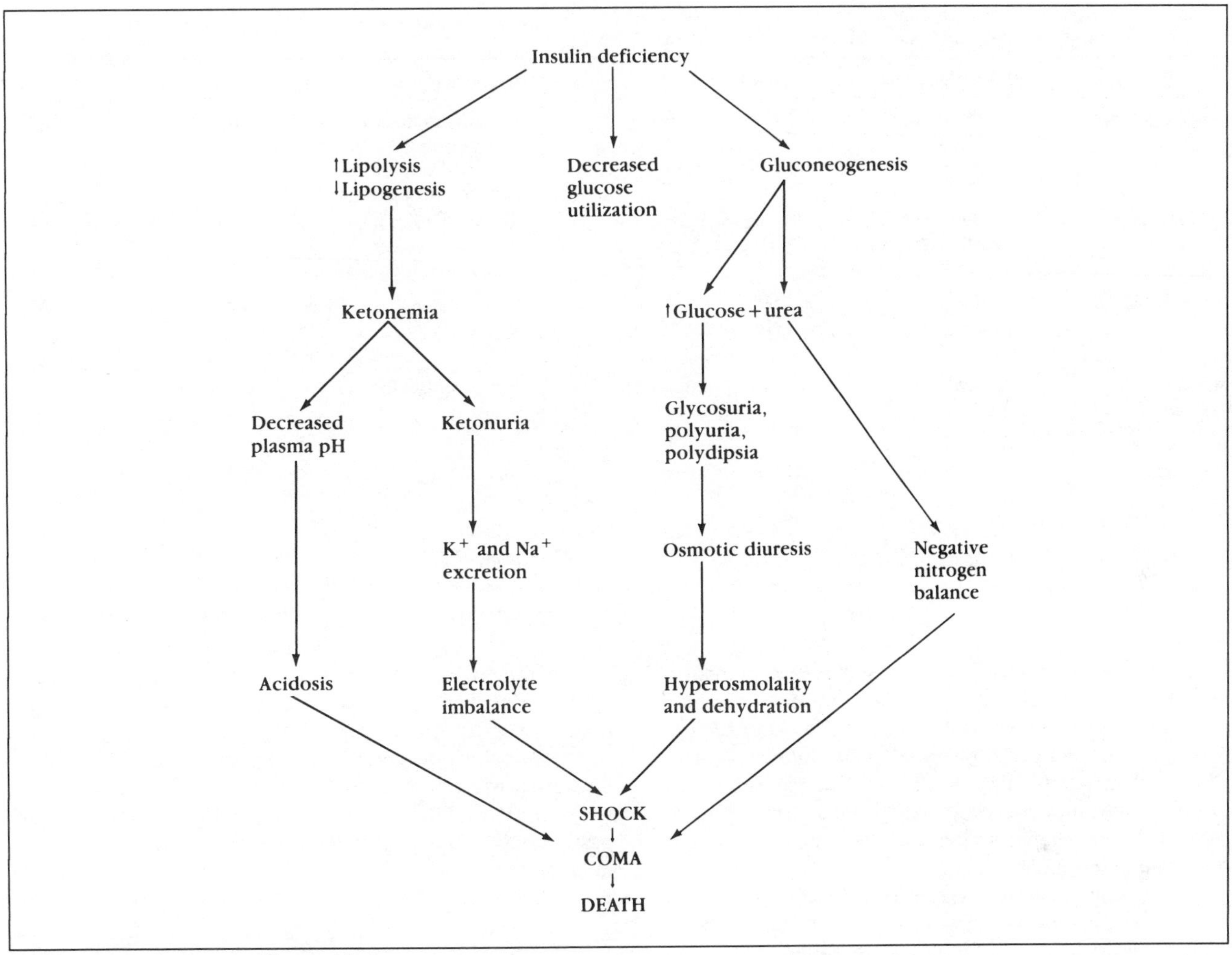

FIGURE 33-9. Pathogenesis of ketoacidosis.

lar coma is not as good as in diabetic ketoacidosis, and death is often attributed to the underlying or associated disease that precipitated the coma. Cases of HHNK coma associated with gram-negative infections were found to have a poor prognosis in a study by Arieff and Carroll [1].

LACTIC ACIDOSIS. When anaerobic glycolysis in the body produces more lactic acid (and some pyruvate) than can be used or converted to glucose, lactic acidosis occurs. It is frequently seen with sustained hypoxia or hypotension (e.g., shock, septicemia, hemorrhage, renal insufficiency, or starvation). Lactic acidosis may develop in diabetic patients in the following situations:

1. Those with complications from phenformin (a hepatic gluconeogenesis inhibitor treatment that has been withdrawn from the market by the FDA). Phenformin alone does not produce lactic acidosis but may precipitate the derangement when the drug accumulates in toxic amounts in patients with unrecognized renal failure.
2. As a spontaneous syndrome.
3. In association with diabetic ketoacidosis or hyperosmolar nonketotic coma.

Lactic acidosis should be suspected in any stuporous or comatose patient in metabolic acidosis. Diagnosis is confirmed by finding a plasma lactate level in excess of 7 mmole/liter with a low plasma bicarbonate, an absence of ketosis, and an anion gap produced by the excess lactate. This condition also bears a high mortality.

INSULIN REACTIONS. Hypoglycemia is a rather frequent metabolic complication of diabetes, although it is largely a complication of insulin therapy. Most diabetic individuals who take insulin experience a hypoglycemic reaction at some time. Reactions result from (1) an overdose of insulin, (2) inadequate food intake, (3) increased amounts of exercise, and (4) nutritional and fluid imbalances due to nausea and vomiting.

The symptoms of hypoglycemia reflect glucose deprivation to the brain. The following physiologic responses occur: (1) epinephrine release (sweating, shakiness, nervous-

TABLE 33-5. Comparison of hypoglycemia, diabetic ketoacidosis (DKA), lactic acidosis, and hyperglycemic hyperosmolar nonketotic coma (HHNK)

	Hypoglycemia	DKA	Lactic acidosis	HHNK
Physical response	Trembly, weak; difficulty talking	Nausea, vomiting; polyuria; polyphagia; polydipsia; headache	Similar to DKA (varied, depending on factors contributing to development)	Similar to DKA
Mental status	Anxious, confused; behavioral changes	Irritable; comatose	Acute changes in state of consciousness; stuporous; comatose	Similar to DKA; stuporous; focal motor seizures
Blood pressure	Normal	Low	Low	Low
Skin	Cold, moist, pale	Hot, flushed, dry	Pallid, dry	Very dry
Mucous membranes	Normal	Very dry	Dry	Extremely dry
Respiration	Normal	Hyperventilation	Hyperventilation	Normal
Urine sugar	0–2+	4+	0–2+	4+
Urine acetone	0	4+	0–2+	0–1+
Blood sugar	40 mg or less	300–800+ mg	80–200 mg	800–2000 mg
Serum ketones	0	4+	0–2+	0–2+
Blood CO_2	24–30	5–16 or less	5–16	18–24
Plasma lactic acid	Normal	Normal	High	Normal
Plasma pH	7.4	7.1–7.3	6.8–7.2	7.4

ness, headache, palpitations, increased blood pressure, heart rate, and respirations), (2) parasympathetic nervous system response (hunger, nausea, eructation), and (3) cerebral function decline (bizarre behavior, dullness of sensorium, lethargy, convulsions, coma). Clinical signs and symptoms may not correlate with blood glucose level. They may occur when a sudden drop occurs, even though the glucose level remains high.

The adrenergic response results in increased liver glycogenolysis to raise blood glucose concentration and stimulation of the reticular activating system to a state of wakefulness and alertness. If the liver glycogen supply is exhausted and glucose is not replaced, convulsions and permanent brain damage result.

Hypoglycemia can also occur independently of insulin. Other conditions—severe *liver disease*, which impairs glycogen uptake and release, *adrenocortical insufficiency*, in which the glucocorticoids (cortisol and cortisone) are unavailable to stimulate gluconeogenesis, and *islet-cell tumors*, which overproduce insulin—can cause low blood-glucose levels. Some medications, such as salicylates, propranolol, MAO inhibitors, and certain sulfonamides contribute to insulin hypoglycemia.

Somogyi described a syndrome of chronic hypoglycemia in persons receiving large amounts of insulin. Some patients have wide variations in blood sugar level that occur when insulin dosage is increased to control elevated blood sugar levels. The exogenous insulin produces hypoglycemia. These patients often have nocturnal hypoglycemia, followed by hormone-mediated hyperglycemia. Epinephrine, adrenal corticosteroids, and growth hormone are secreted as part of the body's mechanism in response to the excessive action of insulin. Epinephrine spurs glycogenolysis in the liver; the corticosteroids stimulate gluconeogenesis in the liver; and hyperglycemia occurs. The blood sugar is usually elevated when checked, even though the patient may experience periods of severe hypoglycemia. If this *rebound hypo-hyperglycemia* is suspected, the insulin dose is slowly reduced, divided into smaller doses, or administered at different times. Table 33-5 offers a comparison between hypoglycemia and different types of coma in diabetes.

Clinical Course

The course of diabetes may be insidious or abrupt. The ketosis-prone insulin-dependent type seen usually in younger persons sometimes undergoes transient remission after onset, but glucose intolerance is unstable or "brittle." The person is very sensitive to changes in exogenous insulin, dietary deviations, growth spurts, unusual physical activity, infection, and stress and is vulnerable to hypoglycemia and ketoacidosis.

Maturity-onset, nonketosis-prone diabetes may have few if any symptoms and follows an insidious course. Thus, the person with nonketosis-prone, non-insulin-dependent diabetes usually does not experience the acute metabolic syndrome, but suffers from other complications (see Table 33-3).

Laboratory Findings

The following laboratory tests are utilized to diagnose and follow the course of diabetes mellitus:

FASTING BLOOD SUGAR (FBS). Normal test values rule out significant diabetic problems but do not completely exclude diabetes, since only approximately 30 to 40 percent of

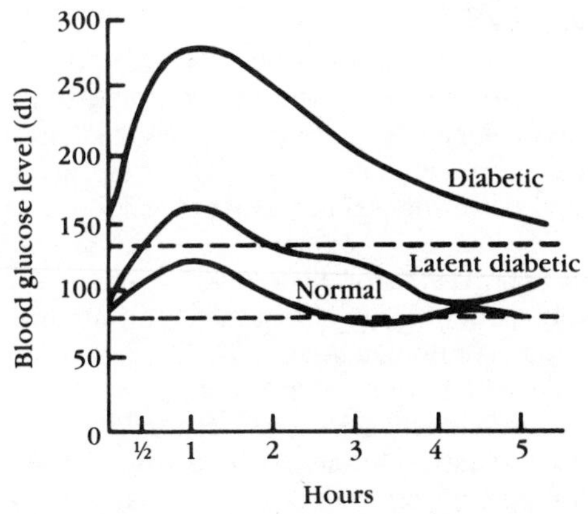

FIGURE 33-10. Glucose tolerance curves.

cases can be diagnosed with a FBS. The fasting blood sugar should be measured in the early morning at least 8 hours after any meal. Normal values are 65 to 100 mg/dl, utilizing a method specific for glucose, or 80 to 120 mg/dl, utilizing a method that measures all blood sugars and reducing substances. A fasting blood sugar above 120 mg/dl should be further investigated with a glucose tolerance test.

TWO-HOUR POSTPRANDIAL BLOOD SUGAR. Values may range from 200 to 2000 mg/dl depending on duration and severity of ketoacidosis. Glucose levels are rarely elevated 2 hours after carbohydrate intake in nondiabetics.

GLUCOSE TOLERANCE TEST (GTT). The GTT is based on the principle that a nondiabetic person can absorb a test amount of glucose from circulation at a faster rate than a diabetic. As demonstrated in Figure 33-10, when a normal fasting person ingests 1 gm glucose per kg of body weight, the blood glucose rises to peak levels of 150 to 160 mg/dl and falls to normal within 2 to 3 hours. The urine usually remains free of glucose.

In the diabetic, the blood sugar peak levels are much higher and the return to fasting levels is delayed 5 to 6 hours because of a lack of insulin response to the glucose.

URINE GLUCOSE. In a normal kidney, the glucose filtered through the glomerulus from the blood is resorbed in the proximal tubule. The renal tubules have a maximum absorptive capacity (renal threshold) of approximately 160 to 180 mg/dl of blood. At blood levels greater than this level, sugar is spilled into the urine and can be detected by screening methods. Glucose may appear in the urine at normal blood levels in persons without diabetes if the ability of the renal tubule to absorb glucose is impaired. Many diabetics, especially those with a history of atherosclerosis, may have a higher renal threshold, which prevents the appearance of glucose in the urine until the blood glucose level is quite high.

URINE KETONES. Ketonuria refers to the loss of ketone bodies, such as acetone, beta-hydroxybutyric acid, and acetoacetic acid, in the urine. This reflects the abnormal oxidation of fats and may be seen in diabetes, glycogen storage disease, starvation, and high-fat diets. Occasionally, ketones will be seen with fever or other conditions that increase metabolic requirements. Accumulation of the acidic ketones in the blood leads to a metabolic acidosis and an acetone smell to the breath.

VOLUME OF URINE IN A 24-HOUR PERIOD. A normal person secretes an average of 1200 to 1800 ml of urine in 24 hours, while the uncontrolled diabetic excretes 2000 ml or more urine in a 24-hour period.

PANCREATIC ISLET-CELL DISEASE

Syndromes associated with hyperfunction of the islets of Langerhans may be caused by (1) diffuse hyperplasia of the islets of Langerhans, (2) adenomas, and (3) malignant islet tumors.

Hyperinsulinism

When hyperplasia or neoplasia of the beta cells occurs, there may be enough insulin secreted to induce hypoglycemia. Most islet cell tumors are benign, but a small percentage are metastasizing malignant tumors. The classic clinical manifestations with demonstrated hypoglycemia that occurs with these pancreatic lesions were described by Whipple. This "triad of Whipple" includes (1) blood sugar levels below 50 mg/dl after an overnight fast; (2) central nervous symptoms of confusion, stupor, and decreased consciousness related to fasting or exercise; and (3) prompt relief of signs and symptoms by administration of glucose [16]. The triad is not specific for patients with hyperinsulinism due to islet-cell disease and may occur in other types of hypoglycemia.

The insulin-producing adenomas, or insulinomas, vary in size from 0.15 to 15.0 cm in diameter and may weigh over 1500 gm. They occur singly or scattered throughout the pancreas and usually appear as encapsulated firm nodules that are distributed throughout the pancreas and compress the surrounding tissue. Histologically, they do not differ from the normal islet cell [16].

Hyperinsulinism may also be caused by hyperplasia of the pancreatic islets, an alteration that occurs in infants born of diabetic mothers. The infant responds to the elevated blood sugar levels of the mother by producing increased numbers of cells and an increase in size of the cells. After delivery, the increased secretion causes serious episodes of hypoglycemia.

Zollinger-Ellison Syndrome (Gastrinoma, Ulcerogenic Tumor)

A syndrome described by Zollinger-Ellison (Z-E) is a clinical condition of peptic ulceration associated with a non-beta-cell islet tumor. The syndrome is characterized by large amounts of gastric secretion of HCl and pepsin. The stimulus for the hypersecretion is attributed to gastrin; hence the tumor is also known as a gastrinoma. Although most of the tumors occur in the pancreas, approximately one-tenth are found in the region of the duodenum or duodenal wall.

Various types of islet cells have been implicated as the causative agents. Gastrin-producing delta cells have been found in tumors and hyperplastic tissue, but it is still unclear whether the delta cell is the distinct agent responsible for the origin of gastrinomas [16].

Microscopically, the tumors resemble islet cells or cancerous tumors. Approximately 50 percent of the cases have metastases located in regional lymph nodes. There may be metastasis to bones, mediastinum, and skin. Death is usually attributed to the effects of the secretion of gastrin from the tumor and its metastases rather than to malignant spread. The tremendous gastric hypersecretion leads to intractable ulcers. The high acidity of the small intestine causes inactivation of pancreatic lipase, and this precipitates bile salts causing fluid and electrolyte imbalance. The large volume of acid gastric juices promotes diarrhea. As a result, many patients develop malsorption syndromes. Alteration in the intestinal mucosa from acidity affects absorption of nutrients. Calcitonin levels are also elevated in patients with Z-E syndrome. This elevation is attributed to stimulation of calcitonin release from the thyroid by gastrin.

Werner's Syndrome (Multiple Endocrine Neoplasia)

The disorder is familial with an autosomal dominant pattern of transmission. Multiple adenomas are found in the parathyroid glands, pituitary, and pancreas. Involving several glands, the disorder is often associated with peptic ulcer and gastric hypersecretion (Zollinger-Ellison syndrome). Both of these disorders have been found in some families, implying that the syndromes are variants of the same mutant gene. Some of the tumors are malignant and the term ***multiple endocrine neoplasia*** (MEN) has replaced the older term *multiple endocrine adenomatosis*.

There are two types of MEN syndromes:

1. Type I consists of tumors or hyperplasia of the parathyroid, pituitary, adrenal cortex, or pancreas and has associated peptic ulceration and gastric hypersecretion.
2. Type II consists of multiple pheochromocytomas (tumors of the adrenal medulla), carcinoma of the thyroid, parathyroid hyperplasia, or adenomas but no peptic ulceration or islet-cell tumors.

Clinical manifestations of MEN include: intractable peptic ulcers, hyperparathyroidism, hyperinsulinism, Cushing's syndrome, and hypertension related to pheochromocytoma [16].

PANCREATITIS

Acute Pancreatitis

Pancreatitis, or inflammation of the pancreas, is characterized by hemorrhage, necrosis, and suppuration of pancreatic parenchyma. The pathologic changes occur in varying degrees of severity and are caused by escape of active lytic pancreatic enzymes into the glandular parenchyma.

INCIDENCE AND ETIOLOGY. This condition accounts for approximately 1 out of every 500 medical and surgical hospital admissions. Acute pancreatitis occurs most frequently in middle life and more in women than in men. Two major causes, *alcoholism* and *gallstones*, are responsible for 50 to 90 percent of cases. In men, pancreatitis is often associated with high consumption of alcohol, but the condition develops only after years of alcohol abuse. Gallstones have been demonstrated in the feces of 40 to 60 percent of persons with acute pancreatitis [16]. Pancreatitis may also occur as a result of surgical trauma, particularly that involving the pancreas and adjoining organs. Other possible causes are hyperparathyroidism, certain drugs (opiates, thiazides, steroids, oral contraceptives, sulfonamides), vascular disease, infection, and nutritional and hereditary factors.

PATHOLOGY. The chemical and pathologic changes characteristic of pancreatitis reflect the destructive lytic effects of pancreatic enzymes (mainly trypsin). What triggers the activation of enzymes and the exact role of the pancreatic enzymes is still being investigated.

The four major histologic alterations in pancreatitis are (1) *necrosis of fat* (lipolysis), (2) *proteolytic destruction of pancreatic parenchyma* (proteolysis), (3) necrosis of blood vessels with ***hemorrhage***, and (4) ***inflammation***. The hallmark of pancreatic necrosis is enzymatic fat necrosis (lipolysis) of the endocrine and exocrine cells by lipase. Fatty acids are released in the process and they combine with calcium and form insoluble salts that precipitate. The deposits may be visible in the pancreas, in the peripancreatic fat, and throughout the abdominal cavity. They are surrounded by areas of hyperemia containing leukocytes.

Trypsin activates the major proteolytic enzymes involved in autodigestion (Fig. 33-11). Trypsin is normally secreted from the pancreas in the form of trypsinogen and is activated in the duodenum (see Chap. 36). The major initiating pathology is the premature activation of trypsinogen in the pancreas. Significant amounts of trypsin, chymotrypsin, and elastase have been detected in the diseased pancreas. The role of two other enzymes, kallikrein and phospholipase A, in the production of the inflammation is being investigated [17].

Elastase exists in high concentrations in granules of acinous cells and is present in pancreatic secretions as an inactive precursor. When activated by trypsin, it causes dissolution of elastic fibers of blood vessels and ducts. Hem-

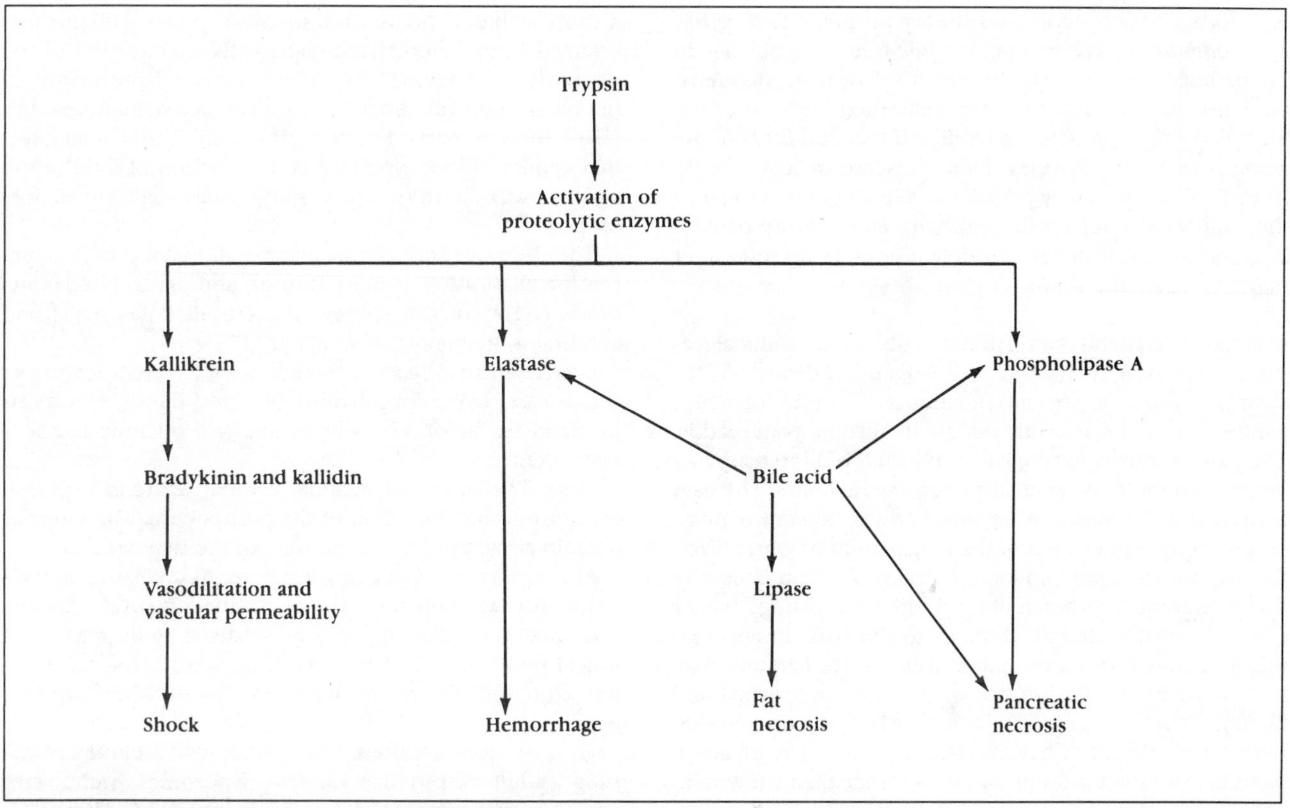

FIGURE 33-11. Pathogenesis of acute pancreatitis. (Adapted from L. H. Smith and S. O. Thier, *Pathophysiology: The Biologic Principles of Disease.* Philadelphia: Saunders, 1981.)

orrhage due to breakdown of elastic fibers of the vessels may be minor or extreme, varying from red blood cells and fibrin clots to large masses of blood over large areas. Kallikrein leads to the release of bradykinin and kallidin (a plasma kinin), which further increase vasodilatation and vascular permeability. Phospholipase A acts on phospholipids with a resultant release of compounds that have strong cytotoxic effects and damage cell membranes. There are inhibitors in the plasma or in the pancreas itself that can quickly inactivate the proteolytic enzymes. Whether deficiencies in the inhibitors are factors in pancreatic disease is unknown [16].

A leukocytic reaction appears around the areas of hemorrhage and necrosis. Secondary bacterial invasion may produce a suppurative necrosis or abscess. Milder lesions may be absorbed or they may calcify or become fibrotic when they are more severe. When fluid is walled off by fibrous tissue during the inflammatory process, a pancreatic cyst known as a pseudocyst is formed.

Several theories are offered to explain the mechanisms and sequence of events leading to activation of enzymes and to pancreatitis.

1. According to the *bile reflux*, or *common channel theory*, there is obstruction of the common channel formed by the common bile duct and the main pancreatic duct, causing a reflux of bile that results in activation of pancreatic enzymes. Many persons with pancreatitis have no common channel and the respective ducts join the duodenum separately. However, bile reflux is seen frequently with pancreatitis, and it is believed to play a role in the inflammatory process.

2. The *hypersecretion-obstruction* theory proposes that rupture of the ducts occurs from active pancreatic secretion in the presence of ductal obstruction of any cause and consequent tearing of cell membranes, permitting leaking of activated enzymes back into the gland.

3. *Alcohol-induced* changes are major factors in the pathogenesis of pancreatitis. Alcohol is a stimulator of pancreatic secretions and also causes duodenal edema of the ampulla of Vater, obstructing flow of secretions. Chronic alcohol ingestion increases the protein concentration of secretions, which leads to formation of protein plugs in the ducts and subsequent obstruction by the precipitates. Alcohol may decrease the tone of the sphincter of Oddi and cause duodenal reflux. Another factor predisposing alcoholics to pancreatitis may be the elevated serum triglycerides found in these patients following a meal [2]. Hyperlipidemia is known to be associated with pancreatitis.

4. Another widely supported theory proposes that *reflux of duodenal secretions* that are bile-free is significant in the pathogenesis of acute pancreatitis. Normally, duodenal contents do not enter the pancreatic duct because of the location of the sphincter of Oddi and mucosal folds of the ampulla of Vater. However, biliary disease or loss of tone from alcohol abuse may permit duodenal contents to enter the pancreatic duct via the sphincter and activate pancreatic enzymes. Gallstones or other lesions in the bile duct may also dilate the sphincter [16].

CLINICAL MANIFESTATIONS. There are no precise clinical features that distinguish pancreatitis from other disorders. *Abdominal pain* is present in almost all cases of acute pancreatitis and frequently occurs in chronic pancreatitis. The pain is usually severe and may reach full intensity in a matter of minutes or gradually over several hours. The pain is frequently localized in the epigastrium, becoming more severe to the right or left of the epigastrium or generalized throughout the upper abdomen. Pancreatic pain is usually steady, boring, and penetrating. Unlike the pain of biliary colic, it radiates straight through to the back in approximately one-half of cases. Individuals are restless and may seek relief by flexing the spine, by bending forward and flexing the knees against the chest, or by lying on one side with knees flexed. Characteristically, the pain of acute pancreatitis lasts for hours and days rather than a few minutes or a few hours.

The pain of pancreatitis is related to ductal swelling, extravasation of plasma and red cells, and release of digested proteins and lipids into surrounding tissue. The pancreatic capsule is stretched by the edema, exudate, red cells, and digestive products. These substances seep out of the gland into the mesentery, causing a peritonitis that stimulates the sensory nerves and causes intense pain in back and flanks when the gland is extensively damaged. During an acute attack, the pain will be generalized over the abdomen because of peritoneal irritation and release of kinins. Large doses of narcotics are avoided because they may induce spasm of the sphincter of Oddi, which aggravates the pancreatitis and further increases pain. As pain increases with the spread of intraperitoneal and retroperitoneal inflammation, a local or diffuse paralytic ileus may occur. Peripheral vascular collapse and shock may rapidly develop. The stretching of the gland may also cause nausea and vomiting.

The extensive injury to tissue, necrosis, and inflammation produce fever in approximately two-thirds of individuals with acute pancreatitis. The fever is due to the absorption of pyrogens into the circulation, but persistent high fever or temperature spikes imply pancreatic abscess or other septic complications [17].

COMPLICATIONS OF ACUTE PANCREATITIS. *Cardiovascular complications.* With massive exudation of plasma into the retroperitoneal space and, in cases of hemorrhage, there is a drop in blood pressure and rise in pulse. This form is referred to as hemorrhagic pancreatitis. Activation of the proteolytic enzyme kallikrein causes liberation of bradykinin and kallidin, which are vasoactive peptides. As a result, there is marked peripheral vasodilatation, which further reduces blood pressure. Accumulation of fluid in the small bowel, "a third space shift," causes additional loss of fluid.

The decrease in intravascular volume along with hypotension diminishes urinary output, and acute tubular necrosis (ATN) of the kidneys may result. Myocardial and cerebral ischemia may also occur [17].

Coagulation defects. Although not a frequent feature of the disease, hypercoagulability of blood due to elevations in platelets, factor VIII, fibrinogen, and possible factor V may occur.

Ileus. The large and small bowel may dilate in a general response to inflammation of the peritoneum. The gut may contain air and fluid, contributing to the hypovolemia.

Pulmonary-pleural complications. Acute pancreatitis is frequently accompanied by a left-sided pleural effusion. This pleural effusion apparently is caused by the retroperitoneal transudation of fluid with markedly elevated amylase into the pleural cavity from the inflamed swollen pancreas.

Other, more serious complications include *shock lung* (adult respiratory distress syndrome), pulmonary edema, and *segmental atelectasis* of lobes of the lung (see Unit IX) [17].

Hypocalcemia. Sharp falls in serum calcium may occur in acute pancreatitis, which are related to extensive lipolysis of peripancreatic mesenteric and peripancreatic fatty tissue, releasing free fatty acids that combine with calcium to form soaps. The parathyroid gland does not rapidly compensate for the abrupt lowering of calcium by the mechanism of soap formation. Neuromuscular irritability and tetany result from severe hypocalcemia.

Acidosis. Lactic acidosis may result from the central hypovolemia, or occasionally ketosis occurs when there is extensive destruction of the gland.

Hyperlipidemia. High serum lipids are often noted during attacks of pancreatitis, especially alcoholic pancreatitis. The plasma may have a creamy appearance.

Pseudocyst. Inflammatory pseudocysts are a frequent complication seen during the recovery period from an episode of severe acute pancreatitis. The cysts are nonepithelial-lined cavities, which contain plasma, blood, pancreatic products, and inflammatory exudate. They are solitary and measure 5 to 10 cm in diameter. They occur as a result of destruction of tissue and obstruction in the ductal system. Pancreatic juice may collect in them and leak into the peritoneal cavity. If large, pseudocysts may impinge on neighboring structures such as the portal vein, causing *acute portal hypertension*, and on the bile duct, causing *jaundice*. Occasionally, the cysts rupture and cause generalized peritonitis [17].

The formation of inflammatory pseudocysts may be associated with pancreatic ascites, which develop from a direct communication between the pseudocyst and the peritoneal cavity. The ascites fluid is high in amylase and resistant to therapy.

Pancreatic abscess. One of the most serious complications of acute pancreatitis, a pancreatic abscess is a collection of purulent and necrotic pancreatic tissue. It occurs if an episode of pancreatitis is severe enough to cause parenchymal necrosis, and if the pancreatic and retroperitoneal tissues become secondarily infected. There are usually several foci of infection rather than a discrete abscess that can be easily drained. A pancreatic abscess may develop in pancreatitis of various etiologies; however, most cases occur in association with alcohol. Incidence is about 3 to 4 percent of all cases of pancreatitis. Fistulization into an adjacent structure with massive bleeding may occur.

Jaundice. Mild jaundice is a common occurrence in acute pancreatitis. The swelling of the head of the pancreas impinges on the common bile duct that passes through it. If there is a compression of the bile duct by pseudocysts, or stones, the jaundice may be more severe.

DIAGNOSTIC TESTS. The cardinal findings of acute pancreatitis are *increases in serum amylase* and *lipase* activities with serum amylase values usually exceeding 250 Somogyi units. Normal serum amylase levels are 60 to 180 Somogyi units/dl; levels above 500 units strongly suggest pancreatitis. Serum lipase activity parallels that of serum amylase and abnormal levels persist for a longer time. Normal serum lipase values depend on the laboratory procedure used, but are generally below 1.5 units/ml. The increased activities occur shortly after onset of disease, almost always within the first 24 hours, and may remain high for weeks. *Leukocytosis* with increased polymorphonuclear leukocytes and a "shift to the left" is frequent. The white blood counts range from 9000 to 20,000 but occasionally rise to 50,000. *Decreases in serum calcium and magnesium* are seen, especially in patients with fat necrosis. Blood calcium levels may fall and remain down for 7 to 10 days. Hypocalcemia below 8 mg/dl is a poor prognostic sign.

Ultrasonic examination of the pancreas is used in severe pancreatitis. This technique may help to confirm a clinical impression, assess degree of resolution of inflammation, and reveal dilatation of common bile duct secondary to obstruction and presence of gallstones.

Computerized axial tomography (CAT scan) may be used if unexplained abdominal pain suggests either pancreatitis or pancreatic carcinoma. This technique may also be used in prolonged pancreatitis or recurrent pancreatitis to rule out a pseudocyst or interductal calculi.

Chronic Pancreatitis

Manifestations of chronic pancreatitis are similar to those of acute pancreatitis except for their chronicity and recurrence. If bouts recur, a state of pancreatic insufficiency may be reached. The pancreas has considerable functional reserve and may meet the body's needs through its secretory functions until 80 to 90 percent of acini and islets are nonfunctional.

In chronic pancreatitis, histologic changes persist even after the etiologic agent has been removed. In the United States, the most common cause of chronic pancreatitis is alcohol abuse. The pathologic changes are characterized by the deposition of protein plugs within pancreatic ductules. As the protein plugs become more diffuse, the ductal epithelium undergoes squamous metaplasia and ulceration. An inflammatory process is set up and fibrous tissue is deposited. Eventually, there is intraductal calcification and marked parenchymal destruction, with only a few islet cells and some acinar tissue remaining.

Exocrine pancreatic insufficiency is manifested by steatorrhea, azotorrhea, and weight loss. Microscopically, the stool exhibits fat globules and striated meat fibers that indicate impaired digestion of fats and proteins. Endocrine pancreatic insufficiency may lead to diabetes mellitus. Abdominal pain is a serious problem in chronic pancreatitis and may be responsible for severe weight loss, malnutrition, and general debility of the affected person.

The predominant complications of chronic pancreatitis that are associated with abdominal pain are pancreatic pseudocyst, stricture and obstruction of the common bile duct or pancreatic duct, and occasionally, a carcinoma of the pancreas.

CARCINOMA OF THE PANCREAS

Carcinoma of the pancreas occurs mainly in the exocrine portion of the gland in the ductal epithelium. Pancreatic cancers have a poor prognosis, causing about 6 percent of all neoplastic deaths in the United States. A significant increase in incidence has been attributed to smoking, consumption of alcoholic beverages, and consumption of fat. Increased risk has also been associated with disease of the gallbladder and bile duct (extrahepatic). Most of the tumors occur in individuals over 60 years of age; they rarely occur before the age of 40.

Clinical symptoms of cancer of the pancreas depend on the location of its site of origin or manifestations of metastasis. Tumors of the head of the pancreas tend to obstruct the bile duct and duodenum and early symptoms of obstructive jaundice occur; whereas carcinoma of the body and tail are less easily recognized clinically and become apparent only when adjacent structures are involved or when metastatic dissemination produces symptoms.

Most carcinomas of the pancreas grow in well-differentiated glandular patterns and are *adenocarcinomas.* About 10 percent assume an *adenosquamous* pattern or an uncommon pattern of extreme anaplasia with *giant-cell formation.* About 0.5 percent arise in cysts and are called *cystadenocarcinoma.* An *acinar cell carcinoma* is occasionally seen in children [16].

Carcinoma of the Head of the Pancreas

These tumors are fairly small lesions with poorly defined margins. They often impinge on the common bile duct and pancreatic duct causing atrophy of the pancreas. The tumors usually extend to the duodenum causing compression and crowding of the common bile duct and ampulla of Vater with distention of the gallbladder.

Carcinoma of the head of the pancreas is usually not a widely disseminated lesion because it produces biliary duct obstruction and jaundice at an early date. Individuals usually die of hepatobiliary dysfunction before the tumor has become widely disseminated.

Carcinoma of the Body and Tail of the Pancreas

These tumors are usually large and invade the entire tail and body of the pancreas; they may even be palpable in the thin individual. Carcinomas of the body and tail spread more extensively than those of the head. They crowd the vertebral column, spread into the retroperitoneal spaces, and may even invade the spleen, adrenals, colon, or stomach. Metastases spread via the splenic vein, which lies on the margins of the organ, to surrounding nodes and the liver. The liver may be enlarged 2 to 3 times its normal size [16].

Clinical Course of Carcinomas of the Pancreas

Carcinomas of the pancreas progress insidiously and are most likely present for months and perhaps years before symptoms appear. Major symptoms include weight loss, abdominal pain, back pain, anorexia, nausea, vomiting, generalized malaise, and weakness. Pain occurs in advanced stages of the disease. Jaundice is seen in about one-half of patients with carcinoma of the head of the pancreas [16].

Laboratory procedures are important in providing clues to the presence of these cancers in their early stages. Approximately 80 to 90 percent of those with cancer of the pancreas have elevated carcinoembryonic antigen (CEA). Levels of this antigen may be helpful in following the course of pancreatic malignancy with titers of greater than 20 mg/ml usually being associated with metastases. As with obstructive jaundice, there are increases of serum bilirubin levels, stools become clay-colored, and urine urobilinogen levels fall. Alkaline phosphatase levels are also elevated [16].

Radiologic procedures can assist in localization of tumors and differentiation of tumors from cysts. CAT scan of the pancreas is helpful in confirming presence of tumor.

Spontaneously appearing phlebothrombosis, also called migratory thrombophlebitis, is seen in carcinoma of the pancreas (Trousseau's sign). Trousseau diagnosed his own fatal disease when he developed migratory thrombophlebitis. The appearance and disappearance of thromboses are seen in other forms of cancer, but the two highest correlations are in pancreatic and pulmonary neoplasms. The thromboses are attributed to confinement to bed and surgical treatment, but thromboplastic factors have been identified in the serum, which lead to a hypercoagulable state due to thromboplastic properties of the necrotic products of the tumor [16].

CYSTIC FIBROSIS (MUCOVISCIDOSIS, FIBROCYSTIC DISEASE OF THE PANCREAS)

Cystic fibrosis, formerly referred to as "mucoviscidosis" or "fibrocystic disease of the pancreas" is a systemic disease of infancy or childhood in which there is an alteration in the secretory process of the exocrine (mucus-producing) glands, resulting in multiple complications in the pulmonary and gastrointestinal tract.

Incidence

Cystic fibrosis (CF) has been recognized clearly as a disease entity only since the late 1930s. However, it is now considered to be a common inherited condition and the most fatal genetic disease in whites. The incidence is between 1 in 1800 and 1 in 1850 in white populations.

Cystic fibrosis is transmitted by the autosomal recessive mode of inheritance. There is no difference in incidence by sex at birth. Chromosome number and structure are normal and carriers of the gene (heterozygotes) show no symptoms of cystic fibrosis. More children with this disease are surviving to adulthood, marrying, and reproducing so that genetic risks are now being considered. Affected persons transmit the gene to all of their offspring, but the children cannot develop the disease (homozygote) unless both parents are carriers.

Pathogenesis

Although the exact cause of cystic fibrosis remains unknown, there is evidence that alteration in function of the exocrine glands results in the elaboration of very viscid mucus. Figure 33-12 illustrates the pathogenesis of cystic fibrosis. A great deal of research is ongoing to determine the biochemical alteration; however, the basic problem is thought to occur at the cellular level, reflecting defects in a protein, a macroglobulin, and an isoenzyme, orginine esterase, which affects epithelial tissue.

The organs most frequently involved are the lungs, sweat glands, pancreas, liver, intestine, reproductive tract, and tear glands. A summary of the pathologic changes occurring in the various organs follows.

GASTROINTESTINAL TRACT. The extent of changes is related to whether secretions are carried to the gastrointestinal tract from cells with narrow necks such as the goblet cells, or from wide-mouthed ducts such as glands in the duodenum, or from narrow ducts such as those in the pancreas, liver, and salivary glands. The thick tenacious secretions tend to cause more problems in longer, narrow ducts with resultant changes in tissues and alterations of function. The

FIGURE 33-12. Pathogenesis of cystic fibrosis.

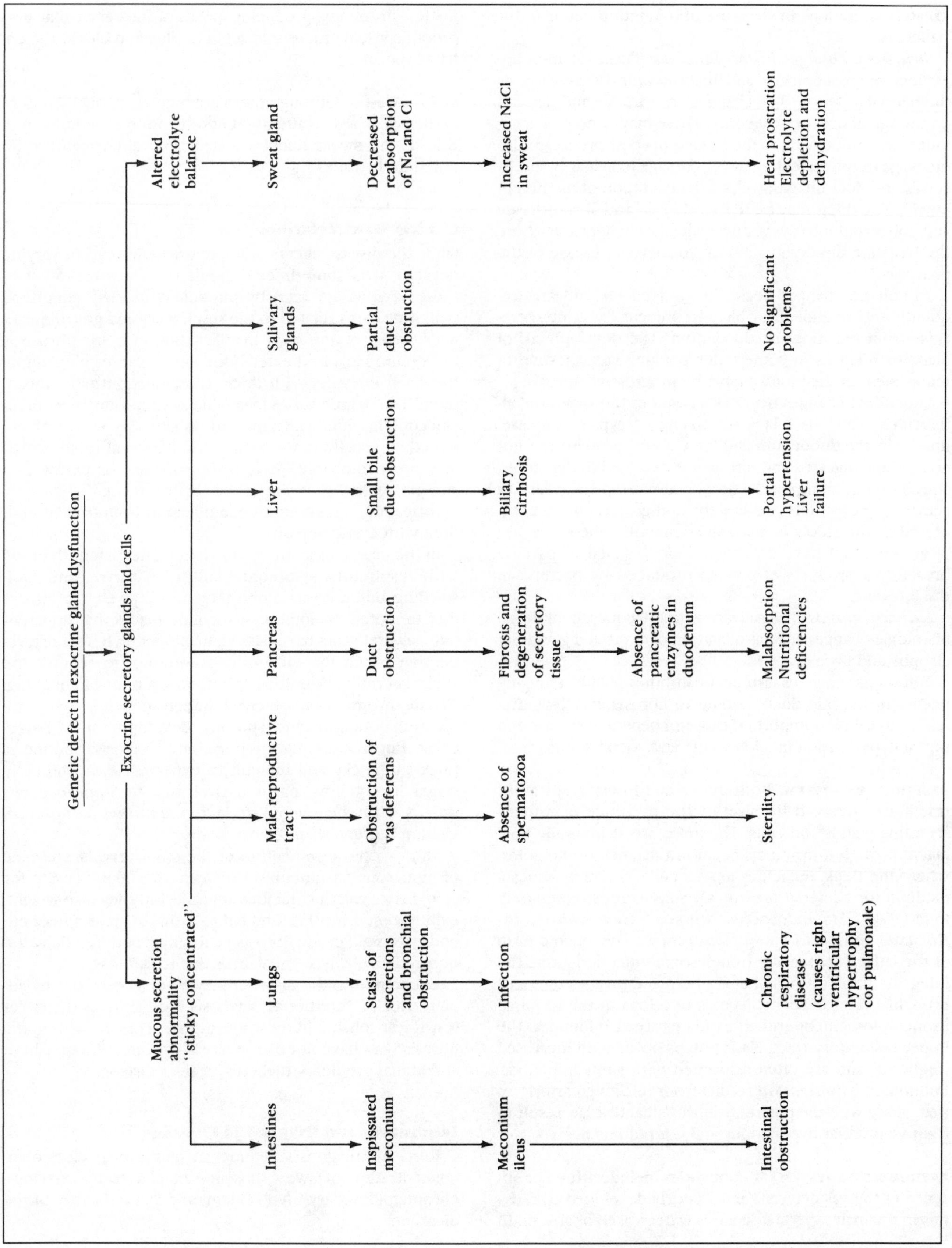

Genetic defect in exocrine gland dysfunction
Exocrine secretory glands and cells
Mucous secretion abnormality "sticky concentrated"
Altered electrolyte balance
Intestines
Inspissated meconium
Meconium ileus
Intestinal obstruction
Lungs
Stasis of secretions and bronchial obstruction
Infection
Chronic respiratory disease (causes right ventricular hypertrophy cor pulmonale)
Male reproductive tract
Obstruction of vas deferens
Absence of spermatozoa
Sterility
Pancreas
Duct obstruction
Fibrosis and degeneration of secretory tissue
Absence of pancreatic enzymes in duodenum
Malabsorption Nutritional deficiencies
Liver
Small bile duct obstruction
Biliary cirrhosis
Portal hypertension Liver failure
Salivary glands
Partial duct obstruction
No significant problems
Sweat gland
Decreased reabsorption of Na and Cl
Increased NaCl in sweat
Heat prostration Electrolyte depletion and dehydration

greatest alterations in structure and function occur in the pancreas.

Structural changes in the pancreas. These changes are evident microscopically and macroscopically as early as the neonatal period. The changes are variable and depend on the age of onset and severity. These may consist of accumulation of mucus or, as the disease process progresses, to blockage of the collecting ducts, damage to acinar tissue, fibrosis and duct dilatations, and degeneration of the parenchyma. The ducts may be replaced by fat and fibrous tissue and converted into cysts. These changes in appearance are the basis for the designation as "fibrocystic disease of the pancreas."

Pathologic changes begin during fetal life and are frequently severe enough by birth to prevent exocrine secretions from reaching the duodenum. The development of diabetes mellitus in some older persons is suggestive of impairment of the blood supply by progressive fibrosis.

Functional changes occur as a result of the structural alterations. There is a lack of enzymes (trypsin, amylase, lipase) in the duodenum and, as a result, proteins are not completely digested and nitrogen is excreted in the stools; starch is not completely broken down and appears as starch granules; fats are largely undigested and are excreted in the stools in excessive amounts. The stools are large, oily, and have a pungent odor caused in part by breakdown products of protein produced by bacteria in the intestine.

Salivary glands. The salivary glands frequently undergo histologic changes such as dilatation of ducts and glandular atrophy and fibrosis.

Pathologic changes also occur in other glands. Plugging occurs in the bile ducts leading to fibrosis and liver dysfunction. CF is an important cause of hepatic cirrhosis and portal hypertension in adolescents and young adults.

RESPIRATORY SYSTEM. Both upper and lower respiratory tracts are involved because of the presence of mucus-secreting glands and cells. The lungs are structurally normal at birth, but problems begin in the small bronchioles, where the thick, tenacious mucus collects and provides a medium for bacterial growth. Organisms most commonly found are *Staphylococcus aureus*, *Hemophilus influenzae*, and *Pseudomonas aeruginosa*. The mucoid form of the latter is especially troublesome. Infection alters the integrity of the bronchial epithelium and invades the peribronchial tissues. Bronchiectasis develops in the terminal bronchioles. Mucopurulent exudates are also found in the upper respiratory tract. Nasal polyps occur with increased frequency and are often associated with sinus infections. Pulmonary hypertension results from thickened arterioles that, along with the obstructive bronchial disease, result in right ventricular hypertrophy and cor pulmonale.

REPRODUCTIVE SYSTEM. Abnormalities include atresia or absence of the vas deferens and a poorly developed epididymis in the male. Spermatogenesis is decreased or absent. In the female, mucus-producing glands of the cervix may also produce viscid mucus that acts as a plug and blocks the entry of sperm.

SWEAT GLANDS. Although there is a high electrolyte content of the sweat and an alteration in resorption of sodium chloride in the sweat ducts, no structural abnormalities are noted in the duct.

Clinical Manifestations

Since the disease affects multiple organ systems in varying degrees, it is sometimes difficult to recognize. Most of these persons are seen by physicians in early childhood with symptoms related to the respiratory and gastrointestinal systems. A very early manifestation of cystic fibrosis is meconium ileus in the newborn, which causes blocking of the small intestine with thick, tenacious, puttylike meconium. The degree varies from a delay in passing meconium (meconium-plug syndrome) to an obvious intestinal obstruction, usually in the area of the ileocecal valve, which may be accompanied by atresia, volvulus, or perforation and peritonitis. Prolapse of the rectum related to chronic constipation is a common complication in untreated children with cystic fibrosis.

In the classic case, the child is seen after 1 month of life with respiratory symptoms, failure to thrive, and foul-smelling, bulky, greasy stools. Any one or all characteristics may be noted. In some cases, symptoms are not apparent until several years have passed. Infants often have a dry, repetitive cough that occurs in an attempt to remove the sticky secretion. Vomiting may follow a bout of coughing. Classic progression of chest infection occurs with increased coughing and sputum, development of barrel chest, finger clubbing, dyspnea, and cyanosis. Sputum is thick and sticky and difficult to expectorate. In the early stages it is yellow, particularly if due to *Staphlococcus aureus*. With the mucoid strain *Pseudomonas aeruginosa*, sputum is greenish and more slimy.

Microscopic examination of the stool reveals presence of numerous fat globules. Children often compensate for stool losses with a voracious appetite, but they lose weight, exhibit tissue wasting, and fail to grow. In areas where humidity is high, cystic fibrosis babies may undergo dehydration and electrolyte imbalances due to salt loss.

Uncommonly, the disorder may be diagnosed during adolescence or adulthood. Diagnosis is difficult, as the sweat test is less reliable in these age groups. Persons with cystic fibrosis who have not had severe chest infection may have abdominal problems, diabetes, or liver disease.

Laboratory and Diagnostic Findings

Criteria for diagnosis include an increase in electrolyte concentration of sweat, absence of pancreatic enzymes, chronic pulmonary involvement, and family history of the disorder.

The *sweat test* is the simplest and most reliable confirmatory method for the diagnosis of CF. Up to 20 years a level of more than 60 mEq/L of sweat chloride is diagnostic of cystic fibrosis. Values between 50 and 60 mEq/L are highly suggestive. Reliable sweat tests are difficult to obtain in the first 3 to 4 weeks of life, as the sweat glands are not yet well developed functionally.

X ray reveals changes in respiratory and gastrointestinal systems. Chest x rays reveal slightly increased diameter of upper chest with overaerated lungs, widespread consolidation, and fibrotic changes. There may be areas of lobar or segmental collapse.

Changes in x-ray patterns of the small intestine are noted in cystic fibrosis as in other malsorptive diseases. Fibrosis abnormalities are also found in barium studies of the duodenum.

Pancreatic deficiency is noted on examination of duodenal contents for pancreatic enzyme activity. Chemical estimation of fat in feces reveals marked steatorrhea. Normal stools should not contain more than 4 gm of fat per day. Stools of children with cystic fibrosis often contain 15 to 30 gm/day.

REFERENCES

1. Arieff, A. I., and Carrol, H. J. Non-ketotic hyperosmolar coma with hyperglycemia: Clinical features, pathophysiology, renal function, acid base balance, plasma-cerebrospinal fluid equilibria and the effect of therapy in 37 cases. *Medicine* (Baltimore) 51:73, 1972.
2. Carmeron, J., et al. A pathogenesis for alcoholic pancreatitis. *Surgery* 77:754, 1975.
3. Cerasi, E., and Luft, R. The plasma insulin response to glucose infusion in healthy subjects and in diabetes mellitus. *Acta Endocrinol.* (Copenh.) 55:278, 1967.
4. Craighead, J. E. The role of viruses and the pathogenesis of pancreatic disease and diabetes and diabetes mellitus. *Prog. Med. Virol.* 19:161, 1975.
5. Danowski, T. S. Hyperosmolar and Other Non-Ketotic Comas in Diabetes. In L. J. Kryston and R. A. Shaw (eds.), *Endocrinology and Diabetes*. New York: Grune & Stratton, 1975.
6. Granda, O. P., and Soeldner, S. S. Genetic, acquired and related factors in the etiology of diabetes mellitus. *Arch. Intern. Med.* 137:461, 1977.
7. Guyton, A. C. *Textbook of Medical Physiology* (6th ed.). Philadelphia: Saunders, 1981.
8. MacMillan, D. R., et al. Seasonal variation in the onset of diabetes in children. *Pediatrics* 59:113, 1977.
9. Meissner, W. A., and Legg, M. A. The Pathology of Diabetes. In A. Marble, et al. (eds.), *Joslin's Diabetes Mellitus* (11th ed.). Philadelphia: Lea & Febiger, 1973.
10. Menser, M. A., et al. Rubella infection and diabetes mellitus. *Lancet* 1:57, 1978.
11. Olefsky, J. M. Insulin resistance and insulin action. *Diabetes* 30:148, 1981.
12. Perley, M. J., and Kipnis, D. M. Plasma insulin responses to oral and intravenous glucose: Studies in normal and diabetic subjects. *J. Clin. Invest.* 46:1954, 1967.
13. Pyke, D. A. Genetics of diabetes. *Clin. Endocrinol. Metab.* 6:1, 1977.
14. Reaven, C. N. Non-ketotic diabetes mellitus: Insulin deficiency or insulin resistance. *Am. J. Med.* 60:80, 1976.
15. Rizza, R., and Gerich, J. E. Somostatin and diabetes. *Med. Clin. North Am.* 62:4, 1978.
16. Robbins, S. K., and Cotran, R. S. *Pathologic Basis of Disease* (2nd ed.). Philadelphia: Saunders, 1979.
17. Smith, L. H., and Thier, S. O. *Pathophysiology: The Biologic Principles of Disease.* Philadelphia: Saunders, 1981.
18. Williams, R. H. *Textbook of Endocrinology* (6th ed.). Philadelphia: Saunders, 1981.

BIBLIOGRAPHY

Anderson, C. N., and Goodchild, M. C. *Cystic Fibrosis: Manual of Diagnosis and Management*. Oxford: Blackwell, 1976.

Anderson, R. A., et al. Effect of exercise (running) on serum glucose, insulin, glucagon and chromium excretion. *Diabetes* 31: 212, 1982.

Anderson, W. A. D., and Scotti, T. M. *Synopsis of Pathology* (10th ed.). St. Louis: Mosby, 1980.

Arieff, A. I., and Carrol, H. J. Non-ketotic hyperosmolar coma with hyperglycemia: Clinical features, pathophysiology, renal function, acid base balance, plasma-cerebrospinal fluid equilibria and the effect of therapy in 37 cases. *Medicine* (Baltimore), 51:73, 1972.

Banks, P. A. *Pancreatitis*. New York: Plenum, 1979.

Biesbroeck, J. J., et al. Abnormal composition of high density lipoproteins in non-insulin-dependent diabetes. *Diabetes* 31: 126, 1982.

Blackard, W. G., and Nelson, N. C. Portal and peripheral vein immunoreactive insulin concentrations before and after glucose infusion. *Diabetes* 19:302, 1970.

Bondy, P. K., and Rosenberg, L. E. *Metabolic Control and Disease.* Philadelphia: Saunders, 1980.

Brandborg, L. L. The Pancreas. In M. H. Sleisenger and J. S. Fordtran (eds.), *Gastrointestinal Disease* (2nd ed.). Philadelphia: Saunders, 1978.

Brown, J., et al. Islet cells grow after transplantation of fetal pancreas and control of diabetes. *Diabetes* 30:9, 1981.

Cameron, J., et al. A pathogenesis for alcoholic pancreatitis. *Surg.* 77 77:754, 1975.

Cerasi, E., and Luft, R. The plasma insulin response to glucose infusion in healthy subjects and in diabetes mellitus. *Acta Endocrinol.* 55:278, 1967.

Craighead, J. E. The role of viruses and the pathogenesis of pancreatic disease and diabetes mellitus. *Prog. Med. Virol.* 19:161, 1975.

Danowski, T. S. Hyperosmolar and Other Non-Ketotic Comas in Diabetes. In L. J. Kryston and R. A. Shaw (eds.), *Endocrinology and Diabetes*. New York: Grune & Stratton, 1975.

Fajons, S. S. (ed.). *Diabetes Mellitus.* DHEW Publ. No. (NIH) 76-854. Washington, D.C.: Department of Health, Education and Welfare, Public Health Service National Institutes of Welfare, 1976.

Felig, P. Pathophysiology of diabetes mellitus. *Med. Clin. North Am.* 55:824, 1971.

Gambill, E. E. *Pancreatitis*. St. Louis: Mosby, 1973.

Gerich, J. E., et al. Prevention of human diabetic ketoacidosis by somatostatin: Evidence for an essential role of glucagon. *N. Engl. J. Med.* 292:985, 1975.

Ginsberg-Fellner, F., et al. HLA antigens, cytoplasmic islet cell antibodies and carbohydrate tolerance in families of children with insulin-dependent diabetes mellitus. *Diabetes* 31:292, 1982.

Goldstein, S., and Podolsky, S. The genetics of diabetes mellitus. *Med. Clin. North Am.* 62:4, 1978.

Guyton, A. C. *Textbook of Medical Physiology* (6th ed.). Philadelphia: Saunders, 1981.

Hermon-Taylor, J. An etiological and therapeutic review of acute pancreatitis. *Br. J. Hosp. Med.* 18:546, 1977.

Howat, H. T., and Sarles, H. S. *The Exocrine Pancreas.* Philadelphia: Saunders, 1979.

Irving, W. J., et al. Clinical and pathogenic significance of pancreatic cell antibodies in diabetes treated and oral hypoglycemic agents. *Lancet* 1:1025, 1977.

Isselbacher, K. J., et al. (eds.). *Harrison's Principles of Internal Medicine* (9th ed.). New York: McGraw-Hill, 1980.

Larson, L. I. Endocrine pancreatic tumors. *Human Pathol.* 9:401, 1978.

MacMillan, D. R., et al. Seasonal variation in the onset of diabetes in children. *Pediatrics* 59:113, 1977.

Malone, J. I., et al. Diabetic vascular changes in children. *Diabetes* 26:7, 1977.

Maugh, T. H. Diabetes: Epidemiology suggests a viral connection. *Science* 188:347, 1975.

Meissner, W. A., and Legg, M. A. The Pathology of Diabetes. In A. Marble, et al. (eds.), *Joslin's Diabetes Mellitus* (11th ed.). Philadelphia: Lea & Febiger, 1973.

Menser, M. S., et al. Rubella infection and diabetes mellitus. *Lancet* 1:57, 1978.

Munger, B. L. The Biology of Secretory Tumors of the Pancreatic Islets. In D. F. Steomer and N. Ereinkel (eds.), *Handbook of Physiology and Endocrinology*. Washington, D.C.: American Physiological Society, 1962.

Olefsky, J. M. Insulin resistance and insulin action. *Diabetes* 30: 148, 1981.

Perley, M. J., and Kipnis, D. M. Plasma insulin responses to oral and intravenous glucose: Studies in normal and diabetic subjects. *J. Clin. Invest.* 46:1954, 1967.

Pyke, D. A. Genetics of diabetes. *Clin. Endocrinol. Metab.* 6:1, 1977.

Raskin, P., and Unger, R. H. Glucagon and diabetes. *Med. Clin. North Am.* 62:4, 1978.

Reaven, C. N. Non-ketotic diabetes mellitus: Insulin deficiency or insulin resistance. *Am. J. Med.* 60:80, 1976.

Rizza, R., and Gerich, J. E. Somostatin and diabetes. *Med. Clin. North Am.* 62:4, 1978.

Robbins, S. L., and Cotran, R. S. *Pathologic Basis of Disease* (2nd ed.). Philadelphia: Saunders, 1979.

Rubenstein, P., et al. Genetics and juvenile diabetes. *N. Engl. J. Med.* 197:1036, 1977.

Selkurt, E. E. (ed.). *Basic Physiology for the Health Sciences.* Boston: Little, Brown, 1975.

Smith, L. H., and Thier, S. O. *Pathophysiology: The Biologic Principles of Disease*. Philadelphia: Saunders, 1981.

Sodeman, W. A., Jr., and Sodeman, W. A. *Pathologic Physiology: Mechanisms of Disease*. Philadelphia: Saunders, 1974.

Sorles, H., and Sahel, J. Pathology of chronic calcifying pancreatitis. *Am. J. Gastroenterol.* 66:117, 1976.

Steiner, D. F. Insulin today. *Diabetes* 26:322, 1977.

Tattersall, R. B., and Fajans, S. S. A difference between the inheritance of classical juvenile-onset and maturity-onset diabetes of young people. *Diabetes* 24:44, 1975.

Unger, R. H. Diabetes and the alpha cell. *Diabetes* 25:136, 1976.

Volk, B. W., and Wellman, K. F. *The Diabetic Pancreas.* New York: Plenum, 1977.

Wagener, D. K., et al. The Pittsburgh study of insulin-dependent diabetes mellitus. *Diabetes* 31:136, 1982.

Witt, K. HHNK: Intercepting a "New Hazard." In P. S. Chaney (ed.), *Managing Diabetes Properly*. Morsham, Penn.: Intermed Communications, 1977.

Williams, R. H. *Textbook of Endocrinology* (5th ed.). Philadelphia: Saunder, 1974.

UNIT 12
DIGESTION, ABSORPTION, AND UTILIZATION OF FOOD

Barbara L. Bullock
GASTROINTESTINAL FUNCTION
HEPATIC FUNCTION

Ann Bavier
MOTILITY AND MOTOR DYSFUNCTION

Concepcion Castro
SECRETIONS AND HYPERSECRETIONS

Francis Monahan
ABSORPTION

Therese Shipps
NUTRITION AND METABOLISM

An understanding of the anatomic and functional activities of the entire gastrointestinal system is essential for the understanding of the pathologies of part or all of the system. The digestion, absorption, and utilization of food require the participation of all of the gastrointestinal organs, including the liver and pancreas. Alterations can occur at any point in the system and affect the entire system. This unit is presented systematically, but the reader must be informed that the entire system works together to accomplish its activities. Chapter 34 includes the normal activities of the gastrointestinal system including the oral tract, stomach, intestines, and other components. Chapter 36 includes the normal liver and the pancreatic exocrine functions. Chapter 35 details alterations in the gastrointestinal system, while Chapter 37 explains alterations in hepatobiliary function. Pancreatic alterations were considered in Chapter 33 (Unit 11). Included in Chapter 37 is a discussion of obesity as a disorder of nutritional balance.

The reader is encouraged to utilize the learning objectives as study guides for chapter content. Each objective can be considered as a study question and answered from the material presented in the chapter. The unit bibliography also gives some guidelines for further study.

CHAPTER 34
NORMAL FUNCTION OF THE GASTROINTESTINAL SYSTEM

LEARNING OBJECTIVES

1. Differentiate between *appetite, hunger,* and *satiety.*
2. Locate the hunger center and the appetite center in the brain.
3. Identify the oral structures that prepare food for later absorption.
4. Describe the function of salivary *ptyalin.*
5. Briefly define *functional syncytium* as applied to the gastrointestinal system.
6. Locate the gastroesophageal or lower esophageal sphincter and briefly describe its functional significance.
7. Clearly locate and describe the function of the gastric glands.
8. Define *chyme.*
9. Identify the four layers of the intestinal wall.
10. Describe the appearance and function of the microvilli.
11. Identify the blood supply, nerve supply, and lymphatic drainage of the gastrointestinal system.
12. Locate the subdivisions of the large intestine.
13. Relate the importance of oral secretions to the process of digestion.
14. Describe the process of swallowing.
15. Clearly delineate the purposes of gastric secretions in digestion.
16. Describe the relationship of nervous and hormonal mechanisms in the process of digestion.
17. Briefly outline the cephalic, gastric, and intestinal phases of gastric secretions.
18. Define and list examples of secretagogues.
19. Describe how the intestines function to inhibit gastric secretions.
20. Specifically describe where nutrients are absorbed in the small intestine.
21. Relate the mechanisms necessary for the absorption of carbohydrates, proteins, and fats.
22. Briefly list the form and mechanism for the absorption of nutrients, vitamins, and minerals.
23. Describe the process of defecation.
24. Briefly explain the role of the large intestine in regulating water balance.

Normal functioning of the human body is dependent on an intact digestive system. In the broadest sense, the gastrointestinal tract is a tubular structure called the alimentary canal, which extends from the pharynx to the anus. Throughout this tubular structure ingested food is processed, digested, and absorbed. The nutrients absorbed may be further processed by accessory organs, utilized for energy, or stored for later use, for energy.

In order for digestion to occur, the vital functions of motility, secretion, and absorption must proceed in a regulated fashion. Finally, by participating in the excretion of waste products, the gastrointestinal system helps to keep the host in a steady, balanced state. The steady state normally provides for a balanced body weight so that ingested nutrients are utilized and the weight of the adult body remains stabilized.

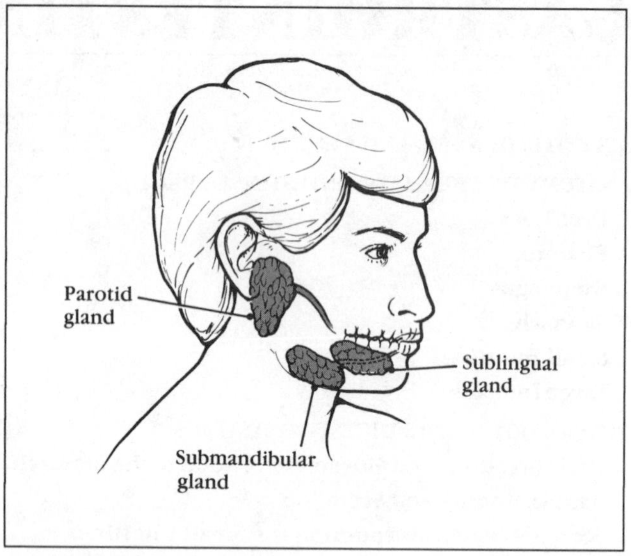

FIGURE 34-1. Salivary glands.

APPETITE, HUNGER, AND SATIETY

Learned patterns of behavior alter the *appetite*, creating a desire for food beyond the needs of the human body. *Hunger* refers to the desire for food that results from the manifest need of the human body for energy. Satisfaction of the feeling of hunger is called *satiety.*

The hunger center is found in the *hypothalamus*, as is the *satiety center,* but these have been shown to be in separate, distinct locations. The feeling of hunger is frequently generated by rhythmic contractions of the stomach, which may cause a painful sensation called hunger pangs. Stimulation from the hunger center is related to the nutritional status of the body. Especially important in this process is the concentration of glucose in the blood. A decreased concentration of blood glucose will intensify the hunger response. The serum fat levels and amino acids also affect satiety. As is discussed on p. 490, distention of the gastrointestinal tract suppresses the hunger center through inhibitory signals.

The *appetite center* is more subtly controlled by the cortical areas and is stimulated by the senses of sight, touch, and smell. Even thoughts of food can stimulate the appetite center. Alterations of appetite for specific foods are conditioned by culture, environment, and socioeconomic living conditions.

ANATOMY OF THE GASTROINTESTINAL TRACT

The distinct purpose of the gastrointestinal tract is carried out through a continuous structure that begins with the oral cavity and terminates with the anal sphincter.

Oral Cavity

The lips, tongue, cheeks, teeth, taste buds, and salivary glands are associated with the oral cavity and contribute to the process of preparing food for absorption later in the system. This preparation includes reduction of size of food particles to manageable sizes, stimulation of salivary glands to increase saliva secretion, and movement of food to the appropriate position for swallowing. Table 34-1 summarizes the oral structures and their participation in the process of preparing food for further digestion.

TABLE 34-1. Participation of the oral structures in process of digestion

Structure	Process
Teeth	Reduce food to sizes appropriate for swallowing; break down dense particles
Tongue	Places food in proper position for swallowing; mixes secretions to moisten food
Salivary glands	Moisten and lubricate foods placed in the mouth; add ptyalin enzyme for digestion of starches
Muscles of mastication, or chewing	Provide movement for the grinding of food to smaller particles; provide more surface area for the digestive enzymes to act

The submandibular, parotid, and sublingual salivary glands (Fig. 34-1) continuously secrete *saliva*, which contains large amounts of water and small amounts of sodium, chloride, bicarbonate, urea, and a few other solutes. Saliva also contains *ptyalin* (salivary amylase), an enzyme that functions to digest starches. The average amounts of salivary secretion range from 1000 to 1500 ml/day. Stimulation for this secretion is relayed to the medulla by the parasympathetic fibers of the facial, trigeminal, glossopharyngeal, and the vagus nerves. Efferent parasympathetic stimulation leads to increased secretion of saliva. Stimulation of the sympathetic system causes localized vasoconstriction and a decrease in salivary secretion.

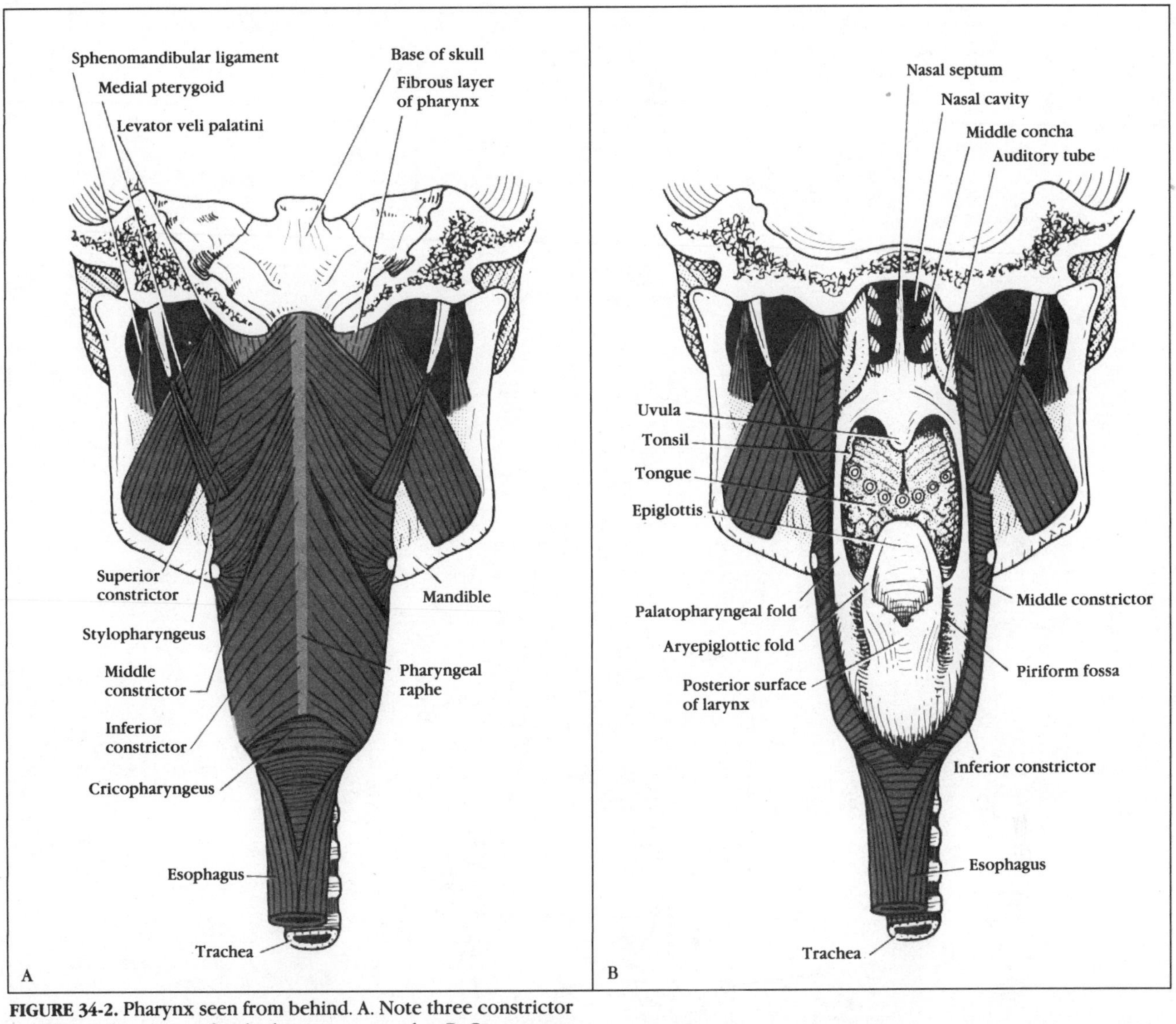

FIGURE 34-2. Pharynx seen from behind. A. Note three constrictor muscles and position of stylopharyngeus muscles. B. Greater part of posterior wall of pharynx has been removed to display nasal, oral, and laryngeal parts of pharynx. (From R. S. Snell, *Clinical Anatomy for Medical Students* [2nd ed.]. Boston: Little, Brown, 1981.)

Pharynx

The pharynx is an important structure for the process of swallowing (Fig. 34-2). It provides for the active movement of food into the esophagus, while closing and sealing off the trachea. Once the swallowing reflex is initiated by voluntary movement of food to the back of the mouth, swallowing continues as a reflex activity.

Esophagus

The esophagus provides a passageway for food from the pharynx to the stomach. It is a muscular, pliable tube, which is easily affected by intrathoracic or intraabdominal pressures or volumes. Mucus-secreting glands along its length secrete mucus to lubricate the bolus of food passing through.

The construction of the smooth muscle of the esophagus and other structures in the alimentary canal has been described as a *functional syncytium* because the smooth muscle fibers lie very close to each other. This construction allows for waves of muscular contraction called peristalsis [1].

Approximately 5 cm above the esophageal entry to the stomach is a narrowed area called the *gastroesophageal*, *cardiac*, or *lower esophageal sphincter* (Fig. 34-3). A sphincter is an opening that has an increased amount of muscle surrounding it. The gastroesophageal sphincter normally remains constricted but relaxes when a peristaltic wave is conducted through it, allowing for passage of

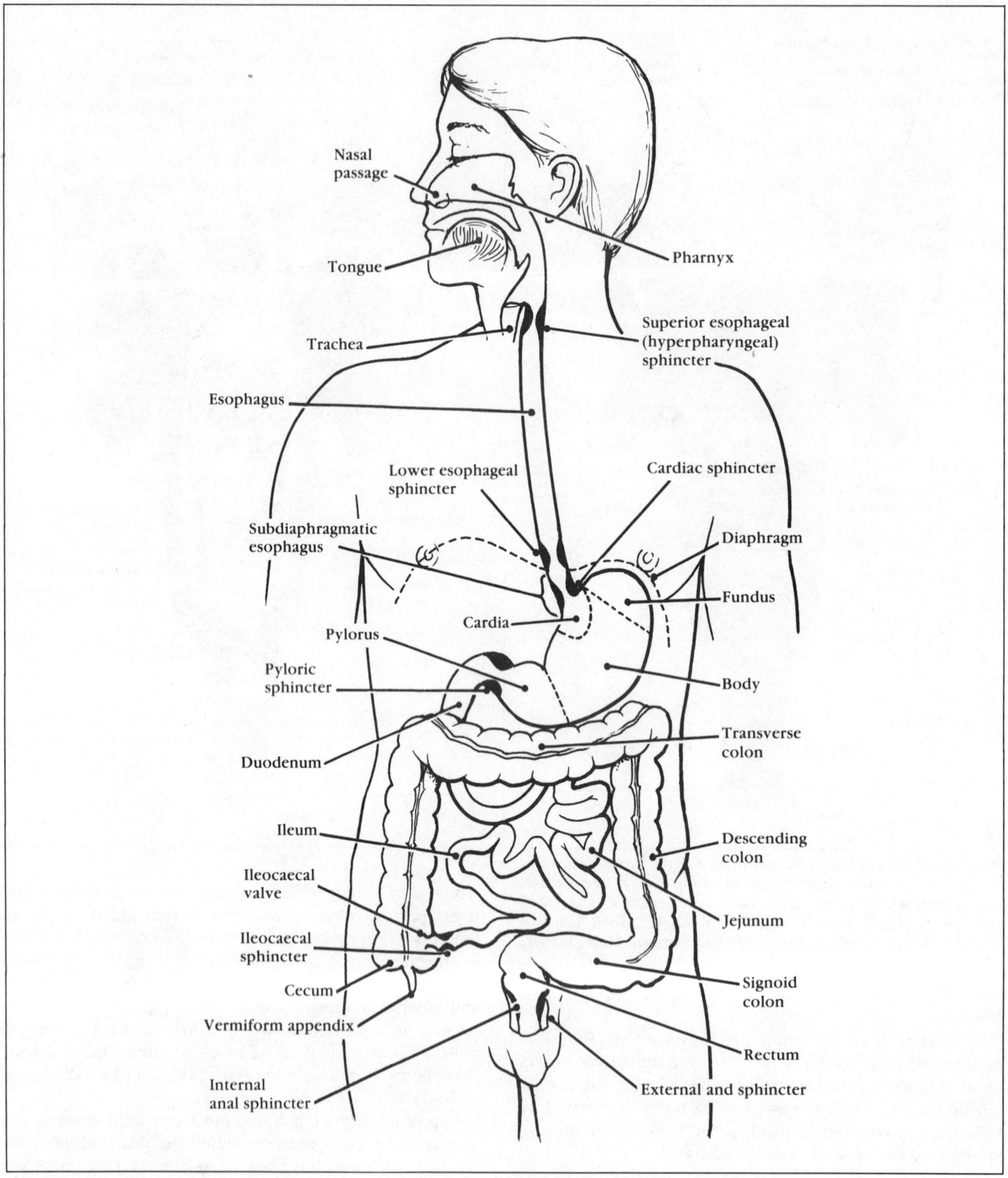

FIGURE 34-3. The digestive system.

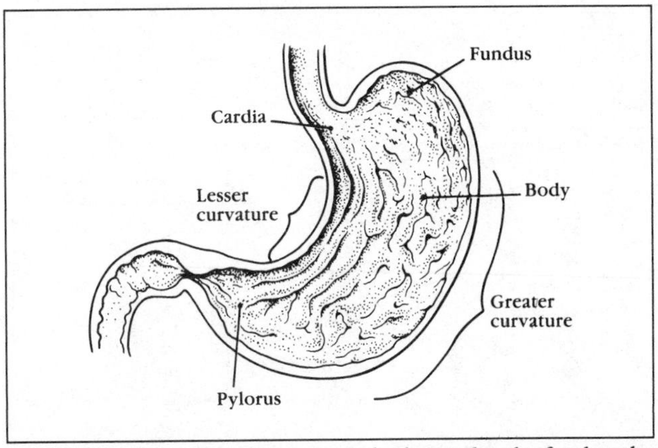

FIGURE 34-4. Segments of the stomach: the cardia, the fundus, the body, and the pylorus. Note the greater and lesser curvatures.

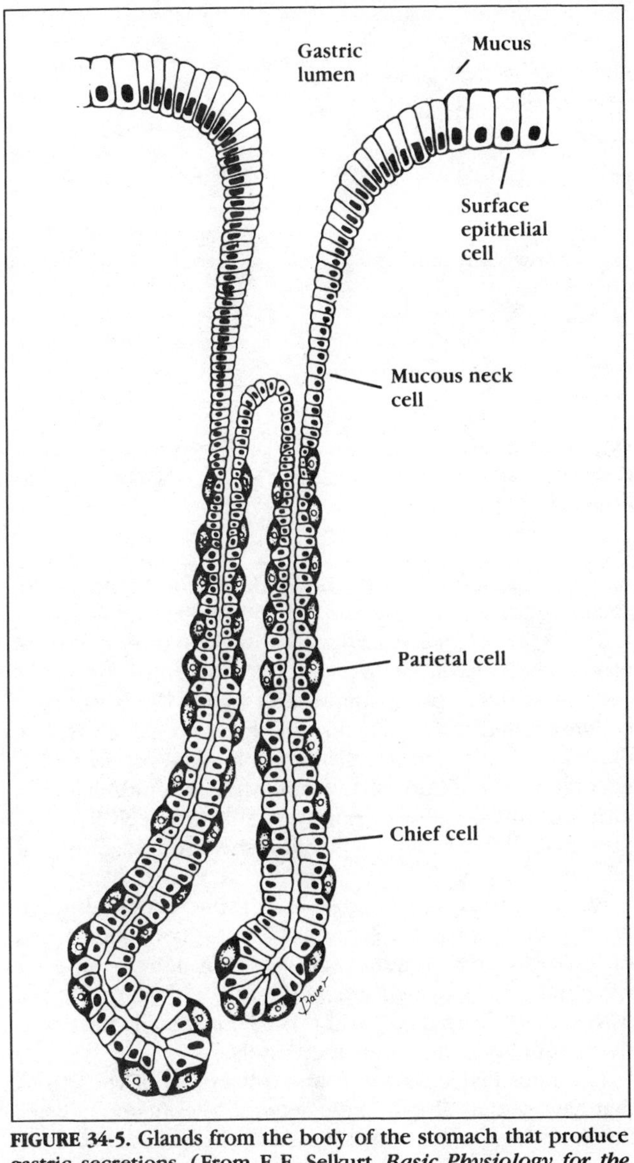

FIGURE 34-5. Glands from the body of the stomach that produce gastric secretions. (From E. E. Selkurt, *Basic Physiology for the Health Sciences* [2nd ed.]. Boston: Little, Brown, 1982.)

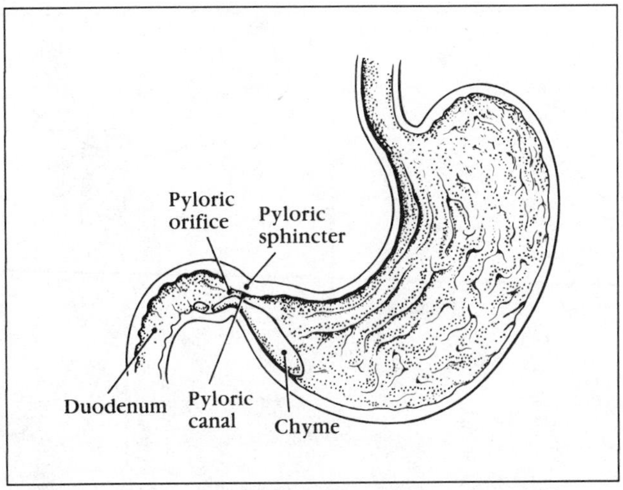

FIGURE 34-6. Movement of chyme through the pyloric sphincter.

food to the stomach. The gastroesophageal sphincter seems to serve in preventing acid reflux into the esophagus.

Stomach

The stomach is a pear-shaped, hollow, distensible organ traditionally divided into the cardia, the fundus, the body, and the pylorus (Fig. 34-4). Figure 34-4 also shows the position of the greater and lesser curvature of the stomach. The upper portion of the stomach is continuous with the esophagus and lies very close to the diaphragm, while the lower portion is continuous with the duodenum through the lower pyloric sphincter.

The interior lining of the stomach lies in mucosal folds called *rugae.* Within the mucosal folds are glands that secrete the gastric juice. Gastric juice is composed of secretions from the *chief cells*, the *parietal cells*, and the *mucous neck cells* (Fig. 34-5). The chief cells secrete the proenzyme *pepsinogen*, which, when activated, functions to digest proteins. The parietal cells secrete *hydrochloric acid*, which has a pH of approximately 0.8. It is believed that these cells also secrete the intrinsic factor, a glycoprotein that binds with vitamin B_{12} and makes it available for absorption in the small intestine [1]. Mucous neck cells secrete large amounts of mucus.

Approximately 1500 to 3000 ml of gastric juice is secreted daily and mixes with the food entering the stomach. The combination of food and gastric juice makes a semiliquid mass, called *chyme,* which is propelled into the small intestine through the pyloric sphincter (Fig. 34-6).

The nervous supply to the stomach is through the intrinsic and the autonomic nervous systems. The intrinsic system begins in the esophagus and continues all the way to the anus. The layers involved in this system include the *myenteric plexus* and the *submucosal plexus*. These control the tone of the bowel, rhythmic contractions, and the velocity of excitation of the gut. The autonomic nervous system (ANS), through the parasympathetic branches, in-

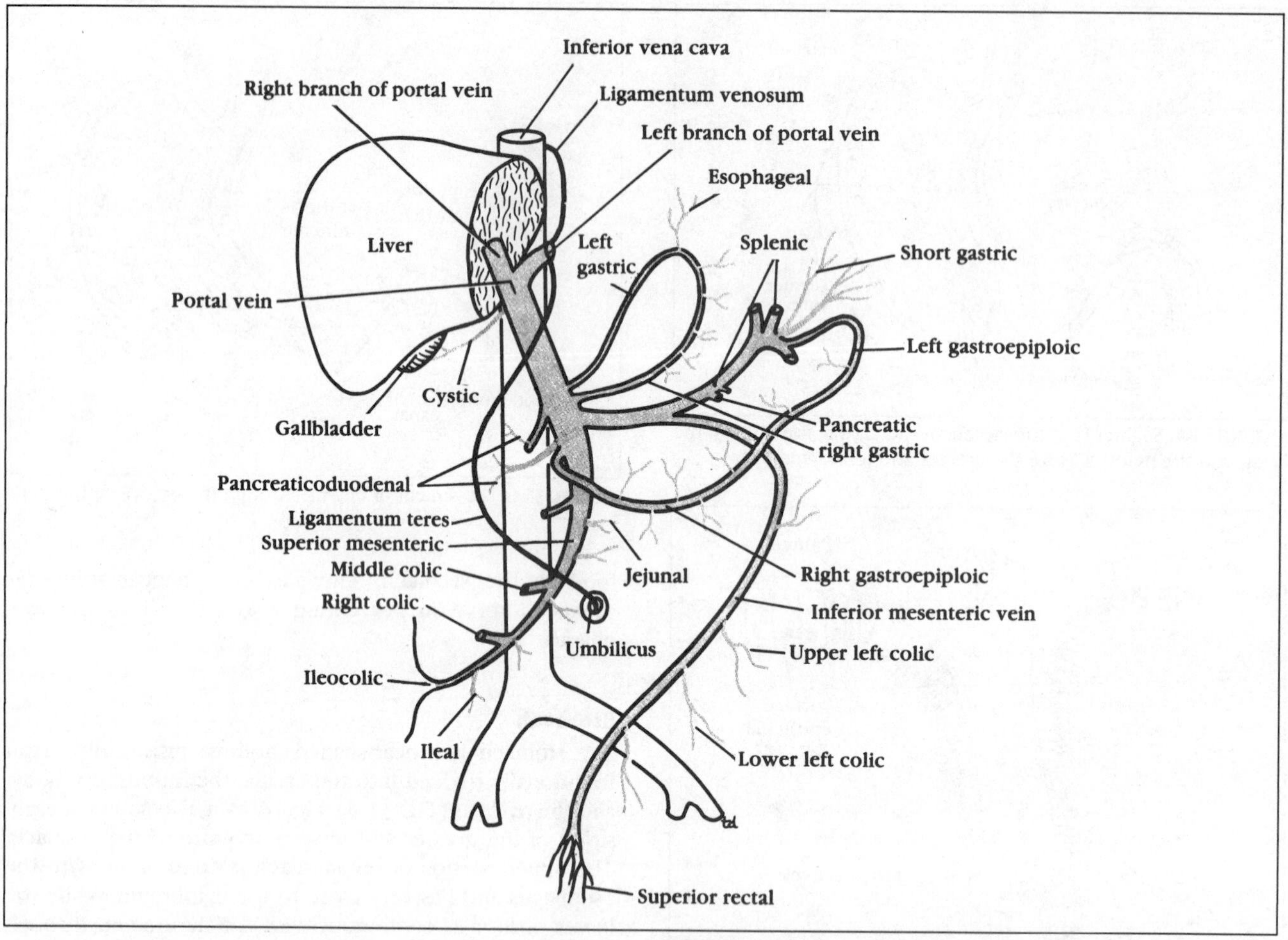

FIGURE 34-7. Venous drainage of the stomach. (From R. S. Snell, *Clinical Anatomy for Medical Students* [2nd ed.]. Boston: Little, Brown, 1981.)

creases excitation, especially in the esophagus, stomach, large intestine, and anal regions. The sympathetic portion of the ANS functions mostly to inhibit activity of the gastrointestinal system.

The arterial blood supply to the stomach comes mainly from the celiac artery. The venous blood is drained through the gastric veins, which connect to and terminate in the portal vein (Fig. 34-7). The stomach has a profuse lymphatic drainage through lymphatic vessels and nodes (Fig. 34-8).

Small Intestine

The small intestine is that portion of the digestive tract that extends from the pylorus to the ileocecal valve. It is approximately 12 ft long in the living subject. Cadaver lengths are longer because the muscles of the intestinal wall are relaxed. The small intestine is divided into sections: the *duodenum*, *jejunum*, and *ileum* (see Fig. 34-3). Absorption and secretion occur throughout the length of the small intestine.

The intestinal wall is composed of four layers: mucosa, submucosa, the muscularis, and the serosa (Fig. 34-9). Fingerlike folds of the mucosa, called *villi*, project into the lumen of the interior of the intestines and increase the absorptive surface by approximately 600-fold (Fig. 34-10).

The *crypts of Lieberkühn* are pitlike structures that lie in grooves between the villi and are composed of absorptive cells and mucus-producing goblet cells. The absorptive cells are columnar in structure and have a brush border on the luminal side. These cells have a marked power for regeneration and differentiate from intestinal epithelial cells into absorptive cells. An intestinal epithelial cell lives approximately 5 days, after which it is shed into the intestinal secretions [2].

Blood circulation to the small intestine occurs through the gastroduodenal, the superior pancreaticoduodenal, and the celiac arteries. Venous drainage is through the superior mesenteric vein, which empties into the portal vein and travels to the liver (Fig. 34-11). The entire small intestine is richly supplied with lymphatic vessels.

The intestinal cells form large quantities of secretions that have a neutral pH. These secretions contain enzymes that function to a limited extent in the breakdown of nutri-

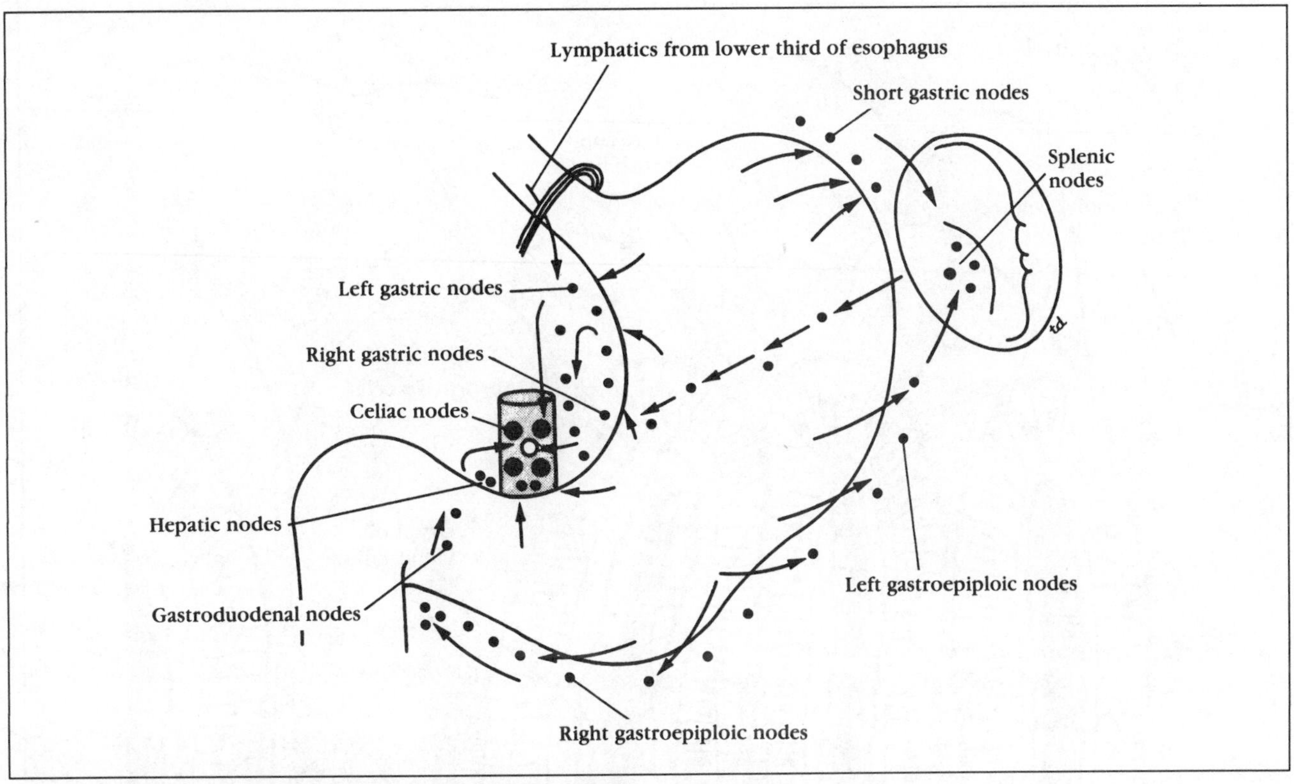

FIGURE 34-8. Lymphatic drainage of the stomach. (From R. S. Snell, *Clinical Anatomy for Medical Students* [2nd ed.]. Boston: Little, Brown, 1981.)

ents. Another important secretion is *cholecystokinin-pancreozymin* (CCK-PZ), which is secreted from the mucosa, absorbed into the bloodstream, and functions in the stimulation of the gallbladder and pancreas (see p. 490).

The liver, gallbladder, and pancreas, considered in greater detail in Chapter 36, are essential organs in the promotion of digestion. Chyme entering the small intestine stimulates CCK-PZ by distention of the small intestine. This hormone in turn stimulates the pancreas to release its enzymatic secretions into the duodenum. The stimulation from this hormone causes the gallbladder to contract and push bile into the small intestine.

Large Intestine

The large intestine begins with the ending of the ileum at the ileocecal valve (Fig. 34-12). The area of meeting is called the cecum. A small structure extends from the cecum called the *appendix*, which is a relatively nonfunctional pouch. The colon portion of the large intestine is subdivided into the ascending, transverse, descending, and sigmoid areas. The large intestine itself begins with the cecum, contains the colon, and terminates in the rectum and anal canal.

An increase in the number of mucus-secreting goblet cells is noted in the large intestine. The mucus material se-

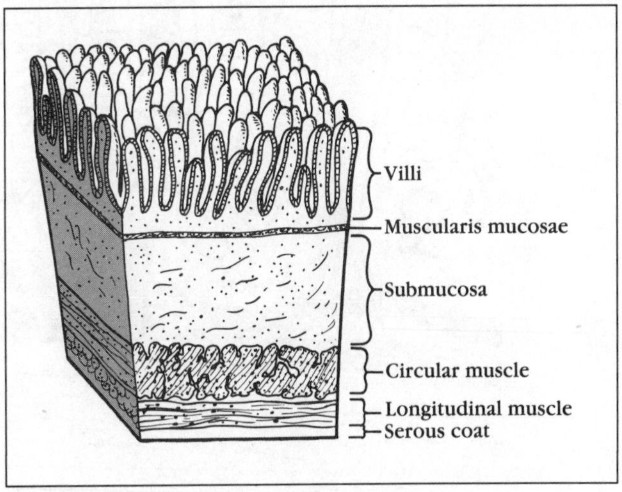

FIGURE 34-9. Layers of the intestinal wall.

creted is important to prevent trauma to the bowel, provide fecal adherent material, and protect the bowel against resident bacteria. Most of the liquid and electrolytes from the semiliquid material of the small intestine are absorbed in the large intestine, especially in the ascending and transverse colon. The resultant feces usually consist of approximately three-fourths water and one-fourth solid matter, of which about 30 percent is dead bacteria. The brown color

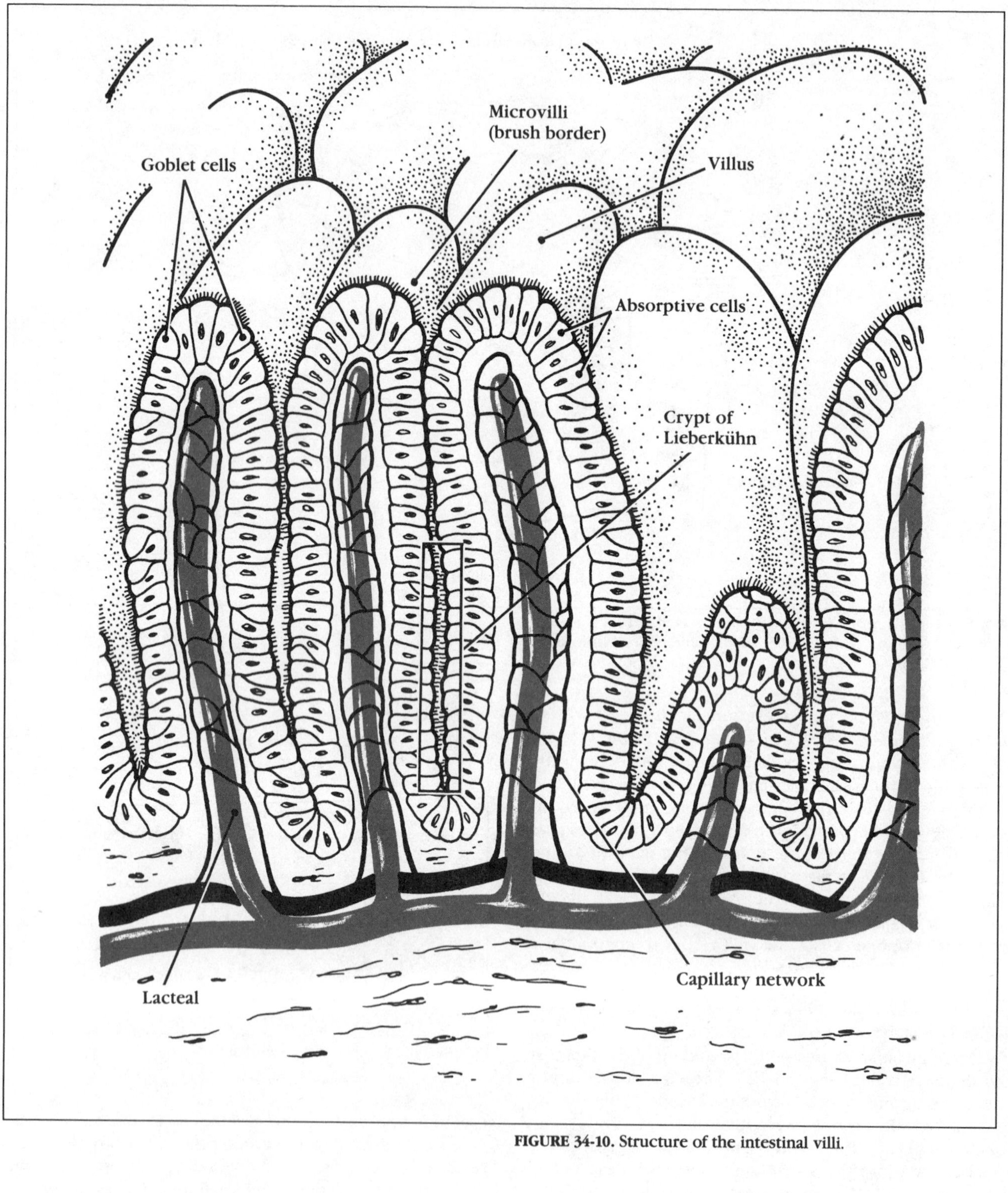

FIGURE 34-10. Structure of the intestinal villi.

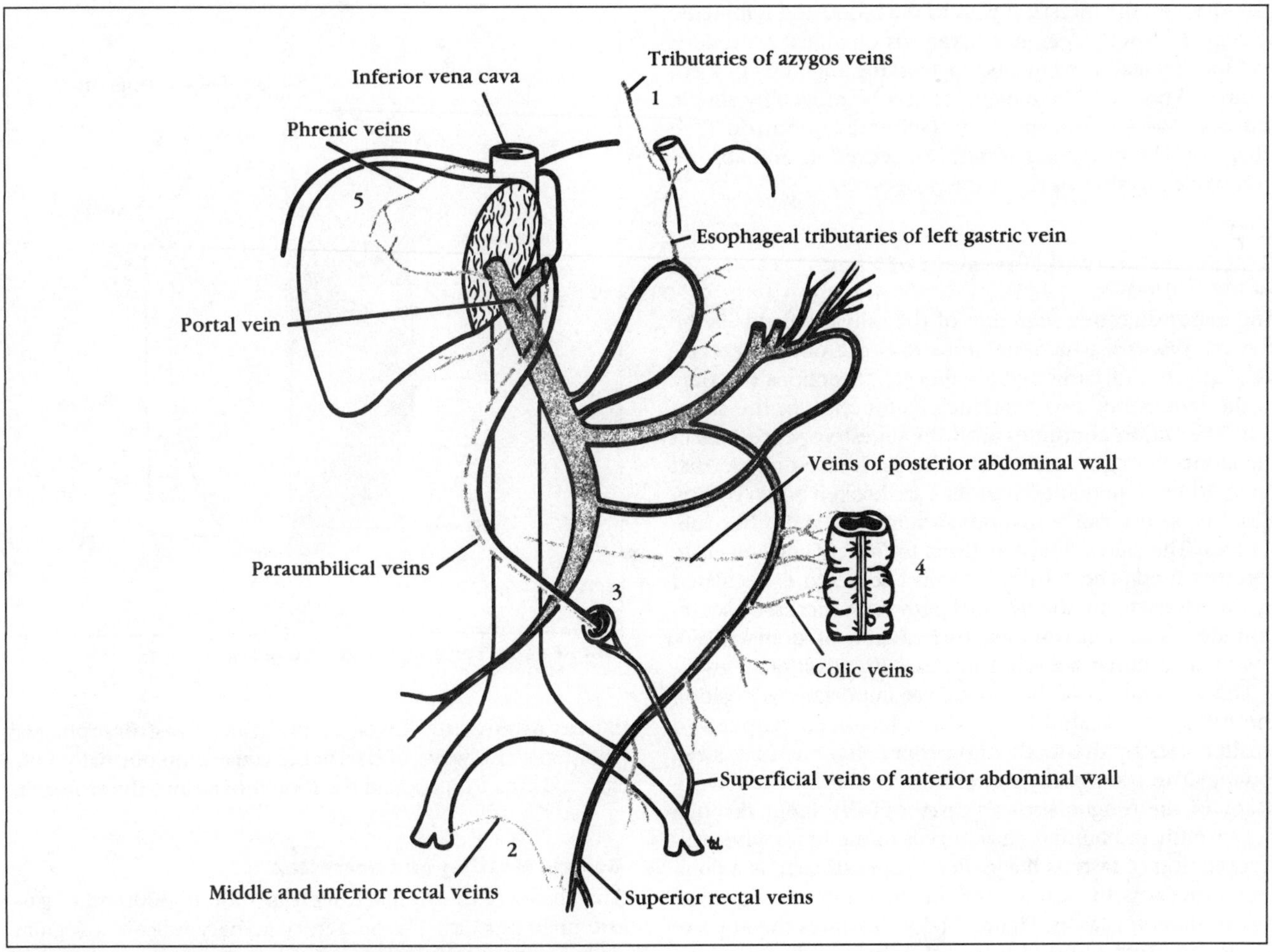

FIGURE 34-11. Venous drainage of the small intestine. (From R. S. Snell, *Clinical Anatomy for Medical Students* [2nd ed.]. Boston: Little, Brown, 1981.)

of fecal material is due to breakdown products of bilirubin called stercobilin and urobilin.

The rectum is approximately 20 cm of the final descending portion of the large intestine and terminates in the anal canal. It is protected from the sigmoid colon by an external sphincter, called the *sphincter ani*, which opens to the outside of the body.

The blood supply to the large intestine is profuse and arises from branches of the superior and inferior mesenteric arteries. The venous drainage is mainly through the mesenteric veins, terminating in the portal veins (see Fig. 34-7). This system is important in the pathology of portal hypertension (p. 524), because the increased portal pressure is reflected in the veins surrounding the esophagus and anal canal.

PHYSIOLOGY OF THE DIGESTIVE SYSTEM

The process of digestion takes substances in one form and breaks them down into molecules that are small enough to

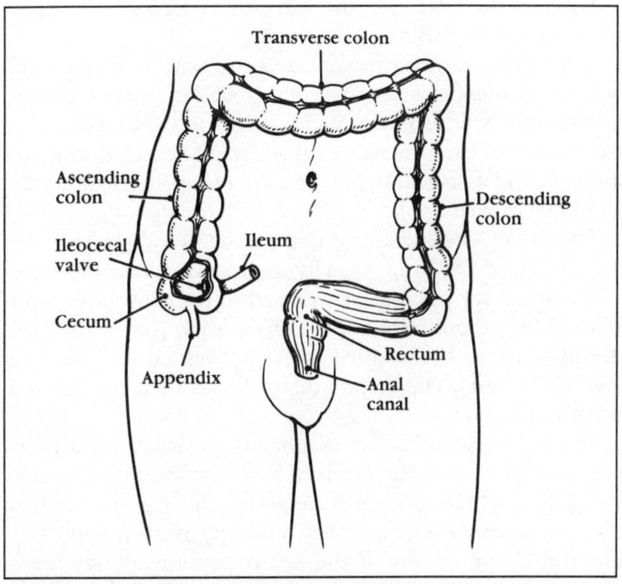

FIGURE 34-12. Segments of the large intestine.

pass through the intestinal wall to the blood and lymphatic system. This activity requires various chemical secretions and mechanical movements, all working together in a coordinated fashion. The molecules may be moved by simple diffusion, active transport, or facilitated diffusion (see Chap. 1). The processes of motility, secretion, and absorption work together to effect the process.

Oral Secretions and Movement of Food to the Stomach

The major digestive secretion of the salivary glands is the enzyme *ptyalin*, which functions to break down starches. This amylase, or carbohydrate digester, functions not only in the mouth but also continues its function in the stomach. The action continues until the digestive secretions of the stomach begin to alter the chyme. It is estimated that up to 30 to 40 percent of starches are broken down by ptyalin. The saliva also contains water, mucus, and other substances. The saliva fluid functions to liquefy and lubricate ingested food. The amount of saliva secreted is regulated by the parasympathetic nervous pathways. Increased secretion also occurs in response to irritation of stomach mucosa, which initiates a reflex increase in salivation.

The movements of the tongue are important to position the *bolus* of ingested food, which has been reduced to smaller sizes by the teeth, into proper alignment for swallowing. The taste buds, scattered over the mucous membrane of the tongue surface, carry sensory input through the seventh and ninth cranial nerves to the brain where interpretation of taste is made. Perception of taste is a complex process with various areas of the tongue being sensitive to different tastes. Figure 34-13 illustrates the areas of the tongue that respond to sweet, salty, and bitter stimulation. The major motor nerve of the tongue is the hypoglossal, which is closely aligned with the vagus nerve. It innervates the extrinsic and intrinsic muscles for tongue movement into various positions.

Swallowing is the key event in the initiation of digestion because it increases esophageal peristaltic motion, causes decreased lower esophageal pressure, and initiates the gastroenteric reflex. This reflex causes small bowel motility to increase and assists in the movement of nutrients along the alimentary canal.

The act of swallowing or deglutition is initiated by the movement of a bolus of food by the tongue to the pharynx. The respiratory passages are closed to prevent movement of food into them. The bolus of food then passes through the pharynx to the esophagus in approximately 1 second (see Fig. 34-14). The respiratory passages then reopen and breathing resumes.

As food passes into the esophagus, peristalsis and pressure changes move the bolus of food toward the stomach. Peristalsis, which occurs throughout the gastrointestinal tract, is a series of sequential muscular movements. The functional syncytium of the entire system allows for a wavelike movement of the smooth muscle. As the food moves toward the lower esophageal or gastroesophageal sphincter, the wave of peristalsis causes the normally constricted area to relax and the food moves into the stomach.

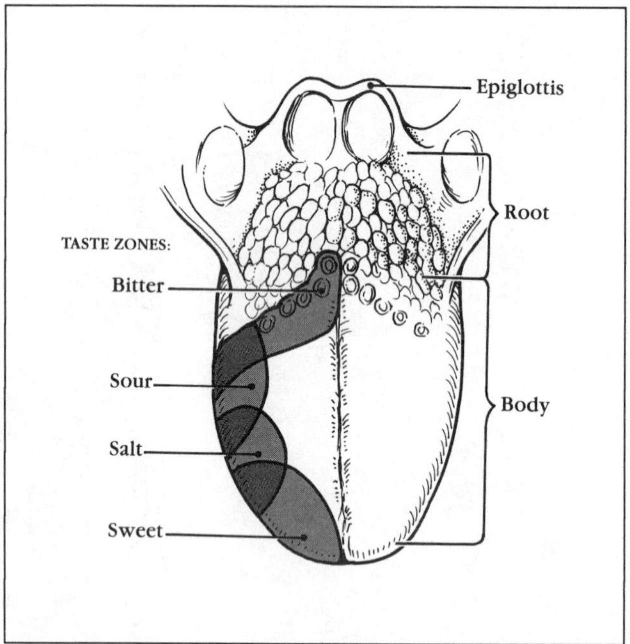

FIGURE 34-13. The tongue and areas of taste.

Gastric Motility and Secretion

The glands of the stomach secrete 1500 to 3000 ml of gastric juice per day. The secretory activity follows a regular daily pattern with the least secretion occurring in the early mornings. The amount of gastric secretion also varies with individual dietary habits, other stimuli that provoke secretions, and the strength of the inhibitory mechanisms.

The gastric juice contains mucus, the intrinsic factor, hydrochloric acid, pepsinogen, and the following electrolytes: sodium, potassium, chloride, and bicarbonate. Certain other enzymes such as gastric lipase, urease, lysozyme, and carbonic anhydrase are also present in the secretions. The three types of cells that make up the gastric glands secrete mucus, pepsinogen, and hydrochloric acid. Figure 34-5 illustrates the appearance and anatomic relationship of these cells.

The parietal cells, found in the fundus and body of the stomach, secrete hydrochloric acid as a highly concentrated juice with a pH of approximately 0.8. A suggested mechanism for the formation of hydrochloric acid is illustrated in Figure 34-15. The theory relating hydrochloric acid secretion to bicarbonate replenishment in the blood is supported by the observation that each H^+ ion secreted is matched by bicarbonate (HCO_3^-) that is returned to the blood. This means that the amount of bicarbonate entering the blood during the gastric secretory phase is directly proportional to the amount of acid se-

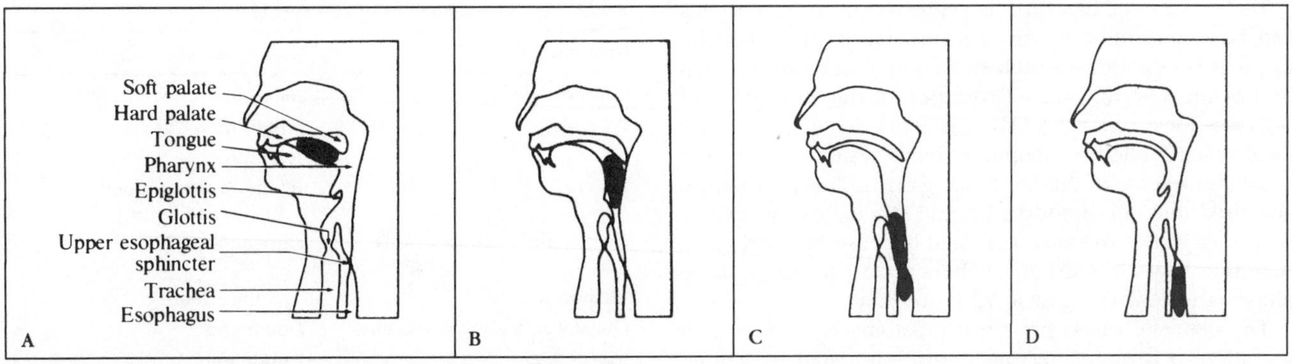

FIGURE 34-14. Passage of a food bolus from the mouth through the pharynx and upper esophagus during a swallow. (From E. E. Selkurt, *Physiology* [5th ed.]. Boston: Little, Brown, 1984.)

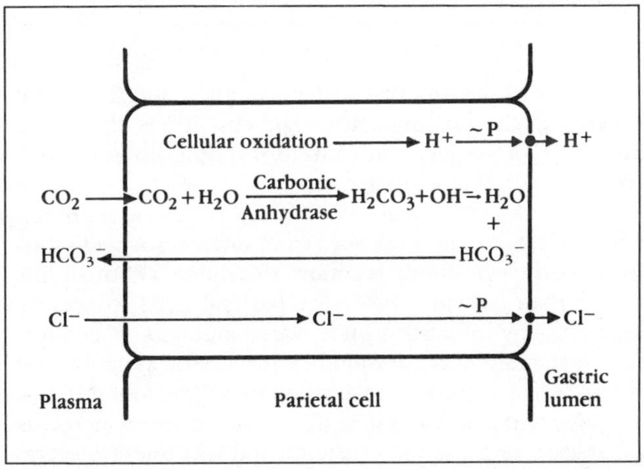

FIGURE 34-15. A possible mechanism for the gastric secretion of HCl. (From E. E. Selkurt, *Basic Physiology for the Health Sciences.* [2nd ed.]. Boston: Little, Brown, 1982.)

creted. Carbon dioxide enters the cell or is formed in the cell during metabolism, reacts with water catalyst by using carbonic anhydrase, and forms carbonic acid. This carbonic acid then dissociates to bicarbonate and hydrogen. The hydrogen ion enters the parietal cell canaliculi by active transport, while the bicarbonate is diffused back into the blood. The chloride ion is also actively transported from the blood to the canaliculi [4]. Only during periods of relative gastric inactivity is adequate carbon dioxide produced to make a small amount of hydrochloric acid. During digestion, the parietal cell takes its needed carbon dioxide from the circulating blood.

Pepsin is the main proteolytic enzyme of gastric juice. It is secreted by the chief cells of the gastric glands in the form of pepsinogen. It has no digestive activity until it is activated into pepsin, which occurs in the presence of hydrochloric acid and previously activated pepsin. Pepsin is most active in a highly acid medium. It functions optimally in a pH of 2 and is almost inactive in secretions with a pH greater than 5.

Mucus is produced by the columnar cells of the surface epithelium and the mucous neck cells of the glands of the cardia, corpus, and pylorus. The surface of the stomach mucosa has a continuous layer of columnar epithelial cells that secretes large amounts of viscous and alkaline mucus to coat the mucosa and provide for a sheet of mucus protection. The epithelial lining of the stomach has remarkable properties of repair and can reproduce itself in 36 to 48 hours. The mucous neck cells secrete a thinner mucus than the other mucus-secreting cells. The amount of this secretion varies with vagal stimulation and irritation. This additional line of defense serves to lubricate the passage of food, absorb pepsin, and wash away noxious substances. Any failure to secrete mucus in adequate quantities to protect the underlying mucosa increases the susceptibility of the mucosa to the action of hydrochloric acid and pepsin [3].

Gastric juices contain the enzymes gastric lipase, gastric amylase, gastric urease, carbonic anhydrase, and lysozyme. Gastric lipase acts primarily on butterfat but has little effect on other fats because bile is needed for the digestion of fats. Gastric amylase does very little for starch digestion. Gastric urease, formed by the bacteria that contaminate the gastric mucosa, splits urea to produce ammonia. Carbonic anhydrase, present in the epithelial cells and in high concentrations in parietal cells, is thought to be produced by the disintegration of desquamated epithelial cells and is essential in hydrochloric acid formation. Lysozyme is a carbohydrate-splitting enzyme found in small amounts in the gastric juice. Its cellular origin is not known but it has been found in increased amounts in persons with gastric ulcers, a reaction thought to be due to the inflammatory reactions from the ulcer [3].

Gastric motility is governed by the peristaltic waves that occur every 15 to 25 seconds and mix the ingested food with the gastric secretions. The end result of this movement and mixing is a thin, highly acidic liquid called chyme. The chyme is moved into the small intestine, mostly because of the higher pressure gradients in the stomach that exceed the duodenal pressure. The acidity and the amount of chyme entering the duodenum helps to regulate the duodenal and pancreatic secretions.

The process of digestion is regulated by both nervous and hormonal mechanisms. The innervation through the vagus nerve excites stomach excretion directly by stimulation of the gastric glands. Distention of the stomach wall activates local reflexes to stimulate gastric secretion. The local reflexes elicit autonomic nervous system activity and cause the release of the hormone, gastrin. This hormone is absorbed into the bloodstream and stimulates the gastric secretory glands to cause a marked increase in gastric acid secretion. Gastric secretion is believed to occur in three phases: the cephalic, gastric, and intestinal.

The cephalic phase prepares the stomach for food and digestion. It is under nervous control, initiated by stimuli such as the sight, smell, or thought of food. Impulses from receptors such as the retina, taste buds, and the olfactory glands travel to the cerebral cortex, and the motor fibers of the vagi of the stomach stimulate the glands of the stomach to secrete juice rich in hydrochloric acid and gastrin.

The gastric phase is initiated when food enters the stomach. The hormone gastrin is released by acetylcholine stimulation of the gastrin-producing cells. The process is triggered by distention of the stomach caused by food and by exposure of the mucosa to certain substances called *secretagogues*. Examples of secretagogues are caffeine and alcohol. The gastrin is absorbed in the blood and stimulates the secretory cells, which produce about two-thirds of the total gastric secretions. Food in the stomach initiates local reflexes in the intramural plexus of the stomach, and vasovagal reflexes stimulate parasympathetic stimulation to increase the secretion. The rate of secretion in response to gastrin continues for several hours while food remains in the stomach. Both the gastrin and vagal mechanisms are important in gastric secretion.

The intestinal phase of gastric secretion is less active than the cephalic or gastric phases but once initiated it may last for 8 to 10 hours while food remains in the duodenum. It is believed that this reflex is carried on by a hormone that is similar but less potent than gastrin. The hormone is thought to be liberated by the intestinal mucosa, absorbed in the bloodstream, and carried back to the secretory cells of the stomach through the circulation.

The intestines also function to inhibit gastric secretion when there are partially digested proteins, acid, fat, or hypertonic solutions in the duodenum. Distention, caused by the presence of food, initiates the *enterogastric reflex*, which slows the influence of the vagus nerve. The purpose of the enterogastric reflex appears to delay stomach emptying until some emptying can occur in the small intestine. Intestinal hormones, especially *secretin* and *cholecystokinin-pancreozymin* (CCK-PZ), oppose the stimulatory effects of gastrin and slow the movement of chyme from the stomach to the small intestine. This inhibitory feedback prevents excessive acid secretion and protects the intestinal mucosa from injury. During the interdigestive phase, while no digestion is occurring in the gastrointestinal tract, the stomach secretes only a few milliliters of gastric juice per hour. Normally, secretions in the stomach follow a steady, dynamic mechanism, regulated by both nervous and hormonal factors that foster structural and functional integrity in the mucosa. Pathologic conditions, drugs and chemicals, or surgery can cause disruption of the balance between secretion and inhibition.

TABLE 34-2. Principal sites of absorption

Nutrient	Absorptive site
Carbohydrates	Jejunum
Protein	Jejunum
Fat	Jejunum
Water	Jejunum; also duodenum, ileum, and colon
Fat-soluble vitamins—A, D, E, K	Duodenum
Vitamin B_{12}	Terminal ileum
Other water-soluble vitamins	Duodenum
Iron	Duodenum
Calcium	Duodenum
Sodium	Jejunum by passive diffusion; ileum and colon by active transport
Potassium	Jejunum and ileum

The best-known chemical stimulant of gastric secretion is *histamine*, which is released from surface mast cells during an antigen-antibody reaction. Histamine, although less potent than gastrin, causes the parietal cells to secrete large amounts of gastric juice. Large amounts of endogenous histamine may be found in the gastric mucosa, and during active secretion small amounts will be found in gastric juice and urine. Physical or emotional stress increases the release of histamine. Caffeine and nicotine are secretagogues that increase the amount and acidity of gastric secretion. Alcohol has been found to stimulate only the amount of gastrin secretion. Aspirin, alcohol, and bile salts alter the permeability of the epithelial barrier and allow back diffusion of hydrochloric acid, which may result in injury to tissue and blood vessels. Aspirin produces changes in the gastric mucosa and decreases the total output of mucus, which reduces its protective effect on the gastric mucosa. There are observations that prolonged administration of large quantities of corticotropic and adrenal steroids increases gastric secretion, which favors the development or recurrence of peptic ulcers [4]. Parasympathetic agents such as acetylcholine, reserpine, and pilocarpine are also secretory stimulants. Insulin, through its hypoglycemic effects, excites the vagus nerve and increases gastric gland activity [2].

Belladonna or its alkaloids — atropine and hyoscine — are secretory depressants acting through a vagal depressant action. Synthetic anticholinergic drugs, such as propantheline bromide (Probanthine), are used to control gastric activity and secretion.

Emotional disruptions have long been recognized as exerting an important influence on the secretory and motor functions of the stomach. Studies seem to indicate that prolonged anxiety, guilt, conflict, hostility, and resentment

TABLE 34-3. Digestive enzymes

Enzyme	Source	Substrate	Products	Remarks
Ptyalin	Salivary glands	Starch	Smaller carbohydrates	
Pepsin	Chief cells of stomach mucosa	Protein (nonspecific)	Polypeptides	
Gastric lipase	Stomach mucosa	Triglycerides (lipids)	Glycerides and FAs	
Enterokinase	Duodenal mucosa	Trypsinogen	Trypsin	Activates or converts trypsinogen to trypsin; trypsinogen hydrolyzed to expose active site
Trypsin	Pancreas	Protein and polypeptides	Smaller polypeptides	Conversion of chymotrypsinogen to chymotrypsin
Chymotrypsin	Pancreas	Proteins and polypeptides (different specificity than trypsin)	Smaller polypeptides	
Nuclease	Pancreas	Nucleic acids	Nucleotides (base + sugar + PO_4)	
Carboxypeptidase	Pancreas	Polypeptides	Smaller polypeptides	Cleaves carboxy terminal end
Pancreatic lipase	Pancreas	Lipids, especially triglycerides	Glycerides, free FAs, glycerol	Very potent
Pancreatic amylase	Pancreas	Starch	2 disaccharide units = maltose	Very potent
Aminopeptidase	Intestinal glands	Polypeptides	Smaller peptides	
Dipeptidase	Intestine	Dipeptides	2 amino acids	
Maltase	Intestine	Maltose	2 glucose	
Lactase	Intestine	Lactose	1 glucose, 1 galactose	
Sucrase	Intestine	Sucrose	1 glucose, 1 fructose	
Nucleotidase	Intestine	Nucleotides	Nucleosides and phosphates (base + sugar)	
Nucleosidase	Intestine	Nucleosides	Base and sugar	
Intestinal lipase	Intestine	Fats	Glycerides, FAs, glycerol	

Note: Enzymes act on each other during and after digestion, but it is only after digestion (after their substrates are removed) that they have any marked effect on each other.

lead to engorgement of the gastric mucosa and increased secretion (see Chap. 4). The significant decrease in gastric secretion after complete vagotomy suggests that hypersecretion is caused by excessive stimulation of the vagus nerve.

Secretion and Absorption in the Small Intestine

The major nutrients are absorbed mostly in the small intestine, with the simpler substances generally being absorbed in the first portion of the small bowel. Substances requiring greater hydrolysis and simplification are absorbed at later points in the small intestine. Table 34-2 shows the specific absorption sites of major nutrients.

Nearly all of the absorption events of nutrients go on in the small intestine. The anatomic structure previously detailed on pages 484–485 provides the mechanism for this to occur. In the small intestine, secretions are received from the pancreas and the liver and are supplemented by intestinal secretions. The *secretions of the small intestine* include enzymes, hormones, and mucus. These substances are listed in Tables 34-3 and 34-4 and include the secretions from the pancreas and the liver. The major effect of all of the enzymes and hormones are detailed in these tables.

All of the secretions work together to digest carbohydrates, proteins, and fats. Absorption depends on the proper hydrolysis of nutrients by secretions that increase the movement from the intestinal lumen to the bloodstream. Formation of pancreatic and biliary secretions is detailed in Chapter 36. The biliary secretions include bile salts, lipids, water, electrolytes, and bilirubin. Of these, bilirubin is a waste product that gives color to the feces. The bile salts exert a detergentlike effect on fats and function to emulsify fat. The pancreatic secretions contain enzymes and large amounts of bicarbonate and water.

The chyme that enters the duodenum is highly acidic because it was mixed with large amounts of hydrochloric acid in the stomach. All of the intestinal enzymes work best in an alkaline medium, which requires neutralization and alkalinization of the chyme. The amount of the alkaline pancreatic secretion has been shown to be closely correlated with the pH of the chyme entering the small intestine.

Chemical and mechanical digestion requires that food be changed into the forms that can be moved by the process of absorption through the mucosal lining cells to the blood

TABLE 34-4. Hormones of digestion

Hormone	Source	Agents that stimulate production	Action
Gastrin	Gastric mucosa (primarily pylorus)	Distention of stomach and some protein derivatives	Stimulates production of HCl
Enterogastrone	Mucosa of small intestine and duodenum	Fats, sugars, or acids in intestine	Inhibits gastric secretion and mobility
Secretin	Duodenal mucosa	Polypeptides, acids, etc. in intestine (duodenum)′	Stimulates pancreas to produce a watery, enzyme-poor juice, with high HCO_3^- content
Cholecystokinin-pancreozymin (CCK-PZ)	Duodenal mucosa	Fats in duodenum	Stimulates pancreas to produce enzyme-rich juice and stimulates gallbladder to contract and release bile

and lymph vessels. The diffusible forms include monosaccharides, amino acids, fatty acids, glycerol, and glycerides [1]. Figure 34-16 shows schematically where materials are absorbed in the entire gastrointestinal system. Nearly all of the nutrients are absorbed in the small intestine and 90 percent of all absorption occurs here. Absorption of the specific nutrients is detailed below.

CARBOHYDRATE ABSORPTION. Carbohydrates are ingested primarily as disaccharides, starches, or polysaccharides. Polysaccharides are hydrolyzed into their component disaccharides by the action of salivary ptyalin and the gastric, intestinal, and pancreatic amylases. Intact disaccharides can be passively absorbed by the small intestine, but relatively few are absorbed in this manner. Most disaccharides are first split into monosaccharides by specific enzymes located in the intestinal microvilli. These monosaccharides are then actively absorbed into the blood capillaries of the villi. Absorption occurs against a concentration gradient and apparently requires active transport, although the method by which this occurs is obscure. It is known that sodium increases cellular permeability to glucose, so that glucose transport is related to the sodium transport system.

PROTEIN ABSORPTION. Protein absorption occurs mostly in the duodenum and jejunum. As a result of gastric pepsin and pancreatic enzymes, 70 percent of the protein ingested in the diet is presented to the intestinal absorptive membrane in the form of small peptides, while 30 percent is in the form of amino acids. The amino acids are immediately absorbed but only a small amount of peptide is absorbed intact. The majority of the peptides are reduced by peptidases in the microvilli to amino acids and then absorption rapidly follows. The sodium transport mechanism also probably provides for amino acid transport. Many amino acids apparently need pyridoxine to aid in transport.

FAT ABSORPTION. Dietary fat consists mainly of long chain triglycerides, which are hydrolyzed intralumenally into fatty acids and monoglycerides. This hydrolysis occurs in the jejunum through the action of lipase. Bile salts and fatty acids aggregate to form *micelles*, which are water-soluble structures. These attach themselves to the surface of the epithelial cells. The fatty acids leave the micelles and enter the cell by diffusion, while the bile salts are released to return to the chyme to aid in the absorption of more fats. When the fats in the duodenum and upper jejunum have been removed, the bile salts are resorbed and eventually

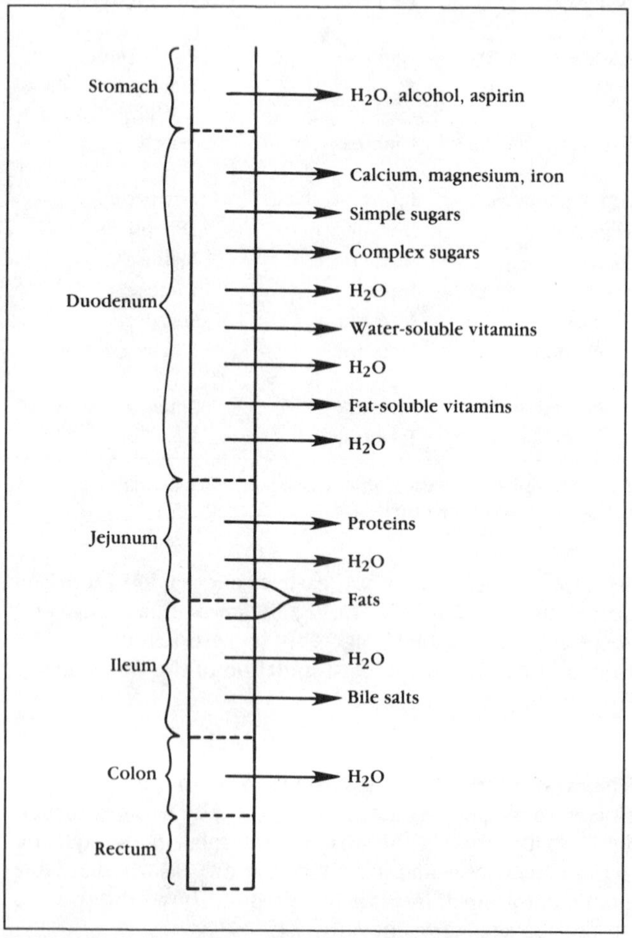

FIGURE 34-16. Absorption of nutrients in the digestive tract.

returned to the liver. The lipids are resynthesized into tryglycerides in the endoplasmic reticulum of intestinal epithelial cells. Molecules of triglycerides then organize into minute fat droplets, which contain small amounts of phospholipid and cholesterol and a protein-coated surface. These droplets, called *chylomicrons*, then pass out of the base of the epithelial cells and enter either the bloodstream or the lymphatic system. Approximately 80 to 90 percent of all fatty acids enter the bloodstream in the form of chylomicrons.

WATER ABSORPTION. Approximately 8 liters of water per day are absorbed from the small intestine into the portal blood. The greatest proportion of this absorption occurs in the jejunum. Water crosses the intestinal cell membrane by passing through the pores of this membrane. The rate of absorption is very great and probably is enhanced by glucose and oxygen. Therefore, active transport may increase water absorption through shifting of other ions.

ELECTROLYTE ABSORPTION. Further water is absorbed in the large intestine. Electrolytes, like water, must cross the intestinal cell membrane by passing through its pores or by utilizing a membrane carrier. Like water, electrolytes are absorbed primarily into the portal blood rather than into the lymphatic system, and a greater absorption rate in the proximal rather than the distal portion of the small bowel is evident. Monovalent electrolytes such as sodium, chloride, potassium, nitrate, and bicarbonate are more easily absorbed than polyvalent electrolytes such as calcium, magnesium, and sulfate.

Most of the *sodium* is absorbed in the jejunum with less being absorbed in the ileum and the colon. The mechanism for this is active transport of sodium from the epithelial cells into the intercellular spaces. This requires a carrier and energy. Increased sodium concentration in the intercellular spaces creates an osmotic gradient for water, which follows the sodium passively. Both sodium and water are finally absorbed into the capillaries of the villi.

Chloride passively moves through the membranes of the duodenum and jejunum. It is actively transported in the large bowel where it is exchanged in close relationship to bicarbonate ions in order to neutralize any acid products in the large intestine.

Potassium appears to move by a passive mechanism down an electrochemical gradient into the epithelial cells. No active transport mechanism for potassium has been demonstrated in the intestines [5].

Calcium is absorbed by active transport throughout the small intestine but most actively in the duodenum. There is increased solubility of calcium salts in the duodenal acid, rather than in the more alkaline medium seen lower in the intestines. The rate of calcium absorption is altered by the level of the parathyroid hormone in the blood (see Chap. 32). Vitamin D is important in the stimulation of the rate of intestinal absorption; is activated by a specific process in the kidney; and then functions to increase calcium absorption.

Most *iron* is absorbed in its ferrous form in the duodenum. An acid medium facilitates iron absorption. Iron uptake is an active process and is facilitated by *ascorbic acid*, which promotes the reduction of the ferric to the ferrous form of iron. The rate of iron absorption is extremely slow but increases when iron deficiency exists and decreases when there is an excessive dietary intake of iron.

The *vitamins* are absorbed primarily in the proximal intestine, except for vitamin B_{12}, which is absorbed in the ileum. Most vitamins are passively absorbed. Some vitamins are stored in the body and some need to be replenished on a regular basis. Vitamin B_{12} forms a complex with the intrinsic factor that, in the ileum, is bound to a specific, unknown receptor in the mucosa and, finally, is absorbed into the blood.

Secretion, Absorption, and Excretion in the Large Intestine

The large intestine functions mainly in the absorption of water, but it also has vital functions in the synthesis of vitamin K and some B-complex vitamins and in the formation and excretion of feces.

The movements of the large intestine are a part of the peristaltic activity initiated on the ingestion of food. The final movement of the large intestine is the *mass peristalsis*, which drives the digested waste material into the rectum. This usually occurs 3 to 4 times per day. The glands of the lining of the large intestine secrete mucus that functions to lubricate the material and protect the lining of the bowel.

Active bacteria in the bowel ferment any remaining carbohydrate and release hydrogen, carbon dioxide, and methane gas and break proteins down into amino acids. The end result of this activity is to give fecal material its odor.

Water (1800–3000 ml) is absorbed daily in the large intestine, along with a few electrolytes. This absorption regulates the consistency of the feces and provides for final water balance in the gastrointestinal system.

Defecation is the process of emptying the rectum and is initiated by distention of rectal walls. The external sphincter is under voluntary control and relaxes when the intraabdominal and intrathoracic pressure increases, pushing the fecal material outside of the body. Increased rectal and intraabdominal pressure may increase the vagal tone and reflexively decrease the heart rate.

REFERENCES

1. Guyton, A. *Textbook of Medical Physiology* (6th ed.). Philadelphia: Saunders, 1981.
2. Jensen, D. *The Principles of Physiology* (2nd ed.). New York: Appleton-Century-Crofts, 1980.
3. McGuigan, J. Peptic Ulcer. In K.J. Isselbacher, et al. (eds.), *Harrison's Principles of Internal Medicine* (9th ed.). New York: McGraw-Hill, 1980.
4. Spiro, H.M. *Clinical Gastroenterology* (2nd ed.). New York: Macmillan, 1977.
5. Tortora, G., Evans, R.L., and Anagnostakos, N. *Principles of Human Physiology.* Hagerstown, Md.: Harper & Row, 1982.

CHAPTER 35
ALTERATIONS IN GASTROINTESTINAL FUNCTION

DISEASES OF THE ORAL CAVITY
- Alterations in the Gums and Teeth
- Oral Mucosal Changes

ESOPHAGEAL ALTERATIONS
- Achalasia
- Gastroesophageal Reflux and Esophagitis
- Hiatal Hernia
- Esophageal Varices
- Carcinoma of the Esophagus

ALTERATIONS IN THE STOMACH AND DUODENUM
- Gastritis
  - *Acute Gastritis*
- Stress Ulcers
- Peptic Ulceration
  - *Gastric Ulcers*
  - *Duodenal Ulcers*
- Gastric Carcinoma

ALTERATIONS IN THE SMALL INTESTINE
- Celiac Disease
  - *Celiac Sprue*
  - *Tropical Sprue*
- Regional Enteritis: Crohn's Disease
- Enteritis

ALTERATIONS IN THE LARGE INTESTINE
- Adynamic or Paralytic Ileus
- Intestinal Obstruction
- Hernias
- Congenital Megacolon or Hirschsprung's Disease
- Diverticula
- Hemorrhoids
- Ulcerative Colitis
- Polyps
- Carcinoma of the Colon

LEARNING OBJECTIVES

1. List the major sources of inflammation of the gums.
2. Define *hamartomatous lesions* of the oral mucosa.
3. Describe the anatomic and functional changes occurring with achalasia.
4. Outline the mechanism for mucosal damage that occurs with esophagitis.
5. List at least two diagnostic procedures that will demonstrate reflux.
6. Describe pathophysiologically a rolling hiatal hernia and a sliding hiatal hernia.
7. Trace the development of esophageal varices.
8. Classify the most common morphologic form of carcinoma of the esophagus.
9. Differentiate between acute gastritis and chronic gastritis.
10. Differentiate the types of peptic ulcerations according to underlying etiology, symptomatology, and relationship to malignancy.
11. Briefly describe the pathology of gastric carcinoma.
12. Describe the pathologic changes that result in malsorption in celiac and tropical sprue.
13. Differentiate between regional enteritis and ulcerative colitis on the basis of etiology, pathology, symptomatology, and course of the disease.
14. Define *adynamic* or *paralytic ileus.*
15. Distinguish between paralytic ileus and bowel obstruction.
16. Define *reducible, incarcerated,* and *strangulated hernia.*
17. Describe the condition called Hirschsprung's disease.
18. Explain why diverticula are commonly seen in elderly persons.
19. List some common conditions that can cause the development of hemorrhoids.
20. List some ways that the American diet may cause carcinoma of the colon.
21. Differentiate between the pathology and symptomatology of carcinoma of the colon arising in different areas of the colon.

DISEASES OF THE ORAL CAVITY

Alterations in the Gums and Teeth

The gums, or *gingiva*, are subject to localized inflammatory diseases or they may react to other systemic diseases or drug therapy. *Gingivitis*, inflammation of the borders surrounding the teeth, may result in pain, bleeding, and destruction of gingival tissue. When this inflammation spreads to the underlying tissues, the bones, or the roots of the teeth, it is called *peridontitis*. This destructive disease state may result in purulent drainage and loss of teeth.

Overgrowth of the gingiva is seen in persons having long-term treatment with phenantoin (Dilantin). Hormonal and metabolic conditions may cause an increased inflammatory response, with enlarged gingiva noted especially at puberty, during pregnancy, and with such conditions as leukemia and thrombocytopenia.

Oral Mucosal Changes

The appearance of changes in the oral mucosa often reflects systemic changes in the body. A variety of conditions may cause changes in the oral mucosa and the manifestations vary. For example, in scarlet fever the tongue becomes bright red (strawberry tongue), while in *Candida albicans* (thrush) localized white lesions of the oral mucosa are seen.

Tumors of the oral mucosa are uncommon but are much like skin tumors, except that many of the tumorous growths are benign, so-called hamartomatous lesions, rather than true growing lesions [9]. The salivary glands may also develop tumorous growths of a benign or malignant nature.

ESOPHAGEAL ALTERATIONS

Although many conditions affect esophageal motility and secretion, only the major alterations are reviewed in this section.

Achalasia

Achalasia is a disorder of esophageal motility (see Fig. 35-1). The combination of decreased peristalsis along with constriction of the lower esophageal sphincter characterize the condition. Degeneration of the myenteric ganglion cells in the esophagus and alterations in vagal tone apparently are the precipitating causes of the disorder. The esophagus becomes distended and may retain several liters of fluid.

This uncommon condition becomes chronic and slowly progressive, causing dysphagia, vomiting, nausea, and weight loss. Lung changes, related to repeated episodes of nocturnal aspiration, may be associated. The amount of swallowing difficulty in the early stages is increased by stress and anxiety. Increasing dysphagia results, and finally even liquids become difficult to swallow.

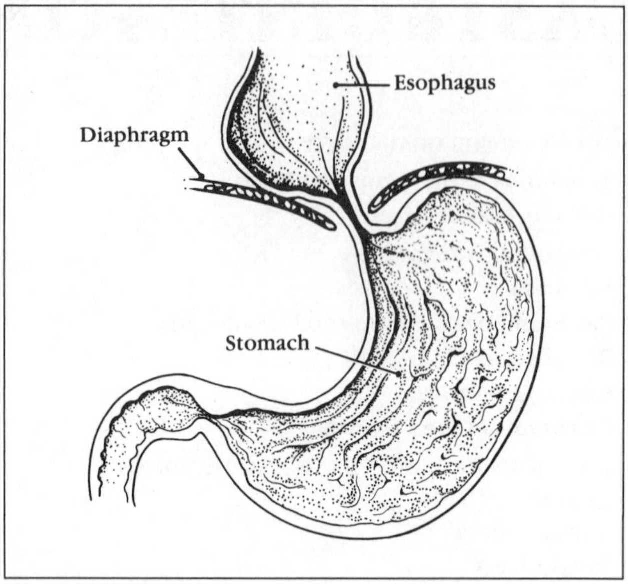

FIGURE 35-1. Schematic representation of location and appearance of achalatic esophagus.

Diagnostic tests usually include a barium swallow that reflects a normally functioning pharynx and cricoesophageal sphincter, but after a few centimeters, peristaltic action stops or decreases to ineffectual motions. The distended, nonemptying lower esophagus is easily visualized as a pouch that narrows into the esophageal-gastric junction (see Fig. 35-2). Although the lower esophageal sphincter does not open in response to swallowing, it may open slightly as food moves into the area and allow some contents to pass through. Frequent follow-up examinations are required because there is a statistical increase in incidence of esophageal carcinoma in these persons. Surgical intervention may be required to decrease the amount of obstruction.

Gastroesophageal Reflux and Esophagitis

Gastroesophageal reflux is the movement of gastric contents into the esophagus. Normally, the lower esophageal sphincter pressure prevents backflow, or secondary peristalsis will move gastric contents from the esophageal mucosa before damage occurs. An incompetent lower esophageal sphincter causing reflux esophagitis is believed to be the primary cause of this condition. Other causes of esophagitis include prolonged gastric intubation, ingestion of corrosive chemicals, uremia, infections, mucosal alterations, and systemic diseases such as systemic lupus erythematosus [9].

Esophagitis, inflammation of the esophageal mucosa, most frequently results from gastroesophageal reflux that may be due to prolonged vomiting or an incompetent lower esophageal sphincter. The mucosal damage is related to the contact time between the esophageal mucosa and

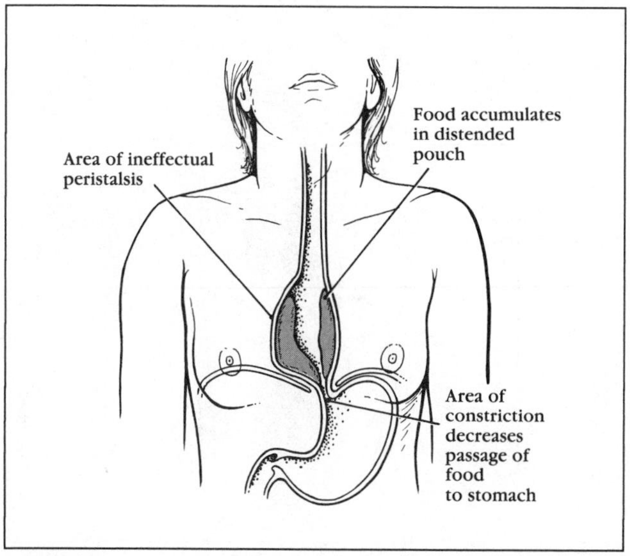

FIGURE 35-2. Nonemptying or poorly emptying lower esophagus resulting from achalasia.

gastric contents, as well as the acidity and quantity of the gastric secretions.

Gastric hydrochloric acid alters the pH of the esophagus and permits mucosal protein denaturation. The pepsin in the gastric secretion has proteolytic properties that are enhanced when the pH is around 2.0. The combination of pepsin and hydrochloric acid increases the capability for damage. Often increased bile salts are associated with the gastroesophageal reflux and act to enhance the effect of the hydrogen ion on the mucosa. This reflux has been shown to cause an inflammation that penetrates to the muscularis layer, resulting in a motor dysfunction and a decrease in esophageal clearance. The end result is increased esophageal contact time, further muscle damage, and an increased amount of reflux [2].

The most common symptoms of esophageal inflammation include heartburn, retrosternal discomfort, and the regurgitation of sour, bitter material. These symptoms are frequently precipitated by ingestion of large amounts of fatty, spiced foods and alcohol. The symptoms correlate with the amount and acidity of reflux. Dysphagia for both solids and liquids increases when severe obstruction occurs. Permanent strictures may develop that make food passage difficult. Irritation of the mucosa may cause bleeding and eventually produce an iron-deficiency anemia. Nocturnal reflux of material into the pharynx may lead to aspiration into the lungs.

Diagnosis is difficult but may be made on clinical, radiographic, and endoscopic appearances. The most effective test of reflux is to measure the pH in the esophagus after instilling 300 ml of hydrochloric acid into the stomach [5]. Biopsy will demonstrate inflammatory changes. Scintiscanning, which involves the swallowing of a radionucleotide, can demonstrate reflux by measuring radioactivity of the esophagus in serial scans.

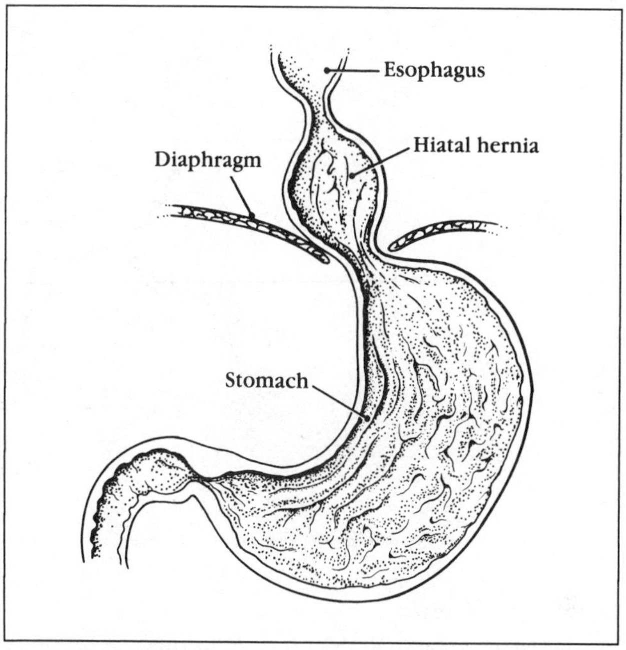

FIGURE 35-3. Schematic representation of location and appearance of hiatus hernia.

Hiatal Hernia

A hiatal hernia is a condition in which part of the stomach protrudes through the opening of the diaphragm (Fig. 35-3). This condition may be continuous or may occur sporadically. The continuous type is called a ***rolling hernia*** and occurs in fewer than 10 percent of persons with this condition. The sporadic type is called a ***sliding hernia*** and occurs in 80 to 90 percent of affected persons on changing position or with increased peristalsis. The stomach is forced through the opening of the diaphragm and moves back to the normal position when the subject assumes an upright position. This type of hernia may be associated with a congenitally short esophagus or may be seen secondarily to postgastritis scarring.

Many patients with hiatal hernia exhibit no symptoms. Symptoms such as heartburn, gastric regurgitation, dysphagia, and indigestion are accentuated by the postprandial supine position, overeating, physical exertion, or sudden changes of posture.

Radiographic diagnosis reveals a hernia. A test to determine the presence of reflux of gastrointestinal material into the esophagus includes instillation of hydrochloric acid into the stomach. When reflux does not occur, the hiatal hernia is considered to be of little clinical importance, and the person usually remains asymptomatic.

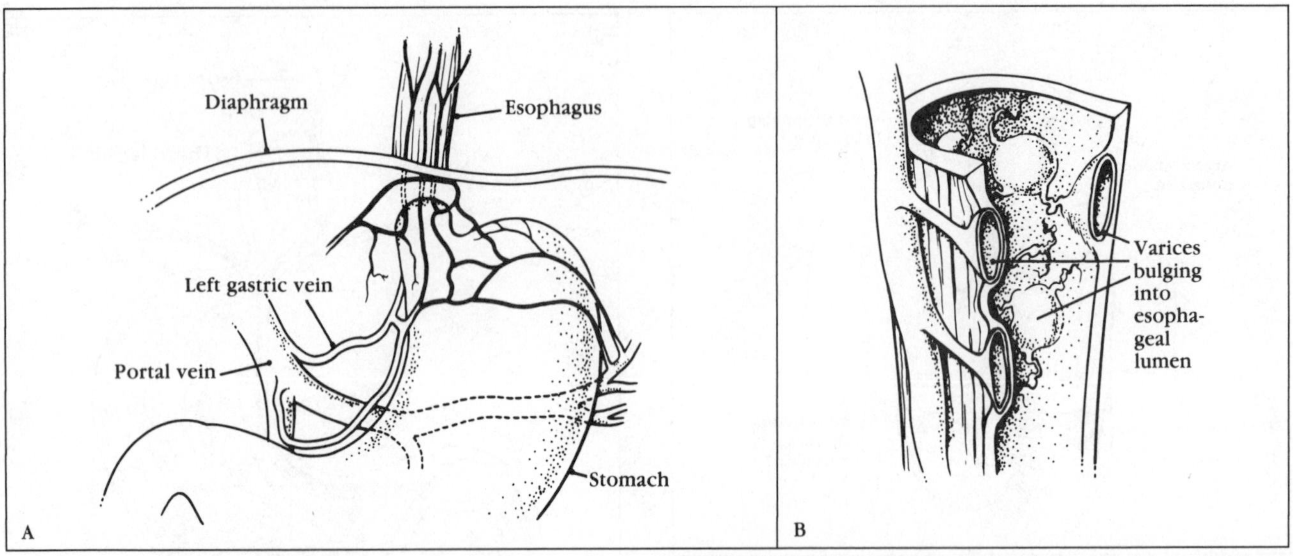

FIGURE 35-4. A. Venous plexus around the esophagus. B. Dilated venous channels from portal hypertension. These varices bulge into the lumen of the esophagus and rupture easily.

Esophageal Varices

Presented in greater detail on p. 524, this condition is closely related to portal hypertension and involves protrusion of the esophageal veins into the esophageal lumen (Fig. 35-4). The distended, thin-walled veins become subject to rupture, a catastrophic event that may occur spontaneously or after vomiting.

Rupture of these vessels creates a very large amount of bleeding into the gastrointestinal system and usually results in large-volume hematemesis. The first bleeding event causes a 40 percent mortality in afflicted persons. Subsequent bleeding events are equally catastrophic [9].

Carcinoma of the Esophagus

About 10 percent of malignancies of the gastrointestinal tract arise in the esophagus; these usually remain asymptomatic until they become surgically unresectable. This type of malignancy usually occurs after the age of 50 and more than 80 percent occur in males. A strong correlation between heavy alcohol intake, cigarette smoking, and esophageal carcinoma has been recorded in the literature [1].

The squamous cell carcinoma is the most common morphologic form. The malignancy may grow around the esophagus at the level of the diaphragm, impinging on the lumen or the tube, or it may cause a bulky, ulcerating tumor mass. The greatest percentage of tumors are located in the middle and lower third of the esophagus.

This disease state is usually asymptomatic for long periods, with the earliest complaint being a mild dysphagia that becomes progressive. Postprandial regurgitation may motivate the affected person to seek medical assistance. Weight loss is a common complaint, but hematemesis and guaiac-positive stools are relatively uncommon. Invasion of surrounding structures may result in back pain, and pressure on respiratory structures may cause varying degrees of respiratory distress.

Definitive diagnosis is through esophagoscopy with biopsy of the tumorous mass. Other diagnostic measures such as barium swallow, chest x ray, and blood tests give additional information.

ALTERATIONS IN THE STOMACH AND DUODENUM

Gastritis

This general term refers to an inflammation of the gastric mucosa that may occur in the presence of an excess of or a complete absence of gastric acid secretion. The classification of *acute* or *chronic gastritis* describes the onset and course of the disease. Chronic gastritis may also be associated with gastric mucosal atrophy, achlorhydria, and peptic ulcerations.

ACUTE GASTRITIS. This form of gastritis is associated with transient inflammation of the gastric mucosa, mucosal hemorrhages, and erosion into the mucosal lining. Acute gastritis is frequently associated with alcoholism, aspirin ingestion, smoking, and severely stressful encounters, such as trauma, burns, central nervous system damage, chemotherapy, or radiation therapy. Erosion of the gastric mucosa can result in a massive gastric hemorrhage. Therefore, acute gastritis may be associated with discomfort or serious outcomes.

Stress Ulcers

When gastric erosions occur, they are multiple and superficial and are found in large areas of the gastric mucosa.

Gastric acid secretion is usually increased, and the erosions often localize in the acid-secreting portion of the stomach. Two mechanisms for production of stress ulcers have been proposed: (1) Mucosal ischemia, relating to lack of blood supply to the gastric mucosa in the poststress period, results from a sympathetic vasoconstrictive action. (2) Enhanced back diffusion of hydrogen ions occurs due to an increased sensitivity of the disrupted gastric mucosa to hydrochloric acid and pepsin. Disruption of the surface mucosal cells occurs, and stimulation of the myenteric plexus leads to a hypersecretion of gastric acid and pepsinogen [4].

The major clinical manifestation of stress ulcers is massive, painless, gastric bleeding. This bleeding, from multiple sites in the gastric mucosa, is very difficult to control. Because of the danger of bleeding following acute stress, preventive measures are routinely used to decrease hydrogen ion secretion and to neutralize gastric acid.

Peptic Ulceration

Peptic ulcers are a group of ulcerative conditions of the gastrointestinal tract that result from an acid-pepsin imbalance. They are thought to develop when the aggressive proteolytic activities of the gastric secretions are greater than the normal protective abilities of these secretions. An increase in acid and pepsin from any cause may produce ulcerations if the protective mechanisms are not adequate. Major factors that alter the mucosal barrier are failure to regenerate the mucous epithelium at a sufficient rate, decrease in the quantity and quality of the mucus, and poor local mucosal blood flow. It has been suggested that vascular occlusion of small nutrient vessels in the mucosa or submucosa causes localized necrosis and subsequent ulcer formation. Peptic activity alone is not responsible for ulcerations; an individual susceptibility to ulceration is essential.

The most frequent site for peptic ulcers is the pyloric region of the duodenum, but ulcers also occur along the lesser curvature of the stomach and in other areas of the stomach (Fig. 35-5). Duodenal ulcers comprise 80 percent of all peptic ulcers. They are 4 times more common than gastric ulcers. Because ulcerative conditions are very common, affecting approximately 10 to 15 percent of the general population, further detail is provided in the subsequent material.

GASTRIC ULCERS. The primary problem with gastric ulcers appears to be a decreased resistance of the gastric mucosa to substances ingested. There is usually a normal or reduced level of hydrochloric acid secretion. True *achlorhydria*, or lack of hydrochloric acid secretion, is rarely seen with these ulcers and when present usually signifies that a gastric carcinoma is present. Because gastric ulcers are often seen in conjunction with gastric atrophy, the secretions may contain mostly water and small amounts of mucus. The intrinsic factor may not be secreted, causing decreased absorption of vitamin B_{12} and *pernicious anemia*.

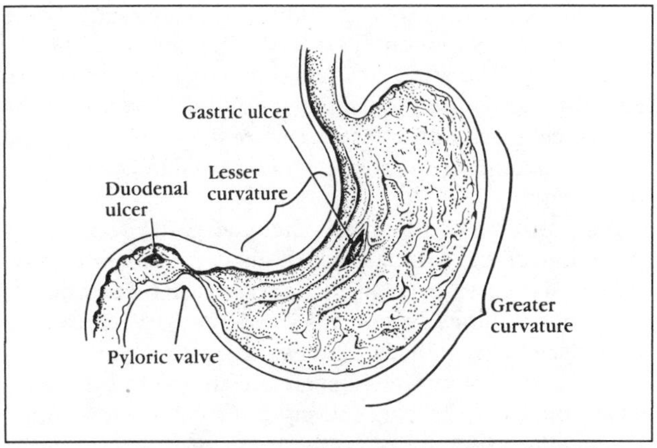

FIGURE 35-5. Common locations for gastric and duodenal ulcers.

Pathologically, gastric ulcers are often associated with atrophy of the gastric glands. Gastritis always surrounds the ulcerated area, which supports the theory that this disease is of an inflammatory nature. The classic ulcer has a sharply punched-out appearance with a smooth, clean base. The mucosa surrounding the ulcers is often edematous. Bleeding may be present if the ulceration erodes through a vessel. Gastric ulcers may be malignant and exhibit a shaggy, necrotic base, as opposed to the smooth base of the nonmalignant ulcer. The incidence of gastric ulcers transforming into malignant ulcers is significant enough to call gastric ulcers "premalignant" and to encourage frequent follow-up in this condition.

Diagnosis of gastric ulcers can be made by a barium upper gastrointestinal series and a direct endoscopy. Benign ulcers frequently localize on the greater curvature of the stomach and are usually smaller than the malignant lesions. If there is associated achlorhydria the ulcer is almost always malignant.

The most common symptom with gastric ulcer disease is epigastric pain. The pain may or may not be relieved by eating or it may be precipitated when food is ingested. Nausea, vomiting, and weight loss are common. Hemorrhage occurs in approximately 25 percent of these cases and is often profound. Perforation of the ulcer into the peritoneal cavity is less frequent than with the duodenal ulcer. Healing and recurrence is common, with lack of healing or failure to decrease in size suggesting gastric malignancy. Healing, with a decrease in the size of the ulcer by 50 percent, should occur in 3 months or less following initiation of therapy [8].

DUODENAL ULCERS. Multiple causes and predisposing factors have been shown that, in combination, upset the balance between the protective mechanism and the acid-pepsin proteolytic action in the duodenal wall. Duodenal ulcers occur in the presence of acid but hyperacidity is not always a significant component. Persons with excessive acid secretion may have an excess secretion of gastrin or gastrin-like substances from the duodenal wall, as well as from the parietal cells. Strong familial history of the disease and type O blood grouping support a genetic weakness theory in this disease.

The emotional factors that increase gastric secretions and influence the pathogenesis of duodenal ulcerations often are shown to precipitate the onset or recurrence of symptoms. Studies have been conducted to identify an ulcer personality, but the findings have not been conclusive [11]. Endocrine factors, such as estrogen and the adrenal steroids, may be contributing factors to the formation of ulcerations.

Duodenal ulcers are usually deep, having a sharp line of demarcation from uninvolved tissue. Most of these ulcerations occur in the first portion of the duodenum, close to the pylorus. The injury to the integrity of the mucosal wall caused by the acid-pepsin imbalance penetrates the entire thickness of the mucosal membrane, including the muscularis mucosa. Healing requires the formation of granulation tissue and scar. Secretory cellular functions are lost in the area of scarring.

A typical duodenal ulcer is a round or oval-shaped, indurated funnellike lesion that extends into the muscularis layer. Duodenal ulcers are frequently found within 1 to 3 cm of the pyloric junction, on either the anterior or posterior wall.

Acute ulcerations may develop on chronic ulcers, and perforations through the duodenal wall in active ulcers results in peritonitis. Erosion of an artery or a vein located at the base of the lesion may cause a hemorrhage. The amount of a hemorrhage depends on the vessel involved, and the effects are related to the rapidity and amount of blood loss.

Scar formation may cause deformity, shortening and stiffening of the duodenum, which may interfere with normal emptying of the stomach. Actual obstruction may result from the stenosis, from spasm, or from edema and/or inflammation.

Clinical manifestations of duodenal ulcerations include a documented pattern of symptoms characterized by remissions and exacerbations of varying periods of time. An attack is frequently triggered by a stressful situation of some nature, and exacerbations have been observed to occur more frequently in the fall and spring seasons.

There is a definite pain-food-relief pattern characteristic of duodenal ulcer. Pain usually develops 90 minutes to 3 hours after eating, often waking the person at night. This pain is immediately relieved by food or antacids. Pain on awakening in the early morning is rare and is thought to be due to decreased gastric secretions [4]. The pain is usually described as steady, boring, burning, aching, or hungerlike, and is localized in the midepigastrium, the right epigastric area, or sometimes in the back. The mechanism of pain in duodenal ulcers is thought to be related to irritation of exposed sensory nerve endings by hydrochloric acid. The pain may result from increased motility or spasm of the muscles at the ulcer site. Rarely, pain is not described and the ulcer is discovered when complications arise.

Other gastrointestinal symptoms include heartburn and regurgitation of sour juice into the back of the mouth. Anorexia is not a usual complaint because the individual seeks relief of pain through eating. Rupture of a duodenal ulcer may occur because of erosion through the duodenal wall and this leads to contamination of the peritoneal cavity. Hemorrhage, as in gastric ulcer disease, may lead to profound blood loss and hypovolemic shock; a slowly bleeding ulcer may be detected by guaiac-positive stools. Localized tenderness around the epigastric area is the only common physical finding on physical examination.

Diagnosis of duodenal ulcerations requires a reliable and accurate history of the characteristic pain. X-ray and fluoroscopic examinations with barium swallow demonstrate ulcer craters and niches as well as outlet deformities. Gastric endoscopy, a direct visualization of the gastric mucosa through a lighted scope, is useful in revealing lesions too small or superficial to be seen on x-ray examination. Tissue for histologic studies may also be taken during the procedure. Gastric juice analysis is especially helpful in persons not presenting typical duodenal ulcer disease to determine the cycle of hydrochloric acid and pepsin secretion. A basal acid output and a maximal histamine stimulation analysis may be done. A basal acid output measures the acidity of gastric secretions without a known or intentional stimulation. Achlorhydria, after histamine stimulation, demonstrates a loss of secretory function and is almost never seen with duodenal ulcerations. A 12-hour nocturnal test provides information regarding secretion during a prolonged basal state. Nocturnal hydrochloric acid and pepsin are higher in persons with duodenal ulcers than in those with gastric ulcers. Zollinger-Ellison syndrome exhibits very high measurements of gastric acid secretion (see Chap. 33). All of the therapeutic approaches for duodenal ulcer disease are directed toward pain relief, promotion of healing, and prevention of complications. Recognition of life-style and factors that precipitate symptoms may assist the individual to comply with therapy and thus help prevent the recurrence of the disease.

Gastric Carcinoma

Ninety to 95 percent of all malignancies of the stomach are classified as carcinomas. The incidence of this malignancy has been steadily declining over the past few decades in the United States, but several countries, especially Japan, Iceland, and Finland, have high incidences. Apparently the development of this malignancy is declining as well in the high-risk countries [7]. Survival rates are poor, with less than 10 percent of those affected surviving for 5 years after diagnosis.

Diet has been implicated in the causation of gastric carcinoma, especially in regard to the nitrates that are used as food preservatives. These convert to nitrites, which convert to nitrosamine, a well-known carcinogen [9].

Genetic or familial linkage is supported by an increased risk among families and the preponderance of blood group A. Gastric carcinoma also affects an older population and is seen associated with atrophic gastritis or polyps of the stomach. Pathologically, carcinomas of this type may arise anywhere on the mucosal surface. Large masses and/or polypoid tumors may grow and cause obstruction to the pyloric outlet. Ulceration may occur, exhibiting a shaggy, necrotic-appearing base. A diffuse form of carcinoma has been identified that causes thickening of the entire stomach wall, the so-called leather-bottle stomach. Distant metastasis is frequent; the sites most often selected are the liver, lungs, ovaries, and peritoneum. These metastases are often present at the time of diagnosis.

The clinical manifestations are often vague and nonspecific, including weight loss, abdominal pain, loss of appetite, vomiting, change in bowel habits, anemia, and guaiac-positive stools. Massive hemorrhage may cause hemorrhagic shock.

The only definitive diagnostic test is gastric biopsy. This is usually obtained through gastric endoscopy and biopsy. Other studies may be helpful; these include a barium study, blood work, and demonstrations of a mass in the gastric area.

ALTERATIONS IN THE SMALL INTESTINE

Most of the events of nutrient absorption go on in the small intestine. Any alteration of the integrity of the small bowel can result in malsorption, whether the source of alteration is motor or mucosal.

Malsorption refers to the inadequate absorption of ingested nutrients and water. Table 35-1 presents an outline of some of the major causes of malsorption. It can be seen that malsorption can be caused by many mechanisms and that the categories are not entirely separate. In other words, many disorders can cause malsorption through multiple mechanisms. Several of the more common disease conditions are discussed in this section. Other related conditions are presented in Chapter 37. Table 35-2 contains a summary of the major laboratory tests commonly used to detect malsorption.

Celiac Disease

CELIAC SPRUE. This disease has many names and is thought to be related to a genetic defect resulting in gluten intolerance. The incidence is greater in women than in men and the onset of symptoms usually occurs in young adulthood.

Histopathologic changes in the absorptive surface in response to exposure to the protein gluten or its breakdown products, found mostly in wheat, are responsible for the

TABLE 35-1. Causes of malsorption

- Incomplete digestion of nutrients
  - Pancreatic insufficiency
  - Primary—deficient production of pancreatic enzymes
    - Chronic relapsing pancreatitis
    - Cancer of the pancreas
    - Cystic fibrosis
    - Extensive pancreatic resection
  - Secondary—defective utilization of pancreatic enzymes
    - Post–Billroth II
    - Zollinger-Ellison syndrome
  - Deficiency of conjugated bile salts
  - Impaired synthesis or release
    - Severe liver disease
    - Extrahepatic biliary tract obstruction
  - Abnormal loss
    - Ileal resection
    - Ileectomy
    - Ileal bypass
    - Severe disease of the terminal ileum
  - Accelerated deconjugation by bacterial overgrowth
    - Surgically created blind loops
    - Fistulas—enteroenteric, enterocolic, gastrojejunocolic
    - Chronic intestinal obstruction due to adhesions or strictures
    - Small bowel diverticula
    - Motor abnormalities except scleroderma
  - Drug-induced precipitation or sequestration
    - Neomycin
    - Calcium carbonate
    - Cholestyramine
  - Inadequate mechanical mixing of chyme with digestive enzymes
  - Post–Billroth II
  - Post–total gastrectomy
- Abnormalities of the absorptive surface
  - Biochemical or genetic
    - Disaccharidase deficiency
    - Abetalipoproteinemia
    - Primary vitamin B_{12} malabsorption
    - Cystinuria
    - Hartnup disease
    - Celiac sprue
  - Inflammatory or infective disorders
    - Tropical sprue
    - Regional enteritis
    - Eosinophilic enteritis
    - Infectious enteritis
- Lack of absorptive surface
  - Intestinal resection
  - Gastroileostomy
- Lymphatic obstruction
  - Whipple's disease
  - Intestinal lymphangiectasia
  - Lymphoma
- Cardiovascular disorder
  - Mesenteric vascular insufficiency
  - Congestive heart failure
  - Constrictive pericarditis
- Endocrine and metabolic disorders
  - Diabetes mellitus
  - Hypoparathyroidism
  - Adrenal insufficiency
  - Hyperthyroidism
  - Carcinoid syndrome

TABLE 35-2. Laboratory tests specific to the detection of malsorption

Test	Normal finding	Meaning of abnormal findings
Fecal fat balance: quantitative determination of stool fat	6 (or fewer) gm of fatty acids extracted from stool in 24 hours	More than 6 gm/24 hours — clinically significant steatorrhea
D-xylose tolerance test	4 gm (or more) D-xylose excreted via the kidneys in 5 hours; or 20 mg (or more) D-xylose/dl of blood in 1–2 hours	Decreased values are found in diseases of the intestinal mucosa and in intestinal stasis; values are normal in pancreatic insufficiency
Schilling test	Greater than 7% of the radioactive vitamin B_{12} is excreted in the urine in 24 hours	Decreased value can indicate (1) lack of intrinsic factor, (2) competition by bacteria, (3) disease of the ileum
With administration of intrinsic factor		Decreased — (2) or (3) above
After 2 weeks of antimicrobial therapy		Decreased — (1) or (3) above
Serum carotene	70 IU/dl of serum	Decreased with malsorption but may also be decreased due to dietary insufficiency or hepatic disease
14C Triolein absorption (breath test)	More than 3.5% of $^{14}CO_2$ appears in breath per hour (6 hr)	Correlates with chemical stool fat

manifestations of a general malsorption syndrome. The mechanism underlying this reaction is not known, but it is theorized that an enzyme deficiency or an autoimmune reaction is occurring. The enzyme deficiency hypothesis, or toxic theory, suggests that specific peptidases are missing either from the brush border or from the cytoplasm of the epithelial cells of the intestinal mucosa, and as a result, gluten is not effectively hydrolyzed to smaller peptides and amino acids. Studies have not demonstrated specific deficiencies and have, in fact, shown that although levels of peptic hydrolases and other brush border enzymes are depressed in untreated cases, they return to normal after treatment with a gluten-free diet [14].

The proposal that gluten or its metabolites initiate a hypersensitivity reaction in the intestinal mucosa is supported by the majority of evidence. Gluten proteins have been shown to have antigenic properties, and circulating antibodies to dietary gluten have been demonstrated in persons having active celiac sprue. The lamina propria of affected mucosa contains mononuclear leukocytes and plasma cells. Serum immunoglobulin levels show elevated levels of IgA with depressed levels of IgM, and corticosteroid therapy has been shown to improve both intestinal absorption and histologic appearance.

Regardless of cause, the mucosal changes are characteristic. The villi are flattened or absent; the epithelium is disorganized and consists of cuboidal rather than the normal columnar cells. The brush border is thickened and the lamina propria is infiltrated with inflammatory cells. Cytoplasmic changes include membrane disruption and rounded mitochondria. All of these changes result in malsorption with impairment of uptake and transport of the nutrients.

The clinical picture includes frequent, foul-smelling, steatorrheic stools. This means that the stools have a fatty or greasy appearance. Loss of body weight and malsorption of fat-soluble vitamins are common. Severe muscle wasting and hypoproteinemia may occur.

Treatment measures support the gluten hypersensitivity reaction in that a dramatic or delayed remission of symptoms occurs when barley, wheat, rye, and oats are removed from the diet. Restoration of the normal mucosal epithelium occurs and malsorption decreases.

TROPICAL SPRUE. This disease differs in etiology from celiac sprue but is usually characterized by identical mucosal changes in the small intestine. It probably results from nutritional and bacterial alterations and is seen in greater incidence in certain tropical areas. Because the mucosal lesions result in malsorption, the clinical picture closely resembles that of celiac sprue. Treatment with folic acid has been shown to be restorative in some cases and antibiotic therapy may be helpful.

Regional Enteritis: Crohn's Disease

This inflammatory disease most commonly affects the terminal ileum, but any portion of the gastrointestinal tract may become involved. The incidence of this chronic inflammatory disease is equal in males and females, is slightly higher in the Jewish race, and exhibits a familial predisposition. Onset is most common between the ages of 15 and 20, with a secondary peak between the ages of 55 and 60 [3].

In this disease, gross inspection of the affected bowel discloses shallow, longitudinal mucosal ulcers, long or short areas of stricture, and a cobblestone appearance of the mucosa (Fig. 35-6). This latter appearance results from interconnecting fissures that cut deeply into the intestinal wall and create islands of mucosa elevated by the existing transmural (full-wall thickness) inflammation and its accompanying edema. The bowel wall becomes congested, thickened, and rigid, with adhesions involving the periintestinal fat. Areas of involvement are localized and interrupted by areas of normal gut. Sometimes several segments of bowel are affected and are separated by normal bowel. These segments are called *skip lesions.* Fistulas to other

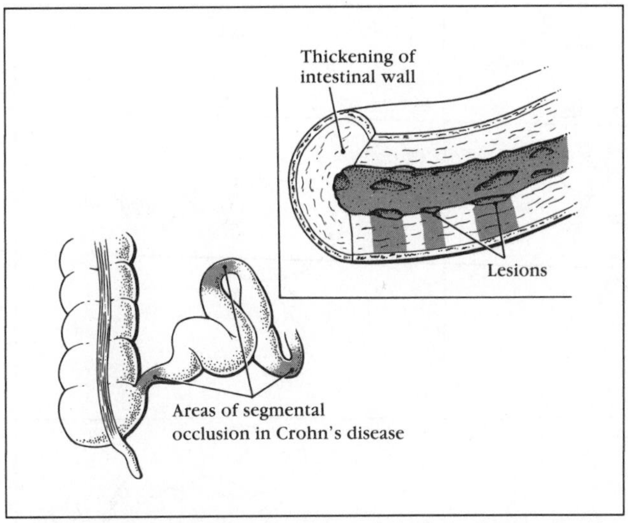

FIGURE 35-6. Schematic appearance of Crohn's disease showing segmental areas of occlusion and transmural involvement of the intestinal wall.

parts of the gastrointestinal tract or other adjacent structures may be present. Microscopically, all layers of the intestinal wall, particularly the submucosa, are edematous and infiltrated with aggregations of inflammatory cells [9]. Characteristic noncaseating granulomas, which have large mononuclear phagocytes and multinucleated giant cells, form in the bowel wall and often are seen in the regional lymph nodes. Dilatation of the lymphatic channels and lymphoid deposits are seen at all levels of bowel involvement.

The inflammatory changes cause functional disruption of the mucosa, producing malsorption, especially of bile salts and vitamin B_{12} whose absorption normally occurs in the jejunum and ileum. Fluid imbalances occur when large segments of ileum are affected.

The strictures and fistulas that occur with this disease predispose the intestine to bacterial overgrowth and abscess formation. Bowel obstruction and peritonitis may be the end result of the formation of strictures and abscesses.

The clinical manifestations of Crohn's disease are variable with diarrhea being a dominant symptom, often accompanied by fever and right lower quadrant or abdominal pain. The apparent linkage with stress and personality factors has been extensively studied with inconclusive results, except that depression and dependency are typical personality patterns. The clinical manifestations are variable, usually beginning with an insidious onset of malaise and diarrhea. As the disease progresses, weight loss, occult blood in the feces, and nausea and vomiting occur. Obstruction and ileus may occur. Fistulas develop in 10 to 15 percent of cases and peritonitis may result from rupture of the fistulous connection.

A significant correlation of this disease with several autoimmune diseases and with adenocarcinoma of the small bowel exists. The chronic debilitating nature of the disease may finally require bowel resection.

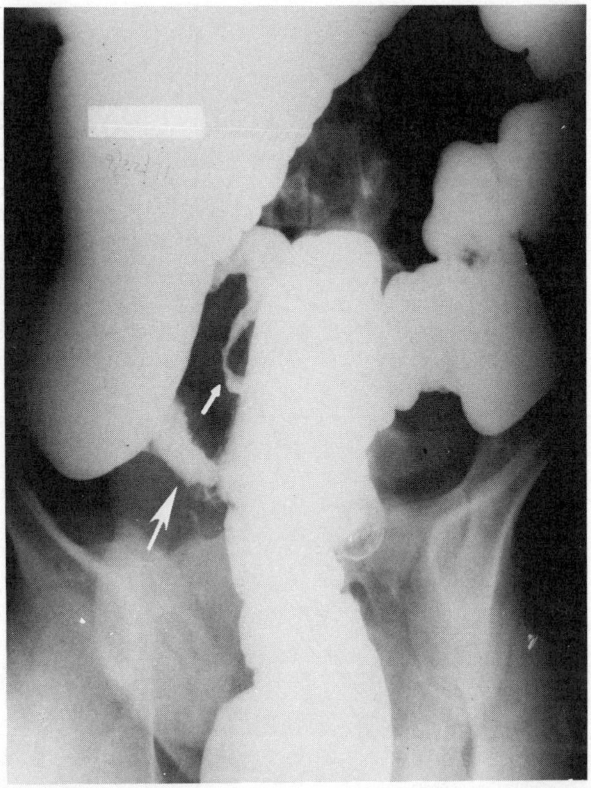

FIGURE 35-7. Crohn's disease. Radiograph of colon showing wide fistula (*larger arrow*) between cecum and sigmoid colon and irregularly narrowed distal ileum (*smaller arrow*). (From J. H. Stein [ed.], *Internal Medicine*. Boston: Little, Brown, 1983.)

Diagnosis of regional enteritis is based on the clinical history, physical examination (which may reveal a right lower quadrant mass), and characteristic radiologic studies. The "string sign" is commonly noted on radiologic studies (Fig. 35-7).

Enteritis

Enteritis, or gastroenteritis, is an inflammatory process that may affect the stomach or small intestine. This condition may be caused by viruses, bacteria, or allergic reactions. When it is due to an organism it may follow the ingestion of contaminated food, especially the contamination by the *Staphlococcus* organism, which produces a toxin that reacts with the small intestinal mucosa. Dysenteries caused by bacteria affect the colon. The pathologic process has varying manifestations that result in abdominal cramping, diarrhea, and vomiting. Fluid and electrolyte imbalance often results. Parasites may localize in the gastrointestinal tract or may invade the circulation. Eosinophilic enteritis is uncommon but may result from an allergy. It is manifested by the accumulation of eosinophils in the gut wall. In general, enteritis causes inflammatory changes in the intestinal mucosa that return to normal when the precipitator of the attack is removed.

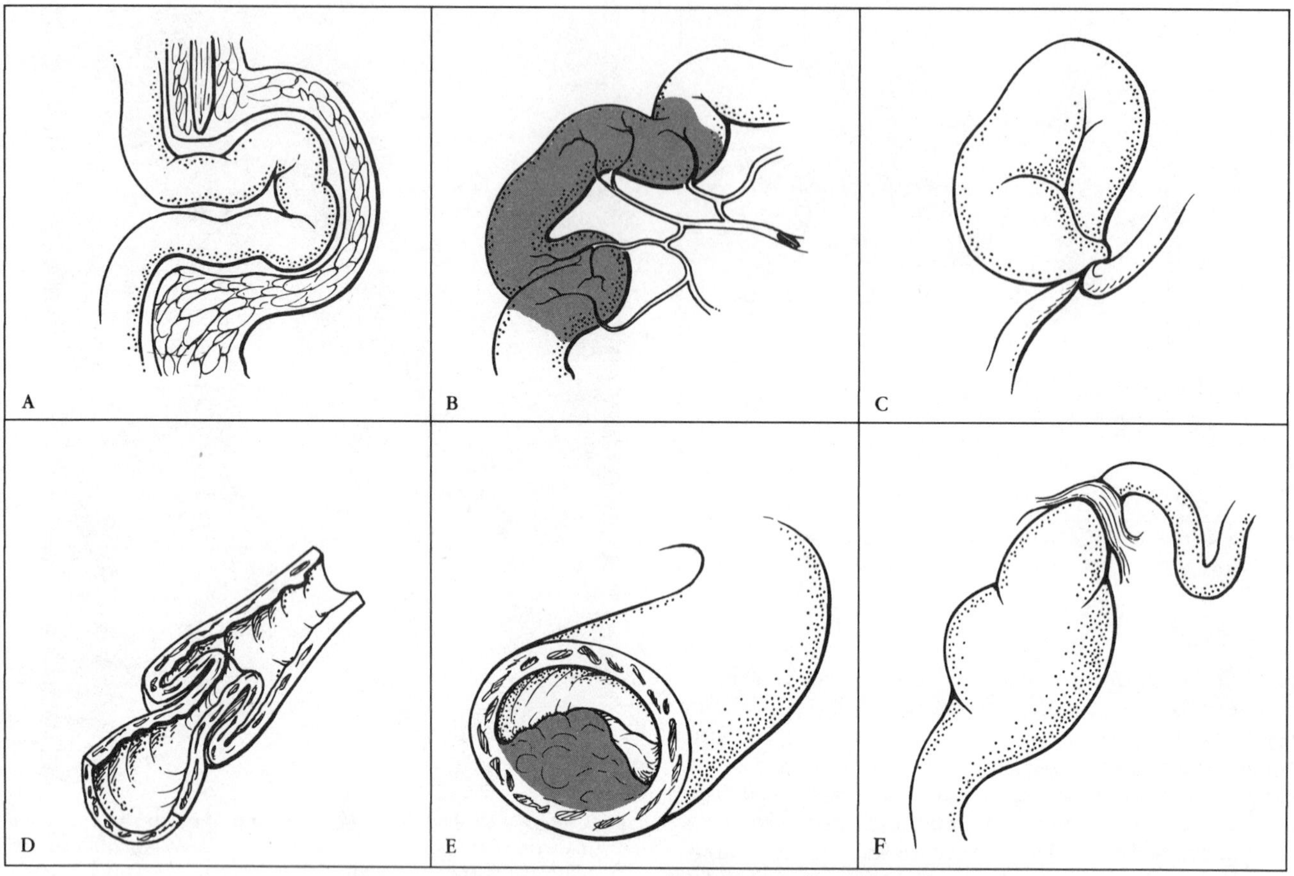

FIGURE 35-8. Illustration of major causes of actual intestinal obstruction. A. Hernia. B. Mesenteric occlusion. C. Volvulus. D. Intussusception. E. Neoplasm. F. Adhesions.

ALTERATIONS IN THE LARGE INTESTINE

Adynamic or Paralytic Ileus

The term *ileus* has come to refer to a functional obstruction of the bowel. Lack of propulsive peristalsis creates an inability to move bowel contents forward, which leads to an absence of bowel sounds and bowel distention. Ileus may be the result of anesthesia, interruption of nerve supply to the bowel, or an abdominal operation. Prolonged ileus may result from intestinal ischemia, abdominal wound infections, electrolyte disturbances, or certain metabolic diseases.

The result of ileus is distention of the bowel with gas and fluid. The process is similar to actual bowel obstruction. If there is associated mesenteric ischemia, necrosis and rupture of the bowel may occur, causing peritonitis. Certain medications, such as morphine and the anticholinergic drugs, have a depressant effect on the nerves of the myenteric plexus of the bowel and may produce an ileus or prolong gastrointestinal motility dysfunction postoperatively. Mesenteric ischemia also may be precipitated by the digitalis preparations, which have been shown to induce vasoconstriction.

Intestinal Obstruction

This term refers to the blockage of the lumen of the bowel by an actual mechanical obstruction. Figure 35-8 illustrates some causes of intestinal obstruction, which include foreign bodies, volvulus, adhesions, intussusception, hernias, ischemia, infarction, and neoplasms of the bowel.

Initially after blockage occurs, gas and air are the primary bowel distenders and the distention occurs proximal to the area of blockage. As the process continues, gastric, biliary, and pancreatic secretions pool. Water, electrolytes, and serum proteins also begin to accumulate in the area. Pooling and bowel distention decrease the circulating blood volume due to a so-called third space shift that moves water into the area proximal to the obstruction and thus decreases plasma volume. Bowel wall edema also interferes with the blood supply to the bowel tissue and depresses normal sodium transport in the mucosa (Fig. 35-9).

Strangulation of a bowel segment may cause bowel necrosis, perforation, and loss of fluid and blood into the inactive bowel. Impairment of blood supply leads at first to increased peristalsis and bacterial invasion of the tissue, finally causing necrosis and peritonitis when intestinal contents are released into the peritoneal cavity. Stasis of the in-

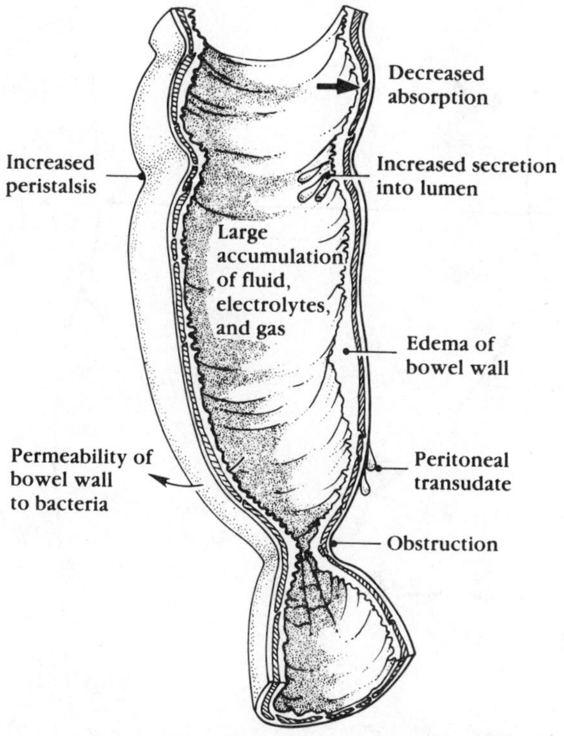

FIGURE 35-9. Pathophysiology of intestinal obstruction and peritonitis. (From P.A. Jones, C.F. Dunbar, and M.M. Jirovec, *Medical Surgical Nursing*. New York: McGraw-Hill, 1978.)

testinal contents provides an area for increased growth of organisms with toxins being released into the tissues, further disrupting the intestinal cellular dynamics. Loss of fluids and electrolytes is a major problem and results in a decreased systemic circulating fluid volume due to the shift from the vascular to the intestinal lumen.

The clinical manifestations include the acute onset of severe, cramping pain that correlates roughly to the area or level of obstruction. Pain may decrease in severity as the distention of the bowel and abdomen increases, which is probably due to impaired motility in the edematous intestine [10]. An increased rate and force of peristalsis causes loud, high-pitched bowel sounds (*borborygmi*) in the early onset period, but these may progress to a silent bowel as the condition persists. Vomiting is almost always present and may be bilious or feculent (having the appearance of feces) depending on the level of the obstruction. Diarrhea may occur if the obstruction is not complete.

Hypovolemic shock is the result of a fluid shift greater than 10 percent of body weight. This has been calculated to be about 700 ml in a person weighing 70 kg [12]. Septicemic shock may also result from contamination of the peritoneum when rupture of the bowel occurs.

Tenderness, rigidity, and fever are usually indicative of peritonitis. Leukocytosis and elevation of the serum amylase are also commonly seen. Distention of the bowel may be noted on x ray, but this does not give conclusive evidence of the cause or exact level of the obstruction.

Hernias

A hernia is a defect in the abdominal wall. It may occur in the scrotal or inguinal area or in the abdominal wall or diaphragm. Incisional hernias occur in a weakened area of a surgical incision. Whatever the cause, the defect allows abdominal structures (e.g., peritoneum, fat, bowel, or bladder) to fill the area, producing a sac filled with the abnormal material. The movement of the abdominal contents into the defect usually occurs when the abdominal pressure increases. If the bulging of the sac occurs intermittently, the hernia is termed a ***reducible hernia.*** ***Incarcerated hernias*** contain abdominal contents all the time, and ***strangulated hernias*** cause necrosis of the abdominal contents due to the lack of blood supply. Necrosis of the bowel then leads to all the clinical manifestations of intestinal obstruction. Figure 35-10 illustrates some of the locations where hernias may be seen.

Congenital Megacolon or Hirschsprung's Disease

This condition is usually manifested in early infancy and is caused by a congenital absence of parasympathetic ganglion cells in the submucosal and intramuscular plexus. Consequently, the bowel becomes greatly dilated with no peristaltic action in the aganglionic area. In megacolon, the aganglionic region remains contracted without reciprocal relaxation, and this produces a functional obstruction. The area most frequently affected is the rectosigmoid.

Hirschsprung's disease is a congenital disorder with a much higher incidence in males than in females. When manifested in early infancy, abdominal distention, constipation, and vomiting are seen. Occasionally this condition is diagnosed in young adults who describe a lifelong problem with constipation.

Megacolon, enlargement of the colon, may also be produced by any process that inhibits bowel evacuation. Among such processes are psychogenic megacolon, which results from ignoring the urge to defecate, some neurologic disorders, fecal impaction, or chronic depression.

The clinical manifestations depend on the degree of aganglionosis or bowel distention. The person is often poorly nourished, anemic, and rarely has production of fecal material. The congenital type is often associated with other anomalies such as Down's syndrome.

Diverticula

The term *diverticula* refers to multiple saclike protrusions of the mucosa along the gastrointestinal tract. Although the terms are loosely used, a *true diverticulum* has all layers of the bowel in its walls while a *false diverticulum* occurs in a weak area of the muscularis of the bowel.

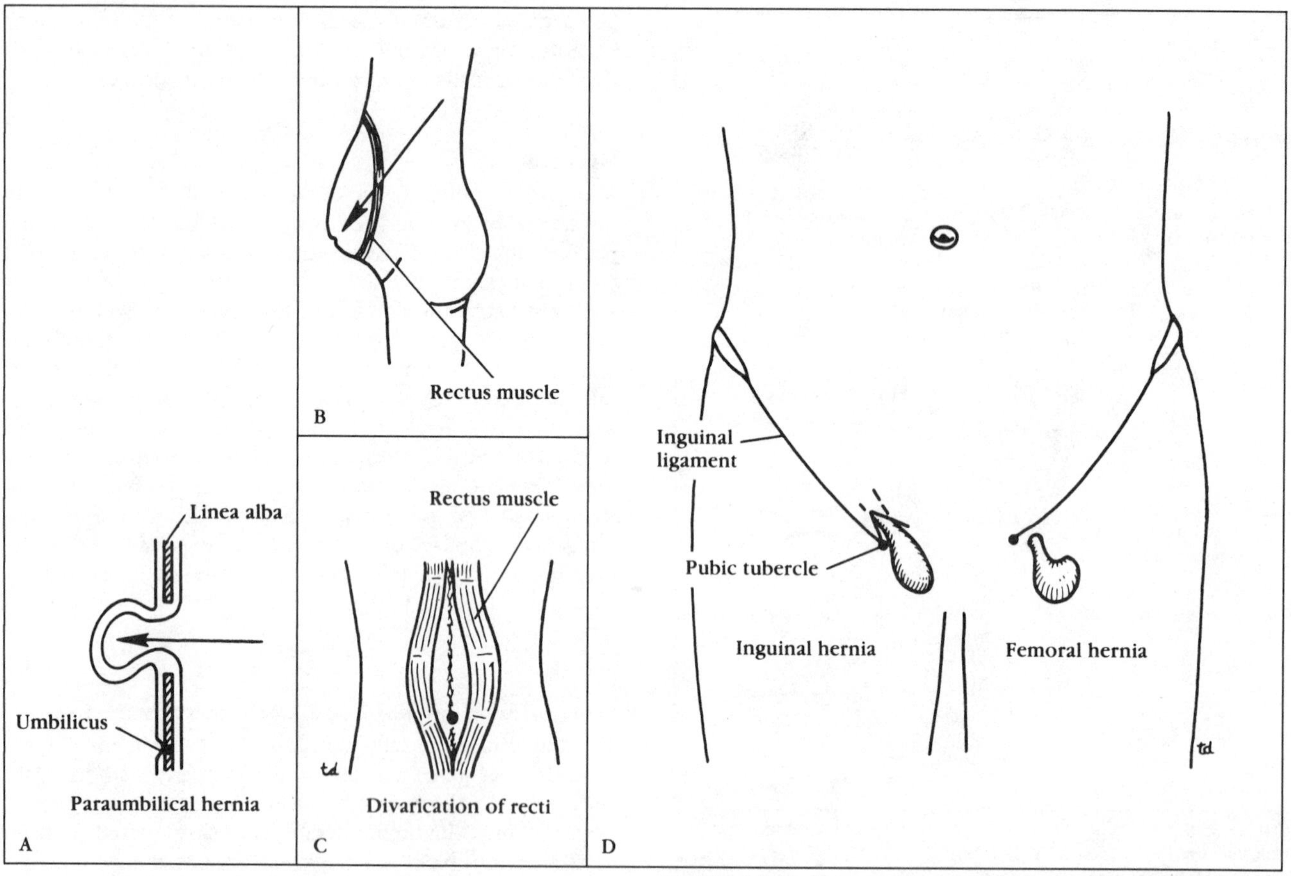

FIGURE 35-10. Types of hernias. A. Paraumbilical. B. Epigastric. C. Divarication of rectus abdominis. D. Inguinal and femoral. (From R. S. Snell, *Clinical Anatomy for Medical Students* [2nd ed.]. Boston: Little, Brown, 1981.)

An example of true diverticular disease is *Meckel's diverticulum,* found in 1 to 2 percent of the population. This sac, located 1 to 3 ft proximal to the ileocecal junction, is formed by persistence of a mesenteric structure that normally closes in fetal life [1]. It may be lined with ileal mucosa or contain other types of gastrointestinal mucosal cells. Complications include gastrointestinal bleeding and inflammation [3]. False colonic diverticula are common and occur most frequently in the sigmoid colon.

Because of the high incidence in elderly persons, it is thought that these weaknesses are related to the blood supply or nutrition of the bowel in the elderly. Lack of dietary fiber or roughage and decreased fecal bulk also have been correlated to this process.

Diverticulosis refers to the presence of diverticula in the colon that are rarely symptomatic. *Diverticulitis* refers to inflammation in or around a diverticular sac that results in the retention of undigested food and bacteria in the sac. This forms a hard mass called a *fecalith* [6]. Rupture of the infected material into the peritoneal cavity may result in peritonitis.

The clinical manifestations of symptomatic diverticular disease vary. Constipation is frequently reported. Fibrosis in the area may develop and cause obstruction by adhesions. The complaint of lower, left-sided abdominal pain may be associated with the signs of peritonitis. The signs of peritonitis include guarding, fever, abdominal rigidity, and rebound tenderness.

Diagnosis by x ray and sigmoidoscopy may not indicate the extent of the problem. Surgery may be performed if the process causes obstruction or perforation.

Hemorrhoids

This term refers to dilatations of the venous plexus that surround the rectal and anal areas. These dilatations are very common and develop in susceptible persons in relation to increased pressure in the venous plexus. Hemorrhoids are often related to other types of abnormalities, especially varicose veins. Predisposition to the disease may result from constipation or pregnancy; bleeding hemorrhoids may be a dangerous outcome of portal hypertension.

The dilated venous sacs protrude into the anal and rectal canals where they become exposed; thromboses, ulcerations, and bleeding develop. They may be painful and irritating. Bright bleeding during defecation or with increased intraabdominal pressure is common. Bleeding in association with portal hypertension may be very profound and even life-threatening (see Chap. 37). Usually, blood loss is insignificant but chronic anemia may be an outcome.

Ulcerative Colitis

This is primarily a disease of the mucous membrane of the colon. Purulent exudate and blood are common and the chronic inflammation may cause bleeding throughout the mucosa. The disease may be confined to the rectum or it may affect segments of the colon or even the entire colon. The bowel fills with a bloody, mucoid secretion that produces a characteristic cramping pain, rectal urgency, and diarrhea. The colon wall becomes thickened and edematous. The process is usually confined to the mucosal layer and rarely affects the muscularis.

Complications of ulcerative colitis include intestinal obstruction, dehydration, and major fluid and electrolyte imbalances. Malsorption is common and the loss of blood in the stools may cause a chronic, iron-deficiency anemia.

There is a significant relationship between ulcerative colitis and cancer of the colon. Ten to 15 percent of persons having ulcerative colitis for more than 10 years will develop colon carcinoma.

The etiology of ulcerative colitis is unknown but some genetic basis has been suggested because the disease occurs in increased incidence in certain families. Other agents such as viruses and specific microorganisms may be implicated and the disease is associated with autoimmune disease. The plasma serum in certain persons with the disease has been shown to have an antibody to the colonic epithelial cells. These factors have led to research into a possible autoimmune nature of this condition.

Clinical manifestations are variable and the disease has periods of remissions and exacerbations. The major classic symptoms include cramping abdominal pain, bloody diarrhea, fever, and weight loss. The affected person usually becomes debilitated. Laboratory findings include anemia, leukocytosis, hypoalbuminemia, electrolyte imbalance, and increased serum alkaline phosphatase. Despite the evident pathologic differences, ulcerative colitis and regional enteritis may be confused clinically. Table 35-3 shows the major differences between the two. Diagnosis of ulcerative colitis is on the basis of the clinical picture, the barium enema, and the sigmoidoscopic appearance of the mucosa.

TABLE 35-3. Major differences between ulcerative colitis and Crohn's disease

	Ulcerative colitis	Crohn's disease
Extent of disease	Mucosa	Entire wall
Ulceration	Extensive, superficial	Patchy, deep
Mesentery	Normal	Thickened
Lymph nodes	Normal	Diseased
Granulomata	Absent	Present (25–75%)
Distribution[a]	Symmetric	Eccentric
"Skip" areas	Never[b]	Common
Diseased rectum	Always[b]	10–20%
Small intestine disease	Never[b]	Usual
Results of surgery	Cure	Frequent recurrence

[a]Radiologically, the entire circumference of the colon is involved in ulcerative colitis, whereas in Crohn's disease only one side may be diseased.

[b]The words "always" and "never" should not be used to describe biologic processes, but here they are probably appropriate.

Source: B. N. Brooke, et al., *Crohn's Disease Aetiology, Clinical Manifestations and Management.* New York: Oxford University Press, 1977.

Polyps

A polyp in the large intestine is a benign growth that protrudes into the lumen of the bowel. The growth begins in the mucosa deep within the crypts of the colonic mucosal glands [9]. The polypoidal cells continue to divide and become hyperplastic growths. When reproductive control is lost throughout the mucosal crypt, a neoplasm results. Polyps are very common in the general population but rarely exceed 5 mm in diameter. The major clinical significance of hyperplastic polyps is that they have potential for becoming neoplastic or adenomatous polyps. Adenomatous polyps may be benign or malignant, and it is very difficult to determine the difference unless there is obvious invasion of the surrounding mucosa. Polyps are usually surgically excised because they have such a close relationship with carcinoma of the colon. In general, the larger the polyp, the greater the risk for malignancy [9]. These growths may be discovered by routine sigmoidoscopy or barium enema and may bleed, causing bright red feces.

Carcinoma of the Colon

This disease accounts for about 20 percent of all deaths due to cancer in the United States. Frequently associated with polyposis of the colon, carcinoma of the colon has a familial tendency and may be associated with dietary factors. Common in both men and women, this disease occurs at all ages but the incidence is greatest at the fifth, sixth, and seventh decades. The incidence is greatest in northwest Europe and North America and lowest in South America, Africa, and Asia.

Dietary investigations have led to the study of animal fat in the diet, anaerobic bacteria of the large bowel, and the fiber content of the diet [9]. Each of these factors may be a partial explanation of geographic differences. The fiber aspect is interesting in that increased bulk in the diet decreases the transit time and also the time of contact between food and bowel. In the average American diet, the transit time may be as much as 4 to 5 days compared to average transit time in African blacks of 30 to 35 hours [9].

The distribution of tumors in the colon is as follows: rectum, 35 percent; sigmoid, 25 percent; descending colon, 5 to 10 percent; and right colon, 10 to 15 percent [9]. The form of the growth depends on the area of origin. Left-sided carcinoma tends to grow around the bowel, encircling it and leading to early obstruction. On the right side, the tumors tend to grow as bulky, polypoid, fungating masses. Either type may penetrate the bowel, cause abscess, peritonitis, invasion of surrounding organs, or bleeding. These tumors do tend to grow slowly, but also remain asymptomatic for long periods of time. Ninety-five percent of carcinomas of the colon are adenocarcinomas that secrete mucin, a substance that tends to aid in the extension of the malignancy. Metastasis may occur to the liver, the lungs, bone, or lymphatic system.

Clinical manifestations depend on the location of the tumor. The affected person may have melena, diarrhea, and constipation; these are the most frequent manifestations of left-sided lesions. Right-sided tumors often cause weakness, malaise, and weight loss. Pain is rare with either type and the tumor mass often is palpated on physical examination. Obstruction of the bowel may be the first sign of the disease. Often at the time of diagnosis some extension of the tumor has occurred, but since the tumors grow slowly, this type of malignancy is considered to be highly curable with early diagnosis.

Diagnosis requires the standard techniques of proctoscopy, barium enema, radionucleotide scanning, and determination of the level of the carcinoembryonic antigen (CEA). This tumor antigen is positive in nearly 100 percent of cases with widespread metastases. The usefulness of the CEA test is being evaluated because normal levels do not rule out malignancy. It can be used to gauge the effectiveness of therapy. "Normal" levels of the CEA are less than 2.5 ng/ml, but it may be elevated in nonmalignant inflammatory disease, especially of the gastrointestinal tract [13].

Prognosis with colorectal carcinoma depends on the extent of bowel involvement, the presence or absence of spread, the differentiation of the lesion, and the location of the lesion within the colon. It is frequently staged by the TNM system as follows [9]:

TIS: carcinoma in situ

T_1: no involvement of the muscle wall, may be polypoid or papillary

T_2: involvement of the muscle wall

T_3: all layers of wall involved with extension to adjacent structures

T_4: same as T_3 with evidence of fistulas

N: refers to the number of lymphatic nodes involved

M: refers to the evidence of metastasis

REFERENCES

1. Anderson, W. A. D., and Scotti, T. M. *Synopsis of Pathology* (10th ed.). St. Louis: Mosby, 1980.
2. Fisher, R. S., and Cohen, S. Gastroesophageal reflux. *Med. Clin. North Am.* 62:3, 1978.
3. Glickman, R. M., and Isselbacher, K. J. Diseases of the Small Intestine. In K. J. Isselbacher, et al. (eds.), *Harrison's Principles of Internal Medicine* (9th ed.). New York: McGraw-Hill, 1980.
4. Greenberger, N. J., and Winship, D. H. *Gastrointestinal Disorders: A Pathophysiologic Approach.* Chicago: Year Book, 1977.
5. Hendrix, T. R. Diseases of the Esophagus. In K. J. Isselbacher, et al. (eds.), *Harrison's Principles of Internal Medicine* (9th ed.). New York: McGraw-Hill, 1980.
6. LaMont, J. T., and Isselbacher, K. J. Diseases of the Colon and Rectum. In K. J. Isselbacher, et al. (eds.), *Harrison's Principles of Internal Medicine* (9th ed.). New York: McGraw-Hill, 1980.
7. MacDonald, W., and Rubin, C. Cancer, Benign Tumors, Gastritis and Other Gastric Diseases. In K. J. Isselbacher, et al. (eds.), *Harrison's Principles of Internal Medicine* (9th ed.). New York: McGraw-Hill, 1980.
8. McGuigan, J. E. Peptic Ulcers. In K. J. Isselbacher, et al. (eds.), *Harrison's Principles of Internal Medicine* (9th ed.). New York: McGraw-Hill, 1980.
9. Robbins, S. L., and Cotran, R. *Pathologic Basis of Disease.* Philadelphia: Saunders, 1979.
10. Silen, W. Acute Intestinal Obstruction. In K. J. Isselbacher, et al. (eds.), *Harrison's Principles of Internal Medicine* (9th ed.). New York: McGraw-Hill, 1980.
11. Spiro, H. M. *Clinical Gastroenterology* (2nd ed.). New York: Macmillan, 1977.
12. Stahlgren, L., and Morris, N. Intestinal obstruction. *Am. J. Nurs.* 77:999, 1977.
13. Wallach, J. *Interpretation of Diagnostic Tests* (3rd ed.). Boston: Little, Brown, 1978.
14. Westergaard, H., and Dietschy, J. M. Normal mechanisms of fat absorption and derangements induced by various diseases. *Med. Clin. North Am.* 58:6, 1974.

CHAPTER 36
NORMAL HEPATOBILIARY AND PANCREATIC EXOCRINE FUNCTION

LEARNING OBJECTIVES

1. Locate the anatomic structures vital to the function of the liver lobule.
2. Describe the unique structure of the liver sinusoids.
3. Identify the cells of the mononuclear phagocyte system in the sinusoids of the liver.
4. Explain the purpose of the dual blood supply to the liver.
5. Describe the role of the liver in protein synthesis and metabolism.
6. Review the relationship of albumin to the colloid osmotic pressure.
7. Identify the factors necessary for the production of the capillary fluid dynamics.
8. State the relationship of protein, ammonia, and urea in the liver.
9. List and describe the purpose of the plasma proteins produced by the liver.
10. Explain why the lymphatic system is important in plasma protein absorption.
11. Outline the role of the liver in fat synthesis and metabolism.
12. Describe how the liver functions in carbohydrate metabolism.
13. Define *proteolysis, deamination,* and *transamination.*
14. Describe the oxidative and conjugative reactions that affect drug and hormone metabolism.
15. Specifically, explain the effect of alcohol on liver function.
16. Define *hepatotoxin*.
17. Describe the process for the conjugation of bilirubin.
18. List and briefly describe the activities of each of the components of bile.
19. List and describe the major liver function tests.
20. Briefly differentiate between the constituents of liver and gallbladder bile.
21. Describe the hormonal and nervous factors that cause the emptying of the gallbladder.
22. Differentiate between endocrine and exocrine secretions of the pancreas.
23. Specifically delineate the actions of the major enzymes in pancreatic secretions.

An understanding of the anatomic and functional activities of the liver is essential to the understanding of alterations exhibited by the liver in pathologic states. Liver function involves the secretion of bile and the formation of many essential substances. The effect of this function on all the metabolic processes of other organs is crucial to the maintenance of a steady balance in the body. A basic review of liver anatomy and physiology and the accessory function of the gallbladder and pancreas is included in this chapter. The reader is referred to the comprehensive materials listed in the unit bibliography for further information.

ANATOMIC CONSIDERATIONS OF THE LIVER

The liver is a large glandular organ weighing approximately 1½ kg in the adult. It is composed of two major divisions, called the right and left lobes. The right lobe has two lobes associated with it, which are called the quadrate and caudate lobes. The multiple units within the lobes that carry out the work of the liver are called the *lobules.* The unique structure and blood flow through the lobules is illustrated in Figure 36-1. An admixture of venous and arterial blood within the *sinusoids,* or capillaries, of the liver lobule provides both oxygen and nutrients for the work of the liver.

The lobules serve as the functional units of the liver and process many substances in the *hepatocytes* or liver cells. The venous blood supply, carried by a branch of the portal vein, moves highly concentrated foodstuffs including fats, carbohydrates, and proteins that have been absorbed from the small intestine. The arterial blood supply contains high concentrations of oxygen. The lobule is composed of sinusoids, rows of cuboidal hepatocytes, bile capillaries, and branches of the hepatic artery and portal vein (Fig. 36-2). Structurally, the sinusoids and surrounding hepatocytes provide a unique processing plant for the raw materials delivered to it from the small intestine.

The sinusoids are lined with cells of the mononuclear phagocyte system, which are called *Kupffer cells.* These cells trap foreign material and function mainly in phagocytosis. The porous endothelial lining allows for the passage of plasma proteins from the sinusoid to a narrow space around the hepatocyte, which is called the "space of Disse" [2]. This space connects with the lymphatic system and allows drainage of plasma proteins and excess fluid (Fig. 36-3).

Within the liver lobules are *canaliculi,* which are the receptacles for bile produced by the hepatocytes (see Fig. 36-2). A meshwork of bile ducts form from the canaliculi and terminate eventually in the common bile duct, which empties into the duodenum during digestion. The gallbladder receives bile from the liver and then stores, concentrates, and releases it into the common bile duct under appropriate stimulation (see p. 518).

The blood supply to the liver is through divisions of the hepatic artery and portal vein, which pass through the complex sinusoidal network to form venules and veins. These finally terminate in the hepatic vein, which empties into the inferior vena cava (see Fig. 36-1). The physiologic tasks that must be performed by the liver require access to a large quantity of the circulation. About 30 percent of the cardiac output flows through the liver each minute, making this organ a large reservoir for blood.

PHYSIOLOGIC CONSIDERATIONS OF THE LIVER

General Information

The liver performs a wide variety of vital, life-sustaining functions. It plays a major role in the synthesis and metabolism of protein, carbohydrate, and fats and also performs the essential function of phagocytosis, which occurs constantly while blood passes through the liver. Many foreign substances, such as pharmacologic agents, are detoxified or changed into different forms as they pass through the liver. The formation and excretion of bile along with the processing of bilirubin into a form that can be excreted are essential liver functions. Specific enzymes are necessary to carry out many activities and these are also synthesized by this organ. Many hormones of the body are detoxified or inactivated by the liver, which also stores many of the vitamins and minerals. The major functions of the liver are discussed in the following section.

Protein Synthesis and Metabolism

Proteins are nitrogen-containing constituents of all cells and tissues in the body and are present in all body fluids except bile and urine. Proteins are essential to the formation of the cell, as well as to enzyme, hormone, immunoglobulin, and blood cell synthesis. All proteins are in a state of constant turnover, making the task of maintenance of body functions an awesome one.

The primary function of protein metabolism is the synthesis of body proteins. Unlike fats and carbohydrates, proteins are not stored, and the size of the amino acid pool is the result of the actual turnover of body proteins and amino acids from exogenous or dietary sources. Synthesis of proteins depends on the availability of amino acids in the pool at any given point in time. The ratio of available amino acids is of extreme importance in that every body protein is made up of specific amino acids in absolute sequences. If one specific amino acid is absent, synthesis of a specific protein is not possible.

SYNTHESIS OF AMINO ACIDS. Of the many amino acids making up human body proteins, 10 cannot be synthesized in adequate amounts to meet the body's metabolic needs. These have been termed *essential amino acids (EAAs)* and are available through dietary intake. EAAs are not all required in the same amounts; rather a ratio of amino acids is utilized. Foods that contain proteins having the correct proportion of EAAs have a high biologic value. Egg albumin is considered to have a nearly perfect mixture; therefore, all other proteins are compared to that mixture. If one EAA is lacking in the diet, a *negative nitrogen* balance occurs. That is, when one or more essential amino acids are miss-

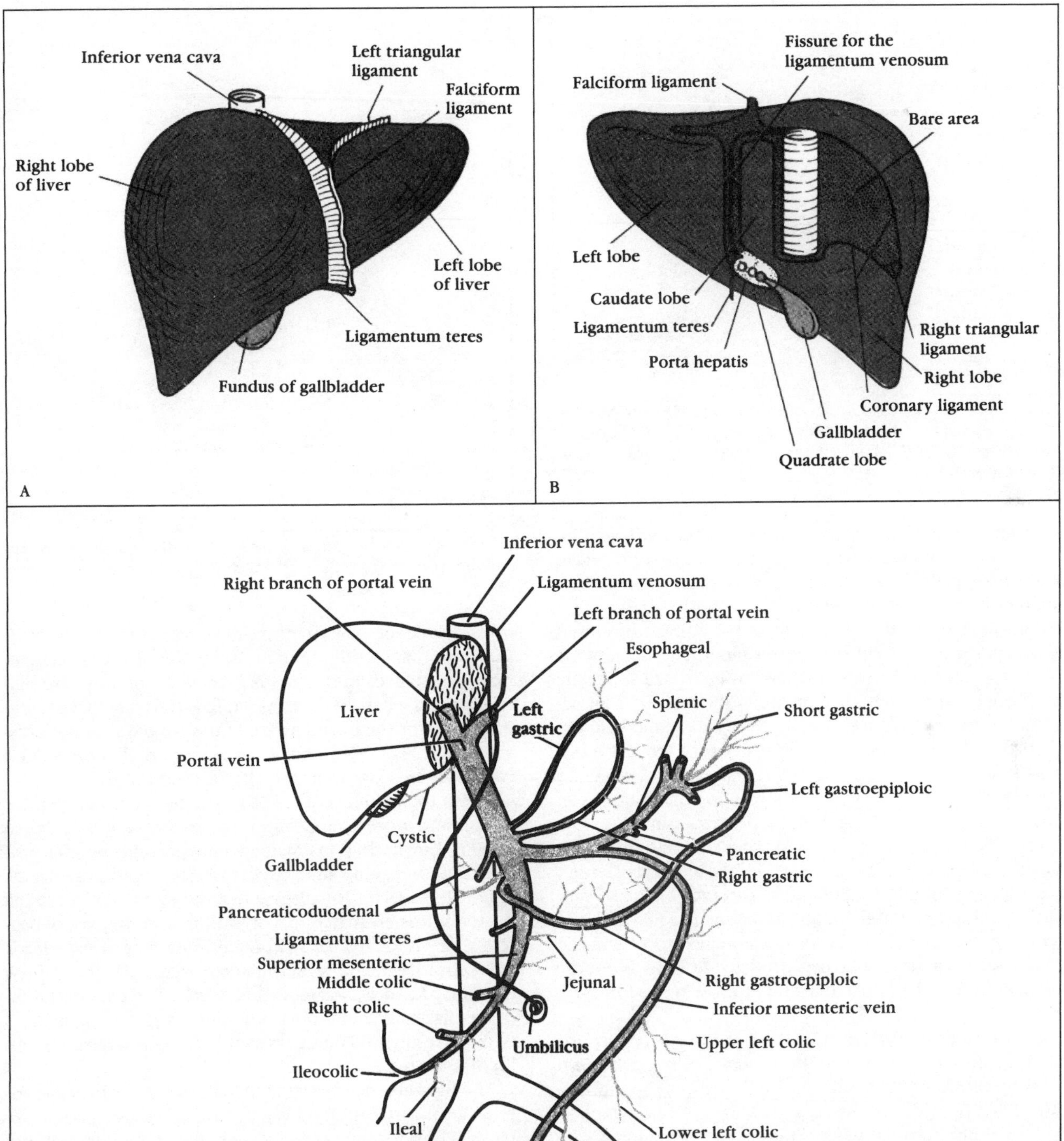

FIGURE 36-1. Macroscopic appearance of the liver. A. Lobes of the liver. B. Posterior surface showing gallbladder and inferior vena cava. C. Blood flow to the liver from the portal vein. (From R. S. Snell, *Clinical Anatomy for Medical Students* [2nd ed.]. Boston: Little, Brown, 1981.)

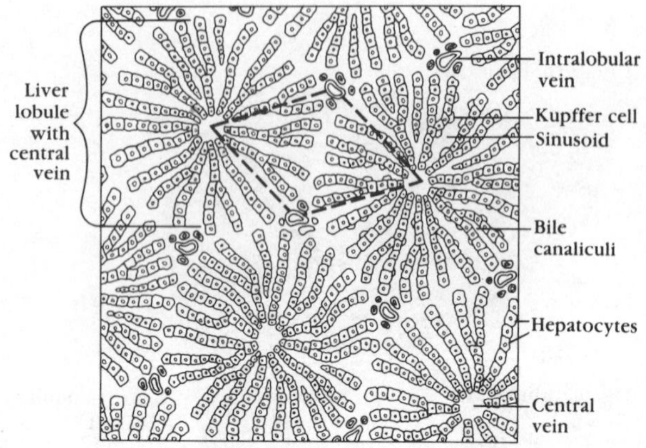

FIGURE 36-2. Schematic diagram of liver lobules. Broken lines indicate liver acinus. (From M. Beyers and S. Dudas, *The Clinical Practice of Medical-Surgical Nursing* [2nd ed.]. Boston: Little, Brown, 1984.)

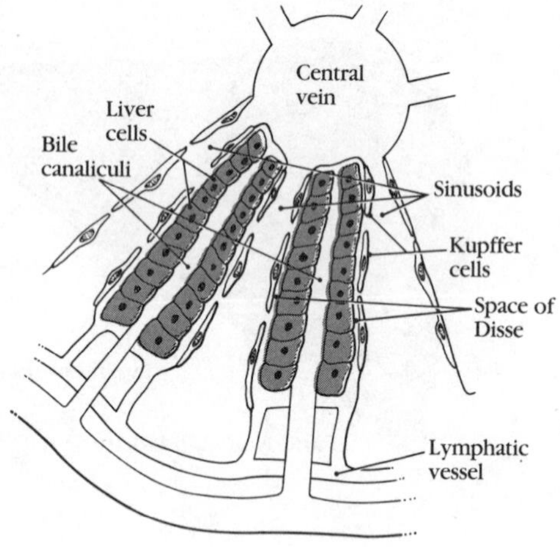

FIGURE 36-3. Another view of liver lobule showing Kupffer cells and the space of Disse through which lymphatic material can flow.

ing from the diet, nitrogen excretion exceeds nitrogen intake. The result is the same as if the total protein intake were inadequate. Loss of body protein occurs and usually is manifested as muscle wasting [7].

The liver plays an active role in the uptake of amino acids from the nutrient-rich portal blood and it converts these to various proteins. The amino acids are relatively strong acids and rarely accumulate in the bloodstream because of protein synthesis by the liver and amino acid excretion by the kidneys. Most amino acids are actively transported through the cell membranes, after which they are converted into cellular proteins, a reaction that requires an enzymatic reaction. These cellular proteins can be rapidly broken down to form amino acids that can be transported out of the cell to the bloodstream [4]. The amount of amino acids in the blood remains quite constant but may vary slightly with diet and the individual person. After the cells have reached their capacity for the storage or proteins, the excess amino acids can be degraded and utilized as energy or changed into fat or glycogen for storage in this form [6].

AMINO ACID METABOLISM. The liver is the major site for amino acid metabolism and the process, called *deamination of amino acids*, results in the formation of ammonia. The liver then converts the ammonia to urea, which is more readily excreted by the kidney than is ammonia. The conversion of ammonia to urea is an important mechanism of the liver resulting in the removal and detoxification of ammonia from the body. Nearly all of the production of urea occurs in the liver; this substance is much less toxic to the central nervous system than is ammonia.

PLASMA PROTEINS. The plasma proteins are large molecules that circulate for the most part in the bloodstream and are mainly synthesized by the liver. All of the albumin, the most abundant plasma protein, is made in the liver. It serves in many bodily functions, including the binding of many substances in the plasma. Examples of these are bilirubin and the barbiturates. Albumin is the principal protein necessary for the maintenance of the colloid osmotic pressure (COP), as described in Chapter 5. It also can effectively bind hydrogen ion and alter the serum pH.

When the amino acid levels of the blood are decreased, the plasma proteins are split to make new amino acids. An equilibrium is thus maintained between the plasma proteins and the amino acids. Decreased levels of amino acids stimulate the liver to increase its production of the plasma proteins. It is estimated that approximately 400 gm of protein are synthesized daily [2]. Significant liver damage leads to hypoproteinemia, which markedly disrupts the colloid osmotic pressure and amino acid levels. The concentration of the plasma proteins normally remains at a constant ratio with more albumin being present in the plasma than globulin (Table 36-1).

The liver also synthesizes the majority of the plasma proteins necessary for blood coagulation. Of these, prothrombin and fibrinogen are the most abundant; however, all the proteins of coagulation are important (see Chap. 16). For prothrombin formation, the liver utilizes vitamin K, the absorption of which depends on the production of bile. Fibrinogen is a large-molecule protein formed entirely by the liver and is an essential factor in the cascade of coagulation.

All of the plasma proteins participate in the production of the colloid osmotic pressure throughout the capillaries of the body. The plasma colloid osmotic pressure (PCOP) is that which retains or pulls fluid into the intravascular

TABLE 36-1. Major liver function tests

Test	Normal level	Abnormalities
Alkaline phosphatase	2–5 BU/ml	↑ Biliary obstruction ↑ Early drug toxicity ↑ Cholestatic hepatitis ↑ Extrahepatic inflammatory condition
Serum glutamic oxaloacetic transaminase (SGOT)	5–40 U/ml	↑ Acute MI ↑ Liver damage and most liver disease ↑ Muscle, pancreas, brain, lung, bowel damage ↓ Some severe liver disease ↓ Diabetic ketoacidosis
Serum glutamic pyruvic transaminase (SGPT)	5–35 U/ml	↑ Markedly in liver necrosis and acute hepatitis ↑ Slightly in MI ↑ Pulmonary, renal, pancreatic injury ↑ Slightly in cirrhosis and chronic liver disease
Lactic dehydrogenase (LDH)	200–680 U/ml	↑ Cardiac injury ↑ Hepatitis, especially LDH isoenzyme 5 ↑ Malignant tumors ↑ Muscle, pulmonary, and renal disease
Serum isocitrate dehydrogenase (ICD)	50–180 Sigma U/ml	↑ Markedly in liver disease
Thymol turbidity and cephalin-cholesterol flocculation	0–5 U/ml 0–2+/48 hours	Both of these tests ↑ in acute liver disease
Bilirubin		
Total	0.2–0.9 mg/dl	↑ Hepatocellular necrosis or damage
Direct	0.1–0.4 mg/dl	↑ Cholestasis due to obstruction
Indirect	0.1–0.5 mg/dl	↑ Hemolytic anemia
Plasma proteins		
Total	6–8 gm/dl	↓ Severe liver disease
Albumin	3.5–5.5 gm/dl	↓ Pyelonephritis and nephrosis
Globulin	1.5–3.0 gm/dl	↓ Malnutrition and protein lack ↓ Chronic inflammation
Fibrinogen	0.2–0.4 gm/dl	↓ Disseminated intravascular coagulation (DIC) ↓ Congenital afibrinogenemia ↓ With depletion of other coagulation factors ↓ With major alteration of hemodynamics in body, e.g., circulatory shock
Prothrombin time	11–16 seconds (control); 80–100% of control	↑ (Prolonged) severe liver disease, especially cirrhosis ↑ Fibrinogen deficiency ↑ Coumadin therapy ↑ Biliary destruction
Partial thromboplastin time	22–37 seconds	↑ (Prolonged) in bleeding disorders, especially of the intrinsic pathway ↑ Heparin therapy ↑ Cirrhosis and severe liver disease
Urine bilirubin	0 mg/24°	↑ Biliary obstruction ↑ Cirrhosis ↑ Hepatitis
Urine urobilinogen	0–4 mg/24°	↓ Biliary obstruction Normal or ↑ cirrhosis
Bromsuphalein (BSP) excretion	5% retention after 45 minutes	↑ Fever ↑ All types liver disease ↑ Specific drugs, e.g., morphine ↑ Acute cholecystitis ↑ GI bleeding
Liver scans		
Colloidal	Uptake of colloid by Kupffer cells	Demonstrates large defects; false negatives seen with small defects
Rose bengal	Uptake of dye by hepatocytes	Area of reduced intake, "hole" in neoplastic or inflammatory cells

TABLE 36-1. (continued)

Test	Normal level	Abnormalities
Gallium	Little uptake of dye by normal cells	Uptake by neoplastic and inflammatory cells
Liver biopsy	Normal hepatocytes	Specific pathology of any material sampled; diagnostic of cirrhosis, malignancy, hepatitis, etc.
Computerized tomography (CT scan)	Normal integrity on image of intraabdominal organs	Differentiate fluid collections in liver from tumors; visualize gallbladder or duct enlargement

Note: ↑ = test results are increased in these conditions; ↓ = test results are decreased in these conditions.

area. Because the plasma proteins are too large to cross the capillary membrane they remain in increased concentrations at the capillary line and produce an osmotic pressure or pull. This has been described as an inward pressure or force. The level of the PCOP remains constant at the arteriolar, capillary, and venular sections of the capillary and provides the major force encouraging fluid to return to the capillary and the intravascular area. This mechanism is illustrated in Figure 36-4, which shows how the plasma proteins prevent a continuous loss of fluid into the interstitial spaces.

The plasma proteins are not easily lost into the interstitial spaces because of their size. When some of these are leaked into the interstitial area, the only route for return to the bloodstream is via the profuse lymphatic drainage found in the interstitial compartment. The lymphatic vessels empty into the lymphatic and thoracic ducts, which empty directly into the superior vena cava.

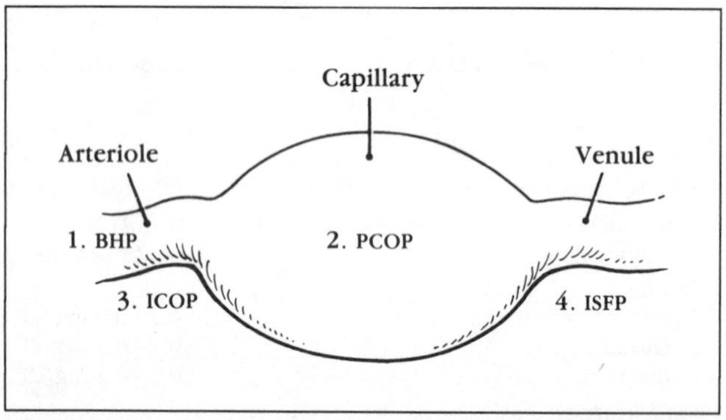

FIGURE 36-4. Schematic diagram of the plasma colloid osmotic pressure (PCOP) in the capillaries. 1. BHP = blood hydrostatic pressure. BHP is generated by the heart and affected by arteriolar tone and intravascular fluid volume. 2. PCOP = plasma proteins in the intravascular compartment. Due to the size of the molecules of plasma proteins, they do not readily diffuse from the plasma to the interstitial spaces. 3. ICOP = interstitial colloid osmotic pressure. ICOP is the pressure exerted by the minute quantities of plasma proteins found in the interstitial spaces. 4. ISFP = interstitial fluid pressure. ISFP is negative.

Fat or Lipid Metabolism

The liver forms almost all of the lipoproteins, which contain mixtures of triglycerides, phospholipids, and cholesterol, as well as protein. Cholesterol is used for the formation of bile salts, which are important in the absorption of fats in the small intestine. It is also used in the formation of the steroid hormones.

Ninety-five percent of the fat ingested daily in the American diet is in the form of triglycerides, which contain both saturated and unsaturated fatty acids. The liver can convert carbohydrates or proteins to fat. Insulin causes the movement of glucose into the cell and promotes fat storage if the glucose is not utilized for energy (see Chap. 33).

Carbohydrate Metabolism

Carbohydrate may be released by the liver in its usable form, glucose, after it has been stored in the form of glycogen. About 5 to 7 percent of normal liver weight is stored glycogen. When blood glucose increases above normal, glycogenesis is stimulated. Conversely, when the blood sugar level falls below normal, glycogenolysis is stimulated.

The liver functions to maintain normal blood glucose levels. After a high-carbohydrate meal, an increased amount of carbohydrate is delivered to the liver, where it is stored and released when the blood glucose begins to drop. The pancreatic hormone *glucagon* is very important in initiating the release of glucose by the liver.

In the process called *gluconeogenesis*, the liver functions to synthesize glucose from other substances, especially proteins. Glucose needs, which cannot be met from glycogen stores or exogenous sources, must be met through this process. This is critically important for the specific cells that cannot use fat for metabolism. These cells include the blood cells and the cells of the kidney medulla. The cells of the central nervous system use glucose preferentially but can adapt to fatty acid oxidation in the form of ketones in 2 to 4 days. During a fasting period, such as between meals and during sleep, the carbon skeleton of amino acids is converted to glucose for energy.

Phagocytosis

The sinusoids of the liver are lined with *Kupffer cells*, which pick up and destroy foreign material circulating through the liver. The portal vein, which circulates the venous blood from the intestine to the liver, carries a higher concentration of toxins and bacteria than other venous blood because of the toxins and bacteria in nutrients absorbed from the intestine.

If the level of bacteria or foreign material in the sinusoids increases, the Kupffer cells become active, proliferate, and destroy the foreign material. This activity is crucial in preventing the spread of organisms to the systemic circulation.

Biotransformation of Foreign Substances

Destruction, biotransformation, and inactivation of foreign substances are carried out in the hepatocyte, and substances are changed to acceptable forms for excretion. Many of the endocrine secretions are inactivated in the liver, and many pharmacologic agents are biotransformed here. Some substances are *conjugated* in the same way as bilirubin with glucuronic acid while others may be inactivated by proteolysis, deamination, or oxidation. *Proteolysis* refers to the breakdown of proteins into simpler substances. *Deamination* means the removal of the amino acids and may involve *transamination* or transfer of this group to another acceptor substance. *Oxidative deamination* causes the release of the amino radical [5].

The oxidative and conjugative reactions function in the biodegradation and/or excretion of foreign substances. It has been found that many drugs affect the reactions of other drugs or hormones and that these interactions, whether they involve speeding up or slowing down the reactions, occur in the hepatocyte. An example is the metabolism of warfarin (Coumadin), the effects of which can be potentiated by aspirin. Phenobarbital increases the activity of drug-metabolizing enzymes and hastens the inactivation of warfarin and other drugs. Many endogenous hormones, especially corticosterone and aldosterone, are inactivated and conjugated for excretion by the liver. The estrogens impair the secretory activity of the hepatocytes and may cause an alteration in the liver function tests.

Acute alcoholic intoxication inhibits drug metabolism by the liver. The chronic alcoholic, however, metabolizes drugs quickly and has an increased tolerance to drugs, unless there is associated liver failure, which appears to cause decreased drug tolerance.

Substances that are directly toxic to liver cells are called *hepatotoxins*. A specific drug that is a known hepatotoxin in excessive dosages is acetaminophen (Tylenol), which causes centrilobular liver necrosis due to the exhaustion of the glutathione to which it is normally conjugated. If, in an overdose situation, a glutathione precursor is given, protection of the subject from permanent liver injury will result. If no treatment is given, the rate of liver failure following overdose is very high and often fatal.

Most liver damage resulting from foreign substances is due to hypersensitivity reactions by hepatic cells after variable exposure to drugs. Some drugs cause jaundice; a notable example is chlorpromazine, which causes cholestasis within the liver. Several other drugs can cause parenchymal necrosis; isoniazid and halothane anesthesia are typical examples [3].

Bile Synthesis

Bile is formed by the liver and stored and concentrated by the gallbladder. The hepatocyte makes bile, which is a liquid material normally composed of bilirubin, the plasma electrolytes, water, bile salts, cholesterol, fatty acids, and lecithin. Several of these constituents are detailed below.

BILIRUBIN. Bilirubin is an excretory product that is excreted from the body only in a specific form called *conjugated bilirubin*. Most of the bilirubin in the body is released in the process of breakdown of red blood cells. The red blood cell gives off its hemoglobin, which further breaks into its component parts, *heme* and *globin*. The globin portion is a protein that probably returns to the intracellular amino acid pool. The heme portion of the hemoglobin is further broken down into bilirubin and iron. The iron is either stored in the form of *ferritin* (a combination of a liver protein called apoferritin and iron), or it is utilized for the production of new hemoglobin. Figure 36-5 summarizes the process.

The bilirubin undergoes several reactions and ends up being bound loosely to albumin, on which it travels to the liver. It is called *unconjugated, fat-soluble*, or *indirect* bilirubin because it cannot be excreted in the bile or through the kidneys. In the liver it is converted to a water-soluble form when it reacts with *glucuronic acid*. In this water-soluble or conjugated form it can be secreted into the bile and excreted by the intestine, or in special circumstances by the kidney. In the intestine, the intestinal bacteria change the excreted bilirubin to *urobilinogen*. Some of this material is resorbed and reexcreted by the liver. Most of the bilirubin is excreted in the feces in the form of urobilinogen, which imparts the dark color to the feces.

In summary, bilirubin must be converted to a conjugated, water-soluble form in order to cross the cell membrane of the hepatocyte and be excreted in the bile. In bile duct obstructions, conjugated bilirubin can cross the membrane of the glomerulus and be excreted by the kidney. Excess bilirubin leads to the condition called jaundice, which is described in detail on p. 522.

BILE SALTS. The bile salts function as detergents and break fat particles into smaller sizes. They aid in making fat more soluble by the formation of special complexes called *micelles*, which are soluble in the intestinal mucosa. The bile salts are formed by the liver with cholesterol precursors; large amounts can be formed and secreted during periods of increased need. The bile salts are also essential for the absorption of the fat-soluble vitamins A, D, E, and K.

ELECTROLYTES. The electrolytes in bile are to some extent resorbed through the gallbladder mucosa because of the

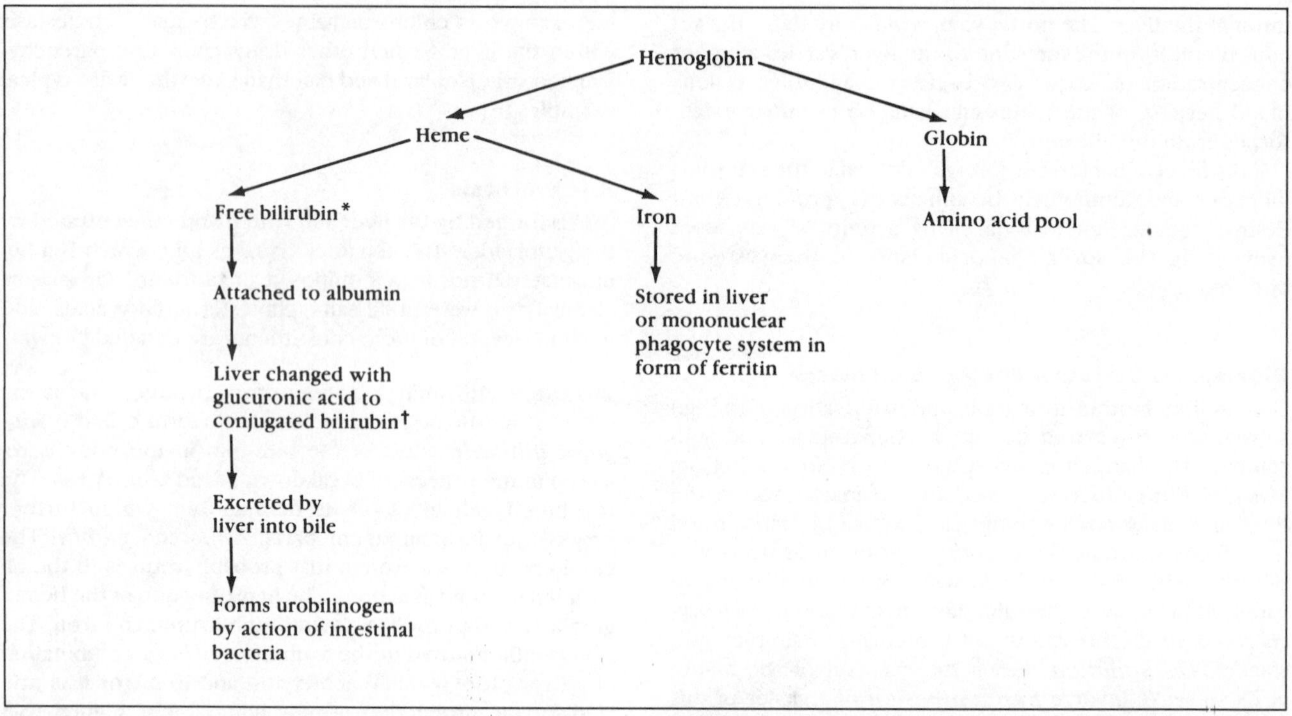

FIGURE 36-5. Fate of hemoglobin. *Free unconjugated, indirect bilirubin persists until the liver changes its form. It is lipid-soluble, water-insoluble, and nonexcretable. †Conjugated, direct, or bilirubin glucuronide is the form after conjugation with glucuronic acid. It is water-soluble, fat-insoluble, and excretable.

concentrating process that occurs in that organ (see p. 518). Substances that are not absorbed become highly concentrated in the gallbladder bile. For example, liver bile contains about 0.04 gm/dl of bilirubin, while gallbladder bile contains about 0.3 gm/dl. Resorption of the water, electrolytes, and free cholesterol in the secreted bile occurs in the small intestine. Cholesterol is excreted through the formation of bile salts and directly in the bile. Imbalance can cause excessive cholesterol in the bile and may cause a predisposition to stone formation (see p. 530).

MAJOR LIVER FUNCTION TESTS

The major liver function tests provide an index of hepatic function and are helpful in establishing a differential diagnosis in intrahepatic and extrahepatic pathology. The tests are summarized in Table 36-1.

Serum Enzymes

The *alkaline phosphatase* of the serum is an enzyme that is manufactured in the liver, kidneys, bone, and other areas and is excreted in bile. Serum levels are elevated in conditions that increase calcium deposits in bone—in viral hepatitis, obstructive jaundice, malignancies, and in many other conditions. Serum levels may be decreased in hypoparathyroidism, pernicious anemia, hypothyroidism, and a few other conditions.

The *serum glutamic oxalacetic transaminase* (SGOT) is an enzyme that is manufactured and concentrated in skeletal muscle, cardiac muscle, and liver. It functions to catalyze certain deamination processes. The SGOT level is increased in acute myocardial infarction, liver disease, muscular diseases, pancreatitis, and other specific conditions.

The *serum glutamic pyruvic transaminase* (SGPT) is an enzyme that is found in high concentrations in the liver, and to a lesser extent, the heart and skeletal muscle. Increased levels occur with all types of hepatic injury.

The *lactic dehydrogenase* (LDH) is found in large quantities in liver tissue. The LDH is elevated significantly in liver damage and also with cardiac and muscular damage. LDH levels are increased with pulmonary embolus, certain malignancies, pernicious anemia, and others. The LDH isoenzymes are isolated into concentrations of isoenzymes 1–5; these vary with specific areas and organs. The isoenzyme LDH-5 is the most specific to liver disease, especially hepatitis.

The *serum isocitrate dehydrogenase* (ICD) is an enzyme that is concentrated in liver tissue. It is specifically seen to be elevated in viral hepatitis, infectious mononucleosis, liver poisons, and to some extent, metastatic carcinoma. It is not elevated in acute myocardial infarction and may provide a differential diagnosis between liver and myocardial disease.

Bilirubin

Bilirubin is measured as a total value and in its conjugated and unconjugated fractions. It measures the ability of the liver to conjugate and excrete bilirubin in the intestine. A high level of unconjugated bilirubin with a normal or high level of conjugated bilirubin usually indicates significant intrahepatic cellular damage, but this report may also be seen with hemolytic jaundice. If there is an increase in the conjugated bilirubin and a normal or slightly increased unconjugated bilirubin level, especially in the presence of dark urine and light stools, almost conclusive evidence of biliary obstruction is provided.

Plasma Proteins

Albumin, the most abundant plasma protein, functions to maintain the plasma colloid osmotic pressure, to synthesize specific amino acids, and to bind certain molecules for transport from one point to another. Albumin levels are evaluated by a process called electrophoresis. Decreased serum albumin, hypoalbuminemia, results from severe hepatocellular dysfunction. The result of albumin depression is an alteration of the COP, leading to systemic edema.

Fibrinogen levels are important in determining the potential for normal blood coagulation. Depletion of this protein occurs in a condition called *disseminated intravascular coagulation* in which precipitation of fibrin in the small vessels and rapid depletion of the clotting factors result (see Chap. 16). Deficiency also may be seen with conditions that can cause fibrinolysis and include such conditions as hemorrhage, burns, poisoning, and cirrhosis.

The *globulins* are important in the production of antibodies and are described in Chapter 9. They also function with albumin in the maintenance of intravascular colloid osmotic pressure. Alteration of the globulin levels occurs with immunosuppression and with chronic inflammations. Elevation or suppression of globulin levels is not a specific sign of liver disease.

Another protein that is measured in liver function screening is *prothrombin*. The prothrombin time reflects prothrombin, fibrinogen, and other factors. A prolonged prothrombin time indicates a deficiency of prothrombin and the other clotting factors or impairment in the uptake of vitamin K. The prothrombin time is a measure of the factors of the extrinsic system and the common pathway of both extrinsic and intrinsic systems (see Chap. 16). The *partial thromboplastin time* (PTT) is a measurement of the factors concerned in the intrinsic clotting pathway and the common pathway and serves as a good screening test for bleeding disorders. The other specific clotting factors can be separately measured and the levels of these may be altered in liver dysfunction.

Urine Bilirubin

Small amounts of bilirubin are usually excreted in the urine in the form of urobilinogen. Conjugated bilirubin can be found in the urine when an excessive amount is not being cleared from the plasma. This finding is common in obstructive biliary tract disease and severe cirrhosis of the liver.

Bromosulphalein Excretion (BSP)

This test measures the ability of the liver to remove a dye from the circulation. Liver injury is probable when more than 10 percent of injected dye remains in circulation after 45 minutes.

Thymol Turbidity: Cephalin Flocculation Tests

These tests are done to determine if a liver disease process is active and are positive in most cases of acute hepatitis. The tests may also be positive with cirrhosis of the liver and biliary tract disease.

Liver Scanning (Scintiscans)

Scans are performed to visualize the position, shape, size, and structure of the liver. The tests involve the injection of specific radiopharmaceutical isotopes, which are taken up by the hepatocytes, by the Kupffer cells, or by neoplasms. Several types of scanning procedures are used, with some isotopes concentrating in neoplasms or in areas of inflammation, while others concentrate in the hepatocytes; areas of abscess or tumor produce a void in the scan.

Reading the liver scan involves looking for areas of increased or no uptake, depending on the isotope used. Agents that are excreted in the bile can be followed for bile duct obstruction, while those having mononuclear phagocytes system affinity are concentrated in the spleen. Changes in the liver scan can also assist in following the course of cirrhosis. Persons with early hepatomegaly will have even distribution of the radiopharmaceutical agent. As the disease progresses, the left lobe of the liver enlarges, the right lobe becomes smaller, and the spleen takes up increased amounts. As liver failure progresses there may be a spotty appearance due to the fibrosis dividing the lobules.

Liver Biopsy

Liver biopsy is utilized to make a precise diagnosis of liver disease and can be beneficial in the diagnosis of hepatitis, cirrhosis, and neoplasms. It may be performed as open biopsy during a surgical procedure or as a needle biopsy utilizing an intercostal approach. In the latter, the material aspirated from the needle is histologically examined for abnormalities. Accurate placement of the needle is imperative for precise diagnosis. Care must be exerted to prevent laceration of the liver and consequent hemorrhage.

Computerized Tomography

This popular procedure provides a radiologic image of the abdominal organs without the injection of dyes or isotopes. It helps in initial evaluation of liver disease in differentiating fluid-filled lesions from tumor-filled areas. The appearance of the surrounding organs and ducts can also be assessed.

GALLBLADDER

The gallbladder is a saclike organ that is attached to the inferior portion of the liver. It receives bile from the liver that has been diverted from the common bile duct (Fig. 36-6). The maximum volume of the gallbladder is 40 to 70 ml, but this gallbladder bile is more concentrated than liver bile. The gallbladder is composed of folds and rugae and can increase its size to accommodate incoming bile. The bile that is stored in the gallbladder is 5 to 10 times more concentrated than liver bile. Approximately 90 percent of the water is continually absorbed by the mucosa. The gallbladder bile electrolyte composition includes an increased concentration of sodium and a decreased amount of chloride and bicarbonate [1].

The gallbladder empties its bile into the common bile duct when a stimulus is received. The major stimulus for this is cholecystokinin (CCK-PZ), a hormone secreted from the duodenal mucosa when fat-containing foods arrive in that area. The CCK-PZ causes bile to move into the intestine by causing contractions of the gallbladder and relaxation of the sphincter of Oddi. The gallbladder also receives stimulation from the autonomic nervous system. The parasympathetic division is the major mediator for contraction of the gallbladder, while stimulation of the sympathetic division causes relaxation of the organ.

Alterations in function of the gallbladder are discussed in Chapter 37. Gallstones and inflammation of the gallbladder are common causes of abdominal pain.

EXOCRINE PANCREATIC FUNCTION

The pancreas is a large organ that lies behind the stomach and extends between the spleen and the duodenum. It is composed of a head, a body, and a tail, which contain the acini cells and the cells of the islets of Langerhans (Fig. 36-7). The exocrine acini cells function to secrete the digestive juices, while the endocrine islet cells secrete hormones that are essential in glucose metabolism. The exocrine functions, or those related to digestion, involve the secretion of pancreatic juice into a system of ducts that empty into the pancreatic duct and, in turn, the ampulla of Vater. The pathologic alterations in the pancreas are included in Chapter 33.

Exocrine Pancreatic Secretion

The cells of the pancreas that secrete pancreatic juice are called *acini cells.* The secretion is composed of an alkaline component and enzymes necessary for digesting proteins, fats, and carbohydrates. The alkaline component contains sufficient bicarbonate ion to cause the pancreatic juice to have a pH of about 8. Up to 2000 ml of juice is secreted daily by the cells. The enzymes contained within the secretion are (1) *amylase*, which hydrolyses carbohydrates to disaccharides; (2) *pancreatic lipase*, which hydrolyses fats to yield glycerol and fatty acids; and (3) the *preproteolytic* enzymes, mainly trypsinogen and chymotrypsinogen, which, when activated, function to hydrolyse proteins to amino acids.

Nervous and Hormonal Regulation of Pancreatic Secretions

The nervous stimulation to the pancreas is mainly through the vagus nerve, which transmits impulses to the pancreas during the cephalic and gastric phases of digestion. This results in the secretion of enzymes by the acini cells. The nervous influences also affect the secretion of the endocrine islet cells.

The hormonal mechanisms are mainly mediated through *secretin* and *cholecystokinin*. When chyme comes into contact with the mucosal cells of the duodenum, the hormone secretin is released, causing the pancreas to secrete large amounts of fluids with large amounts of bicarbonate and few or no enzymes. This alkaline secretion neutralizes the highly acid gastric juice emptied into the duodenum from the stomach, stops the activity of gastrin, and provides an alkalinity of about pH 7, which is optimal for pancreatic enzyme activity. The hormone cholecystokinin (CCK-PZ) also is released from the intestinal mucosa in the presence of food and functions to increase the secretion of pancreatic enzymes from the acini cells. The food distention of the intestinal wall is the apparent stimulus for the release of CCK-PZ.

Protein Digestion

Trypsinogen is converted to the active enzyme trypsin in an alkaline medium through the action of *enterokinase*, which is released by the intestinal mucosa when it comes into contact with the chyme. Trypsin then activates other trypsinogen molecules and triggers the conversion of chymotrypsinogen into chymotrypsin. These proteolytic enzymes then can split proteins into amino acids for absorption in the intestine.

The most important protective mechanisms for the prevention of digestion of the pancreas by the enzymes it secretes are the synthesis of the enzymes in an inactive form and the presence of a *trypsin inhibitor* that is secreted by the same cells that secrete the pancreatic enzymes. This trypsin inhibitor is stored in the cytoplasm of the cells surrounding the enzyme granules and prevents the activation of trypsin, thus preventing activation of the other proteolytic enzymes. When the pancreas becomes damaged or when a duct is blocked, the pancreatic secretion accumulates. It is hypothesized that the trypsin inhibitor is overwhelmed and the pancreatic enzymes become activated to cause acute pancreatitis.

Fat Digestion

The pancreatic lipase is an important ingredient for fat breakdown. It works with the bile salts and helps to break fats into fatty acids and glycerol.

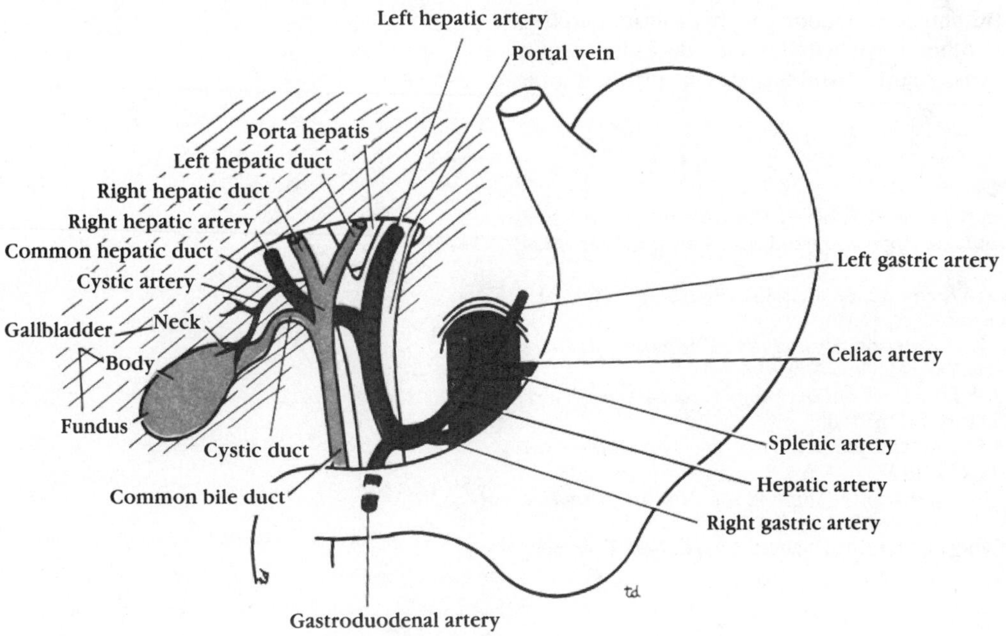

FIGURE 36-6. Appearance and location of gallbladder. (From R. S. Snell, *Clinical Anatomy for Medical Students* [2nd ed.]. Boston: Little, Brown, 1981.)

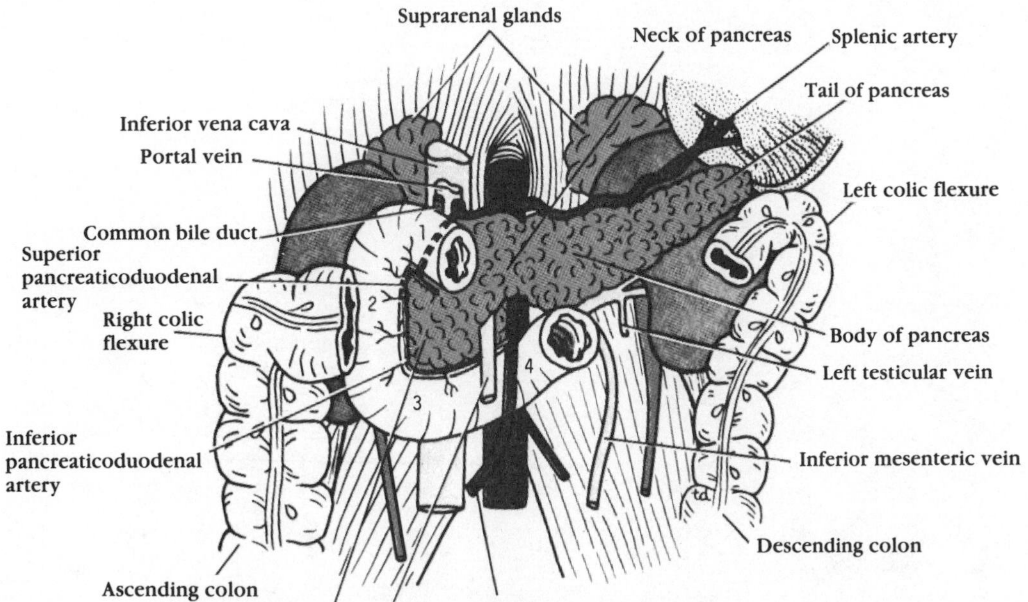

FIGURE 36-7. Appearance and location of the pancreas. (From R. S. Snell, *Clinical Anatomy for Medical Students* [2nd ed.]. Boston: Little, Brown, 1981.)

Carbohydrate Digestion

The pancreatic amylase functions to hydrolyse starches, glycogen, and other carbohydrates into disaccharides. It does not break plant cellulose down into simpler substances.

REFERENCES

1. Greenberger, N. J., and Wenship, D. H. *Gastrointestinal Disorders: A Pathologic Approach* (2nd ed.). Chicago: Year Book, 1981.
2. Guyton, A. C. *Textbook of Medical Physiology* (6th ed.). Philadelphia: Saunders, 1981.
3. Isselbacher, K. J. *Harrison's Principles of Internal Medicine* (9th ed.). New York: McGraw-Hill, 1980.
4. Jensen, D. *The Principles of Physiology* (2nd ed.). New York: Appleton-Century-Crofts, 1980.
5. Pierce, L. Anatomy and physiology of the liver. *Nurs. Clin. North Am.* 12:259, 1977.
6. Schneider, H. *Nutritional Support of Medical Practice.* Hagerstown, Md.: Harper & Row, 1977.
7. Steffee, W. Cancer and protein malnutrition. *Compr. Ther.* 3:30, 1977.

CHAPTER 37
ALTERATIONS IN HEPATOBILIARY FUNCTION

LEARNING OBJECTIVES

1. Define and describe the phenomenon of *jaundice* and its etiology and physiologic effects.
2. Explain how ascites can result from liver failure.
3. Describe the pathologic appearance of fatty liver.
4. Define *portal hypertension*.
5. Relate esophageal varices to portal hypertension.
6. Define the *hepatorenal syndrome*.
7. List the physiologic changes of liver failure.
8. Describe how hepatic encephalopathy and coma can result from liver failure.
9. Explain the major pathologic presentations of cirrhosis of the liver.
10. Define *alcoholic hepatitis*.
11. Differentiate between primary and metastatic carcinoma of the liver.
12. Discuss the etiology, incubation pathology, and clinical presentations of hepatitis A and B.
13. Define *cholelithiasis* and *cholecystitis*.
14. List the major constituents of biliary tract stones.
15. Describe the clinical manifestations of biliary obstruction.
16. Define *obesity*.
17. Differentiate between adult-onset and juvenile obesity in relationship to fat cell accumulation.
18. Describe the major source of lipids and how lipids are transported and metabolized.
19. List at least five chronic health problems that are associated with obesity.

Chapter 36 described how the liver functions in a wide range of intricate metabolic functions. Its large reserve accounts for the lack of clinical signs of dysfunction until large portions of the organ are greatly diseased or damaged. It is estimated that 10 percent of liver function is necessary to sustain life.

This chapter organizes liver and gallbladder dysfunction into general effects of alterations and how these effects apply to specific disease conditions. Common alterations in liver and gallbladder function are included. Obesity resulting from excessive fat metabolism is also included.

GENERAL CONSIDERATIONS IN LIVER DYSFUNCTION

Jaundice

Jaundice refers to the yellowish or greenish hue imparted to a person's skin by something that disturbs the flow of bile or bilirubin (bile pigment). The two most common causes of jaundice are lysis of red blood cells and obstruction in the bile ducts or liver cells. Bilirubin may accumulate in its unconjugated or conjugated form, staining the skin, sclera, and all the tissues of the body. The four major types of jaundice result from (1) impairment of the conjugation process, (2) excessive destruction of red blood cells, (3) interference with the conjugation of bilirubin, and (4) obstructive conditions.

IMPAIRMENT OF THE CONJUGATION PROCESS. This type of impairment may occur in neonatal jaundice when there is a deficiency of *glucuronyl transferase*, an enzyme necessary for the conjugation of bilirubin with glucuronic acid. Frequently occurring with premature infants, this impairment has been successfully treated with phenobarbital, which has been shown to stimulate the essential enzymatic reaction. Improvement in the degree of jaundice usually occurs within days to weeks. In a related condition, the *Crigler-Najjar syndrome*, the glucuronal transferase activity is congenitally absent and unconjugated bilirubin accumulates and crosses the blood-brain barrier. The result is *kernicterus*, which is the deposition of pigment in the basal ganglia of the brain, causing brain damage. Kernicterus only occurs in premature or newborn infants, because the blood-brain barrier becomes impermeable to bilirubin during early infancy.

EXCESSIVE DESTRUCTION OF RED BLOOD CELLS. Excessive destruction of red blood cells causes jaundice through hemolysis. The red blood cells break down into hemoglobin and red cell fragments. Hemoglobin is processed further to heme and globin as described on p. 176, releasing free, unconjugated bilirubin into the plasma. Hemolysis can occur with blood transfusion reactions, after cardiopulmonary bypass, sickle cell anemia, marrow destruction of red blood cells, and some pharmacologic agents. The blood transfusion reaction requires an antigen-antibody reaction to the donor red cells. The red cell is then destroyed in an acute hemolytic reaction.

In *sickle cell anemia*, abnormal hemoglobin and a fragile cell membrane lead to hemolysis and an increase in the amount of free unconjugated bilirubin in the plasma. The precipitating cause of hemolysis is usually hypoxemia, leading to a sickling of the red cell and fragmentation as it passes through tight spaces (see Chap. 14). The liver retains the capability to conjugate bilirubin but it becomes overwhelmed with the free bilirubin and cannot conjugate all that is sent to it.

Bone marrow problems lead to destruction of the red blood cell before they leave the marrow. This condition can be caused by thalassemia or by some pharmacologic agents. An elevation of either or both unconjugated and conjugated bilirubin levels may be seen. Generally classified as bone marrow developmental problems, or *defective erythropoiesis*, are conditions in which the erythrocytes, poorly manufactured, are fragile and of a short life span. These cells hemolyze as they pass through the pulp of the spleen and other tight spaces. The result is that an excess of unconjugated bilirubin is presented to the liver for conjugation. Many drugs can cause hemolysis from drug-induced defective erythropoiesis or as a side effect of the drug. The hemolysis usually results from a hypersensitivity reaction to the drug. Some examples of implicated drugs include chlorpromazine (Thorazine), quinidine, phenacetin (acetophenetidin), sulfonamides, penicillins, cephalosporins, and insulin. Thalassemias refer to a group of congenital diseases involving defective synthesis of hemoglobin leading to an increased propensity for hemolysis.

INTERFERENCE WITH THE CONJUGATION OF BILIRUBIN. A third cause of jaundice is impaired uptake of bilirubin that interferes with the conjugation of bilirubin. The decreased uptake of bilirubin by the hepatic cells is probably due to lack of sufficient glucuronyl transferase to effect the release of the unconjugated bilirubin from the albumin on which it has been carried. This is usually a benign, familial condition, called *Gilbert's syndrome* and occurs in up to 5 percent of the male population [3]. It creates significant jaundice when certain stressful factors create increased metabolism of bilirubin and increased need for the conjugation process. Two types of Gilbert's syndrome have been described, one that involves decreased bilirubin clearance, especially with fasting, and one in which hemolysis can be demonstrated. The first type is more common and has few clinical side effects except for the appearance of transient jaundice.

OBSTRUCTIVE JAUNDICE. Three types of obstructive jaundice have been described: (1) intrahepatic block, or failure of the hepatocytes to function; (2) prehepatic block, in which the unconjugated bilirubin is not being circulated through the liver because of obstruction in the extrahepatic circulation; or (3) posthepatic block, which commonly results from cholestasis as a result of cholecystitis or cholelithiasis.

Intrahepatic obstruction frequently occurs with hepatocellular failure from cirrhotic fibrosis or hepatic scarring.

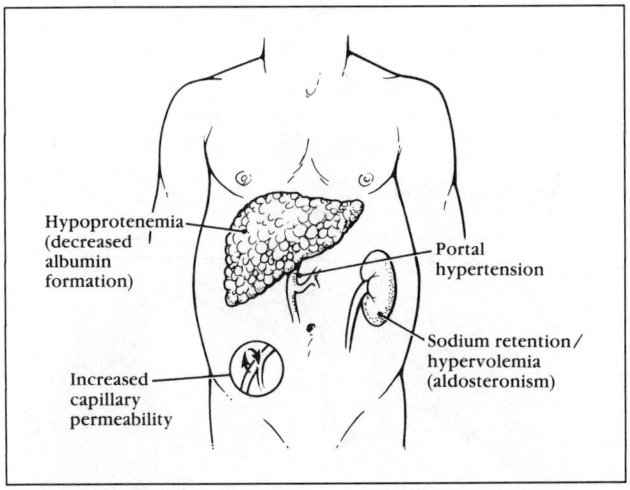

FIGURE 37-1. Factors contributing to the development of ascites.

Some pharmaceutical agents, such as the oral contraceptives and chlorpropamide (Diabenase), have been shown to cause intracellular damage and blockage in certain persons.

Extrahepatic obstructive conditions include gallstones, malignancies of intrahepatic or extrahepatic source, surgical obstruction of the ampulla of Vater, and others. The obstruction limits the excretion of bilirubin in the bile and an excess of conjugated bilirubin accumulates.

The physiologic effects of obstructive jaundice depend on the ability of the liver to conjugate and excrete bilirubin. When the source of the jaundice is hepatocellular failure, increased serum levels of unconjugated bilirubin often result due to the failure of the hepatocyte to produce conjugated bilirubin. Extrahepatic obstruction causes increased levels of conjugated bilirubin with excretion of bilirubin in the urine. As the liver becomes engorged with bilirubin, the function of the hepatocyte diminishes and an increase in the amount of serum unconjugated and conjugated levels will be seen.

Jaundice, caused by conjugated or unconjugated bilirubin, assumes importance in the differential diagnosis of the source and sometimes the severity of the causative condition. Deposition of pigments in the skin lead to the yellowish or greenish discoloration, which may be most noticeable in the sclera of the eyes. In neonates, increased bilirubin levels may lead to kernicterus and neurologic impairment. In adults, the degree of jaundice often correlates with the severity of the liver dysfunction.

Ascites

Ascites refers to the accumulation of fluid in the peritoneal cavity, which usually results directly from increasing portal pressure and/or decreasing plasma protein levels. Sodium retention as a result of aldosterone retention and excessive lymphatic flow may add to the amount of ascitic fluid. Figure 37-1 illustrates the factors that can contribute to the development of ascites.

Portal hypertension, or increased pressure in the portal venous system, can occur because of an intrahepatic block to blood flow through the liver. The resultant increase in capillary pressure leads to a disruption of the normal osmotic force at the capillary line, pushing fluid into the peritoneal cavity.

Decreased plasma proteins, especially albumin, lead to a decrease in the plasma colloid pressure, which decreases the inward forces, or in the resorption pressures, further encouraging fluid to pass into the peritoneal space. Albumin synthesis is depressed in conditions of liver failure.

The ascitic fluid, or transudate, contains large quantities of albumin, the loss of which results in further hypoalbuminemia. Complicating this process is a decrease or depletion of central blood volume as the amount of ascitic fluid increases. A compensatory mechanism of the body is to increase the secretion of aldosterone from the adrenal cortex, leading to retention of sodium and water. The retention indirectly provides more available fluid and increased ascites.

Antidiuretic hormone (ADH), which is synthesized by the hypothalamus and released by the posterior pituitary, also is secreted in greater quantities when the central blood volume is depleted. Increased renal tubular water resorption and increased blood volume result.

It is probable that increased intrasinusoidal pressure within the liver associated with cirrhosis leads to an increase in the lymphatic flow, which, by oozing lymph fluid from the hepatic surface, causes an increase in the ascitic fluid and an increase in the protein concentration of the fluid [7].

Other factors may potentiate this problem but a positive feedback situation results; the compensatory efforts of the body end up being self-defeating and leading the organism away from the steady state. Without intervention the course progressively degenerates, leading to increased ascites.

Ascites causes abdominal swelling that can be evaluated by an increased girth on measurement. The increased intraabdominal fluid may cause pressure on the diaphragm and respiratory difficulties. The ascitic fluid may be removed by peritoneal tapping but frequently reaccumulates rapidly. The associated hypoproteinemia may lead to further ascites along with production of generalized edema. The generalized edema, called *anasarca*, results mostly from a decrease in the plasma colloid osmotic pressure generated from the decreased albumin levels, encouraging fluid exudation into all of the interstitial compartments.

Fatty Liver

Fatty liver refers to the infiltration of the hepatocyte by fat or lipid material. This infiltration by itself usually does not significantly disrupt the physiologic process of the cell, but over a period of time the fatty cell becomes surrounded by fibrous tissue that separates the liver lobules. The pathologic appearance may be described as either micronodular or macronodular. Micronodular infiltration can only be seen with a high-intensity microscope, but macronodular lobules have fat infiltration and fibrosis that are easily seen. Several factors influence the deposition of fat: (1) A diet high in fat may overwhelm the metabolic processes of the liver, leading to increased triglyceride stores. (2) A diet with too little protein, such as with starvation, causes mobilization of fatty acids from adipose tissue. These, in turn, travel to the liver, and fatty infiltration of the hepatocyte results. (3) Alcoholism leads to fat accumulation in the parenchymal cells of the liver and distention of the cytoplasm with fat. In certain areas, the infiltrated cells undergo fibrosis, which increases the likelihood of portal hypertension. Whether alcohol is a direct hepatotoxin or a producer of nutritional inadequacy has been studied. The weight of the evidence supports the claim that it is a hepatotoxic substance. Large amounts of alcohol have been demonstrated to increase accumulation of lipids within the cells, resulting in a liver that weighs 2.0 to 2.5 kg (normal weight is about 1.5 kg) and appears soft and greasy when cut [7]. Alcohol may affect the conversion of fatty acids to lipoproteins in the liver, but the mechanism for its induction is not precisely known.

Clotting Disturbances

Because the liver produces many of the major clotting factors, liver dysfunction of 60 percent or more leads to depletion of these factors and a tendency to bleed. A decrease in the uptake of vitamin K into the hepatocyte leads to decreased prothrombin levels. The major clotting dysfunction results from the depression in the production of prothrombin, but fibrinogen and other clotting factors may also be depressed. The platelet count may be inadequate as a result of hypersplenism, which is a frequent companion to liver failure. In liver failure an increased risk of hemorrhage is always present, especially when it is associated with esophageal varices and portal hypertension.

Portal Hypertension and Esophageal Varices

Obstruction to the blood flow through the liver results in increased pressure in the portal venous system. The term *portal hypertension* refers to high pressures in the portal vein and its tributaries. The blood, meeting resistance in the portal vein, seeks collateral channels around the high pressure areas or through the obstructed liver. In the portal system, the vessels most susceptible to the higher pressure are the esophageal veins and the hemorrhoidal veins (Fig. 37-2). The esophageal veins bulge into the lumen of the esophagus and become thin-walled varices that look like bulging bags on the inner surface of the esophagus. The esophageal varices can become irritated by gastric acidity or by spasmotic vomiting. Irritation from alcohol or other irritants can cause chemical breakdown of the walls of the varices. Any of these situations can result in rupture and massive upper gastrointestinal hemorrhage. The two main factors that encourage the hemorrhage are

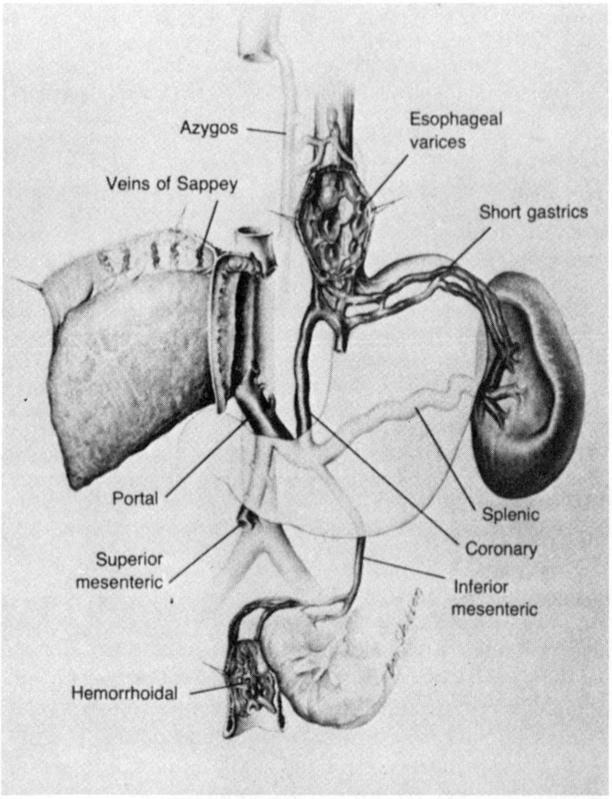

FIGURE 37-2. Esophageal varices and dilated hemorrhoidal veins from portal hypertension. (From W. A. D. Anderson and J. W. Kissane, *Pathology* [7th ed.]. St. Louis: Mosby, 1977.)

depressed formation of clotting factors and high portal pressures. Continued vomiting after the first bleeding event usually results in further bleeding. Rupture of esophageal varices may result in exsanguination and death if it is not treated immediately. Rectal hemorrhoids also may rupture and bleed under pressure, causing a massive amount of bright red rectal bleeding. Anything that can cause increased motility of the lower gastrointestinal tract can increase the risk for hemorrhage from this area.

Collateral channels develop because of the high portal pressure and provide a route for direct shunting of blood from the portal veins to the inferior vena cava, thus bypassing the liver. The shunted blood contains large amounts of ammonia that may precipitate onset of hepatic encephalopathy. The bloodborne bacteria absorbed from the small intestine and normally processed and detoxified in the liver also are shunted directly into the systemic circulation. Various substances that bypass the liver are not metabolized and may accumulate in the body with deleterious effects on the nervous system.

Bleeding from esophageal varices, duodenal ulcers, or other sources may precipitate jaundice and production of ammonia due to the processing and absorption of products of the red blood cell in the intestine. These developments may lead to increased risk of encephalopathy, which, with the bleeding event, may be life-threatening.

Hepatorenal Syndrome

In liver failure, the development of associated renal failure indicates a very poor prognosis. The hepatorenal syndrome seems to be a specific condition that leaves the kidneys almost normal morphologically but functionally impaired. It is diagnosed in person's developing acute renal failure in the presence of significant hepatic disease; frequently it is precipitated by a clinical deterioration such as a gastrointestinal bleeding episode or the onset of hepatic coma [7]. This condition begins suddenly with a decreased urinary output and an elevation in the serum urea nitrogen and the creatinine levels. It is accompanied by an elevated blood ammonia level and increasing jaundice, probably due to the failure of bilirubin excretion in the urine. At autopsy, no permanent morphologic change can be demonstrated in the kidneys. The syndrome seems to be an evolutionary process of functional impairment of the kidney resulting from liver failure.

Liver Failure

Liver failure refers to a constellation of clinical manifestations that are the ultimate outcome of many types of liver disease. The liver has a large reserve and approximately 80 percent of the parenchyma of the liver can be destroyed before clinical signs of liver failure begin. In a series of 60 cases, cirrhosis was the most common cause of liver failure, with viral hepatitis and chemical and drug injury occurring less frequently [3]. All of these conditions cause massive liver damage that leads to a number of characteristic physiologic changes including (1) jaundice, with increased conjugated and unconjugated bilirubin levels; (2) changes in the neurologic status with hepatic encephalopathy and coma; (3) hypogonadism and gynecomastia due to imbalances of the androgen-estrogen levels; (4) palmar erythema with vasodilation in the palms of the hands and feet; (5) spider angiomas of the skin, probably related to clotting disturbances and/or increased portal pressure; (6) fetor hepaticus, a peculiar musty odor of the breath often associated with high serum ammonia levels; and (7) ascites and edema related to portal hypertension and hypoalbuminemia (see Fig. 37-3).

The characteristic wasting of liver disease is manifested by muscular atrophy, weight loss, and loss of plasma proteins and clotting factors. Liver failure frequently causes death from cirrhosis of the liver; recovery depends on the amount of liver damage sustained.

Hepatic Encephalopathy and Coma

Hepatic encephalopathy refers to an alteration in the neurologic status in patients with significant liver disease. The onset may be gradual but more frequently it is precipitated by a major hemodynamic insult in the marginally compensated individual suffering from cirrhosis of the liver. Conditions that may precipitate encephalopathy include bleeding from esophageal varices, ingestion of narcotics or barbiturates, anesthetics, excessive protein intake, electrolyte imbalance, or hemodynamic alterations such as hypovolemia or shock. Anything that can increase the metabolic demands placed on the borderline liver can precipitate liver failure with resultant encephalopathy and coma.

Onset of the neurologic problem is related to the inability of the liver to metabolize the nitrogenous products absorbed from the intestine. These nitrogenous products may include dietary protein or proteins released in gastrointestinal bleeding episodes. The serum ammonia levels are often elevated in encephalopathy, but other substances probably produce the clinical syndrome as well [1]. The liver is believed to produce some substances that are important in normal brain metabolism and these substances may be depressed in liver damage.

Hepatic encephalopathy has been described in terms of discrete stages or phases that are variable in length and may progress insidiously from one level to the next. Advanced hepatic disease is invariably present, frequently complicated by portal hypertension. The onset phase of encephalopathy is heralded by personality changes, including disturbances of awareness, forgetfulness, increased irritability, and confusion. As the condition progresses, a phase having the distinct neurologic patterns of hyperreflexia and asterixis occurs. *Asterixis* is a peculiar "flapping tremor" that can be elicited by dorsiflexion of the hands. Violent, abusive behavior, accompanied by changes on the electroencephalogram (EEG) are often seen. The EEG changes of characteristic symmetric high-voltage, slow-wave patterns are seen 1 to 3 times per second and are imposed on a relatively normal EEG [5]. The progression of the encephalopathy to the coma phase results in absence of the flapping tremor and depression or decline of the wave forms on the EEG. A positive Babinski sign and hyperactive reflexes are seen with the onset of the comatose phase. Persons exhibiting recurrent or progressive forms of this condition have been found to have distinctive changes in the brain tissue with proliferation of the astrocytes and patchy cortical necrosis. When these changes occur, areas of permanent damage result [7].

CIRRHOSIS OF THE LIVER

The term *cirrhosis* is a general term for a condition that destroys the normal architecture of the liver lobules. It has the following three important structural features: (1) destruction of liver parenchyma, (2) fibrous tissue separating the lobules, and (3) formation of regenerative nodules [8]. Cirrhosis is classified according to its causative agent and the resultant pathologic configurations.

The major classifications of cirrhosis are biliary, postnecrotic, Laennec's, and cardiac cirrhosis.

Biliary Cirrhosis

Biliary cirrhosis may be due to an intrahepatic block that obstructs the excretion of bile, or it may occur secondarily

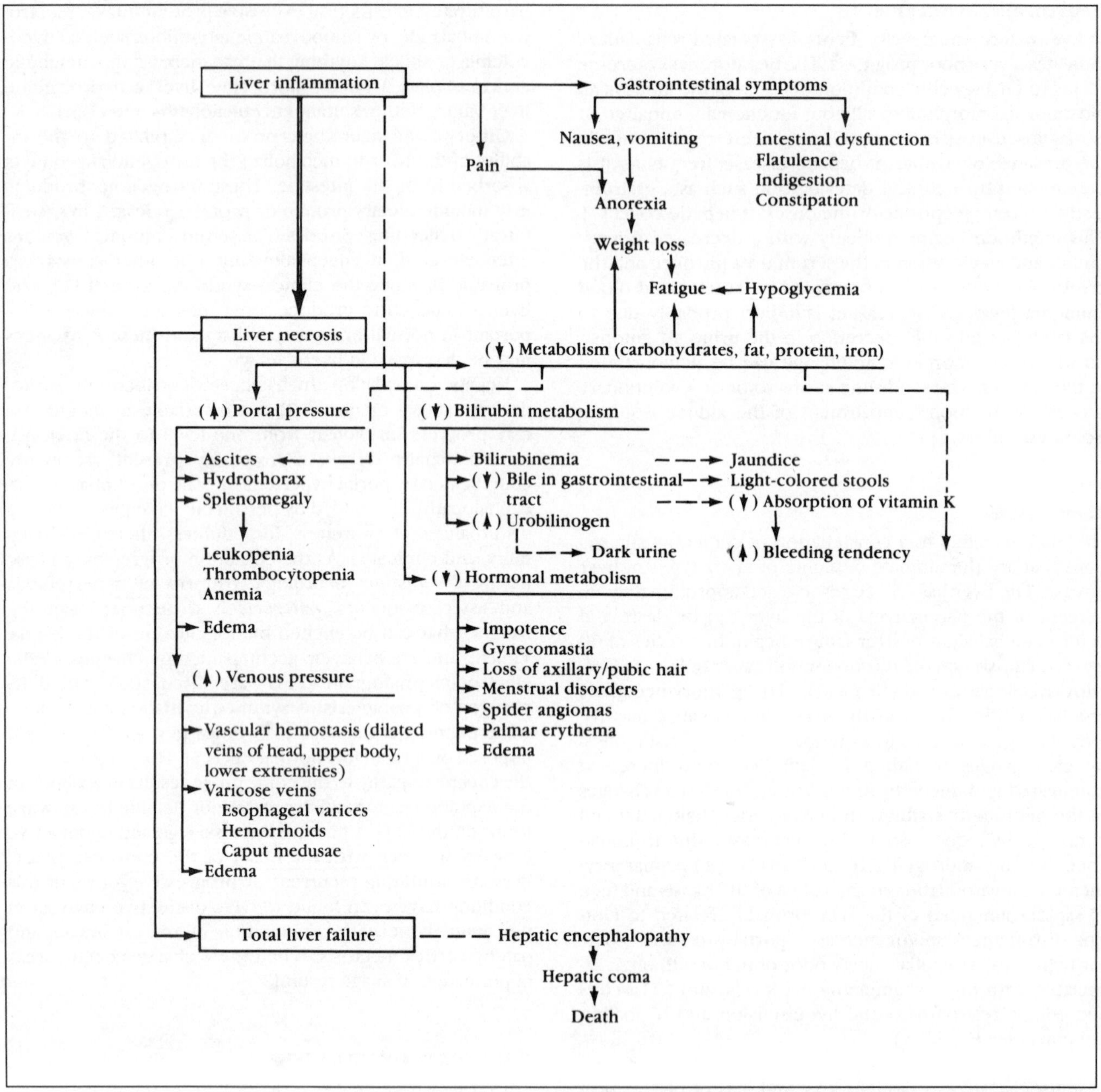

FIGURE 37-3. Progression of liver cell failure. (From W. J. Phipps, B. C. Long, and N. F. Woods, *Medical-Surgical Nursing* [2nd ed.]. St. Louis: Mosby, 1983.)

to obstruction of the bile ducts. The ultimate outcome differs with each type.

Intrahepatic biliary stasis is often called primary biliary cirrhosis and is most frequently seen in women over the age of 40, suggesting an endocrine contribution. Specific and nonspecific immunologic abnormalities have been implicated in this disease based on the demonstration of antibodies and impaired T lymphocyte function [3].

Secondary biliary cirrhosis results from obstruction of the hepatic or common bile duct and produces stasis of bile in the liver. This excess bile may lead to progressive fibrosis, parenchymal cell destruction and regenerative nodules, an apparent reaction of the interlobular bile ducts to the increased amounts of bile within them. Injury, inflammation, and scarring result from the stasis of bile in the lobular compartments [7].

Both intrahepatic and extrahepatic biliary cirrhosis are associated with fibrosis that surrounds hepatocytes and separates the lobules. Scarring and injury are located in close proximity to the interlobular bile ducts.

The clinical course is usually more severe with the primary type than the secondary type because surgical intervention usually relieves the biliary stasis with the latter type. Jaundice may be severe with either type and is associated with bilirubinemia and clay-colored stools. Liver function tests are abnormal with the alkaline phosphatase and cholesterol levels often becoming markedly elevated. When the serum cholesterol exceeds 450 mg/dl *cutaneous xanthomas*—which are nodular swellings filled with cholesterol and tissue macrophages—may appear. Both the conjugated and unconjugated bilirubin levels may increase. As increasing liver damage occurs, all of the signs of hepatocellular failure may appear.

Postnecrotic Cirrhosis

This type of cirrhosis follows massive liver necrosis and involves the destruction of lobules and even lobes of the liver. It may be seen following hepatitis or after exposure to hepatotoxins such as carbon tetrachloride. A period of time after the onset of disease or injury passes when regenerative attempts are made by the liver. The liver may become small and composed of large nodules separated by fibrous bands or scars [3].

Early clinical manifestations include an enlarged, tender liver that is later replaced by a shrunken, nodular liver. Signs of portal hypertension are often present and many problems of liver dysfunction complicate the condition. This type of cirrhosis is suspected in persons who have no history of excessive alcohol ingestion but who have signs of chronic liver disease. Abnormal liver function tests are the rule and a liver biopsy determines the underlying pathology. This condition is also associated with an altered immune system, often with increased immunoglobulins, positive antinuclear antigen tests, and positive LE (lupus erythematosus) cell preparations.

Laennec's Cirrhosis

This disease entity has been shown for the most part to be caused by chronic alcoholism but may be caused by malnutrition and protein depletion. At least 10 to 20 percent of persons who are chronic alcoholics have clinical or morphologic evidence of cirrhosis [3, 7]. A high incidence of the disease is noted in highly civilized countries, among all economic classes, and in all races.

Alcohol has been shown to be a hepatotoxin and induces metabolic changes within the liver, leading to fat infiltration of the hepatocyte and scarring between the lobules. *Alcoholic hepatitis* is commonly associated with Laennec's cirrhosis and may precede the onset of cirrhotic pathology. There is usually a close association between a poor diet and the history of alcohol abuse.

In alcoholic hepatitis, the liver becomes enlarged and hepatocyte degeneration with infiltration by leukocytes and lymphocytes occurs. Intracellular inclusions called *Mallory's bodies,* or alcoholic hyalin, produce the sclerosing hyaline necrosis [1]. The early progression of the disease has an inflammatory character that decreases as the cirrhotic process progresses to the destruction of hepatocytes. Infiltrating fibroblasts and collagen formation lead to early scar formation. Acute exacerbations of alcoholic hepatitis cause inflammation and further damage to the liver parenchyma. As cirrhosis ensues, the liver capsule becomes firm to the touch and regenerative nodules form, resulting in a hobnail appearance. As the pathology progresses, the liver shrinks in size and becomes finely nodular in appearance. The nodules are surrounded by evenly spaced, grayish connective tissue [7]. The liver pathology is usually associated with enlargement of the spleen.

The physiologic results of Laennec's cirrhosis depend on the amount of inflammation, degeneration, infiltration of the cells by fat, and scarring. The liver cell degeneration may lead to portal hypertension and ascites. Jaundice and esophageal varices often occur later in the progression of the disease. All of the complications associated with liver dysfunction may occur depending on the amount of damage the liver has sustained. Some of the more common problems are clotting disorders, hypoproteinemia, signs of biliary obstruction, and gastrointestinal bleeding.

Clinically, cirrhosis of this type appears as an insidious condition causing abnormal liver function tests, fluid retention, ascites, and esophageal varices (Fig. 37-4). With abstinence from alcohol, the liver function tests may return nearly to normal, but excessive ingestion of alcohol or continued poor diet may lead to decompensation.

It has been shown that 80 to 90 percent of patients with significant cirrhosis of the liver die of the disease within 5 years. The progression of the disease can be markedly altered by abstinence from alcohol. Death may be due to liver failure, infection, or gastrointestinal bleeding.

Cardiac Cirrhosis

Cardiac cirrhosis is chronic liver disease caused by right-sided heart failure of long standing and it causes typical cirrhotic changes in the liver. Pathologically, the liver appears swollen, edematous, and dark in color. Fine nodules of regeneration may be seen [2].

In this condition, the liver has served as a reservoir or safety valve for significant amounts of blood for a long period of time. The increased volume and resultant increased pressure leads to those scarring and regenerative changes that are characteristic of cirrhosis.

The clinical appearance is one of acute and decompensating right-sided heart failure that is often refractory to diuretic therapy. Ascites and other signs of portal hypertension may occur. The liver function tests will be abnormal, depending on the degree of impingement on and congestion of the liver parenchyma.

CANCER OF THE LIVER

Tumors of the liver that cause functional impairment and hepatomegaly are almost always malignant. The rare benign tumors are often of the angioma and adenoma classifications.

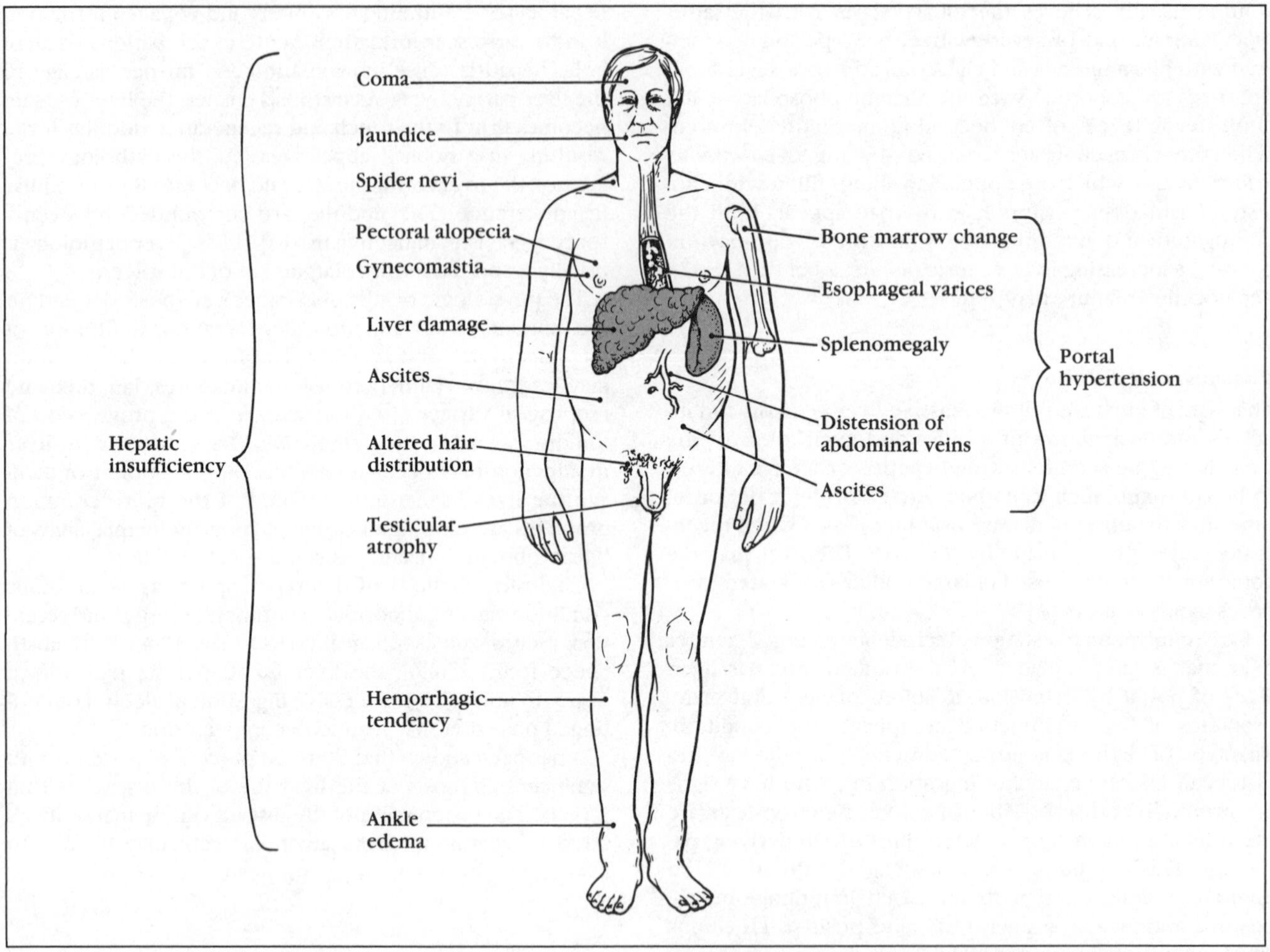

FIGURE 37-4. Clinical effects of cirrhosis of the liver.

Primary Malignancies

Primary carcinoma of the liver is relatively rare and may arise within the hepatocyte, from the canaliculi or small biliary ducts, or it may be of mixed type. The hepatocellular carcinoma accounts for 80 to 90 percent of primary malignancies of the liver [7].

A study of the epidemiology of primary liver tumors shows that they may be related to diet and other types of liver disease, especially hepatitis. In the United States, the incidence of primary liver carcinoma is less than 3 percent, while in some parts of Africa primary liver malignancy may represent 50 percent of all cancers in men and 20 percent in women. Some of the influences that may contribute to its incidence include (1) carcinogenic agents in food, (2) cirrhosis of the liver, (3) viral infections of the liver, and (4) parasitic liver infections [7].

Pathologically, the carcinomatous growth may be limited to one area, occur in multiple nodules, or occur as infiltrates on the surface of the liver [1]. The tumors may secrete different substances, especially bile products. Usually the growth rate is very rapid and terminates in liver failure and death.

Physiologically, tumors of the liver interfere with the normal function of the hepatocyte, but they often create no difficulty until they are far advanced. Biliary obstruction with jaundice, portal hypertension with ascites, and different sorts of metabolic disturbances related to the functional impairment of different hepatocytes result. The metabolic disturbances include hypoalbuminemia, hypoglycemia, and bleeding problems.

Clinically, the affected person will exhibit signs of debilitation, weight loss, and cachexia. Jaundice, ascites, and other signs of liver failure are often related to the progression of the condition and frequently are seen in the terminal state. Tumors of the liver are rarely considered to be resectable. Precise diagnosis is made by biopsy but liver and computed tomography (CT) scans are helpful. Liver function tests reflect the degree of disruption of normal liver function.

Metastatic Carcinoma of the Liver

The liver is very fertile soil for the metastasis of malignancies arising in other areas of the body. Metastasis to the liver is a frequent occurrence with pulmonary, breast, and gastrointestinal tract carcinomas. Other types of malignancies metastasize less readily to the liver.

Physiologically, the liver is vulnerable to metastatic carcinoma because of the large volume of blood it receives each minute, the high nutrient level of its blood, and the large reserve of lymphatic drainage. Development of metastasis usually causes widespread involvement and disruption of liver function. The liver function tests are frequently abnormal, especially the alkaline phosphatase, the serum enzymes, and bromosulfpthalein (Bromosulphalein) retention. The carcinoembryonic antigen (CEA) in the serum, which is increased in the presence of many malignancies, will be increased with many liver malignancies and metastases. The height of the serum levels correlates to some extent with tumor size and degree of metastasis and is seen to decrease markedly after successful treatment.

The clinical course relates to the rapidity of growth of the metastatic lesion and the primary site of the malignancy. There is a rapid decline in the nutritional status with marked cachexia, muscular wasting, and hepatomegaly. Obstruction to bile flow may lead to jaundice and all of the other dysfunctions of liver disease may be present, depending on the amount of liver involvement.

The prognosis following liver metastasis is poor due to the lack of tumor response to treatment and the impossibility of surgical resection of the tumor. The 5-year survival rate has been reported to be less than 5 percent.

ACUTE HEPATITIS

Hepatitis is a condition of inflammation and injury of the liver. It is a reaction of the liver to a variety of conditions, specifically viruses, drugs, and alcohol. This section details acute hepatitis resulting from viral infection.

Acute viral hepatitis is an infectious disease that is caused by at least two strains of viruses, classified as hepatitis A and hepatitis B. These organisms are distinguished by their antigenic properties but both types are transmissible; and the complications that may result can inflict permanent liver damage. Non-A and non-B hepatitis also have been identified on the basis of demonstration of viral antigens. These viruses apparently are transmitted much like hepatitis B.

Hepatitis A

Hepatitis A infection has been shown to result most frequently from fecal-oral contamination by the hepatitis A virus but may also result from the infusion of infected blood. It is more frequently seen in crowded, unsanitary living conditions, has no sex predilection, and is often epidemic in children or young adults. It has been called the "dormitory disease," as epidemics may break out and infect a large number of students in close living situations. This infection may also be transmitted by shellfish, which process and concentrate the contaminated material. Contaminated water has also been implicated as a source for carrying the organism.

Incubation, following exposure, takes about 2 to 6 weeks before clinical signs are evidenced. The antibody level rises quickly after the onset of clinical signs and this level remains elevated for approximately 10 years. In areas such as Costa Rica, where the disease is endemic, 90 percent of the population have anti-HA antibodies by their teenage years [7].

Hepatitis B

Hepatitis B has been shown to result most frequently from viral contamination with the hepatitis B virus. Blood transfusion or needle contamination are common sources of infection but it also may be transmitted by the oral and venereal routes. The high exposure populations for hepatitis B are those exposed to the risks of needle contamination, including persons receiving multiple blood transfusions, personnel and patients in renal dialysis units, drug addicts, and persons taking immunosuppressive medication. Families or other close contacts of any of these individuals may also be at higher risk.

Hepatitis B has a longer incubation period than hepatitis A, averaging 6 weeks, but clinical manifestations can occur up to 6 months after exposure. The hepatitis B organism can be identified by a specific antigen called the *Australian antigen.* Several different particles have been identified, of which the *Dane particle* has been called the hepatitis B particle. This particle is composed of two coats or shells and probably is the intact hepatitis B virus. A specific associated antigen called the ***hepatitis B surface antigen (HBsAg)***, may contain several related antigens that may be used to differentiate hepatitis B from other hepatitis. Through laboratory studies, the hepatitis B virus has been classified as a DNA virus, which means that it utilizes deoxyribonucleic acid (DNA) for specific viral replication [4].

Immunologic Features of Hepatitis A and B

With both hepatitis A and B strains, a nonspecific increase in immunoglobulin gamma (IgG) and immunoglobulin macroglobulin (IgM) occurs. The formation of type specific IgG antibodies has been shown following the infection and may persist for years in the sera. This accounts for the immunity exhibited by patients following hepatitis A infections. Specific antibody to HBsAg has been noted that persists for 6 to 12 months after infection. These antibodies can be seen in 20 to 30 percent of the general population in the United States and probably serve as a protection against infection with the hepatitis B virus [7].

Pathologic Features of Hepatitis A and B

Pathologically, hepatitis A and B are difficult to distinguish, and the pathology may be mild or extensive depending on the severity of the disease. The following three major features are evident: (1) liver cell injury, necrosis, and scarring; (2) regeneration of liver cells with an increased number of mitotic figures, sometimes with crowded, disorganized cells; (3) mononuclear phagocyte system reaction with swelling and reduplication or proliferation of Kupffer cells. The degree of any of the pathologic changes differs according to the severity of the disease and the resolution.

Clinical Course

The clinical course is commonly described in three phases: *prodromal, icteric,* and *recovery.* The development, duration, and severity of the phases depend on the amount of hepatocellular damage. The prodromal phase occurs in the period of time when the person first becomes symptomatic with complaints of anorexia, nausea and vomiting, and many flulike symptoms. It usually precedes jaundice by 1 to 2 weeks. A low-grade fever characteristically occurs with hepatitis A. Dark, bilirubin-positive urine and clay-colored stools may occur 1 to 5 days prior to the onset of jaundice. The icteric phase is heralded by the onset of jaundice and a total bilirubin level of 2.5 mg/dl or greater. The liver becomes enlarged and tender. Laboratory findings may be grossly abnormal. The recovery phase is the period of time when resolution of symptoms occurs. The liver enlargement decreases, but not to normal, and the liver function test findings remain abnormal but recede toward normal. The duration of this period is 2 to 12 weeks and total recovery usually occurs in 3 to 4 months.

The major sequela to hepatitis B is chronic active hepatitis that may lead to liver failure and death. Rare complications may be pancreatitis, pneumonia, peripheral neuropathy, and an increased risk of carcinoma of the liver [3]. The affected person usually suffers the effects of the disease and recovers completely.

GALLBLADDER DISEASE

Cholelithiasis and Cholecystitis

The most common disorders of the gallbladder are cholelithiasis and cholecystitis. Inflammation of the gallbladder is the second most frequent cause of abdominal pain that requires abdominal surgery, the first being appendicitis. Gallstones occur in an estimated 20 million Americans per year, with considerable differences occurring between the races and different socioeconomic groups. Some predisposing factors include an increased incidence in the middle-aged female, in the obese, and possibly with multiparity. Dietary factors, including high fat intake, have long been associated with cholecystitis.

Cholelithiasis refers to biliary tract stones, most of which form in the gallbladder itself. The major constituents of these stones are *cholesterol, calcium bilirubinate,* and *calcium carbonate.* The stones often contain mixtures of these components of bile. Stones comprised primarily of cholesterol account for 80 percent of gallstones in the United States.

CLINICAL MANIFESTATIONS. The clinical manifestations of gallstones occur when the stones migrate to and obstruct the common bile duct. The obstruction causes pain and blockage to the excretion of bile. The visceral pain is precipitated by biliary contractions and is termed *biliary colic.* This pain is not colicky in nature as it is usually perceived as a steady severe aching or pressure in the epigastrium [1].

The obstruction of the bile duct is followed by acute cholecystitis that may be due to increased pressure and ischemia in the gallbladder or to chemical irritation of the organ caused by prolonged exposure to concentrated bile. Primary bacterial infection may cause cholecystitis but in up to 80 percent of cases, obstructive stones in the bile duct are present. Therefore, it is thought that bacterial contamination may either be secondary to the stasis or may result from severe infection such as septicemia. Pancreatic reflux may occur and cause irritation by contact of pancreatic enzymes with the mucosa of the bile duct.

Acute cholecystitis may cause complications with abscesses and/or perforation of the gallbladder. Chronic cholecystitis usually is associated with stones in the biliary ducts and is manifested by fatty food intolerance, nausea and vomiting, and pain following eating.

DIAGNOSIS. The simplest means for diagnosis is the oral or intravenous cholecystogram in which the gallbladder is not visualized. The white blood cell count may be elevated to 10,000 to 15,000. The bilirubin is often increased, causing jaundice. The pain of cholecystitis may mimic myocardial infarction, peptic ulcer, or intestinal obstruction, among other conditions.

OBESITY: A MAJOR DISTURBANCE IN NUTRITIONAL BALANCE

The major nutritional problem in the developed world is the excessive ingestion of sugars, fats, and protein, leading to obesity [6]. Obesity is usually defined as an excess of subcutaneous adipose tissue. The precise definition is difficult but the Framingham Study indicates that a 20 percent excess above ideal weight constitutes a health risk. This means that 20 to 30 percent of the male population and 30 to 40 percent of the female population in the United States suffer from obesity [6].

Eating patterns and appetite are considered on p. 480. Obesity results when the appetite induces a caloric intake above the metabolic expenditure of these calories. Other less common causes of obesity are Cushing's disease, several rare hypothalamic disorders, hyperinsulinemia, and hypothyroidism.

The accumulation of subcutaneous fat tissue may be through an increased number of fat cells or through the enlargement of individual adipocytes (fat cells). Studies indi-

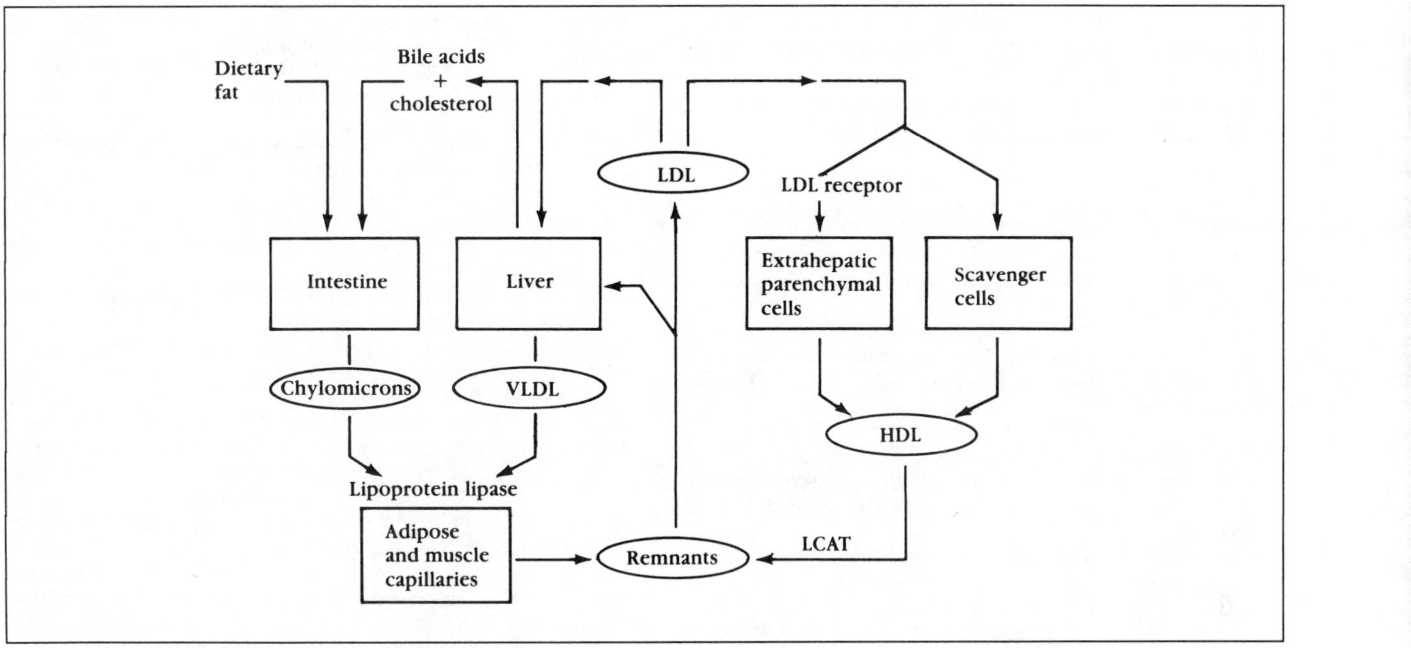

FIGURE 37-5. Model for plasma triglyceride and cholesterol transport in humans. VLDL = very-low-density lipoprotein; LDL = low-density lipoprotein; HDL = high-density lipoprotein; and LCAT = lecithin cholesterol acyltransferase (catalyzes reaction). (From K. J. Isselbacher, et al. [eds.], *Harrison's Principles of Internal Medicine* [9th ed.]. New York: McGraw-Hill, 1980.)

cate that the number of fat cells in the body are laid down during three phases of life: (1) during the last 3 months of gestation, (2) during early childhood, and (3) immediately following puberty [7]. In the adult, an increase in adiposity is primarily due to an increased size of the adipocyte. Studies have also shown that persons with severe obesity problems have a combination of increased size and numbers of adipocytes. When the onset of obesity is in the adult years, it is due to fat cell enlargement and mild to moderate obesity results [7].

Obesity has been linked to the etiology of many diseases; however, it seems to be a contributory factor rather than a causative one. The major diseases of association are hypertension, cardiovascular atherosclerotic disease, diabetes mellitus, pancreatitis, and kidney diseases. Many of these diseases also demonstrate hyperlipoproteinemia, especially in the form of hypercholesteremia.

Lipid Transport

Knowledge of how lipids are transported and the significance of lipoprotein types enhances the understanding of fat deposition in the obese individual. The largest source of lipids are derived from the dietary fats. These are carried in the forms of chylomicrons, very-low-density lipoproteins (VLDLs), remnants of cholestryl esters and triglycerides, low-density lipoproteins (LDLs), and high-density lipoproteins (HDLs). The VLDLs interact with the lipoprotein lipase enzyme, which contributes to the formation of LDL and eventually establishes a cycle by which LDL delivers cholesterol to extrahepatic cells [3, 7]. The production of VLDLs occurs when the liver converts excess carbohydrate to fatty acids and, through another conversion process, forms triglycerides that are the core of the VLDLs. The LDL is the form of most of the total cholesterol of the plasma. This is important in the pathway for the synthesis of steroid hormones as well as in supplying cholesterol to other cells of the body. The HDLs pick up cholesterol, which then reacts with a plasma enzyme, leading again to the formation of LDL (see Fig. 37-5).

In the obese person, when an excess of carbohydrate, fat, or protein is presented to the cell, it can be converted to energy, fat stores, and cholesterol. The fat is broken down to acetate, which, when not needed for energy, is metabolized into fat or adipose stores. Energy production for the most part requires oxygen, while synthesis of fat does not. "It could appear that many individuals supply their cells with too many calories while at the same time these cells do not get enough oxygen. The result is formation of fat within the adipose tissue [6]."

Problems with Excess Fat Production and Storage

Other factors that favor fat production are a decreased thyroid secretion and increased circulating insulin. Thyroid hormones increase the oxidative capability in the Krebs cycle. Excessive insulin leads to fat synthesis and storage.

Obesity, besides being associated with many diseases, increases cardiac workload, can interfere with respiratory excursion, aggravates arthritis and back ailments, precipitates and aggravates varicose veins. Gallbladder disease is associated with obesity and the mortality from cancer has been shown to be increased in persons who are 25 percent or more overweight, especially in breast, colon, and endometrial cancer [7]. In general, obesity is a serious risk factor for many diseases. It can be controlled if the appetite is modified through the hypothalamic appestat and through behavior modification.

REFERENCES

1. Greenberger, N.J., and Winship, D.H. *Gastrointestinal Disorders: A Pathophysiologic Approach* (2nd ed.). Chicago: Year Book, 1981.
2. Hurst, J.W. *The Heart* (5th ed.). New York: McGraw-Hill, 1981.
3. Isselbacher, K.J. Alterations in Gastrointestinal Function. In K.J. Isselbacher, et al. (eds.), *Harrison's Principles of Internal Medicine* (9th ed.). New York: McGraw-Hill, 1980.
4. McElroy, D. Nursing care of patients with viral hepatitis. *Nurs. Clin. North Am.* 12:305, 1977.
5. Netter, F.H. *The CIBA Collection of Medical Illustrations (Vol. 3) Digestive System*. New York: CIBA Pharmaceutical Products, 1957.
6. Ramsey, J.M. *Basic Pathophysiology: Modern Stress and the Disease Process*. Reading, Mass.: Addison-Wesley, 1982.
7. Robbins, S.L., and Cotran, R.S. *Pathologic Basis of Disease* (2nd ed.). Philadelphia: Saunders, 1979.
8. Walter, J.B. *An Introduction to the Principles of Disease*. Philadelphia: Saunders, 1977.

BIBLIOGRAPHY

Altshuler, A., and Hilden, D. The patient with portal hypertension. *Nurs. Clin. North Am.* 12:317, 1977.

Anderson, W.A.D., and Scotti, T. *Synopsis of Pathology* (10th ed.). St. Louis: Mosby, 1980.

Beck, M. Two intestinal tests: One oral, one anal. *Nurs. 81*. 11:20, 1981.

Beeson, P., and McDermott, W. *Textbook of Medicine* (14th ed.). Philadelphia: Saunders, 1975.

Beland, I.T., and Passos, J.Y. *Clinical Nursing Pathophysiological and Pyschosocial Approaches* (3rd ed.). New York: Macmillan, 1975.

Bossome, M.C. The liver: A pharmacologic perspective. *Nurs. Clin. North Am.* 12:291, 1977.

Boyer, C.A., and Oehlberg, S.A. Interpretation and clinical relevance of liver function tests. *Nurs. Clin. North Am.* 12:275, 1977.

Davidson, C.S. *Liver Pathophysiology: Its Relevance to Human Diseases.* Boston: Little, Brown, 1970.

DeCoursey, R.M. *The Human Organism* (4th ed.). New York: McGraw-Hill, 1974.

Delp, M.H., and Manning, R.T. *Major's Physical Diagnosis: An Introduction to the Clinical Process* (9th ed.). Philadelphia: Saunders, 1981.

DiPalma, J.R. How you can prevent GI drug interactions. *RN* 7:63, 1977.

Eisen, H.N. *Immunology* (2nd ed.). Hagerstown, Md.: Harper & Row, 1980.

Ellis, P. Portal hypertension and bleeding esophageal and gastric varices. *Heart Lung* 6:791, 1977.

Fall, D.J. Gastrointestinal Disorders. In S.A. Price and L.M. Wilson (eds.), *Pathophysiology Clinical Concepts of Disease Processes* (2nd ed.). New York: McGraw-Hill, 1982.

Flint, L.M. Trauma: The University of Louisville School of Medicine Symposium. *Heart Lung* 7:247, 1978.

Gilbert, E.F., and Huntington, R.W. *An Introduction to Pathology*. New York: Oxford University Press, 1978.

Greenberger, N.J., and Winship, D.H. *Gastrointestinal Disorders: A Pathophysiologic Approach* (2nd ed.). Chicago: Year Book, 1981.

Gröer, M., and Pierce, M. Guarding against cancer's hidden killer: anorexia-cachexia. *Nurs. 81* 2:6, 1981.

Gröer, M., and Skeleton, M. *Basic Pathophysiology*. St. Louis: Mosby, 1979.

Guyton, A.C. *Textbook of Medical Physiology* (6th ed.). Philadelphia: Saunders, 1981.

Haughey, C. What to say . . . and do . . . when your patient asks about CT scans. *Nurs. 81* 2:72, 1981.

Hegner, B. *Pathophysiology*. Long Beach, Calif.: ELOT, 1980.

Hudak, C., Lohr, T., and Gallo, B. *Critical Care Nursing* (3rd ed.). Philadelphia: Lippincott, 1982.

Hurst, J.W. *The Heart* (5th ed.). New York: McGraw-Hill, 1982.

Isselbacher, K.J. Alterations in Gastrointestinal Function. In K.J. Isselbacher, et al. (eds.), *Harrison's Principles of Internal Medicine* (9th ed.). New York: McGraw-Hill, 1980.

Jenson, D. *The Principle of Physiology* (2nd ed.). New York: Appleton-Century-Crofts, 1980.

Jones, D.A., Dunbar, C., and Jerovill, M. *Medical-Surgical Nursing: A Conceptual Approach* (2nd ed.). New York: McGraw-Hill, 1982.

Junquiera, L.C., and Carneiro, J. *Basic Histology* (3rd ed.). Los Altos, Calif.: Lange, 1980.

Katz, J. Gastrointestinal hormones. *Med. Clin. North Am.* 57:175, 1973.

Kroner, K. Are you prepared for your ulcerative colitis patient? *Nurs. 80* 10:43, 1980.

Lamphter, T., and Robin, A. Upper GI hemorrhage: Emergency evaluation and management. *Am. J. Nurs.* 81:1814, 1981.

Langley, L., and Christiansen, J.B. *Structure and Function of the Human Body*. Minneapolis: Burgess, 1978.

Luckman, J., and Sorensen, K. *Medical-Surgical Nursing: A Psychophysiologic Approach* (2nd ed.). Philadelphia: Saunders, 1980.

McElroy, D. Nursing care of patients with viral hepatitis. *Nurs. Clin. North Am.* 12:305, 1977.

Muir, B. *Pathophysiology: An Introduction to the Mechanisms of Disease*. New York: Wiley, 1980.

Nester, E.W., et al. *Microbiology* (2nd ed.). New York: Holt, Rinehart & Winston, 1978.

Netter, F.H. *The CIBA Collection of Medical Illustrations (Vol. 3) Digestive System*. New York: CIBA Pharmaceutical Products, 1957.

Nursing Grand Rounds: Gastric bypass for morbid obesity. *Nurs. 81* 2:54, 1981.

Pierce, L. Anatomy and physiology of the liver in relation to clinical assessment. *Nurs. Clin. North Am.* 12:259, 1977.

Ramsey, J.M. *Basic Pathophysiology: Modern Stress and the Disease Process.* Reading, Mass.: Addison-Wesley, 1982.

Robbins, S.L., and Cotran, R.S. *Pathologic Basis of Disease* (2nd ed.). Philadelphia: Saunders, 1979.

Selkurt, E.E. *Basic Physiology for the Health Sciences* (2nd ed.). Boston: Little, Brown, 1982.

Shaninpour, N. The adult patient with bleeding esophageal varices. *Nurs. Clin. North Am.* 12:331, 1977.

Shiff, L. *Diseases of the Liver* (4th ed.). Philadelphia: Lippincott, 1975.

Sleisenger, M.H., and Fordtran, J.S. *Gastrointestinal Disease: Pathophysiology, Diagnosis and Management* (2nd ed.). Philadelphia: Saunders, 1978.

Smith, C. Abdominal assessment. *Nurs. 81* 2:42, 1981.

Snell, R. S. *Clinical Anatomy for Medical Students* (2nd ed.). Boston: Little, Brown, 1981.

Sodeman, W., Jr., and Sodeman, W. A. *Pathologic Physiology: Mechanisms of Disease* (6th ed.). Philadelphia: Saunders, 1979.

Sugar, E. Hirschsprung's disease. *Am. J. Nurs.* 81:2065, 1981.

Taylor, P. D. Organ transplantation series: Liver transplantation. *Am. J. Nurs.* 81:1672, 1981.

Thompson, M. Managing the patient with liver dysfunction. *Nurs. 81* 11:100, 1981.

Thorpe, C., and Caprins, J. Gallbladder disease: Current trends and treatments. *Am. J. Nurs.* 80:2181, 1980.

Tobey, L., and Covington, T. Antimicrobial drug interactions. *Am. J. Nurs.* 75:1470, 1975.

Tortora, G., Evans, R., and Anagnostakos, N. *Principles of Human Physiology*. Hagerstown, Md.: Harper & Row, 1982.

Wallach, J. *Interpretation of Diagnostic Tests* (3rd ed.). Boston: Little, Brown, 1978.

Walter, J. B. *An Introduction to the Principles of Disease*. Philadelphia: Saunders, 1977.

Williams, W. J., et al. *Hematology* (2nd ed.). New York: McGraw-Hill, 1977.

Worthington, B. Nutrition symposium. *Nurs. Clin. North Am.* 14:197, 1979.

UNIT 13
MUSCULOSKELETAL FUNCTION

Jennie Lee Moore
MUSCULAR SYSTEM FUNCTION

Joan Williamson
SKELETAL SYSTEM FUNCTION

Thomas Fender
SKELETAL SYSTEM FUNCTION

The musculoskeletal system is often left out of pathophysiology textbooks or is incorporated with other systems of the body. Because this system provides for the framework and for voluntary movement of the body, its inclusion is deemed vital in this text. The muscular system is described in Chapter 38 beginning with the appearance of the muscle cell and progressing to the process of muscle contraction. Smooth muscle physiology is contrasted to that of skeletal muscle, and cardiac muscle structure is reviewed. Common primary muscle abnormalities are described. Chapter 39 describes the architectural framework of the body, especially in relationship to the formation and composition of the bone. No attempt has been made to list all of the bones of the body; the reader is referred to the anatomy texts listed in the unit bibliography for this information. The important disease processes of bone are covered along with traumatic bone and joint injuries. The intent of the material is the discussion of pathophysiology based on normal processes.

The bibliography lists a number of excellent resources for further research. As with each unit, the reader is encouraged to utilize the learning objectives as study guides for chapter content.

CHAPTER 38
NORMAL AND ALTERED FUNCTION OF THE MUSCULAR SYSTEM

LEARNING OBJECTIVES

1. Describe the anatomic components of striated muscle tissue.
2. Define *actin* and *myosin* and their interactions.
3. Discuss the functions of the organelles of the muscle cell.
4. Briefly describe the neuromuscular or myoneural junction.
5. Explain the sliding filament theory.
6. Briefly describe the ratchet theory of contraction.
7. Explain the contraction of a muscle — from the generation of an action potential to the return to the resting state.
8. Describe three ways by which energy is provided to the muscle cell.
9. Define *oxygen debt.*
10. Differentiate between isometric and isotonic contractions.
11. Define *muscle tone.*
12. Compare the anatomy of smooth muscle to that of striated muscle.
13. Trace the progression of an action potential in smooth muscle.
14. Differentiate between spike potentials and slow wave potentials.
15. Describe the two neuromuscular junctions found in smooth muscle.
16. Briefly differentiate between the anatomy of cardiac muscle and that of striated muscle.
17. Define the common problems in muscles: *cramps, twitches, fasciculations, fibrillation,* and *tetany* and *tonic contraction.*
18. Differentiate between adaptive and maladaptive muscular hypertrophy.
19. Describe at least four causes of muscular atrophy.
20. Define *rigor mortis.*
21. Classify the major types of muscular dystrophy.
22. Describe the pathology and clinical course of Duchenne's muscular dystrophy.
23. List the laboratory and diagnostic findings that are helpful in the diagnosis of muscular dystrophy.

The muscles of the human body are well adapted to the work they must perform. Skeletal muscle coordination provides the human being with functions ranging from gross motor activities to fine, precise mobility. Involuntary muscle coordination includes the regular contractions of the heart muscle, the gastrointestinal peristalsis, and other precise essential functions. From the moment of conception, the human body has been programmed to perform with coordination for many years. When alterations in muscular function occur the entire body is affected. This chapter examines the normal process of muscle contraction along with some of the disease processes that may alter muscular functioning.

ANATOMY OF STRIATED MUSCLE

Striated muscle forms the voluntary or skeletal muscular system. Cardiac muscle, which is involuntary, is also classified as striated muscle. Skeletal striated muscle is the predominant type of muscle found in the human body. The muscles are arranged in regular bundles that are surrounded by a sheath of connective tissue called *epimysium*. This structure provides the connective tissue arrangement that binds muscles together and to other structures, while still allowing some freedom of movement.

Description of Muscle Cells

A single muscle is composed of thousands of muscle fibers [7]. The muscle fibers are bundles of long multinucleated cells in which the oval-shaped nuclei are found close to the cell membrane [4]. Bundles of fibers called *fascicles* are embedded in a web of connective tissue called the *perimysium* (Fig. 38-1). Each of the individual muscle fibers is bounded by a network of delicate tissue called *endomysium* [3]. This tissue provides support for the blood vessels and nerves that are adjacent to the muscle fibers.

Muscle cells have a reddish appearance that is due to the presence of the *myoglobin* pigment, an oxygen depot for muscles. The muscles that must maintain activity for periods of time usually contain more myoglobin than other muscles.

Skeletal muscles fibers, whose diameter ranges between 10 and 100 μ, may extend the entire length of the muscle unit or may be joined by connective tissue. Muscle is termed *striated* when it has characteristic markings of regularly appearing bands around the muscle fibers. These bands appear as alternating light and dark areas along the muscle fiber.

The muscle cell contains sarcoplasm, which has many myofibrils, numerous mitochondria, sarcoplasmic reticulum, a t tubule system, numerous sarcoplasmic inclusions, and nuclei very close to the cell membrane. The cell membrane is called the *sarcolemma*.

Myofibrils, Actin, and Myosin

The myofibrils are the contractile units of the muscle. Each myofibril is composed of repeating units called *sarcomeres*, which are composed of contractile proteins called *actin* and *myosin* (Fig. 38-2). This structure is the functional unit of skeletal and cardiac muscle. Actin is a thin filament with twice as many filaments as myosin and has two proteins — *troponin* and *tropomyosin* — associated with it. The myosin filaments, about 1500 per fibril, are thicker and have projections, known as cross bridges, that extend outward toward the actin molecule.

Actin and myosin, lying beside one another, partially overlap, causing the myofibril to have alternate light and dark bands that can be seen only under polarized light in unstained preparations. The light bands containing only actin filaments are called *I bands* while the dark bands containing myosin filaments and part of the actin filaments are called *A bands*. In the middle of the light band is a dark line called the *Z line*. Between the Z lines is the smallest contractile apparatus, the *sarcomere* (Fig. 38-2).

Organelles of the Muscle Cell

The inside of the cell contains *sarcoplasm*, which is the cytoplasm of the muscle cell. Besides containing myofibrils, it contains structural and chemical parts common to all cells (Fig. 38-3). Especially important are the mitochondria, the sarcoplasmic reticulum, the t tubules, electrolytes, and water. Large quantities of potassium, magnesium, and phosphates are found along with enzymatic proteins, bicarbonate, sulfate, and small amounts of sodium, chloride, and calcium.

Mitochondria, found in enormous numbers, provide the energy for contraction. The energy production is through a supply of adenosine triphosphate (ATP), which is mostly formed by the extraction of energy from nutrients and oxygen.

The sarcoplasmic reticulum (SR) is similar to the endoplasmic reticulum of other cells. The major function of the SR appears to be the transport of calcium into the sarcomere unit to initiate muscle contraction (p. 540). The SR is composed of tubules running longitudinally and parallel to the myofibrils. The tubules terminate in closed sacs at the end of each sarcomere, which allow for communication during depolarization and contraction.

The t tubule (transverse tubule) system is closely associated with the SR. It is composed of tubules that extend across the sarcoplasm but open to and communicate with the exterior of the muscle cell.

Neuromuscular or Myoneural Junction

Each skeletal muscle fiber normally receives innervation from a motor nerve. The nerve fiber branches at its end to form a motor end plate or myoneural junction that indents the surface of the muscle fiber membrane (Fig. 38-4). The junction of the axon terminal with the muscle fiber includes the following important structures: (1) the synaptic gutter, the indentation of the fiber membrane where the axon terminal comes in close contact with the fiber; and (2) the synaptic cleft, the small space between the axon and the muscle. Within the axon terminal are synaptic vesi-

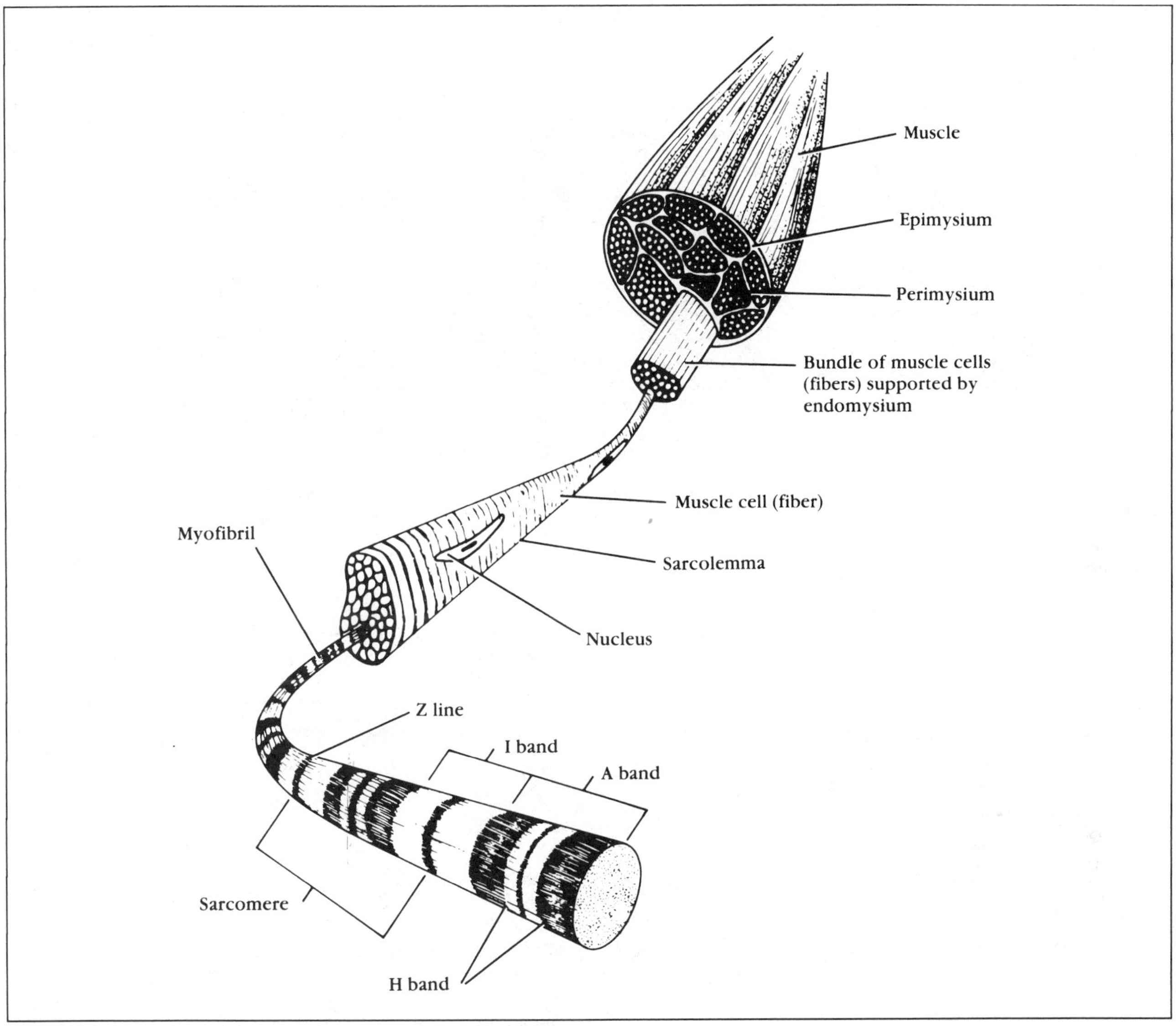

FIGURE 38-1. Structure of striated muscle. (From R. Snell, *Clinical Histology for Medical Students*. Boston: Little, Brown, 1984.)

cles that contain *acetylcholine,* the excitatory chemical transmitter. *Cholinesterase* is present on the surface of the folds of the synaptic gutter and destroys the acetylcholine immediately after the response has been initiated (p. 624).

PHYSIOLOGY OF STRIATED MUSCLE

Sliding Filament Theory

The basis of muscular contraction is the movement or sliding of actin on myosin, which results in a shortening of the entire sarcomere unit. Actin and myosin have been shown to have a strong affinity or attraction for each other, which is inhibited by the proteins troponin and tropomyosin. The structure of myosin facilitates cross linkages with actin, completing the system needed to perform the muscular contraction.

Pure actin filaments bind strongly with myosin when they are in the presence of magnesium ions and ATP, which exist in abundance in the myofibril. When troponin and tropomyosin are added to the thin filament, binding between the actin and myosin filaments is inhibited. When the muscle is at rest, troponin and tropomyosin cover the actin filament so that it cannot bind with myosin. The initiation of the contractile process requires that troponin and tropomyosin be inhibited. When calcium ions are introduced into the sarcomere, troponin and, apparently, tropomyosin are greatly attracted to and bind the ions, leaving actin free to bind with myosin, resulting in contraction. In 1954, A. F. Huxley and associates reported conclusively that when the two sets of filaments (actin and myosin) telescope into each other, contraction takes place [3, 5]. This movement is functionally described as a ratchetlike movement.

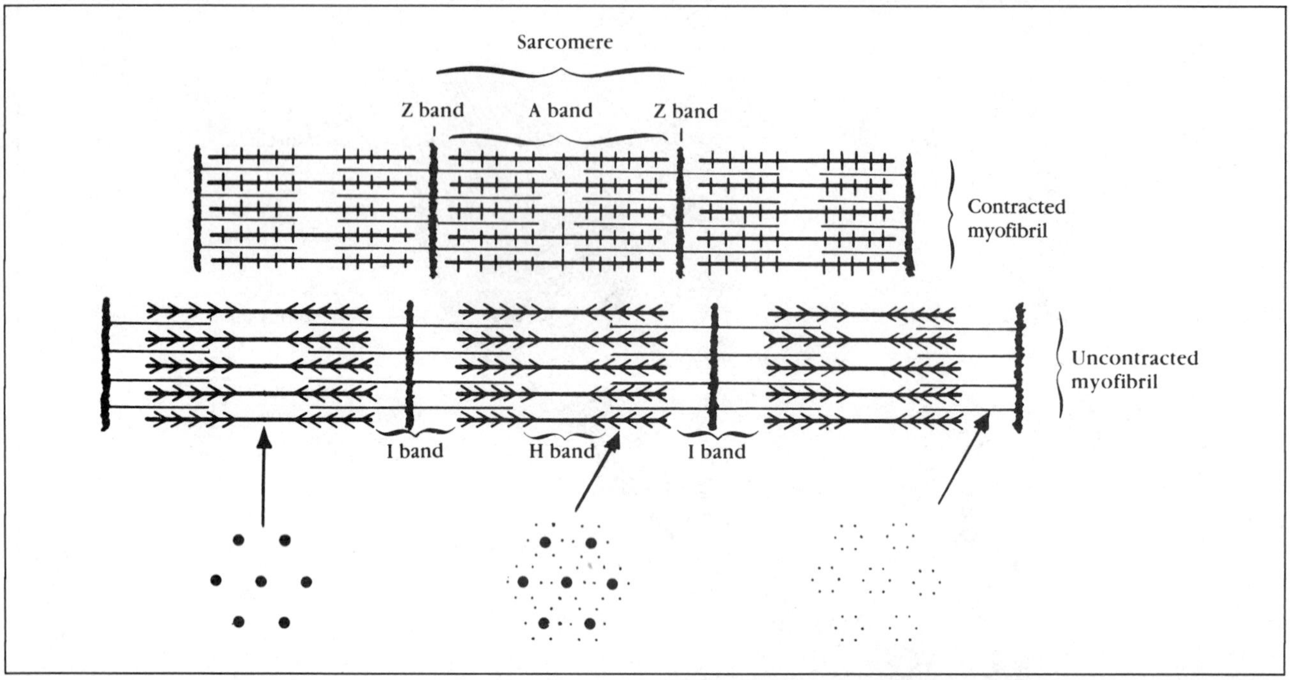

FIGURE 38-2. Portions of contracted and uncontracted myofibrils. The I bands diminish in length in the contracted myofibril. The punctate arrays represent an ultrastructural view of the relationships of thick (myosin) and thin (actin) filaments in cross section through different areas of the sarcomere. A sarcomere is the distance between successive Z bands. (From M. Borysenko, et al., *Functional Histology* [2nd ed.]. Boston: Little, Brown, 1984.)

Ratchet Theory of Contraction

The exact way by which the cross bridges on the myosin interact with the actin is not understood. The ratchet theory proposes that the cross bridges attach to and disengage from active sites on the actin filament (Fig. 38-5). The attachment causes dragging of the actin filament (sliding of actin on myosin). Following this "power stroke," the sites are disengaged and attach to the next active site, pulling the actin filament step by step toward the center of the myosin filament. The cross bridges theoretically operate independently of each other, so that if more cross bridges are in contact with the actin filament, the force of the contraction will be greater [2].

Action Potential Generation and Muscle Contraction

When a stimulus arrives from the nerve axon to the myoneural junction, acetylcholine is released into the synaptic gutter space. This chemical causes the muscle cell membrane to become very permeable to sodium ions. Sodium rushes into the muscle fiber causing a rise in membrane potential or generation of *end plate potential.* The action potential, thus generated, passes down the sarcolemma, depolarizing the t tubule system and causing the release of calcium ions from the SR. Calcium ions, thus released, strongly bind with troponin-tropomyosin, and the sliding of actin on myosin occurs. This is the *contractile phase.*

Calcium must be returned to the tubules of the SR so that troponin and tropomyosin can resume their inhibitory function. This is accomplished by an active *calcium pump* in the walls of the SR. This pump also can concentrate calcium within the tubules and create a depletion of calcium in the myofibrils [2].

The sodium pump also is required for restoration of the sodium-potassium balance and water balance within the cell. This active process is described in Units 1 and 15.

Energy Requirements of Muscle Contraction

Three physiologic reactions provide energy for muscle contraction: the aerobic oxidation of glucose, anaerobic glycolysis, and free energy released from creatine phosphate. These reactions are used to produce ATP.

AEROBIC PROCESS. ATP is a high-energy compound that is supplied mostly through an oxidative process mediated by the mitochondria (see Chap. 1). ATP has been referred to as *energy currency* because it can be made, broken down into adenosine diphosphate (ADP), and then remade by the process of phosphorylation.

CREATINE PHOSPHATE. In the muscle there is a small store of *creatine phosphate* that can rapidly donate its phosphate for energy. This process occurs very rapidly but the stores of creatine phosphate are rapidly depleted. Creatine phosphate is resynthesized in the resting muscle from foodstuffs.

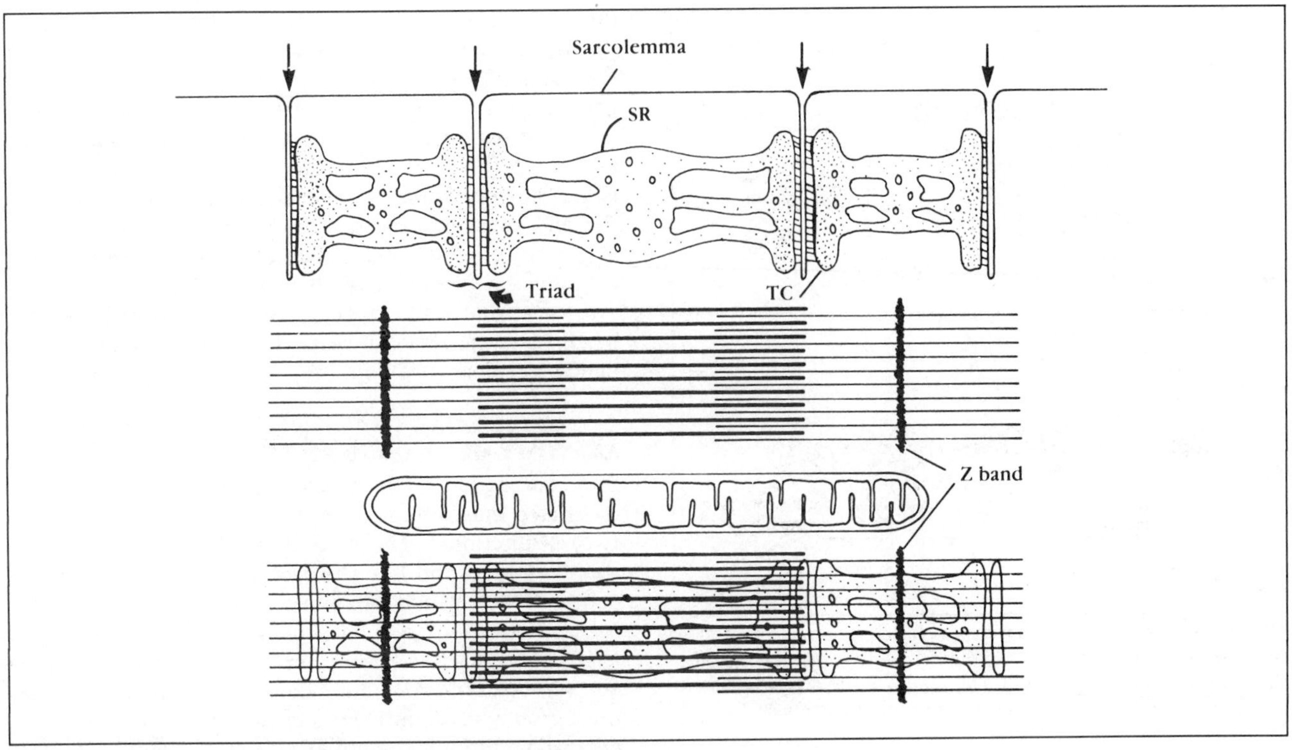

FIGURE 38-3. Thin section of skeletal muscle as it might appear with electron microscopy. Proceeding from the plasmalemma (sarcolemma) inward are the sarcoplasmic reticulum (*SR*), the sarcomere of a myofibril, a mitochondrion separating adjacent myofibrils, and a sarcomere with its associated sarcoplasmic reticulum. The arrows indicate points along the plasmalemma where t tubules invaginate the fiber at the A–I junction of sarcomeres. The terminal cisterns (*TC*) of the SR are associated with the t tubules via short junctional feet, forming the triad where excitation-contraction coupling occurs. (From M. Borysenko, et al., *Functional Histology* [2nd ed.]. Boston: Little, Brown, 1984.)

ANAEROBIC METABOLISM. Anaerobic metabolism provides ATP when the cellular supply of oxygen is insufficient to produce enough ATP to meet the energy requirements of the cell. In the muscular system, it is often utilized when the skeletal muscles are taxed, as in athletic exertion. Without the adequate oxygen supply, the pyruvate does not enter the citric acid cycle to yield carbon dioxide and water, but rather is reduced to lactic acid. The net ATP formed is much less than with oxygen, but it allows the muscle cells to continue their activity for a short period of time.

OXYGEN DEBT. Associated with the entire process of energy and muscle cell contraction is a phenomenon known as the oxygen debt. When muscles are involved in activity, the blood vessels dilate and deliver oxygen to the cells in proportion to the need. When the demand is adequately met, the aerobic metabolism of carbohydrates and fats is accomplished. Sometimes, however, the demand exceeds the rate at which the aerobic process can deliver energy. When this

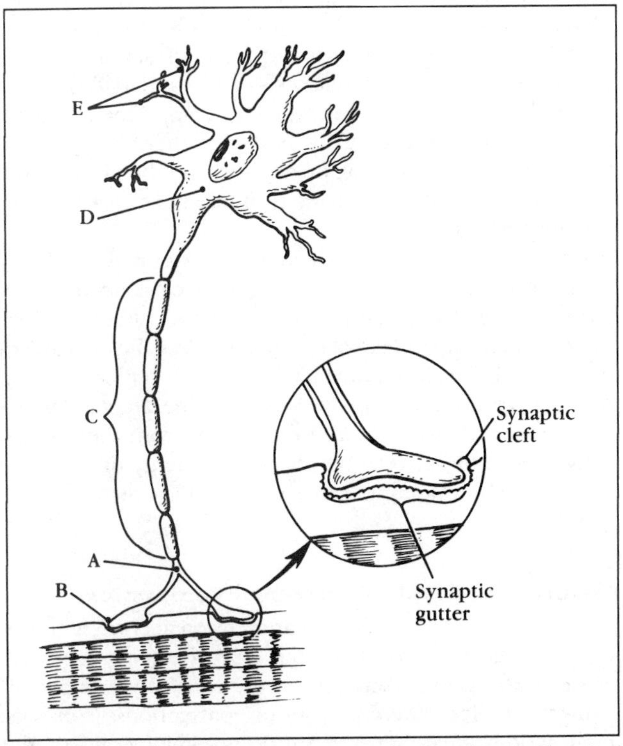

FIGURE 38-4. Myoneural or neuromuscular junction. A. Terminal branching of nerve fibers for the end plates. B. Junction of axon terminal and muscle cell membrane. C. Axon. D. Nerve cell. E. Dendrites.

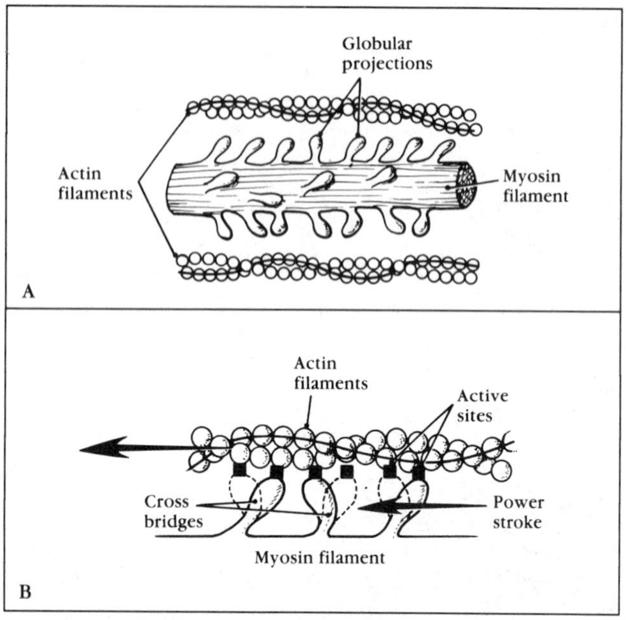

FIGURE 38-5. Ratchet mechanism for muscle contraction. A. The relationship between the myosin filament with its globular projections and the actin filaments. B. The hinges of the myosin filament attach to successive active sites on the actin filaments.

occurs, creatine phosphate is responsible for resynthesis of ATP and ADP. As this supply of creatine phosphate is depleted, anaerobic metabolism of glucose to lactic acid begins. This process results in the resynthesis of creatine phosphate and, hence, resynthesis of ATP and ADP. Because of these events, humans can work far beyond their original muscle capability. Eventually, however, there is more lactic acid produced than can be utilized, and the pH falls to a level so low that the enzymatic response necessary for contraction cannot occur.

Once the intense level of activity has stopped, the body consumes excess amounts of oxygen, as evidenced by the labored breathing seen in runners following a long-distance race. The intake of oxygen oxidizes the excess lactic acid and also aids in the metabolism that replenishes the ATP and creatine phosphate supplies. The amount of excess oxygen that is required to recover from the intense activity is in direct relationship to the energy demands of the body. The amount of oxygen needed is called the oxygen debt.

Isometric and Isotonic Muscular Contractions

Muscles perform work and create tension according to the type of muscle involved and the type of activity required. Muscles are arranged anatomically, electrically, and chemically to provide different types of contractions. *Isometric* contractions create tension but do not involve movement of a load. The muscle fibers do not shorten but tension in the fiber is present. *Isotonic* contractions occur when a muscle contracts against a load and must shorten and remain contracted for the period of time necessary to move the load. Muscles vary according to the work required of the individual muscle. It should be noted that the speed of contraction is matched to the function endowed on the corresponding muscle. Eye muscles, for example, provide fine, precise movement, while large muscles, such as those necessary for posture maintenance, react slowly. The larger, slower muscles have smaller fibers and more capillaries and mitochondria than do faster-moving muscles [2]. These muscles are often called *red* muscles because they contain large quantities of myoglobin.

Muscle tone is the term applied to the tautness seen in healthy muscle tissue at rest. This tone is probably maintained by spinal cord impulses.

ANATOMY OF SMOOTH MUSCLE

The anatomy of smooth muscle differs somewhat from that of striated muscle but the greatest difference between the two is functional. The smooth muscle cell is long and spindle-shaped and has a single nucleus located near the center of the cell. Smooth muscle fibers lack the characteristic striations of skeletal fibers and vary markedly in length. The lack of striations probably is due to a rudimentary sarcoplasmic reticulum and t tubule system. Two distinct groups of smooth muscle have been identified: visceral and multiunit smooth muscle (Fig. 38-6).

Visceral Smooth Muscle

Visceral smooth muscle is found in the walls of the hollow visceral organs, such as the uterus, gut, and bile ducts. The cells are closely aligned and form large sheets of tissue. Because of the close proximity of cells, an action potential spreads cell to cell along the muscle until the entire muscle mass is stimulated.

Multiunit Smooth Muscle

Multiunit smooth muscle is found in the ciliary muscles of the eye and in the piloerector muscles of the skin that cause "goose flesh." The arrangement of cells of this type of smooth muscle is similar to those of striated muscle and it is innervated separately. These muscles contract more rapidly than the visceral smooth muscle.

PHYSIOLOGY OF SMOOTH MUSCLE

Four properties distinguish smooth muscle contractions from other types: (1) the contractile process is relatively slow, with contractions lasting for long periods of time; (2) energy expended during the long contracted states is far less than that of striated muscle; (3) in certain circumstances, such as the delivery of a fetus, the strength of contractions can be very forceful; and (4) a slow relaxation process follows the slow contractile process.

In visceral smooth muscle, electrical excitation proceeds from one muscle fiber to the next without additional release of acetylcholine. This occurs because the tight

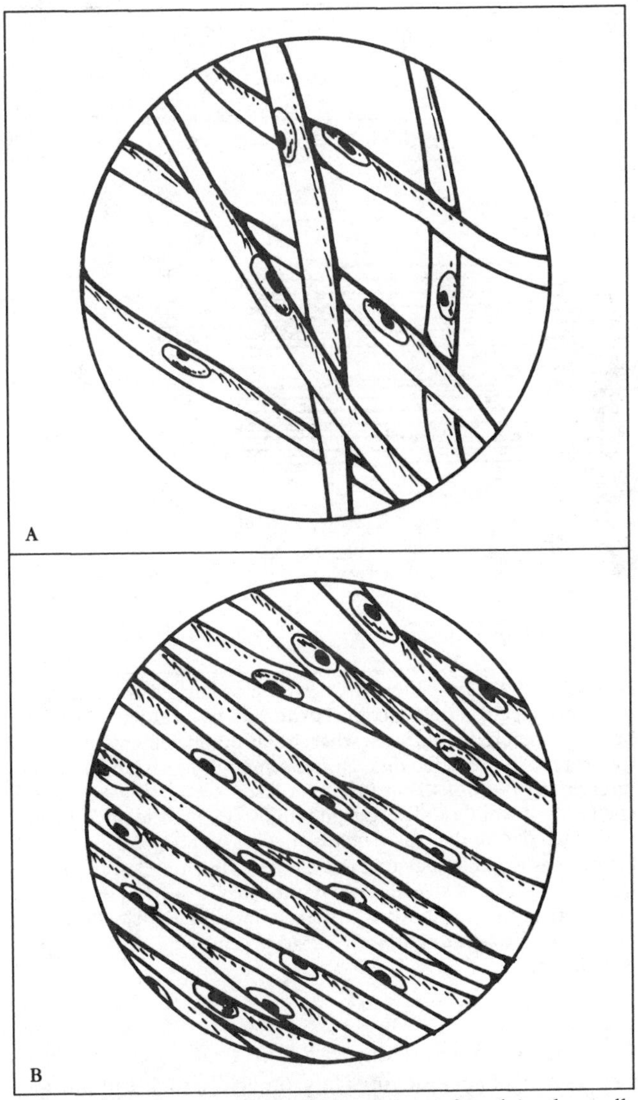

FIGURE 38-6. A. Visceral smooth muscle as found in the walls of hollow, visceral organs. Note close arrangement of fibers. B. Multiunit cells as found in ciliary muscles of the eye, for example. Note the loose arrangement of fibers.

junctions allow the impulse to pass from muscle cell to muscle cell, a syncytial effect.

Action Potentials in Smooth Muscle

SPIKE POTENTIAL. Action potentials develop differently in visceral smooth muscle tissue. The "spike potential," similar to that of striated muscle, can be elicited by (1) electrical stimulation, (2) hormonal action, (3) nerve fibers, and (4) spontaneous generation in the muscle fiber itself.

SLOW WAVE POTENTIAL. The second type of action potential is the *slow wave potential.* Some smooth muscle is self-excitatory with no apparent external stimulation. This is evidenced by rhythmical peristaltic waves. The slow waves apparently contribute to the action potential, a type of pacemaker wave.

Action potentials also may involve *plateaus,* long periods of depolarization, prolonged contraction, and slow repolarization.

Smooth Muscle Tone

Smooth muscle tone relates to the ability of fibers to maintain long-term contraction, which is seen in the peristaltic type of contraction. The smooth muscles of the arterioles exhibit continuous variable degrees of contraction that respond to changing autonomic nervous stimulation.

The degree to which smooth muscle can contract and shorten is much greater than with skeletal muscle. This property allows for changing luminal size in the hollow viscera.

Neuromuscular Junctions of Smooth Muscle

Two types of neuromuscular junctions are seen in the innervation of smooth muscle: (1) the *contact type* in which the nerve fibers come into direct contact with the muscle cells, and (2) the *diffuse type,* which occurs when nerve fibers never come into direct contact with the smooth muscle fibers. The contraction of the muscle may be initiated by nerve impulses (through transmitter substances), chemical agents, changes in the muscle itself, and even local stretch or distention.

Smooth muscle has a nerve supply for inhibition and one for excitation. The transmitters for this — acetylcholine and epinephrine—are secreted by the autonomic nervous system. The response to the chemical transmitters varies, but generally, if acetylcholine excites an organ, norepinephrine acts as an inhibitor and vice versa (see p. 644).

ANATOMY OF CARDIAC MUSCLE

Prior to advancements in microscopic technology, cardiac muscle cells were thought to form a morphologic syncytium. A light microscope reveals cardiac tissue to have cross striations with unique dark bands encircling the fibers at random sites. Seemingly, the cells are incomplete and branch into one another forming a continuous mass of protoplasm. However, use of the electron microscope reveals that cardiac muscle cells are netlike in appearance, with fibers running together, spreading apart, and again running together in no apparent pattern. The dark bands that can be seen with the light microscope are abutting bands of tissue encircling the cardiac fibers (Fig. 38-7). They have been labeled *intercalated disks* and are located at the site of the Z bands. Although each cardiac fiber branches and anastomoses with other fibers, a plasma membrane actually encases each fiber. Each cell has a single, centrally located nucleus. An abundance of elongated mitochondria are found close to the myofibrils in cardiac tissue. As in skeletal cells, myofibrils and the contractile proteins (actin and myosin) are present.

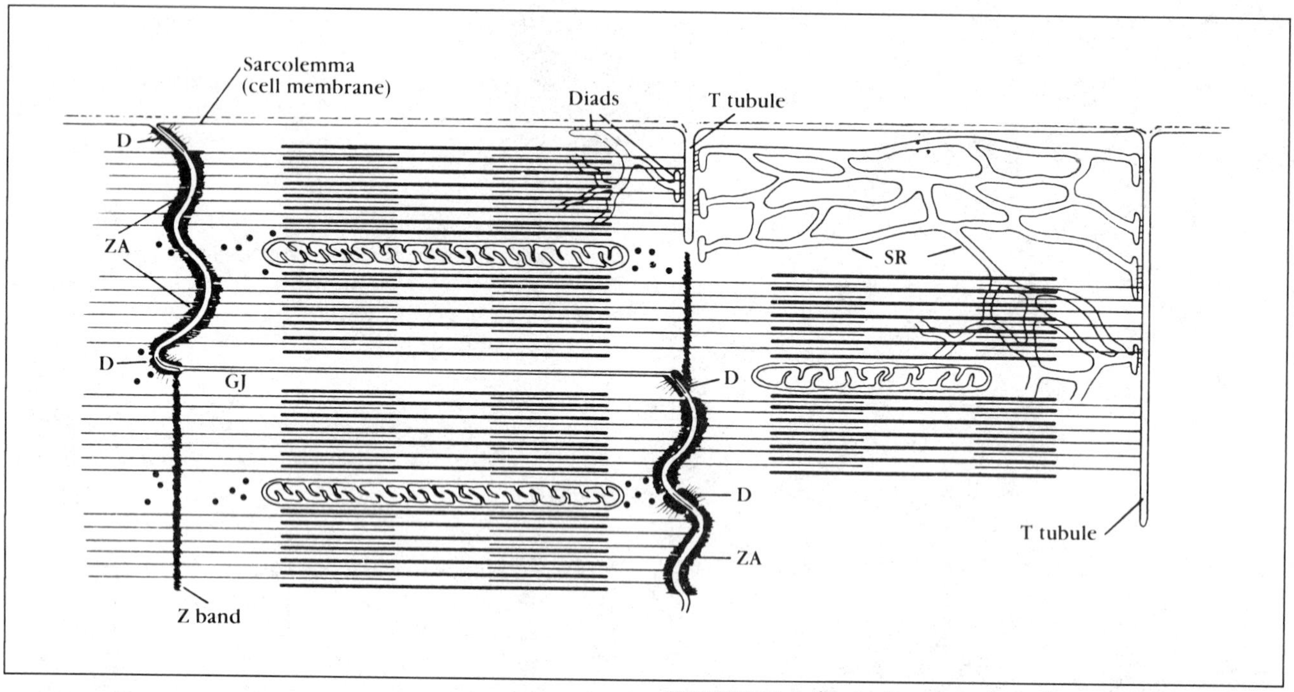

FIGURE 38-7. A thin section through cardiac muscle as it might appear with electron microscopy. Portions of two cardiac muscle fibers are depicted in the area where their plasmalemmas associate to form the intercalated disk. Desmosomes (*D*) provide structural integrity to the disk. Thin filaments insert into the fascia adherens (*ZA*) of the disk. The gap junctions (*GJ*) are located in the horizontal part of the disk. The disk occurs where a Z band would have been. T tubules occur at the Z lines. The sarcoplasmic reticulum (*SR*) forms a sleeve around the myofibrils, but here it is depicted alone to show its pattern more clearly. (From M. Borysenko, et al., *Functional Histology* [2nd ed.]. Boston: Little, Brown, 1984.)

Structural differences between skeletal and cardiac tissue are apparent. A sarcoplasmic reticulum is present in cardiac muscle, but it is very rudimentary in comparison to the sarcoplasmic reticulum of skeletal muscle. The t tubules, however, are 5 times larger in cardiac tissue than in skeletal tissue and are lined with mucopolysaccharide filaments. These filaments seem to trap calcium ions that are used by the sarcoplasm once an action potential has been initiated. Since the terminal cisternae found in skeletal tissue are missing in cardiac tissue, scientists believe that the t tubules function as reservoirs for calcium in cardiac muscle as the terminal cisternae do in skeletal tissue.

Mycocardial muscle fibers are structured in such a way that the atria and ventricles, when normal and intact, react individually as syncytial units. The specialized conductive units—the sinoatrial (SA) node, the atrioventricular (AV) node, the bundle of His, and the Purkinje fibers—work in concert to cause cardiac contraction. The physiology of cardiac contraction is described in detail in Chapter 17.

ALTERATIONS IN MUSCLES OF THE BODY

Common Problems in Muscles

CRAMPS. Cramps, or spasms, are frequent occurrences in the skeletal muscles. They may be associated with motor system disease, metabolic disease such as uremia, tetanus, and electrolyte depletion, especially of sodium, potassium, and calcium. Muscle cramps are often reported at night or during rest and may be due to lowered blood sugar levels at night. Dehydration also may cause cramping, especially if associated with sodium depletion. Cramps are involuntary spasms of specific muscle groups in which the muscle becomes taut and painful. They may be seen in the calf, thigh, hip, or any other major muscle group. Visible fasciculation may also be seen before and after the cramp.

STRAIN. Various degrees of muscle damage may be diagnosed as strain, which usually results from overuse. Strains most frequently occur at the most susceptible part of the muscle-tendon unit and may be very painful or associated with tendonitis.

TWITCHES, FASCICULATIONS, AND FIBRILLATION. These reactions are the result of spontaneous discharge of motor units and single muscle fibers. Twitches occurring at rest may be associated with motor neuron disease and peripheral neuropathies. A fasciculation refers to the involuntary contraction of a single motor unit. It may occur in normal persons and causes visible dimpling or twitching of the skin. Fasciculations may occur rhythmically, starting and stopping for no apparent reason. Fasciculations during contraction of a muscle indicate excessively irritated muscles and may be seen years after poliomyelitis or a degenerative nervous system disease. Continuous fasciculations, called *myokymia*, of unknown etiology may involve all of the voluntary muscles. The spasms may be abolished or alleviated by curare, succinylcholine, and diphenylhydantoin [7]. Fasciculation is often confused with fibrillation, which results from the contraction of single muscle fibers and appears when the motor unit of the axon is destroyed [7].

TETANY. This spasmotic condition most frequently results from hypocalcemia and hypomagnesemia. It is probably due to unstable depolarization of the distal segments of the motor nerves [1]. Hyperventilation may precipitate the condition by lowering serum carbon dioxide, reducing the ionized calcium.

Hypertrophy

Hypertrophy, an enlargement of individual muscle fibers, is an adaptive condition of the cells in the body to an increased demand for work. The cardiac and skeletal muscle cells apparently cannot regenerate to adapt to a need for increased function. They adapt by enlargement of individual fibers. Various nutrients such as ATP, creatine phosphate, and glycogen increase in concentration within the cell when there is need for increased work.

Most hypertrophy is considered to be adaptive hypertrophy that results when resistance is continually applied to the muscle walls. A weight lifter or athlete increases the work load through specific muscles that increase size and strength up to a physiologic limit.

Cardiac hypertrophy is a common result of arterial hypertension, aortic valvular stenosis, and coarctation of the aorta. The hypertrophy increases the force of the cardiac contraction, which can maintain cardiac output for long periods of time. Initially, this is considered to be an adaptive mechanism, but it may become maladaptive if the nutritional needs of the hypertrophied ventricle outstrip the blood supply from the coronary arteries.

Atrophy

Atrophy refers to the decrease in muscle mass due to diminution of the size of the myofibril. Atrophic muscles can result from such diverse factors as aging, immobilization, chronic ischemia of the muscles, malnutrition, and denervation [6]. *Disuse atrophy* is the term used to describe wasting of muscle tissue due to lack of muscle stress, an example of which is atrophic changes occurring after a bone fracture and treatment with casting.

Ischemia causes the cessation of an adequate blood supply so that the oxygen and nutrients required for cellular maintenance are diminished. Eventually, ischemic changes may result in infarction of the ischemic tissue.

Denervation causes atrophic muscular changes that become irreversible. The loss of normal neural stimulation and reduction of muscle tone seem to be the major factors in the atrophic change, rather than lack of weight bearing. If a muscle cell is reinnervated within 3 to 4 months, full function can be restored. After this time some of the muscle fibers become permanently atrophied, and after 2 years muscle function is rarely restored.

Atrophy of muscle tissue may also occur in malnutrition or wasting diseases such as cancer, cirrhosis of the liver, and so forth. The muscle does not receive adequate nutrition and consequently protein wasting occurs.

Rigor Mortis

Rigor mortis is a state of muscular contraction that occurs approximately 2 to 4 hours after somatic death. It results from the lack of production of ATP, which finally allows calcium release and actin-myosin interaction. The contracture becomes intense and the joints become fixed into immovable positions. This state continues for approximately 48 hours, after which gradual autolysis of muscle protein causes the onset of muscle and tissue flaccidity.

PATHOLOGIC PROCESSES AFFECTING THE SKELETAL MUSCLES

Muscular Dystrophies

The muscular dystrophies (MD) are a group of genetically determined, progressive diseases of specific muscle groups. The specific syndromes are classified mainly by the distribution of involved muscles. Classification may also be made by pattern of inheritance, age of onset, and speed of progression [6]. Several members of the same family may be affected, with males predominating and females carrying the genetic abnormality.

DUCHENNE'S MUSCULAR DYSTROPHY. This genetic recessive disorder is almost exclusively seen in males. It is characterized by early development of motor difficulties, inability to walk, symmetric weakness of the arms, and enlargement of the muscles of the calves. Intellectual impairment is common.

The progression of the disease usually is characteristic with lower extremity weakness progressing upward and finally affecting the head and chest muscles. The characteristic pseudohypertrophy of the calf muscle is due to infiltration of the muscle fiber with fatty deposits. The muscle becomes significantly weakened. Weakness of the back muscles results in lordosis. Respiratory or cardiac failure often causes death.

Prognosis in this disease is very poor with death usually occurring before the age of 20. Prior to that time, increasing disabilities require much medical assistance.

ADULT FORMS OF MUSCULAR DYSTROPHY. Adult forms of MD such as the Becker, limb-girdle, facioscapulohumeral, and myotonic forms have a later onset and differ somewhat by the pattern of muscle involvement, heredity, and rate of progression.

LABORATORY AND DIAGNOSTIC TESTS. Most persons with any form of MD have an elevation in the enzymes normally found in the muscles. These include the creatine phosphokinase (CPK), lactic dehydrogenase (LDH), glutamic transaminases, and glucose phosphate isomerase. All of the findings indicate abnormal muscle plasma membranes [6]. Lymphocyte abnormalities have been described in persons with MD.

Electron myography reveals weak electrical currents present in the muscle cell. Muscle biopsies are abnormal due to presence of fatty tissue deposits in the cell.

Myasthenia Gravis (MG)

MG is a disease related to the inability of the neuromuscular junctions to effectively transmit nerve impulses to the muscle cells. It is discussed in more depth on p. 734.

REFERENCES

1. Adams, R. D., and Bradley, W. G. Other Major Muscle Syndromes. In K. J. Isselbacher, et al. (eds.), *Harrison's Principles of Internal Medicine* (9th ed.). New York: McGraw-Hill, 1980.
2. Guyton, A. *Textbook of Medical Physiology* (6th ed.). Philadelphia: Saunders, 1981.
3. Huxley, H. E. The double array of filaments in cross-striated muscle. *J. Biophys. Biochem. Cytol.* 3:631, 1957.
4. Junquiera, L. C., and Carneiro, J. *Basic Histology* (3rd ed.). Los Altos, Calif.: Lange, 1980.
5. Murray, J. M., and Weber, A. The cooperative action of muscle proteins. *Sci. Am.* 230:58, 1974.
6. Robbins, S. L., and Cotran, R. S. *Pathologic Basis of Disease* (2nd ed.). Philadelphia: Saunders, 1979.
7. Young, R. R., Bradley, W. G., and Adams, R. D. Diseases of Striated Muscle. In K. J. Isselbacher, et al. (eds.), *Harrison's Principles of Internal Medicine* (9th ed.). New York: McGraw-Hill, 1980.

CHAPTER 39
NORMAL AND ALTERED STRUCTURE AND FUNCTION OF THE SKELETAL SYSTEM

LEARNING OBJECTIVES

1. Name the three types of bone cells and give the functions of each.
2. Differentiate between intramembranous and endochondral ossification in bone formation.
3. Describe the gross anatomy of the femur as a typical long bone of the body.
4. Describe the blood supply to a bone, including the nutrient and periosteal arteries.
5. Give examples of long, short, flat, and irregular bones.
6. Describe epiphyseal bone growth in children.
7. Name the factors that retard and the factors that accelerate bone growth.
8. Explain the calcium-parathyroid feedback mechanism.
9. Relate calcium and parathyroid levels to vitamin D absorption and manufacture.
10. Discuss the feedback mechanism for calcitonin and calcium.
11. Explore the relationship between the levels of sex hormones, age, and bone formation.
12. Discuss the effects of weight bearing on bone formation.
13. Identify the three classifications of joints and give examples of each.
14. Differentiate between tendons, ligaments, and bursae.
15. Describe the clinical syndrome of osteogenesis imperfecta.
16. Describe the polyostotic form of fibrous dysplasia (Albright's syndrome).
17. Describe Paget's disease of bone.
18. Discuss the skeletal manifestations of the hormone problem in Von Recklinghausen's disease.
19. Name five types of persons at high risk for developing osteoporosis.
20. Identify the usual pathogenesis of rickets or osteomalacia.
21. Compare rickets and scurvy in regard to etiology and physical findings.
22. Describe the pathology of avascular necrosis of the head of the femur.
23. Describe the course of osteomyelitis from beginning infection to the chronic stage.
24. Describe the bone alterations when tuberculosis and syphilis affect the bone.
25. Describe the physical changes of scoliosis.
26. List some possible causes of a congenitally dislocated hip.
27. Explore theories of causation of rheumatoid arthritis (RA).
28. Describe the joint pathology of rheumatoid arthritis.
29. Discuss how rheumatoid arthritis affects other systems of the body, e.g., heart, lungs, eyes, and nerves.
30. Name the joints most commonly affected with degenerative changes.
31. Describe the metabolic disorder responsible for gout.
32. List the most common inflamed bursae and relate the common cause.
33. Define a *complete, comminuted, compression, depressed, stress,* and *avulsion fracture.*
34. Describe the process of fracture healing.
35. List five factors that will modify the healing process of fractures.
36. Differentiate between delayed union, nonunion, and malunion.
37. Relate the symptoms of anterior compartmental syndrome.
38. Describe basic differences between benign and malignant bone tumors.
39. Name three benign tumors arising from cartilage tissue and three from bony tissue.
40. Compare and contrast the sarcomas of cartilaginous origin with those of osteogenic origin regarding symptoms, gross pathology, survival rate, and incidence.
41. Define *Ewing's sarcoma,* including incidence and survival rate.
42. Discuss the skeletal involvement and symptoms of persons with multiple myeloma.

NORMAL STRUCTURE AND FUNCTION OF BONE

In the world we live in, almost everything has a framework. The framework of the human body is the skeletal system. This system of more than 206 bones protects internal organs, provides for support and movement through its muscle attachments, serves as a storehouse for mineral supply, and manufactures blood cells. A living, dynamic tissue, bone contains a blood, nerve, and lymph supply while providing for the constant movement of calcium, phosphorus, and other minerals into and out of the bloodstream.

Bone is a living, collagenous protein into which complex calcium salts have been implanted. The organic matrix of bone, called *osteoid*, is made up primarily of collagen (protein), some polysaccharides, and lipids. The implanted salts, which consist of calcium carbonate ($CaCO_3$), and calcium phosphate ($Ca_3[PO_4]_2$), form a substance that is a hard crystalline salt. The organic matrix of bone provides for *tensile strength* (resistance to being pulled apart), while the mineral deposits provides *compressive strength* (resistance to being crumbled). This combination, like reinforced concrete, gives bone the tensile strength of white oak, and a compressive strength greater than granite [6].

Bone Formation

CELLULAR COMPONENTS. Bone tissue is constantly being formed and reformed. This modeling is facilitated by three types of cells found in living bone that have to do with bone formation and resorption. It is believed that these cells, the *osteoclast*, the *osteoblast*, and the *osteocyte*, are different phases of the same cell [4]. The sequence with which these cells are formed is as follows:

1. Mesenchymal stem cell (from the bone marrow or the periosteum) forms osteoclasts.
2. Osteoclasts form osteoblasts.
3. Osteoblasts form osteocytes.

Osteoclasts are the cells that resorb bone, either by secreting an acid that demineralizes the bone around it, or by actually phagocytosing the bone and ingesting it into the cytoplasm. They live from a few hours to a few days, and whether or not bone formation or bone resorption predominates depends on hormonal and other factors that affect the life span of the osteoclasts [5].

Osteoblasts are the bone-forming cells that secrete collagen, which immediately calcifies into bone. Osteocytes are the living bone cells residing in the lacunae of compact bone.

INTRAMEMBRANOUS OSSIFICATION. Bone formation begins in early fetal life. The fetal skeleton is composed mostly of hyaline cartilage that undergoes ossification. The swapping of the cartilaginous material with bone, begun during fetal life, continues until after puberty. There are two main types of bone formation: intramembranous ossification and endochondral ossification. The more simple and direct type of bone formation is the *intramembranous ossification*, which occurs in the flat bones of the face and skull. In the cartilaginous fetal structure, osteoblasts secrete organic material that calcifies; from this center of ossification, small bone spicules build up an interlacing network on which more bone is developed. Eventually, the osteoblasts become trapped in small spaces called *lacunae* and become osteocytes. The spongy bone developed is then covered by layers of compact bone.

ENDOCHONDRAL OSSIFICATION. This is the process by which the long bones of the body are formed. The "baby skeleton," which is cartilage, is transformed into bone by ossification, which begins in the center of the shaft, the *diaphysis*, and in each end, the *epyphysis*, of the bone. This bone formation spreads, and with it the destruction of cartilage, until only two thin strips of cartilage are left at either end of the bone (the epiphyseal plate), which will remain until bone growth and maturation are accomplished. As spongy bone is formed within, marrow is formed in the spaces and the marrow cavity takes its place in the center of the bone. The osteoblasts on the outside of the bone form layers of hard, compact bone. The perichondrium, which is the layer surrounding the early cartilage, becomes the periosteum, and as more layers of compact bone are laid circumferentially, osteoclasts make the marrow, or medullary cavity, larger in order to support the larger bone (Fig. 39-1).

Bone Structure

MICROSCOPIC STRUCTURE. All bone occurs in three structural forms: cortical or compact bone (hard surface area), cancellous or spongy bone, and medullary bone (inner core). The microscopic structure of *compact bone* consists of multiple, parallel, longitudinal canals, the *haversian canals,* which contain blood vessels, lymphatics, and nerves. Around each canal are several layers, or rings, of bone called *lamellae*. Connecting the haversian canals with the lamellae are minute canals called *canaliculi*, which carry oxygen and nutrients to the bone cells. Each canal with its contents and surrounding lamellae is termed a *haversian system* (Fig. 39-2). Directly under the periosteum and surrounding the medullary canal, several thicknesses of lamellae are laid down surrounding the entire shaft with hard thickness. The haversian systems run parallel to each other and longitudinally from metaphysis to metaphysis, and are connected transversely by tubes called *Volkmann's canals*. Blood vessels from the periosteum enter the bone and pass through these canals to enter and leave the haversian system.

CANCELLOUS AND MEDULLARY BONE. Cancellous bone is found in flat bones and in the ends of long bones and is a collection of *trabeculae*, or beams of bone, which gives it a spongy appearance and adds strength due to the many interlacing parts (Fig. 39-3). The spaces in between these

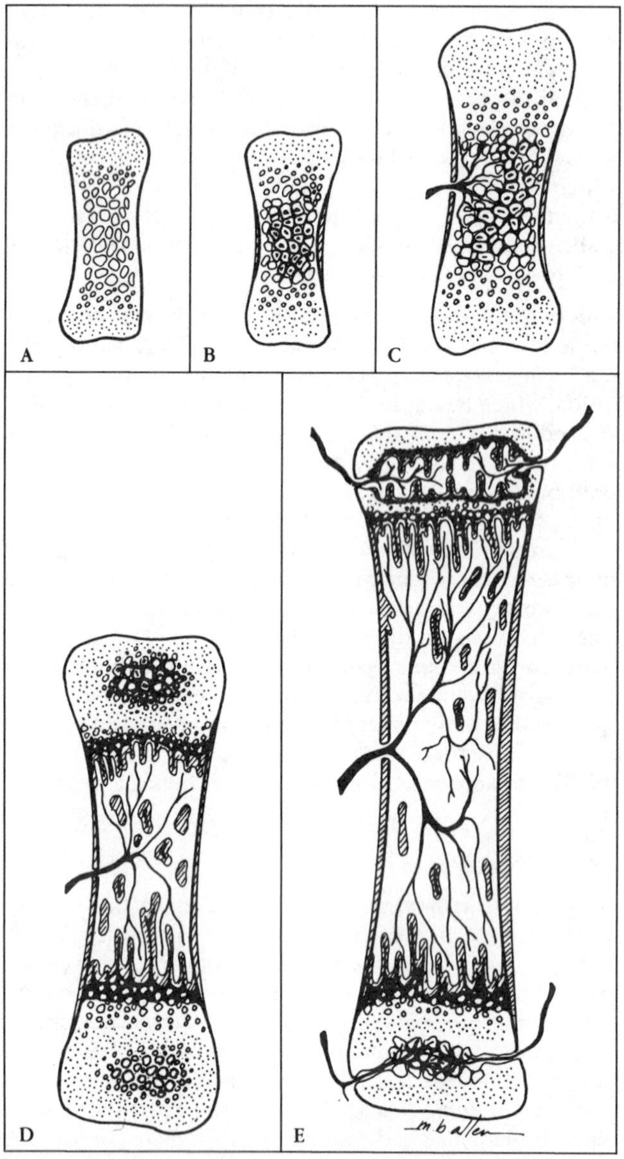

FIGURE 39-1. Some major events in the formation of a long bone organ by endochondral ossification. A. Hyaline cartilage model; hypertrophy of central chondrocytes. B. Hypertrophied chondrocytes begin to die due to initiation of matrix calcification; formation of the bone collar. C. Invasion of blood vessels and pluripotential osteoprogenitor cells; resorption of calcified cartilage matrix to form exposed surfaces for bone tissue apposition in primary center of ossification. D. Growth of bone organ and formation of marrow cavity via cartilage proliferation at epiphyseal ends, bone tissue apposition at calcified cartilage surfaces, and resorption in diaphyseal cavity; initiation of secondary center of ossification above; elongation of bone collar. E. Further growth of bone organ; formation and development of secondary center of ossification above leaving cartilaginous epiphyseal plate separating epiphysis from diaphysis; appearance of additional secondary center of ossification below; growth in girth of bone organ by concomitant bone tissue apposition on outer diaphyseal surface and resorption from inner surface. Black, calcified cartilage; black arborizations, blood vessels; parallel diagonal lines, bone tissue. (From M. Borysenko, et al., *Functional Histology* [2nd ed.]. Boston: Little, Brown, 1984.)

TABLE 39-1. Anatomic terms in common use

Process	A general term for any bony prominence
Spine or spinous process	A sharp prominence
Tubercle	A rounded prominence on a bone
Tuberosity	A protuberance on a bone
Trochanter	A large process, e.g., below the neck of the femur
Crest	A ridge, or linear prominence, e.g., iliac crest
Condyle	A rounded protruding mass that carries an articular surface, e.g., knuckle
Head	The top or beginning, the most prominent part, e.g., the enlargement beyond the constricted part as in the femoral head
Sinus	A cavity within a bone
Foramen	A hole or opening in a bone
Axial skeleton	The 80 bones composing the skull, vertebral column, sternum, and ribs
Appendicular skeleton	The 126 bones composing the upper and lower extremities
Proximal	Near the origin of the limb
Distal	Away from the origin of the limb
Medial	Nearer to the midline of the body
Lateral	Farther from the midline of the body

trabeculae are filled with bone marrow. The red marrow actively participates in the formation of red blood cells, and in the adult is found in the cancellous bone of the ribs, sternum, vertebrae, and pelvis. Red marrow is found in many bones in infants and is gradually converted to yellow marrow, so-named because it is composed of fat cells. Most long bones of the adult contain yellow marrow rather than red. ***Medullary bone*** is simply a continuation of cancellous bone and is the central area of bone filled with marrow, blood, and lymph vessels.

NERVE AND BLOOD SUPPLY. Because bone is living tissue, nutrients must be supplied and waste material removed. Total bone blood flow has been estimated at from 200 to 400 ml/minute [4]. Small bones usually have a single artery and vein entering them, with large bones having several. The chief artery, which enters near the middle of the shaft of long bones, is called the ***principal nutrient artery*** (see Fig. 39-1E). After piercing the shaft and reaching the medullary canal, it branches into ascending and descending branches ending in sinusoidal capillaries. The artery and its branches supply the marrow and cortex, as well as the haversian systems.

Nerve supply to bone is sparse and found mainly in the periosteum. Both afferent (sensory) fibers and sympathetic fibers are present, with the autonomic ones accompanying and controlling the dilatation of bone blood vessels. Pain of

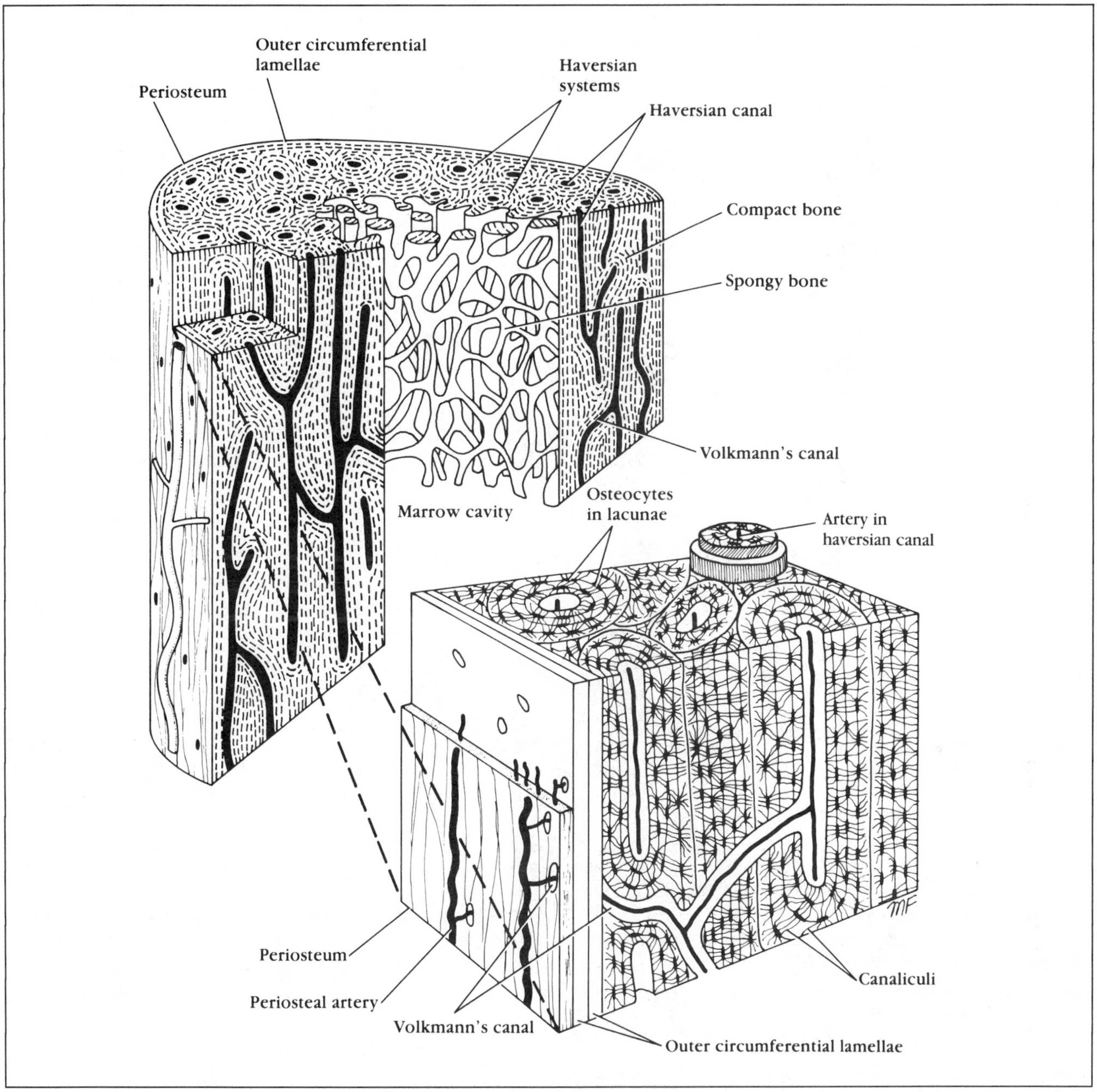

FIGURE 39-2. Compact bone tissue in histologic section. (From R. Snell, *Clinical Histology for Medical Students*. Boston: Little, Brown, 1984.)

bone tumors is thought to arise from the afferent fibers, but the pain of a fracture is largely due to pain fibers in the surrounding soft tissue and periosteum [6].

Types of Bones

The most common classification of bones divides them into long, short, flat, and irregular bone. Table 39-1 provides common anatomic terms that may be helpful to the reader.

LONG BONES. Long bones are the bones of the extremities, which have an elongated shape. The bone includes *epiphyses*, or ends, which are knobby areas containing cancellous bone, the *diaphysis*, which composes the shaft or long portion, and the *metaphysis*, which contains the epiphyseal plate and newly formed bone. In the adult, the metaphysis and epiphysis are continuous. The outer and inner surfaces of bone are covered with specialized connective tissue. The dense, white, fibrous membrane wrapping the

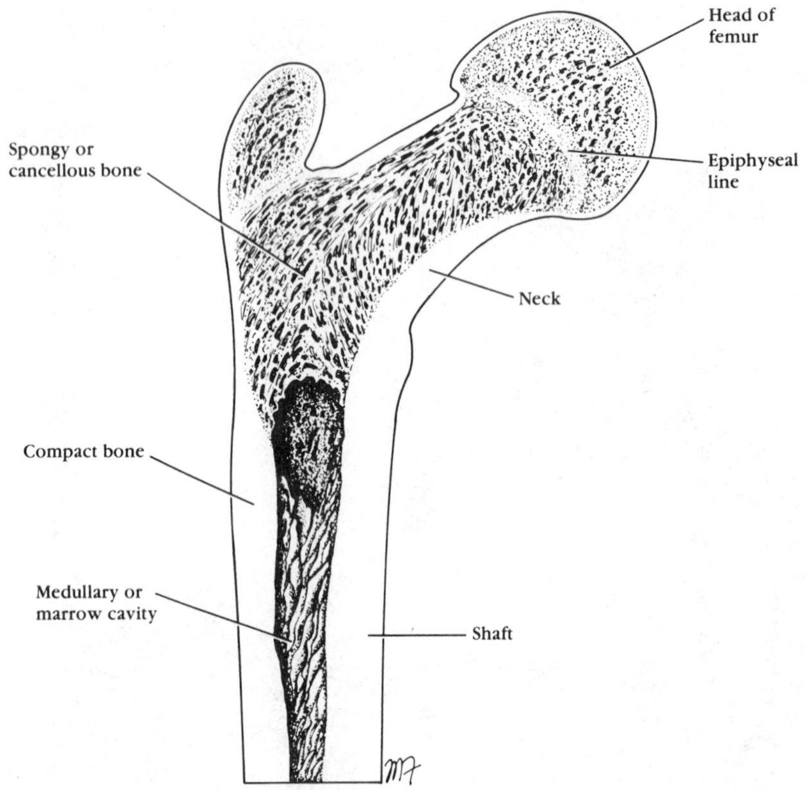

FIGURE 39-3. Bone structure. Note the differences in the three forms of bone structure: spongy, compact, and medullary. (From R. S. Snell, *Clinical Histology for Medical Students*. Boston: Little, Brown, 1984.)

outside is called the *periosteum* and is composed of two layers. The outer layer, the *fibrous layer,* has relatively few cells and is made up of fibrous tissue. The inner layer, the *marrow* cavity, is very vascular and has an osteogenic function. In addition to supplying a site of attachment for tendons and ligaments, the periosteum is richly supplied with nerves and blood vessels, which is important in the nourishment of the bone. Long bones form most of the appendicular skeleton, such as the femur, humerus, and phalanges (Fig. 39-4).

SHORT BONES. *Short bones*, such as the bones in the wrist, are cube-shaped and consist of cancellous bone enclosed in a thin case of compact bone. These often are found in combination with other short bones.

FLAT BONES. The bones of the skull, the ribs, scapulae, and sternum are examples of *flat bones*. These bones, with a largely protective function, consist of two plates of hard compact bone covering a thin layer of cancellous bone. These bones, especially the ribs and sternum, are important sites for blood formation.

IRREGULAR BONES. The other bones are placed in the category of *irregular bones* because they are irregular in shape; they are similar in formation to the short bones. The vertebrae and the ossicles of the ear are examples of irregular bones.

Bone Growth and Factors Affecting Bone Growth

LOCATION OF BONE GROWTH. The epiphyses, or ends, of the long bones are separated from the shaft by the epiphyseal plate, which is responsible for the longitudinal growth of bone. On the distal side of this plate, osteoblasts are constantly secreting the bone matrix, which immediately becomes ossified, increasing the length of the bone. At the same time, on the proximal side of the epiphyseal plate, new cartilage is being formed. During puberty, ossification exceeds cartilage formation; gradually the cartilaginous epiphyseal plate becomes completely ossified and linear bone growth ceases. This epiphyseal closure occurs about 3 years earlier in women than it does in men, in whom bone length ceases to increase at about the age of 20 [6].

As bones are growing longitudinally, they are also

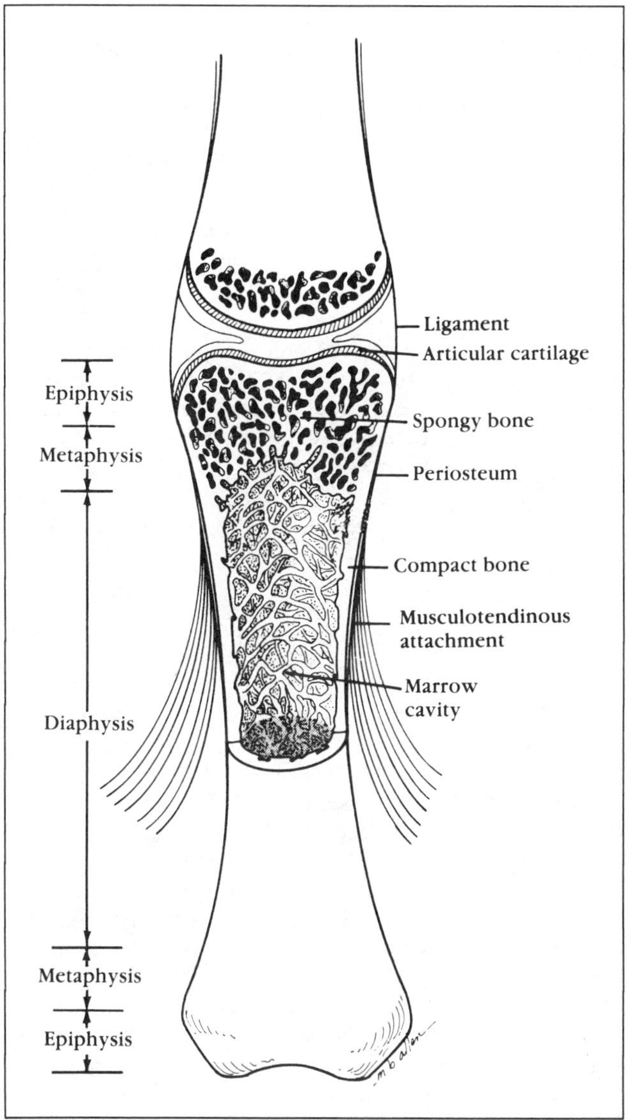

FIGURE 39-4. A bone organ and some of its relationships. (From M. Borysenko, et al., *Functional Histology* [2nd ed.]. Boston: Little, Brown, 1984.)

increasing in circumference. Osteoblasts on the inner surface of the periosteum deposits layers of new bone, while osteoclasts in the area next to the medullary cavity are making the canal larger to fit the larger bone.

Bone growth is affected by many factors, including the diet, hormones, and the environment.

CALCIUM, PHOSPHORUS, AND PARATHYROID HORMONE. The exact mechanism that causes calcium to deposit and new bone to form remains a mystery. However, certain nutritional, endocrine, and environmental states must exist in order for bone formation to occur in an orderly fashion. Adequate amounts of calcium and phosphorus must be present in the plasma and interstitial fluid that bathes the osteoblasts in order for new bone to be formed. Calcium and phosphate are supplied in the diet, mainly in milk and meats. Phosphate is absorbed with calcium. When calcium is absorbed in abundance, so is phosphate. These minerals are excreted from the body in the feces and urine.

Normal plasma calcium concentration is 10 mg/dl with a very narrow acceptable range of 9.2 to 10.4 mg/dl. This is controlled by powerful feedback mechanisms. When the serum calcium ion concentration is high, *parathyroid* hormone virtually ceases to be secreted. This results in a lowered serum calcium level (see Chap. 32). Conversely, when serum calcium levels are lowered, parathyroid hormone secretion increases, which expands vitamin D activity and absorption of calcium in the intestinal tract. Parathyroid hormone promotes the formation of osteoclasts and retards the production of osteoblasts. The net result is to increase the resorption of bone, causing the short-term effect of elevating serum calcium levels. Parathyroid hormone increases renal tubular resorption of calcium and decreases the resorption of phosphate ions.

VITAMIN D. Vitamin D increases calcium absorption in the intestinal tract and affects bone absorption and deposition. It is taken in the diet and is formed in the skin by the action of ultraviolet rays of the sun. Through a series of events in the liver and the kidneys, vitamin D is converted to a substance called 1,25-dihydroxycholecalciferol, which is the active form of the vitamin. Parathyroid hormone is also necessary for this conversion. The most important effect of 1,25-dihydroxycholecalciferol is to form calcium-binding protein in the cytoplasm of the intestinal and epithelial cells [5]. The greater the quantity of these cells, the greater the absorption of calcium. Vitamin D is virtually ineffective in renal failure, which causes a decrease in the intestinal absorption of calcium. Parathyroid hormone increases when the serum calcium levels drop, which increases 1,25-dihydroxycholecalciferol formation by the kidney and leads to increased calcium absorption. These negative feedback mechanisms are important in ensuring an optimal amount of calcium and phosphate in the plasma. Lack of either calcium or active vitamin D over a period of time can considerably hamper ongoing bone formation and remodeling.

CALCITONIN. Calcitonin is a hormone that is produced and secreted by parafollicular cells of the thyroid gland. It has the opposite effect of parathyroid hormone on the plasma calcium concentration; that is, it causes a rapid decrease in calcium levels. The immediate effect of the hormone is to decrease osteoclast activity and increase that of the osteoblast. A more prolonged effect is to reduce the quantity of osteoclasts being formed from the mesenchymal stem cells. The effect of calcitonin is more significant in children than in adults because they have a more rapid rate of bone remodeling. Increased calcitonin secretion is triggered by an increase in plasma calcium levels. The resulting decrease in serum calcium levels provides a second feedback mechanism for the control of blood calcium.

SEX HORMONES. *Estrogen* has an osteoblastic stimulating activity. At puberty, a young girl will have a rapid growth spurt before the epiphyseal plate closes, which is attributed to estrogen. Girls, therefore, stop growing taller a few years before their male counterparts. Throughout the premenopausal period, estrogen promotes bone formation with the accompanying increase in calcium and phosphorus absorption. In the postmenopausal woman, osteoporosis can be caused by the lack of estrogen, which decreases bone matrix.

Testosterone, in the male, increases bone length and thickness, and at the same time enhances epiphyseal closure. Lack of testosterone in the elderly man can cause osteoporosis. *Glucocorticoids* cause an increase in protein breakdown in all tissues of the body. Since bone matrix is a protein product, an increase in steroids, as in Cushing's disease, can decrease matrix formation and weaken the bones, causing osteoporosis. Steroids also have the specific effect of depressing osteoblastic activity [5].

As was described earlier, two-thirds of the volume of bone is made up of osteoid organic material. Because all living tissues contain protein, anything that causes a decrease in protein in the body, such as starvation, will retard bone formation.

Lack of vitamins A and C also decrease the ground substance in bone and lead to decreased bone formation. Persons having long-term heparin therapy develop osteoporosis, because heparin apparently speeds up the breakdown of collagen material [15].

Growth Hormone

The anterior lobe of the pituitary gland secretes the growth hormone (somatotrophic hormone), which causes a linear increase in long bones by increasing cartilage formation, widening the epiphyseal plates, and increasing the amount of matrix laid down in the ends of the long bones (see Chap. 30). An increase in growth hormone in the growing person can cause giantism. In the adult, whose epiphyseal plates are closed, the characteristic bone and soft tissue deformities of acromegaly result. Pituitary insufficiency can result in dwarfism in the child.

Weight Bearing

It has long been observed that atrophy of muscle and bone demineralization occur when a limb is immobilized. Weightlessness experienced by astronauts was noted to cause loss of bone calcium and bone weakness [12]. Physical compression stimulates osteoblastic deposition in bone, probably by generating an electrical potential. This potential at the compression site stimulates osteoblastic activity and increases bone formation. Electrical signals can also stimulate epiphyseal growth [14]. Studies in animals show that increased activity leads to an increase in bone mass while inactivity, especially in the growing animal, leads to a decrease in bone mass, decrease in the length and thickness of bones, and irregular articular surfaces and epiphyseal lines [14]. Local skeletal mass increases in the bones most used in physical exertion such as tennis, weightlifting, and dancing. Increased physical activity seen in young girls in recent years may eventually cause larger bones and a decreased incidence of osteoporosis in later life [7]. A summary of factors affecting bone formation is found in Table 39-2.

TABLE 39-2. Factors that affect bone formation

Facilitate	Retard
Calcium	Hyperthyroidism
Phosphorus	Vitamin deficiency
Estrogen	Starvation
Calcitonin	Diabetes
Vitamins D, A, and C	Steroids
Growth hormone	Inactivity/immobility
Exercise	Heparin

NORMAL STRUCTURE AND FUNCTION OF JOINTS

Types of Joints

Even though individual bones are hard and inflexible, the human body can have graceful flowing movements. Any motion, whether in writing a lesson or playing football, is brought about by the simultaneous movement of several *articulations*, or joints. Almost all of the bones of the body are joined to each other in one way or another. Some permit a range of motion and some allow none at all. Joints are classified in several ways, but the most common method is to group them according to the degree of movement they permit as follows: *synarthroses,* immovable joints; *amphiarthroses*, somewhat movable joints; and *diarthroses,* freely movable joints. Joints may also be classified according to the material that connects them, e.g., cartilaginous, fibrous, and synovial joints [6].

Using the degree of movement classification, the subgroups and their types are described in this section (Fig. 39-5). Synarthroses provide little movement, a rigid surface, and especially include the bones of the skull. The sutures of the cranial bones are joined together by fibrous tissue and interlocking projections and indentations. These joints are not completed at birth and an infant has six gaps, or *fontanelles*, between bones. *Synchondrosis*, another type of immovable joint, is cartilage joining two bony surfaces. An example of synchrondrosis is the "joint" between the epiphysis and diaphysis of long bones that disappears following puberty. A third type of synarthrosis is a *gomphosis* (nail), which resembles a peg in a hole, an example of which is a tooth in the jaw.

Amphiarthroses are joints that permit very limited motion. A symphysis is a joint where the bones are connected by disks of fibrocartilage. Examples are the symphysis pubis and the intervertebral disks between the verte-

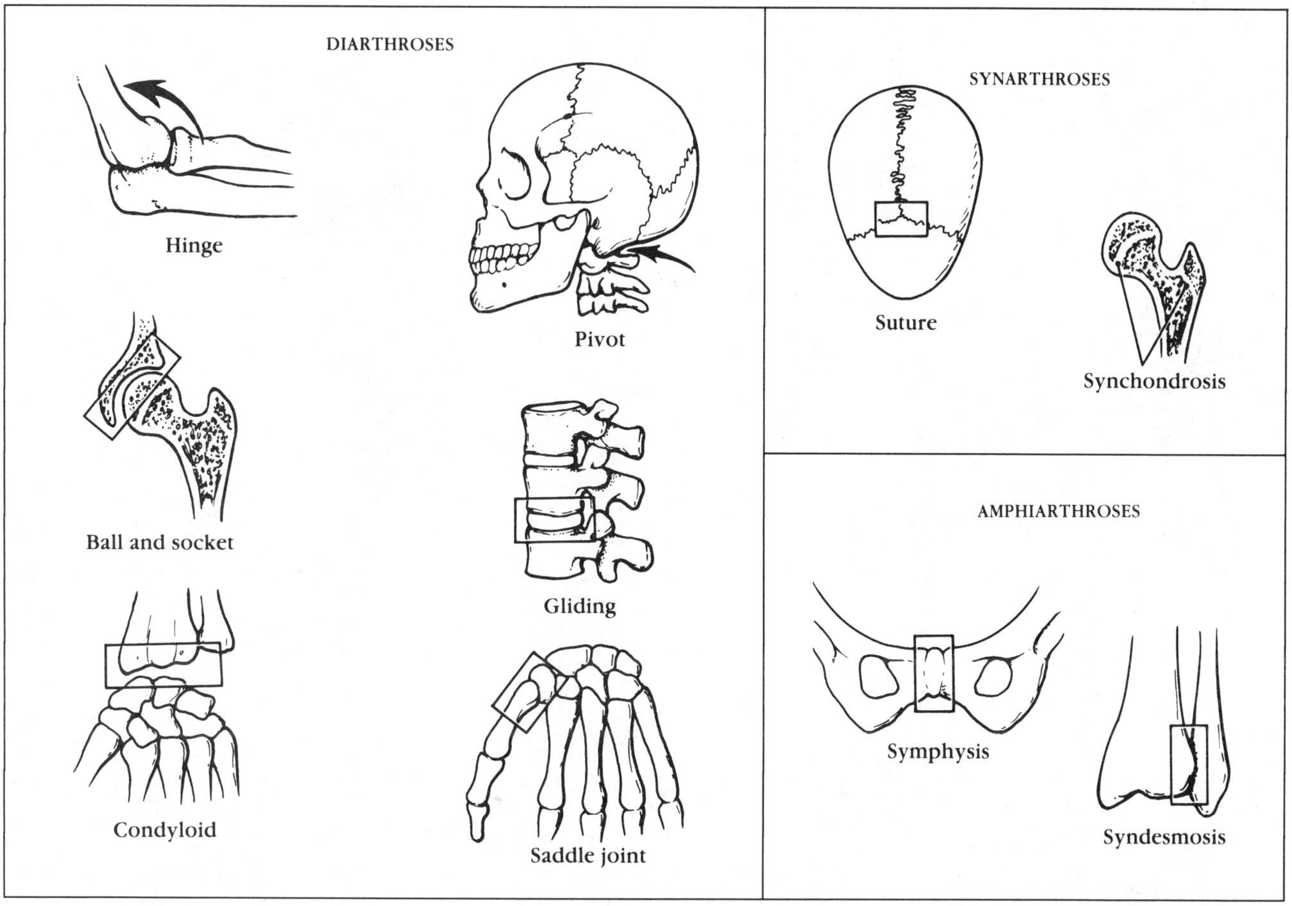

FIGURE 39-5. Types of joints based on degree of movement.

brae. One can see the benefits of such flexibility of the pelvis in childbirth, and flexibility of the backbone with any movement. A *syndesmosis* is a slightly movable joint in which the bones are connected by ligaments permitting some bending and twisting; an example is the articulation between the tibia and fibula.

Diarthroses are often called *synovial* joints and are freely movable joints that require lubrication to reduce the friction and abrasion that occur when one surface moves on another. The articulating surfaces of the bone are covered by a white, slick hyaline cartilage, and the entire joint is surrounded by an articular capsule that is filled with a viscous synovial fluid. The inner layer of this capsule is a slippery, smooth membrane, while the outer layer is a tough, fibrous membrane. This inner, or *synovial*, membrane is rich in capillaries and cells and is composed of secreting and phagocytic cells. The secretory cells produce the synovial fluid that contains water and protein [12]. The glucose level of the fluid is similar to that of serum. The chief function of this fluid is to lubricate and supply nutrients to the cartilage. The excess protein in the fluid is returned to the blood via the lymphatic systems that drain the area. Synovial joints are supplied with sensory nerves that cause pain when there is swelling of the joints.

The synovial joints permit a variety of motion and are typed according to the shape of the articulation and the motion it facilitates (Fig. 39-6).

Classification of Synovial Joints

BALL AND SOCKET JOINTS. These joints allow the greatest degree of motion and are formed by a bone fitting into a cup-shaped cavity of another bone. Examples are the hip and shoulder joints.

CONDYLOID JOINTS. An oval-shaped articular surface fits into an elliptical cavity. These joints allow much movement, similar to the ball and socket, but abduction-adduction is limited. An example is the wrist between the radius and carpal bones.

HINGE JOINTS. This type of joint permits movement in one plane only. The surface of one bone is convex, the other concave and they fit together smoothly. Examples are the knee, elbow, and finger joints.

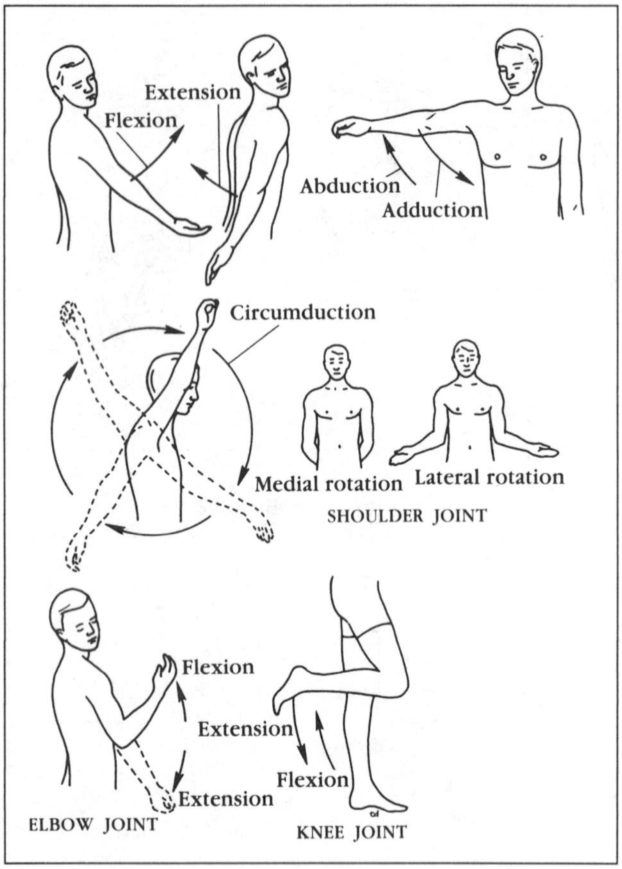

FIGURE 39-6. Some anatomic terms used in relation to movement. (From R. S. Snell, *Clinical Anatomy for Medical Students*. Boston: Little, Brown, 1981.)

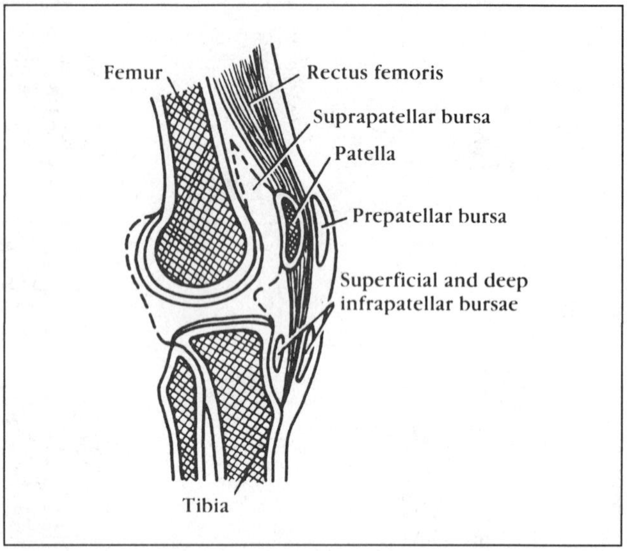

FIGURE 39-7. Four bursae related to the front of the knee joint. (From R. S. Snell, *Clinical Anatomy for Medical Students*. Boston: Little, Brown, 1981.)

PIVOT JOINTS. These joints allow for rotation and supination and pronation. Examples are the atlas and axis joints of the head and the juncture between the head of the radius and the radial notch of the ulna.

SADDLE JOINTS. The articular surface of one bone is concave in one direction and convex in another while the other bone is just the opposite, so that the two sides fit together smoothly. An example is the carpometacarpal joint at the base of the thumb.

GLIDING JOINTS. The bone surfaces are flat or only slightly curved thus permitting sliding movement in all directions. Examples of this type of joint are the carpal bones of wrist and the intervertebral joints.

All movements of joints may be classified as (1) gliding movement, producing some bone displacement; (2) angular movement, in which the angle between bones is changed; and (3) rotation, a twisting of a body part [12]. Table 39-3 summarizes the movements of the joints and how they can be altered.

Bursae

Bursae are small flat cavities that are lined with synovial membrane and filled with synovial fluid [12]. The chief functions of bursae are to reduce friction between moving parts; for this reason, they are generally found between bones, tendons, and ligaments that move against one another. There are 50 named bursae in the body, with many other smaller ones. They are typically flattened, collapsed spaces containing just enough fluid to keep them moist (Fig. 39-7). Bursae are in the shoulder, elbow, hip, heel, and knee.

Ligaments and Tendons

Ligaments and tendons are structures composed of connective tissue that serve to hold the body together. There are two types of ligaments; those that connect viscera to each other and those that connect one bone to another [6]. Tendons, on the other hand, always connect voluntary muscle to another structure.

Ligaments are composed of distinct bands of connective tissue. The yellow ones are elastic (vertebral column ligament) and allow for stretching. The white ligaments, such as at the knee, do not stretch and provide stability.

Tendons are actual extensions of muscles and attach muscles to bones or to other tissues. The thick collagenous tissue has fibers that run in one direction so it can withstand a great deal of pull. These parallel bundles give tendons a glistening, shiny white appearance. As a part of broad and flat muscles, they tend to have the same general appearance, and similarly, when they are part of a long

TABLE 39-3. Joints commonly affected by disease

Name of joint	Type of movement	Normal movements	Effects of alterations
Vertebral	Diarthrotic (may be classified as synarthrotic, cartilaginous, amphiarthrotic)	Bending, stretching, twisting of entire column; slight movement between vertebrae	Pain when moving or lifting; stiffness; low back pain
Clavicular	Diarthrotic	Elevating, protracting, retracting	Pain; inability to move shoulder forward or backward; unable to lift shoulder
Shoulder	Diarthrotic (ball and socket)	Flexion, extension, abduction; rotation; circumduction of upper arm	Pain; stiffness; immobility; heat; inability to lift objects; cannot bring arm in toward body; range of activity curtailed
Elbow	Diarthrotic (hinge and pivot joint)	Flexion, extension; supination of lower arm and hand; pronation of lower arm and hand	Immobility; pain; stiffness; heat; activities of daily living greatly diminished; swelling
Wrist	Diarthrotic	Flexion, extension; abduction of hand; adduction of hand	Pain; stiffness; swelling; common complaints of inability to do common activities of daily living such as cooking, opening lids, various grooming activities; may complain of dropping things
Hand	Diarthrotic	Flexion, extension, abduction, adduction, circumduction of thumb; thumb and finger apposition; flexion, extension, limited abduction and adduction of fingers; flexion, extension of fingers	Pain; swelling; stiffness; drops objects; deteriorating writing; ability to perform activities of daily living greatly diminished (buttoning clothes, tying knots or bows, combing hair, etc.)
Hip	Diarthrotic (ball and socket)	Flexion; extension; abduction; adduction; rotation; circumduction	Pain; stiffness; immobility; heat; limping; loss of range of motion; inability to put on garments that require lifting the legs; cannot climb stairs
Knee	Diarthrotic (hinge)	Flexion; extension; slight tibial rotation	Pain; stiffness; swelling; immobility; limping, falling; redness, swelling; heat
Ankle	Diarthrotic (hinge)	Dorsiflexion; plantar flexion	Pain; stiffness; immobility; limping; unusual discomfort with shoes; foot drop
Foot	Diarthrotic	Flexion; extension; gliding; inversion; slight abduction, adduction	Pain; stiffness; immobility; avoidance of standing and walking; shoes ill-fitting

Source: J. Moore. Unpublished material. Used by permission of the author.

slender muscle, they are cordlike. The long, hard, cordlike tendons running into the hands and feet have been termed *leaders*. Tendons that cross bones or other tendons are lubricated by nearby bursae or the tendon sheath that surrounds them. Tendons receive sensory fibers from muscle nerves, nearby deep nerves, and overlying superficial nerves. Blood supply to tendons is scarce and it is for this reason that injured tendons heal slowly.

FRACTURES AND ASSOCIATED SOFT TISSUE INJURIES

Fractures are most commonly defined as a break in continuity of bone. A fracture is a rupture of living tissue and is normally the result of trauma. Thus, a fracture may have associated extensive soft tissue damage with hemorrhage into muscles and joints, dislocation and rupture of tendons, nerve damage, and disruption of blood supplies.

A fracture occurs when a force (energy) is imposed on a bone that is greater than it can absorb. Fractures are described in terms of types and directions of fracture lines (Fig. 39-8).

Classification of Fractures

Simple fractures are those that do not disrupt the skin overlying the bone. A *compound fracture* disrupts the overlying skin.

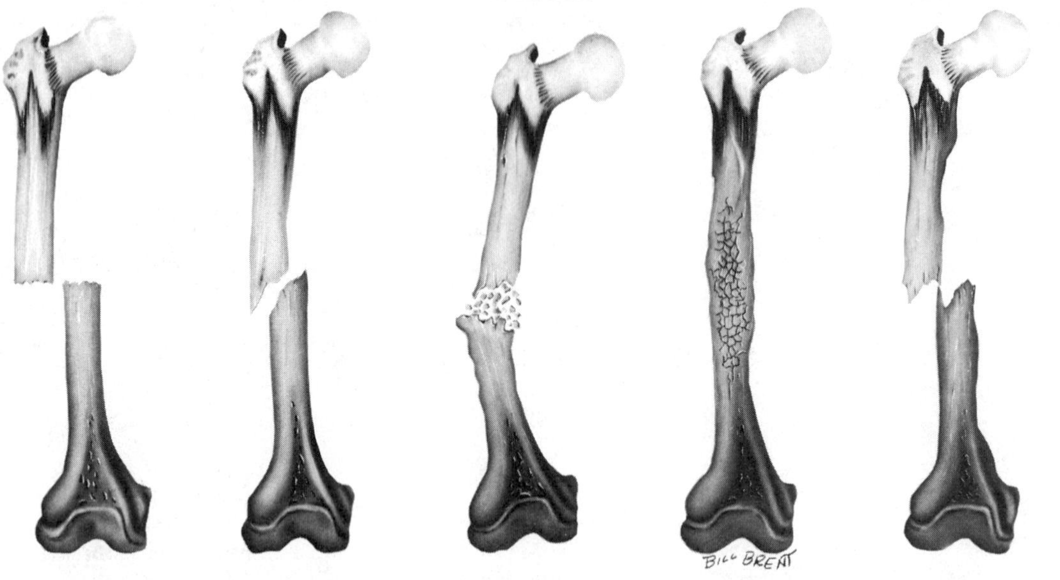

FIGURE 39-8. Some terms used for different types of fractures. (From N. Caroline, *Emergency Care in the Streets* [2nd ed.]. Boston: Little, Brown, 1983.)

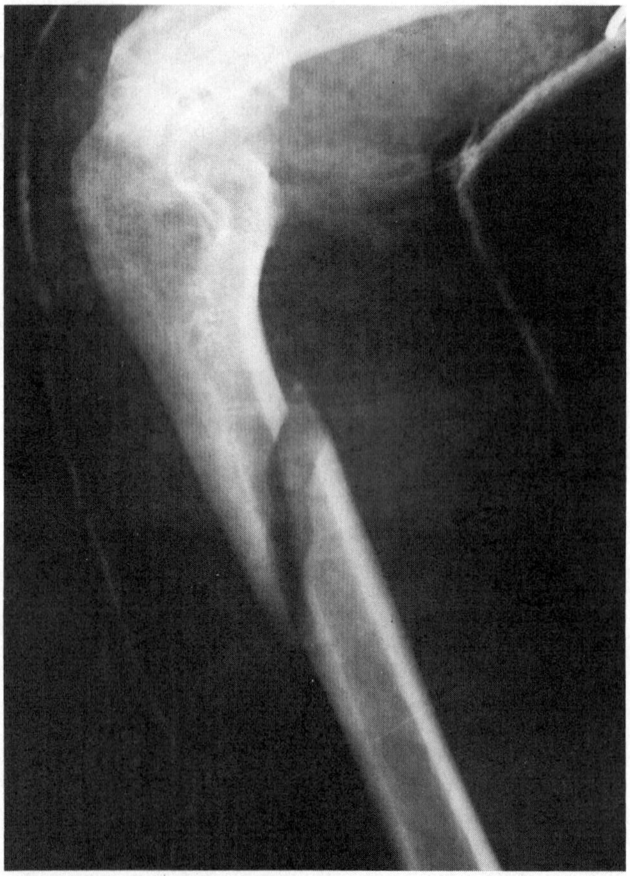

FIGURE 39-9. A complete fracture of the humerus.

Fractures are either *complete*, in which there is a complete interruption in the continuity of bone, or *incomplete*, with some part of the bone intact (Figs. 39-9 and 39-10). If a bone is fractured in such a manner as to produce three or more bone fragments, it is called a *comminuted* fracture (Fig. 39-11). An *impacted fracture* is one in which one fragment of bone is imbedded in the substance of the other. A fracture characterized by crushed bone is called a *compression* fracture and usually involves the spinal column (Fig. 39-12). A *depressed* fracture, frequently seen in skull fractures, occurs when the bone is driven inward. Repeated mechanical stress and strain can result in a *stress* fracture (Fig. 39-13). *Pathologic fractures* occur from diseased bone with little external force or with trivial trauma. Severe twisting or straining may cause a tendon or ligament to pull its bony attachment completely off the main part of the bone producing an *avulsion* fracture.

Directions of fracture lines may be described as longitudinal, transverse, oblique, or spiral (Fig. 39-14). Other descriptive terms also include overriding, angulation, and displacement (Fig. 39-15).

In general, soft tissue damage is greatest when a direct force is applied over the area that is fractured, but is usually decreased when the force that breaks the bone is applied distal to the fracture. Table 39-4 lists mechanical forces and types of fractures that may be associated with them. These relate primarily to the long bones.

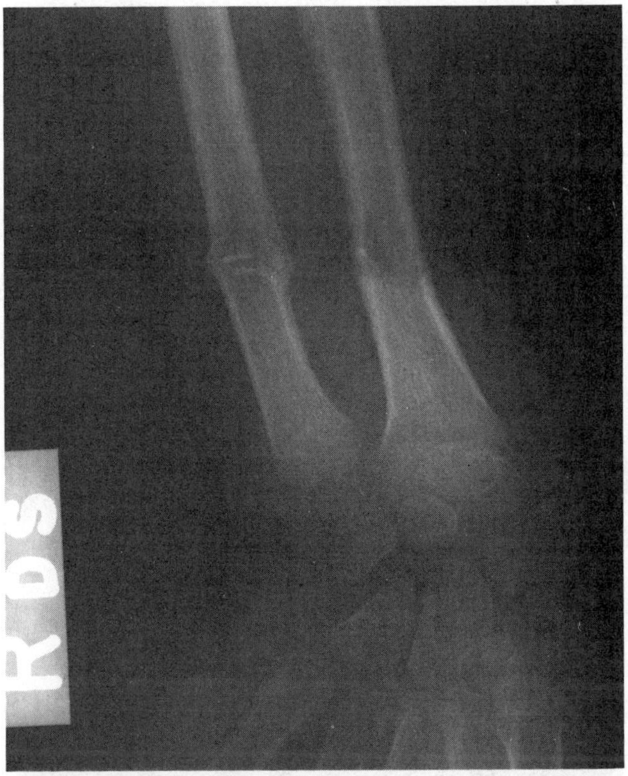

FIGURE 39-10. A greenstick fracture of the radius and ulna is an example of an incomplete fracture that usually occurs in children.

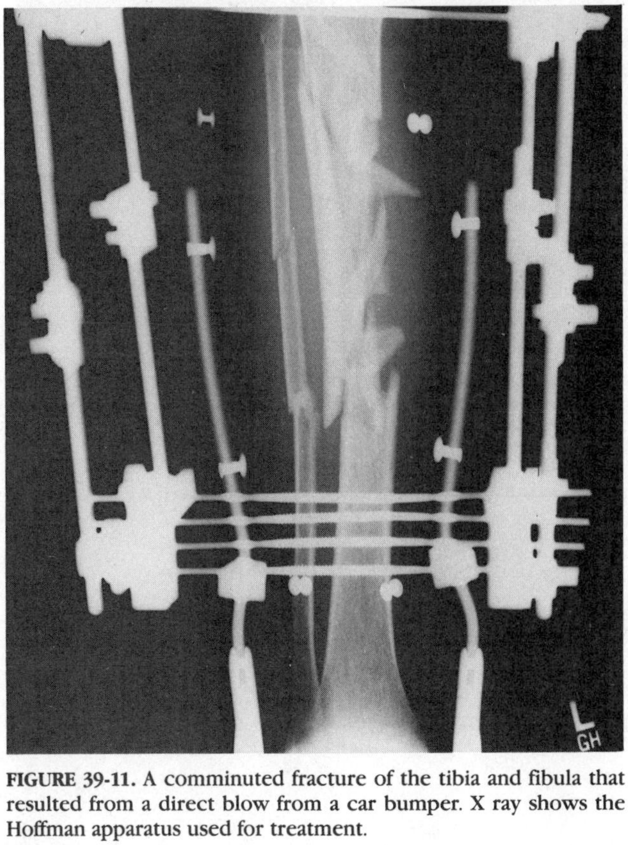

FIGURE 39-11. A comminuted fracture of the tibia and fibula that resulted from a direct blow from a car bumper. X ray shows the Hoffman apparatus used for treatment.

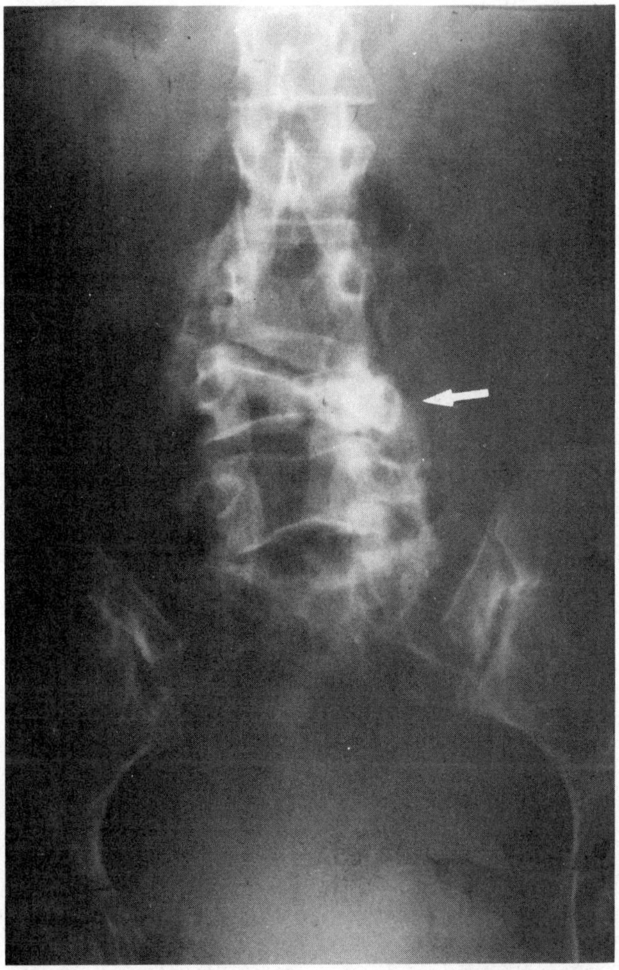

FIGURE 39-12. Compression fracture of the fourth lumbar vertebra.

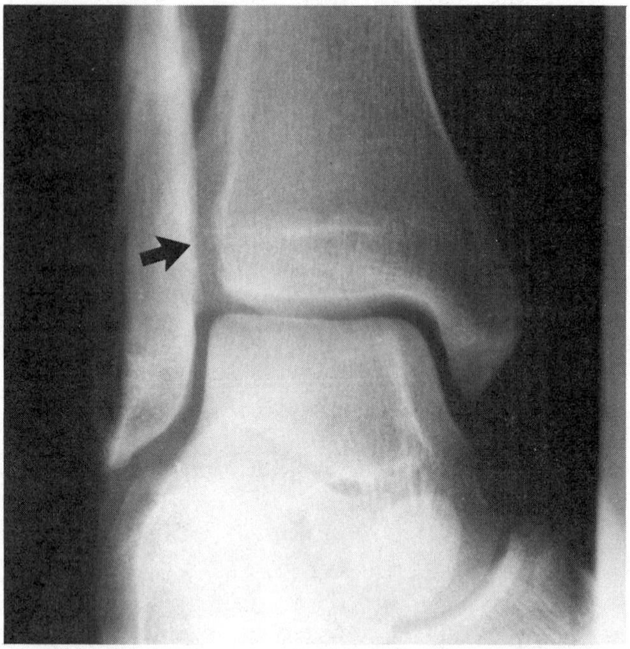

FIGURE 39-13. Stress fracture of the fibula in a distance runner.

TABLE 39-4. Mechanical forces and related fractures of long bones

Force	Resulting fracture
Twisting	Spiral
Angulation	Transverse
Angulation with axial compression	Transverse with separate triangular piece (butterfly)
Twisting, angulation, and axial compression	Short oblique
Direct blow	Transverse
Crushing blow	Comminuted

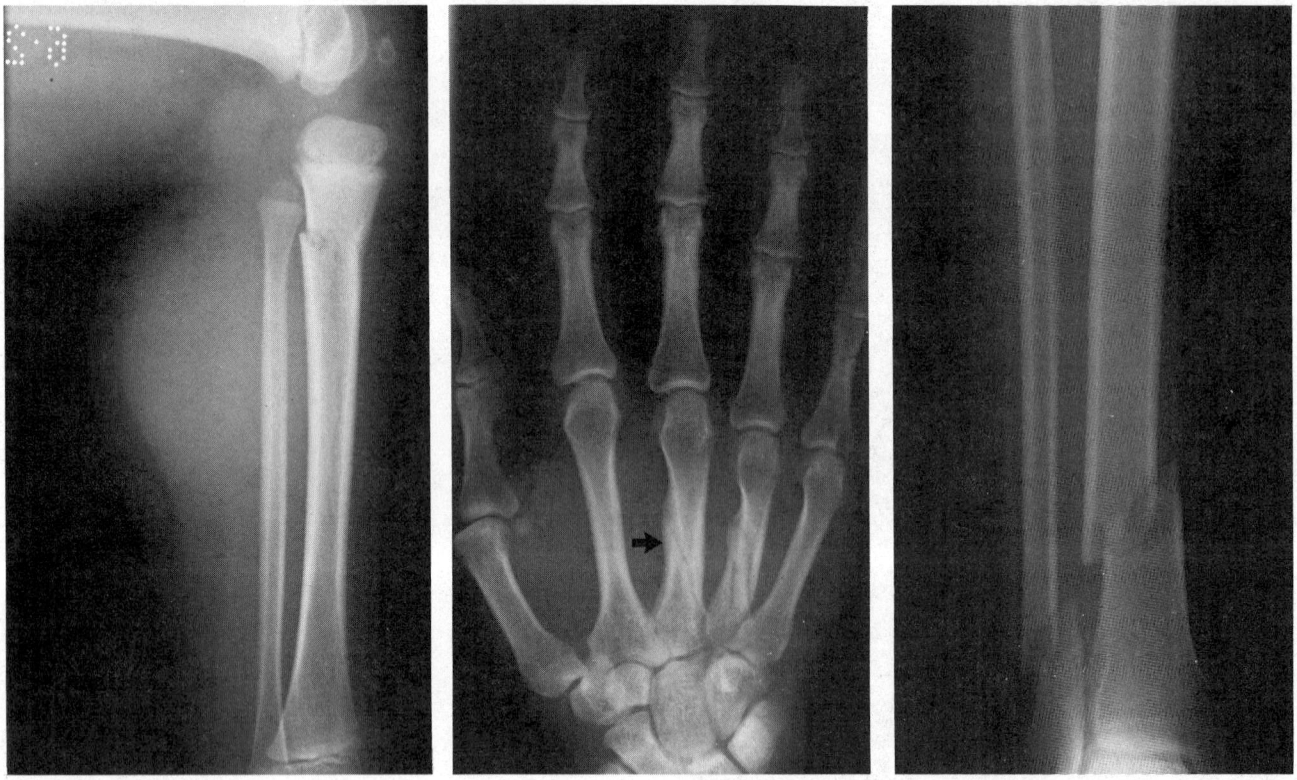

A B C

FIGURE 39-14. A. Transverse fracture of the tibia. B. Oblique fracture of the third and fourth metacarpals. C. Spiral fracture of the tibia and fibula.

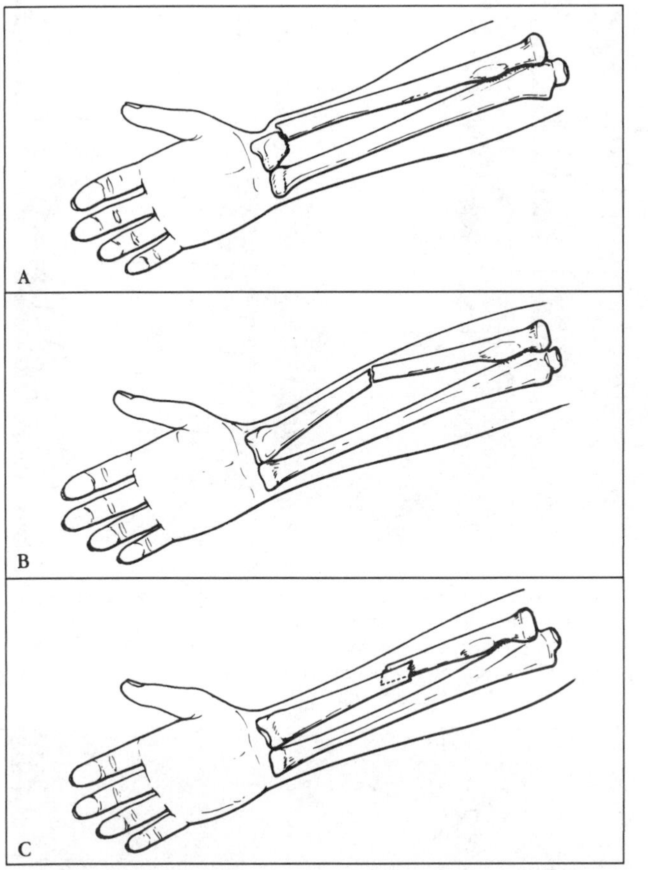

FIGURE 39-15. Descriptive terms indicating types of fractures. A. Displacement. B. Angulation. C. Overriding.

Fracture Healing

It normally takes a good deal of force to break a bone and there is often associated soft tissue damage. Once a fracture has occurred, there is rupture of blood vessels and periosteum, with the seeping of blood into the fracture site from the fragments. This is called the *fracture hematoma.*

The specialized bone cells, the osteoclasts and osteoblasts, become active to form new bone. This reaction begins distal to the fracture site. That is, in undamaged periosteum, osteogenic cells multiply and give rise to osteoclasts and osteoblasts. This reaction progresses toward the fracture.

At the same time, in the medullary canal, the giant-cell form of macrophages form a line of demarcation between viable bone and necrotic bone. This area of demarcation is followed by the proliferation of both osteoblasts and osteoclasts.

The soft tissue response is much like that of the medullary canal. From the surrounding tissue, fibroblasts are formed that follow a line of demarcation toward the fracture site. Fibroblasts may differentiate into osteoblasts and chondroblasts and participate in the healing process. Within 1 week, new bone and cartilage are laid down forming a temporary *callus.* This secures the fragments, but provides no rigid strength. In the following weeks, bone spicules increase and join together to form what is known as provisional callus or *procallus* [10]. It obtains its maximum size in 3 weeks.

The procallus creates a balloon shape over the fracture site and extends well past the fracture. As the fracture continues to heal, new bone spicules proliferate and at the same time are remodeled by osteoblastic and osteoclastic activity [10].

The remodeling process is controlled by the weight bearing and muscle stresses put on the bone. That is, through the bone formation and resorption process bone returns to an architecturally sound state. *Wolff's law* describes this as a feedback system in which local instability stimulates bone formation and lack of stress stimulates bone resorption [1]. In a period of a year, a simple bone fracture will resume an almost normal appearance if aligned correctly (Fig. 39-16).

CONDITIONS THAT MODIFY THE HEALING PROCESS. Because the healing of fractures is a continuous, sequential process, any interruption at a given point may result in modification of the healing process. This may be the result of inadequate immobilization, poor blood supply, distraction of fragments, interposition of soft tissue, or infection.

When the bone is completely transected, *immobilization* is required. The purpose of immobilization is to rigidly hold the fracture fragments in place. Any movement of the bone fragments could rupture the fracture hematoma. If the hematoma is ruptured by fragment movement, it serves to reverse the healing process, because bleeding into the fracture site will reoccur, thus prolonging the healing process. Immobilization is the first line of defense in ensuring a solid union.

A poor *blood supply* to the traumatized area can also modify the healing process. All tissues of the body need nutrition provided through the bloodstream to maintain life. In order for the surrounding soft tissue and bones to heal, there must be an adequate blood supply to provide the needed nutrition.

Position or *aposition* also can affect the healing process. *Distraction* is a term used to describe a situation where the fracture fragments are pulled apart from each other and there is no bony contact. This may be caused by skeletal traction applied to align fragments or by muscle pull on individual fractures. The distraction, if great enough, may cause excessive tension on the capillaries and decrease the vital blood supply. An increased fracture gap must be bridged with granulation tissue, which increases healing time. When the healing time is increased, the chance of nonunion also increases. Distraction of fracture fragments also is associated with the complication of separation of the fracture fragments by soft tissue that seals off the surface of one or both bones. This is known as *interposition of soft tissue.* If one or both of the fragments become covered with soft tissue, the hematoma is unable to form, and formation of granulation tissue becomes inhibited. This leads to a poor osseous union (Fig. 39-17A).

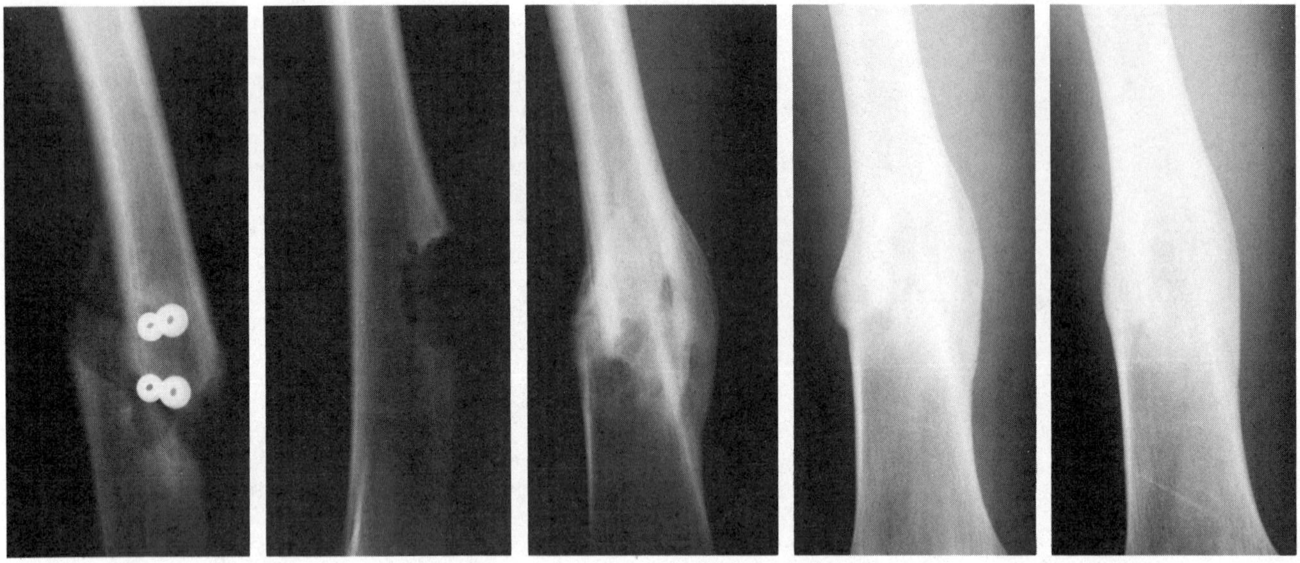

A B C D E

FIGURE 39-16. A. The sequencing of bone healing and remodeling is demonstrated in a 13-year-old boy with a chondromyxoid that was removed surgically. B. It was followed 1 month later by a pathologic fracture that was repaired. C. A procallus forms. D. Osteogenesis. E. Bone remodeling.

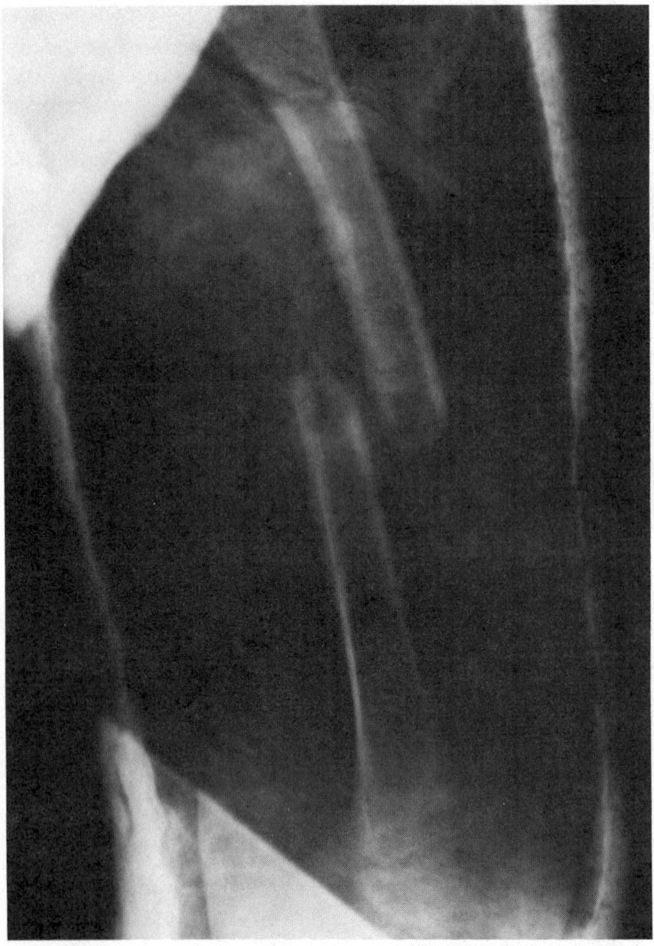

A

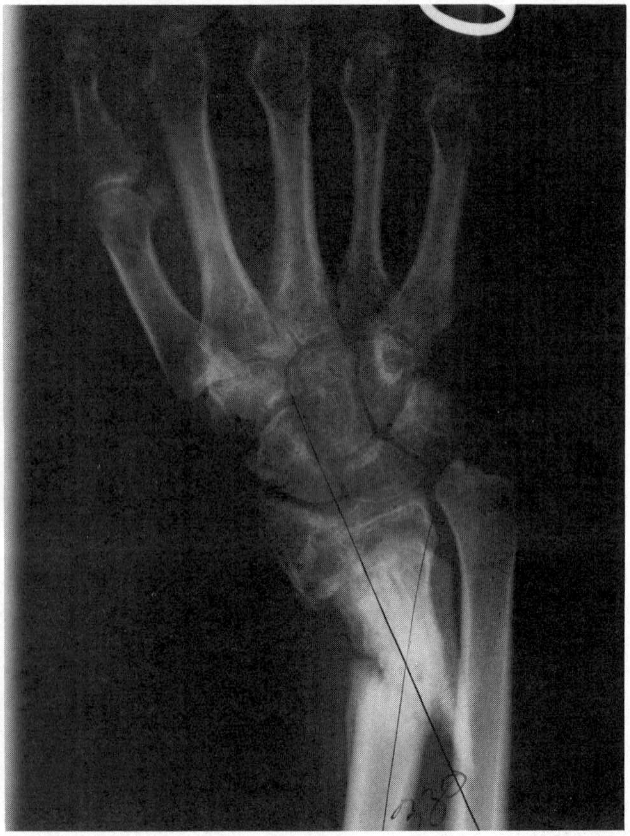

B

FIGURE 39-17. A. Loss of apposition in this fractured femur increases the likelihood of soft tissue interposition and delayed or nonunion. B. Malunion of the radius due to poor alignment during the healing process.

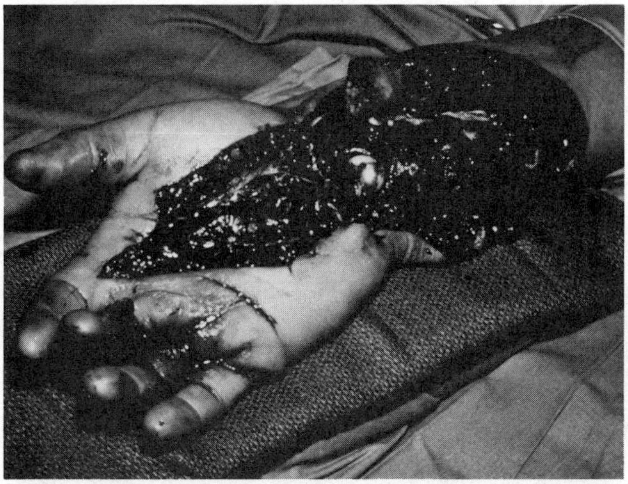

FIGURE 39-18. Compound fracture of the radius and ulna with extensive soft tissue damage.

Compound fractures open internal structures to various microorganisms; therefore, *infection* becomes the major complication of bone healing of this type of fracture. The open area is a rich culture medium for infection in the tissues or for osteomyelitis (Fig. 39-18). If osteomyelitis does occur, the healing process is retarded by destruction of newly forming bone and interruption of blood supply.

Delayed union is a term used to denote an increased healing time. Although each person heals at a different pace, there is general consistency of average time needed to completely heal a fracture. A delayed union normally results from a breakdown in the early stages of healing, i.e., inadequate immobilization, breakdown in hematoma formation, and/or poor alignment. Infection at the fracture site delays union, usually until the infectious process is stopped.

Nonunion occurs when there is a failure of the fragments to unite, usually occurring from infection and movement. Infection causes continuous bleeding and breakdown of osteoid matrix. Movement at the fracture site causes repeated bleeding episodes and decalcification at the fragment ends; it may cause the fracture gap to increase to the point where the ends no longer touch, leading to a permanent nonunion.

Malunion refers to union of the fragments in a position that modifies function. The wrist fracture in Figure 39-17B was allowed to heal in poor alignment and resulted in shortening of the extremity and alteration of function.

ALTERATION IN NERVE FUNCTION DUE TO BONE TRAUMA. Soft tissue injuries such as laceration of a major artery, the insidious compartmental syndrome, disabling tendon avulsion, or serious visceral injury are associated with fractures, and if left untreated, lead to alteration of function (Fig. 39-18).

Sometimes a fracture causes an injury to adjacent structures. The fragments may rupture and compress nerves that may also be damaged by dislocation or direct trauma. Axillary nerve, radial, and peroneal nerve damage are described as compartmental syndromes.

The axillary nerve may be damaged by fractures or dislocations around the shoulder or by penetrating wounds and direct blows. The axillary nerve is composed of C5 and C6 fibers and is a branch of the posterior cord of the brachial plexus. It emerges at the level of the humerus head and winds around the neck of the humerus. It supplies the deltoid and teres minor muscles. The deltoid muscle is used as an abductor for the shoulder; therefore, lack of ability to abduct the shoulder indicates damage to the axillary nerve.

The radial nerve is commonly injured in spiral fractures of the humerus. It may be completely severed, impaled on a fracture fragment, or entrapped between the fragments. Lacerations of the arm and proximal forearm, and gunshot wounds are also common causes for radial nerve injury. Temporary nerve damage may also result from direct pressure from crutches or by hanging an arm on the back of a chair. The radial nerve is composed of the fibers from C6, C7, C8, and sometimes, T1. It is primarily a motor nerve that innervates the biceps, supinates the forearm, and extends the wrist, fingers, and thumb. Therefore, it can be summarized that injury would result in inability to extend the elbow or supinate the forearm. A typical wrist drop occurs that includes inability to extend the fingers. Complete return of function can be expected in most persons with temporary nerve damage. In others, function may not return for as long as 3 months to a year. When return of function does not occur, surgery is usually indicated, but it should be noted that the radial nerve has the greatest ability to regenerate compared to all other large nerves. This is probably because the radial nerve is primarily a motor nerve that is involved mainly in gross muscle movements.

Peroneal nerves are divided into common, superficial, and deep peroneal nerves. Injury to the common peroneal nerve can be used as an example of how direct trauma may cause alterations in function. The common peroneal nerve emerges from the popliteal fossa and encircles the fibula neck. Damage may be the result of a direct blow, e.g., a baseball bat applied to the fibula head with or without the presence of fractures. The result is a foot drop deformity, in which the foot returns to normal in a few hours if the nerve is not ruptured.

Compartmental Syndromes

Compartmental syndromes are not a common complication of fractures and affect the forearm and tibia primarily. These syndromes are commonly referred to as Volkmann's ischemia and anterior tibial compartmental syndromes. *Volkmann's ischemia* (volar compartmental syndrome) usually is related to the common supracondylar fracture of the humerus in children. Fracture of the tibia is common in anterior compartmental syndrome.

The compartments of the leg and forearm are composed of bones, muscles, nerves, and other associated structures encapsulated by the fascia and the skin, thus making a closed space. When injury occurs, the pressure builds within the compartment due to bleeding and soft tissue reaction. When the swelling reaches a point where the fascia will permit no further outward enlargement, the increasing pressure is directed inward and compresses blood vessels and other components of the compartment. When tissue pressure increases to equal the diastolic pressure, the microcirculation ceases. Within 30 minutes, damage to nerves begins that will result in irreversible functional loss if allowed to persist for 12 hours. Muscles require an abundant blood supply and when the microcirculation is severely compromised the muscles become ischemic, with onset of necrosis in 2 to 4 hours that becomes irreversible in 12 hours. *Anterior compartmental syndrome* is heralded by pain in the anterior aspect of the tibia, paresthesia over the distribution of the deep peroneal nerve, and pain on passive dorsiflexion of the toes. The area appears swollen and blisters may develop on the skin. If allowed to proceed unchecked, paralysis, anesthesia, contractures, foot drop, and gangrene may develop, which in turn may lead to the loss of limb.

Volkmann's ischemia produces a disturbing contracture if untreated. Pain is the predominant symptom; it is referred to the palmar area with exacerbation of pain with passive extension of fingers. Some degree of sensory loss in the fingers occurs in the early stages. Formation of contractures described as clawlike deformities of the hand, wrist drop, and paralysis then result.

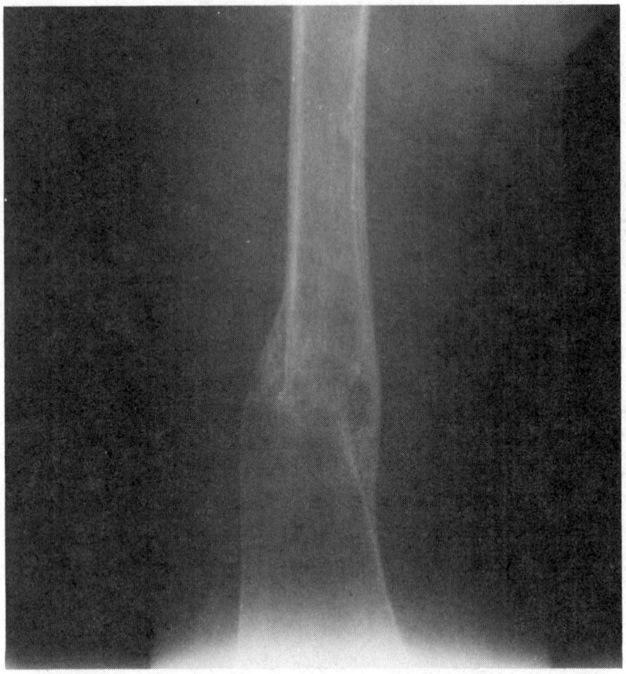

FIGURE 39-19. Osteogenesis imperfecta in an infant with a pathologic fracture of the femur. Note the thin cortical bone with a transparent medullary area.

Other Associated Soft Tissue Traumas

Tendons may also be damaged as a result of fractures. When ligaments and tendons are involved in fractures, avulsion fractures may result. Damage to the extensor tendon of the distal phalanx can serve as an example. When a fracture occurs, it avulses (pulls apart) a small piece of bone to which the tendon is attached, leading to the inability to extend the distal phalanx. If left untreated, a mallet deformity may result. If tendon damage caused by fractures is left untreated, it may lead to dysfunction of its bony attachment.

Visceral damage, or damage to internal organs, may also occur from fractures. Examples include fracture of the pelvis in which the bladder is ruptured, and rib fractures causing perforation of the lung.

ALTERATIONS IN BONE DEVELOPMENT

Osteogenesis Imperfecta

Osteogenesis imperfecta is a hereditary disease in which defective connective tissue formation leads to extremely fragile bones. Homozygous infants with the recessive trait are most severely affected and mortality is high in the first year of life. In this type, the bones of the skull and face are poorly ossified with numerous fractures appearing in the long bones. Death during childbirth may occur due to trauma to the brain, which is relatively unprotected by the soft, membranous skull. The dominant trait produces a less severe type called *osteogenesis imperfecta tarda* (Fig. 39-19). This clinical syndrome is characterized by brittle, thin bones with deformities caused by multiple fractures, dwarfism with deformed extremities, and slow physical development. Mental development is usually normal. Associated features are relaxed ligaments, a high incidence of hernias, and fragile skin. Blue sclera is characteristic and is thought to be due to defective fibrous tissue of the sclera enabling the color of the choroid to show through.

Osteopetrosis (Marble Bones, or Albers-Schönberg's Disease)

Osteopetrosis is a familial disease characterized by overgrowth and sclerosing of bone. Although the bones are heavy and thick, they tend to break rather than bend, and multiple fractures often occur. When this disease is due to a recessive trait, it is termed *malignant osteopetrosis* and can cause death in utero or in early life. The autosomal dominant trait causes less severe problems that may not be diagnosed until adulthood. The pathologic changes include an increase in cortical bone to nearly twice its normal density with the growth being almost exclusively endochrondral; crowding of the marrow cavity, often with complete marrow obliteration, results. Signs and symptoms of the disease relate to the skeletal malformations and the defects in hematopoiesis. Optic nerve impingement due to failure of modeling of the skull can result in blindness. Deafness can occur due to overgrowth of bone in the middle and inner ear. Cranial nerve palsies, nystagmus, and hydrocephalus may also be present. The teeth usually erupt late, develop cavities early, and often give rise to osteomyelitis of the jaw. Anemia can be profound due to the small marrow spaces and the enlarged liver and spleen are sources of extramedullary hematopoiesis. As in osteogenesis imperfecta, treatment is only palliative, but those who reach adulthood can look forward to a relatively normal life span.

Fibrous Dysplasia of Bone

This disorder, which is characterized by a replacement of cancellous bone by fibrous tissue, can affect one bone, (monostotic), or many bones (polyostotic). The fibrous lesion begins in the medullary canal and spreads to the cortex with cancellous bone and marrow being replaced by yellow gray fibrous tissue. The cortex is thin and bowing deformities and fractures are common. If this disease occurs in the monostotic form, the lesion grows slowly, but eventually deformity occurs unless the mass is surgically removed. Many times the polyostotic form of the disease is accompanied by extraskeletal signs and is called Albright's syndrome.

ALBRIGHT'S SYNDROME. This form is differentiated by a precocious puberty in females, café au lait pigmentation of the skin over the bone involvement, and a predominant unilateral bone deformity, especially of the skull and long bones. When the facial bones are affected, asymmetry of the face with distortions of the nose, jaw, and even severe displacement of an eye may occur. Although fibrous dysplasia has no proven genetic links, the multisystem involvement of the polyostotic form does suggest some basic genetic defect. Any other etiology remains a mystery.

Paget's Disease

As early as 1877, Sir James Paget described a disease of chronic bone inflammation causing softening and bowing of the long bones. Paget's disease existed in ancient times as evidenced by the study of bones in archaeologic collections. Evidence of the disease has been found in the skull of American Indians and even the Neanderthal skull.

The disease is rarely seen in people under 40 years of age, with men and women being equally affected. The frequency of the disease has ranged statistically from 0.1 to 3.0 percent. The latter figure includes subclinical cases in which the disease was discovered microscopically on autopsy. The possible causes of the disease are many but no exact etiology has been defined. Paget, himself, thought the disease was due to a chronic infection, and he called the affliction "osteitis deformans." Other etiologic investigation includes hormonal dysfunction, autoimmune states, vascular disorders, and neoplastic diseases. The most recent speculation is that the disease is caused by a latent virus. Nuclear inclusions, characteristic of a long-standing virus, have been found in the osteoclasts of individuals with Paget's disease [13]. The disease occurs late in life, which allows time for a long period of latency.

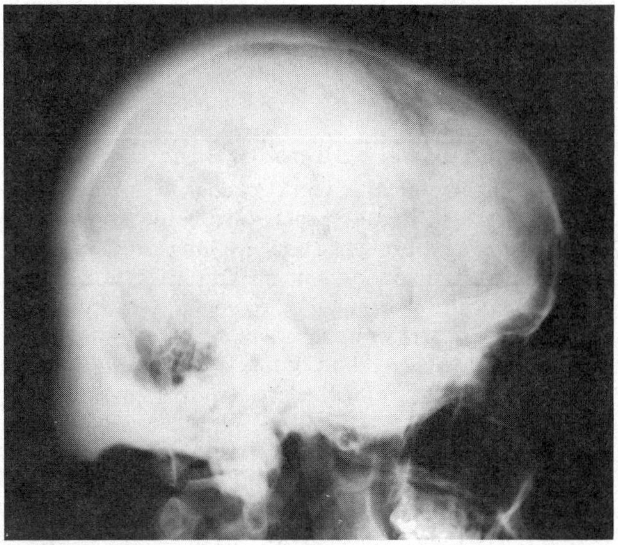

FIGURE 39-20. Paget's disease of bone. Punched-out areas in the skull represent areas of resorption and remodeling that occur simultaneously.

Pathologically, Paget's disease is characterized by resorption of bone followed by rapid overgrowth, a phenomenon that can occur in different stages in the same person and even in the same bone. The histologic features are usually described in phases. The initial phase, the osteolytic or destructive phase, is marked by extensive resorption of existing bone, with the presence of numerous multinucleated osteoclasts [8]. The "mixed" or active phase occurs when the osteoclasts destroy the ordered lamellar bone and osteoblasts respond to the bone destruction by rapid disposition of vascular connective tissue and remodeled lamellar bone. At this time, the area appears to be highly vascular with cement lines forming at sites where the lamellae are erratically joined, giving a mosaic appearance that may completely replace the preexisting bone [13]. The osteoblastic or sclerotic phase of the disease occurs when bone formation outstrips bone resorption, with lamellar bone as the predominant ingredient. The bone size and thickness are increased primarily in the head, femur, humerus, and scapula. This bone is soft, poorly mineralized, and subject to fractures (Fig. 39-20).

The clinical features progress slowly and the bone deformities can be considered part of the "normal" aging process by the individual. The long bones of the legs become bowed and the pelvis misshapen. The thorax shortens causing a loss of height. The bones of the skull are often affected, causing symptoms of vertigo, headache, and progressive deafness due to compression of the eighth nerve. In the early stages of the disease, pain in the affected bones may be experienced. Increased vascularity of the rebuilding bone, along with cutaneous vasodilatation, can produce warmth over affected bone, requiring an increase in cardiac output [8]. No cure exists for Paget's disease, but newer therapies utilize calcitonin to increase bone remodeling. Mithramycin, a cancer drug, may also be used, which suggests that the etiologic basis is a virus-induced neoplastic process [11].

Von Recklinghausen's Disease of Bone

Osteitis fibrosa cystica, or von Recklinghausen's disease of bone, is characterized by progressive resorption and destruction of bone brought about by long-standing hyperparathyroidism. Parathormone (PTH) excretion causes calcium and phosphorus to be removed from bone (see p. 553). Hyperplasia, or neoplasia of the parathyroid glands may cause a hypersecretion of this hormone and thus demineralization of bone. Secondary hyperparathyroidism, as in chronic renal insufficiency, causes a decreased conversion of vitamin D to its active form in the kidney and decreased calcium absorption in the intestine. The low serum calcium stimulates PTH secretion. In the early stages of both primary and secondary hyperparathyroidism changes in bone resemble osteomalacia or osteoporosis. However, with advanced disease, there is osteoclastic resorption of bone, which is replaced by fibrous tissue in the marrow spaces. The cancellous and cortical bones undergo thinning with resultant deformities. In focal areas of bone resorption, large fibrous scars develop, yielding minute to very large cysts, called *brown tumors*. These nonmalignant granulomas receive the brownish color from degeneration and hemorrhage into the site. Fractures and joint pains result that will be reversed if the levels of PTH are reduced.

Osteoporosis

Osteoporosis, or osteopenia, exists when there is reduction in both bone matrix and mineralization, resulting in soft bones that fracture quite easily. Because bone remodeling, with bone resorption being balanced by bone formation, normally occurs throughout life, anything that either increases resorption or decreases formation will cause a loss of bone mass. The rate of resorption follows the surface-volume mass of bones. Therefore, because the trabeculae are composed of sheets of bone and have more surface volume than cortical bone, they are lost more rapidly. This loss leads to an increased incidence of fractures in the weight-bearing bones where trabecular bone predominates. The vertebral bodies, the radial head, and femoral neck are examples of this type of bone. Likewise, resorption is accelerated on the endosteal surfaces of trabecular bone while bone formation is occurring at the periosteal surfaces, thus leading to wider bones with a thinner, more porous cortex. The ratio of bone mineral to matrix formation is constant but there is simply a reduction in both. This contrasts with osteomalacia where the matrix is normal but the mineralization is deficient.

Osteoporosis may be caused by genetic, nutritional, mobility, drug-related, hormonal, and age factors. Deficiencies in protein, vitamin C, vitamin D, vitamin A, and calcium can lead to reduced matrix and mineralization. Estrogen and testosterone stimulate osteoblastic activity so that with menopause, the incidence of osteoporosis increases. Women with artificially induced menopause seem to develop the disease faster than women with normal, more slowly declining hormonal levels. Other endocrine changes, such as diabetes mellitus and thyrotoxicosis, wherein protein synthesis is decreased and catabolism increased respectively, also cause osteoporosis. Cushing's disease with its protein catabolic loss has the same bone results as prolonged steroid therapy. Prolonged therapy with heparin and certain cancer drugs, may lead to osteoporosis. X-ray irradiation, as well as that resulting from radioactive materials, may affect bone by damage to the osteoblasts. Immobility of a limb and prolonged bed rest can also cause bone loss (see pp. 554–555).

The incidence of osteoporosis is significant in people over 40, and it is agreed that bone loss predominates over bone production in all persons past the age of 35. Osteoporosis appears to be an exaggeration of the aging process and is quite rare in younger people. The greater incidence encountered in aging women seems to be the effect of estrogen deficiency.

Clinical manifestations are related to fractures and/or pain. Back pain due to a collapsed vertebra may be sudden and severe, or chronic and aching if compression has occurred over a period of time. Fractures may result from trivial trauma, often affecting the hip or long bones. Gradual loss of stature and spinal deformities with increased dorsal kyphosis are common.

The course of osteoporosis is dependent on the cause. Small amounts of estrogen in postmenopausal women have been found to retard the process but the drug will not arrest the problem. Prevention of significant osteoporosis can be achieved by diet and activity levels that increase the bone mass.

Rickets/Osteomalacia

Rickets is a disease in the infant or growing child that usually is caused by a lack of vitamin D. Osteomalacia in the adult results in similar pathologic features that may have the same etiologies as rickets. The primary pathology consists of a lack of mineralization of bone with a relative increase in uncalcified osteoid. The normal time for osteoid to become calcified is about 6 to 10 days, but in osteomalacia, the time interval lengthens to several months [10]. Due to the lack of mineralization, the bones are soft and will bow and break easily. Because bone formation in the growing child is most accelerated at the ends of the long bones, the epiphyseal tissue in rickets is softer with the normally sharp, narrow line of ossification being replaced by a wide irregular zone of soft gray tissue. Bowed legs and deformities of the costochondral junction (rachitic rosary) and thorax (pigeon breast) along with defective tooth enamel are evidence of rickets. In the adult, osteomalacia is displayed by mineral changes and pain in the lumbar vertebrae, the pelvic girdle, and the long bones

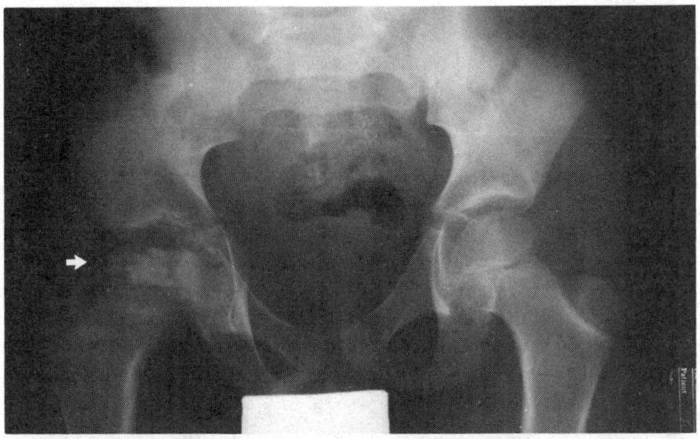

FIGURE 39-21. Legg-Calvé-Perthes disease. Flattened femoral bone is a result of necrosis.

of the lower limbs. Deformities can also occur in adults when the muscles and tendons change the shape of the softened bone.

Scurvy

Vitamin C (ascorbic acid) is necessary for the production of the collagen of fibrous tissue and of bone matrix. A deficiency of vitamin C leads to scurvy, which is characterized by hemorrhages, anemia, and bone and teeth changes. Hemorrhages can occur in any organ and can vary from tiny petechiae to large hematomas. Bone disturbances are evidenced by a defective osteoid and a relative increase in bone resorption over formation. This leads to a decreased density of bone. Bleeding, spongy gums, and loose teeth are common. Scurvy in infants usually does not appear until after 6 months of age and it takes from 3 months to a year of severe vitamin C deficiency to produce scurvy in an adult.

Avascular Necrosis

The word *osteochondrosis* refers to a set of conditions affecting the epiphyseal region of bone in children during the growth period. The pathology involved is brought about by an avascular necrosis in the area that causes the bone of the epiphysis to soften and die (Fig. 39-21). Various names have been ascribed to avascular necrosis occurring in specific areas, but the designation *Legg-Calvé-Perthes disease* is the most familiar. The onset of the condition appears to be growth related. Until the ages of 3 and 4 years, the predominant blood supply to the femoral head comes across the growth plate from the metaphysis of the femur with other supply from the lateral epiphyseal vessels. At about 4 years of age, the growth plate begins to block the metaphyseal blood supply and full development of the ligament artery supply to the femoral head occurs when the child is 7 or 8. This leaves a period of time when the blood supply to the femoral head is dependent on the lateral epiphyseal vessels.

Precipitating causes of avascular necrosis may be trauma, infections, or inflammation. In the 2- to 4-year course of the disease the following stages occur: (1) Avascular necrosis causes the bone of the femoral head to soften and die, but the cartilage surrounding it, nourished by the synovial fluid remains viable. (2) Blood vessels from adjacent viable tissue grow in through the neck of the femur and begin the slow process of removing dead bone a little at a time, a process called "creeping substitution." (3) Areas of resorbed bone are filled with new bone and ossification occurs. All three of these stages — necrosis, removal of dead bone, and reossification — may be occurring simultaneously within the same bone. Children may complain of aching pain and limited motion early in the disease, but later processes remain painless.

Osgood-Schlatter disease usually occurs in boys from 10 to 15 years of age and is characterized by a painful, tender and enlarged tibial tubercle. It is caused by a pull of the patellar tendon on the tibial tubercle epiphysis. Serial x rays show changes due to aseptic necrosis that results from avascular changes. Like Legg-Calvé-Perthes disease, pain disappears shortly after onset but the tibial tubercle may remain enlarged.

INFECTIOUS DISEASES OF BONE

Osteomyelitis

Osteomyelitis occurs when the bone and bone marrow are invaded by pyogenic organisms. Infection of bone can come about in three ways: (1) by direct expansion from a neighboring focus, (2) by direct contamination, as with compound fractures or open wounds, and (3) by hematogenous spread from distant sites of infection (infected tonsils, boils, upper respiratory infections) [10]. The latter condition occurs most frequently in children and young people under the age of 21.

The causative organisms may be the hemolytic *Staphylococcus*, the streptococci, coliform bacteria, *Pneumococcus, Gonococcus,* or any bacterial or fungal agent. The infecting organism enters the bone through the nutrient or metaphyseal vessels and moves into the medullary canal. Vascularity increases, causing edema. Polymorphonuclear leukocytes accumulate in the area. In a few days, thrombosis of local vessels occurs and ischemia results. Portions of bone tissue die. Pus in this confined space is under pressure and is pushed out through Volkmann's canals to the surface of the bone. It then spreads subperiosteally and can enter the bone at another level, or burst out into the surrounding tissue. In infants, before the epiphyseal cartilage seals off the metaphysis, spread can go directly to the joint and cause a suppurative arthritis. In older individuals, if joint involvement does occur, it does so through subperiosteal spread. The dead bone is separated from viable tissue and granulation tissue forms beneath the area of dead bone and infection. The necrotic bone, isolated from viable tissue, is termed *sequestra* [10]. New bone forms from the elevated periosteum. This bone, called the *involucrum*, envelopes the granulation tissue and sequestrum. Small sinuses permit the pus to escape.

In chronic osteomyelitis, the granulation tissue becomes scar tissue and forms an impenetrable area around the infection. New area of bone develops to further isolate the area. The process is characterized by chronically draining sinuses with organisms that are resistant to normal antibiotic therapy.

The person with acute osteomyelitis appears acutely ill with fever, chills, and leukocytosis. The affected limb becomes very painful; the pain is often described as a constant throbbing. Redness and swelling usually occur over the site and sensitivity to the touch is characteristic. X-ray evidence can be seen after about 10 days and reflects bone destruction. Blood cultures are usually positive for the specific causative organism; massive antibiotic therapy usually arrests the disease.

Tuberculosis

Tuberculosis is a systemic disease caused by the tubercle bacillus; which spreads through the body via lymphatic or hematogenous routes (see Chap. 23). Skeletal involvement is rarely seen now due to adequate therapy but when it occurs it is often caused by seeding of the bacillus in the marrow cavity. The infection causes destruction of bone tissue and caseous necrosis that may enter the joint cavities or occur under the skin as an abscess with draining sinuses. Tubercular skeletal lesions usually do not wall themselves off so invasion of joints and intervertebral disks may cause many deformities. Tuberculosis of the spine, called *Pott's disease,* most frequently occurs in children and can lead to kyphosis, scoliosis, or the "hunchback" deformity.

The onset of skeletal tuberculosis, in contrast to acute pyogenic osteomyelitis, is insidious, beginning with vague descriptions of pain. Complications of tuberculosis of the spine include paraplegia and meningitis. Tuberculosis of the hip and knee joint have a greater incidence in children.

Syphilis

Congenital or acquired syphilis of the bone is rare in the United States. In congenital syphilis, the spirochetes are delivered to the bones by the fetal bloodstream. Osteogenic function is inhibited by the spirochetes. The epiphyseal plate is severely damaged and may actually be separated from the metaphysis. Bone syphilis is marked by endarteritis and periarteritis and reactive bone formation occurs from viable surrounding periosteum. Granulation tissue between the periosteum and cortical bone is laid down. In the tibia, a resulting deformity, called the "saber shin" deformity gives a curved appearance to the anterior portion of the bone.

Acquired syphilis may also cause osteochondritis or periosteitis; there is a possibility that frank syphilitic lesions will appear within the medullary canal. The skull and vertebrae, as well as the long bones, can be affected in acquired syphilis.

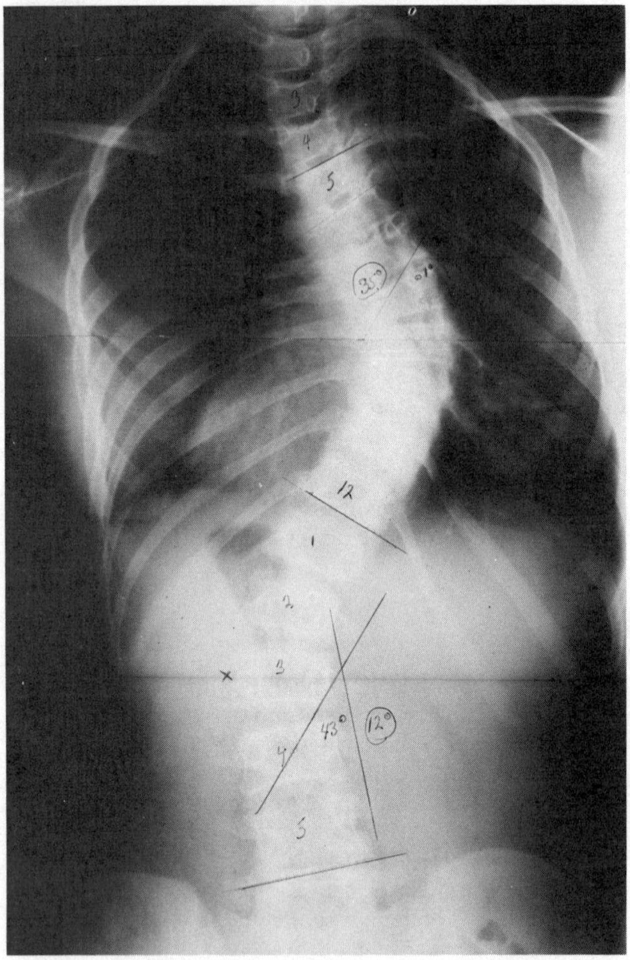

FIGURE 39-22. Scoliosis of the spine with a thoracic primary curve and a compensatory curve in the lumbar spine. Vertebral bodies are marked at the approximate beginning and end of each curve and are used to measure the degree of curvature.

ALTERATIONS IN SKELETAL STRUCTURE

Scoliosis

Scoliosis is a lateral curvature of the spine, and most commonly is called idiopathic adolescent scoliosis. Thought to be genetic, this deformity most frequently affects young girls. The curvatures are classified according to location and consist of a primary, fixed curve with compensatory curves above and below the original (Fig. 39-22). The deformity occurs slowly and is accelerated by the preadolescent growth spurt. The shoulder blade protrudes, the level of the iliac crest becomes unequal, and the curvature appears to be exaggerated when the individual bends over. In general, the younger the age when the curvature is noticed and the higher up in the thorax it occurs, the poorer the prognosis. Severe scoliosis can affect the heart and lungs by restrictive action but may be markedly improved by surgical procedures.

Clubfoot (Talipes)

Clubfoot deformities, the most frequent of the orthopedic congenital deformities of the lower extremities, occur with greater frequency in boys. Two-thirds of cases involve unilateral deformities that may be caused by genetic and environmental factors. The usual presentation is with the talus pointing downward and the foot adducted. The clinical varieties are termed *easy* and *resistant*, with the easy cases responding to strapping and stretching alone while the resistant cases require surgical intervention.

Congenital Dislocation of the Hip

Congenital dislocation of the hip is probably caused by a combination of genetic and environmental factors. Genetic factors are linked to both joint laxity and acetabular dysplasia. Also, the pregnant woman secretes a ligament-relaxing hormone just prior to delivery of a full-term infant that crosses the placental barrier and enhances joint laxity. This fact accounts for the relatively rare incidence of hip dislocation in premature infants. Other environmental factors include intrauterine malposition and swaddling practices in the neonatal period in some cultures.

Pathologically, the acetabulum is defective and the femoral head is completely out of the joint, being posterior and superior to the acetabulum. Most frequently, this is a unilateral occurrence. On examination, one sees asymmetric groin skin creases, with the affected leg being shorter than the other. The leg cannot abduct completely; when the leg is extended and flexed at the hip, a click, called Ortolani's click, may be felt or heard. Because the femoral head must be in correct alignment with the acetabulum for the bones and joint to grow and develop normally, early detection is necessary. Reduction after the age of 6 is almost impossible and secondary bone changes occur that cause the child to walk with a typical lurching gait. The younger the age of treatment, the more likely that complete hip function will be restored.

ALTERATIONS IN JOINTS AND TENDONS

As discussed earlier, the joints function to allow mobility of the body. The synovial joint is most affected by alterations. Recent studies have shown that this type of articular cartilage, which receives lubrication and nutrition from the synovial fluid, has many microscopic spaces filled with water, causing it to be elastic and able to "bounce back" despite subjection to daily compression [9].

Arthritis

The most frequent joint diseases are in the arthritis group, which attack 1 out of every 20 to 30 Americans and constitute a financial and health problem of considerable magnitude. Arthritis simply means inflammation of a joint, and it occurs in many forms. *Suppurative* arthritis implies an infection of the joint with pyogenic organisms; *tuberculous arthritis* is a joint inflammation that is secondary to tuberculosis. The most crippling of the arthritis group is *rheumatoid arthritis* (RA), which has many forms. The discussion that follows includes RA and osteoarthritis.

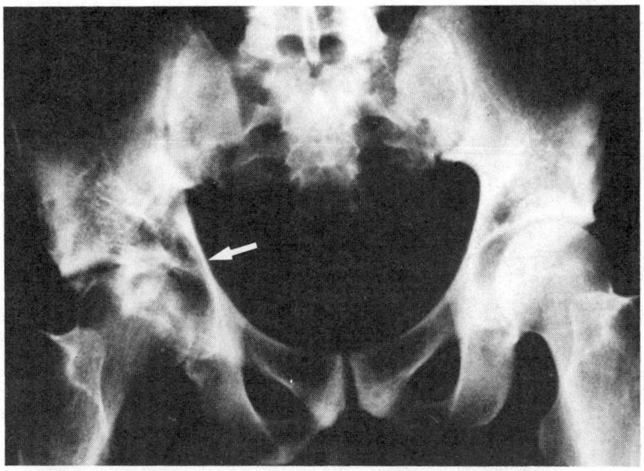

FIGURE 39-23. Rheumatoid arthritis of the right hip.

RHEUMATOID ARTHRITIS. This chronic inflammatory disease has been studied extensively in order to uncover an etiologic agent. Theories have been supported in recent years involving an infectious cause or an autoimmune response. Hard evidence to support the infectious disease theory has been lacking, but a significant body of knowledge seems to back the immune response theory. Antibodies, known as *rheumatoid factor* (RF), have been demonstrated in the sera of almost all individuals with RA. Synovial lymphocytes produce an IgG, which is targeted as being foreign, and production of IgG and IgM anti-immunoglobulin result. These anti-immunoglobulins are actually the rheumatoid factor. By binding with IgG, the antigenic target, the resulting complex causes activation of the complement system in the joint. The RF titer is in direct relationship to the severity of the disease, although the actual stimulus for the formation of RF is unknown. The numerous T lymphocytes in the joint may become sensitized to the joint collagens, causing an immunologic response, one enhanced by the release of lymphokines and presence of prostaglandins [3, 10]. Increased physical or emotional stress has always been recognized as a precipitator of acute exacerbations but the mechanisms for the stress interaction is unknown.

Joint destruction is the primary pathology of RA and may affect any synovial membrane in the body. Joint inflammation with effusion is accompanied by capsular and periarticular soft tissue inflammation causing swelling, redness, and painful motion of the joint. Proliferative synovitis persists and the synovium becomes a thickened, hyperemic, densely cellular membrane, called a *pannus*, which in-

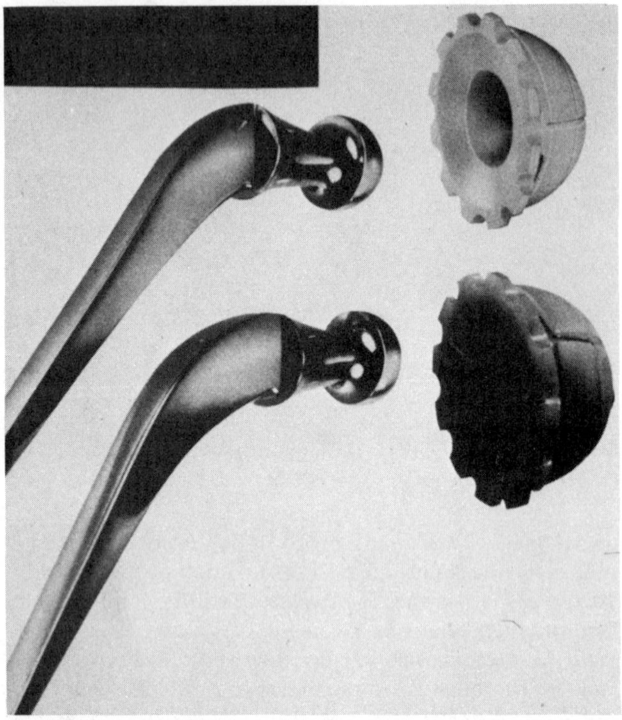

FIGURE 39-24. Stainless steel femoral head and shaft fits into the artificial acetabulum, which is glued into correct placement.

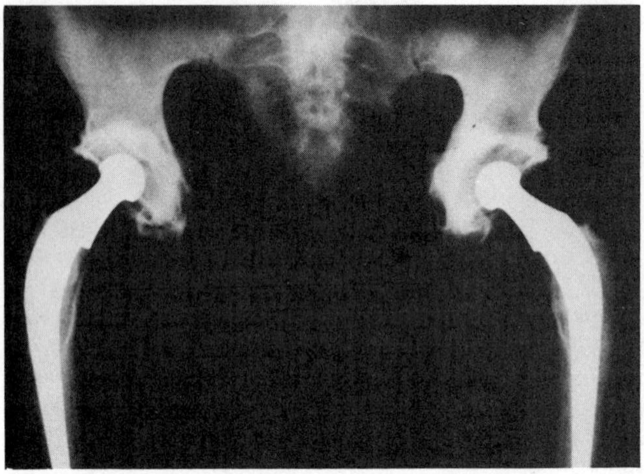

FIGURE 39-25. Total hip replacement with ball and socket.

vades and erodes surrounding cartilage and bone. Joint motion causes bleeding within the cavity. Fibrin clot with formation of granulation tissue fills the joint space. The pannus formation destroys the articular cartilage and underlying bone, resulting in loss of motion. Figure 39-23 shows an almost totally destroyed right hip joint caused by RA. The muscles that pull across the joint give rise to flexion and extension and subluxation deformities. Subcutaneous rheumatoid nodules, which are areas of necrosis surrounded by lymphocytes and plasma cells, are found in about one-fourth of the patients.

The fluid aspirated from the joint is thin and cloudy with an elevated white cell count. The lysosomal enzymes released from these neutrophils may be a factor in cartilage destruction. As the acute inflammatory process subsides, granulation tissue becomes scar tissue and eventually bone, causing a true ankylosis (fixed, stiff joint). Local degenerative muscle is gradually replaced by fibrous tissue and the involved bones show osteoporosis.

Rheumatoid arthritis is a systemic disease, but its effects are less frequent on other areas of the body. The small and large arteries anywhere in the system can develop acute necrotizing vasculitis with thrombosis. The vasculitis can cause the vascular insufficiency of Raynaud's phenomenon or obliterative vasculitis from intimal proliferation. The manifestations of cardiac disease include conduction disturbances, myocarditis, and valvular impingement [3]. In the lungs, the patient may exhibit pleuritis or interstitial pneumonitis. The eye may show uveitis, keratoconjunctivitis, or chronic inflammation. Neuropathies, skeletal muscle inflammations, and spleen and liver enlargement may result.

RA affects females in a ratio of 3 : 1 over males with most individuals being between 20 and 50 years of age. The onset can be vague or acute. Fatigue, fever, and malaise may precede actual joint pain, or high fever and aching joints may herald the onset of the disease. Joint stiffness is more noticeable in the morning or after rest. The erythrocyte sedimentation rate is elevated. Exacerbations are common and often cause increasing damage with further stiffness and deformities. Surgical procedures to replace dysfunctioning joints are often required (Figs. 39-24 and 39-25).

Variants of rheumatoid arthritis include *juvenile rheumatoid arthritis* and *ankylosing spondylitis*. The onset of juvenile RA is usually abrupt with chills and high fever, or it may appear insidiously with typical joint stiffness of one or more joints. The joint pathology is like the adult form, and subcutaneous lesions may also be present. Fortunately, over one-half of these young persons have a complete remission. Some of the others suffer permanent deformities.

Ankylosing spondylitis, or Marie-Strümpell disease, is a variant of RA with a genetic linkage that involves the sacroiliac joints, the spine, and adjacent soft tissue. Cartilage and bone destruction result in fibrous and bony ankylosing of the spine, giving the patient the typical stiff or "poker spine." Ninety percent of cases are men between the ages of 20 and 40. An elevated erythrocyte sedimentation rate (ESR) is characteristic, but rheumatoid factor (RF) and antinuclear antibodies (ANA) are not seen in this disease.

OSTEOARTHRITIS. The term *osteoarthritis* is misleading because inflammation is not a usual component of this condition. The designation *degenerative joint disease* more clearly defines the problem. The incidence usually is age-related with most of those affected being over 50 years old. Joints have a limited way in which to respond to the compressive forces in day-to-day living. In osteoarthritis, it has been found that the matrix in the articular cartilage has been depleted, thus "unmasking" the basic collagen structure. Normally, the matrix spreads compression stress hydrostatically, but with its depletion the collagen fibers may rupture, causing flaking, fissuring, and erosion of the articular cartilage. These alterations are characteristic of the disorder. The bone immediately under the affected area shows proliferation of fibroblasts and new bone formation. Periosteal bone formation also increases at the joint margins and at the site of ligament or tendon attachments, which causes the formation of bone spurs or ridges, called *osteophytes*. The synovial capsule decreases in size, and movement is limited. Degenerative joint disease generally affects joints that are under much pressure, especially the spine, fingers, knees, hips, and shoulders. Pain and stiffness after resting are generally relieved by walking, but permanent ankylosing of the joints may occur. Persons who have occupational stress, are obese, or have faulty posture have a greater incidence of the problem. Trauma, such as sports injuries to a joint at an early age, can render the individual more susceptible to osteoarthritis with advancing years. Studies have shown a *wear-and-tear* process with increased incidence in joints under greater stress.

Gout

Gout is often a hereditary disorder of uric acid metabolism characterized by hyperuricemia. It may be primary or secondary. Primary gout involves an inborn error in metabolism and genetic links have been established. Ninety-five percent of those affected with primary gout are male. Secondary gout occurs whenever some superimposed condition either increases the production of uric acid or decreases its excretion. Diseases characterized by a rapid breakdown of cells (such as leukemia), hemolytic anemia, cytolytic agents, and drugs that decrease excretion of urates (e.g., thiazides and mercurial diuretics) have all been implicated in secondary gout.

The incidence of primary gout exceeds that of secondary gout by about 20 to 1. In the body, uric acid is made by the enzymatic breakdown of tissue and dietary purines. In gout, either the enzymes are increased or the feedback mechanism is faulty, so that an abnormally large amount of uric acid in the blood is produced. In primary gout, the kidneys may become dysfunctional and cause a decreased excretion of uric acid. The result of this is an increased uric acid content in all of the body fluids. At an excessive point, uric acid crystals precipitate into the joint fluids, the kidneys, the heart, the earlobes, and the toes. The mass of urate crystals surrounded by inflammation with lymphocytes, plasma cells, and macrophages is called a *tophus*. Tophi may clump together and form large plaquelike encrustations that invade the articular surface and underlying bone causing deformities. Gout is described in three stages:

Stage 1: A high blood uric acid concentration is noted but the individual is usually asymptomatic.

Stage 2 is characterized by acute gouty arthritis with redness, swelling, and exquisite tenderness over the toes, fingers, wrists, ankles, knees, and other joints. Attacks and remissions are common for many years.

Stage 3: The disabling joint disease is compounded by renal changes with renal stones, colic, and hypertension being common.

Atherosclerosis becomes a problem in almost half of cases of gout, and death occurs most frequently from myocardial infarction or renal failure.

Bursitis

Bursae are enclosed sacs containing a small amount of fluid that also serves to lubricate and cushion joints. Inflammation of a bursa is common and may be caused by unusual use of a part, by trauma, infection, or rheumatoid arthritis. The inflammation results in an excess production of fluid in the sac causing distention of the sac and pain. Commonly affected bursae are: (1) the prepatellar bursae, of which the cause is kneeling (housemaid's knee or nun's knee), (2) the olecranon bursae, subject to the repeated trauma of leaning on one's elbows (bartender's elbows), and (3) the bursa located on the plantar aspect of the heel, which is subjected to repeated pressure (postman's heel).

Baker's Cyst

Baker's cyst is a firm, cystic mass found along the medial border of the popliteal space. These cysts, found mostly in children, are believed to be caused by fluid distention of the bursal sac associated with local muscles. Some cysts communicate directly with the joint cavity. Swelling is usually the only symptom, and surgical excision, although possible, is not often necessary.

Tumors of Joints

SYNOVIAL SARCOMA. Tumors of joints are uncommon, but may occur on the tendon sheath, the bursae, and around the joints. Primitive mesenchymal cells, rather than synovial membrane cells form the primary tumor. A gray white mass invades along muscle and fascial planes, and although the tumor is slow-growing, it can metastasize into the lung, bone, and brain.

Tenosynovitis

Tenosynovitis is an inflammation of the tendon sheath and the enclosed tendon primarily affecting the wrist, shoulder, and ankle. This condition is thought to be use-related, and occupational stresses, such as typing and heavy labor, may precipitate it. Synovial fluid and fibrin constituents within the tendon sheath may cause adhesions. These inflammations cause extreme pain on movement and may exhibit heat and redness or inflammation. Bacterial invasion of pyrogens and tuberculosis also have been implicated as causes of tenosynovitis.

Fibromatosis

Palmar fibromatosis denotes a chronic hyperplasia of the fascia in the palm of the hand, leading to fibrosis and a particular deformity called Dupuytren's contracture. The fingers, most often the ring and little fingers, contract into a fixed, flexed position. Usually bilateral, this condition is most frequently found in middle-aged men with heredity believed to be a major factor in causation.

Plantar fibromatosis is similar to palmar fibromatosis, but it usually does not cause contractures. Nodular masses of fibrocytes arise from the plantar fascia, usually on the medial side of the foot. Trauma is thought to be causative.

BONE TUMORS

Tumors in the skeletal system can be either primary or secondary. Primary lesions of the bone can be benign or malignant. Of these, benign tumors are much more common and usually are self-limiting. Malignant tumors of the bone, although rare, are devastating and often fatal. Diagnosis is made by a careful history, location, and radiographic appearance.

Benign bone tumors are usually slow-growing, noninvasive, and well localized. Adolescents or young adults are usually affected more frequently and the tumor growth stops when the adolescent's skeletal system reaches maturity. Because of the noninvasive characteristics, benign tumors cause little or no pain and are often found secondarily to another complaint or a pathologic fracture.

Malignant neoplasms grow rapidly, spread and invade irregularly, and cause pain. Adolescents and young adults are most commonly affected. These tumors metastasize into other parts of the body and are usually fatal unless there is early diagnosis and treatment.

Secondary tumors of the skeletal system are usually from primary sites in the breasts, lungs, kidneys, or other body systems. As the primary lesion grows and invades surrounding tissue, clumps of cancerous tissues are carried by the blood and lymphatic system to the bone, where they continue to grow and cause destruction.

The growth of tumors in the bone often causes increased radiodensities due to increased osteoblastic activity within the tumor. This can be seen on x ray, which is helpful in diagnosis. Some tumors exhibit a translucent-appearing bone on x ray, indicating increased osteoclastic activity.

Classification of Tumors

CHONDROGENIC TUMORS. Chondrogenic tumors are those whose origin is in the cartilage tissue. The most common benign tumor is the *osteochondroma*. Many of these tumors are asymptomatic and are only found accidentally because of an injury to the area. Osteochondromas form a long mass produced by progressive endochondral ossification of a growing cartilaginous cap. The tumor is basically osseous and protrudes from the cortex of the bone with or without a stalk. The caps are usually cauliflower-shaped (Fig. 39-26) and occur mainly in persons between the first and second decades of life. The growth of the tumor parallels that of the adolescent and once the epiphyses have closed, growth of the tumor normally stops. Multiple osteochondromas may occur when more than one bone is affected, with each growth having the same characteristics as the single osteochondroma.

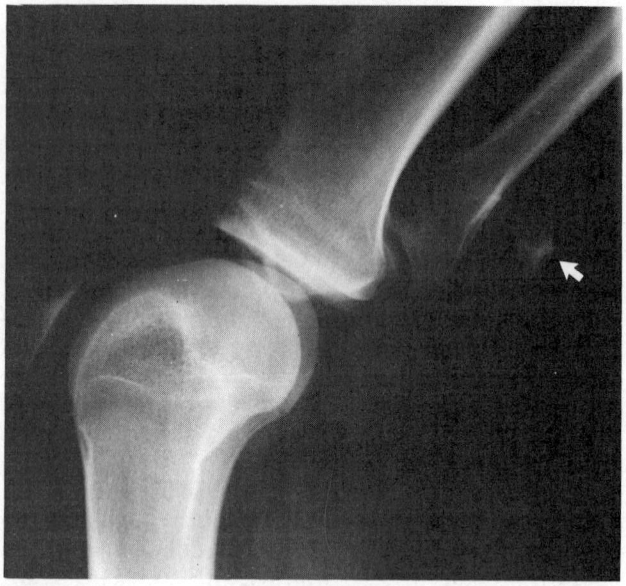

FIGURE 39-26. Typical osteochondroma of the fibula.

Osteochondromas rarely will undergo malignant change and become an osteosarcoma. This transformation occurs more frequently with multiple osteochondromas and occasionally follows the surgical removal of an osteochondroma. The most common site for the tumorous mass is the metaphyseal region of long bones, specifically the femur and tibia, but it can affect any bone that develops by endochrondral ossification.

Endochondroma is the term used to describe a tumor when it only involves the medulla and is encapsulated by an intact cortex. It commonly affects the small bones of the hands and feet and also may affect ribs, sternum, spine, and long bones of persons between the ages of 20 and 30 years. This tumor usually affects the phalanges of the hand, producing a central area of rarefaction (decreasing density and weight) (Fig. 39-27). Normally discovered when a fracture is found after a trivial injury, the tumor appears on x ray as a well-defined translucent area with the cortex intact and areas of calcification.

Benign chondroblastoma closely resembles giant-cell tumors and affects mainly persons under the age of 20, or before epiphyseal closure. Giant-cell tumors are rare under 20 years of age. Histologically, chondroblastomas differ from giant-cell tumors in that they contain foci of calcifica-

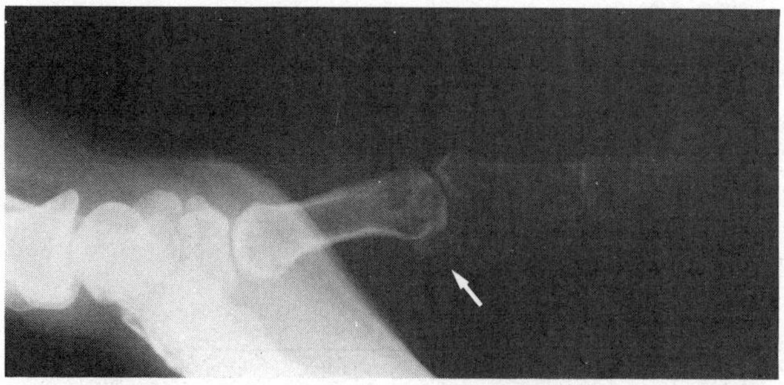

FIGURE 39-27. Endochondroma of the thumb.

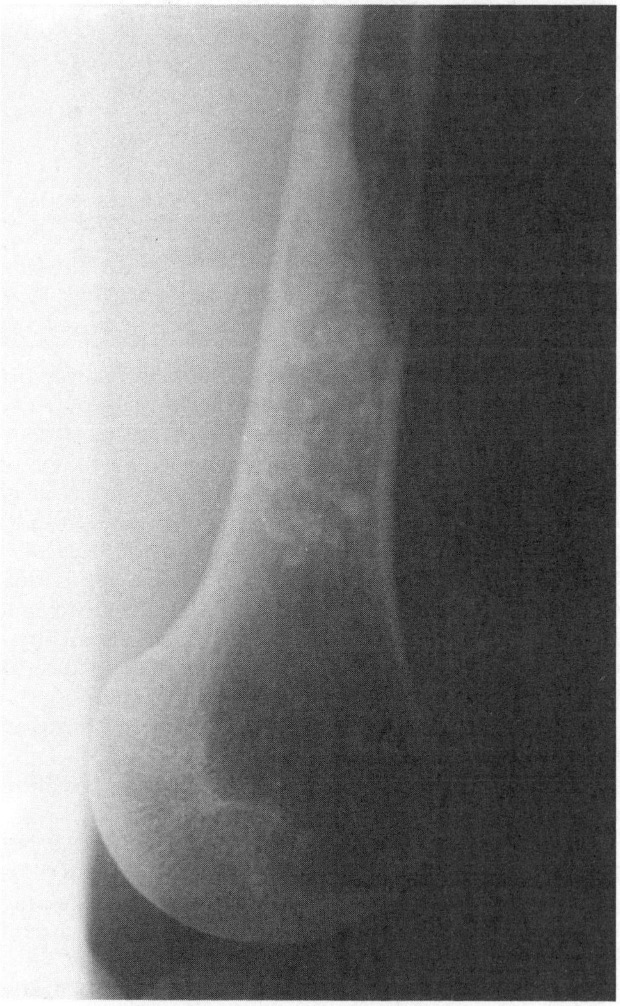

FIGURE 39-28. Chondrosarcoma of the humerus. Mixed lytic and sclerotic areas give patchy appearance to bone.

tion, trabeculae of osteoid tissue, and well-developed bone, as well as more or less well-defined areas of cartilaginous matrix that are not usually present in giant-cell tumors. Chondroblastomas are virtually always benign, localized lesions that do not recur and do not invade.

Localized pain may be experienced and this is often referred to the adjacent joint region. A wasting of muscle

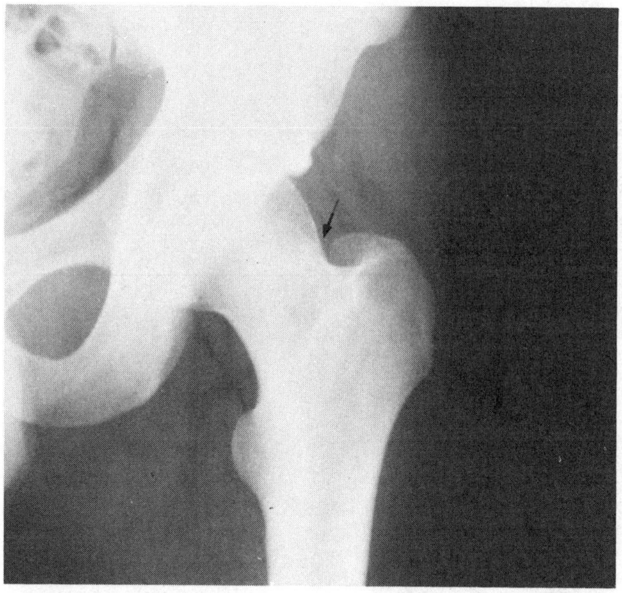

FIGURE 39-29. Osteoid osteoma. Note small transport area indicated by arrow representing the central nidus.

mass due to disuse caused by pain and limping may also be observed.

On x rays, an area of central bone destruction is clearly demarcated by surrounding normal bone. There may be margins of increased bone density with mottled areas of calcification within the lesion. The tumor almost always involves the epiphyses and frequently the adjacent metaphyses, which can also be seen on x rays [2].

Chondrosarcomas can be divided into three groups: primary chondrosarcomas, secondary chondrosarcomas, and mesenchymal chondrosarcomas. Secondary chondrosarcomas are those that arise from benign chondrogenic origin as described earlier. Chondrosarcomas represent only about 7.6 percent of all malignant bone tumors and occur more frequently in men than women [10]. This tumor is primarily one of adulthood and old age, although secondary chondrosarcoma may affect the young individual.

Chondrosarcomas usually originate in the trunk and the upper ends of the femur and humerus, but can occur in virtually any bone of the body.

Physical symptoms may include pain, swelling, and a palpable mass due to the active invasive growth of the tumor. Those tumors located in the trunk and long bones may be evidenced only by pain, which makes radiographic findings important. The usual radiographic findings include mottled areas of calcification and areas of osseous destruction (Fig. 39-28).

Even when treated with wide resection, recurrence has been encountered even after 10 years. The overall survival rate of 65 to 70 percent for 5 years is not indicative of a cure because metastases may occur many years after initial diagnosis and treatment.

OSTEOGENIC TUMORS. *Compact osteoma* is a benign tumor composed of dense bone with a well-circumscribed edge.

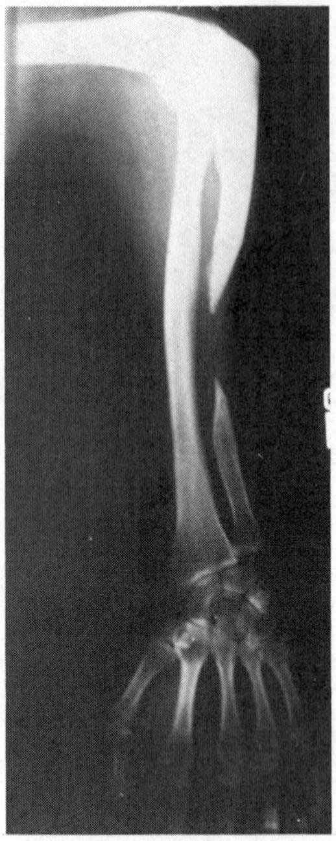

FIGURE 39-30. Osteogenic sarcoma. Note the complete destruction of the ulna.

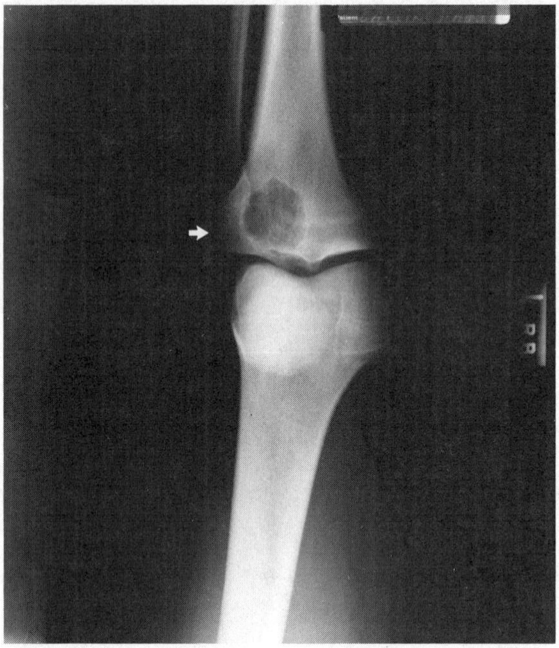

FIGURE 39-31. Giant-cell tumor of the tibia (*arrow*).

It is frequently found in the cortical surface of bone of the skull and paranasal sinuses. Symptoms are caused from impingement on the brain or air sinuses. Affected persons often complain that the tumors cause cosmetically unacceptable appearances.

Osteoid osteoma most commonly affects the femur and tibia but can affect any bone in the body except the skull. It is usually located in the diaphyses of long bones. It occurs predominantly in males between the ages of 5 and 25 years. The tumor consists of a well-rounded central nidus that is sharply demarcated from a surrounding zone of bone. The nidus may range from a few millimeters to a centimeter and consists of osteoid tissue and trabeculae (Fig. 39-29). The tissue is a reddish-gray color and is granular to the touch. It may be removed because it causes localized pain, especially at night.

Benign osteoblastoma is a rare benign tumor that is sometimes confused with osteoid osteoma or even giant-cell tumors. This benign growth occurs more frequently in males in the first three decades of life. It has a marked predilection for the spinal cord.

Pain is a cardinal symptom, usually due to the pressure on adjacent structures, such as the spinal cord or nerve roots. The pain seems to lack the intrinsic severity of that caused by an osteoid osteoma and may be referred to a site distant from the tumor; there may be weakness or even paraplegia.

There is not a characteristic radiographic appearance. In some cases, one may see bone destruction that is more or less demarcated from normal bone. When the tumor is in a long bone, it may take on the appearance of an osteoid osteoma with a sclerotic border except that the nidus may be many times longer. Surgical removal usually relieves the spinal column and nerve root compression.

Osteogenic sarcoma (osteosarcoma) is the most common primary malignancy of the bone. It is a tumor of mesenchymal cells that produce osteoid [10]. It has an affinity for the young and a 2 : 1 male to female ratio, with its peak occurrence during the second decade of life. Radiation and oncogenic viruses have been explored in the etiology of this disease [10]. When this lesion does occur in later years of life, it is usually related to Paget's disease. Irradiation treatment for other tumors has also been indicated in the causation of osteogenic sarcoma in later life.

To be classified as a true osteogenic sarcoma, an osteoid substance must be produced. The tumor may show a predominance of elements with osteoid, chondroid, or fibromatoid differentiation [2].

Osteosarcomas usually occur in long tubular bones, but the skull, maxilla, spinal column, and clavicle, as well as other bones, are also affected. The femur and tibia are the most frequently affected sites. The humerus, ilium, mandible, and ribs follow in decreasing order of frequency. Over the age of 25, flat bone and long bone incidence is nearly equal [10]. Osteogenic sarcomas are normally located at approximately the distal femur and proximal tibia. When the humerus is affected, it usually affects the shoulder.

Osteogenic sarcomas have been divided into subdivisions such as periosteal, sclerotic, lytic, central, telangiectatic, and so forth. This section limits the discussion to *sclerosing osteogenic sarcoma* and *osteolytic osteogenic sarcoma*, which produce quite different x rays.

The sclerosing variety forms a large amount of osseous neoplastic tissue that causes considerable reactive bone

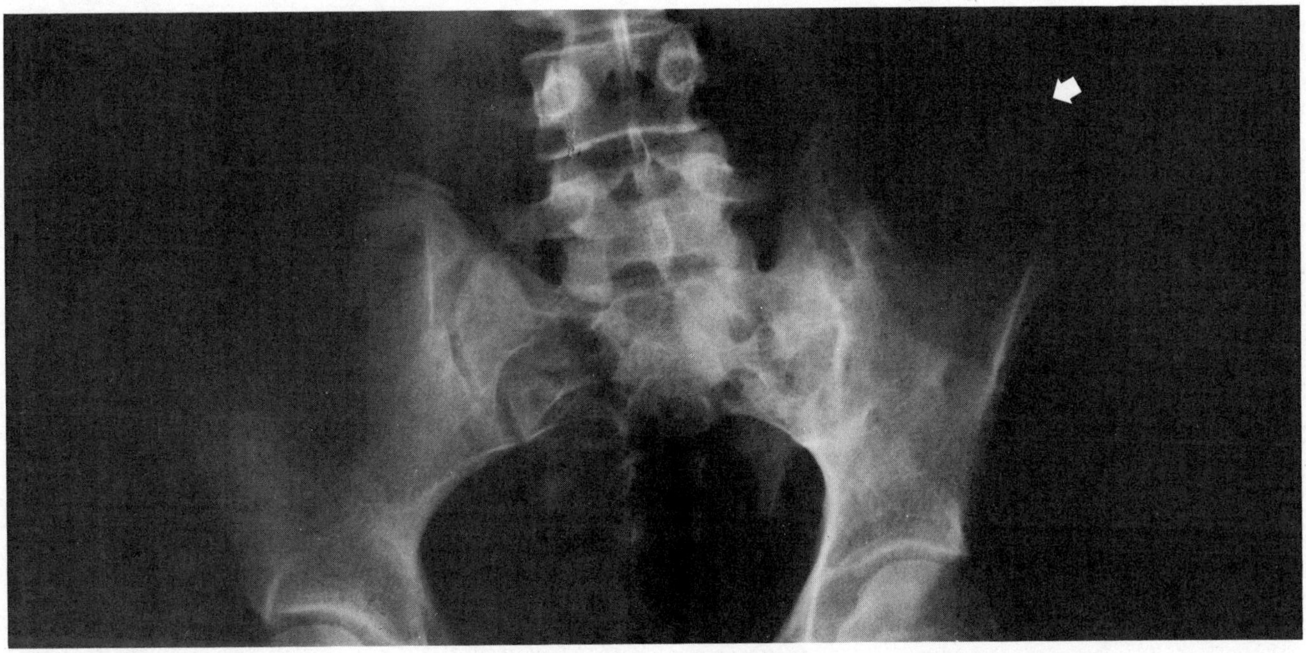

FIGURE 39-32. Ewing's sarcoma. Note that the top of the ischium has been carved out by tumor.

formation and produces dense growths. The growth may protrude as far down as the articular cartilage, but this cartilage seems to form a barrier to further spread. Penetration of the cortex is almost invariable, often lifting up the periosteum. Periosteal elevation in combination with cortical bone formation produces an acute angle that can be seen on x ray, known as Codman's triangle. The central region of the growth tends to be the most densely sclerotic with increased density of the enveloped cortical bone.

The osteolytic mass is composed mostly of sarcomatous connective tissue stroma with minimal amounts of osteoid matrix. The osteolytic type is a bulkier tumor because it is faster growing [10]. It also involves the medullary canal but has a fleshy consistency with areas of hemorrhage, necrosis, and cystic changes. There is more destruction of cortical bone, and more involvement of the soft tissue (Fig. 39-30). Small foci of calcification are seen, but microscopically, it appears as a soft tissue neoplasm [10].

Local swelling and tenderness with a large mass may be initially presented. Distal swelling and large distended veins are often noted. The 5-year survival rate even after surgical excision was 20.3 percent and the 10-year rate was 17.3 percent in a reported study [2].

Giant-cell tumors are poorly understood, apparently malignant distinct neoplasms. Cases of seemingly benign giant-cell tumors have been reported to undergo malignant transformation. For this reason, a histomorphic grading system has been developed, with grade I as benign and grade III as malignant [10]. Unfortunately, this system is not always accurate.

Multinucleate giant cells are not the neoplastic element within these tumors; rather, the background mononuclear fibroblasticlike mesenchymal cells determine the biologic behavior of these lesions. The giant cells may be osteoclastic in origin or analogous to foreign body giant cells derived from histiocytes [10].

Giant-cell tumors generally affect individuals between the ages of 20 and 40 and tend to decline. The peak occurrence is in the third decade of life, affecting females more than males. Most giant-cell tumors are found in the epiphyses of long bones with over one-half of the lesions arising close to the knee in the distal femur and proximal tibia; other sites are the sacrum, vertebrae, humerus, and radius as well as other bones [2].

Giant-cell tumors usually begin their formation within the cancellous bone. As they grow and invade, the cortex may be thinned or even broken, but new reactive bone usually preserves the cortex. The expansion of the tumor in the epiphyses classically forms a clublike deformity. X-rays reveal a somewhat translucent area at the end of the long bones with a thin cortex (Fig. 39-31).

Ewing's sarcoma, although rare, is one of the most lethal bone tumors. Approximately 90 percent of individuals affected are under the age of 30, with the greatest number occurring in the second decade of life. It has a marked predilection for males with a 2 : 1 ratio [10]. The long tubular bones are most commonly affected, with the innominate bones — the pelvis, ischium, ribs, scapula, and sternum — following in order, and then virtually any other bone in the body (Fig. 39-32).

Ewing's sarcoma, like many other invasive tumors, has symptoms of pain, a tender mass, and venous distention. Some patients may have anemia, temperature elevation, and sometimes leukocytosis that supports an inflammatory etiology [2]. Ewing's sarcoma generally has its origin in the medullary canal, growing outward and causing a lytic area on x rays. Some spicules of bone may be seen, but this is reactive bone and not part of the neoplasm. Elevation of the periosteum is typical, followed by periosteal bone formation, which on x rays creates what is known as an onion-skin appearance.

Hematogenic Tumors

Multiple myeloma is the most common neoplasm of the bone. The neoplasm is composed of plasma cells showing variable degrees of differentiation. This condition is further described in Chapter 15, but the skeletal effects are emphasized in this section.

Multiple myeloma affects women and men equally, rarely occurs before age 50, and has its peak incidence at the fifth and sixth decade. It has a predilection for the vertebral column, but ribs, skull, pelvis, and virtually any bone in the system may be affected. Multiple myeloma appears as multifocal destructive bone lesions throughout the skeletal system producing what appear to be rounded punched-out areas on x ray [10]. These areas may be up to 5 cm in size with no surrounding zone of sclerosis. Pathologic fractures of the vertebrae are common.

The affected individual has a history of pain that is often referred to the spinal column. Neurologic symptoms occur because of compression of vertebral bodies or compression of nerve roots due to extension of the neoplasm. Weakness, loss of weight, hemorrhagic disorders, and renal involvement are also associated with multiple myeloma. Hypercalcemia, hyperuricemia, and presence of Bence Jones proteins in the urine are frequently found.

REFERENCES

1. Apley, A. *System of Orthopaedics and Fractures* (5th ed.). London: Butterworth, 1977.
2. Dahlin, D. *Bone Tumors.* Springfield, Ill.: Thomas, 1967.
3. Fudenberg, H. H., et al. *Basic and Clinical Immunology* (3rd ed.). Los Altos, Calif.: Lange, 1980.
4. Ganong, W. *Review of Medical Physiology* (10th ed.). Los Altos, Calif.: Lange, 1981.
5. Guyton, A. *Textbook of Medical Physiology* (6th ed.). Philadelphia: Saunders, 1981.
6. Hollingshead, W. *Textbook of Anatomy* (3rd ed.). Hagerstown, Md.: Harper & Row, 1974. P. 21.
7. Kleerekoper, M., Tolia, K., and Parfitt, A. Nutritional, endocrine and demographic aspects of osteoporosis. *Orthop. Clin. North Am.* 12: 550, 1981.
8. Krane, S. M. Paget's disease of bone. *Clin. Orthop.* 127:24, 1977.
9. Mankin, H. J. The reaction of articular cartilage to injury and osteoarthritis. *N. Engl. J. Med.* 291:1285, 1974.
10. Robbins, S. L., and Cotran, R. *Pathologic Basis of Disease* (2nd ed.). Philadelphia: Saunders, 1979.
11. Ryan, W. Treatment of Paget's disease of bone with methramycin. *Clin. Orthop.* 127:106, 1977.
12. Silverstein, A. *Human Anatomy and Physiology.* New York: Wiley, 1980.
13. Singer, F., and Mills, B. The etiology of Paget's disease of bone. *Clin. Orthop.* 127:37, 1977.
14. Steinberg, M., and Trueta, J. Effects of activity in rat bone growth. *Clin. Orthop.* 156:59, 1981.
15. Vaughan, J. *The Physiology of Bone.* London: Oxford, 1975.

BIBLIOGRAPHY

Albright, J., and Miller, E. (eds.). Osteogenesis imperfecta. *Clin. Orthop.* 159:1, 1981.

Anderson, W., and Scotti, T. *Synopsis of Pathology* (10th ed.). St. Louis: Mosby, 1980.

Apley, A. G. *System of Orthopaedics and Fractures* (5th ed.). London: Butterworth, 1977.

Arnstein, A. R. Recent progress in osteomalacia and rickets. *Ann. Intern. Med.* 67:1296, 1967.

Babock, J. L., and Wray, J. B. Analysis of abduction in shoulder and deltoid paralysis due to axillary nerve injury. *Clin. Orthop.* 68:116, 1970.

Brown, P. W. The time factor in surgery of upper-extremity peripheral nerve injury. *Clin. Orthop.* 68:14, 1970.

Byers, P. D. Solitary benign osteoblastic lesions of bone: Osteoid osteoma and osteoblastoma. *Cancer* 22:43, 1968.

Clark, J. M. *Orthopaedics Science of Fractures.* Washington, D. C.: Butterworth, 1964.

Clawson, D. K., and Frederick, A. M. Compartmental syndromes. *Clin. Orthop.* 113:2, 1975.

Clissold, G. K. *The Body's Response to Trauma: Fractures.* New York: Springer, 1973.

Dahlin, D. C. *Bone Tumors: General Aspects and Data on 3,987 Cases* (2nd ed.). Springfield, Ill.: Thomas, 1967.

Eaton, R. G., and Green, W. T. Volkmann's ischemia volar compartments syndrome of the forearm. *Clin. Orthop.* 113:58, 1975.

Edmonson, A., and Crenshaw, A. N. *Campbell's Operative Orthopaedics* (6th ed.). St. Louis: Mosby, 1980.

Enneking, W. F., and Springfield, D. S. Osteosarcoma. *Orthop. Clin. North Am.* 8:785, 1977.

Fraumeni, J. F., Jr. Stature and malignant tumors of bone in childhood and adolescence. *Cancer* 20:967, 1967.

Frost, H. M. *Orthopaedic Biomechanics.* Springfield, Ill.: Thomas, 1976.

Ganong, W. F. *Review of Medical Physiology* (9th ed.). Los Altos, Calif.: Lange, 1979.

Gartland, J. *Fundamentals of Orthopaedics.* Philadelphia: Saunders, 1974.

Grabbiani, G. Synovial sarcoma. *Cancer* 28:1031, 1971.

Guyton, A. C. *Textbook of Medical Physiology* (6th ed.). Philadelphia: Saunders, 1981.

Harris, W. The natural history of fibrous dysplasia. *J. Bone Joint Surg.* 44:207, 1962.

Harrison, M., and Burwell, R. Perthes' disease: A concept of pathogenesis. *Clin. Orthop.* 156:115, 1981.

Hollingshead, W. H. *Textbook of Anatomy* (3rd ed.). Hagerstown, Md.: Harper & Row, 1974. P. 21.

Ibsen, K. H. Distinct varieties of osteogenic imperfecta. *Clin. Orthop.* 50:279, 1967.

Jaffe, H. The classic Paget's disease of bone. *Clin. Orthop.* 127:4, 1977.

Kleerehoper, M., Talia, K., and Parfitt, A. Nutritional endocrine and demographic aspects of osteoporosis. *Orthop. Clin. North Am.* 3:550, 1981.

Krane, S. M. Paget's disease of bone. *Clin. Orthop.* 127:24, 1977.

Leffert, R. D. Brachial plexus injuries. *Orthop. Clin. North Am.* 2:399, 1970.

Lutwak, I. Current concepts of bone metabolism. *Ann. Intern. Med.* 80:630, 1974.

Macnab, I., and Rorabeck, C. H. The pathophysiology of the anterior tibial compartmental syndrome. *Clin. Orthop.* 113:52, 1975.

Mankin, H. J. The reaction of articular cartilage to injury and osteoarthritis. *N. Engl. J. Med.* 291:1285, 1974.

Mankin, H. J., and Lipiello, L. Biochemical and metabolic abnormalities in articular cartilage from osteo-arthritic human hips. *J. Bone Joint Surg.* 52A:424, 1970.

McDuffie, F. Etiology and pathogenesis of rheumatoid arthritis: Current lines of investigation. *Orthop. Clin. North Am.* 2:601, 1971.

McKenna, R. J. Osteogenic sarcoma arising in Paget's disease. *Cancer* 17:42, 1964.

Milgram, J. W. Radiographical and pathological assessment of the activity of Paget's disease of bone. *Clin. Orthop.* 127:43, 1977.

Narakas, A. Surgical treatment of traction injuries of the brachial plexus. *Clin. Orthop.* 133:71, 1978.

Price, S. A., and Wilson, L. M. *Pathophysiology: Clinical Concepts of Disease Processes* (2nd ed.). New York: McGraw-Hill, 1982.

Robbins, S., and Cotran, R. *Pathologic Basis of Disease* (2nd ed.). Philadelphia: Saunders, 1979.

Russell, W. D. A clinical and pathological staging system for soft tissue sarcomas. *Cancer* 40:1562, 1977.

Ryan, W. Treatment of Paget's disease of bone with methromycin. *Clin. Orthop.* 127:106, 1977.

Silverstein, A. *Human Anatomy and Physiology.* New York: Wiley, 1980.

Singer, F., and Mills, B. The etiology of Paget's disease of bone. *Clin. Orthop.* 127:37, 1977.

Steinberg, M., and Trueta, J. Effects of activity on rat bone growth. *Clin. Orthop.* 156:59, 1981.

Vaughan, J. *The Physiology of Bone.* London: Oxford, 1975.

UNIT 14
PROTECTIVE COVERINGS OF THE BODY

Pam Appleton

NORMAL STRUCTURE AND FUNCTION OF THE SKIN
TRAUMATIC ALTERATIONS IN THE SKIN

Joan Buffalino

ALTERATIONS OF SKIN INTEGRITY
INFECTIONS
SCALING DISORDERS
CANCER

Helen Ptak

BURN INJURY TO THE SKIN

The skin is one of the largest organs of the body but its function is often taken for granted. Chapter 40 discusses the protective and complex metabolic activities of skin. Chapter 41 describes common inflammatory processes, tumors, and traumatic alterations in skin integrity.

The reader is encouraged to consider that the skin functions as a dynamic regulating organ for body temperature and fluid balance and for prevention of microbial invasion. Utilization of the learning objectives as a study guide outline will help in the study of this important organ.

CHAPTER 40
NORMAL STRUCTURE AND FUNCTION OF THE SKIN

LEARNING OBJECTIVES

1. Discuss the embryonic development of the skin.
2. Describe the characteristics of the layers of the epidermis.
3. Describe the life cycle of the epidermal cell.
4. Discuss the chemical properties of the epidermis.
5. Describe the production of melanin.
6. List the layers of the dermis.
7. State the components of the dermis.
8. Discuss the function of the dermis.
9. Describe the structure and function of the subcutaneous tissues.
10. List the epidermal appendages.
11. Describe the process of sweat production and its function in heat regulation.
12. Compare the structure and function of sweat and sebaceous glands.
13. Discuss the growth and development of hair.
14. Describe the blood and nerve supply to the skin.
15. State the role of the skin in vitamin D production.

The skin is one of the largest organs of the body, with a surface area of 1.8 sq m in the average adult. This surface area increases 7 times from birth to maturity. The skin's consistency ranges from the thick, tough, yet pliable covering of the body to the thin, delicate mucous membrane of the mouth, nose, and eyelids. This chapter discusses the formation, structure, and function of the skin.

ANATOMY AND PHYSIOLOGY OF THE SKIN

The skin is composed of three major layers that are, from the surface inward, the epidermis, the dermis, and the subcutaneous tissues (Fig. 40-1). These layers have the following functions: (1) protection against the external environment, (2) maintenance and regeneration of layers, (3) secretion of protective substances, (4) participation in defense against foreign substances, (5) preservation of the internal fluid environment, (6) participation in excretion of wastes, (7) assistance in regulating body temperature, and (8) production of vitamin D.

Epidermis

LAYERS OF THE EPIDERMIS. The main layers of the epidermis, from the dermis to the surface, are the stratum germinativum, stratum spinosum, stratum granulosum, stratum lucidum, and the stratum corneum (Fig. 40-2).

The deepest layer, the stratum germinativum or the *basal layer,* is one cell thick and lies in contact with the dermis. Within the basal layer are basal cells, which are cuboidal or columnar in appearance, have oval nuclei, and are united to each other by desmosomes or bridges. These cells are attached to a basement membrane by tonofibrils or half-desmosomes. The epidermis is also attached to the dermis by interlocking irregularly shaped processes of basal cells with corresponding dermal processes that extend different depths into the dermis. Processes are found in varying numbers throughout the skin. For example, the eyelid has few processes, while the nipple has a complex system of ridges, and the fingertips have parallel ridges to form cavernous valleys and tunnels [4]. The highly individualized patterns of fingerprints are the result of these valleys. In the normal epidermis, mitosis of new basal cells is limited to the basal layer. During regeneration, mitosis continues upward into the squamous layer.

Throughout the basal layer are dispersed melanocytes, which form melanin, and are responsible for pigmentation of the skin. These cells are wedged between the basal cells. When stained, melanocytes have clear cytoplasm and small dark nuclei.

The stratum spinosum layer contains cells with a polygonal shape. Bridges hold the cells together. As these cells move toward the surface they begin to flatten. Within the cells fibril or keratin precursors make a tridimensional framework throughout the cytoplasm.

The stratum granulosum is from two to four cells thick and lies directly above the stratum spinosum. The cells become diamond-shaped and are filled with keratohyalin

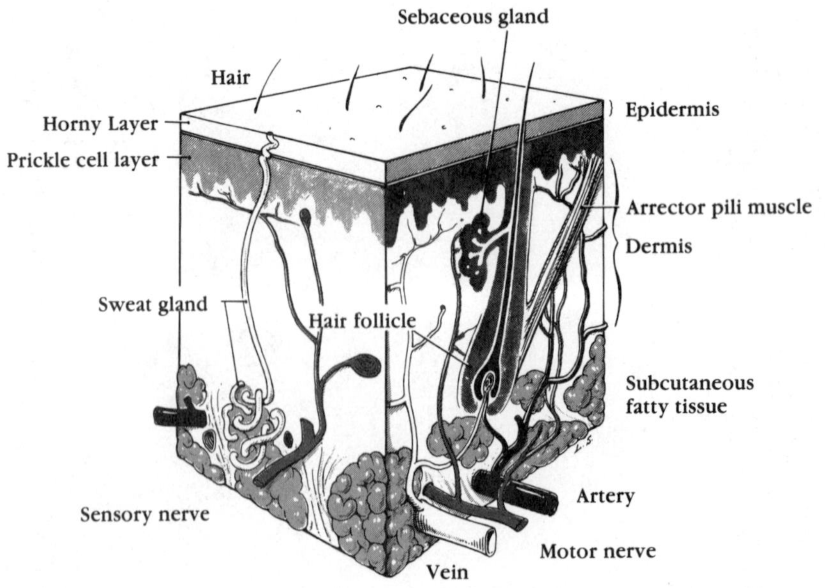

FIGURE 40-1. Structure of the skin. (From J. Sana and R. Judge, *Physical Assessment Skills for Nursing Practice.* Boston: Little, Brown, 1982.)

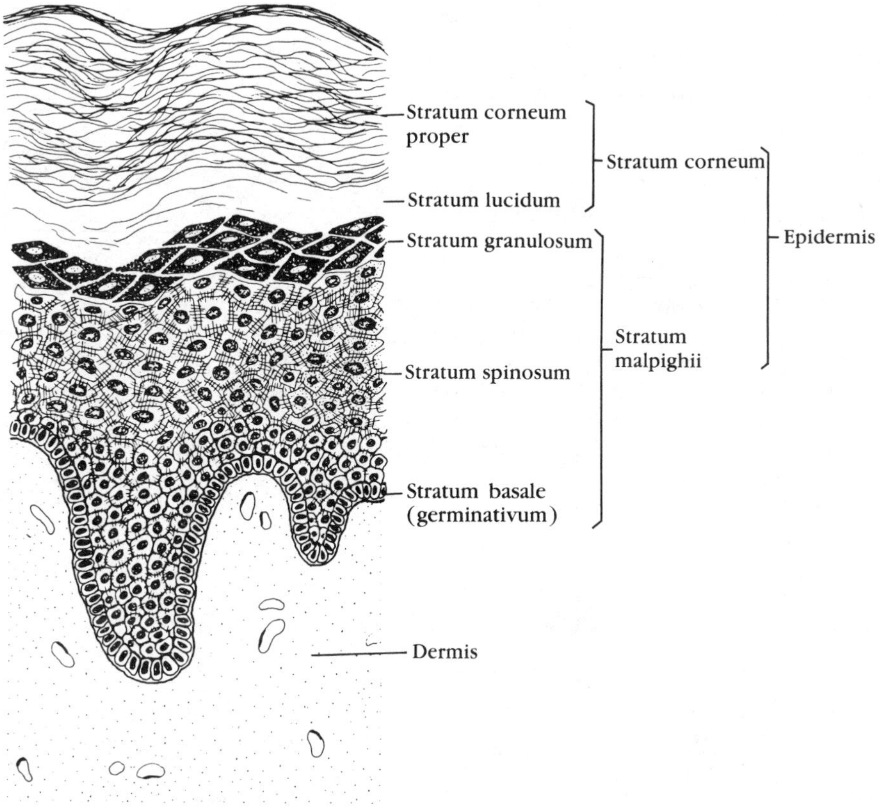

FIGURE 40-2. The epidermis of "thick skin" in vertical histologic section, with its various layers. (From M. Borysenko, et al., *Functional Histology* [2nd ed.]. Boston: Little, Brown, 1984.)

granules (hematoxylin granules). During keratinization, keratohyalin granules form the interfibrillary substance that cements keratin fibers together.

The stratum lucidum is not present in all skin sections but is seen with thick epidermis, such as in the palms of the hands and soles of the feet. This layer provides a friction surface.

The horny layer, stratum corneum, varies in thickness from 0.02 mm on the forearm to 0.5 mm or more on the soles of the feet (see Fig. 40-2). The cells of this layer are flat, have no nuclei, and constitute the keratin layer. Keratin is a tough fibrous protein that resists chemical change. The function of the stratum corneum is to shield the body from environmental damage and maintain the internal milieu. The low permeability exhibited by these cells retards water loss and prevents entrance to most toxic agents. The horny cells are continuously being shed, making way for new cells.

LIFE CYCLE OF EPIDERMAL CELLS. The life cycle of an epidermal cell involves three phases: mitosis, keratinization, and exfoliation. Epidermal cells are continuously formed in the basal or germinative layer at a rate commensurate with the constant loss. New cells move from the basal layer to the stratum corneum in a random fashion, which is influenced by the rate of keratinization and by the time that each cell left the basal layer. Transit time from basal layer to surface is anywhere from 12 to 25 days. An increase in mitotic rate occurs within 24 to 36 hours after an injury.

Mitosis is affected by two major factors: the diurnal cycle and the hormones. Mitosis seems to occur at a greater rate during periods when the body is at rest or asleep. Hormonal influences include androgens, which function in the formation of hair follicles and sebaceous glands, and estrogen, which aids in the formation of the vaginal epithelium. Mitosis may be inhibited by adrenalin, which is increased during a time of wakefulness, so that mitosis seems to be greatest during rest or sleep.

The second phase in the epidermal cell life cycle is keratinization. As the epidermal cell from the basal layer moves toward the surface, it loses its ability to experience mitosis. Instead, it begins to synthesize fibrillar and amorphous proteins, keratin, and membrane-coating granules. The cell finally loses its nucleus and cellular organelles, becomes part of the stratum corneum, and is shed. The fibrillar proteins make up the fibrils in the epidermal cell and give the stratum corneum strength and chemical inertness. As the cell moves toward the surface, more and more fibrils form, until they make up 50 percent of the protein in stratum corneum cells. Amorphous proteins that make up the other 50 percent in stratum corneum cells are imbedded in a matrix and are without definite structure. Membrane-coating granules are formed and align near the apical part of the cell membrane. They fuse with the membrane, break it, and discharge their contents into the intercellular spaces in the granular layer of the stratum Malphighii. The function of membrane-coating granules is not clear, but they may serve to bind cells together.

As the epidermal cell moves closer to the surface, keratohyalin granules form. These granules are seen in cells immediately below the horny layer. When cells reach the horny layer, a thickening of the cell membrane occurs. The nucleus and organelles disintegrate and are eliminated from the cell.

At the end of keratinization, cornified cells are cemented together in varying thickness. Cells at the surface are shed, resulting in exfoliation, which is the last phase in the life of an epidermal cell (Fig. 40-3).

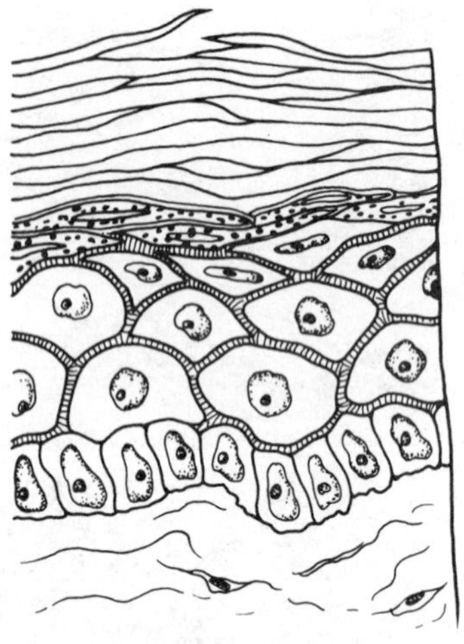

FIGURE 40-3. Life cycle of the epidermal cell.

CHEMICAL PROPERTIES OF THE EPIDERMIS. The epidermis contains carbohydrates and various enzymes that influence skin cell activity. In normal skin, small amounts of glycogen are present, scattered in various areas of the body, such as in the scrotum and scalp and in cells surrounding pilosebaceous and sweat gland openings. After the skin has been traumatized, there is an increase in the amount of glycogen found in the epidermis.

The epidermis also contains glucose, which diffuses easily into the cells, the amount depending on the serum glucose levels. Eighty to ninety percent of the energy in epidermal cells is derived from adenosine triphosphate (ATP) generated through respiration and glycolysis. Intense glycolytic activity in the presence of oxygen is a specific feature of the epidermis, which is especially important during wound healing and skin regeneration.

Enzymes found in the epidermis that influence all activity include alkaline phosphatase, acid phosphatase, and esterases. Alkaline phosphatase is not found in normal epidermal cells but is present in a damaged epidermis and disappears after healing. Acid phosphatase is found in the normal epidermis. Esterases seem to help facilitate cell migration [4].

SKIN PIGMENTATION. The color of the skin is the responsibility of melanocytes originating in the germinative layer of the epidermis and in the hair follicle. The main function of melanocytes is the synthesis of pigment granules, or melanosomes. The main component of melanosomes is melanin, which ranges in color from light yellow to black.

The melanocyte is classified as a connective tissue cell [2]. It appears in the basal layer of the epidermis as a *clear cell* before it begins to produce melanin. Functioning melanocytes contain organelles of pigment granules, the melanosomes.

The melanocyte produces and disperses melanin to keratinocytes (keratinizing basal cells) and hair cells. Melanin is a biochrome of high molecular weight and is produced by oxidation of the amino acid tyrosine with tyrosinase. It forms with a protein matrix in the melanosome to make a melanoprotein. As more melanoprotein is formed, the melanosome grows to become a melanin granule and eventually loses the activity of the enzyme tyrosinase.

Formed melanin is transferred to keratinocytes by active phagocytosis of the distal end of the dendritic processes of the melanocyte. The amount of melanin in these melanocyte dendrites determines the skin color. In light-skinned individuals, melanin is found primarily in the basal layer of the epidermis. In dark or black-skinned individuals, melanin is found throughout the epidermis, including the outermost horny layer. Melanogenesis increases after exposure to ultraviolet light or x rays. After exposure, the melanocytes in the basal layer increase activity, become larger, develop longer dendrites, and produce more melanin. Melanocytes may increase in number after exposure to ultraviolet light [2]. The melanin acts as a protective screen to protect the deep layers of the epidermis and the dermis from too much solar ultraviolet radiation [4].

The control of skin pigmentation is genetic and hormonal. Genes control the number and shape of melanocytes in the epidermis and the hair follicle. Hormonal influences have been demonstrated through the study of hyperpigmentation as noted in cases of hyperpituitarism and Addison's disease. Estrogen, progesterone, and melanocyte-stimulating hormone (MSH) play a part in increased pigmentation in various areas of the body during pregnancy. The exact hormonal mechanism for increasing pigmentation is not known.

Dermis

The dermis, or *corium*, lies between the epidermis and subcutaneous tissues (see Fig. 40-1). It consists of a matrix of loose connective tissue, a fibrous protein embedded in an amorphous ground substance. The dermis is traversed by blood vessels, nerves, and lymphatics and is penetrated by epidermal appendages. The mass of the dermis accounts for 15 to 20 percent of total body weight [4].

LAYERS OF THE DERMIS. There are two main layers in the dermis: (1) the finely textured papillary dermis and (2) the deeper, thicker, coarsely textured reticular layer. The papillary layer lies directly beneath the epidermis. It is composed of thin fibers of collagen, reticular fibers, branching elastic fibers, fibroblasts, abundant ground substance, and capillaries. When the epidermis is removed, the upper surface of the papillary layer forms a negative image of the underside of the epidermis. The reticular layer lies beneath the papillary layer and extends to the subcutaneous tissue. This layer is mainly composed of thick collagen bundles enmeshed in a network of coarse elastic fibers. The reticular layer is responsible for the strength and toughness of the skin. There are fewer reticular fibers, blood vessels, fibroblasts, and ground substance in this layer than in the papillary layer [5]. Sensory nerve endings, hair follicles, sweat and sebaceous glands, and some smooth muscle are found in the reticular layer. The combined layers of the dermis vary in thickness, being thinnest over the eyelid and thickest over the back [5].

COMPONENTS OF THE DERMIS. The two layers of the dermis are composed of varying amounts of collagen, elastic and reticular fibers, and ground substance. Collagen fibers are of tropocollagen, a triple helix of polypeptide chains, which makes up most of the dermis. The molecules form fibers that unite into bundles. These bundles are slightly extensible and wavy, allowing for a certain amount of stretching of the skin. The collagen content is thickest in the lower portion of the dermis.

Elastic fibers are composed of microfibrils and elastin. The elastic fibers are abundant in human skin, being entwined with collagen in the reticular layer of the dermis and extending into the papillary dermis. These fibers help anchor the epidermis to the dermis and anchor blood vessels, along with arrectores pilorum muscles. These fibers can be deformed by a small force and recover their original dimensions.

Reticular fibers are young, finely formed fibers of collagen. They are found within and under the epidermal basement membrane and also help to anchor the epidermis to the dermis.

Ground substance is present in small amounts in normal skin. It is the structureless portion of connective tissue lying outside of cells, fibers, vessels, and nerves that holds all these items together. Ground substance is composed of water, electrolytes, glucose, plasma proteins, neutral and acid mucopolysaccharides, and mucoproteins.

CELLULAR COMPONENTS OF THE DERMIS. The three major cells that are found in the dermis are (1) fibroblasts, (2) macrophages, and (3) mast cells. *Fibroblasts* are the most abundant of these cells; they secrete procollagen, proelastin, microfibrillar proteins, elastin, and components of ground substance [4]. *Macrophages* probably develop from the blood monocyte and can be fixed or ameboid cells that help rid the dermis of foreign substances and cell residue. Macrophages participate in the immune response and are vital to wound healing, inflammation, tissue resorption, and recycling of tissue components (see Chap. 8). The *mast cells* are found in perivascular connective tissue and their microscopic appearance shows the cytoplasm to be filled with large metachromatic granules. Under certain physical and chemical conditions, these cells degranulate. Such conditions include exposure to cold, heat, x rays, ultraviolet light, toxins, certain peptides, and protamine sulfate. When degranulation occurs, the substances of heparin and histamine are released. Heparin prevents blood clotting and, in small amounts, accelerates lipid transportation. Histamine increases capillary permeability, contracts smooth muscle, increases chemotaxis, produces an itching sensation, and increases gastric hypersecretion [4].

FUNCTIONS OF THE DERMIS. The dermis provides the main protection of the body from external injury. Its flexibility allows joint movement and localized stretching, but resists tearing, shearing, and local pressure. When skin is at rest, the protective collagen network is slack. When exposed to tension, the skin "gives" until the slack is taken up. Skin kept taut for long periods of time becomes fatigued, and stretching results. This is exhibited by the stretch marks of striae gravidarum (a pinkish-white or gray line seen where skin has been stretched by pregnancy, obesity, tumor, etc.), which is irreversible. The skin also becomes thinner when compressed under force and will well up around the source of compression. Pressure damage may occur from a duration of pressure and distribution of force. More damage is done as a result of long pressure, but severe point pressure can damage underlying and cutaneous tissues.

The dermis also provides the necessary substratum on which the epidermis receives nutrients and grows. It serves as a barrier to infection by way of hyaluronic acid in the ground substance, which acts as a barrier to bacterial penetration [4]. The hyaluronic acid also binds water and helps maintain dermal turgor. The skin may also function as a water and electrolyte storage organ. Dermal concentrations of cations are slightly above the concentration in the blood, so that cations "stored" in the dermis may be tapped to maintain normal blood cation levels.

Subcutaneous Tissues

The third major layer of skin is the subcutaneous tissue. This tissue appears loose-textured, white, and fibrous. Fat and slender elastic fibers are intermingled. Subcutaneous papillae jut into the dermis. These are larger and more dispersed than dermal papillae. It is through these that blood vessels and nerves enter the upper layers of skin.

The subcutaneous tissue layer contains blood and lymph vessels, roots of hair follicles, secretory portions of sweat glands, cutaneous and sensory nerve endings, and fat. Sub-

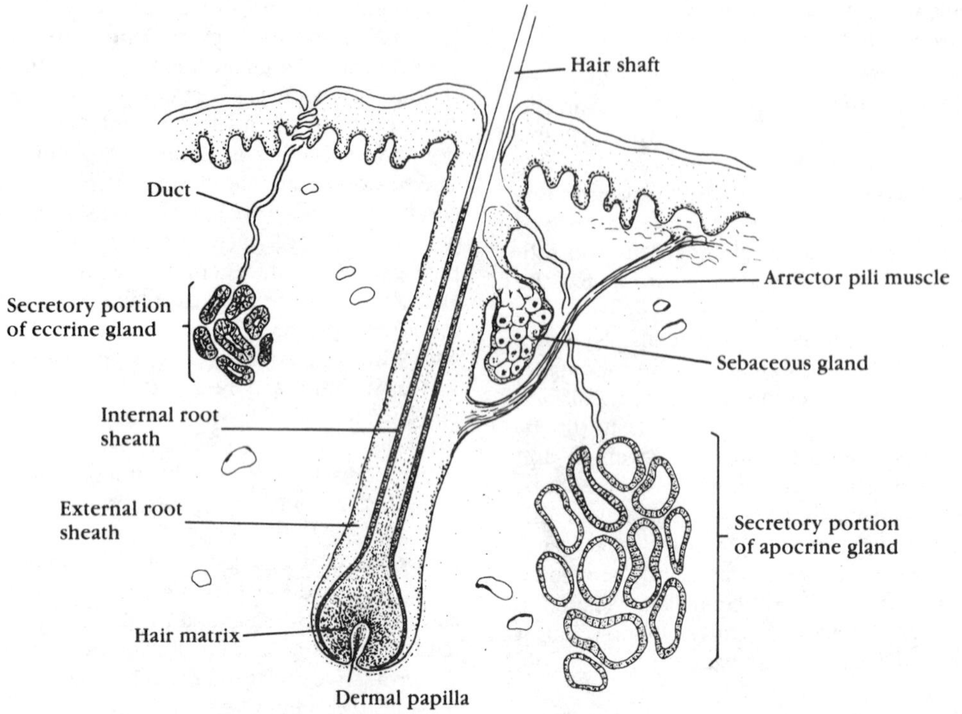

FIGURE 40-4. Some cutaneous appendages. (From M. Borysenko, et al., *Functional Histology* [2nd ed.]. Boston: Little, Brown, 1984.)

cutaneous fat varies in amount throughout the body and is absent in the eyelids, penis, scrotum, nipple, and areola. The unequal fat distribution between males and females is partially a result of hormonal influence. Strands or sheets of white, fibrous connective tissues support the fat tissue.

The subcutaneous tissue contains voluntary and involuntary muscles. Voluntary muscle is found on the scalp, face, and neck. Involuntary smooth muscle is found in the dartos muscle of the scrotum and in the muscle tissue of the areola and nipple [6]. Subcutaneous tissue serves the purposes of heat insulator, shock absorber, and caloric-reserve depot.

Epidermal Appendages

The sweat glands, sebaceous glands, hair, and nails compose the epidermal appendages. These extend through varying layers of the skin (Fig. 40-4).

SWEAT GLANDS. There are two types of sweat glands: eccrine and apocrine. The *eccrine* sweat glands are found all over the body and are more numerous in the thick skin. They open to the surface epidermis and descend through the dermis to just above the subcutaneous layer of the skin. These glands are especially prominent on the soles of the feet, palms of the hand, and axilla.

The eccrine gland is a simple coiled tubular gland that may be divided into four segments. The lowermost or secretory portion has two layers of cells. Of these, myoepithelial cells make up the outer layer and contract to facilitate sweat release. The inner layer, composed of clear large cells and dark small cells, contains glycogen and polysaccharides, respectively. The secretory layer is one cell layer thick. In ascending order, the remaining portion of the eccrine unit includes the coiled dermal duct and a straight dermal duct, which opens on the surface of the epidermis through the spiraled intraepidermal duct (see Fig. 40-4). The coiled and straight dermal ducts are two cell layers thick and are composed of cuboidal basophilic epithelium. The duct narrows as it ascends to the surface and widens again as it becomes the intraepidermal spiral duct. The cells lining the spiraling duct are keratinized but have no melanin.

The purpose of the eccrine gland is to produce sweat to aid in temperature regulation of the body. Sweat is formed in the secretory coil of the eccrine unit. The solution here is isotonic or slightly hypertonic and contains lactate with small amounts of bicarbonate. In the dermal duct, sodium, chloride, and water are resorbed. As sweat exits onto the epidermis it is hypotonic. As the sweat rate increases, sodium and chloride concentrations in the sweat also increase, whereas potassium, lactate, and urea decrease. Not all eccrine glands function all of the time, but they respond promptly to heat stress. The amount of sweat produced depends on the amount of heat to which the person is exposed. Two to three liters of sweat per hour may be produced in an adult exposed to extreme heat conditions. Eccrine sweat is a colorless and odorless hypotonic solution that is 99 percent water, with 1 percent solutes such as sodium chloride, potassium, urea, protein, lipids, amino acids, calcium, phosphorus, and iron. The specific gravity is 1.005, and the pH ranges from 4.5 to 7.0.

The skin plays a passive and an active role in control of body temperature. Passively, skin serves as a barrier to the external environment. Actively, the eccrine units, along with the cutaneous blood vessel network, participates in regulatory heat exchange. The sweat glands cool the surface of the skin with the liquid sweat that evaporates, causing further cooling. The cutaneous vessels dilate or constrict to dissipate or conserve body heat. The control of this process is in the hypothalamus, the neural thermostat.

The hypothalamus is stimulated by changes in surface and blood temperatures. An increase in body temperature of 0.5°C causes the hypothalamus to send a message by way of cholinergic fibers of the sympathetic nervous system to the sweat glands, which pour sweat onto the body surface, causing cooling when it evaporates.

Heat is the primary stimulus to eccrine sweat production, but other physiologic stimuli can stimulate sweating. Gustatory sweating occurs on the face and scalp after eating spicy foods. Emotional stress causes sweating on palms, soles, axilla, and forehead that may extend to the whole body.

The apocrine sweat glands are found in the axilla, around the nipples, the anogenital region, the external ear canal (ceruminous glands), in the eyelids (Moll's gland), and in the breast (mammary glands). These glands make a secretion with an unknown function in humans. In animals, the secretion serves to attract an animal of the opposite sex. The glands remain small in size until puberty, when they begin secreting.

Apocrine gland ducts empty into the pilosebaceous follicle above the entrance of the sebaceous gland duct (see Fig. 40-4). This gland begins as a tubular structure, but it ends in a straight duct. The coiled secretory gland is located in the lower dermis or subcutaneous tissues. The straight duct empties into the hair follicle. The apocrine coil has a larger diameter than the eccrine coil. The inner secretory layer of the coil is one cell layer thick. Surrounding the secretory cells are myoepithelial cells, basement membrane, and elastic and reticular fibers. The straight ductal portion of the gland has two cell layers with no myoepithelium and merges with the epithelium of the hair follicle.

Apocrine sweat has a milky color and contains protein and carbohydrates. In the duct, the sweat is sterile and odorless. Only after reaching the surface, where it contacts bacteria, does the sweat take an odor. Two steps are involved in the production of sweat from the apocrine glands, secretion and excretion. Sweat is secreted continuously and fills the duct before being excreted. When the duct is full, peristaltic waves produced by the myoepithelium propel the secretion outward. Excretion may be stimulated by emotional stress and pharmacologic agents, such as epinephrine.

SEBACEOUS GLANDS. Sebaceous glands arise as an epithelial bud from the outer root sheath of the hair follicle. The glands are found throughout the body, except in the palms of the hands and soles and dorsa of the feet. Since these glands develop as buds from the root sheath, they are almost always associated with hair follicles, but are also found in some hairless skin, such as that of the nipples, prepuce, labia, and glans penis. The size of the gland is inversely proportional with the diameter of the hair in the follicle. They are largest where hair is small or absent, such as on the forehead and nose, chest, and back.

Several lobules compose the gland. The lobules are surrounded by a thin, vascular fibrous tissue capsule in the dermis. The cells next to the capsule provide the germinative layer and correspond to the germinative cells of the basal layer of epidermis (see Fig. 40-4). The germ cells change, taking up and filling with lipid, become bloated, disintegrate, and their content of lipid and cell debris is discharged into the sebaceous duct as sebum. Other components of sebum include phospholipid, esterified cholesterol, triglycerides, and waxes. The sebum is then evacuated to the follicle and to the surface. Sebum is what produces oily skin; it lubricates the hair and skin and prevents drying. Sebaceous glands are holocrine glands, because they have no lumen and form secretions from decomposition of cells.

HAIR. Human beings are covered with hair in all areas except the palms, soles, dorsum of digits, lips, glans penis, labia, and the nipple. There are different types of hair. Primary hair or lanugo is found on the human fetus and infant. These same fine hairs may be found on the adult as vellus hairs. An example is the bald man who has fine vellus hair present. In the adult, coarse pigmented hair is best developed on the scalp, beard, chest in men, pubic, and axillary areas.

Hair varies morphologically and biologically on different parts of the body. It also varies in structure, length, rate of growth, and response to stimuli. For instance, sex hormones govern hair growth in the pubic and axillary regions as part of the secondary sex characteristics. Sex hormones do not govern other hair growth. Morphologically, hair is divided into four types: straight, wavy, helical, and spiral, depending on the angle of the hair follicle.

The hair originates in the hair follicle and may be considered one structure, with the follicle developing from the fetal epidermis. The hair and follicle can be divided into three sections: infundibulum, isthmus, and inferior portion. The infundibulum is the uppermost portion of the hair follicle and extends from the orifice down to the opening of the sebaceous gland. The isthmus, or middle portion, lies between the sebaceous duct and the erector muscle. The inferior portion is the section from the muscle to the base

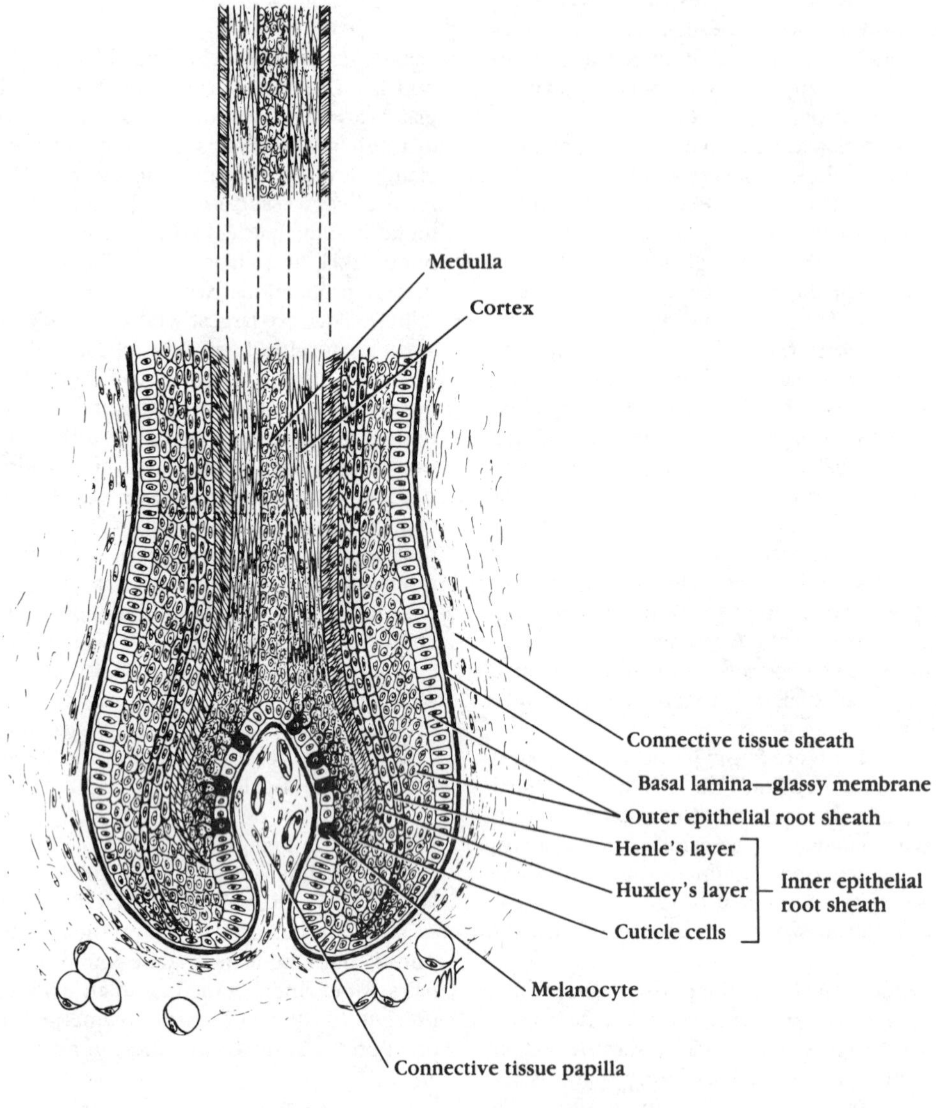

FIGURE 40-5. Detailed structure of a hair shaft and a hair follicle in longitudinal and cross sections. (From R. Snell, *Clinical Histology for Medical Students*. Boston: Little, Brown, 1984.)

of the follicle. The hair bulb lies at the lower end of the follicle and encloses an ovoid-shaped, vascular papilla of connective tissue. The matrix cells of the bulb surround the papilla as it juts upward into the bulb (Fig. 40-5). At an outlet at the distal end of the bulb, the papilla emerges and is continuous with the connective tissue sheath that surrounds the follicle. The hair bulb is covered with concentric layers of tissue. A thin outer root sheath encloses the hair bulb. A basement membrane of reticular fibers and neutral mucopolysaccharides lies against the outer root sheath. A fibrous sheath lies next to the basement membrane and is composed of collagen and fibroblasts. Melanocytes are present in the bulb and in the outer root sheath. The color of hair depends on the amount and distribution of melanin within it. The hair matrix cells differentiate into six layers. The single-cell outer layer cornifies first and lies next to the outer root sheath. Other layers from the outside include a two-cell thick layer of Huxley, cuticle of the inner root sheath, cuticle of the hair, hair cortex, and hair medulla [5].

The matrix cell's mitotic activity is very great, with the hair matrix being replaced every 12 to 24 hours. The hair and inner root sheath interface, so that they grow at the same rate. When the hair and inner sheath reach the level of the isthmus, the inner sheath disintegrates, and the outer sheath begins to cornify. As the hair reaches the surface

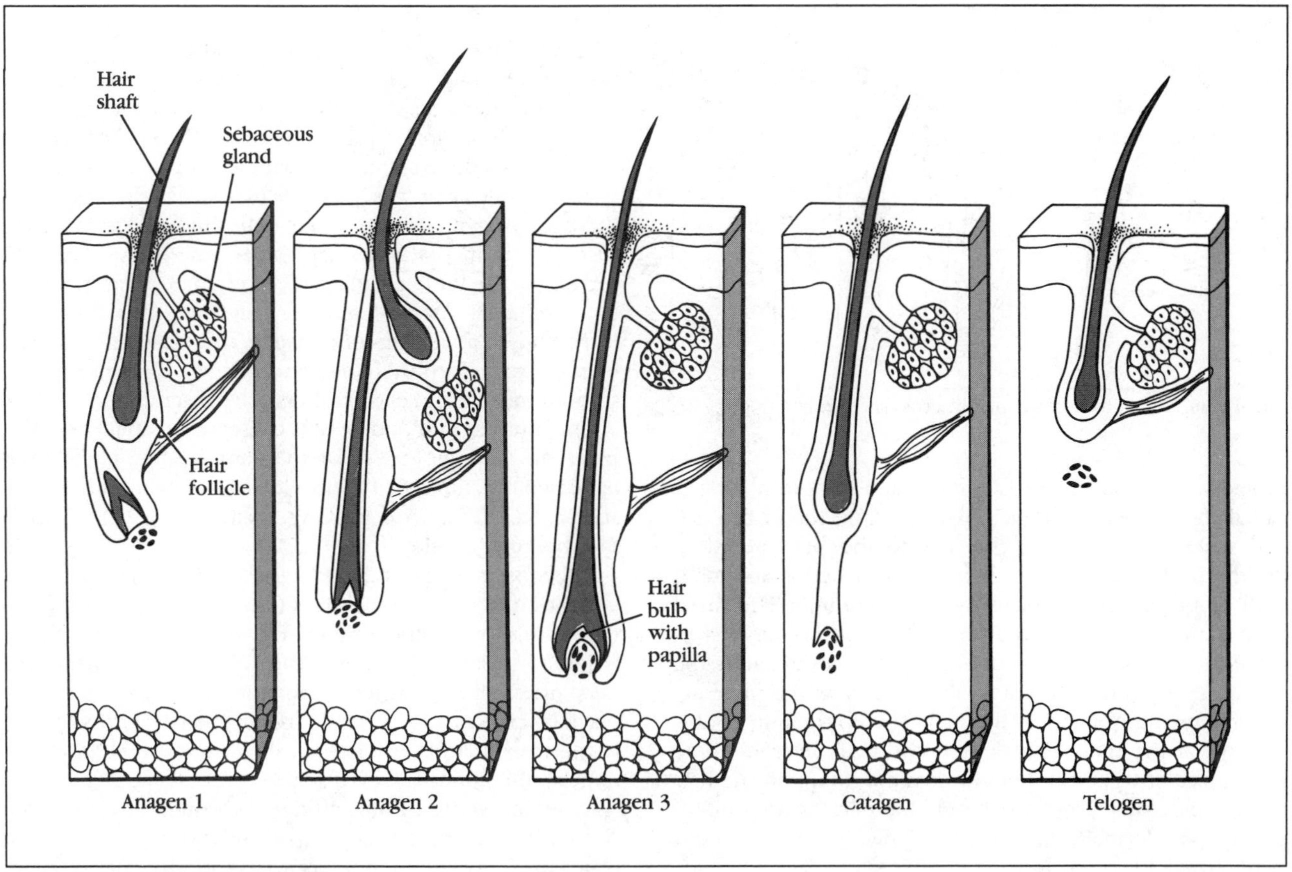

FIGURE 40-6. Growth cycle of hair.

opening of the follicle, it is called a hair shaft and is a dead cornified structure extending out from the follicle. The hair shaft now has three components left over from the original six of the matrix: the outer cuticle, the cortex, and the inner medulla. The medulla is sometimes absent in human hair. The cortex is composed of tightly packed keratinocytes lying parallel along the length of hair. The cuticle surrounds the hair in overlapping squames.

The growth of hair occurs in cycles: *anagen* (growing), *catagen* (involuting), and *telogen* (resting). Anagen begins when a papilla joins with cells that enclose it. The papilla juts into the hair bulb and new matrix cells in the bulb begin to form a hair and push toward the surface. As it pushes to the surface, the old hair in the follicle is loosened, pushed out, and is lost. At the end of anagen, the hair follicle contains the infundibulum, the isthmus, and the inferior portion. In catagen, the inferior disappears, the outer root sheath cornifies around the bulbous end of the hair shaft, melanin synthesis ceases, and the bulb turns white. A cord of epithelial cells replaces the inferior portion and connects the papilla to the bulb. In telogen, the epithelial cord shrinks away from the papilla and disconnects; the epithelial cells of the cord are undifferentiated and wait to join a new papilla and begin anagen (Fig. 40-6) [5]. Each hair follicle operates independently; therefore each hair may be in a different phase of the cycle from its neighbor. The life cycle of hair through the three stages varies in different parts of the body. Scalp hair—which is in anagen from 3 to 10 years, in catagen 3 weeks, and in telogen 3 months—has the longest growth period of any hair on the body. The longer the growing period, the longer the hair. Scalp hair grows 0.35 mm daily [5]. Factors such as nutrition, light, hormones, and temperature influence hair growth. The phases of the hair cycle may be influenced by illness, which may place growing-phase hairs into resting-phase hairs that can be more easily lost or shed.

Hair is needed to screen the nasal passages, protect the scalp and eyes from sun and sweat, and provide a means of sexual attraction [5].

Attached to the hair follicle is the arrector pilorum muscle, a smooth muscle attached to connective tissue hair sheath and inserted in the dermal papilla. Contraction of this muscle erects hair, squeezes out sebum, and creates goose flesh during the spasm.

NAILS. The nail is composed of specialized layers of epithelial cells and serves as a protective covering at the end of fingers and toes (Fig. 40-7). The rectangular nail plates on the dorsal surfaces of the ends of fingers and toes are composed of closely welded cells of cornified epithelium, are semitransparent, and allow the pink of the vascular nail bed

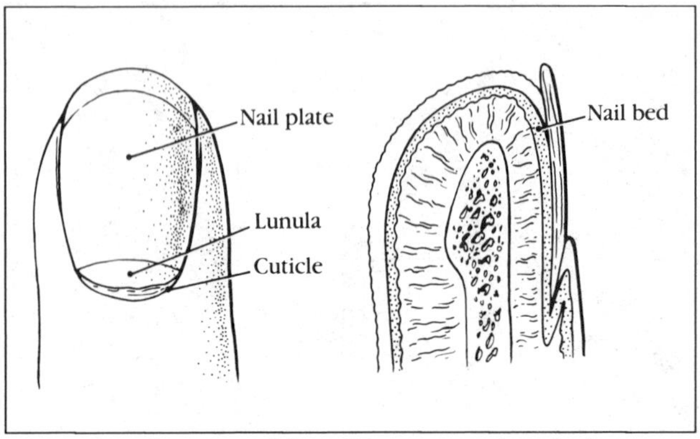

FIGURE 40-7. Structure of the nail in cross section of a finger.

to show. Each nail plate is surrounded by a fold of skin called the nail wall. The nail plate rests on top of the nail bed where fibers attach the nail to the periosteum of the distal phalanx of each digit. The nail bed is abundant with blood vessels and sensory nerve endings. The distal edge of the nail is freely movable. The proximal edge is attached firmly at the nail root. At the base of the nail is the lunula. This white half-moon–shaped area is the most actively growing portion of the nail. The epithelium in this portion of the nail is thick, and the cells here become keratinized with harder keratin than that found in the hair or the epidermis. From the lunula the nail grows longitudinally over dermal ridges of the nail bed at a rate of about 1 mm/week [3].

Blood Supply

Blood supply to the skin varies in different parts of the body, depending on factors such as the type of skin perfused, the thickness of the skin's layers, and the types and number of skin appendages. Common to skin throughout the body is a deep subdermal arterial plexus and a superficial subpapillary plexus. The vascular structures arise from the mesenchyme. Endothelial cells line all parts of the vasculature. In the small capillaries, one endothelial cell surrounds the lumen. Collagen or reticular fibers ensheath the capillaries. Arterioles have an intima, smooth muscle layer, and an adventitia of collagen and elastic fibers. Venules consist of epithelium and collagen. In larger veins, smooth muscle and elastic fibers are present.

The number of blood vessels is greater than necessary to meet the biologic needs of the skin tissues. The vessels have two functions: (1) to provide oxygen and nutrients to skin cells, along with moving wastes, and (2) to aid in thermal regulation.

The vessels are arranged in a three-dimensional network consisting of the two plexuses (deep and superficial) and the vessels that connect them (Fig. 40-8). The deep plexus is joined to larger vessels in the subcutaneous layer. The deep plexus lies in the lower portion of the dermis. The superficial plexus lies beneath the papillary dermis. A network of capillaries reaches up into the dermal papilla to nourish the upper layers of skin.

A second route of blood flow is through arteriovenous shunts located in the upper part of the reticular dermis (Fig. 40-9). These shunts, known as *glomi*, play a major

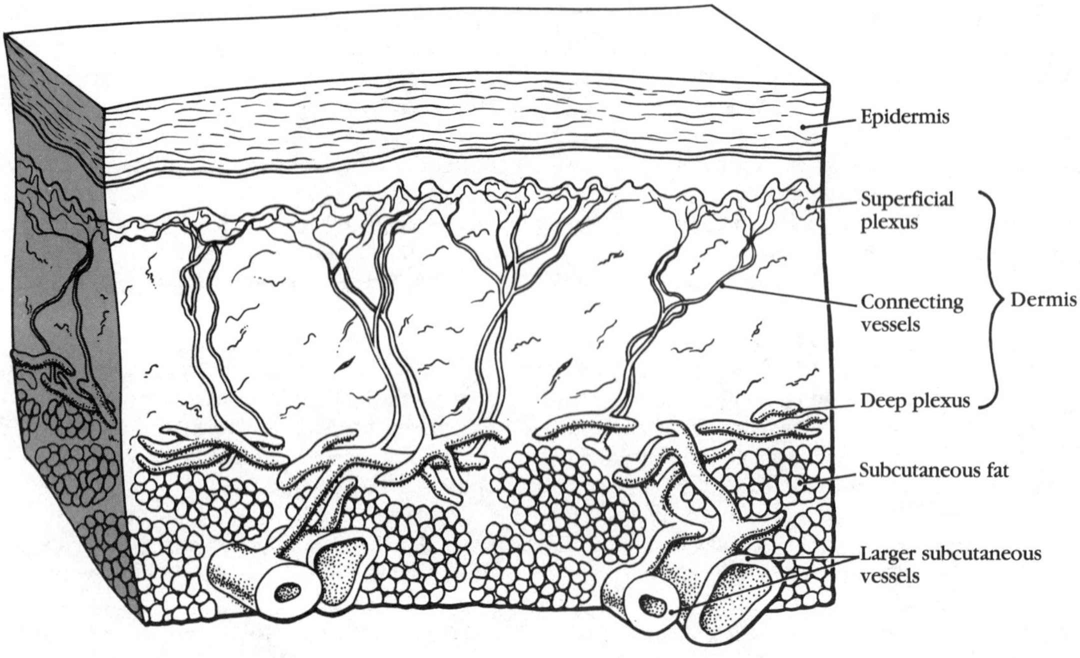

FIGURE 40-8. Blood vessels of the subcutaneous tissue.

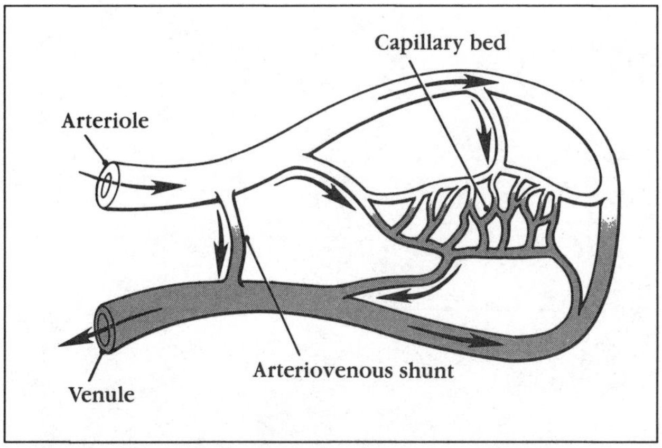

FIGURE 40-9. Blood flow through arteriovenous shunts.

role in heat regulation. They are present throughout the skin but are particularly prevalent in the pads and nail beds of fingers and toes, soles and palms, ears, and center of the face. The shunts enable blood to bypass the capillaries and increase blood flow. The plexuses and arteriovenous shunts are controlled by the sympathetic nervous system and respond to various chemical agents, such as epinephrine and histamine.

Nervous Control

The skin is a major sensory organ. Dermal nerve endings receive stimuli from touch, pressure, temperature, pain, and itch. The nerve endings are most numerous on palms, soles, fingers, and mucocutaneous areas of lips, glans penis, and clitoris.

The sensations of temperature, pain, and itch are perceived by unmyelinated nerves ending in the dermal papilla and surrounding hair follicles. Meissner's corpuscles receive touch stimuli and lie in the papillary derma on the palms and soles. They consist of myelinated and unmyelinated nerve fibers. Pacini's corpuscles are responsible for sensing pressure and are found on the soles, palms, nipples, and genital and perianal regions. These encapsulated end organs of myelinated and unmyelinated fibers swiftly send messages to the central nervous system. Mucocutaneous end organs are found in regions such as lips, genitalia, tongue, gums, eyelid, and perianal areas. These organs probably perceive general sensory stimuli and are found in the subpapillary dermis. Myelinated nerves enter the end organ, lose their myelin, and form numerous networks.

The mucocutaneous end organs, Meissner's and Pacini's corpuscles, are specialized sensory nerve end organs in areas of modified hairless skin. The remainder of skin over the body is supplied with sensory and autonomic nerve fibers located in the dermis. Sensory nerves are myelinated up to their terminal branches, are large in diameter, and extend toward the epidermis or hair follicle. These nerves arise from the spinal cord, return via the dorsal root ganglia, and receive sensations of temperature, pain, and itch on the unmyelinated nerve ends. Autonomic nerves to the skin are motor, and they do not always have a myelin sheath. Branches of nerves from the sympathetic nervous system innervate blood vessels, arrector pilorum muscles, and eccrine and apocrine glands. Autonomic adrenergic stimulation of arteriolar muscle produces vasoconstriction.

Vitamin D Synthesis in the Skin

Vitamin D is an essential fat-soluble vitamin in the body that, when activated, aids in the absorption of calcium and phosphate in the intestine. The activated form of vitamin D (1,25-dihydroxycholecalciferol) is commonly referred to as vitamin D hormone. Vitamin D hormone also mobilizes calcium from the bone compartment to support plasma calcium concentration. Current evidence suggests that vitamin D hormone improves renal absorption of calcium but not of phosphate. It therefore improves mineralization of bone by increasing plasma calcium and phosphate concentrations to support forming bone [1].

Vitamin D hormone is not a single compound but is a family of compounds, the two most important of which are vitamin D_2 and D_3. Vitamin D_3, or cholecalciferol, is produced in the skin when it is exposed to ultraviolet irradiation. The skin cells contain 7-dehydrocholesterol in the epidermis. Ultraviolet light penetrates the epidermis and causes 7-dehydrocholesterol to undergo photolysis to form previtamin D, which over a period of a few hours isomerizes to form vitamin D_3. Vitamin D_3 is then transported in the blood bound to serum protein. It is converted in two steps to vitamin D hormone and may then be stored in the liver and in body fat [1]. Vitamin D_2, ergocalciferol, is the therapeutic form of vitamin D and is transported to the liver and kidney where it is converted to vitamin D hormone.

REFERENCES

1. DeLuca, H. F. *Vitamin D: Metabolism and Function.* New York: Springer-Verlag, 1979.
2. Lever, W. F. *Histopathology of the Skin.* Philadelphia: Lippincott, 1967.
3. Luckmann, J., and Sorensen, K. C. *Medical-Surgical Nursing: A Psycho-Physiologic Approach.* Philadelphia: Saunders, 1980.
4. Montagna, W., and Parakhal, P. F. *The Structure and Function of Skin.* New York: Academic, 1974.
5. Moschella, S. L., Pillsbury, D. M., and Hurley, H. J. *Dermatology* (vol. 1). Philadelphia: Saunders, 1975.
6. Woodburne, R. T. *Essentials of Human Anatomy.* New York: Oxford University Press, 1978.

CHAPTER 41
ALTERATIONS IN SKIN INTEGRITY

LEARNING OBJECTIVES

1. List the questions used to obtain an adequate history of the skin.
2. Describe the pathophysiology of the inflammatory response.
3. State the two types of skin sensitivity responses.
4. Explain the pathophysiologic process that results in acne.
5. List and describe the three types of dermatitis/eczema disease.
6. List examples of the complications of atopic dermatitis.
7. State the cause and precipitating factors of herpes simplex.
8. Describe the presentation and course of the varicella virus.
9. Discuss the mechanism of activation of herpes zoster, its target population, and persons at greater risk.
10. Discuss the cause and treatment of warts (verrucae).
11. Describe the presentation of rubeola.
12. State the instance in which rubella has serious complications.
13. Review the common characteristics of impetigo.
14. List the common organism causing folliculitis.
15. Explain the use of systemic antibiotics in treatment of the furuncle and carbuncle.
16. Provide examples of fungal diseases of the skin.
17. List the predisposing factors for superficial fungus of the skin.
18. Compare the two examples of scaling disorders of the skin and their treatments.
19. State and discuss briefly the types of benign skin tumors.
20. List two premalignant skin lesions.
21. Differentiate the three types of malignant skin tumors.
22. Compare and contrast the differences between partial- and full-thickness burns.
23. Describe the changes that occur in the skin as a result of thermal therapy.
24. Discuss the systemic changes that occur as a result of burn injury.
25. State the cause, type of injury, and effects of electrical and chemical burns.
26. Discuss the critical factors in the formation of decubitus ulcers.
27. Describe the various stages of decubitus formation.
28. Discuss the skin changes resulting from abrasions, incisions, puncture wounds, and lacerations.

Discussion of the pathophysiology of the skin and its diseases must be preceded by the appreciation of descriptive terms used to characterize skin lesions and a comprehension of the inflammatory process that heralds the disease. A systematic approach to the lesions prepares one for an assessment of the extent of disease.

The approach to skin lesion identification begins with a simple but specific investigative process. Questions are directed to obtain a history and include the following: (1) presentation and characteristics of the lesion, (2) distribution of multiple lesions, (3) length of time present and recurrence, (4) history of medications taken, both systemically and topically, (5) familial history of disease, and (6) environmental or personal exposure to hazardous material. Once the history is obtained, assessment of the lesion is necessary. Visible body areas must be inspected along with areas frequently overlooked, such as skin folds, scalp, hands, and feet.

Table 41-1 lists the basic nomenclature utilized to describe lesions. Figure 41-1 shows the appearance of the various lesions. Description of a lesion may require a combination of these terms.

TABLE 41-1. Terminology used in describing lesions

Macule—circumscribed spot, nonpalpable, not raised above level of the skin (e.g., freckle)
Papule—circumscribed, solid lesion, elevated above level of skin, palpable up to 5 mm in largest diameter (e.g., acne pimple)
Nodule—circumscribed, solid, elevated lesion of the skin over 5 mm in diameter (e.g., pigmented nevus)
Vesicle—circumscribed, elevated lesion of the skin, containing fluid, over 5 mm in diameter (e.g., blister)
Bulla—circumscribed, elevated lesion of the skin containing fluid, over 5 mm in diameter (e.g., large lesion of contact dermatitis due to poison ivy)
Pustule—circumscribed, elevated lesion of the skin up to 5 mm in diameter containing pus (e.g., acne pustule)
Wheal—circumscribed, red white transient elevation of skin approximately 0.5 to 10.0 cm in diameter, formed by local edema (e.g., common hives)
Lichenification—thickening and exaggeration of normal skin markings and furrows, usually due to persistent scratching
Squamous or scaly—having dried, then epithelial horny lamellae, usually resulting from imperfect cornification

Source: S. Robbins and R. Cotran, *Pathologic Basis of Disease*. Philadelphia: Saunders, 1974. P. 1379.

INFLAMMATION

A skin lesion is the result of the body's response to injury, which generates inflammation. Sources of injury include bacteria, virus, temperature extremes, and chemical or mechanical irritants.

Inflammation causes alterations in the surrounding blood vessels and adjacent tissues. Redness or erythema is the hallmark of inflammation. An irritant causes injury to the site, which results in an increased vasculature, with fluid exuding, and edema. Pressure from the edema or chemical irritation from the release of various mediator substances causes pain by irritation of the nerve fibers present in that area. The duration of the inflammatory response is variable.

Skin Sensitivity

Although afterward referred to as a disease, *urticaria* and *angioedema* can also be classified as a reaction to injury or a facet of the allergic reaction.

URTICARIA. This is a vascular reaction manifested by transient erythema or whitish swellings (wheals) of the skin or mucous membranes [1]. Skin changes or lesions are the result of increased vascular permeability, resulting in localized areas of edema. Resolution of edema may begin within several hours. These lesions are often pruritic and sting. *Acute urticaria* can be defined as a cutaneous vascular reaction that evolves over a short period, from days to several weeks. It resolves completely. *Chronic urticaria* lasts for at least 2 months and may persist for years. It also may go away and then recur.

The etiologies of urticaria are numerous and can include such components as foods; inhalants; drugs; injectants (e.g., blood, vaccines); chemicals; and mechanical and environmental irritants.

Treatment involves removal of the causative agent. Antihistamines are often used. Alleviation of irritating factors, elimination diets, and prevention and treatment of dry skin may be of benefit.

ANGIOEDEMA. Angioedema is a reaction that involves edema not only of the superficial skin but also of the subcutaneous tissues. The differences between urticaria and angioedema are degree and location. Angioedema can be described as giant wheals, often involving the mucous membranes. Angioedema can cause many physical symptoms (including severe respiratory distress), especially when it affects the larynx; this complication constitutes a medical emergency.

COMMON INFLAMMATORY DISEASES OF THE SKIN

Acne

Acne vulgaris is a common chronic inflammatory disease of the sebaceous glands and hair follicles of the skin, also known as the pilosebaceous ducts (Fig. 41-2). The occurrence of this disease is based on two factors: (1) accumulation of sebum, which is the fatty secretion liberated by the breakdown of sebaceous cells, and (2) an irritation of the area around the hair follicle, leading to a perifolliculitis.

The exact etiology is still unknown, but it may be due to either increased activity of the sebaceous glands or the inability of the material secreted to escape through a narrow opening. The resulting inflammation is precipitated by the combination of sebum, bacteria, and subsequent fatty acid release. The latter is caused by the hydrolytic action of the lipases, which are furnished by the bacteria on the sebum itself. The inflammatory reaction, with resulting edema,

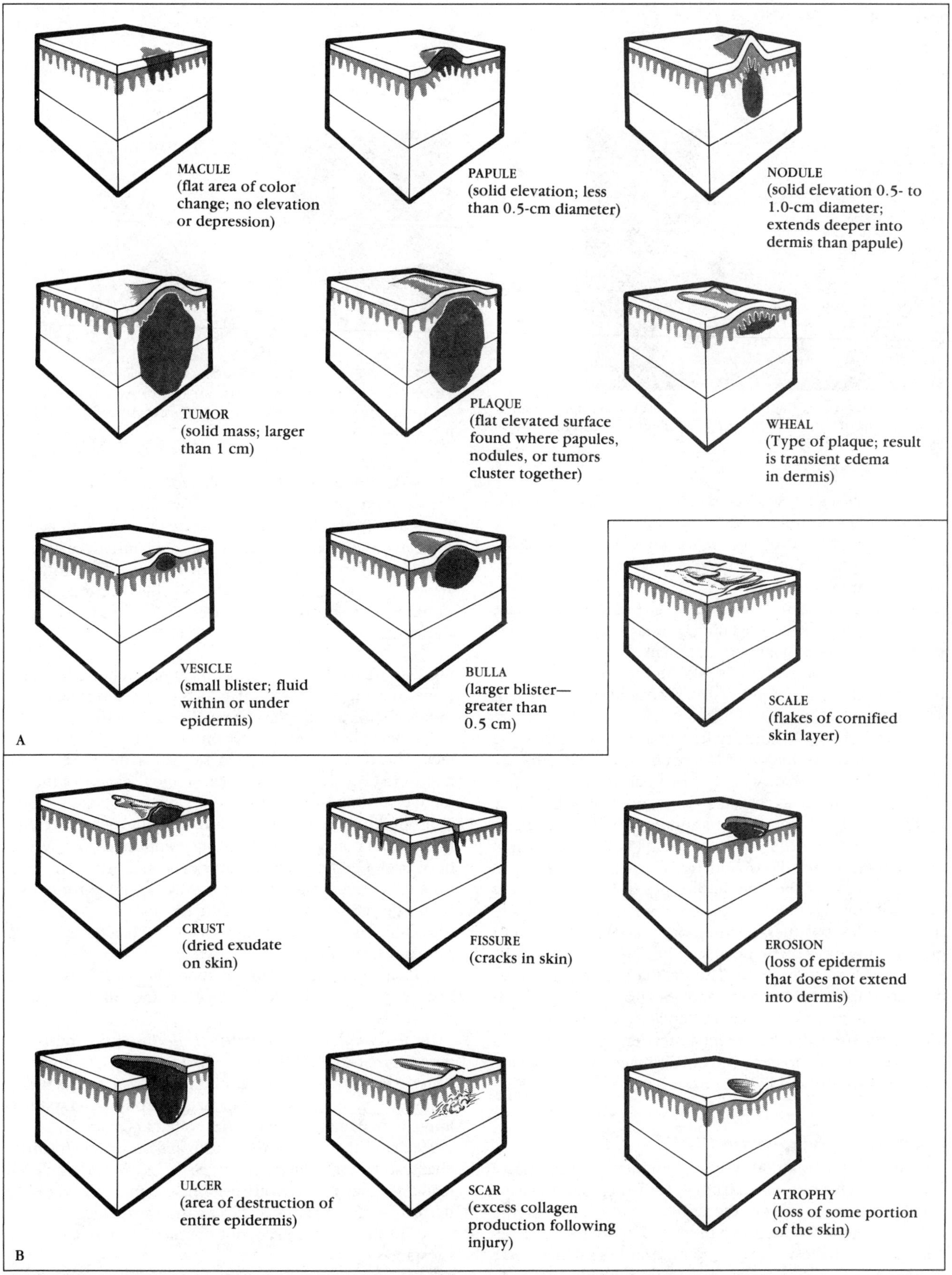

FIGURE 41-1. A. Primary skin lesions and their characteristics. B. Secondary skin lesions and their characteristics. (From J. Sana and R. Judge, *Physical Assessment Skills for Nursing Practice* [2nd ed.]. Boston: Little, Brown, 1982.)

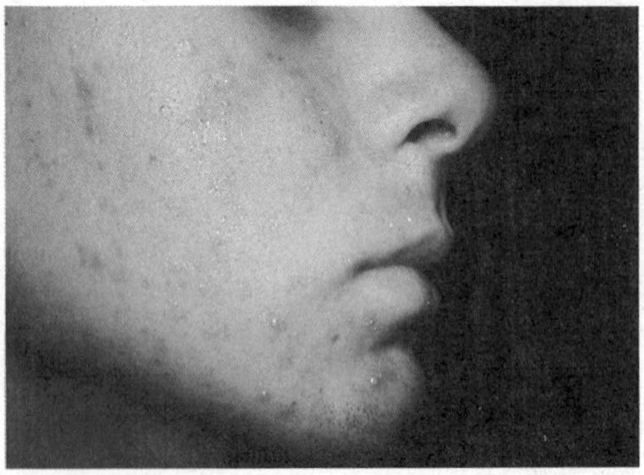

FIGURE 41-2. Acne: papules, pustules, and scarring. (From K. Arndt, *Manual of Dermatologic Therapeutics* [3rd ed.]. Boston: Little, Brown, 1983.)

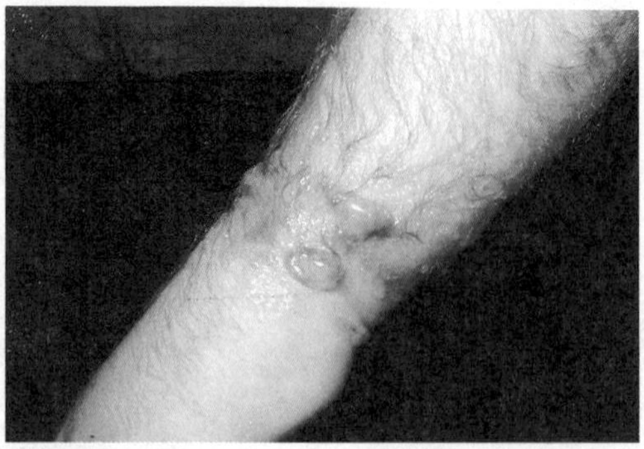

FIGURE 41-3. Contact dermatitis from leather (watchband). (From K. Arndt, *Manual of Dermatologic Therapeutics* [3rd ed.]. Boston: Little, Brown, 1983.)

probably causes the sebaceous follicle to perforate its wall and develop a perifolliculitis.

The development of acne is dependent on several factors: heredity, use of oil-based cosmetics or skin treatments, ingestion of drugs (e.g., steroids, androgens), and the presence of bacteria. Sebaceous glands are hormonally controlled, and the androgenic hormones may function to increase sebaceous gland development and secretion.

The location of the lesions follows the area of predominant pilosebaceous glands—the face, chest, back, neck, and upper arms.

The early noninflammatory lesions are of two types, the white and black comedones. The white comedo occurs in a closed excretory duct with a very small, possibly microscopic, opening that prevents drainage. This lesion may lead to an inflammatory process and give rise to a papule or pustule. The black comedo (blackhead) is a widely dilated follicle filled with a discolored, horny material plugging an excretory duct of the skin. Both types of lesions obstruct the emptying of sebum to the surface and may develop into small papules, pustules, nodules, or cysts. With time, most pustules and cysts open, drain, and heal. If severe, these lesions may lead to scarring. The prevalence of acne is increased during adolescence and early adulthood, but is usually self-limited. The central theme of medical treatment involves reducing the inflammation of the pilosebaceous glands by fostering free drainage of the gland, avoiding rupture, and limiting bacterial growth.

Hidradenitis Suppurativa

Although not a common disease, hidradenitis suppurativa is a severe chronic inflammatory disease of the apocrine glands. It usually affects the axillae, but can affect the anogenital area. It begins as a reddened, tender subcutaneous nodule. The lesion may suppurate and drain or resolve spontaneously. If this recurs, sinuses can develop that can result in extensive scarring.

Treatment ranges from topical antibiotics for mild cases to systemic antibiotics for more advanced lesions. Surgical incision and drainage may be required for acutely inflamed nodules.

DERMATITIS/ECZEMA. *Dermatitis* and *eczema* are terms that are used interchangeably. These skin conditions constitute the superficial inflammatory diseases of the skin. Morphologically, the changes of acute and chronic dermatitis are specific and recognizable as particular to dermatitis. The main classifications discussed in this section include: contact dermatitis, atopic dermatitis, and seborrheic dermatitis.

CONTACT DERMATITIS. This classification includes inflammations that are the result of contact with external agents, either chemical allergens or mechanical irritants.

The morphology of the lesion begins in the area of contact. The shape of the lesion simulates the area of local exposure (Fig. 41-3). The irritant removes some of the protective mechanisms of the skin, such as lipids and other hydrophilic material, and causes varying degrees of dryness. When contact is with strong compounds, or there has been prolonged use, lesions may evolve. If exposure is continued, acute dermatitis can progress to the chronic form. In most circumstances, complete tissue repair is possible, if the irritant is removed and permanent changes in the skin have not taken place.

Contact dermatitis can be subdivided into two types: primary irritant contact dermatitis and allergic contact dermatitis.

In *primary irritant contact dermatitis*, there is a nonallergic skin reaction from irritant exposure. Repeated or lengthened contact by a mild irritant such as detergent is necessary to cause skin damage. Strong irritants cause immediate damage when initial contact is made.

Mechanical irritation is due to inflammation from mechanical factors, such as large-size particles of certain materials that cause pruritus. One example is wool. The dermatitis that results is due to the mechanical "scratchiness" of the irritant itself, not the mediation of a chemical substance.

There has been an increase in the incidence of chemically caused contact dermatitis. A basic substance, such as water, can indirectly be a chemical irritant through prolonged exposure and removal of the skin's protective barriers. Soaps and detergents increase the drying and facilitate the irritating action of water. Other chemicals and medica-

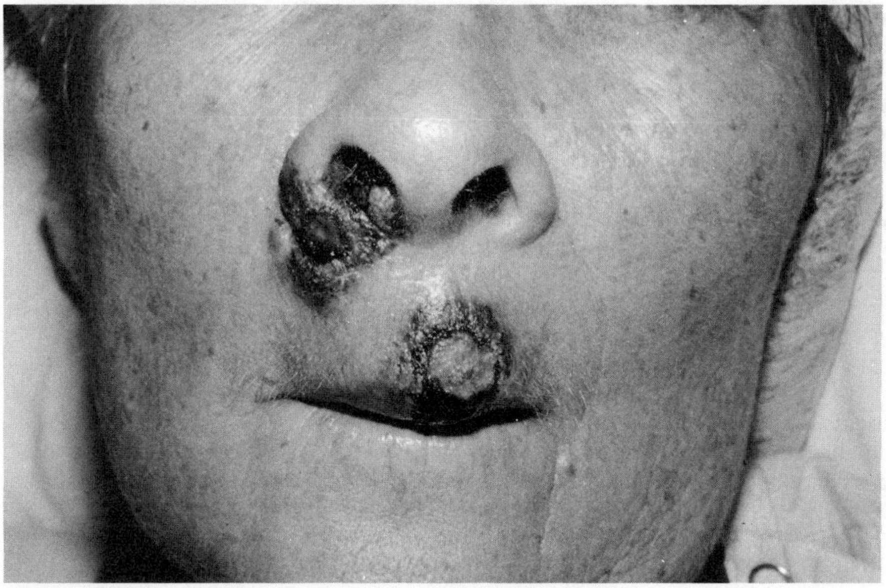

FIGURE 41-4. Lesions caused by the herpes simplex virus. (From K. Rosen, et al., *The Nurse's Atlas of Dermatology*. Boston: Little, Brown, 1983.)

tions may cause an irritant dermatitis. Various biologic irritants, including human excrement, saliva, and tears, result in dermatitis after prolonged contact. Biologic irritants can also cause a predisposition to the development of yeast and bacterial infections, compounding the problem.

Allergic contact dermatitis is the presentation of a delayed hypersensitivity dermatitis. It results from exposure of a previously sensitized individual to contact allergens. Some of the causes include poison ivy antigens, many industrial chemicals, various drugs, and some metals.

Removal of the sensitizer is necessary for treatment. Identification of the causative agent can be accomplished by a history, patch testing, or a use test. Unless severe, medical treatment includes soaks and corticosteroid creams. When dermatitis becomes severe and frequent, systemic steroids may be required.

ATOPIC DERMATITIS. This is a highly specific disease that results from a hereditarily determined lowered threshold to pruritus and is characterized by intense itching [1]. It may appear as a small papule, but there is evidence that scratching is the major factor producing the lesion. The intense scratching will develop into erythema, weeping, scaling, and lichenification. The histology is that of a nonspecific dermatitis. It occurs in areas of flexion and extension, such as the popliteal space, antecubital fossa, and neck area.

The list of exacerbating factors includes sudden changes in weather, psychologic stress, contact with wool, furs, and primary irritant chemicals.

Many complications can develop with atopic dermatitis, including an increase in the severity of viral infections. Affected persons should not be vaccinated against smallpox, as disseminated vaccinia can develop and cause a generalized infection of the skin. These persons are also prone to bacterial and fungal infections, ocular complications, and allergic contact dermatitis.

Treatment involves palliation through reduction or control of precipitating events and symptomatic relief of pruritis. Topical agents afford some relief. The prognosis is difficult to determine, but studies have demonstrated that the length of disease is long, although the frequency of attacks is less after adolescence.

SEBORRHEIC DERMATITIS. This inflammatory, erythematous, and scaling disease predominates in areas of the body that have numerous seborrheic glands. Often it is compared to dandruff, which is the noninflammatory counterpart, or mild form. It occurs as an accelerated epidermal, immature growth. This entity involves not only the scalp, but also eyebrows, portions of the forehead, bridge of nose, and the trunk. Treatment includes antiseborrheic shampoos and topical agents.

VIRAL INFECTIONS OF THE SKIN

Herpes Simplex

Categorized as a virus, herpes simplex is also known as a fever blister or "cold sore." It is caused by type 1 herpes simplex virus. Its initial presentation is as an acute grouped eruption, with erythematous and vesicular characteristics; it later becomes purulent and crusting. Distribution may occur to any area of the body, but the most frequent areas are the lips, perioral, and genital areas; the lesions may be painful and pruritic (Fig. 41-4). Resolution usually occurs within 2 weeks.

It is believed that first exposure to infection occurs by the fifth year of life, but is not often observed. Nevertheless, the person has developed antibodies to the virus. A small percentage of children have primary gingivostomatitis or vulvovaginitis as a result. Recurrence may occur throughout life as a result of either reactivation of the virus or reinoculation and may be precipitated by stress-producing factors, such as fever, excessive sun exposure, common cold, or injury.

Herpes progenitalis has become a frequently seen infection of the genital area and is believed to be caused by the type 2 herpesvirus. Studies in process are investigating a relationship of this virus to cervical cancer.

Since no cure has been discovered, treatment of herpes simplex is aimed toward symptomatic relief with bland topical therapy. Prevention can only be aimed at avoiding the identified precipitating factors.

Varicella

Otherwise known as chickenpox, this disease is caused by the herpes zoster virus. An airborne, highly contagious virus in the prodromal and vesicular stages, it affects children more frequently than adults.

The varicella virus has an incubation period of 10 to 20 days. The prodromal stage often begins with moderate fever and malaise. Pink papules, 2 to 4 mm in size, are surrounded by a reddened halo that later dries and crusts. Lesions are usually seen in groups. Distribution of the lesions on the face, scalp, trunk, and arms is common. Generalized symptoms of headache, moderate fever, anorexia, and malaise may continue after the lesions present. Varicella in the adult is much more severe than in children.

Treatment for the usual varicella in children is aimed at keeping the skin lesions dry and relieving pruritus with lotion as necessary.

Herpes Zoster

This is also a varicella virus; it is often referred to as "shingles." This acute inflammatory disease occurs when the person undergoes an activation of the dormant varicella virus. It usually occurs in the elderly population, but it can occur in any age group. In the older person, pain usually precedes the lesion by 1 to 2 days.

The initial presentation is one of erythema and discomfort, followed in 1 to 7 days by grouped vesicles along a unilateral dermatome (Fig. 41-5). These vesicles later crust and clear in approximately 2½ weeks.

Severe pain can result, and persistence is a feared complication. Although uncommon, a generalized herpes zoster can result, a condition usually associated with a systemic malignancy of the lymphoma group [3].

Warts (Verrucae)

Verrucae, or warts, are viral infections of the skin. There are three main types: verruca vulgaris (common wart), verruca plantaris (plantar wart), and condyloma acuminatum (venereal wart). It is believed that these are variations of the same virus.

The etiology of warts is not clearly understood, but they can be transmitted by contact from person to person. They are benign lesions and are frequently seen at sites of injury or along a break in the skin.

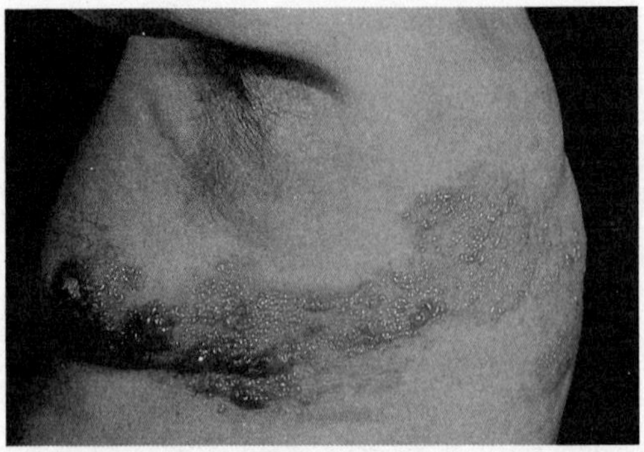

FIGURE 41-5. Herpes zoster. (From K. Arndt, *Manual of Dermatologic Therapeutics* [3rd ed.]. Boston: Little, Brown, 1983.)

Verruca vulgaris occurs as a raised, well-circumscribed growth with an irregular gray surface, frequently seen on the hands. Although treatment is often unsatisfactory, surgical removal, electrosurgery, and cryosurgery have been used. Many warts will resolve without treatment.

Verruca plantaris differs from the common wart by its location and the effect that pressure has on the lesion. The wart tends to grow on the soles of the feet, and pain is frequent, resulting from the irritation of walking. As a result, the wart tends to grow inward.

Condylomata acuminata are lesions established primarily in warm, moist anogenital areas. Also known as venereal warts, they do not necessarily stem from sexual contact. These growths present as large lesions, pinkish or purplish projections with a rough surface.

Rubeola (Measles)

Rubeola is a highly contagious viral infection caused by a myxovirus. The incubation period is approximately 10 to 14 days. Its course usually begins with fever and symptoms of upper respiratory infection that occur 6 to 7 days after inoculation and last 24 hours. The disease then enters what is known as the invasion phase, with symptoms of high fever, chills, malaise, headache, photophobia, and dry cough. These symptoms last for 4 to 7 days. Lesions begin as inflammation or petechiae of the soft palate, followed by Koplik's spots, which are blue white spots surrounded by a bright halo over the buccal mucosa. A macular eruption appears on the face, upper extremities, and trunk.

Rubella

Also known as German measles, this common acute infectious disease is caused by a myxovirus. The incubation period ranges from 12 to 25 days and begins with malaise and mild fever approximately 4 to 5 days before lesions appear. Lesions are small, irregular pink macules and papules that appear initially on the face, spreading to the entire body. These lesions fade rapidly within 2 to 3 days. Adenopathy of the superficial cervical and posterior auricular glands is common.

Rubella is serious in pregnant women, especially in the first trimester, when transmission to a fetus results in fetal

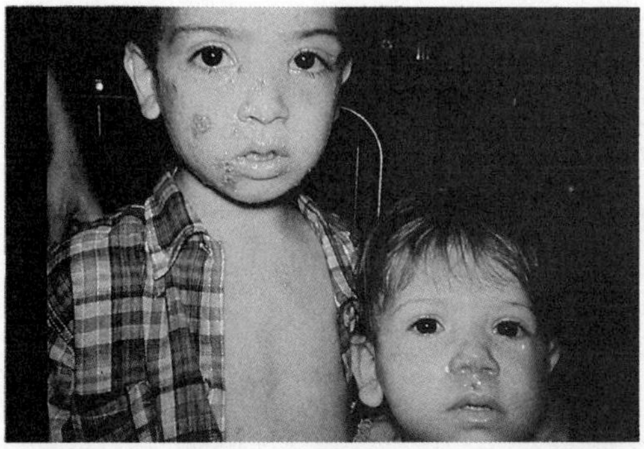

FIGURE 41-6. Impetigo. (From K. Arndt, *Manual of Dermatologic Therapeutics* [3rd ed.]. Boston: Little, Brown, 1983.)

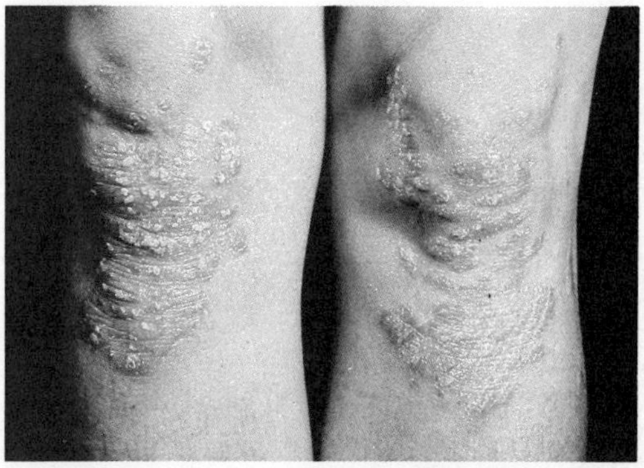

FIGURE 41-7. Psoriasis. (From K. Arndt, *Manual of Dermatologic Therapeutics* [3rd ed.]. Boston: Little, Brown, 1983.)

anomalies. A titer is available to assess immunity. Vaccination is used with school-aged children and, with caution, in women of child-bearing age with low rubella titers.

BACTERIAL INFECTIONS OF THE SKIN

Impetigo

This is an acute bacterial infection that occurs superficially on the skin as serous and purulent vesicles that later rupture and form a golden crust (Fig. 41-6). It frequently occurs in children, but persons in ill health are also predisposed to it. A common location for presentation is the face, but it also may involve the extremities.

Causative organisms include β-hemolytic streptococci and coagulase-positive staphylococci. It is autoinoculous and can be transmitted between humans. Influencing factors include poor hygiene, tropical climates, and improper sanitation. A serious complication is glomerulonephritis, which may not be prevented by antibiotic treatment.

Folliculitis

This bacterial infection of the skin originates within the hair follicle. Staphylococci are the usual causative organisms. It appears as a pustule located at the opening of the hair follicle, predominantly on the scalp and extremities. The basic lesion is a reddened macule or papule surrounding the hair follicle. Predisposing factors include poor hygiene and maceration. Folliculitis can extend into the deeper skin layers if not treated promptly, and systemic antibiotics may be necessary.

Furuncle and Carbuncle

A *furuncle,* also known as a "boil," frequently develops from a preceding staphylococcal folliculitis and is usually located in body areas containing hair follicles. Irritation, maceration, and lack of good hygiene are predisposing factors in its development. This lesion presents as a nodule that is usually tender and red. It frequently remains tense for 2 to 4 days, becomes fluctuant, and later drains purulent material [1].

A *carbuncle* is a larger staphylococcal abscess that drains through various points of the lesion. Several cases of furuncles and almost every case of carbuncles require systemic antibiotic therapy.

FUNGAL DISEASES OF THE SKIN

Fungal diseases of the skin can be classified in three groups: superficial, intermediate, and deep. The superficial diseases result in what is commonly known as ringworm (tinea capitis), athlete's foot (tinea pedis), "jock itch" (tinea cruris), and tinea versicolor. These fungal diseases are primarily caused by dermatophytes that invade the superficial layers of the epidermis, hair, and nails. They are characterized by areas of scaling, erythema, and frequently vesicles and fissures [10].

Moisture, heat, and maceration are predisposing factors for growth; consequently, lesions appear in areas between toes, axilla, nails, and the groin. Treatment involves local therapy, and with certain resistant fungi, griseofulvin, a fungicidal and fungostatic antibiotic, is used.

Intermediate fungal diseases invade both the superficial and deeper tissues. Moniliasis caused by *Candida albicans* is an example.

Deep fungal infections invade deeper structures of living tissue and include diseases such as sporotrichosis, candidiasis, histoplasmosis, and aspergillosis. The reader is referred to Chapter 7 for further discussion of these diseases.

SCALING DISORDERS OF THE SKIN

Psoriasis

Psoriasis is a disease that results from hyperplasia of the epidermal layer of the skin, causing formation and shedding of the keratin scales (Fig. 41-7). Thus, the clinical presentation is of sharply defined erythematous plaques, covered by silvery white, loosely adherent scales.

The precise etiology is not determined, but genetic determination and environmental factors play a significant role in its development. It is viewed as a chronic disease with much diversity in its location, severity, and frequency of its appearance. Factors that often precipitate its exacerbation include local trauma, sun exposure, infection, and stress [11].

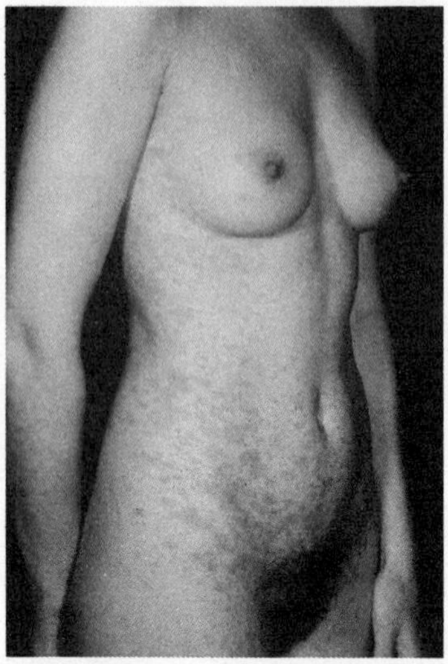

FIGURE 41-8. Pityriasis rosea. (From K. Arndt, *Manual of Dermatologic Therapeutics* [3rd ed.]. Boston: Little, Brown, 1983.)

It can be found in all ages and is often distributed over the knees, elbows, scalp, and lumbosacral skin. Involvement of the nails is exhibited by pitting and dimpling. Psoriasis has a strong association with arthritis. A serious but rare condition known as pustular psoriasis also can occur, which manifests with high fever, elevated white blood cell count, electrolyte imbalance, and malaise. This condition can be fatal.

In the usual presentation, psoriasis can be controlled and remission is possible. Avoidance of local skin injury, infection, and stress. Good nutrition and avoidance of excessive weight gain improve the control of this disease.

Pityriasis Rosea

This is a common, acute disease of the skin, usually affecting the adolescent and young adult. Its course is self-limited and is thought to be infectious in nature, possibly caused by a virus.

Clinical manifestations often follow a prodrome of malaise, fatigue, and headache. The first lesion, known as the "herald plaque," is a single, oval, ringlike plaque that is later followed by lesions that are usually flat, erythematous patches covered by a fine scale; they resemble the primary plaque, but are smaller (Fig. 41-8). Lesions are often pruritic. Distribution is most frequently on the neck, trunk, and arms.

SKIN TUMORS

Tumors of the skin can be divided into two basic categories, benign and malignant. Characteristics of benign tumors include structural differentiation and they are usually composed of well-differentiated cells. These lesions are slow-growing, and growth may stop entirely [8]. Malignant lesions show disorganization and abnormalities. They frequently grow rapidly and infiltrate surrounding tissues. Metastasis is common, depending on the origin of the tumor.

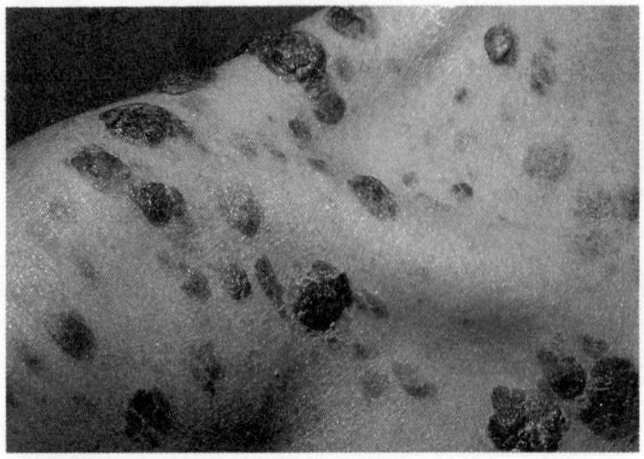

FIGURE 41-9. Seborrheic keratoses. (From K. Arndt, *Manual of Dermatologic Therapeutics* [3rd ed.]. Boston: Little, Brown, 1983.)

Benign Tumors

SEBORRHEIC KERATOSIS. Seborrheic keratosis is the most common tumor in the elderly. A strong predisposing factor is prolonged exposure to the sun. The cutaneous manifestation is a lesion, slightly raised, light brown, and sharply demarcated; pigmentation may become deep and thick (Fig. 41-9). These lesions are covered with a greasy crust, which is loosely attached. Locations include trunk, shoulders, face, and scalp. Malignant transformation is quite uncommon. Most of these lesions do not require treatment unless they pose cosmetic difficulties or cause suspicion of malignancy.

HEMANGIOMA. Hemangioma is a benign tumor of newly formed blood vessels. There are many different types. A strawberry hemangioma frequently appears as a dome-shaped, fully red, soft lesion with sharply demarcated edges. It has a tendency to grow slowly and usually regresses completely.

The *port-wine stain*, or nevus flammeus, is a congenital vascular malformation [7]. These lesions are usually unilateral and located on the face and neck. They appear as flat, red patches. Unfortunately, they grow as the child grows and do not regress.

Cavernous hemangiomas are usually not congenital. The location includes both the skin and subcutaneous tissues, and presentation depends on the extent of the lesion, varying from round or flat to bright red or deep purple in color.

KERATOACANTHOMA. Keratoacanthoma is a benign, cutaneous tumor with a central crater. Because it resembles squamous cell carcinoma, lesions are removed and sent for pathologic examination.

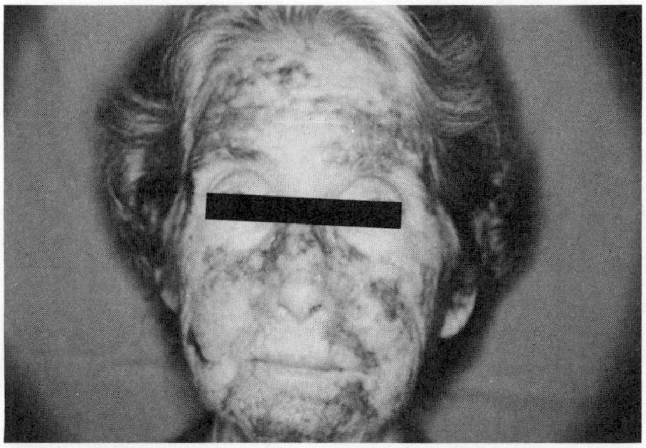

FIGURE 41-10. Note the smooth surface and pearly border of basal cell carcinoma. (From K. Rosen, et al., *The Nurse's Atlas of Dermatology*. Boston: Little, Brown, 1983.)

ACTINIC KERATOSIS. Actinic keratosis is a premalignant lesion. Common names include "senile" or "solar" keratosis. They are sharply demarcated, rough lesions, red to brown or gray in color. At high risk to develop lesions are fair-skinned persons whose skin easily burns with sun exposure. Age of onset is related to the amount of sun exposure. Treatment is necessary, since a number of these lesions will progress to squamous cell carcinomas. A variety of methods can be used to destroy them, including curettage, electrodesiccation, cryotherapy, topical chemotherapy, and excisional biopsy.

Leukoplakia is also a premalignant lesion occurring on the mucous membranes. This lesion is often seen in elderly persons, especially women.

Malignant Disorders

BASAL CELL CARCINOMA. Basal cell carcinoma is also known as basal cell epithelioma and is the most frequent type of skin cancer. It tends to occur in older persons, and the majority of lesions appear on sun-exposed areas. Persons who have had x-ray treatment in the past are at increased risk. Although it rarely metastasizes, treatment is necessary, for it may become locally destructive and can erode into a vital area.

Characteristically, the carcinoma has a smooth surface with a pearly border, often with ulceration of its center (Fig. 41-10). Usually, multiple telangiectasias are visible [10]. Treatments include cryotherapy, curettage, and electrodesiccation, a topical chemotherapy.

SQUAMOUS CELL CARCINOMA. Squamous cell carcinoma is a malignant lesion that can affect both the skin and mucous membranes. It most frequently occurs in sun-damaged areas or areas exposed to radiation or burns.

Characteristically, it appears as a rough, hyperkeratotic nodule with an indurated base (Fig. 41-11). It may ulcerate and can metastasize. Surgical excision is the treatment of choice. In some instances, curettage and electrodesiccation, irradiation, and chemosurgery can be used.

MALIGNANT MELANOMA. Malignant melanoma is a cancer arising from the melanin-producing cells. This malignancy is associated with an increased risk of invasion and metastasis. Risk of development of the disease is increased with exposure to the sun. Recognizing the lesion early is important, since prognosis is dependent on such factors as early removal, size, type, and extension of the lesion. All nevi

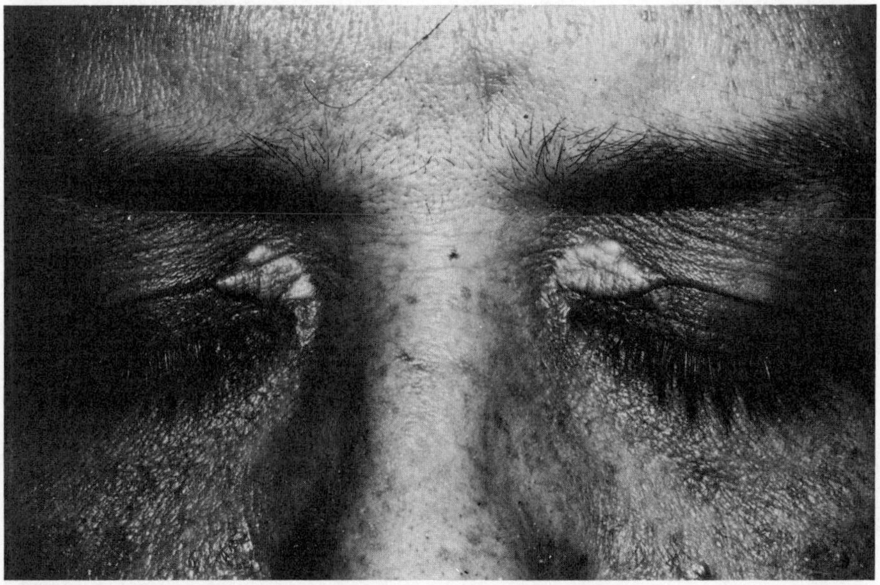

FIGURE 41-11. The characteristic look of squamous cell carcinoma. (From K. Rosen, et al., *The Nurse's Atlas of Dermatology*. Boston: Little, Brown, 1983.)

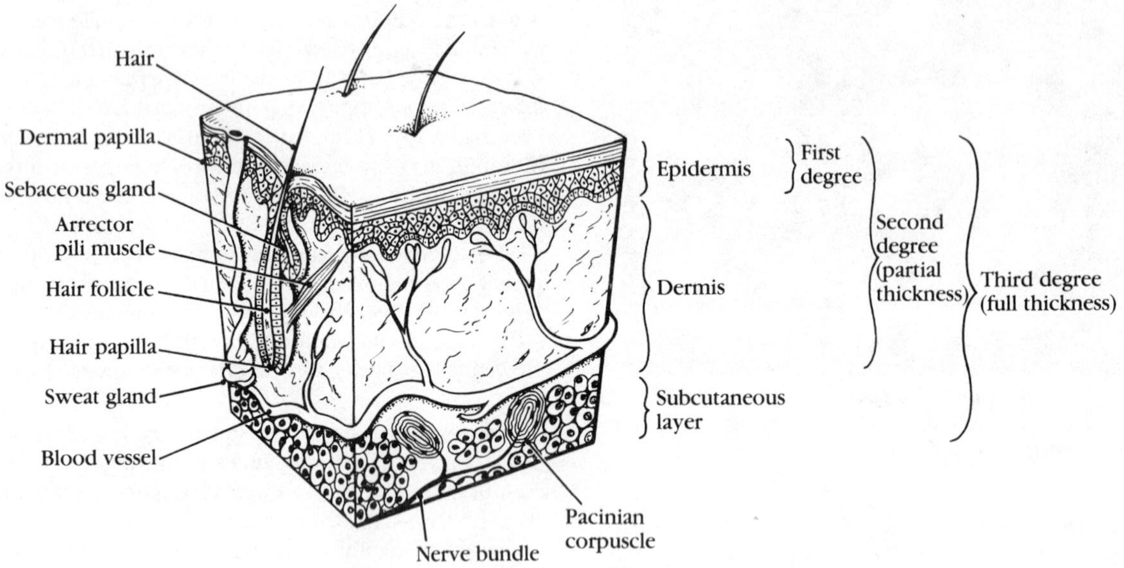

FIGURE 41-12. Areas affected by first-, second-, and third-degree burns.

TABLE 41-2. Classification of burns

Degree	Tissue	Appearance	Symptoms	Resolution
First				
Partial thickness	Epidermis	Red, pink, slight edema	Pain	Epidermis peels in 3–6 days; itch, redness in a week or so; no scar
Second				
Partial thickness				
Superficial	Epidermis and upper dermis	Mottled pink to red; blistering; edema; moist	Sensitive	Heals in 10–14 days without grafting; no scar if no infection or trauma to wound
Deep dermal	Epidermis, dermis to subcutaneous tissue	Varies: white, tan, cherry red; red area blanches; dark, coagulated capillary streaks; blister and moist, or dry	May or may not be sensitive; if hair follicle present, hair does not pull out	Has potential to heal spontaneously over several months; may be excised or grafted
Third				
Full thickness	Epidermis; dermis; subcutaneous layer; no viable epithelial cells remain	White, tan, brown, black, deep cherry red; red areas do not blanch; wet or dry; sunken; eschar; coagulated capillaries	Anesthetic; hair pulls out	Grafting required after debridement
Fourth				
Full thickness	Epidermis; dermis; subcutaneous layer; fascia; muscle; bone	Blackened; depressed; bone-dull and dry	Hair pulls out	Grafting required

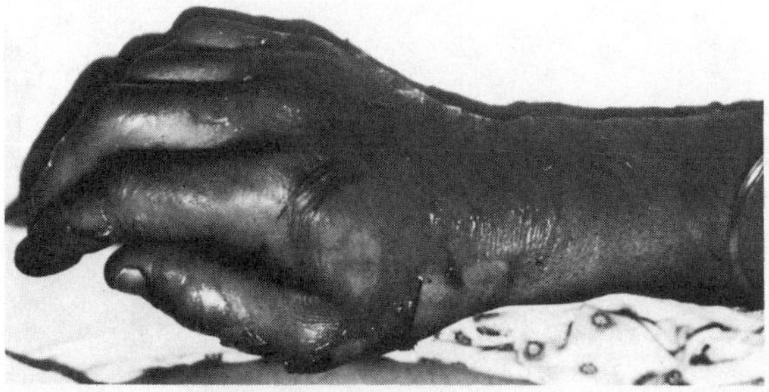

FIGURE 41-13. Partial-thickness burn injury. (From C.V. Kenner, C.E. Guzzetta, and B.M. Dossey, *Critical Care Nursing*. Boston: Little, Brown, 1981.)

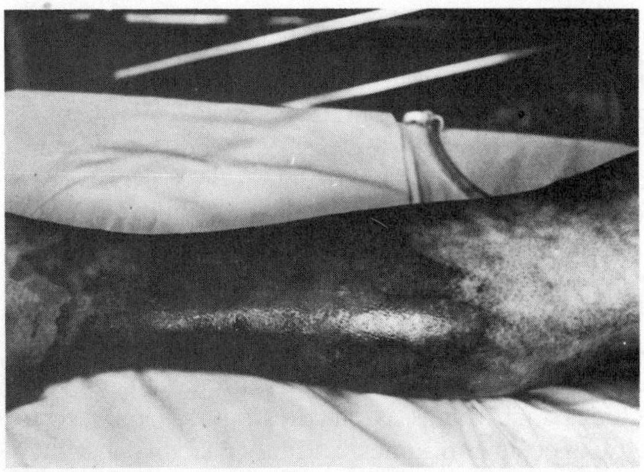

FIGURE 41-14. Full-thickness burn injury. (From C.V. Kenner, C.E. Guzzetta, and B.M. Dossey, *Critical Care Nursing*. Boston: Little, Brown, 1981.)

should be inspected regularly, and self-examination should be taught. The significant characteristics are variable colors and irregular borders and surfaces. Nevi may have brown or black pigmentation with shades of red, white, or blue. Small satellite lesions 1 to 2 cm away from the primary lesion may be seen. Only a small percentage (20%) of these malignancies occur on nevi that have been present for a period of time. Usually, a new nevus is described that rapidly undergoes malignant changes. These are most common on the legs of women and the chests and backs of men.

TRAUMATIC ALTERATIONS IN THE SKIN

Burns

Burn injuries occur in every age group of both sexes. When burn injury does occur, the trauma involves not only the skin tissue but also involves the whole body. Burns may be classified as first-, second-, third-, or fourth-degree burns. A more precise classification may be made on the basis of partial-, deep dermal, or full-thickness injury. It is often difficult to ascertain the depth of burn injury in the initial postburn period. To further complicate matters, a partial-thickness injury may convert to a deep dermal or full-thickness injury as a result of burn wound sepsis and microcirculatory insufficiency with delayed degeneration of deep epithelial appendages. As time progresses, the depth and extent of the burn become more apparent.

PARTIAL-THICKNESS BURNS. Each degree of burn wound depth has various characteristics. Partial-thickness burns include first- and second-degree and deep dermal injuries (Table 41-2). The first-degree burn involves the epidermis (Fig. 41-12). This burn may be caused by exposure to sunlight, brief exposures to a heat source, splashed hot liquid, high-intensity short-duration explosions, or chemical and electrical injury. A first-degree burn is pink to red in color, painful, and slightly edematous. The epidermis peels in 3 to 6 days, with itching and redness persisting a week or more. The wound leaves no scar when healed [6].

The second-degree partial thickness burn may be superficial or deep dermal. The superficial burn involves the epidermis and dermis, while the deep dermal burn extends down to the subcutaneous tissues. These burns result from intense flash heat, hot liquid, contact with hot objects, chemicals, or electrical injury. The superficial second-degree burn has a mottled pink to red color (Fig. 41-13). The deep dermal burn varies in color. It is mottled with more white than red, a dull white, tan, or cherry red. The red areas blanch and refill. Dark streaks of coagulated capillaries may be seen. The superficial second-degree burn exhibits blistering and subcutaneous edema, is moist and very sensitive. This burn will heal in 10 to 14 days without grafting. If it does not become infected or traumatized, then usually no scar forms. In the deep dermal burn, if epidermal appendages are intact, the burn has the potential to heal spontaneously without grafting, since viable skin cells are present in the appendages. The deep dermal wound may be blistered and moist or it may be dry; it may or may not be sensitive; if a hair follicle remains, the hair will not pull out. If the deep dermal burn is allowed to heal spontaneously, it takes several months. The epithelium produced is extremely thin and may break down easily; the burn may convert to a full-thickness burn if it becomes infected. Many deep dermal burns are excised and grafted [6].

FULL-THICKNESS BURNS. The third-degree burn is a full-thickness injury with no viable epithelial cells present. The causes may be the same as for first- and second-degree burns. The wound's appearance may vary, being white, tan, brown, black, and/or deep cherry red. The red areas in this burn do not blanch. The burn may be wet or dry and have a sunken appearance. It is covered with a leathery covering called eschar. A black network of coagulated capillaries may be seen. This wound is anesthetic and hair pulls out easily. Grafting is required to close the wound [6] (Fig. 41-14).

The so-called fourth-degree burn is also a full-thickness injury and involves the subcutaneous fat layer, fascia, muscle, and bone. This burn appears black and depressed. If bone shows through, it appears dry and dull. Grafting is also necessary to close this wound. If a graft is required over bone, small perforations are made in the bone to the marrow. Granulation buds grow from these holes, coalesce, and form a bed to accept the graft [6].

The degree of burn just discussed depends on the temperature of the heat source and the duration of exposure to that source. The severity of the injury is dependent on the size of the burned area, the depth and location of the burn, the age of the victim, the presence of concomitant illness or injury, and the psychologic status of the victim. In further assessing the burn situation, it is helpful to know the circumstances surrounding the injury. Important information includes such things as place of injury, exposure to electricity, exposure to fumes, and other factors that may complicate the recovery.

CHANGES AS A RESULT OF BURN INJURY. When skin is burned, many changes occur. Protein in cells is denatured, and enzymes are inactivated. The tissue becomes coagulated, desiccated, or carbonized, depending on the temperature of the heat source and the time of exposure to the source. Even with mild heat, the normal metabolic activity of a cell is altered. Burns caused by long exposure to low-intensity heat are characterized by major changes in deeper tissues.

The stratum corneum is the water vapor barrier in the body. When it is destroyed, large amounts of fluid are lost. In a deep wound, the fluid loss is greater and often continues until the wound finally is closed, usually by grafting.

Burns extending down to and damaging the stratum germinativum will not regenerate if all parts of this layer are destroyed. Heat extending to the "cement" that binds the epidermis to the dermis causes the epidermis to loosen; lost fluid fills in the space, and a blister develops. When new epidermis is formed beneath the blister, the blister dries and peels off.

The dermis, made of collagen fibers, elastin, and mast cells, is damaged when exposed to high degrees of heat. The epidermal appendages, if intact, contain epidermal cells in the external sheath of the hair follicle. Glands can grow out and form new epithelium. When the burn extends to the subcutaneous tissues, the collagen fibers that normally anchor the dermis to the subcutaneous layer now hold the leathery burn eschar in place. The bacteria that form under the eschar release enzymes that lyse the collagen fibers, making it easier to remove eschar. The melanocyte in the epidermis does not regenerate well, and in deep burns, the skin color usually does not return. As blood vessels are damaged from the thermal injury, color changes occur in the burn. In sunburn, the vessels in the subpapillary and papillary plexi dilate, causing reddening. In a severe burn, coagulation of vessels causes the area to lose redness and be whiter, with the vessels themselves coagulating into blackened lines in the wound. Plasma leaks from damaged blood vessels and provides the fluid for blisters. Lymph vessels, compressed by the edema from the burn wound, become permeable as a result of the heat injury and cannot drain the affected area. Escharotomy or fasciotomy may help decompress lymph and blood vessels (Fig. 41-15).

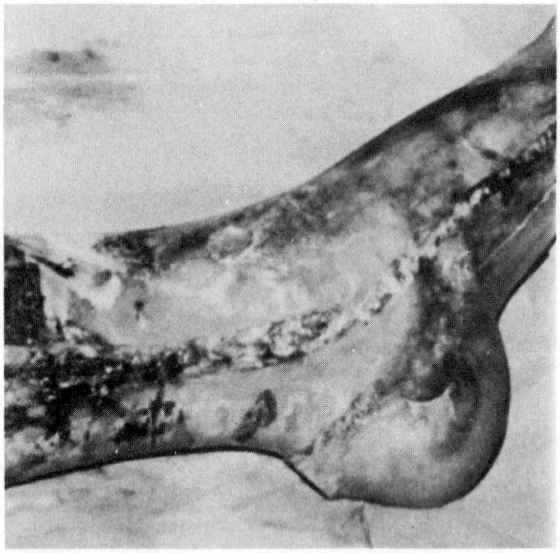

FIGURE 41-15. Escharotomy site. (From C. V. Kenner, C. E. Guzzetta, and B. M. Dossey, *Critical Care Nursing*. Boston: Little, Brown, 1981.)

SYSTEMIC CHANGES DUE TO BURN INJURY. There are many changes that occur throughout the body as a result of burn injury. Changes in the circulatory system account for color changes and the edema of burn injury. Contraction of the skin capillaries causes blanching. The wound appears white if the superficial dermis is coagulated. Later, when arterioles and capillaries dilate, the wound appears red. The capillaries lose protein-rich fluid through their abnormally permeable walls into the surrounding tissues, creating the most characteristic feature of the burn wound, *edema*. Normally, plasma and interstitial fluid are chemically similar, except for blood cells and large plasma proteins, which make the colloid osmotic pressure greater in the blood. After burn injury, colloid leaks out of the damaged capillaries and into the interstitial spaces. Colloids are plasma proteins, such as albumins and the globulins. The loss of protein-rich fluid decreases the colloid osmotic pressure difference between capillary plasma and tissue fluid exudate. There is also an accompanying rise in intracapillary pressure as a result of capillary dilatation and increased blood flow of the inflammatory process. The loss of colloid from capillaries is termed *capillary sieving* [1]. The amount of sieving is correlated with the severity of the burn. The more severe the burn, the more colloid lost. Increased capillary permeability also increases in tissues around the burn and other areas of the body, as well [2].

The permeability of tissue cells in and around the burn seem to allow abnormal interchange of fluids and electrolytes between cells and interstitial fluid. A limiting factor for extravasation of fluid is increased tissue pressure. Tissue pressure increases as fluid loss increases and reaches a point where the tissue will hold no more fluid.

The depth of the burn affects the volume and composition of edema fluid. In first-degree burns, protein loss is insignificant and edema slight, because vasodilatation is the only circulatory change. A second-degree burn has more severe capillary damage and more tissue damage. At first assessment, the surface area of burn is easily seen, but the depth is not always immediately apparent. Large volumes of fluid can escape beneath the wound before swelling is seen. The third-degree burn has a large injury to skin and area beneath and around the burn, which accounts for extensive fluid losses.

The edema can be displaced by pressure, can move to dependent areas, and can spread beyond the burn. The rate of edema formation depends on temperature of the heat source, duration of exposure, area of the burn, and the time since injury. It is difficult to ascertain fluid loss by the amount of visible edema, because fluid losses occur deep in the wound and beneath it. Eschar does not give with edema pressure, and large amounts of fluid collect beneath it, putting pressure on underlying tissues. The pressure is relieved by escharotomy.

Studies show that fluid losses occur rapidly in the period immediately after the burn and decline in about 48 hours. The fluid loss slows when the capillary endothelium returns to its normal state, the tissue pressure is in balance with capillary hydrostatic pressure, or when capillary stasis occurs. The resorption of edema in minor uncomplicated burns occurs chiefly by the lymphatic system and takes approximately as long as it took the edema to form. Lymphatics also drain larger burns, but this process may take weeks.

The protein lost from plasma varies in amount from one burn to another. Albumin and globulin are lost, with greater amounts of albumin lost than globulin, owing to the smaller size of albumin. Immediately after the burn, the concentration of protein in the plasma increases, because there is a greater loss of water and electrolytes along with the protein loss. Compensatory mechanisms exist to counteract the fluid loss: Interstitial fluid in unburned areas is absorbed by the blood; blood vessels in the spleen and unburned skin constrict, reducing the space the remaining blood volume must fill; and fluid is absorbed by the gut. Thirst may be intense. In minor burns, these mechanisms suffice. In major large burns, fluid and colloid must be replaced [2].

Hemoconcentration is a sequel to capillary fluid loss. The fluid portion of the blood is lost to the tissues, allowing the cellular elements to concentrate. The hematocrit rises, the blood flow becomes sluggish, compromising tissue nutrition and oxygenation. A thrombosis may sometimes be present.

Water and electrolytes shift back and forth across normal capillary walls. Burn injury alters the shifts by increasing capillary permeability causing protein loss and altered colloid osmotic pressure. Potassium is released from severely injured cells, causing serum potassium elevation and cardiac arrhythmias (see Chap. 5). Sodium increases in burn tissue, taking water with it [2]. When the burn victim begins diuresis after 48 hours or so, potassium and sodium are excreted. Careful monitoring of electrolyte levels is important, so replacement therapy may be initiated and electrolyte concentrations of replacement fluids may be reduced, as in the case of sodium.

In some burns, there is a substantial loss of red blood cells, intensifying the effects of plasma loss. This loss is usually seen in deep burns and seems to be a gradual process. The loss of red blood cells is due in part to the hemolysis of red blood cells in the burned area, which results in hemoglobinemia and hemoglobinuria soon after the burn occurs. Free hemoglobin in the plasma indicates a severe burn. For 24 to 48 hours, delayed hemolysis of partially damaged red blood cells occurs. Further decrease in red blood cells results from thrombosis and sludging. Anemia is seen as a result of red cell loss, as well as from bleeding during burn debridement and other causes.

Fluid is further lost as insensible water loss from evaporation from the burn wound surface and through the respiratory system. The respiratory loss is greater when a tracheostomy is required. Each gram of evaporative water removes 0.580 kcal of heat from the body [2].

Signs and symptoms of fluid deficiency include thirst, restlessness, and disorientation. Plain water given to relieve thirst may lead to water intoxication. Solutions with balanced electrolytes must be given to avoid this problem. Fluids are usually given intravenously, because of the problem of vomiting following burn injury. Changes in the central nervous system are useful in following the progress of therapy. Restlessness is an early indication that fluid replacement therapy is ineffective. Disorientation in the first 24 hours usually means that more intensive therapy is needed.

The loss of fluid to burn wound edema and insensible fluid loss reduce circulatory blood volume and can result in reduced cardiac output and inadequate tissue perfusion. Tissue hypoxia may result, causing a shift to anaerobic cellular metabolism. Acidosis and irreversible burn shock can occur. The acid-base balance is disrupted, because the buffering mechanism is upset by fluid shift in the body compartments, hyperventilation, and reduced renal function. Blood urea levels may rise if excessive protein catabolism has occurred or large amounts of nitrogen are released from burned tissue in the presence of oliguria [6].

The respiratory system is often altered by burn injury, by inhalation injury, and by therapy. Heat exposure and irritants cause swelling and tissue breakdown. Respiratory tissues are irritated by gases from burning materials, such as carbon monoxide. Altered circulation may lead to inadequate pulmonary circulation. Hypoxia may result from the decreased amount of oxygen circulating. Aspiration pneumonia may develop from vomiting episodes. Tracheal or laryngeal obstruction may result from edema in the head and neck region, causing pressure against the trachea and larynx. Also, inflamed linings of trachea and larynx swell and block the airway. Edema under tight eschar in burns of the torso restricts chest movements, which also may lead to respiratory problems. Finally, pulmonary emboli are always a danger as a result of changes in the vasculature, sepsis, and immobilization.

Physical findings in the respiratory system include singed nasal hairs and reddened or dark pharynx; irritation and heat damage to respiratory tissue may lead to respiratory stridor, dyspnea, and copious secretions, often carbonaceous. Deep full-thickness burns of the face also cause burning of pharyngeal tissues. Laryngeal edema, focal erosion, focal laryngitis, and necrosis may be seen. Edema may be exhibited in hoarseness. Respiratory problems that may occur during the course of therapy include pneumonia, atelectasis, obstruction from mucous plugs, and septic emboli from infected venosections.

The gastrointestinal tract is also affected in burn injury. Changes that occur here include acute stress (Curling's) ulcers, gastric dilatation, paralytic ileus, and bleeding.

Acute gastric and duodenal ulcers in burn patients are morphologically identical to acute stress ulcers in nonburn patients. Acute stress ulcers in patients with and without burns are mostly gastric [2]. These ulcers occur in 20 to 30 percent of persons with total body surface burns. Ulcers may be found in the stomach, the duodenum, or both. The anatomic location of stress ulcers differs from that of the peptic and duodenal ulcers not caused by stress. Stress gastric ulcers are found in the fundic mucosa, versus the pyloric mucosa of other gastric ulcers. Stress duodenal ulcers are found posteriorly, rather than anteriorly. Stress ulcers in burns have multiple foci when occurring in the stomach, and a single focus when they occur in the duodenum.

Gastric ulcers are generally smaller than duodenal ulcers. Gastric ulcers of 2 to 3 mm are difficult to see during gastroscopy, or even autopsy, but these ulcers are deep enough to cause significant bleeding. Many ulcers are hidden in the folds of the rugae. Stress ulcers exhibit a relative lack of inflammatory response, which may be due to the fact that many of these ulcers occur in the terminal stages of burn illness. Many of these stress ulcers are colonized with gram-negative bacilli. Vascular congestion and submucosal edema are often present. No single theory is held concerning pathogenesis of Curling's stress ulcers. They are similar morphologically to steroid-induced ulcers, but the pathogenesis of acute stress ulcers is different from that of peptic ulcers. Bleeding and perforation are common complications [2].

Gastric dilatation and paralytic ileus may appear early after burn injury. These problems are neurologic in origin, may be secondary to fear or pain, or may occur as a result of hypovolemia or sepsis.

Liver dysfunction often occurs with burn injury. Factors that contribute to liver dysfunction include bacterial infection, lack of proper nutrition, drugs, anesthesia, blood transfusions, leading to viral or serum hepatitis, and hepatic hypoxemia. Hepatic hypoxemia seems to be a result of a decrease in circulating fluid volume. The necrosis that results is usually minimal and focal, of a fatty nature, and reversible.

The kidney changes seen in burn injury may be permanent or temporary. Temporary kidney changes are manifested by oliguria, which results from a decreased glomerular filtration rate from the decreased circulatory volume. Blood urea nitrogen (BUN) and creatinine levels are elevated, and an increase in the antidiuretic hormone may be seen. Tubular damage may occur when the kidney is presented with an increased amount of protein breakdown products from the burn. If there is a history of prior kidney disorder, or if the person does not receive adequate treatment, permanent damage may occur. Hematuria may be seen as a result of damaged red blood cells. Death may result from acute renal insufficiency, despite adequate treatment.

Stress also causes an enhanced secretion of adrenocortical hormones. The adrenal medulla secretes large amounts of epinephrine and norepinephrine.

Problems in coagulation may occur after severe burn injury and may result from the burn, from complications secondary to the injury, or from therapy. Abnormalities seen include a decrease in the platelet count, a decrease in clot retraction time, a fall in PTT and prothrombin times, elevated fibrinogen levels, presence of a heparinlike material circulating, which causes prolonged thrombin clotting times, and depression of the prothrombin level. These defects seem to occur in large burns involving large body surface areas, as well as in smaller burns. Consumption or use of clotting factors plays a role in coagulopathies. Coagulopathies, such as disseminated intravascular coagulation (DIC), are treated with transfusions of platelets, fresh frozen plasma, whole blood, fibrinogen concentrations, and other clotting factors. Many patients die because of coagulopathies.

ELECTRICAL BURN INJURY. A variety of lesions occur as a result of electrical burn injury. Six factors play a part in determining the extent of electrical injury: (1) type of current, (2) voltage of current, (3) resistance of body tissues, (4) value of current that flows through the tissues, (5) pathway of the current through the body, and (6) duration of the contact with the electrical source [2].

The type of current, direct or alternating, has an effect on the injury. Direct current does not produce the same contraction of muscle, and low-voltage direct current is not as dangerous. High-voltage direct current is often fatal.

Alternating current seems to produce more muscle contraction at low voltages and is more dangerous than at higher voltages. Low voltage means less than 500 volts, and high voltage is greater than 500 volts. Low-tension injuries occur at home and are likely to involve children and infants [5]. The high-tension injury more commonly occurs in adults working with high-tension lines or equipment. These injuries have a high mortality, often due to cardiac arrest.

The body tissues offer varying degrees of resistance to electrical current. The resistance of tissues, in order of least to greatest, is as follows: nerve, blood, muscle, skin, tendon, fat, and bone. Skin resistance varies from person to person. The epidermis is nonvascular and offers high resistance when it is dry but, when wet, the moisture decreases resistance and enhances the flow of current. The dermis offers low resistance because of its highly vascular nature [2].

Thin skin is less resistant than thick skin, making the palms and soles more resistant. Usually, the greater the skin resistance, the greater the local burn, and the less the skin resistance, the more the internal injury. Current in contact with skin eventually causes blistering. Blisters are moist and conduct current through the skin along the tissues of least resistance, blood vessels, and nerves. Vessel walls are damaged and thrombi occur, often at a site far from the site of the electrical injury, making it difficult to evaluate the full extent of injury at the initial evaluation.

Electric current may flow through the heart, producing ventricular fibrillation and often immediate death. High-voltage current often travels to the respiratory center of the brain, causing respiratory arrest and death [2].

The value of the alternating current flowing through the body determines the resulting injury. Contact with a circuit produces muscle contraction, which may be severe enough to prevent the victim from releasing himself or herself from the source of current. If cardiac or respiratory arrest does not occur, and the victim remains conscious, he or she may complain of ringing in the ears and deafness for a time, or visual disturbances such as flashes and brilliant luminous spots.

The pathway through the body is also important in determining the extent of injury. The longer the contact, the greater amount of damage.

The injury in electrical burns may be one or more of three types: (1) entry and exit wounds of electrical injury, (2) electrothermal burns (flash or arc burns), and (3) flame burns. The entry wound occurs at the contact site with the current. It may be small or large and usually appears as an ischemic, yellow white, coagulated area, or it may be charred. It is dry, painless, and the edges are well-defined [11]. However, the extent of damage may be far greater than is seen on the surface. Necrosis of subcutaneous tissues and muscle from arterial thrombi may occur, or lack of thrombosis may cause hemorrhaging. Damage may be due to heat from the passage of current or due to the action of the current itself [11].

The exit wound appears as a blow-out type of injury caused by arcing current between victim and a nearby ground [4]. It is a dry area with depressed edges. This exit wound is usually less severe than the entry wound.

Electrothermal burns are from the heat of the current passing near, but not through, the skin. The depth of the wound depends on the closeness to the electrical source. These are mainly associated with high-tension current. The electric arc leaping from the high current has a temperature of 2500°C [2].

Flame burns occur when heat from an electric current ignites clothing. This burn may cause more serious injury than the electric injury itself.

The tetanic contractions that lock the victim to the electric source may cause fractures and dislocations of joints. Cataracts often develop months to years after an electrical injury involving the head area.

Abdominal injury may occur as a result of electrical injury to the abdomen. The extent of injury is difficult to determine at first. Abdominal symptoms may not occur until days after the injury.

Renal involvement seems to be more prevalent in electrical injury than in thermal injury. The damage may be caused by the initial electric shock, direct current damage to the kidney and/or kidney vessels, from abnormal protein breakdown in the damaged tissue, or a combination of all three [2].

CHEMICAL BURN INJURY. Chemical burns result from exposure to acid and/or alkali chemicals. Most lethal burns result from military conflict or from an industrial accident. Domestic and laboratory accidents or criminal assault usually result in smaller areas of damage [2]. The injury may result from chemical changes, as well as from thermal injury to the tissues, depending on the nature of the chemical. Chemical changes in tissues include denaturation, precipitation, alkalization, edema, separation of the epidermis from the dermis, disorganization of epidermal appendages, widening and coalescence of collagen bundles. The concentration and duration of exposure determine the extent of damage.

Acid burns more frequently occur in industrial plants as immersion injuries. The acid burn is often a result of splattering or spilling of an acid substance. The wound is painful and persists because of the chemical action. The depth and appearance of the burn vary, depending on the amount of acid and the time of exposure. Systemic changes in acid burns are rare, but inhalation of acid fumes may occur. Treatment of acid burns is best accomplished by initial dilution of the acid.

Alkali burns result from chemical irritation from a highly alkaline substance. Phosphorus burns are painful and often occur as a result of warfare. Phosphorus melts at body temperature and penetrates into tissue. When exposed to air, the wound smokes; in the dark, the wound glows bluish-green. Copper sulfate is used to treat these burns by inactivating the phosphorus. The chemical is then removed surgically. Caution must be used in working with

TABLE 41-3. Chemical burns: pathophysiology and treatment

Type	Mechanism	Appearance	Treatment		
			Cleanse	Neutralize	Debride
Acid burns					
Sulfuric Nitric Hydrochloric Trichloroacetic	Exothermic reaction; cell dehydration; protein precipitation	Gray, yellow; brown, black; soft to leathery eschar	Water	Sodium bicarbonate	Debride
Phenol			Ethyl alcohol	Sodium bicarbonate	Debride
Hydrofluoric			Water	Sodium bicarbonate; magnesium oxide; glycerin paste; calcium gluconate	Debride
Alkali burns					
Potassium hydroxide Sodium hydroxide	Exothermic reaction; cellular dehydration; saponification of fat; protein precipitation	Erythema and blister; soapy, thick eschar; painful	Water	Acetic acid or ammonium chloride	Debride
Lime			Brush off lime powder	Acetic acid or ammonium chloride	Debride
Ammonia	Same as above, plus laryngeal and pulmonary edema	Gray, yellow; brown, black; deep; soft leathery texture	Water	Acetic acid or ammonium chloride	Debride
Phosphorus	Thermal effect; melts at body temperature; runs and ignites at 34°C	Gray blue green; glows in dark; depressed, leathery eschar	Water	Copper sulfate	Debride and remove phosphorus particles

Source: K. Arndt, *Manual of Dermatologic Therapeutics* (3rd ed.). Boston: Little, Brown, 1983.

copper, as its use may result in copper toxicity with massive hemolysis of red blood cells and acute renal tubular necrosis. Table 41-3 summarizes the important chemical burns.

Complications of all types of burn wounds include infection, contractures from scarring, renal failure, ulcers, liver failure, pneumonia, urinary tract infection, and acidosis. The incidence of complications increases with the severity of the burn.

Decubitus Ulcers

The word *decubitus* derives from the Latin *decumbo*, meaning "lying down." During the late nineteenth and early twentieth centuries, people with decubitus ulcers were those with wasting diseases, such as tuberculosis, osteomyelitis, and chronic renal failure. Now, people at risk for decubiti are those with problems that alter mobility, i.e., people with spinal cord injuries; elderly people who are incontinent; or people who are bed- or wheelchair-bound. Decubiti are significant health problems, because they increase the length of hospitalization, increase health care costs, and increase the chances of death.

Four critical factors play a role in decubitus formation: (1) pressure, (2) shearing forces, (3) friction, and (4) moisture. Pressure is the most critical factor, and decubiti may accurately be called pressure sores.

Pressure is not evenly distributed over the body when lying or sitting. It is greatest over bony prominences, and it is over these areas that decubiti develop.

There exists a balance between interstitial pressure and solid tissue pressure to make a total tissue pressure of zero. With an increase in external pressure over an area, the interstitial fluid pressure increases, increasing total tissue pressure. As a result, increased capillary and arteriolar pressure occur, causing filtration of fluid from capillaries. Edema and autolysis of cells follow. As the pressure continues, lymph vessels are occluded, resulting in an accumula-

TABLE 41-4. Classification of decubiti

Stage	Layers of skin	Wound appearance	Systemic changes	Resolution
Stage 1	Partial thickness	Irregular; warm; erythema; pain; edematous	None	Reversible with relief of pressure and local cleansing
Stage 2	Partial thickness Epidermis Dermis	Shallow skin ulcer; edges distinct; fibrosis; skin color changes	None	Reversible with relief of pressure and local cleansing
Stage 3	Full thickness Epidermis Dermis Subcutaneous layer	Thick epidermal ulcer margin; light and dark pigmentation; skin layers distorted; drains foul-smelling fluid	Infection; fat necrosis; loss of fluid and protein; fever; dehydration; anemia; leukocytosis	Relief of pressure; systemic treatment with IV fluids; diet; medications; debridement and wound graft
Stage 4	Full thickness Epidermis Dermis Subcutaneous fat Fascia Muscle Bone	Large open area; bone shows through	Osteomyelitis; sepsis; joint dislocation; toxic; fatal	Radical surgery to remove necrotic areas and amputations; general support measures (IVs; diet; medications)
Closed	Subcutaneous tissue and deeper	No external sign until later, when skin ruptures; inside appears as a stage 3 or 4 wound; bursalike cavity with necrotic debris	Infrequent infection	Wide excision; removal of bursa sac; flap graft with muscle

tion of anaerobic metabolic wastes and tissue necrosis [9]. The duration and magnitude of pressure are key factors in the amount of tissue damage that may occur. With high pressure, it takes less time for tissue necrosis to occur. Constant pressure of 70 mm Hg for more than 2 hours produces irreversible tissue damage. If pressure is intermittently relieved, minimal tissue change is noted.

The sliding of adjacent tissue layers provides a progressive relative displacement of tissues. These shearing forces may be seen when the head of the bed is raised and the torso of the person slides down, exerting pressure to the sacrum and deep fascia, while the posterior sacral skin is fixed. The shearing force in the deep superficial fascia stretches and angulates blood and lymph vessels, causes thrombosis, and undermines the dermis. The subcutaneous fat layer lacks tensile strength and is vulnerable to the mechanical shearing force. The friction of two surfaces that are in contact move across each other. This action removes the outer protective stratum corneum and hastens the onset of ulceration. Friction occurs when a person is dragged across bed sheets. The so-called sheet burn occurs as a result of friction.

Genitourinary and gastrointestinal wastes and perspiration irritations macerate the skin, softening it and making it more vulnerable to pressure sore formation.

CLASSIFICATION OF DECUBITI. Decubiti may develop in stages and in categories (Table 41-4). In stage 1, the sore is reversible. The sore resembles an abrasion where the epidermis is abraded, exposing the underlying dermis. An acute inflammatory response occurs; the wound is irregular in shape, is red, warm, and indurated, and is painful in a normally innervated person. Relief of the pressure and local cleansing usually resolve the problem in 5 to 10 days.

A stage 2 decubitus ulcer is also reversible. As pressure continues, the entire dermis is affected. The wound appears as a shallow, full-thickness skin ulcer with distinct edges, early fibrosis, and skin color changes. The inflammatory response is present. Relief of pressure and local cleansing will allow the wound to heal.

In stage 3, the decubitus is extended downward, and the epidermis, dermis, and subcutaneous tissues are involved. This full-thickness skin defect spreads peripherally, because the fascia underlying the subcutaneous layer is resistant to pressure. A small broken area may appear on the surface, with a larger area occurring beneath. The epidermis thickens and rolls over the wound edge toward the ulcer base. The ulcer has a dark-light pigmentation. The skin layers are completely distorted, and the wound begins to drain foul-smelling fluid (Fig. 41-16). Systemic problems begin to occur in a stage 3 decubitus ulcer. As in a full-thickness burn injury, there is loss of fluid and protein [9]. The person may experience fever, dehydration, anemia, and leukocytosis.

In a stage 4 wound, the fascia underlying the subcutaneous tissue is penetrated and undermining of the wound is rapid. Complications include osteomyelitis of bone, sepsis, joint dislocations, and release of toxins. The situation may

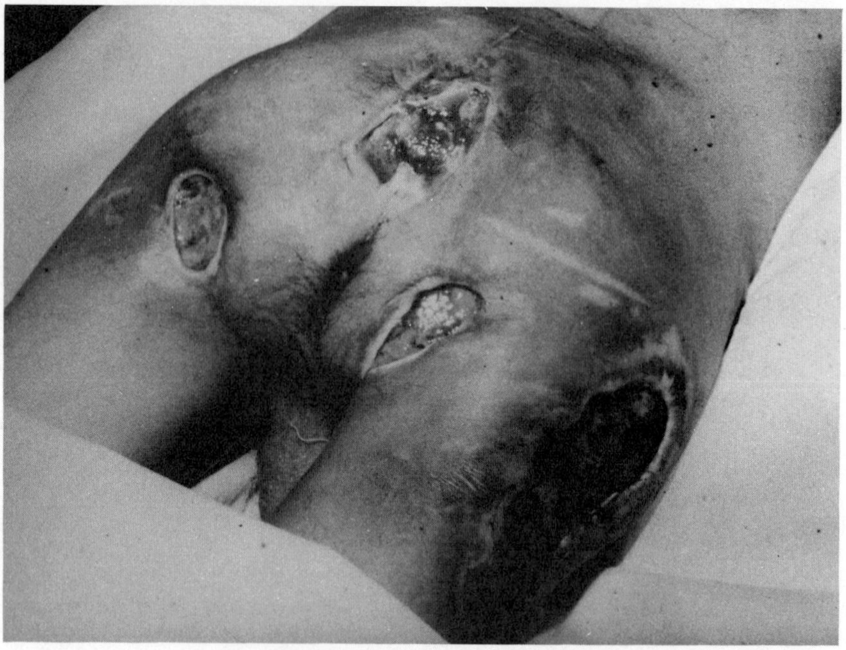

FIGURE 41-16. This sacral ulcer, because of widely undermined edges produced by shearing forces, communicates with ischial and trochanteric ulcers bilaterally. (From M. B. Constantian, *Pressure Ulcers*. Boston: Little, Brown, 1980.)

become fatal [9].

A closed decubitus has no external opening but, inside, may act and appear as a stage 3 or 4 lesion. These decubiti occur after long pressure insults with shear stress. A bursalike cavity forms and is filled with debris from the necrosis of subcutaneous and deeper areas. This type of decubitus often occurs over ischial tuberosities. Eventually, the overlying skin ruptures.

Other Trauma

Other traumas to the skin include abrasions (scrapes), incised wounds (as an incision), puncture wounds, and lacerations (cuts). An abrasion is a superficial open wound in which the outer surface layers of skin are scraped off. Nerve endings are exposed, and there is minimal bleeding. There is often foreign material on the wound that should be removed, and the wound should be cleansed. This type of wound normally heals spontaneously. An incision is a clean, straight-edged wound; it bleeds freely, goes through all layers of skin, and heals cleanly when sutured. Puncture or stab wounds are deeper than they are wide and are caused by knives, pins, needles, spikes, and so forth. Damage to underlying structures may be present, with concealed blood loss. A laceration is a cut or tear of tissues and is unlikely to heal without treatment [12].

REFERENCES

1. Arndt, K. *Manual of Dermatologic Therapeutics* (3rd ed.). Boston: Little, Brown, 1983.
2. Artz, C.P., and Moncrief, J.A. *The Treatment of Burns.* Philadelphia: Saunders, 1969.
3. Beeson, P., McDermott, W., and Wyngaarden, J. *Cecil Textbook of Medicine* (15th ed.). Philadelphia: Saunders, 1979.
4. Feller, I., and Archambealt-Jones, C. *Nursing the Burned Patient.* Ann Arbor: National Institute for Burn Medicine, 1973.
5. Hunt, J.L. Electrical Injuries of the Upper Extremity. In R. Salisbury and B. Pruitt (eds.), *Burns of the Upper Extremity.* Philadelphia: Saunders, 1976.
6. Jacoby, F. G. *Nursing Care of the Patient with Burns.* St. Louis: Mosby, 1976.
7. Levene, G.M., and Calnan, D.C. *Color Atlas of Dermatology.* Chicago: Year Book, 1974.
8. Moschella, S.L., Pillsbury, D.M., and Hurley, H.J. *Dermatology.* Philadelphia: Saunders, 1975.
9. Reuler, J., and Cooney, T. G. The pressure sore: Pathophysiology and principles of management. *Ann. Intern. Med.* 94:661, 1981.
10. Robbins, S., and Cotran, R. *Pathologic Bases of Disease* (2nd ed.). Philadelphia: Saunders, 1979.
11. Salisbury, R.E., and Pruitt, B.A. *Burns of the Upper Extremity.* Philadelphia: Saunders, 1976.
12. Spittell, A.J. *Clinical Medicine.* Hagerstown, Md.: Harper & Row, 1982.

BIBLIOGRAPHY

Arndt, K. *Manual of Dermatologic Therapeutics* (3rd ed.). Boston: Little, Brown, 1983.

Balinsky, B. I. *An Introduction to Embryology* (5th ed.). Philadelphia: Saunders, 1981.

Baur, P.S., Parks, D.H., and Larson, D.L. The healing of burn wounds. *Clin. Plast. Surg.* 4:389, 1977.

Beeson, P., McDermott, W., and Wyngaarden, J. *Cecil Textbook of Medicine* (15th ed.). Philadelphia: Saunders, 1979.

Bickley, H. *Practical Concepts in Human Disease* (2nd ed.). Baltimore: Williams & Wilkins, 1980.

Bryant, W. Wound healing. *Clin. Symp.* 29:1, 1977.

Carpenter, N. H., Gates, D. J., and Williams, H. T. Normal processes and restraints in wound healing. *Can. J. Surg.* 20:315, 1977.

Cohen, I. K., and Diegelmann, R. F. The biology of keloid and hypertrophic scars and influence of corticosteroids. *Clin. Plast. Surg.* 4:297, 1977.

Crouch, J., and McClintic, J. R. *Human Anatomy and Physiology.* New York: Wiley, 1976.

Guyton, A. *Textbook of Medical Physiology* (6th ed.). Philadelphia: Saunders, 1981.

Hayes, H., Jr. A review of modern concepts of healing of cutaneous wounds. *J. Dermatol. Surg. Oncol.* 3:188, 1977.

Ketchum, L. D. Hypertrophic scars and keloids. *Clin. Plast. Surg.* 4:301, 1977.

Larson, C., and Gould, M. *Orthopedic Nursing* (9th ed.). St. Louis: Mosby, 1978.

Levene, G. M., and Calnan, D. C. *Color Atlas of Dermatology.* Chicago: Year Book, 1974.

Levenson, S. M., and Seifter, E. Dysnutrition, wound healing, and resistance to infection. *Clin. Plast. Surg.* 4:375, 1977.

Miller, F. N. *Peery and Miller's Pathology* (3rd ed.). Boston: Little, Brown, 1978.

Montandon, D., D'Andrian, G., and Gabbiani, G. The mechanism of wound contraction and epithelialization. *Clin. Plast. Surg.* 4:325, 1977.

Moschella, S., Pillsbury, D., and Hurley, H. *Dermatology.* Philadelphia: Saunders, 1975.

Nicoletis, C., Bazin, S., and LeLous, M. Clinical and biochemical features of normal, defective and pathologic scars. *Clin. Plast. Surg.* 4:347, 1977.

Ninikoski, J. Oxygen and wound healing. *Clin. Plast. Surg.* 4:361, 1977.

Price, S., and Wilson, L. *Pathophysiology: Clinical Concepts of Disease Processes* (2nd ed.). New York: McGraw-Hill, 1982.

Purtilo, D. *A Survey of Human Diseases.* Reading, Mass.: Addison-Wesley, 1978.

Robbins, S., and Cotran, R. *Pathologic Basis of Disease.* Philadelphia: Saunders, 1974.

Rosen, K., et al. *The Nurse's Atlas of Dermatology.* Boston: Little, Brown, 1983.

Sabiston, D. C. *Davis-Christopher: Textbook of Surgery* (11th ed.). Philadelphia: Saunders, 1977.

Salisbury, R., and Pruitt, B. *Burns of the Upper Extremity.* Philadelphia: Saunders, 1976.

Sana, R., and Judge, R. *Physical Assessment Skills for Nursing Practice.* Boston: Little, Brown, 1982.

Selye, H. *The Stress of Life* (2nd ed.). New York: McGraw-Hill, 1978.

Spittell, J. A. *Clinical Medicine.* Hagerstown, Md.: Harper & Row, 1981.

Walter, J. *An Introduction to the Principles of Disease* (2nd ed.). Philadelphia: Saunders, 1982.

Williams, D. F., and Harrison, I. D. The variation of mechanical properties in different areas of a healing wound. *J. Biomech.* 10:633, 1977.

UNIT 15

NEURAL CONTROL

Reet Henze
NORMAL STRUCTURE AND FUNCTION OF THE CENTRAL AND PERIPHERAL NERVOUS SYSTEM
ADAPTATION AND ALTERATION IN THE SPECIAL SENSES
TRAUMATIC ALTERATIONS

Gretchen McDaniel
TUMORS AND INFECTIONS OF THE CENTRAL NERVOUS SYSTEM

Karen Jones
DEGENERATIVE AND OTHER ALTERATIONS IN THE NERVOUS SYSTEM
EPILEPSY

M. S. Megahed
Pearl Rosendahl
ALTERATIONS IN SENSATION
DISTURBANCES OF CONSCIOUSNESS
ALTERATIONS IN HIGHER CORTICAL FUNCTION

June Larrabee
ALTERATIONS IN MOVEMENT

The nervous system is incredibly complex and must be approached from an adequate basic knowledge of neural control. This approach considers the complicated system of connections and interconnections that allow for perception and movement. The advanced nervous system allows for the achievement of complicated thought and reasoning powers. Chapter 42 begins the discussion with the normal structure and function of the nervous system. Chapter 43 adds the normal and altered function of the special senses. Chapter 44 details some alterations that affect higher cortical functions, especially cerebrovascular accident, aphasia, agnosia, and epilepsy. Chapters 45, 46, and 47 detail traumatic alterations, tumors and infections, and degenerative alterations respectively. Each chapter presents specific diagnostic tests that may be helpful in delineating these alterations.

An attempt has been made to discuss neural pathology in sufficient depth for understanding without requiring a complete textbook on the topic.

The most useful approach to the nervous system shows how alterations in specific areas can disrupt function. Frequently the location of the alterations rather than their size, finally determines how much functional difficulty will occur. The reader is again encouraged to utilize the learning objectives to organize study and to acquire a firm grasp of the material in Chapter 42 before considering the pathophysiology of the system.

CHAPTER 42
NORMAL STRUCTURE AND FUNCTION OF THE CENTRAL AND PERIPHERAL NERVOUS SYSTEMS

LEARNING OBJECTIVES

1. Identify the components of the neuron.
2. Describe variations in neuron morphology.
3. Discuss classification of neurons according to function.
4. Explain the events occurring with axon injury and regeneration.
5. Define *membrane potential*.
6. Discuss the events of the action potential.
7. List the major types of nerve fibers and their characteristics.
8. Identify factors influencing conduction velocity in nerve fibers.
9. Identify factors that increase neuron membrane excitability.
10. Identify factors that decrease neuron membrane excitability.
11. Define *sensory receptors.*
12. Explain types of sensory receptors.
13. Discuss the phenomenon of receptor adaptation.
14. Contrast receptor potential and generator potential.
15. Define *synapse.*
16. Discuss the events occurring at the chemical synapse.
17. Discuss characteristics of neurotransmitters.
18. List the major structures of the central nervous system in hierarchical order from spinal cord to cerebral cortex.
19. Identify the major functions of the central nervous system structures.
20. Trace the major ascending and descending spinal tracts.
21. Identify the major information transmitted by the ascending and descending spinal tracts.
22. List the components of the peripheral nervous system.
23. Differentiate between the structure and function of the somatic efferent and of the visceral efferent fibers.
24. Contrast the functions of the sympathetic and parasympathetic divisions of the autonomic nervous system.
25. Differentiate between adrenergic and cholinergic effector organs.
26. Describe the function, formation, and flow of cerebrospinal fluid.
27. Discuss the function of the blood-brain barrier.
28. List the major arteries supplying blood to the brain.
29. Discuss the factors responsible for cerebral vasomotor control.

Humans interact with the environment through the nervous system perceiving and responding to the stimuli that continually impinge on them. An incredibly complex system of connections and interconnections of nerve cells functions to provide this perception, interim processing, and response. In addition, unique characteristics of humans that endow the ability to think, feel, reason, and remember evolve from these complex interacting neuronal networks of the human brain.

THE NEURON

The neuron (Fig. 42-1) is the structural and functional unit of nerve tissue, having the capability of generating and conducting electrochemical impulses. Its cellular and cytoplasmic components and metabolic activities maintaining cell life are similar to those of other cells. The distinctive cellular shapes of neurons and their structural synapses that allow transmission of impulses from one neuron to another are unique to the nerve cells. Unlike other cells, the mature neuron is unable to reproduce itself. Centrosomes are lacking in the neuron and, therefore, neurons are incapable of mitosis, if the cell body dies, the entire neuron dies. However, under certain circumstances, *axons,* the processes of peripheral nerves, regenerate if the cell body is preserved.

Incoming signals to the neuron body are transmitted by *dendrites,* which are short projections from the cell body of the neuron. Dendrites, along with the cell body, contain *Nissl particles,* which are involved in cell protein synthesis and contain much of the ribonucleic acid (RNA) of the cytoplasm.

A fibrous *axon*, or nerve fiber, originates from the *axon hillock* of the cell body (perikaryon) and transmits signals from the cell body to various parts of the nervous system. These long fibers differ from dendrites in their branching and in composition of their outer membrane. Some axons are myelinated while others exist without a myelin sheath. Myelin is a fatty layer that surrounds the nerve fiber. The *myelin sheath* is interrupted by periodic gaps known as the *nodes of Ranvier.* Axon collaterals or fibers may emerge from these gaps. Exchange of metabolites takes place between the axon and the extracellular environment at the nodes. The nodes of Ranvier are found in both the central and the peripheral nervous system neurons; however, they are much easier to identify in the peripheral nervous system. *Schwann cells* are found along the peripheral axons and produce the myelin sheath of lipoprotein that encase the fiber. Some of these cells produce numerous concentric wrappings around the central core axon and give the axon its characteristic white color (Fig. 42-2). Unmyelinated fibers contain Schwann cells but lack the concentric wrappings. The outermost thin layer of myelin of the myelinated fibers is known as the *neurolemma* of the axon. This neurolemma is lacking in the myelinated fibers within the spinal cord and brain. Myelin provides a protective, nutritive, and conductive function for the axon.

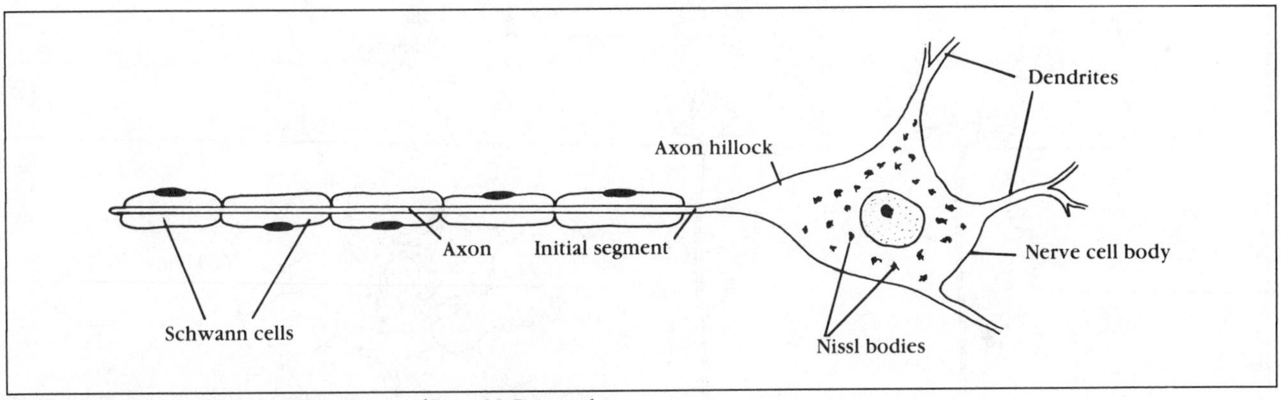

FIGURE 42-1. Neuron with myelinated axon. (From M. Borysenko, et al., *Functional Histology* [2nd ed.]. Boston: Little, Brown, 1984.)

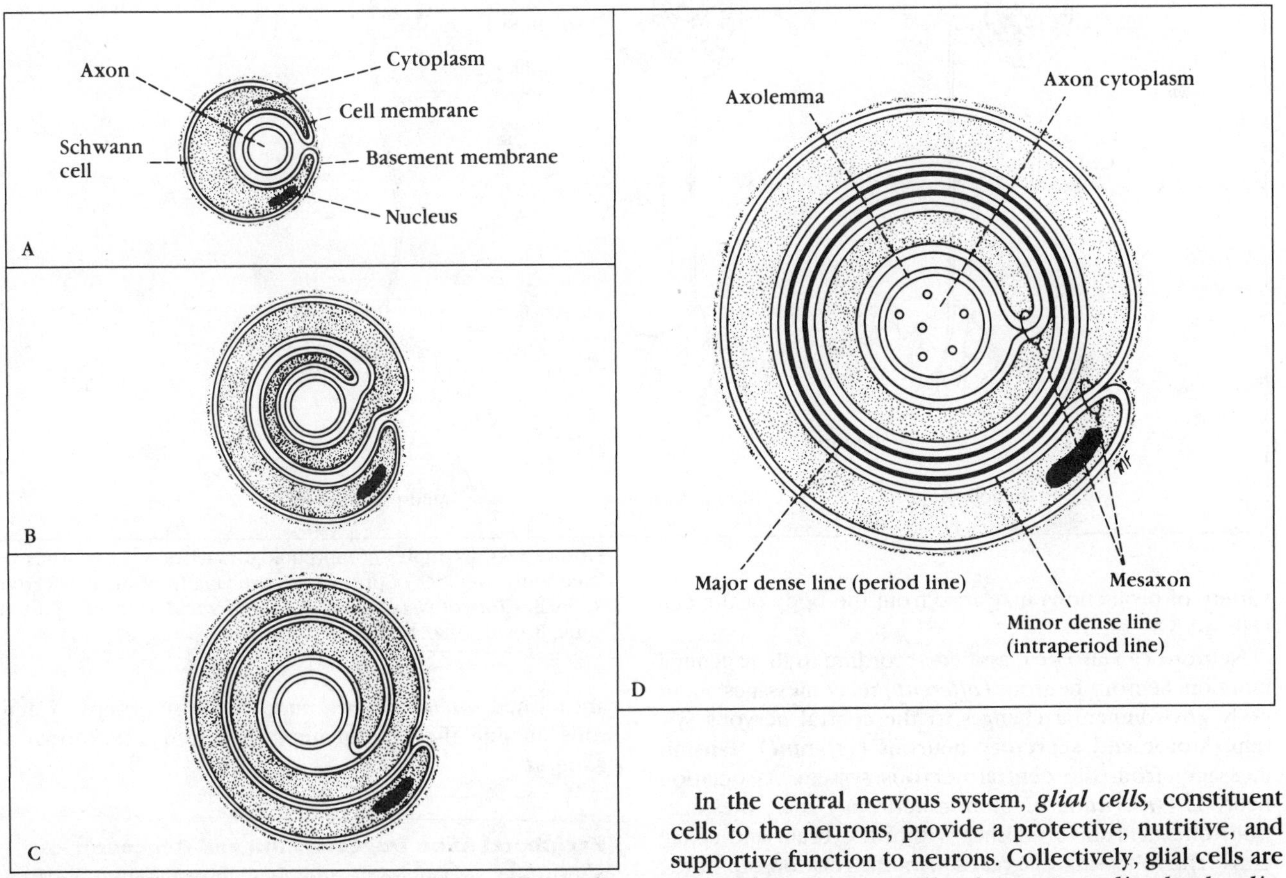

FIGURE 42-2. Schematic representation of evolution of the myelin sheath of an axon. A. Schwann cell engulfs the axon, B. surrounds it, and C. wraps tight concentric layers (myelin sheath). D. Appearance of mature axon and myelinated sheath. (From R. Snell, *Clinical Neuroanatomy for Medical Students.* Boston: Little, Brown, 1980.)

In the central nervous system, ***glial cells,*** constituent cells to the neurons, provide a protective, nutritive, and supportive function to neurons. Collectively, glial cells are referred to as ***neuroglia. Astrocytes, oligodendroglia, microglia,*** and ***ependymal*** are different types of glial cells [6]. Astrocytes, the most plentiful of the glial cells, provide structural support and nourishment for the neurons. Oligodendroglia form myelin along axons and the microglia have phagocytic properties. Ependymal cells line the ventricles of the brain and central canal of the spinal cord.

The billions of neurons in the nervous system may be identified according to their *morphology* and *function.* A

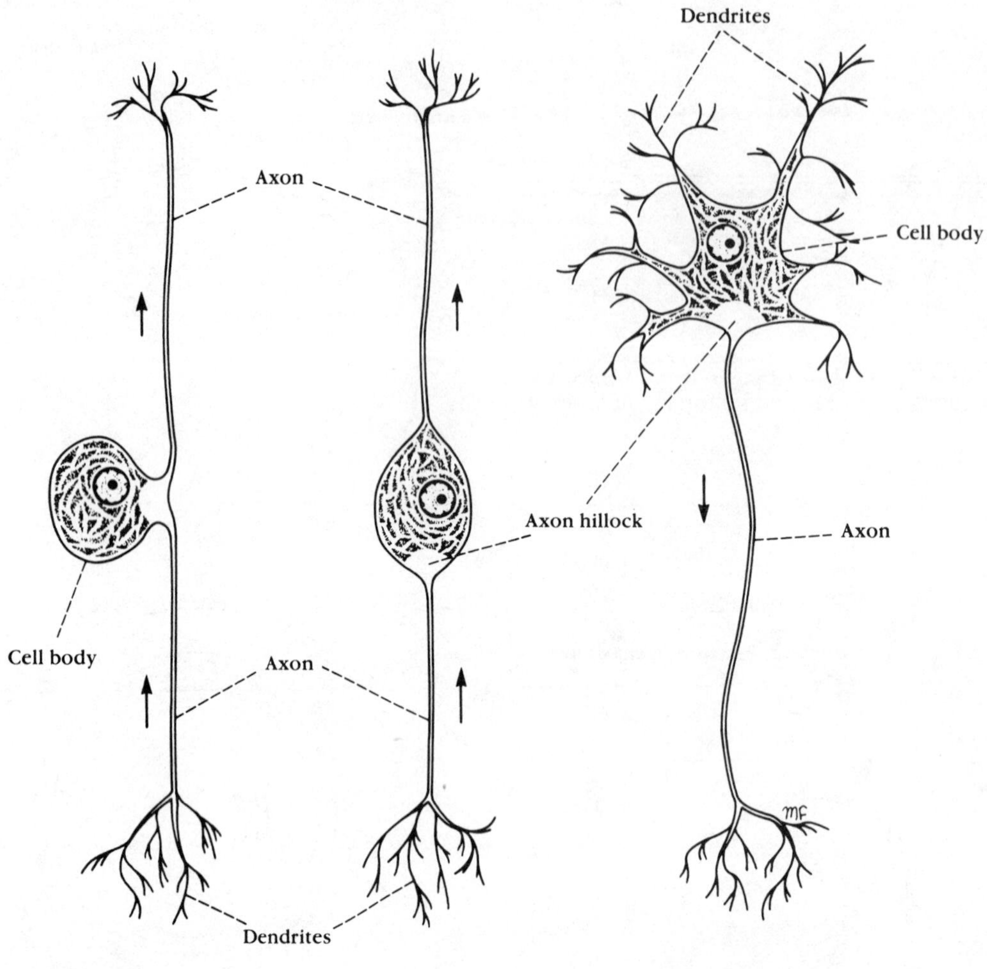

FIGURE 42-3. Examples of morphologic variations in neurons related to the number of projections evolving from the cell. (From R. Snell, *Clinical Neuroanatomy for Medical Students*. Boston: Little, Brown, 1980.)

variety of projections may arise from the body of the cell (Fig. 42-3).

Neurons can also be classified according to their general function. Sensory neurons (*afferent*) relay messages about body environmental changes to the central nervous system. Motor and secretory neurons (*efferent*) transmit messages from the central nervous system. Association neurons (*internuncial* or *interneurons*) relay messages from one neuron to another within the brain and spinal cord. The following diagram shows the relationship of the afferent, association, and efferent neurons and their fibers as sensations are perceived from the somatic and visceral tissue and transmitted to glands and muscles.

		CNS		
Somatic Visceral	Afferent → fibers	Interneurons	Efferent → fibers	Glands Muscles

Clusters of neurons within the central nervous system are termed *nuclei*, or *gray matter*. Those groups of neurons outside the central nervous system are known as *ganglia*.

Peripheral Axon Degeneration and Regeneration

A crushed or severed axon of a peripheral nerve fiber triggers certain processes within a few hours of injury. Changes in the axon distal to the injury (*wallerian degeneration*) are particularly dramatic, since that portion has been severed from the metabolic control of the cell body. Initially the distal portion swells and the terminal neurofilaments hypertrophy. The myelin sheath shrinks and retracts at the nodes of Ranvier where the remaining nerve fiber becomes exposed. The axon gradually disappears and

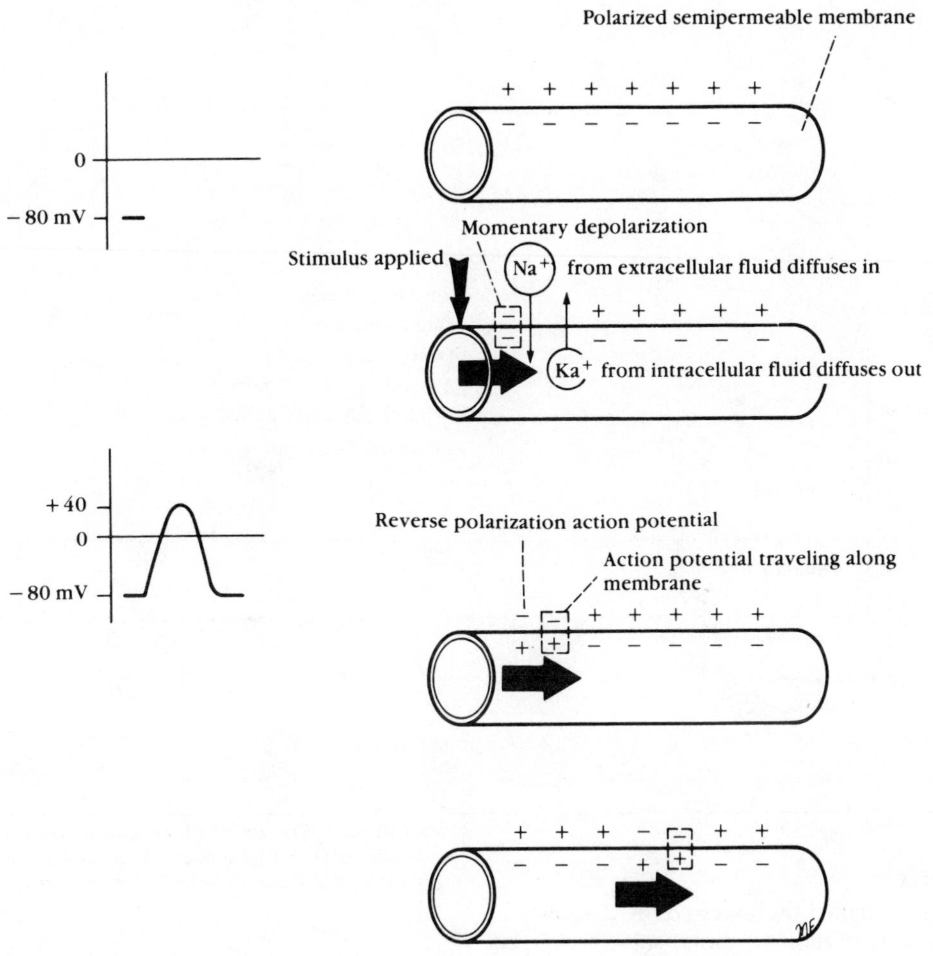

FIGURE 42-4. Summary of electrical changes occurring in the axon during an action potential. (From R. Snell, *Clinical Neuroanatomy for Medical Students*. Boston: Little, Brown, 1980.)

the myelin disintegrates into fragments and is phagocytized by the Schwann cells.

Changes are also seen proximal to the injury, both in the axon and the cell body itself. Degenerative changes similar to those in the distal portion of the axon are seen at the proximal portion for a few millimeters from the injury. The changes observed in the cell body are in response to repair of damages. The cellular cytoplasm swells and the nucleus is eccentrically placed toward the cell wall. Chromatolysis of basophilic substances (Nissl bodies), suggestive of increased protein synthesis, takes place and the number of mitochondria increase. Injured neurofibrils (delicate threads projecting into the axon from the cell body) will attempt to grow back into their original placements and begin sprouting from the proximal portion of the injured axon within 7 to 14 days from injury. If the fibrils are successful in finding their way into the neurolemma, they will grow at a rate of 3 to 4 mm per day. The remaining Schwann cells form a sheet of myelin around the restored neurofibril and the nodes of Ranvier are reformed as the nerve regenerates. Regeneration of injured nerves in the central nervous system is more difficult due to glial (supportive tissue) scarring, which frequently inhibits new fibrils from reaching their destinations.

EXCITATION AND CONDUCTION IN NEURONS

Membrane Potential

Membrane potentials are generated because of a disparity between cations and anions at the semipermeable cell membrane. Specific proteins at the cell membrane allow the movement of ions and facilitate the existence of the nerve cell potential and impulse propagation. These proteins include *cell membrane pumps* and *channels.* Pumps maintain appropriate ion concentrations in the cell side of the membrane by actively moving these against concentration gradients. Channel proteins provide selective paths for specific ions to diffuse across the cell membrane.

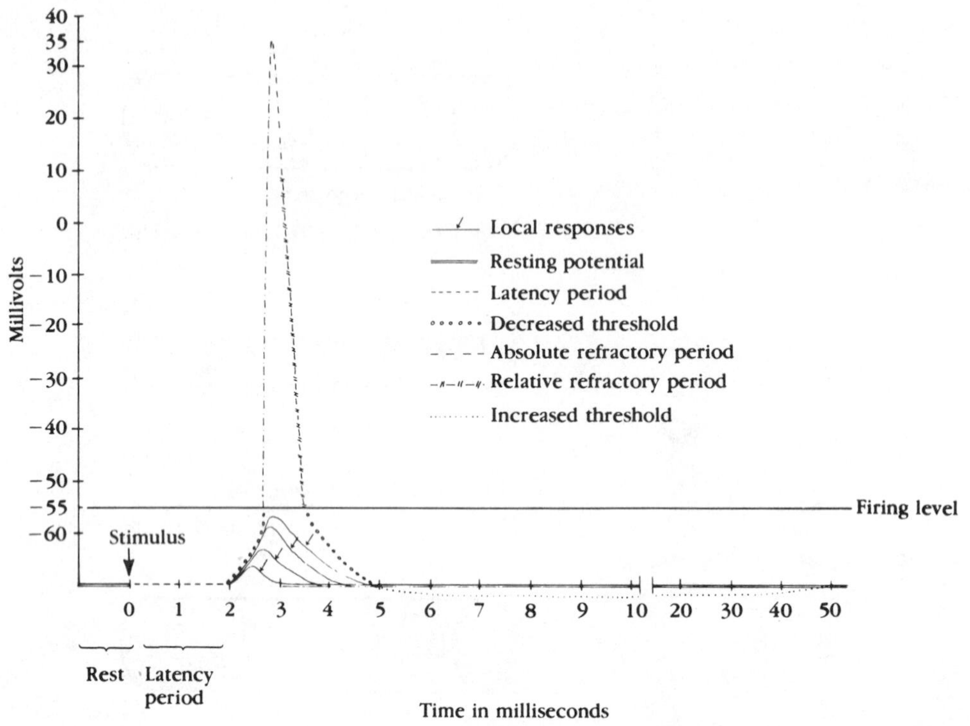

FIGURE 42-5. The action potential and associated refractory periods. (From D. R. Dickson and W. Maue-Dickson, *Anatomical and Physiological Bases of Speech*. Boston: Little, Brown, 1982.)

Resting Potential

During the resting potential the inner cell wall surface is negatively charged in relation to the positively charged outer surface (Fig. 42-4). The extracellular fluid has a much higher sodium concentration than the intracellular fluid whereas potassium concentration is much higher within the cell. The inside of the cell contains many anions that are too large to pass across the cell membrane. These attract the positively charged sodium ions, some of which leak through the sodium channels of the cell membrane. Should this movement continue unchecked, the influx of the positively charged ions into the cell would soon result in electroneutrality in the cell. To counterbalance this diffusion of ions, a strong active transport system (sodium pump) pumps out sodium that has leaked into the cell and helps maintain the appropriate sodium concentrations on both sides of the cell membrane (see Chap. 1).

The higher intracellular concentration of potassium ions is maintained primarily through its passive movement. Potassium diffuses across the cell membrane through its channels with more ease than sodium. A weaker potassium pump also moves some potassium from the extracellular to the intracellular fluid. More sodium is pumped out of the cell than potassium into the cell, three sodium ions for each two potassium ions. This is how the resting cell membrane maintains electropositive charges on the outer surface. In this state the cell is said to be *polarized*. The inner surface remains electronegative and maintains a resting potential of approximately −70 to −90 mV. Lacking a stimulus, the resting potential can remain unchanged for long periods of time [3].

Action Potential Propagation

Unique to nerve, muscle, and gland cells is the change that can occur in a resting cell membrane potential when the cells are stimulated by electrical, chemical, or mechanical means. The stimuli produce a sudden increase in cell membrane permeability to sodium. A very brief, positive potential within the cell results.

A sequence of physiochemical events last about 1 msec and is called the *action potential* (see Fig. 42-4). In response to a stimulus the cell membrane becomes much more permeable to sodium ions that rush into the cell through the opened sodium channels and cause the initial spike potential (Fig. 42-5). Due to the positive changes carried into the cell by sodium a change in the voltage occurs inside the axon from approximately −70 mV at resting potential to about +40 mV at the height of the spike. This phase of the action potential identified as *depolarization*, travels in both directions along the entire fiber.

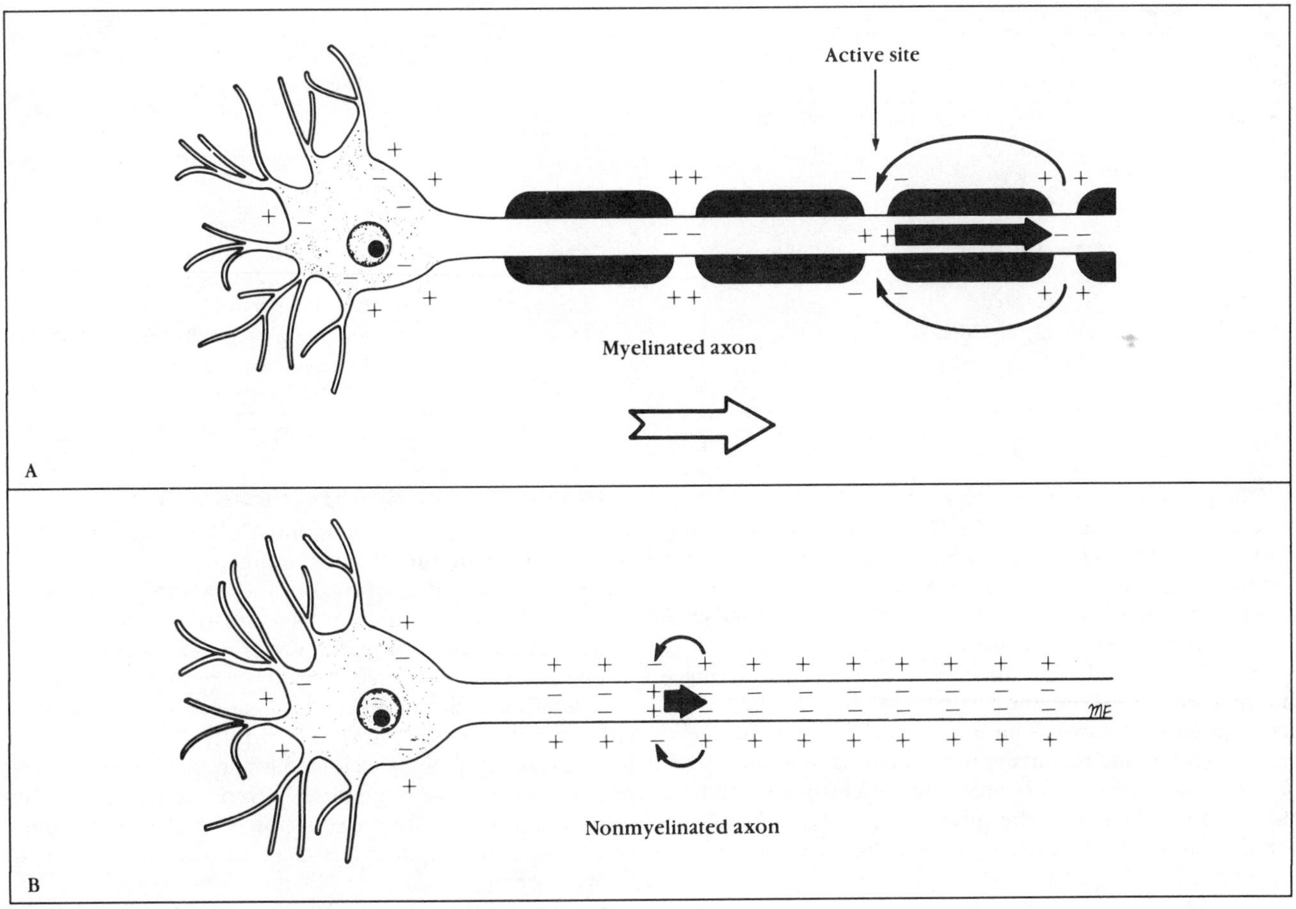

FIGURE 42-6. Propagation of the action potential along A. myelinated and B. unmyelinated axon. (From R. Snell, *Clinical Neuroanatomy for Medical Students*. Boston: Little, Brown, 1980.)

The influx of sodium is limited because permeability of the cell membrane to sodium is transient and the channels formerly open to sodium close. During a very brief time, called the *absolute refractory period*, the nerve cell responds to no further stimulus. Following the absolute refractory period, the *relative refractory period* occurs during which time the cell gradually resumes its excitability and is able to respond to stronger than normal stimuli. As the sodium permeability decreases, potassium permeability increases and there is an efflux of potassium from the cell, which is reflected by the negative afterpotential shown in Fig. 42-5. The efflux of potassium allows the inside of the cell to become more negative once again. This period of return to original potential is called the *repolarization phase.*

Finally, the cell membrane becomes less permeable to potassium and the sodium pump transports sodium out of the cell. This pump is reflected by a "positive" afterpotential. Simultaneously, potassium shifts into the cell through both membrane channels and pumps, returning the fiber to its original potential. The terminology "positive" and "negative" afterpotentials are labeled as such because they were first measured outside the nerve fibers rather than inside. Modern terminology expresses these in terms of *inside* rather than *outside* potentials.

Depolarization, in response to the stimulus, progresses along the nerve fiber and is self-propagating (Fig. 42-6). As the current flows along the adjoining resting membrane, it increases the permeability of the membrane to sodium and thus depolarizes this area. The current flow is continuous until the action potential has propagated the entire length of the axon, very much like a flame travels the fuse of a firecracker [7].

Characteristics of the Action Potential

The lowest point at which a stimulus can elicit excitation of a fiber is known as the *threshold potential*, and its value differs with various types of nerve cells. For most neurons, the threshold potential is about 15 mV above the resting potential. For example, if the resting potential of a neuron is −80 mV, its threshold potential would be about −65 mV.

Once the threshold potential is reached, the stimulus will travel until total depolarization of the axon is accomplished. The commencement of depolarization ensures propagation of the impulse along the entire axon, irrespective of changes in the stimulus that originally initiated

TABLE 42-1. Major nerve fiber classification

Fiber type	Sheathing	Diameter (μm)	Conduction speed (m/sec)	Function
A fibers				
Alpha	Myelinated	10–18	120	Somatic motor, muscle proprioceptors
Beta	Myelinated	5–10	70	Motor and rapid sensory touch, kinesthesia
Gamma	Myelinated	1–5	30	Motor to muscle spindle, rapid sensory (touch, pressure)
Delta	Myelinated	2–5	12–30	Pain, temperature, pressure
B fibers	Thinly myelinated	3	15	Automatic preganglionic transmission
C fibers	Unmyelinated	1–3	2	Automatic postganglionic transmission

it. This phenomenon is known as the "*all or none*" law, which applies to excitable cells. The impulse propagation continues at the same speed and intensity and remains unchanged by increasing stimulus intensity. However, a stronger stimulus increases the frequency of the impulses that will be initiated during the relative refractory period.

Nerve trunks contain many neurons, which have varying independent threshold and velocity values, and the total action potential known as the *compound action potential* may depend on the number of neurons firing. A weak stimulus activates only a few neurons, while a strong stimulus excites more neurons. The total action potential of the nerve trunk is the summation of the active neuron action potentials.

Conduction Velocity in Nerve Fibers

The velocity of nerve conduction is influenced by the myelinization and diameter of the axon. Myelin acts as an effective insulator and inhibits electrochemical conduction. Therefore, the current passes over the myelin, through the extracellular fluid, and enters the nodes of Ranvier at 1- to 2-mm intervals where the membrane is permeable to the ions. This type of current propagation is known as *saltatory conduction*, implying a leaping or hopping phenomenon [3] (Fig. 42-6A).

The myelin sheath enhances current conduction velocity as capacitance is reduced, which results in a reduced number of charges propagating the length of the fiber. The heavily myelinated large motor fibers transmit impulses at approximately 100 m/sec. In contrast, small unmyelinated fibers may conduct impulses as slow as 0.5 m/sec.

The diameter of the fiber is an additional important factor contributing to nerve conduction velocity. Velocity is increased in large-diameter nerve fibers due to lower internal resistance and a quicker depolarization time. Table 42-1 presents the relationship of nerve fibers to conduction velocities.

Factors Increasing Membrane Excitability

Extrinsic and intrinsic conditions affecting the permeability of the sodium ion can have profound effects on cell excitability. Certain drugs can alter the sodium permeability so that facilitory and inhibitory mechanisms of the cell can no longer function normally. Veratrine, an alkaloid compound, for example increases sodium permeability at the cell membrane and thus greatly enhances impulse generation in response to minimal stimuli. Because of the hyperexcitability of the cell membrane that veratrine produces, ingestion of large doses is reflected clinically by central nervous system excitation, muscular twitching, seizures, total body pruritus, paresthesia, and cardiopulmonary arrest.

Another mechanism increasing nerve cell membrane excitability is a low extracellular calcium level. Normally, calcium binds with some of the sodium channels and thereby reduces the movement of sodium across the membrane. With less calcium bound to the sodium channels, the movement of sodium becomes less restricted. This increased cell permeability to sodium results in progressively more excitable neuronal tissue that is manifested clinically by a wide range of signs including paresthesia, muscular twitching, carpopedal spasms, laryngeal stridor in children, bronchial spasms, tetanic spasms, and convulsions.

Factors Decreasing Membrane Excitability

On the other hand, increased calcium levels in the extracellular fluid decrease membrane excitability by reducing the membrane permeability that inhibits sodium passage through its channels. Calcium has high protein-binding power as well as positive charges that facilitate its repulsion of sodium at the cell membrane. This results in an inhibitory or stabilizing effect on the cell membrane. Clinically, excess serum calcium levels are reflected by central nervous system depression.

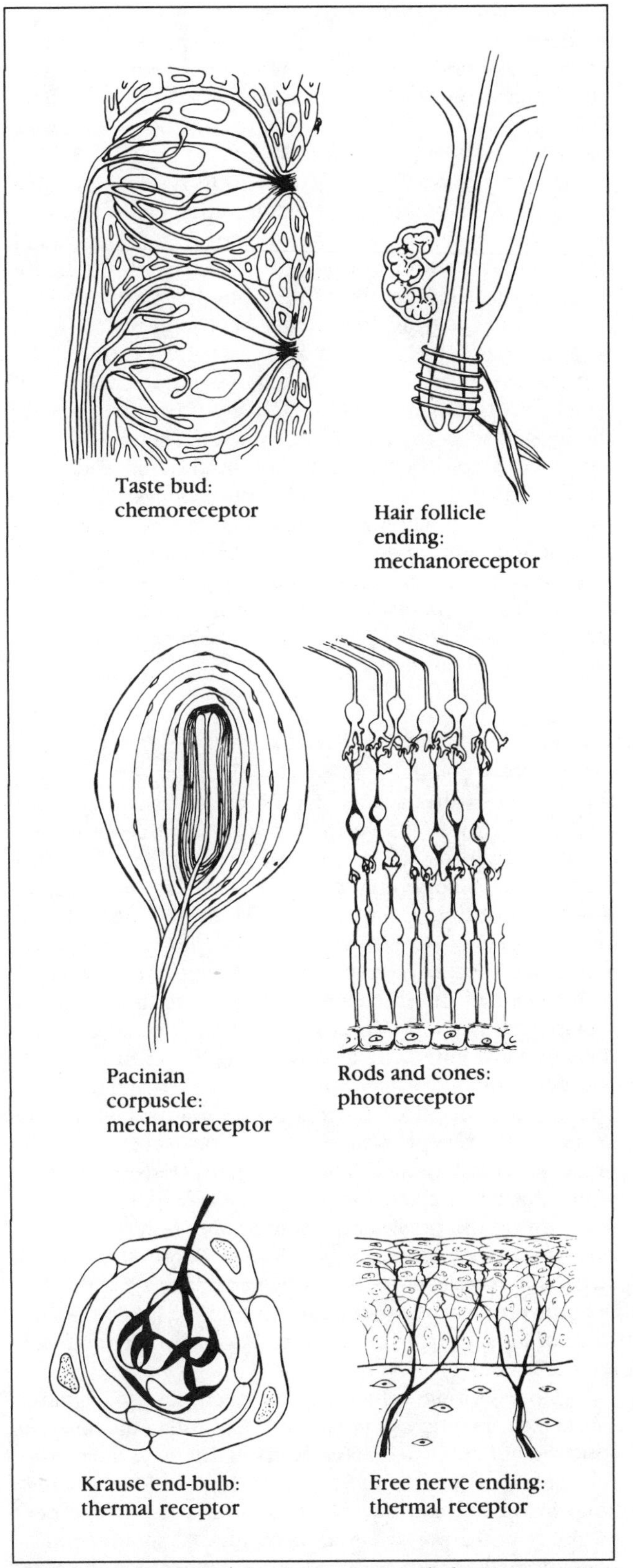

FIGURE 42-7. Examples of variations in morphologic composition of somatic sensory receptors. (From D. M. McKeough, *The Coloring Review of Neuroscience.* Boston: Little, Brown, 1982.)

Decreased levels of potassium in the extracellular fluids also decrease the membrane excitability by increasing the resting potential of the membrane. The resting potential is dependent on a constant concentration of potassium. The effect of a low extracellular potassium level is reflected clinically by depressed neuromuscular excitation, generalized weakness and fatigability of all muscles, diminished or absent reflexes, and paralytic ileus.

Local anesthetics such as lidocaine and tetracaine are other examples of factors that can interfere with the initiation and transmission of the action potential. Depolarization is prevented by decreasing the membrane permeability to sodium and the negative potential necessary for a propagated discharge does not develop or pass through the anesthetized area. The ease of anesthetization is related to nerve fiber size. Small fibers associated with temperature and superficial pain sensations are most easily anesthetized. Large fibers transmitting sensation of deep pain, touch, and pressure are anesthetized with more difficulty.

RECEPTORS

Characteristics of Receptors

Sensory receptors are specialized nerve cells that respond to specific information from the internal and external environment; the information is then transmitted to specific areas of the central nervous system for interpretation. This is accomplished through conversion of various forms of natural energy from the environment into action potentials in neurons. Common to all receptors is this *transduction* of energy. Energy, converted by receptors, includes mechanical energy by *mechanoreceptors,* thermal energy by *thermoreceptors,* light energy by *photoreceptors,* and chemical energy by *chemoreceptors.* Receptors that respond to physical and chemical tissue deformation are known as *nociceptors. Exteroreceptors* give information about the external environment and *interoceptors* and *proprioceptors* are sensitive to internal impulses and changes. *Teleceptors,* such as those found in the eye and ear, provide information from a more distant environment.

Receptor cells exhibit a wide range of morphologic and sensitivity differences [3] (Fig. 42-7). Some have free nerve endings with coils, spirals, and branching networks and may be found throughout the body and detect pain, cold, warmth, and crude touch. Some receptor cells are encased in variously shaped capsules and detect tissue deformation. Each receptor cell has adapted to respond to one specific type or modality of stimulus at a much lower threshold than do other receptors. This response is referred to as *adequate stimulus.* Each nerve tract terminates at a specific point in the central nervous system where interpretation of that specific stimulus is made. The response remains the same no matter how the receptor is stimulated.

When a constant stimulus has been applied to a receptor for a period of time, the frequency of action potentials initiated in the sensory nerve decreases. This phenomenon is known as *adaptation.* There is a wide variation in sensory organ adaptation. The pressure applied to a pacinian corpuscle results in a receptor potential that adapts rapidly. The fast adapting receptors are called *phasic* receptors. In contrast, the muscle spindles and receptors for pain adapt very slowly. These receptors are known as *tonic* receptors.

Receptor Potential

The modalities of sensation are converted by the specific receptors into electrical energy by action potentials through graded potential changes. The receptor responses are not an all-or-nothing event like the action potentials of neurons, but rather the magnitude is dependent on the intensity of the stimulus. As the magnitude of the stimulus is increased, the receptor potential increases. Receptor potentials are stationary, producing a local flow of current that spreads electrically to surrounding areas of the cell through a change of ionic conductance of the membrane of the nerve terminal. The ionic permeability change initiating the receptor potential depends only on the stimulus, not on conductance changes through the function of the membrane potential as brought about in the action potentials. Because the receptor potential is not dependent on the membrane potential, it does not regenerate and remains stationary at the transducer area of the nerve terminal. If the receptor potential is great enough, the axon is depolarized and an action potential is triggered at the first node of Ranvier.

The mechanisms that generate receptor potentials vary with receptors [3]. For example, deformation generates receptor potential in the pacinian corpuscles, and chemicals initiate receptor potentials in the rods and cones of the eye. Because most receptor terminals are minute in size and difficult to study, less information is available about their activity than about the action potentials.

THE SYNAPSE

The relay of information concerning our environment takes place through a succession of neurons in contact with each other. These areas of contact are known as the *synapses.* The terminal portion of the presynaptic axon, the *bouton* or *knob*, may synapse with the cell body, dendrites, axons of other nerve cells, or with muscle or gland cells. Transmission of impulses at the synapse can be through chemical or electrical means. Chemical synapses, by far the most common, involve the release of a chemical substance in response to a stimulus. This substance has an excitatory or inhibitory effect on the postsynaptic cell membrane. The electrical synapses found in invertebrate and lower vertebrates are fused synapses for the purpose of propagation of uninterrupted impulses. The discussion of synapses here is limited to the chemical synapses.

Electron microscopy has considerably enlightened our knowledge of the synaptic characteristics and properties in recent years. Anatomically there is wide variability in the structure of synapses in various parts of the human nervous system. Likewise, there exist a variety of functional differences.

The presynaptic fiber terminates in an enlarged knob called the *synaptic bouton*, *knob*, *end-foot*, or *button*. This presynaptic bouton is divided from the postsynaptic membrane by a narrow cleft of about 200 to 300 Å known as the *synaptic cleft*. The presynaptic bouton contains stored particles of a transmitter substance that is released at the synapse in response to a stimulus. Vesicles open and empty the transmitter substance that then excites or inhibits the postsynaptic neuron. Mitochondria in the presynaptic bouton provide the adenosine triphosphate (ATP) for synthesizing the released substance that is continually regenerated. For example, the common transmitter substance, acetylcholine, when activated by the enzyme cholinesterase, is reduced to choline and acetic acid. This substance is resorbed by the terminal bouton and, with the enzymatic assistance of choline acetylase, is resynthesized to acetylcholine, which is stored in the presynaptic vesicles until the next adequate stimulus.

Conduction of impulses through synapses is unidirectional. That is, impulses can be transmitted only through terminal boutons of presynaptic membranes to postsynaptic membranes.

Events at the Chemical Synapse

As previously noted, the presynaptic terminal bouton contains vesicles with packets of appropriate transmitter substances. A very low level of spontaneous release of this transmitter substance occurs in the "resting" synapse. This causes spontaneous mini-depolarizations at the synapse. When an action potential spreads to the presynaptic bouton, as shown in Figure 42-8, the depolarization of the membrane triggers release of this transmitter substance. It is thought that the trigger release at the terminal bouton requires calcium ions. This theory is supported by observations that low extracellular calcium levels result in diminishing the amounts of transmitter substance being released. The neurotransmitter substance then attaches to the postsynaptic receptor sites and the postsynaptic membrane potential is modified. The neurotransmitter substance not taken up by the postsynaptic receptors may be taken up by the presynaptic bouton and stored or inactivated by monoamine oxidase (MAO). Some of the unattached neurotransmitter is inactivated at the synaptic cleft or at the postsynaptic membrane by enzymes. Additionally, some of the free neurotransmitter is lost through extracellular diffusion.

The presynaptic release of an excitatory transmitter substance can initiate depolarizing response in the postsynaptic membrane that is referred to as the *excitatory postsynaptic potential* (EPSP) [2]. The EPSP is graded, nonpropagative, and the result of an increase in the permeability of the postsynaptic membrane to sodium, potassium, chloride, and calcium ions. Sodium ions flow in across the membrane and decrease the negativity of the

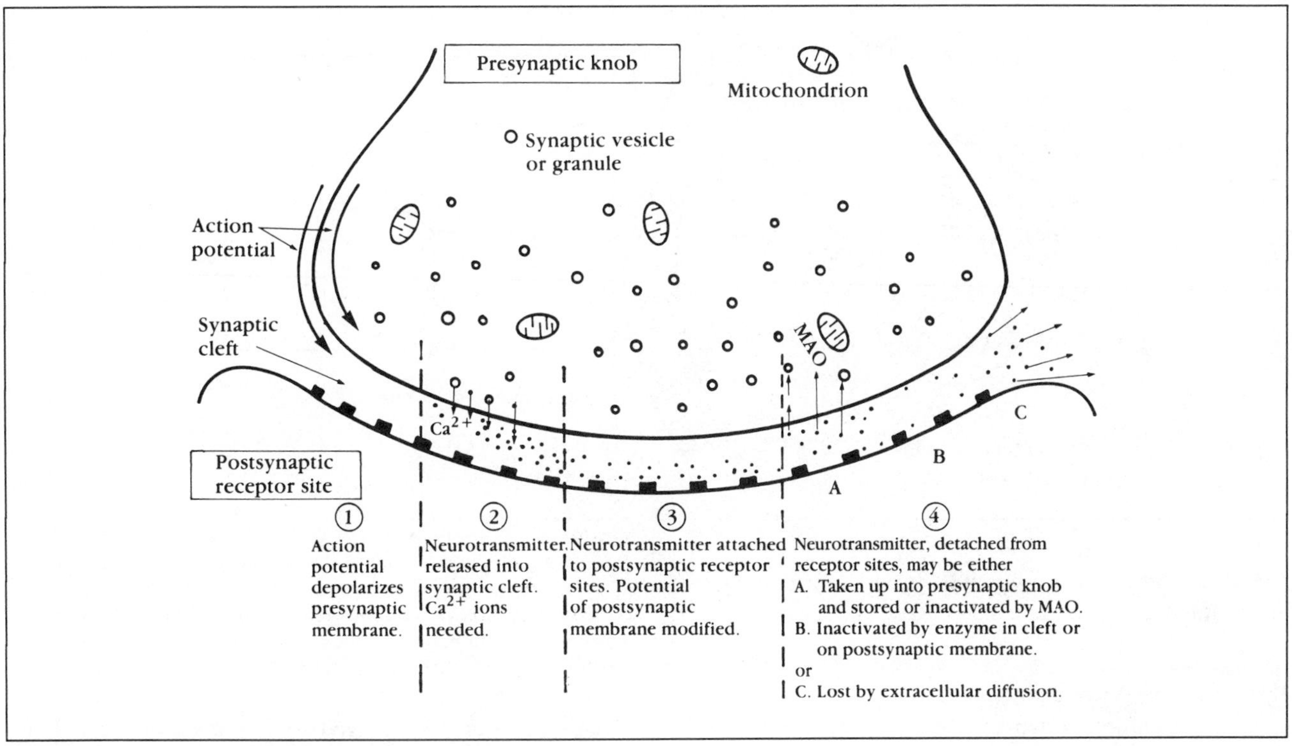

FIGURE 42-8. Events occurring at the chemical synapse. (From A. Lewis, *Mechanisms of Neurological Disease*. Little, Brown, 1976.)

postsynaptic cell. The threshold voltage change produced in a motoneuron during depolarization in an EPSP is approximately 13 mV, from a resting potential of −70 to −57 mV.

The activity of one terminal bouton is not significant enough to initiate an action potential in the postsynaptic cell. It requires many active terminals discharging spontaneously to elicit an action potential. This phenomenon is known as *summation* [7]. Thus, the amplitude of the EPSP depends on the number of activated synapses, and if a sufficient number are firing, an action potential results.

It has been shown that the threshold is the lowest on the motoneuron at the axon hillock, and the thresholds of the cell body and dendrites are considerably higher. Therefore, action potentials initiated in most neurons originate in the axon hillock.

Some synapses release an inhibitory transmitter, thought to contain gamma-aminobutyric acid (GABA) at the postsynaptic membrane. This produces a limited permeability to potassium and chloride. Potassium effluxes as chloride influxes and no corresponding inflow of positive sodium ions occurs. This increases the negativity of the already negative postsynaptic cell and a state of hyperpolarization results. This is called an ***inhibitory postsynaptic potential*** (IPSP) [2]. The permeability change is very brief as active transport of chloride out of the cell restores resting potential rapidly. Like the EPSP, the IPSP is graded and does not propagate. During the IPSP, the cell is less excitable as the membrane potential is more negative and increased excitatory activity is needed to reach the threshold level.

Facilitation

Many presynaptic terminals converge on each postsynaptic neuron. A certain number of action potentials must be transmitted simultaneously in order for a sufficient amount of neurotransmitter to be released to produce an action potential in the postsynaptic membrane. If an insufficient amount of a neurotransmitter is released the postsynaptic membrane is excitatory, although not to threshold level, and it is said to be facilitated. It is above resting potential but below threshold value, and thus very receptive to another stimulus that can activate it with ease.

Presynaptic Inhibition

In addition to the IPSP previously discussed another form of inhibition, called presynaptic inhibition, has been shown to occur throughout the nervous system. Though concentrated in the peripheral afferent fibers, this type of inhibition occurs at the presynaptic bouton and no change is observed in the postsynaptic membrane. An inhibitory terminal acts on the presynaptic bouton, which greatly reduces the voltage of the action potential, thus reducing the excitability in the membrane of the bouton by reducing the amount of transmitter substance released. It is thought that presynaptic inhibition provides for a control mechanism of sensory inflow so that less important input is

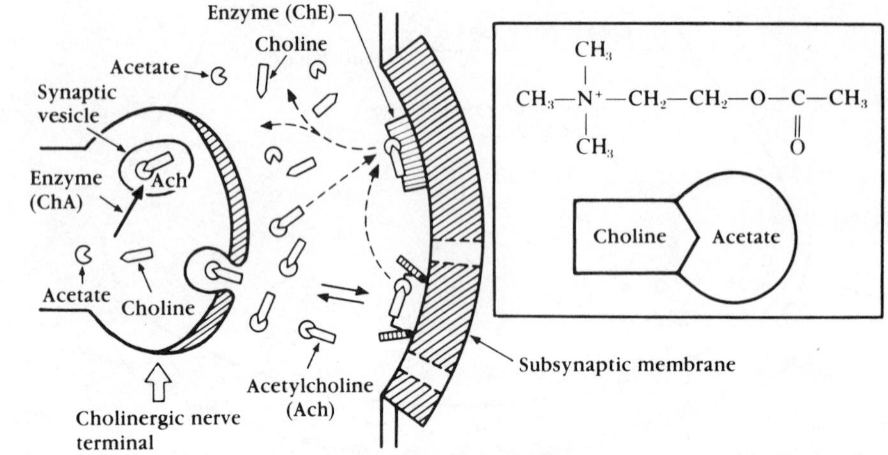

FIGURE 42-9. Acetylcholine (ACh) exocytosis. Acetylcholine formed in presynaptic bouton through enzyme action of choline acetylase on acetate and choline. ACh is removed from the cleft by action of enzyme cholinesterase (ChE), which is present in subsynaptic membrane. (From E. Selkurt, *Basic Physiology for the Health Sciences* [2nd ed.]. Little, Brown, 1982.)

eliminated and the major signal is relayed more clearly to the central nervous system.

Divergence and Convergence

Extremely complex networks of neurons exist in the nervous system. Extensive interactions among neurons are mediated through highly organized circuit connections. As axons emerge from the cell body, they divide and subdivide into many collateral branches that synapse with varying numbers of other neurons. This presynaptic division is known as *divergence.* For example, the fibers of afferent neurons entering the spinal cord generally divide and subdivide into collateral branches that supply terminal boutons to many other postsynaptic spinal neurons. As a result, no one fiber contributes to an action potential but rather many fibers cooperatively produce the innervation. The repetitive subdivision strengthens the afferent information, which is made available to various parts of the central nervous system through the process of divergence.

Likewise, most postsynaptic neurons receive terminal boutons from presynaptic fibers. This postsynaptic anatomic phenomenon is known as *convergence.* Thousands of axons may converge on a single neuron and the EPSP is dependent on sufficient amplitude of the active boutons converging upon it.

Neurochemical Transmitter Substances

Presynaptic bouton vesicles contain specific chemical substances that either excite or inhibit other cells when released into the synaptic cleft. Some transmitter substances are found only in the specific parts of the nervous system, while others are widely dispersed. Only a few neurochemical transmitters have been identified with certainty, and it is thought that many more will be found in the future. The identification of these substances has been very difficult because of the complexity of the nervous system fiber structures.

Substances are considered to be neurochemical transmitters if they have the following general characteristics:

1. Are released by the presynaptic bouton on stimulation
2. Contain an enzyme in the presynaptic bouton for transmitter synthesis
3. Produce excitation or inhibition in the postsynaptic cell
4. Have a mechanism demonstrated that diminishes the effects of the transmitter

Acetylcholine and norepinephrine are two well-established neurochemical transmitters [4]. The activity of acetylcholine as a neurochemical transmitter at the neuromuscular junction is well understood. The terminal bouton of cholinergic nerve fibers contains vesicles, each of which contain about 10,000 molecules of acetylcholine. A vesicle fuses with the presynaptic membrane and results in the release of acetylcholine. This process is known as *exocytosis* (Fig. 42-9). It is thought that the fusion of the vesicle to the presynaptic membrane is brought about by a sudden, transient increase in the concentration of calcium ions in the terminal bouton. The nerve impulse at the terminal bouton opens calcium channels to allow their flow into the bouton to facilitate exocytosis. The exact mechanism of the calcium activity in exocytosis is still unknown. When the fused vesicle has discharged its acetylcholine at the presynaptic membrane, it is reclaimed by the bouton and restored with acetylcholine for its future use. This synthesis of acetylcholine occurs in the bouton in the following manner:

$$\text{Acetyl-coenzyme A (acetate)} + \text{choline} \xrightarrow[\text{ATP}]{\text{choline acetyltransferase}} \text{acetylcholine}$$

The acetylcholine that crossed the synaptic cleft binds with an acetylcholine receptor on the postsynaptic membrane. This receptor is a channel protein that, in the presence of acetylcholine, lowers its energy state to an open conformation allowing opening of the channel and the passage of sodium and potassium ions. Thus, a postsynaptic potential or voltage change is produced. The chemically gated postsynaptic potentials differ from action potentials of neurons in that their amplitude is smaller, their duration longer, and they are graded in accordance with the amount of transmitter released.

Within 2 or 3 msec of its release into the synaptic cleft, after it has depolarized the postsynaptic membrane, acetylcholine is hydrolyzed by the enzyme acetylcholinesterase:

$$\text{Acetylcholine} \xrightarrow[\text{water}]{\text{acetylcholinesterase}} \text{choline} + \text{acetate}$$

Acetylcholinesterase is found abundantly in the membrane of the terminal bouton.

Insights into neurotransmitters and their inhibiting enzymes have been gained through the use of various pharmacologic agents that act on or compete with these substances. For example, the muscle relaxant curare competes with acetylcholine for receptor sites at the postsynaptic membrane. Thus, acetylcholine cannot bring about the membrane permeability for depolarization. Some drugs, such as nicotine, simulate acetylcholine action. Drugs such as neostigmine and physostigmine inactivate the enzymatic action of acetylcholinesterase. Magnesium affects acetylcholine release. Elevated magnesium levels inhibit acetylcholine release by competing with the calcium ions that are necessary for acetylcholine release.

Norepinephrine is the transmitter substance at all postganglionic sympathetic fibers except those innervating sweat glands and skeletal muscle vasculature. The formulation of this substance occurs through a series of steps catalyzed by enzymes with the initial active transport of tyrosine from the circulation into the nerve terminals as follows:

$$\text{Tyrosine} \xrightarrow{\text{tyrosine hydroxylase}} \text{dopa} \xrightarrow{\text{dopa-decarboxylase}}$$

$$\text{dopamine} \xrightarrow{\text{dopamine beta-hydroxylase}} \text{norepinephrine}$$

$$\xrightarrow{\text{phenylethanolamine } N\text{-methyltransferase}} \text{epinephrine}$$

A nerve impulse initiates the release of norepinephrine into the cleft. Termination of norepinephrine activity at the receptor is achieved primarily through its uptake into the terminal bouton and transport back into the vesicles for reuse. In addition, a small amount of norepinephrine is inactivated by the activity of monoamine oxidase (MAO), and a small amount of norepinephrine escapes the terminal bouton uptake and enters the systemic circulation, where it is primarily metabolized by the liver into vanillylmandelic acid (VMA) and excreted in the urine. Disease states exhibiting increased production of catecholamines characteristically show increased VMA urinary excretion. Minute amounts of released norepinephrine, which escapes uptake and the metabolic breakdown in the liver, appear unchanged in the urine.

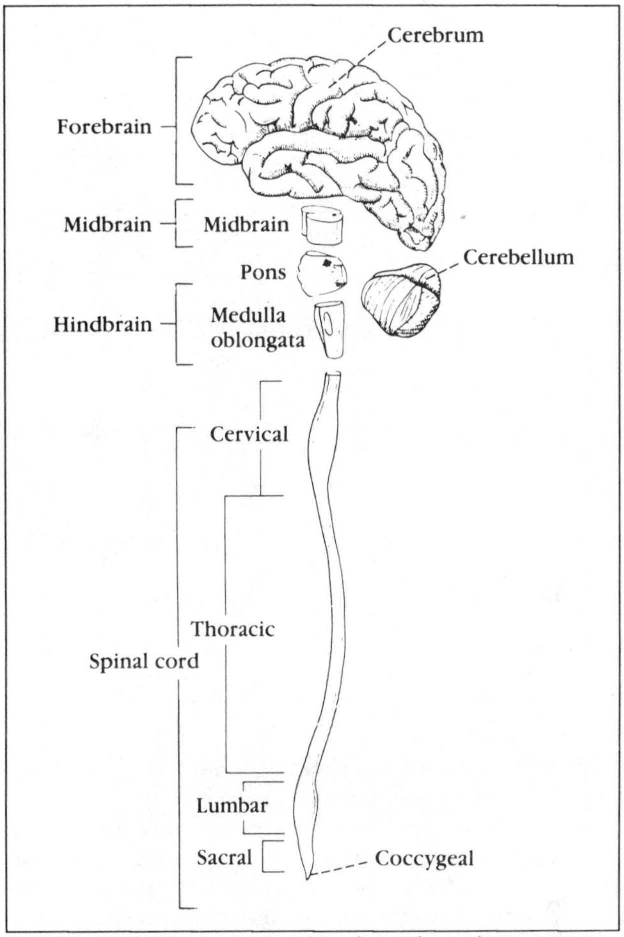

FIGURE 42-10. The brain develops from three distinct regions called the hindbrain, the midbrain, and the forebrain. (From R. Snell, *Clinical Neuroanatomy for Medical Students*. Boston: Little, Brown, 1980.)

THE CENTRAL NERVOUS SYSTEM

Phylogenetic Development

The human nervous system has a complex major processing system that lends control in a hierarchical manner. The highest level is the cerebral cortex, and the lowest, or most rudimentary, is the spinal reflex arc.

One can identify in the embryonic brain three distinct regions: the *rhombencephalon* or *hindbrain*, the *mesencephalon* or *midbrain*, and the *prosencephalon* or *forebrain* (Fig. 42-10). The most sophisticated activities and complex subdividing occur in the prosencephalon, which includes the cerebral hemispheres, the basal ganglia, and olfactory tract. This portion of the brain is also called the *telencephalon* or *endbrain*. The "deep inside" component of the prosencephalon is the *diencephalon*. Optic tracts traverse the prosencephalon and terminate in the optic nerves of the retina at the inferior surface of the forebrain.

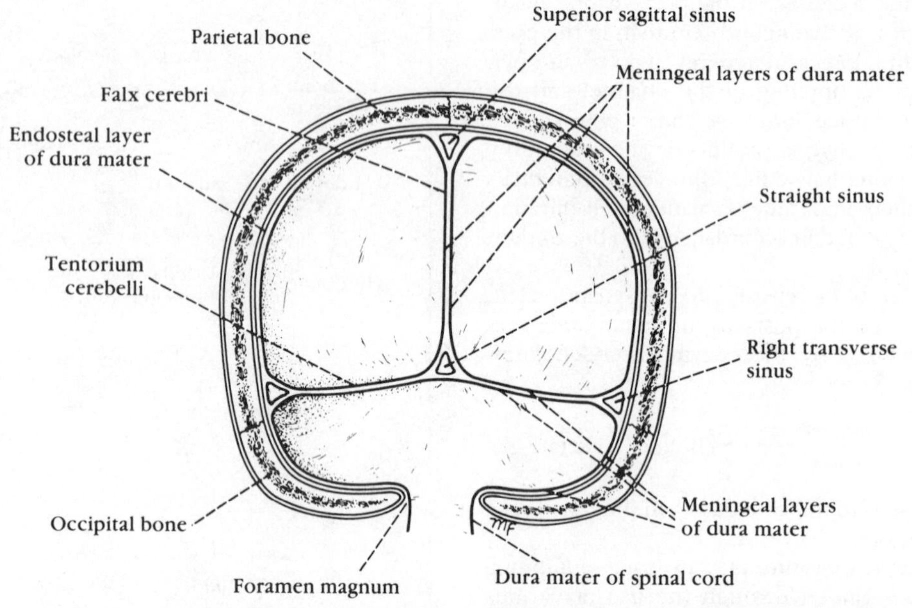

FIGURE 42-11. Relationship of intracranial contents with the foramen magnum. (From R. Snell, *Clinical Neuroanatomy for Medical Students*. Boston: Little, Brown, 1980.)

The diencephalon includes structures such as the thalamus, the hypothalamus, the subthalamus, and the subthalamic nucleus. In addition, the pituitary complex evolves from the hypothalamus. The mesencephalon connects the forebrain with the hindbrain; anteriorly it comprises the cerebral peduncles and posteriorly the corpora quadrigemina (also known as superior and inferior colliculi).

Below the mesencephalon is the rhombencephalon, which surrounds the fourth ventricle and comprises the pons and medulla oblongata. Extending from the rhombencephalon posteriorly is the cerebellum; the spinal cord extends inferiorly.

Protective Coverings of the Brain and Spinal Cord

Protection is afforded the brain and spinal cord by bony coverings, the meninges, and the cerebrospinal fluid. The brain is encased within the skull, which in the adult is a nonflexible structure comprised of several fused bones. Three depressions in the base of the skull are known as the anterior, middle, and posterior fossae.

A major opening, the foramen magnum, is at the base of the skull and allows for information processing between higher and lower centers (Fig. 42-11). At birth, openings within the skull known as the *fontanelles* can be noted. These generally close by 18 months of age.

The spinal cord is encased in the vertebral column, which consists of 24 movable vertebrae: 7 cervical, 12 thoracic, and 5 lumbar, and the fused 5 sacral and 4 coccygeal vertebrae (Fig. 42-12). Intravertebral disks separate each of the vertebrae. The central cartilaginous portion of the intervertebral disk is known as the *nucleus pulposus* and the outer fibrous capsule as the *anulus fibrosus*.

Additionally, the brain and spinal cord are protected by three connective tissue membranes called the *meninges*: the *dura mater,* the *arachnoid*, and the *pia mater* (Fig. 42-13). The dura mater is a thick, tough, nonelastic fibrous membrane that lies directly below the skull. Its extension between the cerebral hemispheres is known as the *falx cerebri*; and between the cerebrum and cerebellum it is known as the *tentorium cerebelli.* Likewise, the dura mater together with the arachnoid and pia mater extends through the foramen magnum and lines the vertebral column. The *epidural space* is that between the inner surface of the skull and the dura mater. The space between the dura and arachnoid is known as the *subdural space.* A network of small blood vessels traverses this space. The arachnoid, consisting of fibrous, weblike tissue, is the middle layer of the meninges wherein the cerebrospinal fluid circulates and is resorbed. The area below the arachnoid membrane containing the cerebrospinal fluid is known as the *subarachnoid* space. The innermost layer, the *pia mater*, is a delicate, vascular, lacelike membrane directly adherent to the brain and spinal cord. The arachnoid layer projects small extensions called *arachnoid villi* into the dura mater that resorb cerebrospinal fluid into the blood. Larger blood vessels lie in the subarachnoid space and branch into smaller vessels that pass through the pia mater as they enter the brain tissue.

The Spinal Cord Processing System

The spinal cord serves as a transmitter of more complex signals at the higher centers and responds spontaneously to

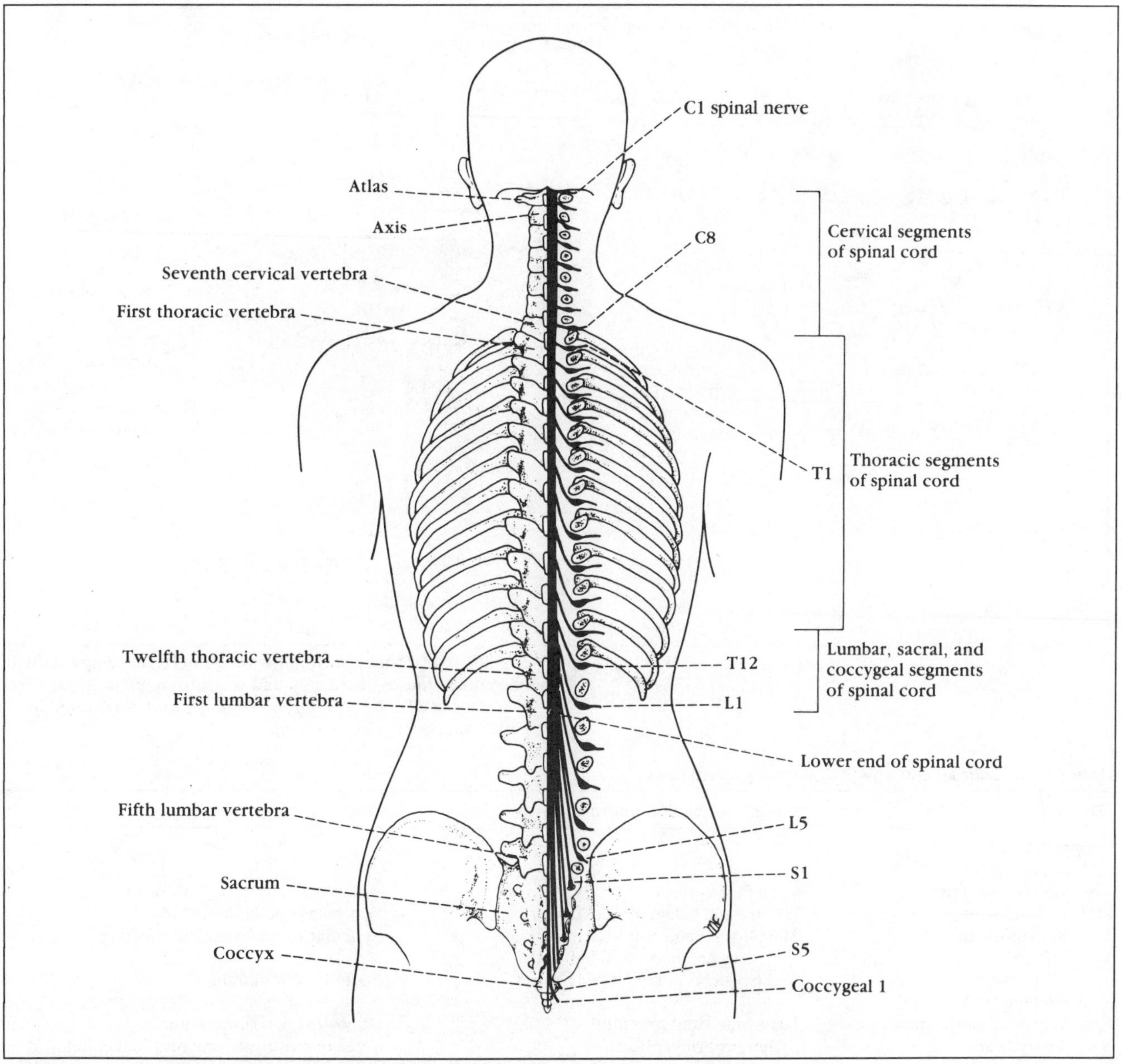

FIGURE 42-12. Relation of vertebral segments of cord with actual vertebrae. (From R. Snell, *Clinical Neuroanatomy for Medical Students*. Boston: Little, Brown, 1980.)

local sensory information with automatic motor responses called *reflexes*. It is approximately 42 to 45 cm long in the adult and is segmented into cervical, thoracic, lumbar, and sacral sections. Signals are received and transmitted through 31 pairs of spinal nerves, which are named for their corresponding vertebral level. However, segments of the spinal cord do not correspond with the vertebral levels (Fig. 42-12). The spinal cord is approximately 25 cm shorter than the vertebral canal and ends at the level of the first or second lumbar vertebra in the adult. It emerges from the base of the skull, the *foramen magnum*, and continues to the coccyx where it ends in a tapered filament called the *filum terminale*. Together, the lower nerve roots of the spinal cord are called the *cauda equina*.

The spinal cord enlarges at the lower cervical vertebrae and again at the lower thoracic vertebrae. These enlargements denote the origins of the *brachial* and *lumbar plexuses*, respectively. The cell bodies are located in the inner butterfly-shaped gray portion of the spinal cord and the ascending and descending projection nerve fibers form the outer white area. Major ascending and descending tracts and their transmissions are presented in Table 42-2. A small opening in the middle of the spinal cord is called the *central canal*. It is lined by ependymal cells and contains cerebrospinal fluid. Spinal nerves enter the cord at the dorsal root (somatic sensory and visceral) and emerge at the ven-

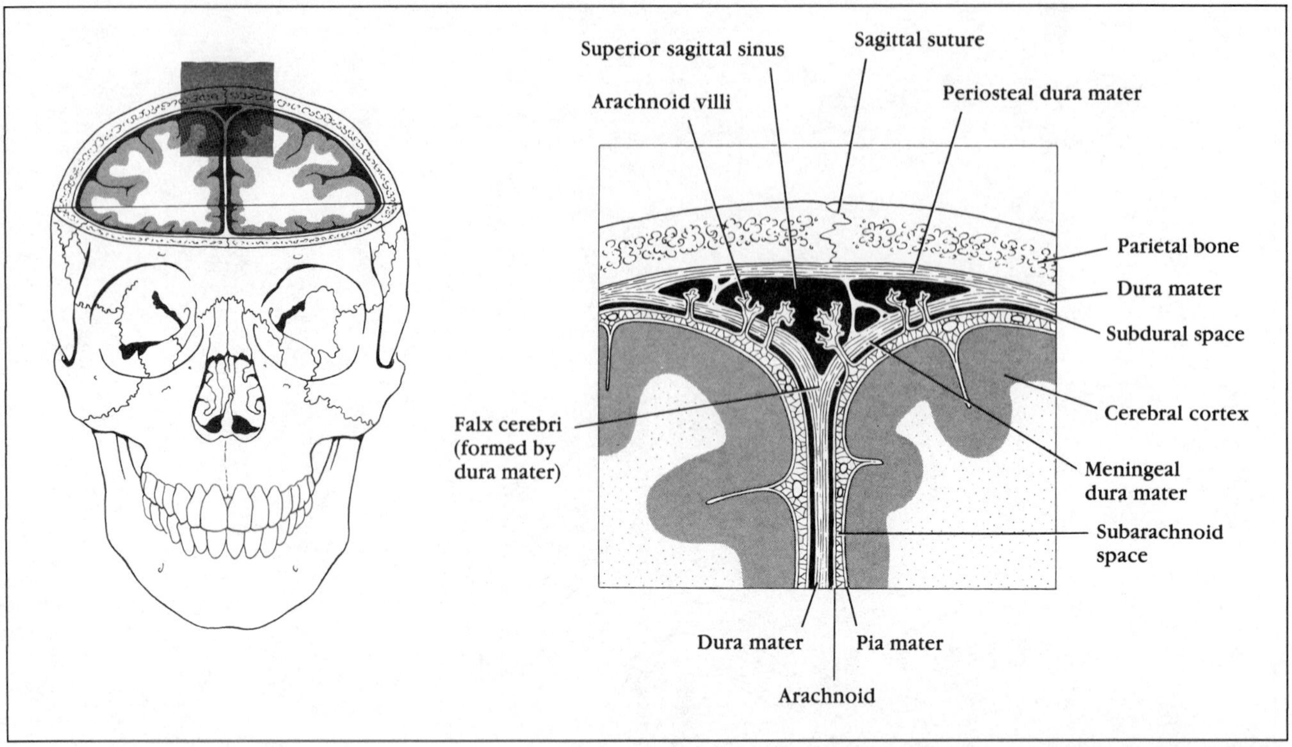

FIGURE 42-13. Frontal section showing the relationships of the dural venous sinuses, meninges, and the subarachnoid space. (From A. Spence and E. Mason, *Human Anatomy and Physiology*. Menlo Park, Calif.: Benjamin/Cummings, 1979.)

TABLE 42-2. Major ascending and descending spinal tracts

Tracts	Major transmission information	Origin
ANTERIOR WHITE COLUMN		
Descending (motor)		
Ventral corticospinal	Voluntary movement	Pyramidal cells of motor cortex
Vestibulospinal	Posture and balance reflexes	Vestibular nuclei in medulla
Reticulospinal	Muscle tone controls activity of autonomic nervous system	Reticular of midbrain and medulla
Tectospinal	Audiovisual reflexes	Roof of the midbrain
Ascending (sensory)		
Ventral spinothalmic	Light touch and pressure	Opposite posterior column
Spinoolivary	Reflex proprioception	Anterior marginal zone of spinal column
LATERAL WHITE COLUMN		
Descending (motor)		
Lateral corticospinal	Voluntary movement	Contralateral pyramidal cells of motor cortex
Rubrospinal	Muscle tone, head and upper trunk movement	Red nucleus of midbrain
Olivospinal	Facilitative and inhibitory reflexes	Inferior olivary nucleus
Ascending (sensory)		
Dorsal spinocerebellar	Reflex proprioception to cerebellum	Ipsilateral dorsal nucleus
Ventral spinocerebellar	Reflex proprioception to cerebellum	Posterior white column
Lateral spinothalamic	Pain temperature tactile sensations	Contralateral dorsal column
POSTERIOR WHITE COLUMN		
Descending (motor)		
Fasciculus interfascicularis	Integration and association	Intraspinal and dorsal root
Ascending (sensory)		
Fasciculus gracilis	Both transmit vibration, discriminative tactile senses, joint position, kinesthetic sensations	Posteromedian septum of low spinal cord
Fasciculus cuneatus		Posterior nerve roots of thoracocervical cord

Source: D. G. Chusid, *Correlative Neuroanatomy and Functional Neurology* (17th ed.). Los Altos, Calif.: Lange, 1979. P. 69.

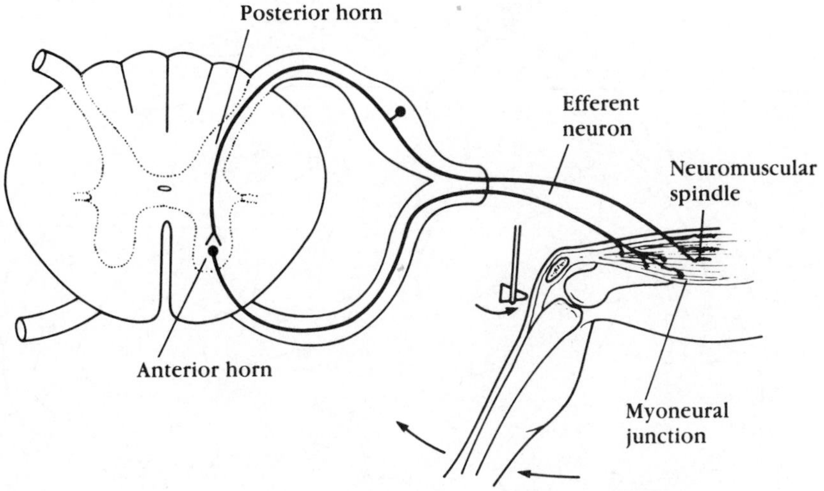

FIGURE 42-14. A monosynaptic reflex arc. (From R. Snell, *Clinical Neuroanatomy for Medical Students*. Boston: Little, Brown, 1980.)

tral root (motor and autonomic) [5] (Fig. 42-14). The cell bodies of efferent motor fibers are located in the ventral horn and the cell bodies of the afferent sensory fibers are situated outside the spinal cord in the dorsal root ganglion. Contact between the afferent and efferent fibers is made within the spinal cord through interneurons.

REFLEX ARC. A fundamental concept in understanding the function of the nervous system is the *reflex*, which, in its simplest form, occurs in the spinal cord. A stimulus from the external environment produces an immediate stereotypical reflex response from the central nervous system. For this response to occur, the following mechanisms must be functional: an afferent neuron with its receptor, an area for the synapse transmission to occur (one or more central neurons), and an efferent neuron with its effector organ. The impulse passes from receptor to effector and commands a quick organ response. This simple chain of neuronal activity is known as a *reflex arc* and, at its most elemental level, is a monosynaptic process, consisting of only one synapse and two neurons (see Fig. 42-14). Most reflexes result from many more synaptic interconnections and are referred to as *polysynaptic reflexes.* The reflex activity encountered at higher levels in the central nervous system is considerably more complex.

Low Brain Processing System (Rhombencephalon)

The next level of processing in the central nervous system is that of the rhombencephalon regions. The major components of these regions are the medulla oblongata, the pons, and the cerebellum (Fig. 42-15). The processing encountered at this level occurs at the unconscious level and influences such vital activities as respiratory, cardiac, and vasomotor control.

MEDULLA OBLONGATA. The medulla extends directly from the cervical spinal cord and lies below the pons and fourth ventricle. It is an important relay center as major ascending and descending tracts travel through and many decussate (cross over) here at the pyramid. Some tracts have their terminal stations here. The reticular formation, a network of interconnecting neurons, extends from the upper spinal cord through the medulla to the midbrain and on to diverse parts of the mesencephalon, diencephalon, and prosencephalon. The medulla contains nuclei that project the ninth through twelfth cranial nerves (see p. 639). Other nuclei here control respiratory, cardiac, vasomotor, and reflex activities. The central canal from the spinal cord begins to emerge as the fourth ventricle in the upper part of the medulla.

PONS. The pons is continuous with and superior to the medulla, lying inferior to the cerebellum. The pons contains the fourth ventricle. In addition to bridging the medulla and midbrain, it also bridges the two cerebellar hemispheres. The pons joins the *superior, middle,* and *inferior cerebellar peduncles* that provide transmission to and from the cerebellum. The pons contains nuclei for the fourth through eighth cranial nerves (see Chap. 45). Respiratory regulation from the pons comes from its pneumotaxic center. The reticular formation continues its ascent through this region.

CEREBELLAR PROCESSING. The cerebellum (Fig. 42-16), directly above the pons and medulla and inferior to the occipital portion of the cerebrum, processes and transmits information concerning the adjustments of current body movements and maintenance of posture and equilibrium. It does this through the information it receives from the motor cortex of the cerebrum via the corticocerebellar pathway, and from the various sensory receptors via the *anterior* and *posterior spinocerebellar* tracts. The

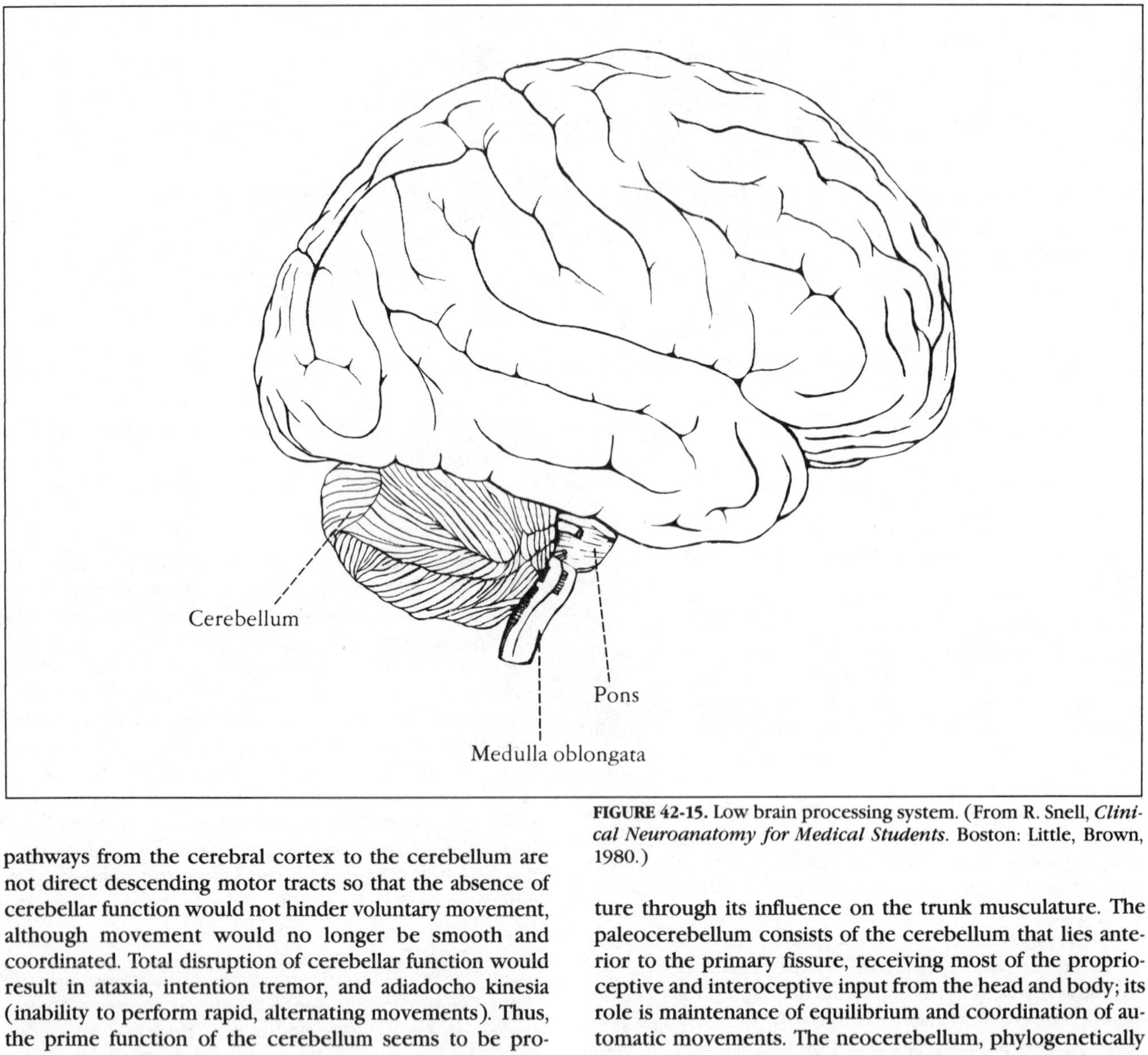

FIGURE 42-15. Low brain processing system. (From R. Snell, *Clinical Neuroanatomy for Medical Students*. Boston: Little, Brown, 1980.)

pathways from the cerebral cortex to the cerebellum are not direct descending motor tracts so that the absence of cerebellar function would not hinder voluntary movement, although movement would no longer be smooth and coordinated. Total disruption of cerebellar function would result in ataxia, intention tremor, and adiadocho kinesia (inability to perform rapid, alternating movements). Thus, the prime function of the cerebellum seems to be processing and adjusting body movements but not initiating the movements. It senses possible discrepancies in movement and signals activation in appropriate parts of the brain for corrective measures.

Additional significant tracts relaying information to the cerebellum include the spinoreticular tract via the reticular area of the brainstem and the spinoolivary tract via the inferior olivary nucleus. Fiber efferent tracts originate in various cerebellar nuclei and transmit information to the cerebral motor cortex, basal ganglia, red nucleus, reticular formation, and vestibular nuclei.

As noted in Figure 42-17, the cerebellar structures are divided into three principal lobes: the *archicerebellum* (flocculonodular lobe), the *paleocerebellum* (anterior lobe), and the *neocerebellum* (posterior lobe). The archicerebellum is integrated with the vestibular system and is concerned with muscle tone, equilibrium, and posture through its influence on the trunk musculature. The paleocerebellum consists of the cerebellum that lies anterior to the primary fissure, receiving most of the proprioceptive and interoceptive input from the head and body; its role is maintenance of equilibrium and coordination of automatic movements. The neocerebellum, phylogenetically the newest, consists of the cerebellum between the primary fissure and the posterior fissure. It is concerned with coordination of voluntary movements and has extensive connections with the cerebral cortex.

Disorders of the cerebellum are evidenced by symptoms denoting motor system dysfunction. These include disorders such as ataxia, hypotonia, tremor, and asthenia. The cerebellum exerts ipsilateral influence; the right side of the cerebellum influences the right side of the body and the left side of the cerebellum influences the left side of the body.

Midbrain (Mesencephalon) Processing System

The midbrain extends from the pons and projects briefly between the two cerebral hemispheres. It is a major motor and sensory fiber pathway between the higher and lower

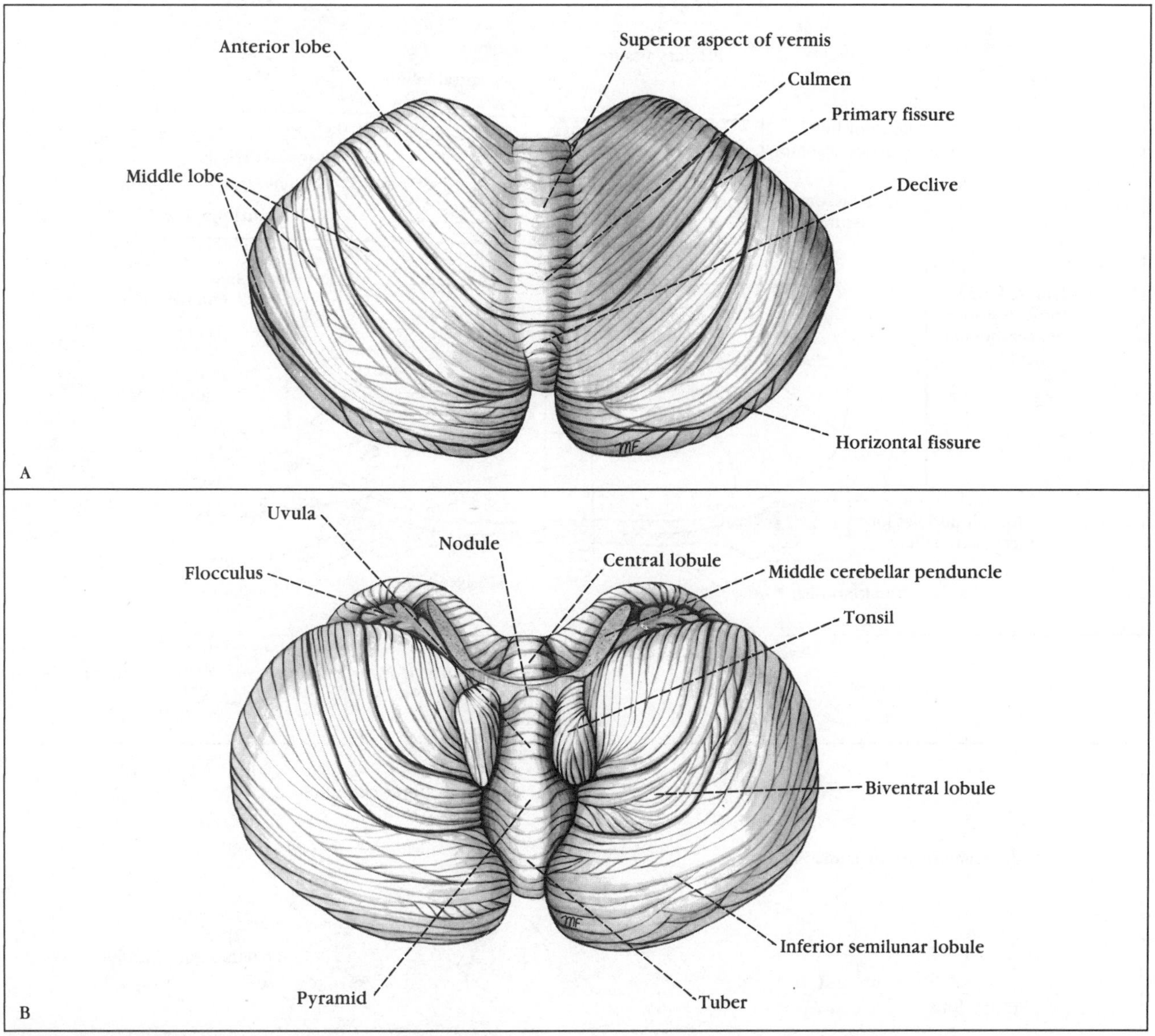

FIGURE 42-16. The cerebellum. A. Superior view. B. Inferior view. (From R. Snell, *Clinical Neuroanatomy for Medical Students.* Boston: Little, Brown, 1980.)

centers. The nuclei for third and fourth cranial nerves originate in this region. The *aqueduct of Sylvius*, a small channel between the third and fourth ventricle, lies in the midbrain. The reticular formation in this region contains *substantia nigra nuclei* and the *red nuclei.* The *superior colliculi*, a reflex center for eye and head movement, and the *inferior colliculi*, which relays nuclei for the auditory pathway, are contained in this area. The superior and inferior colliculi comprise the *corpora quadrigemina.*

Diencephalon Processing System

The diencephalon region arises from the midbrain and is considered to be a part of the forebrain. It lies directly under the cerebral hemispheres and encases the third ventricle. Included in this area are structures of the epithalamus, thalamus, hypothalamus, and subthalamus.

THALAMIC PROCESSING. The thalamus is a major center for processing sensations relaying these to higher stations of the brain. Input from all sensoria except that for olfaction are processed here. Numerous afferent nerve tracts from lower levels transmit information to the specific relay nuclei of the thalamus. The thalamus contains three sections, *lateral*, *medial*, and *anterior*, which are divided by the *internal medullary lamina.*

The reticular activating system continues its upward projection to the thalamic nuclei. From the thalamic nuclei, fibers project diffusely cortical relationship in activation is known as the *diffuse thalamocortical system* [3].

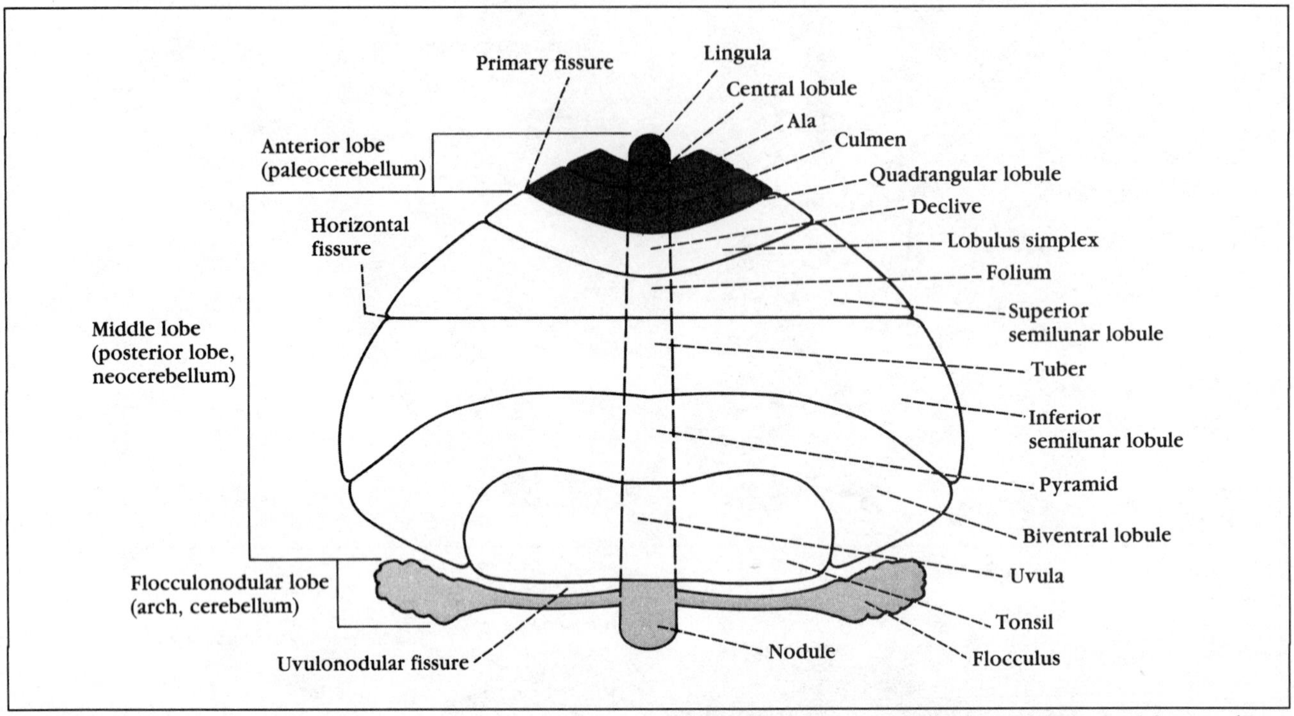

FIGURE 42-17. Main cerebellar lobes, lobules, and fissures. (From R. Snell, *Clinical Neuroanatomy for Medical Students*. Boston: Little, Brown, 1980.)

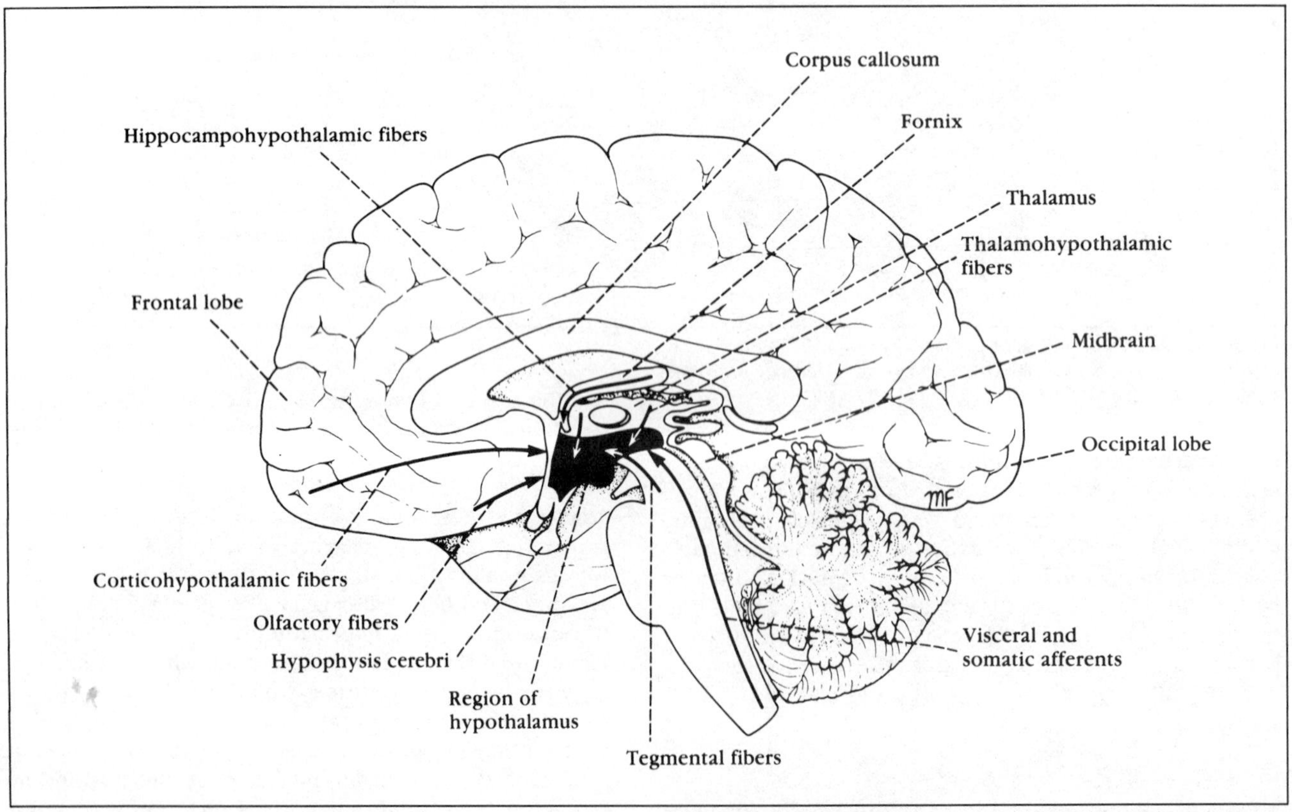

FIGURE 42-18. Sagittal section of brain, showing main afferent pathways entering hypothalamus. (From R. Snell, *Clinical Neuroanatomy for Medical Students*. Boston: Little, Brown, 1980.)

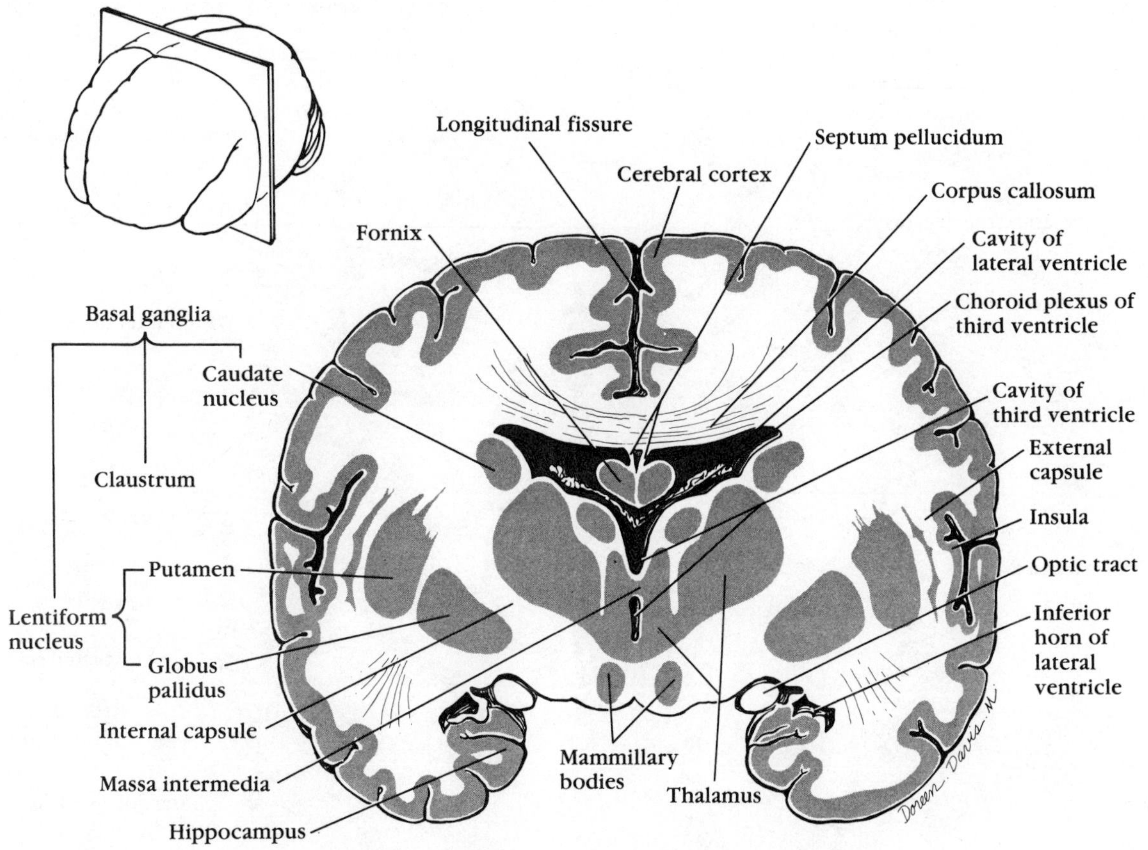

FIGURE 42-19. Frontal section of the cerebrum and diencephalon showing the cerebral cortex (gray matter) surrounding the white matter and the basal ganglia deep within the white matter. (From A. Spence and E. Mason, *Human Anatomy and Physiology.* Menlo Park, Calif.: Benjamin/Cummings, 1979.)

This system activates the first two layers of neurons of the cortex by partially depolarizing superficial cortical dendrites, resulting in increased facilitation of the cortex. Axons of the optic tract synapse in the lateral geniculate body, which projects from the thalamus. The fibers projecting from the lateral geniculate body pass posteriorly and terminate in the visual cortex.

HYPOTHALAMIC PROCESSING. The hypothalamus lies in the walls and floor of the third ventricle and extends to the superior border of the pons. It consists of a group of nuclei with specific functions that are divided into the anterior and posterior portions. The pituitary stalk connects the hypothalamus to the pituitary gland, which provides the route for its neuroendocrine control (Fig. 42-18).

Major processing of internal stimuli evoking the autonomic nervous system is concentrated in the hypothalamus. The functions that maintain the internal milieu processed by the hypothalamus include blood pressure, heart rate, respiratory rate, body temperature, water metabolism, and body fluid osmolality, feeding behavior, and neuroendocrine activity. The hypothalamus is a focal structure of the *limbic* system, which is composed of structures associated with autonomic function, emotion, and learning. Because of the vital functions processed here, the destruction of the hypothalamus results in death. The majority of the hypothalamic activity occurs at an unconscious level, but excessive stimulation may evoke a conscious response. An example of this is a person who is chilled and whose conscious awareness of cold initiates some activity to conserve heat.

Responses to emotions of fear, anger, and excitement reflected by increased pulse rate, increased respiratory rate, increased gastric acidity, and sweating are communicated from the hypothalamus. Prolonged stimulation of the hypothalamus may result in hypertension or ulcers.

The *epithalamus* consists of the pineal body, the habenular nuclei, stria medularis, and the posterior commissure. It is found in the region above the thalamus and contains the roof of the third ventricle. Olfactory impulses are relayed through this region and visual reflexes are associated with certain fibers in the posterior commissure. The function of the pineal gland in the adult is uncertain, although it becomes visible on skull x rays due to calcified material called brain sand, which accumulates with age. It can provide useful information in the identification of space-occupying lesions.

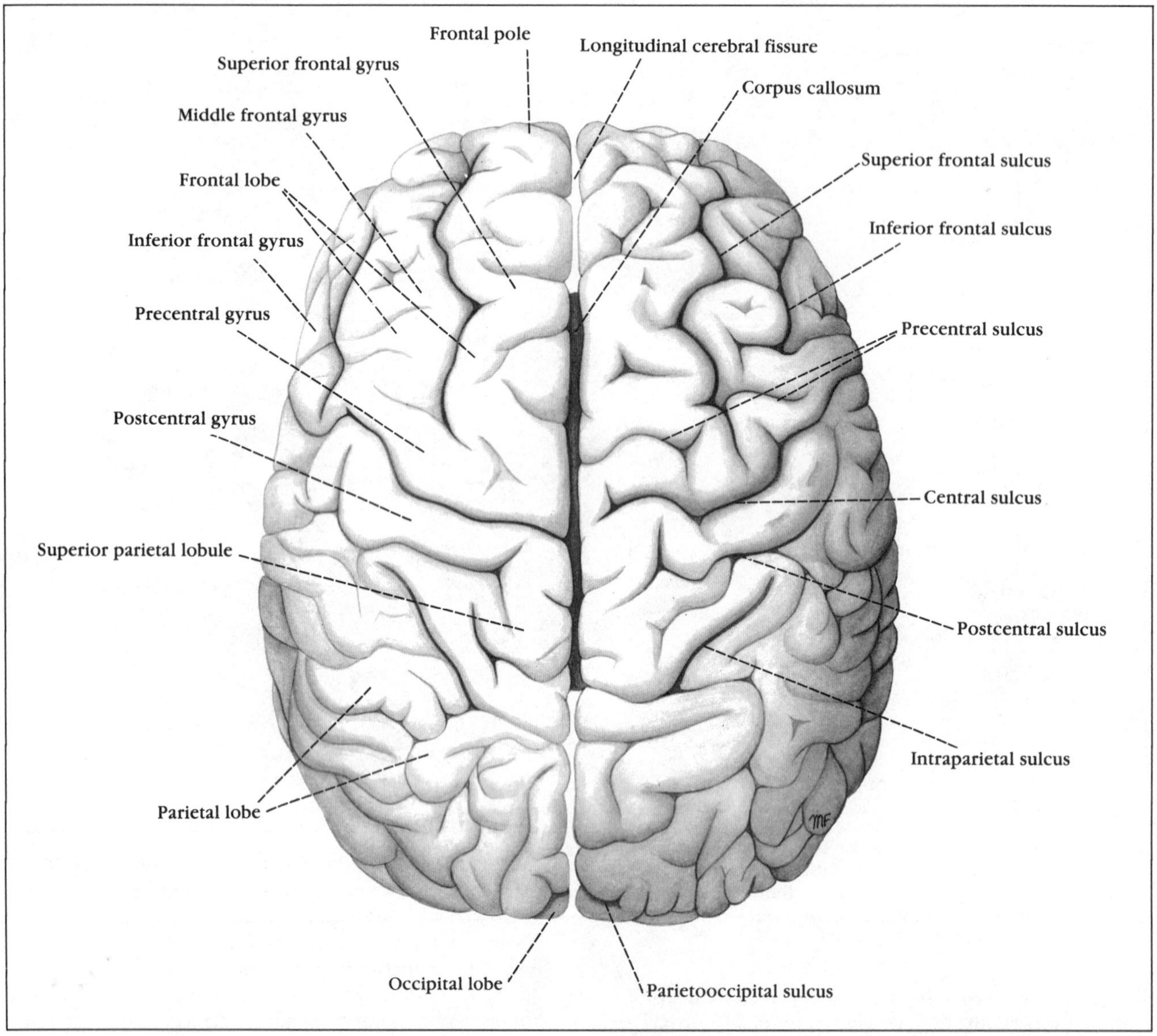

FIGURE 42-20. Superior view of cerebral hemispheres. (From R. Snell, *Clinical Neuroanatomy for Medical Students.* Boston: Little, Brown, 1980.)

BASAL GANGLIA PROCESSING. The basal ganglia (Fig. 42-19), situated deep within the cerebral hemispheres, are responsible for motor control and information processing in the extrapyramidal system. The basal ganglia include the *caudate nucleus*, *putamen*, and *globus pallidus*. These nuclear masses have complex interconnections with the *subthalamic nucleus*, *red nucleus*, and *substantia nigra*. The claustrum and amygdaloid body, considered by some authors to be part of the basal ganglia, are not directly involved in motor control. The basal ganglia are intimately related to the thalamus through circular neural pathways controlling motor function. They inhibit muscle tone by transmitting inhibitory signals to the bulboreticular facilitory area and excitatory signals to the bulboreticular inhibitory area. Lesions in the basal ganglia result in an overactive facilitory area and underactive inhibitory area.

Gross intentional movement that is carried out without conscious thought is regulated by the caudate nucleus and putamen (collectively called the *striate body*). Striate body transmissions are sent to the globus pallidus and relayed on to the ventrolateral nucleus of the thalamus and then on to the cerebral cortex. From the cortex the information travels via the pyramidal and extrapyramidal tracts to the spinal cord. Other impulses travel to the globus pallidus and then on to the substantia nigra and on to the reticular formation where the final route transmits down through the reticulospinal tract. The globus pallidus relays impulses via a similar feedback circuit to the ventrolateral nucleus of the thalamus and on to the cerebral cortex, and finally to

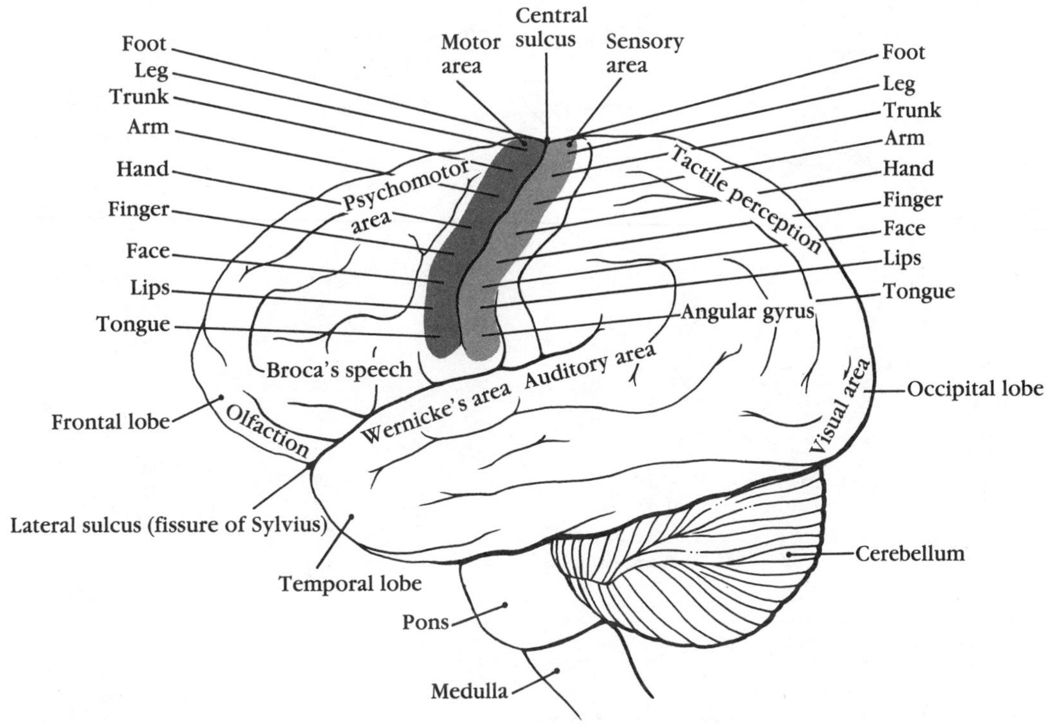

FIGURE 42-21. Topographic organization of functions of control and interpretation on the precentral and postcentral gyrus.

the pyramidal and extrapyramidal tracts to the spinal cord. It also transmits via shorter circuits to the reticular formation and on to the reticulospinal tract of the spinal cord.

The subthalamus nucleus, red nucleus, and substantia nigra are closely related to the globus pallidus and striate body. Their interactions are extremely complex and little is known of their exact interconnections. Their extensive interaction further controls and coordinates motor function.

The neurons transmitting to the globus pallidus and striate body from the substantia nigra are inhibitory through *dopamine* secretion [1].

Dysfunction or lesions in the region of the basal ganglia are manifested in tremor, ballism, athetosis, and torticollis (see pp. 737–739).

Forebrain (Prosencephalon)

Anatomically, the highest and largest portion of the brain, the cerebrum, is thought to be phylogenetically related to the thalamus through its closely associated structure and function. All areas of the cerebral cortex have afferent and efferent fibers interconnecting with specific areas of the thalamus. As previously noted, this relationship is affirmed through the diffuse thalamocortical system.

The gray cerebral cortex is composed of five basic types of neurons: pyramidal cells, stellate cells, fusiform cells, horizontal cells, and the cells of Martinotti. The pyramidal and the stellate cells are the most common. Pyramidal cells have pyramid-shaped bodies with axons that extend into the subcortical white matter. The stellate cells have a star-shaped body with short axons and dendrites. The horizontal cells lie entirely on the horizontal plane with axons and dendrites that are parallel in direction to the cortical surface. Polymorph or multiform cells may be modified types of pyramidal cells with a wide variety of shapes and contours. The dendrites often extend into the cortical layers while the axons project into the white matter. The cells of Martinotti are multipolar with short branching dendrites and myelinated axons. These cells may be modified stellate cells.

The white matter of the cerebral hemispheres is composed of three types of myelinated nerve fibers: projection, transverse, and association. Projection fibers connect the cerebral cortex with lower centers of the brain and spinal cord; transverse fibers connect the two cerebral hemispheres; and association fibers provide interconnections within the same cerebral hemisphere.

The cerebrum appears as a series of convolutions (*gyri*) and grooves (*sulci*) that are instrumental in identifying the structural and functional geography of the cortex. The deeper grooves, called *fissures*, assist in establishing the

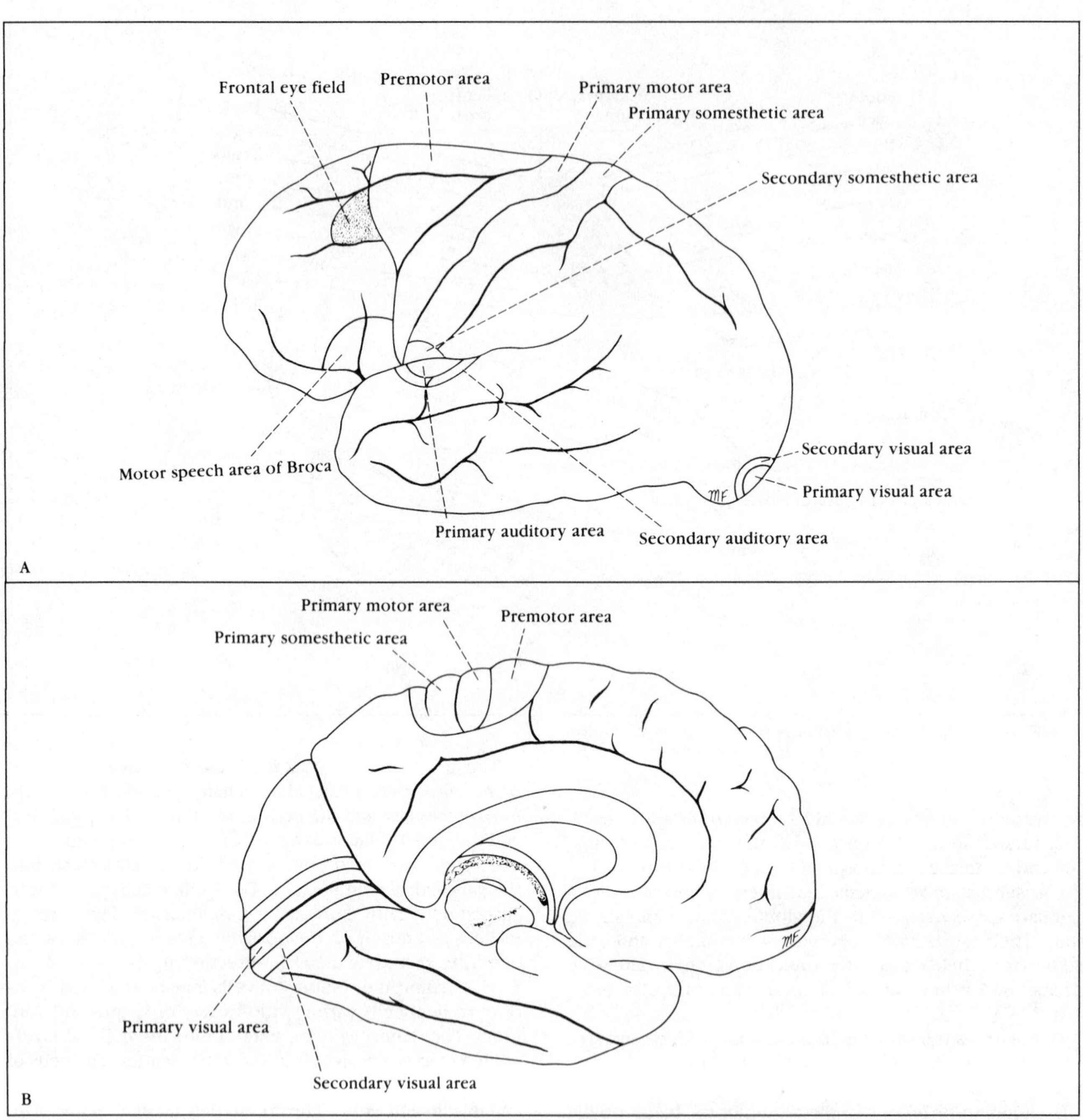

FIGURE 42-22. Functional localization of the cerebral cortex. A. Lateral view of left cerebral hemisphere. B. Medial view of left cerebral hemisphere. (From R. Snell, *Clinical Neuroanatomy for Medical Students.* Boston: Little, Brown, 1980.)

major cerebral regional divisions; the *frontal*, *parietal*, *temporal*, and *occipital* lobes. Likewise, the two cerebral hemispheres are distinguished from each other by a deep fissure, the *longitudinal fissure* (Fig. 42-20). The cerebral hemispheres, which exhibit *contralateral* body control, are divided by continuation of the dura mater known as the *falx cerebri*, which projects into the longitudinal cerebral fissure. Directly inferior to the longitudinal cerebral fissure, the fibers of the corpus collosum join the hemispheres. In the great majority of the population the left hemisphere is dominant in the interpretive functions.

In addition to its anatomic superiority, the cerebral cortex maintains the highest level of information processing in the human. Some functional areas are localized; others are more general and widely dispersed. The significant localized functional areas include the primary motor projection and sensory projection areas. The motor projection area is located on the anterior wall of the central sulcus and adjacent to the precentral gyrus (Fig. 42-21). This area controls voluntary skeletal muscle movements of the contralateral body. The sensory projection area (somesthetic area) is found on the postcentral gyrus and receives input from the thalamic-projected sensations of the contralateral side of the body.

Other rather well localized functions processed in the cortex include visual, hearing, olfaction, and somatic interpretations. The mental and intellectual activities in humans are processed and interpreted in widely dispersed association areas of the cortex.

A brief review of the cerebral hemisphere lobes follows. The *frontal* lobe extends from the central sulcus (fissure of Rolando) forward and from the lateral fissure (fissure of Sylvius) upward. It contains the motor strip, premotor area, Broca's speech center, and association areas related to higher mental functions and behavior. The *parietal* lobe lies between the central sulcus and the parietooccipital fissure. It extends laterally to the lateral fissure. Angular, postcentral, and supramarginal gyri are significant landmarks in the parietal lobe. Primary and secondary somesthetic areas are contained here as are many sensory association fibers. Interpretations of feeling and hearing are made here. Additionally, body image recognition evolves from the parietal lobe.

The *occipital* lobe lies posterior to the parietal lobe and is divided from the cerebellum by the parietooccipital fissure. Primary visual centers and visual association areas are contained in the occipital lobe. The *temporal lobe* extends downward from the lateral fissure and posteriorly to the parietooccipital fissure. Auditory centers, auditory association area (Wernicke's), smell interpretation, and memory storage are contained in the temporal lobe (Fig. 42-22).

TABLE 42-3. The cranial nerves

Number	Name of nerve	General function
I	Olfactory	Impulses for sense of smell
II	Optic	Impulses for vision
III	Oculomotor	Impulses for motor control and sensation for four eye muscles and upper eyelid elevator
IV	Trochlear	Impulses for movement of major eyeball muscle
V	Trigeminal	Impulses for mastication muscles and some facial sensations
VI	Abducent	Impulses for movement and muscle sense of eyeball
VII	Facial	Impulses for hyoid and facial muscles, salivation, cutaneous and taste sensation
VIII	Vestibulocochlear (acoustic)	Impulses for equilibration, static sense, and hearing
IX	Glossopharyngeal	Impulses for salivation, movement of pharynx, heart and some unstraited muscles, and sensations of skin, taste, and viscera
X	Vagus	Motor impulses to a number of muscles such as the heart and viscera and sensation from the pharynx, thorax, and abdominal structures
XI	Accessory	Impulses to the straited muscles of the pharynx and shoulder
XII	Hypoglossal	Motor impulses to the tongue, a number of skeletal muscles and viscera, and sensation from skin and viscera

THE PERIPHERAL NERVOUS SYSTEM

The peripheral nervous system includes the nerve tissue outside the brain and spinal cord. It is composed of paired spinal nerves and cranial nerves as well as the multiple ganglia and plexuses that are associated with visceral innervation. Every spinal nerve contains a dorsal (afferent) and ventral (efferent) root. The afferent nerve cells lie within the dorsal root ganglion and their fibers innervate through spinal nerves and through plexuses of the visceral nervous system. The efferent cell bodies lie within the ventral gray column of the spinal cord and innervate through ventral roots of all spinal nerves to the skeletal muscle and through ventral roots of spinal nerves of the thorax, upper lumbar, and middle sacral region to the viscera.

The cranial nerve nuclei are contained in the brainstem. The physiologic anatomy of the cranial nerves is not as clearly delineated as that of the spinal nerves. Some cranial nerves have only sensory components, some only motor components, and others contain both. The names and general functions of the cranial nerves are presented in Table 42-3. Function and dysfunction of the cranial nerves is further described in Chapter 45.

The Afferent Division (Sensory)

The afferent or sensory division of the peripheral nervous system detects, transmits, and processes environmental information from internal and external sources through a variety of specific receptors. The somatic afferent fibers carry impulses from the skin, the skeletal muscles, joints, and tendons to the central nervous system. The *visceral afferent* fibers carry impulses from the viscera to the central nervous system.

The receptors of afferent fibers transmit to the central nervous system by numerous converging fibers through peripheral nerves. As a result of this convergence of neurons, injury to a nerve fiber does not result in clearly defined sensory deficits. Rather, the area that responds in an altered manner is vaguely defined.

The areas in the skin innervated by specific spinal nerves are commonly called *dermatomes*. Traditionally, these have been arranged to correspond to the spinal cord segments. Thus, a rather loose topographic division of these segments includes the 8 cervical, 12 thoracic, 5 lumbar, and 5 sacral cord regions. Dermatomes are more specifically mapped according to the segmentation of individual dorsal roots (Fig. 42-23).

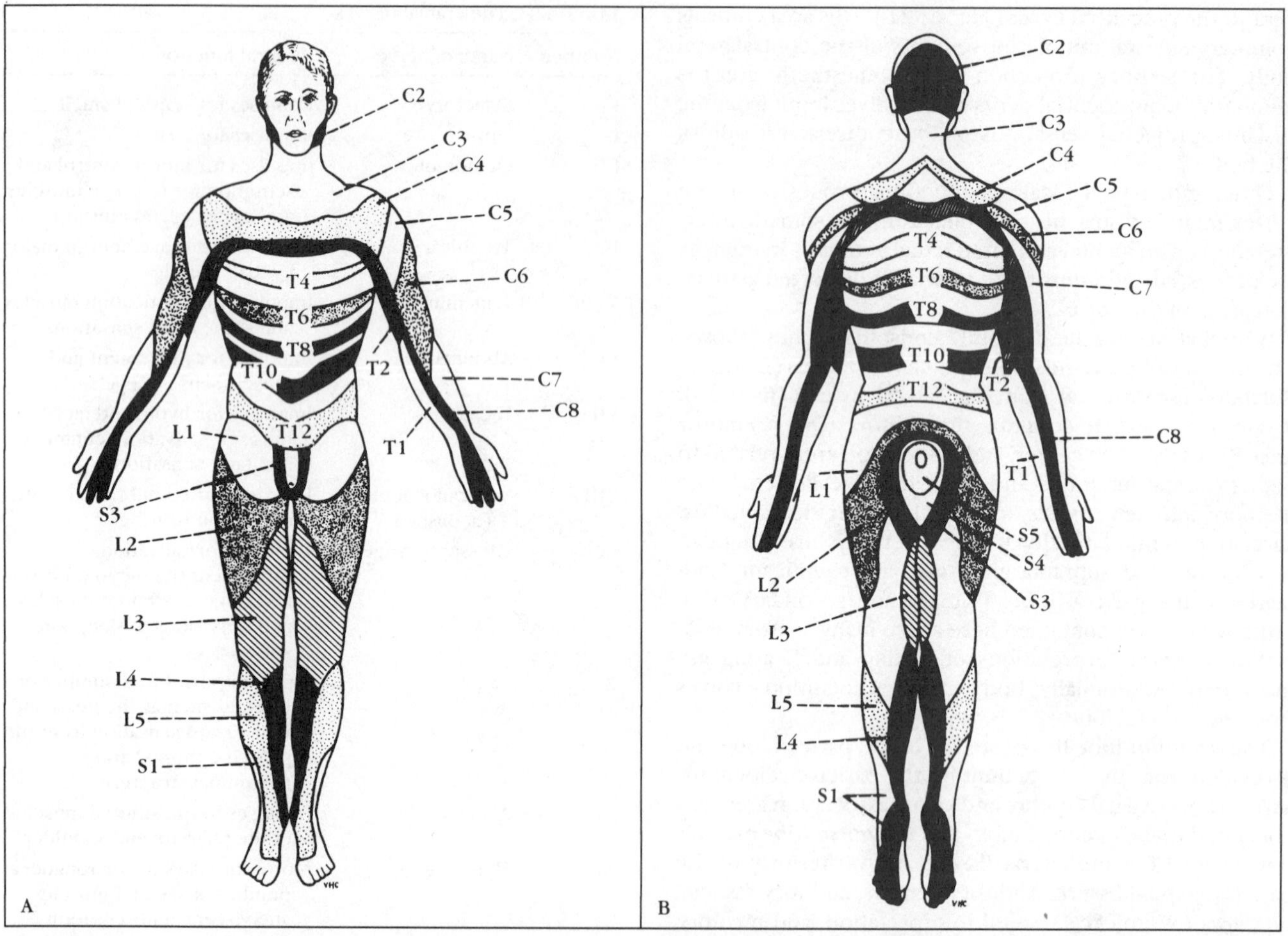

FIGURE 42-23. A. Dermatomes on the anterior aspect of the body. B. Dermatomes on the posterior aspect of the body. (From R. Snell, *Clinical Neuroanatomy for Medical Students*. Boston: Little, Brown, 1980.)

The afferent fibers carrying sensory data enter the spinal cord via the dorsal roots and become dispersed according to function. Fibers associated with pain and temperature transmission are anatomically related and ascend through the *lateral spinothalamic tract* to the posterior ventral nucleus of the thalamus. The *ventral spinothalamic tracts* contain fibers from receptors that are sensitive to touch and pressure (Fig. 42-24). From here they proceed to the somesthetic region of the cerebral postcentral gyrus. Impulses from muscles, tendons, ligaments, and joints (proprioceptive fibers) disperse in a variety of tracts. Some simply cross the cord to the anterior horn (stretch reflex). Others synapse with the posterior gray column and ascend the spinocerebellar tracts to the cerebellum, while yet others ascend via the posterior white columns, decussate at the medial lemniscus, and continue to the posterior ventral nucleus of the thalamus. The ascent from this region continues to the sensory cortex at the postcentral gyrus. Figure 42-22 identifies the somesthetic projection areas on the postcentral gyrus. It is significant that the body areas that contain more sensory receptors are accorded a larger area on the surface of the sensory cortex. For example, the face and fingers, which are prolific with receptors, occupy a larger neuronal area in the cortex than does the large body area of the trunk with its comparatively smaller receptor population.

As noted earlier, an important component of the afferent division is the thalamus, primarily because almost all sensory systems convey impulses to its specific nuclei via either the dorsal column or anterolateral tract. Together with the thalamus, the cortex plays an important role in conscious perception of sensory stimuli occurring distantly from it. The thalamus provides perception of touch and pressure, whereas more complex discrimination sensations such as texture, size, and weight of objects are interpreted by the cortex.

The Efferent Division (Motor)

Voluntary and involuntary body activities initiated by the efferent division are transmitted as a response to the stimuli the central nervous system has received from the afferent division. These responses may be through the innervation of smooth muscles, cardiac muscle, and glands. This

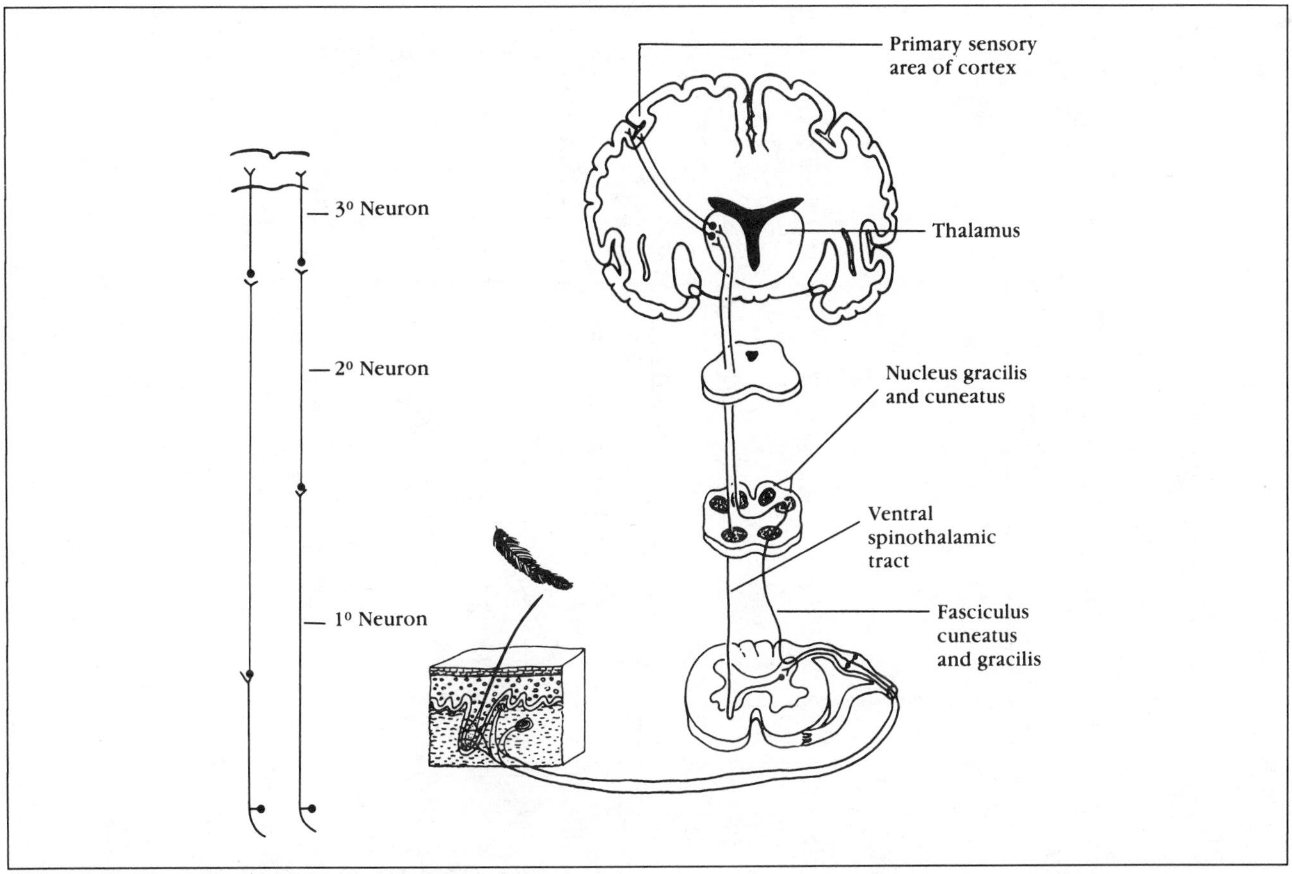

FIGURE 42-24. Touch-pressure pathways ascending to the thalamus via the ventral spinothalamic tract. Information is transmitted through a continuous neuron chain. (From L. Langley and J. Christensen, *Structure and Function of the Human Body*. Minneapolis: Burgess, 1978.)

transmission arrives via the autonomic nervous system and is referred to as the *visceral efferent system*. The skeletal muscles, tendons, and joints receive innervation from the central nervous system via the *somatic efferent system*. The somatic responses at the lowest level occur in the spinal cord and are transmitted through the spinal reflex arc from each spinal segment. These responses are automatic and spontaneous.

The efferent fibers emerge from the ventral horn nuclei (motor horn cells) and transmit impulses through the spinal nerves. It is significant to note that both efferent and afferent fibers are transmitting concurrently in most peripheral nerves and, thus, injury to one of these nerves results in both a sensory and motor deficit.

The efferent fibers receive their impulses from simple spinal reflex circuits or more complicated descending pathways from higher centers. The significant higher centers that play an important role in the relay of efferent responses to the periphery include the precentral gyrus (motor cortex), basal ganglia, brainstem, and cerebellum. The fibers that transmit from these areas do so through two principle tracts, the pyramidal and extrapyramidal tracts.

PYRAMIDAL AND EXTRAPYRAMIDAL SYSTEMS. The pyramidal tract (Fig. 42-25), both lateral and ventral, originates in the motor cortex (precentral gyrus) of the cerebrum in large pyramid-shaped cells, called Betz cells. It transmits, uninterrupted, in a descending manner through the basal ganglia and brainstem. The area where it joins other projection fibers, between the basal ganglia and the thalamus, is known as the *internal capsule*. In the brainstem, the tract decussates and projects through a structure known as the *pyramid*. The crossed fibers then continue to descend as the *lateral corticospinal tract*. A few fibers continue to descend without decussation via the *ventral corticospinal tract*. The fibers of the pyramidal tract compose the *upper motor neuron*. The pyramidal fibers synapse with segmental anterior horn cells (motor neurons) which, in turn, synapse with peripheral efferent fibers innervating specific muscles, tendons, and joints. The neurons innervating skeletal muscle are known as the *lower motor neuron* [1].

The remaining efferent fibers that do not traverse the pyramid in the brainstem are known to be part of the *extrapyramidal systems*. Unlike the pyramidal tract, the extrapyramidal tracts do not continue to the cord uninterrupted. The system is more complex and is considered by some authors to be a functional rather than an anatomic entity. Many of the fibers descend from the cortex directly to specific areas in the basal ganglia and brainstem

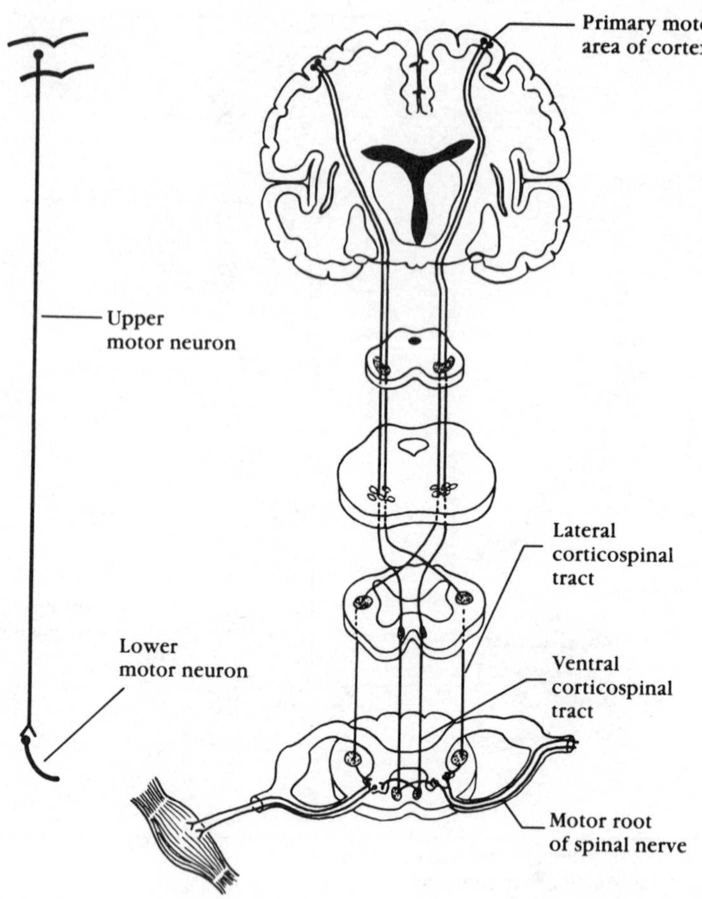

FIGURE 42-25. Pyramidal motor pathways originating at the primary motor area. The lateral corticospinal tract crosses at the level of the medulla and the ventral corticospinal tract descends uncrossed. The pyramidal tract is composed of the upper motor neuron and the lower motor neuron. (From L. Langley and J. Christensen, *Structure and Function of the Human Body.* Minneapolis: Burgess, 1978.)

while others make intermediate synapses. Several extrapyramidal tracts originate in the brainstem and are named for the site of their origin. These include the *vestibulospinal tract* from the lateral vestibular nucleus in the medulla, the *rubrospinal tract* from the red nucleus in the midbrain, the *tectospinal tract* from the roof (superior colliculus) of the midbrain, and the *reticulospinal tract* from the reticular formation in the pons and medulla. The majority of the extrapyramidal fibers decussate with the reticulospinal tract. In addition to the named extrapyramidal tracts, important fibers of this system originate in the cerebellum and the vestibular apparatus.

The pyramidal tract processes information regarding voluntary movement dealing with precise and specific activities of muscles, whereas the extrapyramidal tracts provide the "supporting" type of movement that accompanies the more precise movements afforded by the pyramidal tract. For example, the gross movements necessary to engage in the activity of writing are influenced by the extrapyramidal tracts. Included here are such movements as might be necessary for proper body positioning, particularly of the upper arm and shoulder, in order to engage in writing activity. The more precise movement of holding the pencil effectively is controlled by the corticospinal tract.

THE AUTONOMIC NERVOUS SYSTEM

Autonomic fibers project innervations from the central nervous system to smooth muscles, cardiac muscle, and glands in an involuntary manner. These fibers differ from somatic efferent fibers in that they consist of a double neuron chain from the central nervous system to the visceral effectors, whereas the somatic efferents transmit through one neuron. Visceral efferent fibers transmit in spinal nerves and in several cranial nerves. Visceral efferent innervation frequently accompanies somatic efferent activity. For example, a jogger receives innervation from the somatic efferent fibers to provide the skeletal muscle re-

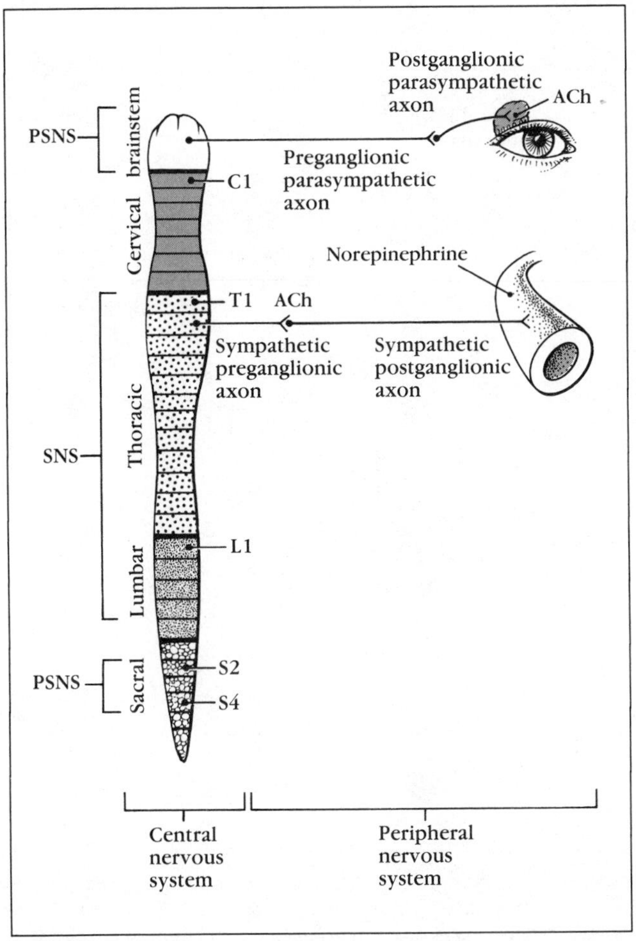

FIGURE 42-26. Schematic overview of the origins of sympathetic (SNS) and parasympathetic (PSNS) nervous systems with corresponding major transmitter substances at the synapses: acetylcholine (ACh) and norepinephrine (noradrenalin).

sponses required in the jogging activity, and simultaneously the somatic efferent system innervates the cardiac and smooth muscle. The somatic efferent responses can be observed readily, whereas the visceral efferent responses are less obvious.

In addition to the autonomic efferent fibers certain afferent fibers are sometimes assigned to the autonomic nervous system. These are found in spinal nerves as well as in certain cranial nerves and innervate receptors in the viscera, the thorax, as well as the walls of the blood vessels.

The autonomic nervous system consists of two functionally distinct divisions, the *sympathetic* and the *parasympathetic* (Fig. 42-26). Many visceral effector organs have a dual nerve supply, one from the sympathetic division and another from the parasympathetic division. The sympathetic division assists the body into action during physiologic and psychologic stress by supportive activities, such as increasing the heart and respiratory rates and mobilizing glucose from glycogen stores to supply the skeletal muscles with additional energy. The parasympathetic division provides a counterbalance for a sympathetic division. Nerve cells of both divisions of the autonomic nervous system group outside the central nervous system in structures known as *autonomic ganglia.* Cell fibers that terminate with a synapse at these ganglia and retain the cell body within the central nervous system are the *preganglionic neurons.* Conversely, nerve cells having cell bodies in the ganglia and axons extending to the organs and glands are known as the *postganglionic neurons.*

The sympathetic system has a chain of paired ganglia on either side of the spinal cord, extending its full length. These ganglia are connected on each side by nerve trunks and together are referred to as the right and left *sympathetic chain* or *sympathetic trunk.* In addition to these paired sympathetic ganglia, single ganglia exist in the abdominal and pilar region where preganglionic neurons from both sides terminate without synapsing in the sympathetic chain. These are known as *collateral (prevertebral) ganglia* and include the celiac and superior and inferior mesenteric ganglia. The parasympathetic ganglia are located in the proximity of the effector organs.

The Sympathetic Division (Thoracolumbar)

The cell bodies of the short preganglionic sympathetic neurons arise from the sympathetic motoneurons of the intermediolateral horns of the spinal cord between the first thoracic vertebra and fourth lumbar vertebra (see Fig. 42-26). The fibers of these neurons pass through the intervertebral foramina in conjunction with respective spinal nerves. Shortly the sympathetic fibers (preganglionic) depart from the spinal nerve and enter a sympathetic chain through the white rami communicantes (Fig. 42-27). They may synapse here immediately with a postganglion neuron or pass directly through the sympathetic chain to synapse with a single sympathetic ganglion, or pass up or down the sympathetic chain and synapse at a different level.

Some postganglionic sympathetic fibers, after having synapsed in the sympathetic chain, pass back into the spinal nerve via the gray rami communicantes and accompany the spinal nerve to innervate blood vessels, sweat glands, and arrector pili muscles in the skin.

The Parasympathetic Division (Craniosacral)

The autonomic fibers that evolve from the cranial and sacral portions of the central nervous system compose the parasympathetic nervous system (see Fig. 42-26). Somatic efferent fibers in the cranial region arise in conjunction with the oculomotor (third), facial (seventh), glossopharyngeal (ninth), and vagus (tenth) nerves. The vagus transmits the majority of the parasympathetic impulses through its wide distribution in the thoracic and abdominal viscera. The remaining cranial nerves innervate organs of the head. The sacral fibers arise from the anterior roots of the second, third, and fourth sacral spinal nerves. Most of the preganglionic fibers transmit without interruption to the

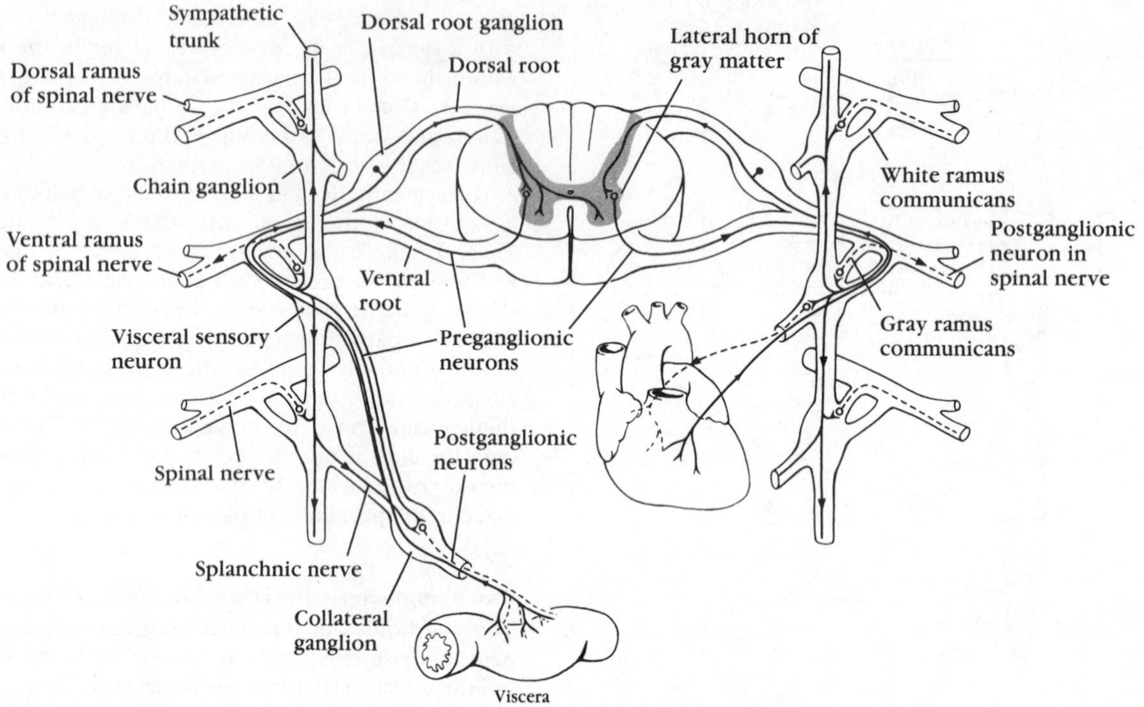

FIGURE 42-27. Sympathetic fibers emerge from the spinal cord in conjunction with respective spinal nerves and transmit to autonomic ganglia via white rami. (From A. Spence and E. Mason, *Human Anatomy and Physiology*. Menlo Park, Calif.: Benjamin/Cummings, 1979.)

organs they innervate where they synapse with the parasympathetic ganglia that are located in the area of the effector organ. In contrast to the sympathetic fibers, the parasympathetic preganglionic fibers are long and the postganglionic fibers short.

Transmitter Substances of the Autonomic Nervous System

Chemical mediation is necessary for neuronal transmission between neurons and between neurons and their effector organs. Excitation results from chemical release of transmitter substances between preganglionic and postganglionic neurons and their effectors in the autonomic nervous system. The transmitter substance in the autonomic nervous system from the preganglionic neurons to the postganglionic neurons in both the sympathetic and parasympathetic nervous systems is *acetylcholine*. Acetylcholine (ACh) continues to be the transmitter substance from the parasympathetic postganglionic neurons. Because of the secretion of ACh these fibers are known as *cholinergic* and their receptors are cholinoceptive.

The primary transmitter substance secreted by the postganglionic fibers of the sympathetic nervous system to its effector organs is *norepinephrine* (NE). The fibers are referred to as *adrenergic* and terminate on *adrenoceptive* receptors (alpha and beta). A few of the fibers of the postganglionic sympathetic nervous system secrete ACh at their terminal fibers, including fibers to sweat glands and postganglionic sympathetic vasodilator fibers to skeletal muscle vasculature. A single postganglionic sympathetic nerve may innervate thousands of receptor sites. This is demonstrated by the diffuse response to the sympathetic nervous system excitation in contrast to the more localized responses characteristically seen with parasympathetic activity.

Receptor Substances of the Effector Organs

The effector organs secrete substances that react with terminal bouton secretions. The exact nature of these substances is uncertain at this time. It has been theorized that the combination of the autonomic nervous system transmitter substance and receptor substances alters the permeability of the cell membrane to certain ions. This alteration may result in changes in membrane potential eliciting either action potentials or tonic effects. In addition to changes in the cell membrane, receptor substances may initiate chemical reactions within the cell.

TABLE 42-4. The effects of sympathetic and parasympathetic stimulation on effector organs

Organ	Sympathetic stimulation	Parasympathetic stimulation
Eye		
Radial muscle of iris	Dilates	
Sphincter muscle of iris		Constricts
Heart		
SA node	Increases rate	Decreases rate
Atria	Increases contractility	Decreases contractility
Ventricles	Increases contractility, conduction, automaticity	
Blood vessels	Generally constricts, dilates coronary arteries	None
Lungs		
Bronchial muscle	Dilates (relaxes)	Constricts
Bronchial secretions	Decreases	Increases
Bronchial vessels	Contracts	None
Skin		
Sweat glands	Copious generalized secretion	Slight localized secretion
Intestine		
Motility	Decreases	Increases
Sphincters	Contracts	Relaxes
Liver	Glycogenolysis	None
Gallbladder and ducts	Relaxes	Constricts
Pancreas		
Acini cells	None	Secrete
Islet cells	Inhibit alpha-receptors, stimulates beta-receptors to secrete	Secrete
Salivary glands	Thick secretions	Thin secretions
Fat cells	Lipolysis	None
Bladder		
Detrusor muscle	Relaxes	Contracts
Trigone	Contracts	Relaxes
Penis	Ejaculation	Erection
Basal metabolism	Increased	None
Adrenal cortex	Increased secretion	None
Mentation	Increased	None

Stimulation and Inhibition Action of the Autonomic Nervous System

The actions of the sympathetic and parasympathetic nervous system on various receptor organs are summarized in Table 42-4. The dual actions are a cooperative effort to maintain a constant internal environment in response to the ever-changing external world. General responses of the sympathetic nervous system are activated under emergency situations to provide internal adjustments that facilitate an appropriate response by the body. For example, in response to stressful exercise, the cardiovascular system is stimulated by the sympathetic system to increase cardiac output by increasing heart rate in order to provide additional perfusion to skeletal muscle, brain, and liver, while simultaneously reducing the blood supply to the viscera. The parasympathetic system, in contrast, promotes activities that maintain body function from day to day, including digestion and elimination.

The visceral effectors that receive stimulation from both the sympathetic and parasympathetic systems generally receive antagonistic stimulation. An example of this includes the effect on bronchial secretions. Sympathetic stimulation decreases bronchial secretions and these are increased by parasympathetic stimulation. In another example, the sympathetic system dilates the pupil while the parasympathetic system constricts it. The dual system does not function consistently in a cooperative balance, as some organs receive innervation primarily from only one system. Examples include the innervation of smooth muscles of the skin, hair, sweat glands, and cutaneous blood vessels from the sympathetic system alone. The detrusor muscle of the bladder receives parasympathetic innervation only.

The inibitory actions of the autonomic nervous system occur both directly and indirectly on the effector organs. For example, vagal stimulation (parasympathetic) slows the heart through a direct inhibitory action of the cholinergic postganglionic neurons on the sinoatrial node. On the other hand, vasodilation of the peripheral arterioles occurs indirectly through a decrease in impulse transmission in the sympathetic effector fibers.

While most organs and viscera receive innervation from both sympathetic and parasympathetic systems, one of these generally has an inhibitory effect and the other an excitatory effect. However, there is no consistent rule of thumb for guidance as to which system stimulates and which system inhibits.

Effects of Sympathetic and Parasympathetic Stimulation on Various Structures

LACRIMAL GLANDS. The parasympathetic system vasodilates and stimulates secretion of the lacrimal glands through the postganglionic axons from the sphenopalatine ganglion via the maxillary division of the fifth cranial nerve. The preganglionic axons originate in the superior salivatory nucleus and follow the route of the seventh cranial nerve. The sympathetic system has a vasoconstrictive effect on the lacrimal glands and transmits its impulses through preganglionic neurons, which originate from the intermediolateral cells in the thoracic spinal column, and through postganglionic neurons of the superior cervical ganglion; the impulses reach the glands via the maxillary division of the fifth cranial nerve.

EYE. Pupillary constriction and near vision accommodation are accomplished through parasympathetic stimulation. The oculomotor nucleus sends preganglionic axons via the oculomotor nerve to the ciliary ganglion. From here the postganglionic axons reach the ciliary muscle and constrictor muscle of the iris via the ciliary nerve. When pupils are reflexively stimulated with light, the pupillary opening decreases and reduces the amount of light reaching the retina.

The sympathetic stimulation dilates the pupil, constricts vessels, elevates the eyelid, and provides far vision accommodation. The preganglionic axons of fibers accomplishing these activities originate in the thoracic spinal segments and ascend via the sympathetic chain to the superior cervical ganglion where they synapse with the postganglionic neurons. The postganglionic axons travel via divisions of the fifth nerve to the dilator muscles of the iris (levator palpebrae superioris), and radial fibers of the ciliary muscle. Innervation of blood vessels of the retina, orbit, and conjunctiva are accomplished in the same manner.

SALIVARY GLANDS. The superior salivary nucleus projects the preganglionic axons for the submaxillary and sublingual glands, and the inferior salivary nucleus projects preganglionic axons for the parotid gland. The axons from the superior salivary nucleus travel via a branch of the seventh cranial nerve to the submaxillary and sublingual ganglia, and those from the inferior salivary nucleus travel via a branch of the ninth cranial nerve to the otic ganglia. From the submaxillary and sublingual ganglia axons project to their glands and from the otic ganglia to the parotid gland via the fifth cranial nerve. The parasympathetic system activates these glands to vasodilate and secrete.

The sympathetic system vascoconstricts and promotes secretion of salivary glands. Its preganglionic axons ascend from the upper thoracic spinal cord to the superior cervical ganglia to synapse with the postganglionic neurons. These axons reach the glands along the external carotid and external maxillary arteries.

HEART. The overall effect of the parasympathetic system on the heart is of deceleration. Its stimulation of the heart decreases its effectiveness; however, in the process it does slow the metabolism and oxygen requirements, and thus provides some rest for the cardiac muscle. The parasympathetic preganglionic fibers pass from the dorsal motor nucleus of the vagus and synapse with the postganglionic neurons through the vagal trunk at cardiac plexus ganglia in the atrial walls.

In contrast, the sympathetic system increases the overall activity of the heart, produces both positive chronotropic and inotropic effects, and dilates the coronary arteries. In essence, the sympathetic system makes the heart more effective, although it simultaneously increases work load and metabolic requirements. The upper thoracic spinal cord provides the origin of the preganglionic neurons, which project their axons from the ventral roots and white rami to the sympathetic chain. The postganglionic neurons emerge from higher thoracic and lower cervical ganglia and travel to the cardiac plexus.

BRONCHI. The bronchi are constricted by the parasympathetic system. The origin of the parasympathetic neurons and the course of their preganglionic and postganglionic fibers are similar to those of the parasympathetic fibers innervating the heart. The preganglionic fibers synapse with the postganglionic fibers in the pulmonary plexus. The axons of the postganglionic cells terminate in the bronchi and blood vessels.

The sympathetic system dilates the bronchi. The neurons originate in thoracic segments 2 through 6 and their axons enter the pulmonary plexus in a manner similar to that of the parasympathetic system.

ESOPHAGUS. The parasympathetic system exerts the main autonomic influence over the function of the esophagus. The stimulation causes contraction of smooth muscle of the esophagus, increasing its overall activity in propelling ingested materials along its course. This stimulation comes from various branches of the vagus nerve.

ABDOMINAL VISCERA, GLANDS, AND VESSELS. The parasympathetic system stimulation promotes peristalsis and increase in secretion by the various gastrointestinal glands. The preganglionic fibers originate from the vagus and synapse with the postganglionic fibers of the various visceral organs in their intrinsic plexus.

In contrast, the sympathetic system inhibits peristalsis and enhances vacoconstriction. The lower thoracic and upper lumbar cord segments provide the origin of the preganglionic neurons. Their axons traverse the splanchnic nerves to synapse with the postganglionic neurons in the prevertebral ganglion plexus. Innervation is provided to the visceral smooth muscle and blood vessels.

PELVIC VISCERA. The parasympathetic system stimulation assists in urination and defecation by contraction of the bladder and lower colon. In addition, erection is facilitated by the parasympathetic system. The parasympathetic system neurons accomplishing these functions originate in the sacral cord segments and their axons transmit to the various organs.

The sympathetic system stimulation promotes contraction of the vesical sphincter, vasoconstriction, and ejaculation. The preganglionic neurons originate in the lower thoracic and upper lumbar segments and travel along the splanchnic nerves similarly to those of the abdominal viscera. The postganglionic fibers travel along the hypogastric nerves of the organs innervated.

PERIPHERAL VESSELS AND SWEAT GLANDS. The major effect of the autonomic nervous system on the peripheral and deep vessels is through stimulation of the sympathetic system. This stimulation results in vasoconstriction of cutaneous vessels as well as deep visceral vessels. Sweat glands secrete in response to sympathetic stimulation. However, the postganglionic fibers to the sweat glands are cholinergic in contrast with other sympathetic fibers that are adrenergic. For this reason, many sources classify sweat secretion as a sympathetic function.

ADRENAL MEDULLA. In response to sympathetic stimulation, the adrenal medulla secretes epinephrine and norepinephrine into the circulating blood, which reaches all cells and produces an excitatory effect. This mechanism is part of the diffuse sympathoadrenal system, which is activated in response to stress. In addition to the stimulatory effect on the nervous system, epinephrine and norepinephrine affect metabolism through glycogenolysis in the liver and skeletal muscle and mobilization of fatty acids. Distinct effects of circulating epinephrine and norepinephrine on heart function include an increased force and rate of contraction, as well as increased excitability of the myocardium. Norepinephrine produces vasoconstriction in most organs, whereas epinephrine has a dilating effect on the vessels of the liver and skeletal muscle. Other effects observed in response to circulating epinephrine and norepinephrine include an increased mental acuity, inhibition of the gastrointestinal tract, and pupillary dilation. Thus, the circulating catecholamines released by the adrenal medulla have functions similar to those of the adrenergic nerve discharges and, indeed, enhance their action. The effects of the circulating catecholamines linger as their metabolism or removal from blood takes longer than it does in those released at the adrenergic nerve terminals.

Minimal secretion of epinephrine and norepinephrine occurs at basal conditions as in sleep; however, during increased activity and stress, or when adrenergic stimulation is increased in such conditions as pain, cold, hypoglycemia, and emotional excitement, secretion is considerably increased. This stimulation is transmitted to the adrenal medulla via the hypothalamic nervous centers as well as direct sympathetic innervation of the medulla.

To distinguish the effects of epinephrine and norepinephrine on receptor cells, two distinct receptor catecholamine substances have been identified. These are *alpha-receptors,* which mediate vasoconstriction and are acted on by both norepinephrine and epinephrine, and *beta-receptors,* which mediate vasodilation and actions to increase the rate and strength of the cardiac function. The latter are acted upon by epinephrine. Alpha-receptors are dispersed widely in various organs but predominate in the precapillary sphincters of smooth muscles of blood vessels. Beta-receptors predominate in the heart, coronary arteries, liver, and brain.

AUTONOMIC REFLEXES. In response to certain environmental conditions, autonomic reflexes maintain the internal environment appropriate to the demand, that of either action or repair. For the most part the actions occur at an unconscious level and involve functions such as control of pupillary size, cardiovascular status, and variations in respiratory and gastrointestinal and genitourinary systems.

THE VENTRICULAR AND CEREBROSPINAL FLUID SYSTEMS

Function of Cerebrospinal Fluid

The cerebrospinal fluid (CSF) that circulates in the subarachnoid space around the brain and spinal cord (Fig. 42-28), provides an important supportive and protective mechanism for the central nervous system. Along with support from blood vessels, nerve roots, and fine fibrous arachnoid trabeculae, the brain is directly encased within the subarachnoid cerebrospinal fluid and receives buoyance from it which prevents stretching of the vessels and nerve roots in response to acceleration of the head. The average weight of the adult brain is approximately 1450 gm in the air, although in the buoyant CSF bath its weight is reduced to approximately 50 gm. This buoyancy allows for a relatively effective suspension of the brain and assists in preventing lethal damage under everyday traumas.

The *pneumoencephalography* procedure demonstrates the effects of CSF deficiency on the brain. This diagnostic procedure to visualize structural elements of the brain requires that the CSF be removed and replaced by air. Thus, the weight of the brain rests on the vascular, nervous, and meningeal structures and results in a severe headache which is greatly intensified by the slightest jarring of the head.

In addition to its mechanical function, CSF provides a medium for passage of substances between blood and the extracellular fluid of the brain. It probably functions in the nourishment of brain tissues and removal of the metabolites of nerve cell function.

Formation and Absorption of CSF

The production, circulation, and resorption of CSF occurs continuously. Its principal formation site is in the *choroid plexuses* of the lateral ventricle with most of the remainder being formed in the third and fourth ventricle (Fig. 42-29). Choroid plexuses consist of capillary tufts that are surrounded by cuboidal epithelium (Fig. 42-30). CSF is produced through filtration, diffusion, and active transport from the blood. In the adult human, approximately 500 ml of fluid is produced per 24 hours and approximately 125 ml is circulating at any given time. However, wide fluctuations may occur in the amount produced during any given 24-hour period (Table 42-5). Sodium ion is actively transported across the epithelial cells into the CSF from the blood. This results in a greater osmotic force in the CSF so that to maintain osmotic equilibrium water passively follows the ions. Thus, water is extracted from the capillaries and is responsible for the secretory function of the choroid plexus. Facilitated diffusion allows transportation of glucose in both directions.

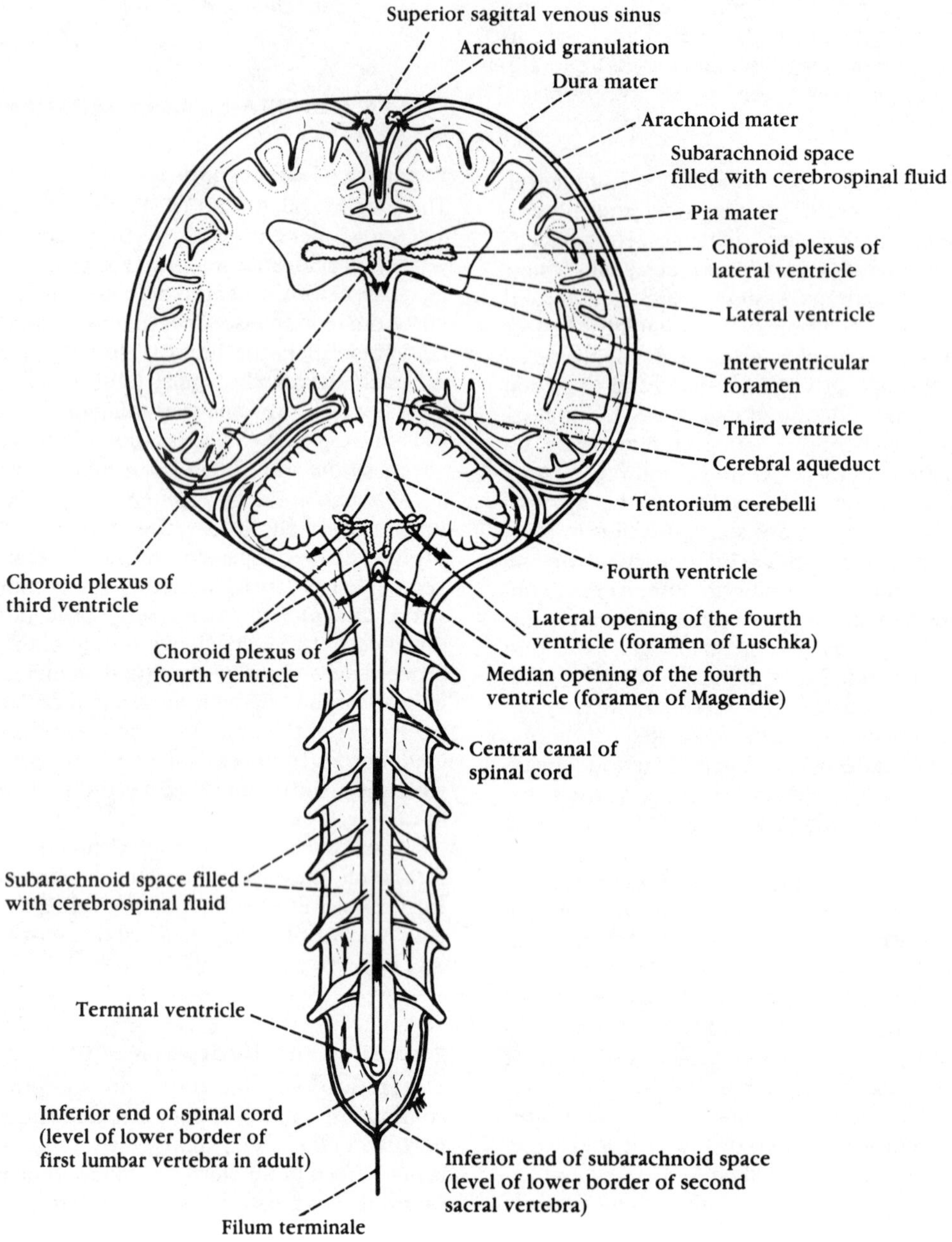

FIGURE 42-28. Formation and circulation of cerebrospinal fluid. (From R. Snell, *Clinical Neuroanatomy for Medical Students*. Boston: Little, Brown, 1980.)

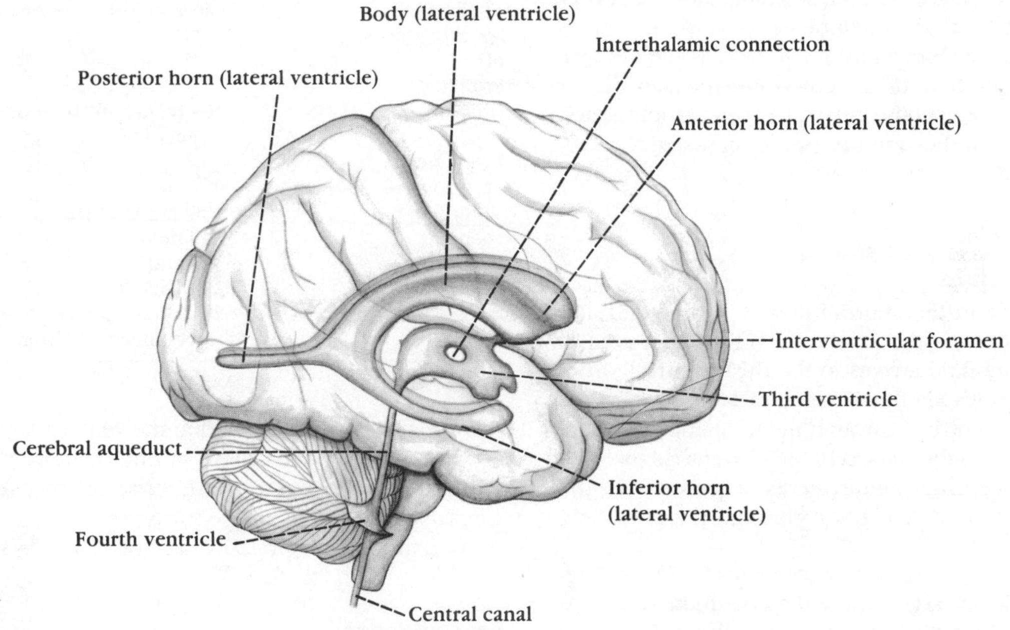

FIGURE 42-29. The lateral third and fourth ventricles. (From R. Snell, *Clinical Neuroanatomy for Medical Students*. Boston: Little, Brown, 1980.)

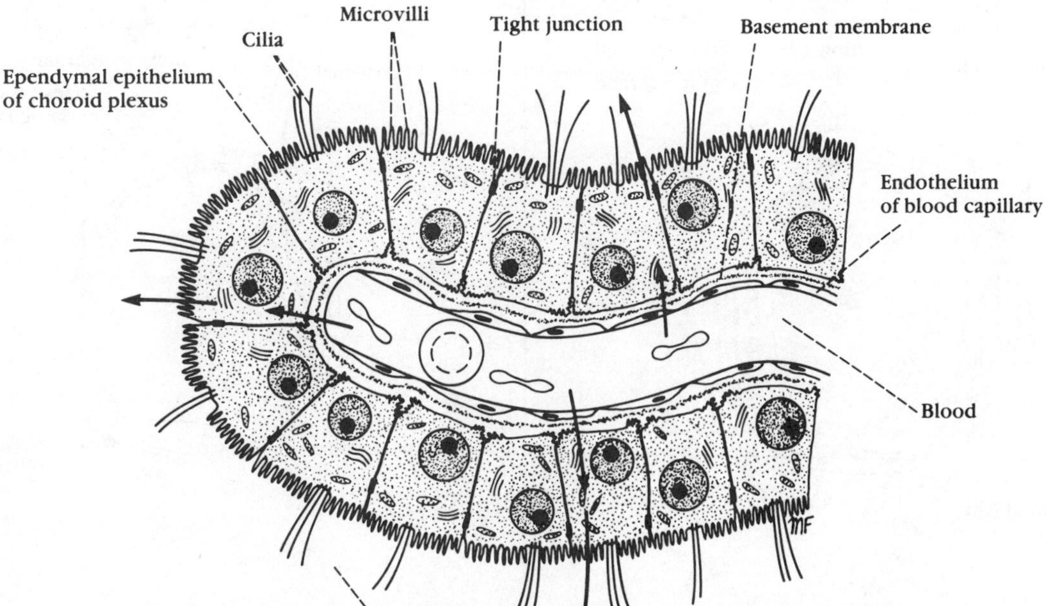

FIGURE 42-30. Microscopic structure of choroid plexus. (From R. Snell, *Clinical Neuroanatomy for Medical Students*. Boston: Little, Brown, 1980.)

CSF is absorbed into the venous circulation through *arachnoid villi* (see Fig. 42-13), or granulations that project from the cerebral subarachnoid space into the venous sinuses. The passive absorption of CSF takes place because the hydrostatic pressure of the CSF is greater than that of venous blood in the venous sinuses. Certain particles, such as red blood cells and creatinine, pass unimpeded through the arachnoid villi.

Flow and Obstruction of Flow of Cerebrospinal Fluid

The origin of CSF in the choroid plexus of the ventricles and its normal flow to the arachnoid villi is illustrated in Figure 42-28. The fluid arrives in the third ventricle from the lateral ventricles via the foramen of Monro and flows on to the fourth ventricle through the foramina of Magendie and Luschka into the subarachnoid cisterns. As the fluid flows over the cerebral hemispheres, it passes into the sagittal sinus for rapid resorption through the arachnoid villi.

Interference along the pathway of the flow of CSF will result in ventricular enlargement and a condition known as *hydrocephalus.* Two distinct types of hydrocephalus are the *communicating type* and the *noncommunicating type.* If CSF flows freely between the ventricles and lumbar subarachnoid space, it is known as *communicating hydrocephalus* and a blockage within the ventricular system that prevents free flow of CSF from one or more ventricles is referred to as *noncommunicating hydrocephalus.* Ventricular dilation results in both types and this leads to increased intracranial pressure (see pp. 732–733).

TABLE 42-5. Normal values of cerebrospinal fluid

Appearance	Clear, colorless, odorless
Specific gravity	1.007
pH	7.35
Protein	15–45 mg/dl
Glucose	40–80 mg/dl (60% of serum glucose level)
Lymphocytes	0–5
Erythrocytes	0
Chlorides	120–130 mEq/L
Sodium	140 mEq/L
Potassium	3.0 mEq/L
Bicarbonate	23.6 mEq/L
Pressure	80–180 mm H_2O (in side recumbent position)

Brain Barrier

Brain cell function is dependent on a closely controlled environment. Not all circulating substances in the blood pass freely to the brain or CSF. This occurs either because their

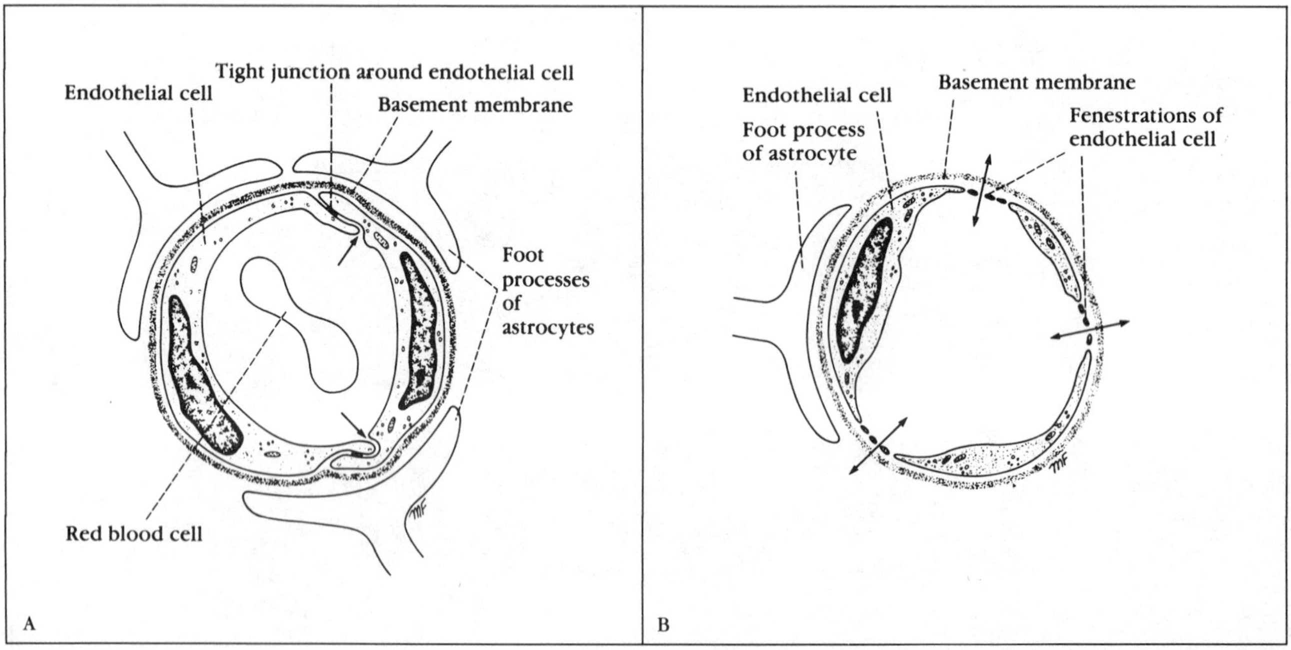

FIGURE 42-31. Blood-brain barrier. A. Cross section of blood capillary of central nervous system in area where blood-brain barrier exists. B. Cross section of blood capillary of central nervous system where blood-brain barrier appears to be absent. Note presence of fenestrations in endothelial cells. (From R. Snell, *Clinical Neuroanatomy for Medical Students.* Boston: Little, Brown, 1980.)

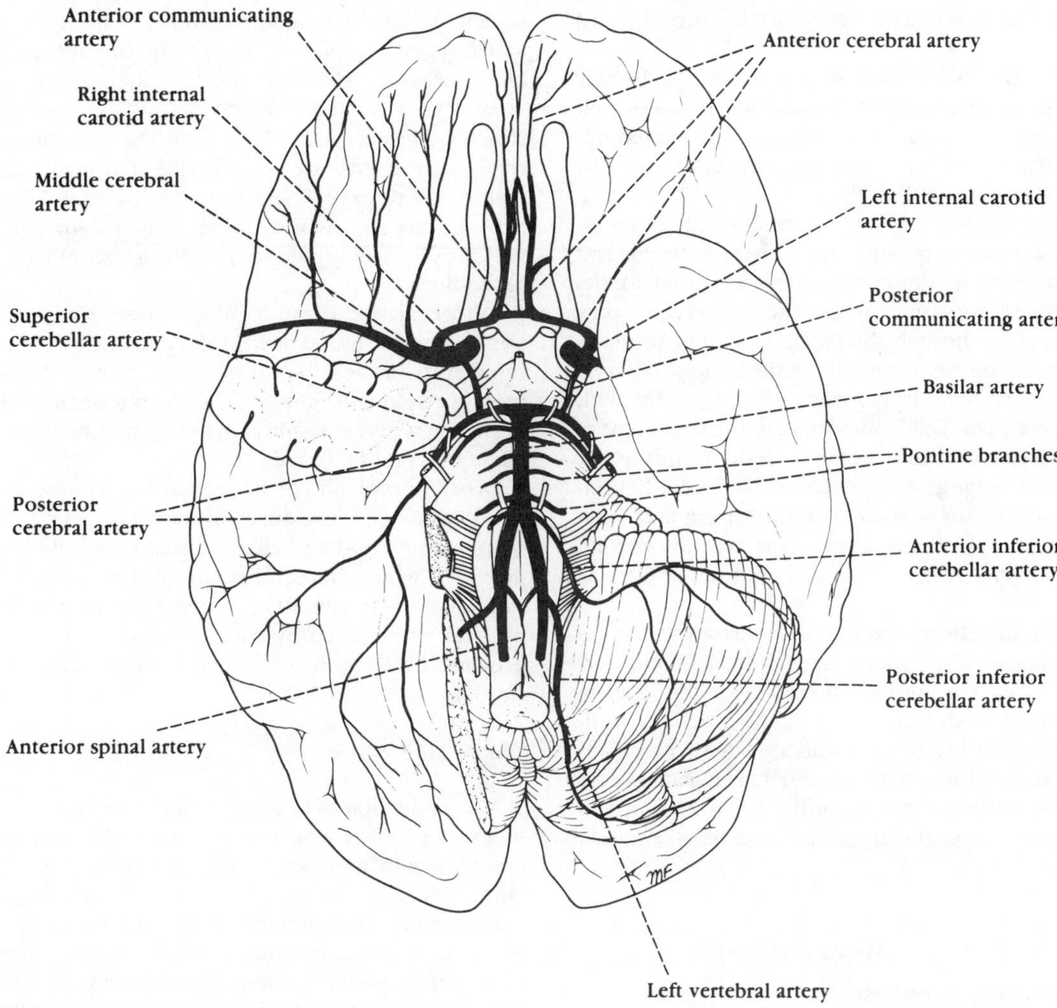

FIGURE 42-32. The arteries on the inferior surface of the brain. Note the formation of the circulus arteriosus (circle of Willlis). (From R. S. Snell, *Clinical Neuroanatomy for Medical Students*. Boston: Little, Brown, 1980.)

molecules are too large or the molecules they bind with are too large to cross the CNS membranes. This has been demonstrated with the injection of certain acidic dyes such as trypan blue, which stains other body tissues but not most brain tissue. The molecules these dyes bind with are too large to enter the brain or CSF. Substances pass into the brain from the blood via capillaries to the extracellular space of the brain, or by the way of the choroid plexus into the CSF from which small amounts are passed into the brain. Barriers exist between the blood and brain and between the blood and the CSF.

The materials separating the various cerebral compartments, in essence, are responsible for the entrance and exit of materials to and from the CSF and brain. The choroid plexus and the brain parenchyma (except the hypothalamus) provide the barriers for free movement of substances into the brain. Molecular size, charge, and lipid solubility affect the rate of diffusion across the cerebral membranes and cells. The small molecules and lipid-soluble substances penetrate more rapidly than large molecules and water-soluble polar compounds. Plasma proteins are excluded from the central nervous system because of their large molecular size. Nonionized substances pass more readily into the brain and CSF than ionized substances. Substances that penetrate rapidly into the CSF and brain include water, carbon dioxide, and oxygen.

The endothelia of capillary cells of the brain overlap and are fused together by tight junctions, creating a common thickened basement membrane with adjacent glia and neurons. This dense basement membrane, in conjunction with an additional layer of neuroglial cells surrounding the capillaries, restricts diffusion of large molecular substances between the blood and brain (Fig. 42-31). This capillary structure is equated with the blood-brain barrier. The blood-CSF barrier exists as a result of the secretory function of the choroid plexus. This is evidenced by different concentrations of certain substances in the CSF and in plasma indicating a selective transport by the choroid plexus.

A weaker barrier is afforded by the brain-CSF barrier through the ependymal lining of the ventricular system and its adjacent glial cells. These structures provide some limitation in the transfer of fluids and chemical substances to the interstitial fluids from the CSF.

The brain barriers serve as a protection for the brain by inhibiting potentially toxic substances from entering and facilitating entrance to those substances essential for its metabolism. Substances, such as glucose and oxygen, pass to the brain rapidly through the capillary system to maintain constancy of the environment for the central nervous system neurons. Certain drugs penetrate the barrier with more ease than others. This is important in the treatment of central nervous system infections as certain antibiotics, such as chlortetracyclines and penicillin, have very limited access to the brain; others, such as erythromycin and sulfadiazine enter readily. Because proteins are not readily available for binding, drugs generally do not accumulate in the CSF.

Radiotherapy, infections, and tumors interrupt the brain-barrier systems and allow transport of materials that normally are not readily accorded entrance. For this reason, tumor localization with brain scanning is effectively utilized. Intravenous radioactive substances are injected into the patient and monitored with a scanner. The gamma rays emitted by the substance are recorded on x-ray film and appear as dark areas in the regions of the barrier breakdown.

BRAIN BLOOD SUPPLY AND REGULATION

Arterial and Venous Circulation

The brain receives the blood supply from the *internal carotid* arteries anteriorly and *vertebral* arteries posteriorly. As the internal carotid arteries ascend into the brain, they eventually branch into the *anterior* and *middle cerebral* arteries. The vertebral arteries ascend and become the *basilar* artery at the pons level. The basilar artery terminates in the right and left posterior cerebral arteries, which supply the posterior regions of the cerebrum. The anterior and posterior cerebral arteries are joined by smaller communicating arteries and form a ring known as the *circle of Willis* (Fig. 42-32). The blood supply to both cerebral hemispheres is identical, although anomalies are common and, for the most part, clinically insignificant. The venous system drains the blood from the cerebrum and cerebellum via deep veins and *dural sinuses* that ultimately empty into the *internal jugular* veins.

Autoregulation and Vasomotor Control

The healthy brain has the ability to maintain a fairly constant blood flow (approximately 750 ml/minute) even within widely fluctuating physiologic conditions. Significant factors influencing cerebral blood flow (CBF) constancy include metabolic variations in the carbon dioxide and oxygen levels and changes in the systemic arterial blood pressure. Cerebral arteries dilate in response to increases in carbon dioxide tension and decreases in oxygen tension that increase CBF levels. The vasodilation allows removal of excess carbon dioxide and may facilitate the restoration of oxygen levels toward normal. The effects of hypercapnia and hypoxia have a significant effect on the vessel caliber and thus on the intrinsic control of cerebral blood flow.

Autoregulation of the cerebral vessel size allows a relatively constant blood flow in the presence of wide fluctuations in the arterial blood pressure. A mean arterial blood pressure below 60 mm Hg results in a decreased cerebral perfusion whereas marked hypertension has essentially no effect on cerebral blood flow.

Other factors affecting cerebral blood flow include cerebral perfusion pressure, intracranial pressure, cardiac output, and blood viscosity. Normal cerebral blood flow is provided when the cerebral perfusion pressure (CPP) is maintained between 40 to 130 mm Hg. Cerebral perfusion pressure is obtained by subtracting the mean intracranial pressure (ICP) from the mean systemic arterial pressure (MAP):

$$CPP = MAP - ICP$$

Autoregulation of cerebral blood flow ceases to function when the CPP is less than 40 mm Hg. When the ICP increases significantly and equals the MAP, CPP and CBF become zero. Marked reduction of CBF is seen when intracranial pressure rises rapidly to about 35 mm Hg. Cerebral blood flow is compromised when cardiac output is decreased by one-third. Increased blood viscosity decreases CBF, and decreased blood viscosity increases CBF.

REFERENCES

1. Clark, R. G. *Essentials of Clinical Neuroanatomy and Neurophysiology* (5th ed.). Philadelphia: Davis, 1975.
2. Eccles, J. C. *The Understanding of the Brain*. New York: McGraw-Hill, 1973.
3. Guyton, A. *Textbook of Medical Physiology* (6th ed.). Philadelphia: Saunders, 1981.
4. Iverson, L. I. The chemistry of the brain. *Sci. Am.* 241:134, 1979.
5. Nauta, W. J., and Feirtag, M. The organization of the brain. *Sci. Am.* 241:88, 1979.
6. Snell, R. S. *Clinical Neuronatomy for Medical Students.* Boston: Little, Brown, 1980.
7. Stevens, C. F. The neuron. *Sci. Am.* 241:54, 1979.

CHAPTER 43
ADAPTATIONS AND ALTERATIONS IN THE SPECIAL SENSES

LEARNING OBJECTIVES

1. Identify the structures of the eye.
2. State the normal intraocular pressure.
3. Trace the visual pathways from the optic disk to the occipital lobe.
4. Discuss the mechanism of image formation in the eye.
5. Define *refraction index*.
6. Explain the process of accommodation.
7. Discuss factors that influence the pupillary aperture.
8. Identify function of rods and cones.
9. Discuss the initiation of receptor potential of the retina.
10. Explain the trichromic theory of color vision.
11. Contrast myopia and hypermetropia.
12. Define *astigmatism*.
13. Discuss the pathologic basis of the hemianopsias.
14. Identify the structures of the ear.
15. Trace sound conduction through the ear and the fiber pathways to the auditory cortex.
16. Differentiate between conduction deafness and sensorineural deafness.
17. Discuss the role of the vestibular system position and movement changes.
18. Identify three tests that might be utilized to detect hearing loss.
19. Locate the primary sensations of taste on the tongue.
20. Trace taste pathways from innervation of taste bud to cerebral cortex.
21. Discuss pathogenesis of taste disturbance.
22. Identify the receptor cell for the sense of smell.
23. Discuss adaptation of smell receptors.
24. Identify potential causes of anosmia.

The senses of vision, hearing, taste, and smell provide humans with the means to perceive the environment and respond in a way that supports adaptation and, at times, even survival. The receptors of the eye, ear, tongue, and nose are stimulated and messages are transmitted to specific regions of the cerebral cortex for processing. Alterations in the function of the special senses, particularly vision and hearing, can result in varying physiologic, psychologic, sociologic, and economic difficulties. The alterations in special senses are multitudinous; the reader is referred to special texts for additional materials.

VISION

Structure and Function

The eye is a complex peripheral structure that transmits vision to the visual area of the occipital lobe of the cerebral cortex. It nestles in the orbit, a cone-shaped cavity with fragile walls composed of the frontal, maxilla, zygomatic, sphenoid, ethmoid, lacrimal, and palatine bones. The thinness of the orbital wall makes this area particularly susceptible to fractures. The eyeball occupies the anterior portion of the orbital cavity; its principle structures are identified in Figure 43-1. The area of the orbit not occupied by the eyeball is filled with fascia, fat, nerves, blood vessels, muscle, and the lacrimal gland. Six extrinsic muscles, most of which arise from the apex of the orbit and insert into the scleral lining, allow for the movement and rotation of the eyeball. These include the superior rectus, inferior rectus, medial rectus, lateral rectus, superior oblique, and inferior oblique muscles. Innervation for these muscles arrives from the third, fourth, and sixth cranial nerves.

The three layers of the eyeball are the *sclera, choroid,* and *retina.* The outermost supportive and protective layer, the sclera, is composed of dense fibrous tissue and forms a white opaque membrane around the eyeball except at the cornea, where it becomes transparent. It is through this transparent area that light rays enter the eye to stimulate the rods and cones. The second, or middle, layer of the eyeball is the vascular choroid. The exchange of nutrients takes place in this heavily pigmented layer. The ciliary muscle, which is important in facilitating the light and accommodation reflex, lies between the sclera and choroid layers. The choroid also contains the *iris,* the center of which is the *pupil.* The sphincter and dilator muscles of the iris, together with the ciliary muscle, are known as the intrinsic muscles of the eye and control the amount of light admitted into the eye. The innervation to these muscles comes from the third cranial nerve and the superior cervical ganglion. The crystalline lens, which is suspended by the suspensory ligament from the inner surface of the ciliary body, bends the rays of light so that they are projected properly on the retina. The *anterior chamber* is a fluid-filled space anterior to the iris and lens. The *posterior chamber,* posterior to the iris and fluid-filled as well, together with the anterior chamber assists in maintaining a constant pressure in the eyeball. Normal intraocular pressure is between 20 and 25 mm Hg. *Glaucoma* results if drainage of this aqueous humor is insufficient through the canal of Schlemm. *Vitreous humor,* which is soft and gelatinous, fills the space behind the lens and helps maintain the shape of the eyeball.

The third layer of the eyeball, the retina, consists of two parts, the outer pigmented layer being attached to the choroid, and the inner layer consisting of a synaptic series of nervous tissue. The *macula lutea,* a yellowish spot near the center of the retina, encompasses a small depression in its center called the *fovea centralis.* This is an area consisting only of cones and projecting the most acute vision. Medial to the fovea centralis is the optic disk, or blind spot. It is at this whitish spot that the optic nerve exits from the eyeball. Because this area contains no sensory receptors, it is known as the *physiologic blind spot* of the retina. Increased intraocular pressure is reflected in the optic disk by a cupped disk, that is, a disk that appears pushed backward. In contrast, increased intracranial pressure produces the opposite effect, an optic disk that is pushed inward, called a choked disk, or *papilledema.*

The blood supply for the retina enters through the central artery, a branch of the ophthalmic artery, which enters the eyeball with the optic nerve and runs with it to the retina where it divides in the middle of the disk into superior and inferior branches. The veins in the eyeball are anatomically related to the arteries and empty into the ophthalmic veins.

Visual Pathways

The ganglionic cell axons of the retina emerge from the optic disk as the optic nerve. Axons from the nasal half of each eye cross in the optic chiasm and terminate in the opposite occipital lobe. Axons from the temporal half of each eye do not cross but terminate on their respective sides [3] (Fig. 43-2).

Image Formation

The refractive surfaces of the cornea and lens initiate the mechanism for image formation. These surfaces and the aqueous and vitreous humors encountered within the eye provide varying densities for the light to pass through. This accounts for the refractive phenomenon. If a light ray passes into a more dense medium, it is bent toward the perpendicular and the speed of transmission is slowed. A lighter medium bends the light ray away from the perpendicular and speeds its transmission. The degree of light impediment, or the power of a substance to bend light, is its *refractive index* [4]. The refractive index of air is 1.0; of water, 1.33; of the cornea, 1.38; and of the crystalline lens, 1.40.

Light strikes the cornea at different angles and is bent in different amounts, depending on the curvature and refractive indices of the interposed structures. Refraction of light occurs at the corneal interface, the aqueous humor, and crystalline lens and is projected on the retina in an inverted

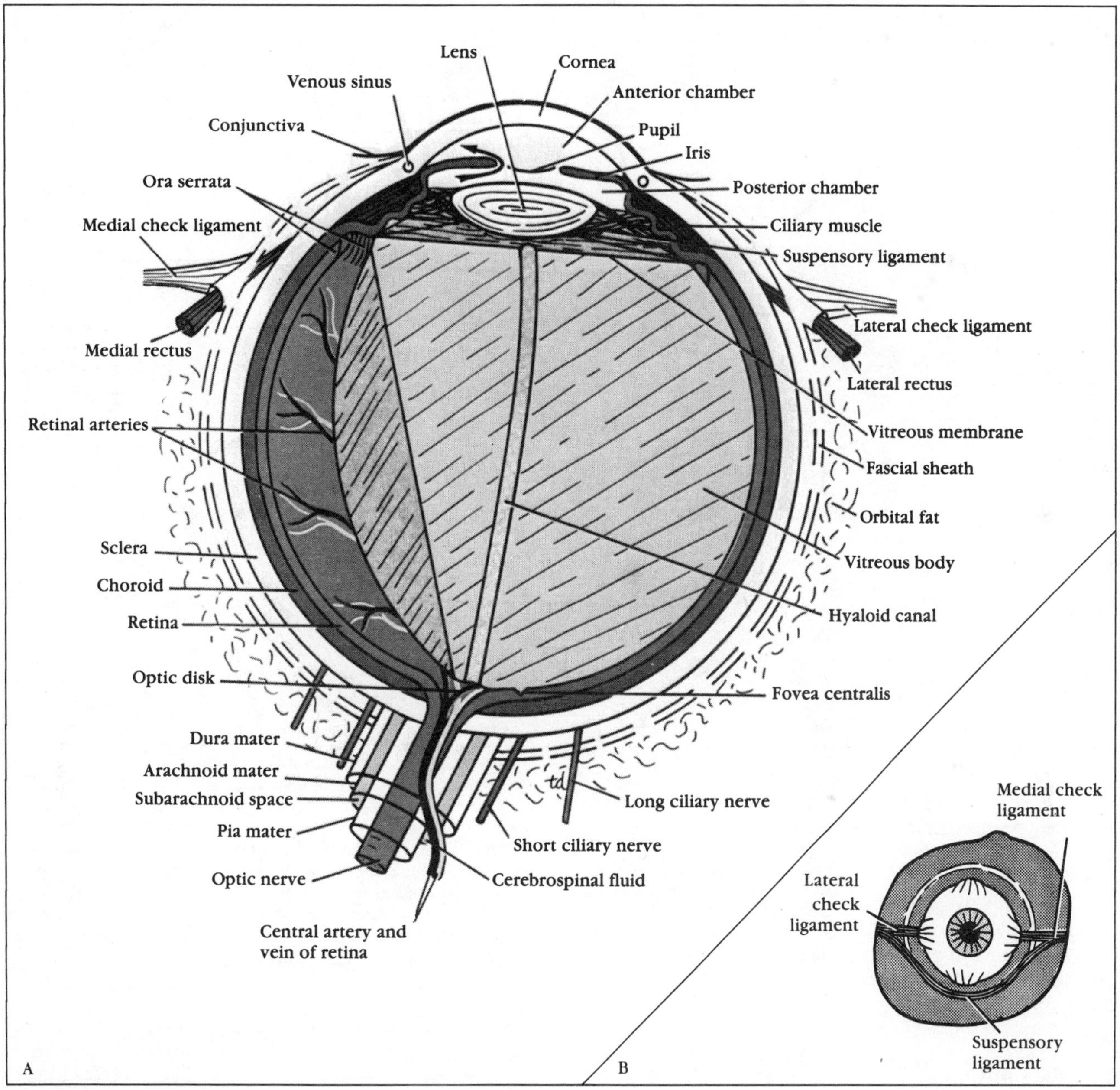

FIGURE 43-1. A. Horizontal section through eyeball and optic nerve. Note that central artery and vein of retina cross subarachnoid space to reach optic nerve. B. Check ligaments and suspensory ligament of the eyeball. (From R. Snell, *Clinical Anatomy for Medical Students* [2nd ed.]. Boston: Little, Brown, 1981.)

and reverted manner that is perceived by the brain as upright.

Accommodation

Adjustments for distant vision are made by the lens. Normally, parallel light rays from distant objects are focused on the retina. The ciliary muscle contracts to increase the curvature of the lens to view objects closer to the eye. This is the process of *accommodation.* The closest point at which a person can clearly focus an object is called the *near point.* This point recedes with advancing age. For example, the near point for a normal eye of an 8-year-old child is approximately 8.6 cm; for a 20-year-old it is 10.4 cm; and for a 60-year-old it is approximately 83 cm from the eye. Ocular convergence and pupillary constriction are associated with the accommodation reflex. The increased curvature of the lens increases its power, shortens the focal length, and focuses near objects on the retina.

The accommodation reflex is mediated by the third cranial nerve through parasympathetic postganglionic fibers. The stimulus that triggers the accommodation response is

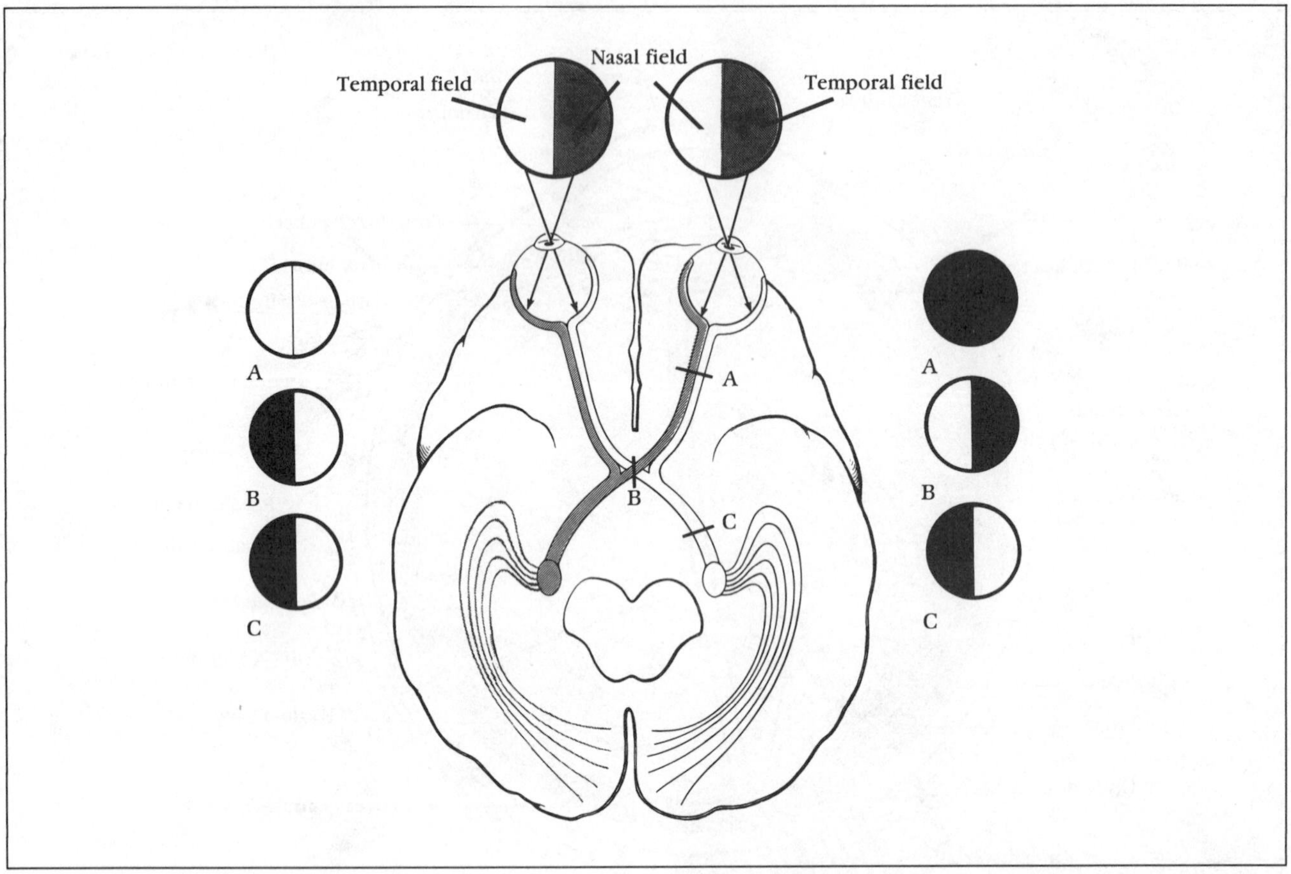

FIGURE 43-2. The visual pathway. On right and left are maps of visual fields with areas of blindness darkened to show the effects of lesions in each location. A. Lesion of optic nerve (loss of vision, right eye). B. Midline lesion of optic chiasm (bitemporal hemianopsia). C. Lesion of the right anterior optic tract; blindness for objects in left half of each field of vision (left homonymous hemianopsia). Lesions can occur at other locations along the visual pathway, causing a variety of patterns of visual field losses. (From J. Sana and R. Judge, *Physical Assessment Skills for Nursing Practice* [2nd ed.]. Boston: Little, Brown, 1982.)

perception of an image out of focus. The parasympathetic impulses on the ciliary muscle must, therefore, increase progressively to maintain the image in focus continually.

Progressive age reduces the efficiency of accommodation due to the loss of elasticity of the lens, and the eye may remain focused almost permanently on a constant distance. This deterioration of old age is known as *presbyopia*. This condition is readily corrected with proper bifocal lenses for far and near vision.

Pupillary Aperture

The iris controls the amount of light that enters the eye through the action of its two sets of smooth muscles, the sphincter and dilator muscles. *Miosis* is accomplished through the contraction of the sphincter muscle, and *mydriasis* is facilitated through the contraction of the dilator muscle. Innervation for these muscles comes from the postganglionic parasympathetic neurons in the ciliary ganglion. The preganglionic neurons transmit to the ganglion via the third cranial nerve. The innervation for the dilator muscle arrives from the sympathetic postganglionic neurons of the superior cervical ganglion, and reaches the eye through a series of progressively smaller arteries.

The pupillary aperture in the human eye can vary from 1.5 to 8.0 mm in diameter. In the normal eye the pupillary aperture is a reflex response to change in the light intensity encountered by the eye. Pupils constrict in response to increased light intensities and dilate to decreased light intensities (pupillary light reflex). If illumination enters only one eye, both pupils constrict. This simultaneous constriction of the contralateral eye is referred to as the *consensual light reflex*. Photoreceptors of the retina, including rods and cones, are receptors for the light reflex.

Emotional states of alarm produce pupillary dilation. This reaction is initiated by stimulation of the sympathetic fibers and the inhibition of the parasympathetic fibers. Darkness inhibits the parasympathetic supply and results in pupil dilation.

Light reflex of the pupil and miosis of accommodation are not identical mechanisms and can occur independently of the other. An example of this occurs with the *Argyll Robertson* pupil, which may be seen as a complication of

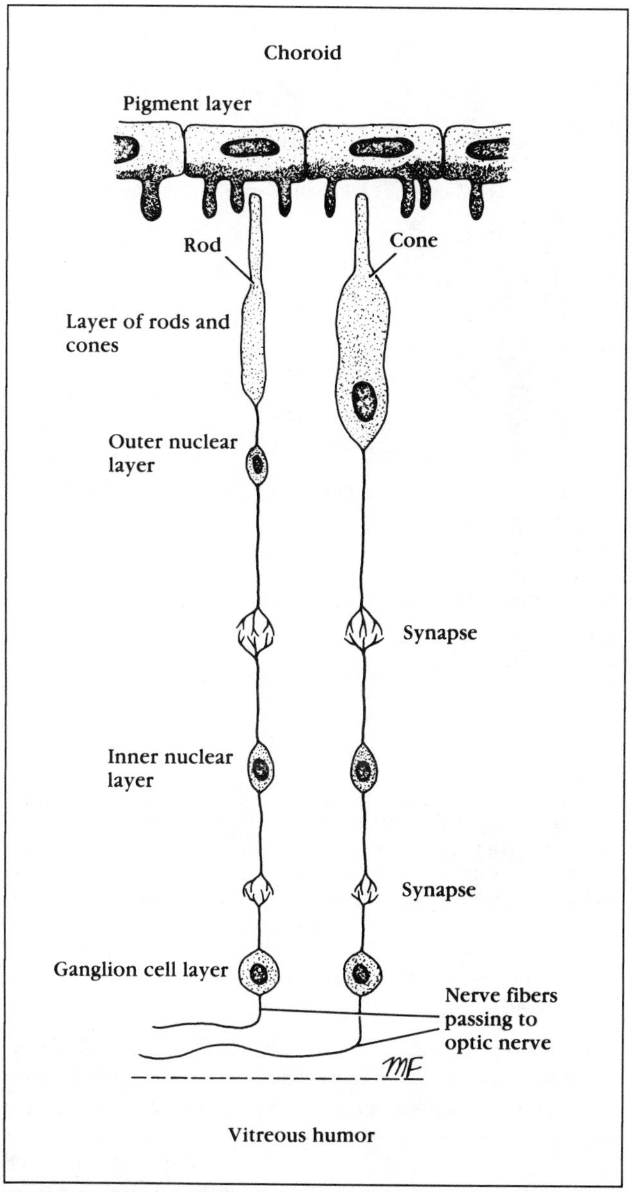

FIGURE 43-3. Rods and cones.

syphilis. In this phenomenon the pupil remains constricted and unresponsive to light but does respond to the accommodation mechanism.

Physiology of Vision

Rods and *cones* are receptors of the retina and have distinctly different morphologic compositions and functions (Fig. 43-3). The cones mediate daylight vision, allowing perception of detail and color of objects. The rods mediate night vision, allowing visualization of outlines of objects without revealing color or detail. The rods, however, are very sensitive to movement of objects in the visual field.

The retina is formed by numerous layers of cells, fibers, and ganglia (Fig. 43-4). The nerve cells found in the retina include bipolar cells, ganglion cells, horizontal cells, and amacrine cells. The rods and cones, which are adjacent to the pigment epithelium of the choroid, synapse with the bipolar cells which, in turn, synapse with dendrites of the ganglion cells. Horizontal cells connect receptor cells (rods and cones), and amacrine cells connect ganglion cells to each other. The axons of the ganglion cells converge to form the fibers of the optic nerve, which is easily recognized through ophthalmoscopic examination of the *optic disk*. The *fovea centralis* is composed of tightly packed cones that connect individually to the optic nerve, whereas in other parts of the retina they share fibers with many other rods and cones. The pigmented layer of the retina is the outermost layer, which decreases light reflexion. This pigment layer is directly adjacent to the choroid and receives much of its nutritive needs from the choroid vascular supply. Melanin is the black pigment that gives this layer its characteristic dark color.

As light passes through the layers of the retina to reach the light-sensitive portion of the rods and cones, light energy is absorbed by the pigment *rhodopsin*, or *visual purple*. Rhodopsin is a light-sensitive protein and aldehyde of vitamin A compound contained in rods that breaks down when light reaches it. This is the initial activity in generator potential production. The breakdown of rhodopsin can be visualized by the color change in the dark adapted retina from a dark purple to a lack of color on exposure to light. The breakdown of rhodopsin results in the formation of a protein, *scotopsin*, and a *carotene* pigment, *retinene* [2]. In darkness, scotopsin and retinene recombine through a series of intermediary steps and form rhodopsin again, which once again is photoexcitable.

$$\text{Rhodopsin} \underset{\text{dark}}{\overset{\text{light}}{\rightleftharpoons}} \text{retinene} + \text{scotopsin} \dashrightarrow \text{generator potential}$$

The knowledge about the pigments in the cones is somewhat speculative at this time. Reflexion densitometry has demonstrated the presence of pigments in the foveal region of the retina that peak in the blue green and red parts of the spectrum. This is accomplished by shining light in the eye and measuring the intensity of energy at different wave lengths in the light reflected from the retina. In this manner the amount of light absorbed by the visual receptor cells can be determined. *Erythrolobe* is a pigment identified in the fovea that absorbs light in the red part of the spectrum; *chlorolobe* is a pigment absorbing light in the green part of the spectrum in the fovea. A third cone pigment, *iodopsin*, which is a violet-sensitive substance, has been isolated from the retinas of chickens and is also thought to exist in the human eye cones. Recently a pigment receptor for blue substances has also been identified. The composition of the cone pigments is similar to rhodopsin, although in varying degrees. Thus, cone pigments absorb a variety of colors to different extents, and color-

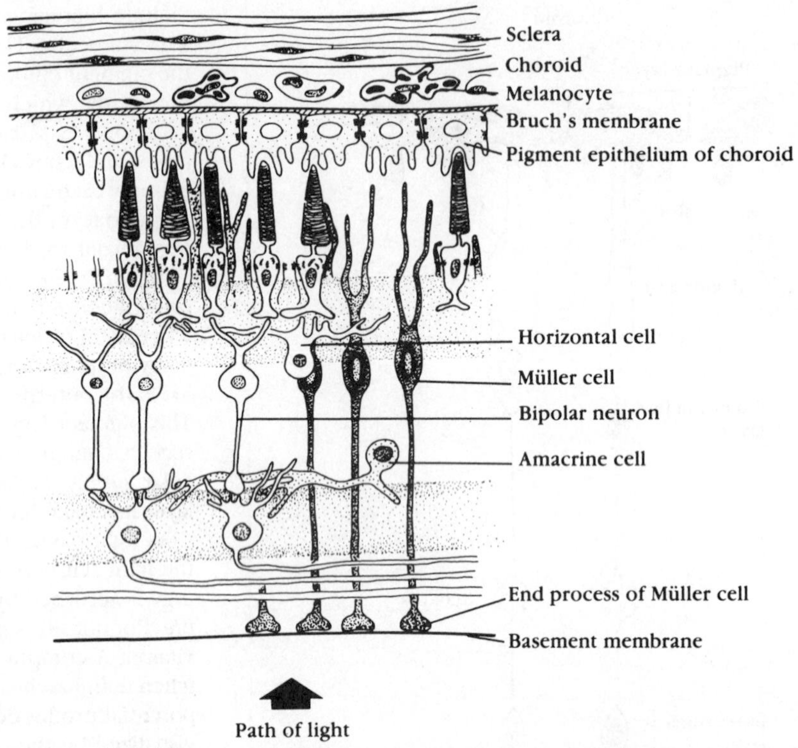

FIGURE 43-4. Highly schematic diagram of the retina, showing the nine layers of the retina and their connections, using a few cells of each type as an example. Note that light must pass through the entire thickness of the retina before it finally triggers a photochemical reaction in the rod and cone outer segments. This "backward" retina is typical of all vertebrates. (From M. Borysenko, et al., *Functional Histology* [2nd ed.]. Boston: Little, Brown, 1984.)

dependent nerve impulses result. These impulses are interpreted by the visual cortex as color sensations.

The photochemical decomposition that occurs in response to light striking either the cones or rods produces a receptor potential that remains for the duration of the stimulus. The receptor potentials of the retina differ from other receptor potentials in that a hyperpolarization is produced rather than a depolarization. Each optic nerve fiber connects with many receptors via ganglionic cells. The number of receptor cells on the retina is much greater than the number of fibers in the optic nerve. This convergence on ganglionic cells allows summation to occur, so that light falling on different parts of the retina together may cause excitation. Thus, the more rods and cones excited, the more intense the signal. The ganglion cells receive the excitation impulses from the rods and cones via the bipolar cells.

The ganglionic cells produce synaptic depolarization and stimulate threshold spikes that are all or nothing and are propagated along their axons to the lateral geniculate body. Three types of responses are observed in ganglionic cells: One fires only in response to light stimulus on the retina and is known as the *on fiber;* another discharges only in response to light off and is known as the *off fiber;* the third type, the most numerous, responds to both light on and off and is called the *on-off fiber*.

The horizontal cells transmit inhibitory impulses laterally from rods and cones to bipolar cells and become most important in detecting visual contrasts and color differentiations. Amacrine cells have a very transient inhibitory effect on the ganglionic cells in response to stimulation from bipolar cells and possibly rods and cones. Amacrine cells transmit, signaling a change in retinal illumination. The neural pathways from the retina to the visual cortex are identified in Figure 43-2.

Color Vision

The differentiation of wave lengths of the visible spectrum allows the human eye to detect color in the environment. The precise mechanism that is responsible for color detection has been theorized by numerous researchers throughout the past century. Most of the research seems to be based on the *trichromatic theory* of color vision. This theory assumes that there are three variations in cones, each containing a different photochemical substance. One type of cone is responsible for red color, another for blue, and the third for green [2]. This theory, known as the *Young-Helmholtz* theory, named after its originators over a century ago, is a widely accepted explanation for color vision today. Each of these cones gives rise to a distinct impulse that travels to the visual cortex of the occipital lobe. Red, blue, and green are colors that may produce any color in the spectrum by correct proportionate mixture. When all of the cones are stimulated equally, the sensation of white results. In contrast, when no stimulation of the three types of cones occurs, black is experienced. Other color perceptions are as a result of the combined stimulation of the three types of cones to varying degrees.

In summary, color vision evolves from the spectral sensitivity of cones and is most highly developed in the fovea where a concentration of cones is found. Each cone is maximally stimulated by a specific color. Color information is transmitted to the brain via common cone pathways of the optic fibers and the transmission of specific colors is monitored by the stimulation of horizontal cells.

Color Blindness

Color blindness is observed in the general public by the inability to distinguish red from green. It may be a hereditary or an acquired phenomenon. When a certain group of color receptors are not present in the retina, all colors appear the same in the range of missing cones.

Assessing individuals for color blindness can be accomplished with numerous tests. Most commonly used tests are the polychromatic charts and the yarn-matching tests. The former presents a chart with multiple look-alike colored spots in a figuration that a person with normal vision can easily identify. These charts are known as the *Ishihara* charts. The yarn-matching test involves asking the person to match a skein of yarn with yarn from a pile of variously colored yarn.

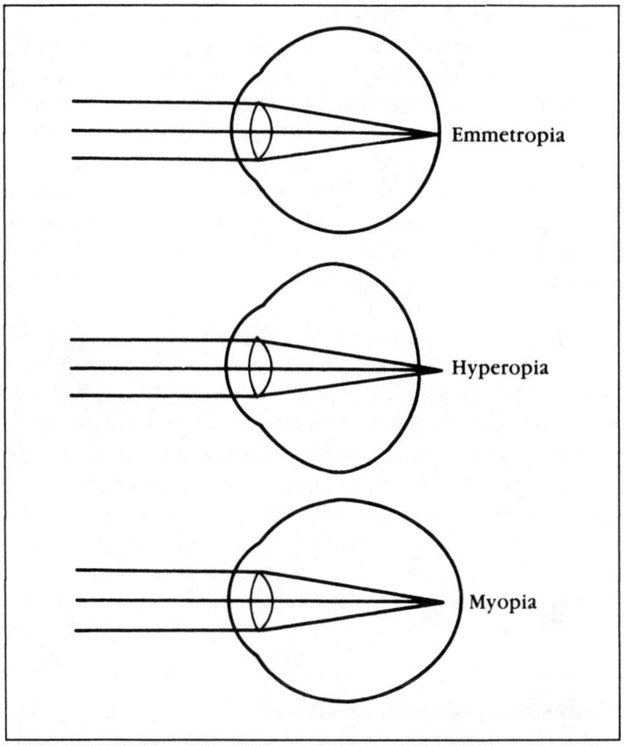

FIGURE 43-5. Common defects in the optical system of the eye. Emmetropia is normal refraction. A shortened eyeball gives rise to hyperopia (farsightedness). An abnormally long eyeball may characterize myopia (nearsightedness). Adjustments should be made in the lens selection on the ophthalmoscope for these anatomic differences. (From R. Judge, G. Zuidema, and F. Fitzgerald, *Clinical Diagnosis: A Physiologic Approach*. Boston: Little, Brown, 1982.)

Dark Adaptation

The eye is said to be *dark adapted* after a period of time in darkness. This decline in visual threshold is at its maximum after approximately 20 minutes in the dark environment. When one returns into the light environment, the uncomfortably bright light requires the eye to adapt to light again. This adaptation takes about 5 minutes and is called *light adaptation*. Dark adaptation occurs, in part, as rhodopsin stores are rebuilt in the rods and some similar, yet unknown, process occurs in the cones [2]. Dark adaptation is most effectively secured by avoiding exposure to light. When visual acuity is necessary in a dark environment, such as for viewing a fluoroscopy screen and x-ray films, red goggles may be worn in bright light to avoid having to wait 20 minutes for adaptation. The light wavelengths in the red part of the spectrum allow cone vision to continue while stimulating rods only to a slight degree.

Only the periphery of the retina of the human eye is sensitive to light in the dark adapted eye and, therefore, the sensitivity to darkness is much greater in the rods than the cones. However, rods are not exclusively responsible for dark adaptation. Because of the presence of both rods and cones in the human eye, dark adaptation takes place in two stages. First, a small increase in sensitivity, which is accomplished in about 7 minutes, is attributed in dark adaptation of cones. Following this, a less rapid, but quantitatively greater rod adaptation occurs.

Refraction Defects

Normal refraction (*emmetropia*) occurs when the relaxed eye is capable of clearly focusing distant parallel light rays on the retina (Fig. 43-5). Nearby vision requires contraction of the ciliary muscle to bring the object to focus. Defects of vision are present if the light rays converge either in front of or behind the retina, or if the eyeball is abnormally shaped [2].

Myopia (nearsightedness) is a result of an object focusing in front of the retina due to an increased anteroposterior diameter (see Fig. 43-5). Myopic individuals cannot focus distant objects sharply, but as they move closer to the object, it becomes more focused and eventually falls on the retina. The excessive refraction of myopia is readily corrected by a *concave* diverging lens, which produces a longer than normal focal point.

Hypermetropia (farsightedness) occurs with an abnormally short eyeball; the parallel light rays are focused beyond the retina in the relaxed eye (see Fig. 43-5). Through the action of the accommodation mechanism, the hypermetropic person can focus on distant objects. As objects move closer to the eye, images become blurred and the accommodation phenomenon can no longer compensate. The near point in this individual is abnormally distant. Hypermetropia is corrected by utilizing the refraction of light rays through a *convex* lens and shortening the normal focal point.

Astigmatism is a defect of the curvature of the cornea and lens, producing refractive errors where parallel light rays are imperfectly focused on the retina. Clear focusing requires a spherical cornea and lens on all meridians. In the presence of irregular curvature of these structures, light striking peripheral areas is bent at different angles and is not focused on a single point on the retina. Astigmatism can be corrected with lenses that are cut from a piece of cylindrical instead of spherical glass. The axis of the cylinder is placed approximately in relation to the meridian of the eye lens.

Other Disturbances of Vision

Decreased visual acuity may be associated with various lesions, syndromes, drug therapies, and nutritional deficiencies. Specific types of visual impairments result from lesions in different locations along the visual pathways [1]. Some of these are identified in Figure 43-2. Blindness in one-half of the visual field is known as *hemianopsia*. As there are many different types of hemianopsia, one usually finds the term further localized such as *bitemporal hemianopsia*, denoting blindness in the temporal visual fields of both eyes. The term *unilateral hemianopsia* is used to refer to blindness in one-half of the visual field in one eye; *homonymous hemianopsia* refers to loss of one-half of the visual field in both eyes, opposite the side of the visual pathway lesion in the brain.

Scotomas are abnormal blind spots in the visual field. These may exist with a person's knowledge (positive scotomas) or without his or her knowledge (negative scotomas). Scotomas may result from vascular disease, toxic effect of certain drugs, nutritional deficiencies, and with glaucoma. Various visual field defects may result from *retrobulbar neuritis* involving the optic nerve. This defect is commonly associated with multiple sclerosis.

Papilledema (choked disk) is most commonly seen with increased intracranial pressure due to brain tumors, trauma, hemorrhage, infections, and other causes. *Diplopia*, double vision, results from an eye muscle imbalance between the two eyes, resulting in image reception at different spots on each retina.

Optic atrophy results in decreased visual acuity. *Primary optic* atrophy such as that associated with multiple sclerosis or tabes dorsalis does not produce papilledema. *Secondary optic atropy* resulting from neuritis, glaucoma, or increased intracranial pressure is associated with papilledema. *Degeneration of the retina* may result from drug therapy (particularly the phenothiazine group), from infections, and from various metabolic or endocrine disorders.

Cerebral tumors, aneurysms, vascular diseases, infections, or degenerative processes may produce visual defects, producing a variety of symptoms associated with a specific region. Defects may result in ocular movement, visual acuity, or interpretation of what is seen.

Measurement of Visual Acuity

Individual visual acuity, the degrees to which a person can recognize contours and details of objects, can be readily measured. This can be determined by use of charts such as the *Snellen letter chart*. The subject is asked to read the chart from the distance of 20 feet and identify the smallest line that can be seen. This is tested with each eye, one at a time. The results are recorded as a fraction, with 20 as its numerator for the distance from which the person views the chart. The denominator is the distance from which the smallest line is seen. Normal visual acuity is considered to be 20/20.

Visual acuity is dependent on a number of factors, including brightness of the stimulus, density of the receptor cells, state of the cones, contrasting illumination between background and the stimulus, and the length of exposure to the stimulus.

HEARING

Structure and Function

The ear is a mechanoreceptor; it is sensitive to rapid changes in pressure that are transmitted to its fluid medium. In essence, the ear is a mechanical transducer as sound at various frequencies is converted into nerve impulses that are transmitted into the central nervous system for interpretation. Sound is conducted through air, ossicles, and fluid and is measured in number in vibrations per second, which are recorded as *cycles per second* (cps) or *Hertz* (Hz). The human ear is able to perceive frequencies to 20,000 cps or Hz. The aging process reduces the number of frequencies perceived. The greatest sensitivity of the human ear is in the 1000- to 4000-Hz range.

In addition to the hearing function of the ear, its receptors also mediate a sense of position and equilibrium.

Sound Conduction Through the Ear

The ear is anatomically segmented into the *outer, middle*, and *inner* ear (Fig. 43-6). The outer ear funnels sound waves to the *tympanic membrane* (eardrum). Its canal is an S-shaped 3-cm tube that is supplied with ceruminous and sebaceous glands as well as hair follicles. The canal has resonance properties as sound waves are reflected from the tympanic membrane and may enhance or dampen incoming waves. The external canal is lined with squamous epithelium, cartilage, and bone that provide support in maintaining its patency.

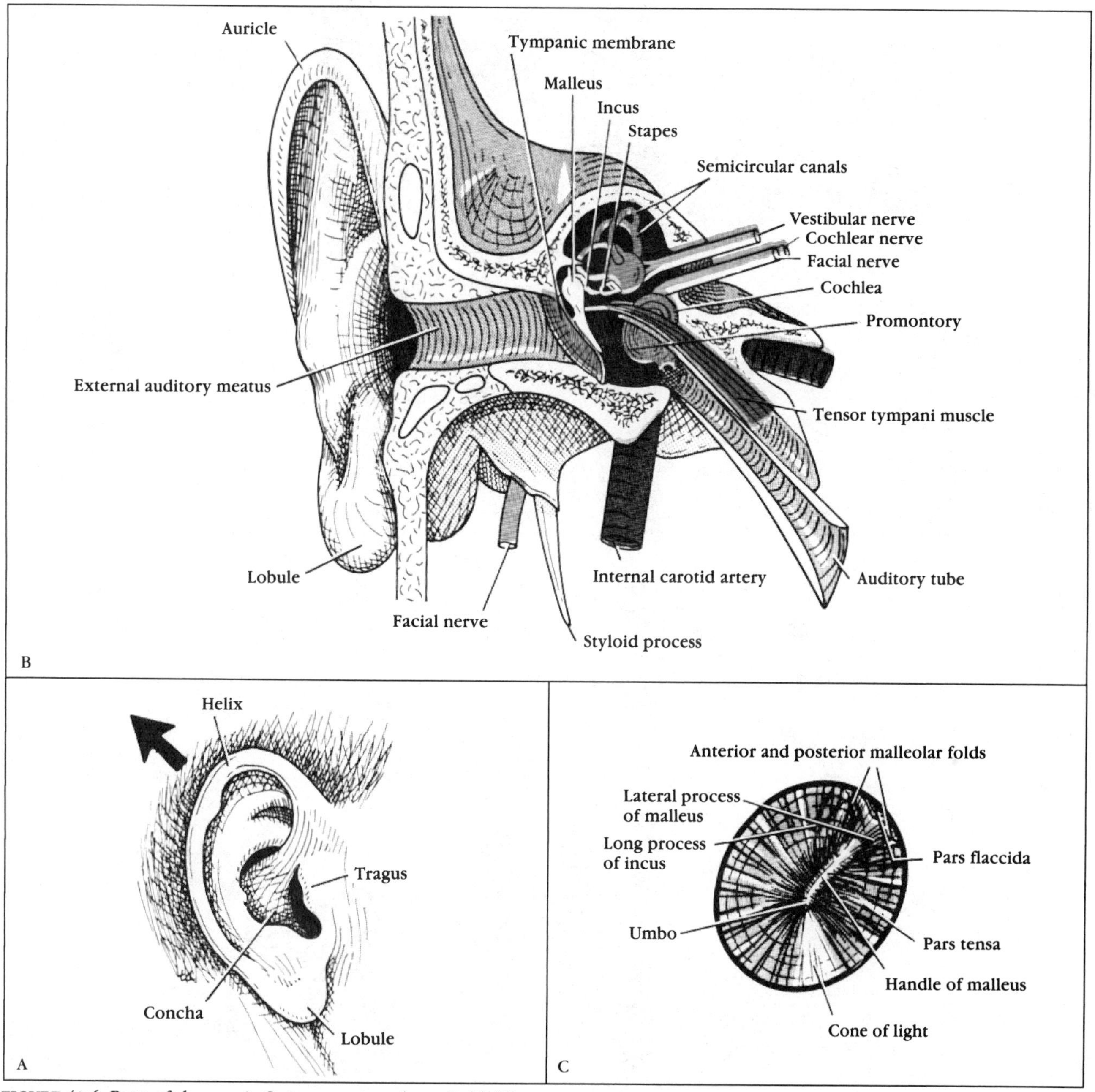

FIGURE 43-6. Parts of the ear. A. Outer or external ear. B. Middle ear component. C. Inner ear components. (From R. Snell, *Clinical Anatomy for Medical Students* [2nd ed.]. Boston: Little, Brown, 1980.)

At the terminal end of the external ear is the tympanic membrane, which separates it from the middle ear. This fibrous tissue vibrates freely with all audible sound frequencies and transmits these to the three auditory ossicles of the middle ear, the *malleus, incus,* and *stapes.* The middle ear with its three ossicles is situated in an air cavity of the temporal bone. It communicates with the nasopharnyx by means of the auditory or eustachian tube; the mucous membrane that lines the middle ear continues to line the pharynx as well as the air cells of the mastoid. The auditory tube also serves to equalize pressure in the middle ear with that of atmospheric pressure. Swallowing and yawning open the tube; high atmospheric pressures tend to close the tube. Microorganisms from the oropharynx often travel through the auditory tube to the middle ear, causing infections in this area.

The manubrium of the malleus is attached to the tympanic membrane, and its short process articulates with the incus to produce vibratory movements in the stapes, which

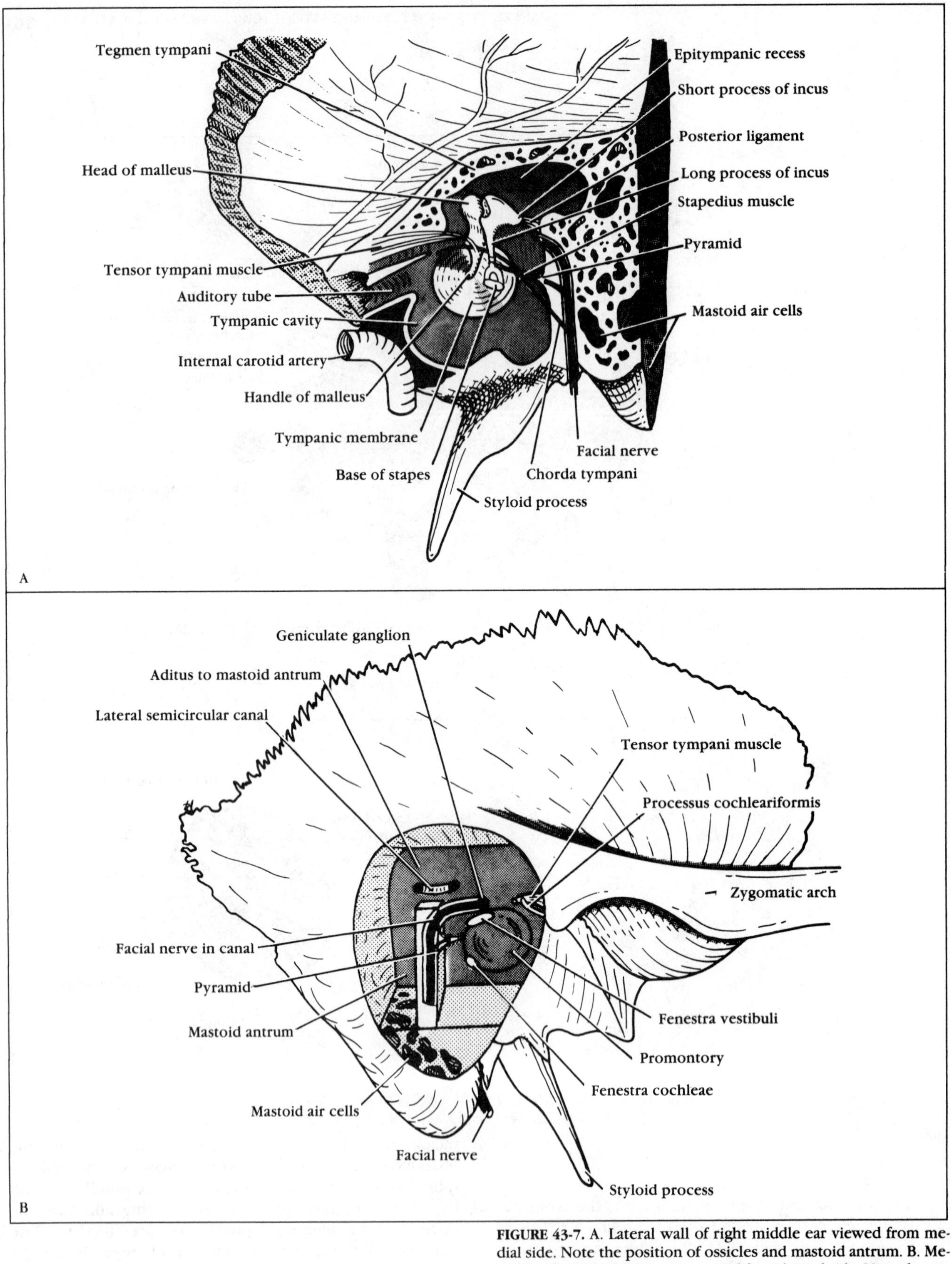

FIGURE 43-7. A. Lateral wall of right middle ear viewed from medial side. Note the position of ossicles and mastoid antrum. B. Medial wall of right middle ear viewed from lateral side. Note the position of the facial nerve in its bony canal. (From R. Snell, *Clinical Anatomy for Medical Students* [2nd ed.]. Boston: Little, Brown, 1981.)

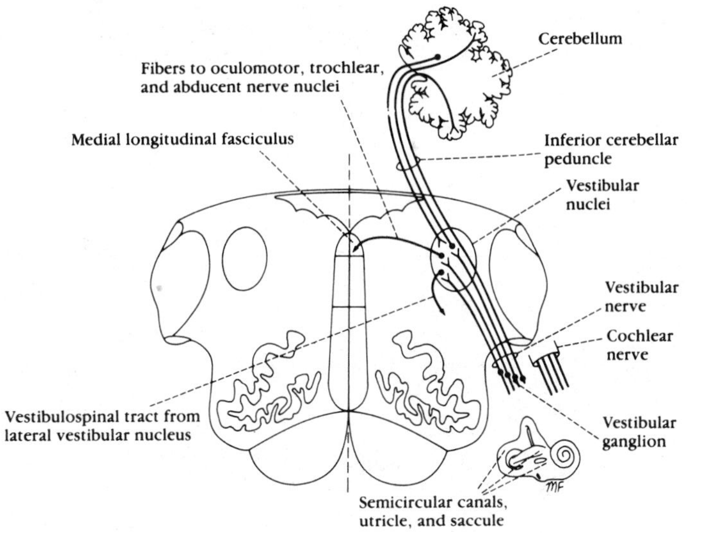

FIGURE 43-8. Vestibular nerve nuclei and their central connections. (From R. Snell, *Clinical Neuroanatomy for Medical Students*. Boston: Little, Brown, 1980.)

is attached to the walls of the oval window (Fig. 43-7). The *tensor tympani* and *stapedius muscles* of the middle ear prevent the bones from transmitting excessive vibrations by pulling on the bones to decrease contact with the tympanic membrane and oval window.

The inner ear is encased in the petrous part of the temporal bone and mediates sound induced nerve impulses, position orientation, and balance. It is composed of two labyrinths, one within the other. The outer labyrinth is bony and separated from the inner membranous one by perilymph fluid; it contains the cochlea, vestibule, and the three semicircular canals. The membranous labyrinth contains a fluid called *endolymph*. The anterior portion of the membranous labyrinth contains the cochlea, which receives the sound waves from the oval window. The cochlea, a small shell-shaped structure, is divided into three chambers by the *basilar* and *Reissner's* membranes. These chambers are the *scala vestibule, scala tympani*, and *cochlear duct*. Posteriorly, the cochlea opens into the osseous vestibule, which, in turn, extends to the three semicircular canals.

The *organ of Corti*, located on the basilar membrane, contains the receptor cells of audition. These are hair cells that generate nerve impulses in response to sound vibrations from the oscillations of the oval window. Impulses that arouse the dendrites of the cochlear division of the acoustic nerve are transmitted to the hearing center in the temporal lobe of the cortex. The various frequencies of sound generate different patterns of vibrations and allow sounds to be discriminated from each other. The subjective interpretation of the frequency of sound waves results in the recognition of *pitch*. The higher frequencies are identified as higher pitch. In addition to frequency discrimination of pitch, the location of the stimulation of the cells on the basilar membrane affects pitch. Low-frequency sounds generate greater activity of the basilar membrane near the apex of the cochlea, and high frequency sounds activate the basilar membrane near the base of the cochlea. Other frequencies fall between these extremes. This explanation of pitch discrimination is known as the *place theory*.

The amplitude of vibrations affects the perception of loudness at a constant frequency in that greater amplitude produces greater loudness. However, this does not hold true when two sounds of different frequency are contrasted simultaneously, as auditory sensitivity is a function of frequency. Thus, frequency and amplitude are both significant in determining the perception of loudness in two or more simultaneous sounds.

Hearing Pathways

The axons of bipolar neurons from the cochlea enter the pons and divide into the dorsal and ventral cochlear nuclei. Second-order neurons cross here and ascend via the lateral lemniscus to the inferior colliculus from which they transmit to the medial geniculate body and on to the auditory cortex in the temporal lobe via the auditory radiations (Fig. 43-8).

The auditory cortex provides for recognition of tone patterns, analysis of characteristics of sound, and localization of sound. Low-frequency tones are recognized anteriorly and high-frequency tones posteriorly in the auditory cortex. Neurons throughout the auditory cortex respond to onset, duration, and direction of stimulus.

The auditory association area lies inferiorly to the primary auditory center and is thought to associate auditory information with other sensations as well as different sound frequencies with each other. Lesions in this area in the human prevent comprehension of the meaning of sounds heard. Words can be heard but not comprehended.

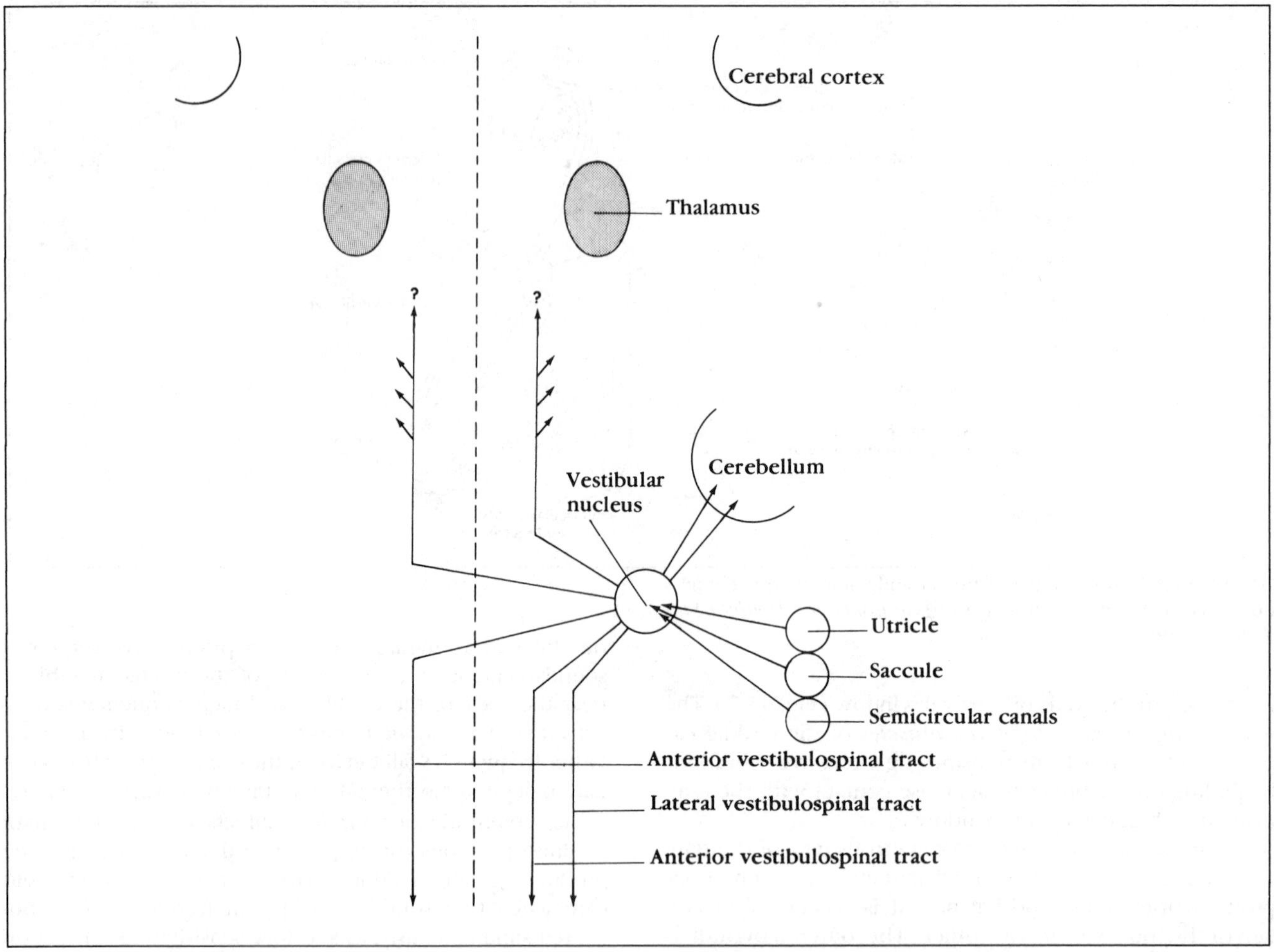

FIGURE 43-9. Pathways of the vestibular nerve. (From D. R. Dickson and W. Maue-Dickson, *Anatomical and Physiological Bases of Speech*. Boston: Little, Brown, 1982.)

The direction of sound origin is facilitated by detection of sound arrival in the two ears. One ear can receive information before the other and the closer ear to the sound source receives a louder sound.

Hearing Loss

Hearing loss can result from problems of the central hearing mechanisms or the peripheral pathways. Peripheral hearing loss involves impairment of sound transmission in the external and middle ear and is referred to as *conduction deafness*. Neural pathway lesions produce *sensorineural deafness*.

Conduction deafness can result from an external canal obstructed by cerumen or foreign objects, a damaged tympanic membrane, or immobility of the tympanic membrane or ossicles secondary to chronic otitis media. *Otosclerosis* results in conduction deafness by immobilization of the stapes in the oval window.

Sensorineural deafness can be caused by chronic therapy with certain antibiotics in the mycin group, pathology in the hair cells of the cochlea, or disease processes in the auditory nerve pathway.

The Vestibular System

Disorders of coordination may result from the vestibular system through the labyrinthine and righting reflexes. Lesions may occur in the labyrinths, the vestibular nerve, the vestibular pathways within the brainstem, the cerebrum, or the cerebellum. Figure 43-9 shows the pathways of the vestibular nerve and its interconnections with the cerebellum, parts of the labyrinths, and the cerebrum. The vestibular system functions to maintain equilibrium to preserve head position and to direct the gaze of the eyes.

The vestibular portion of the eighth nerve has its peripheral endings on the hair cells of the maculae of the *utricle* and *saccule* and on the cristae in the ampullae of the three *semicircular canals* (Fig. 43-10). The utricle and saccule record linear acceleration and static phenomena; and the semicircular canals record angular acceleration. Recent evidence implies that the utricle may be more related to the semicircular canals' vestibular functions, while the saccule has a closer association with hearing.

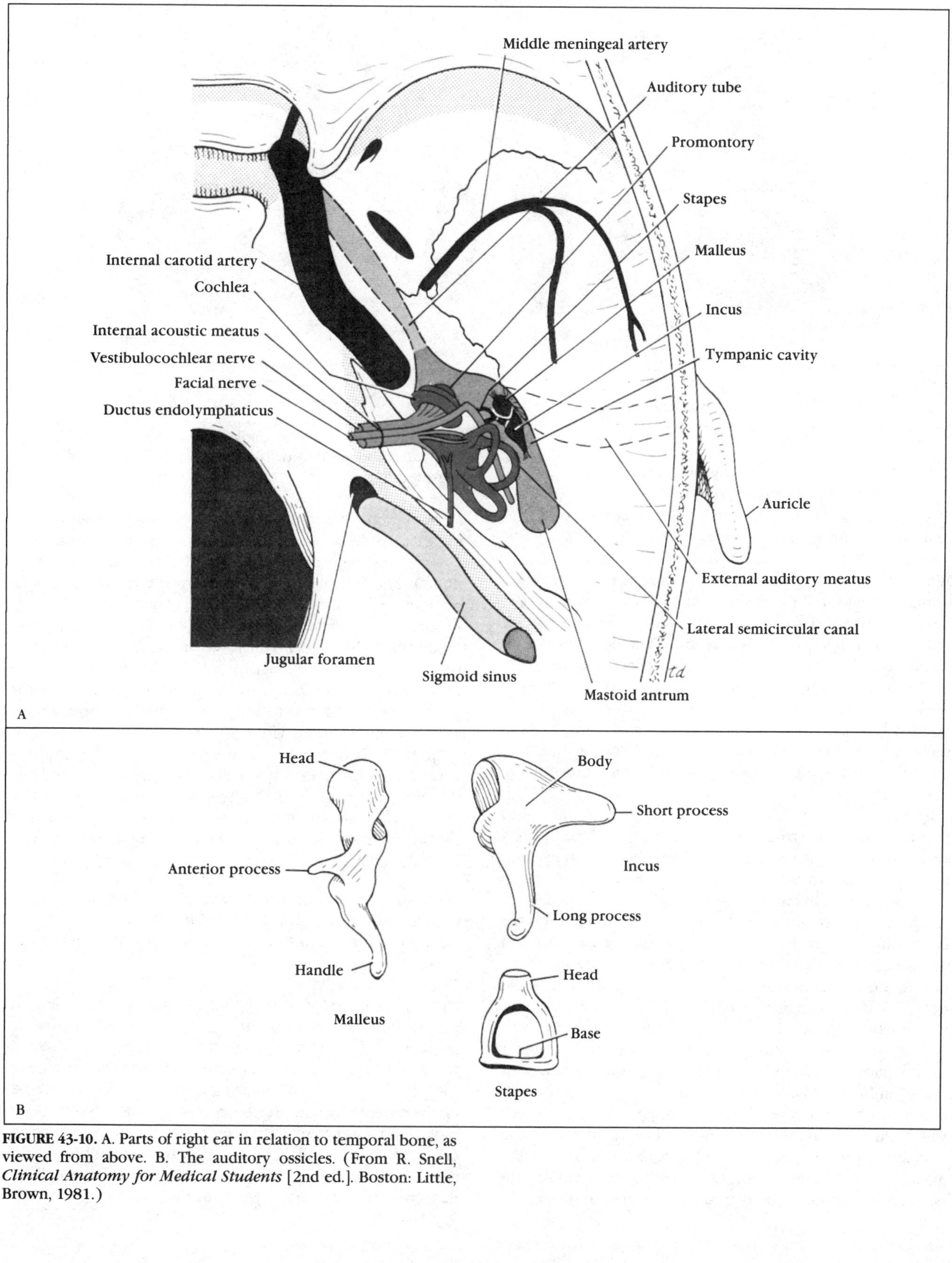

FIGURE 43-10. A. Parts of right ear in relation to temporal bone, as viewed from above. B. The auditory ossicles. (From R. Snell, *Clinical Anatomy for Medical Students* [2nd ed.]. Boston: Little, Brown, 1981.)

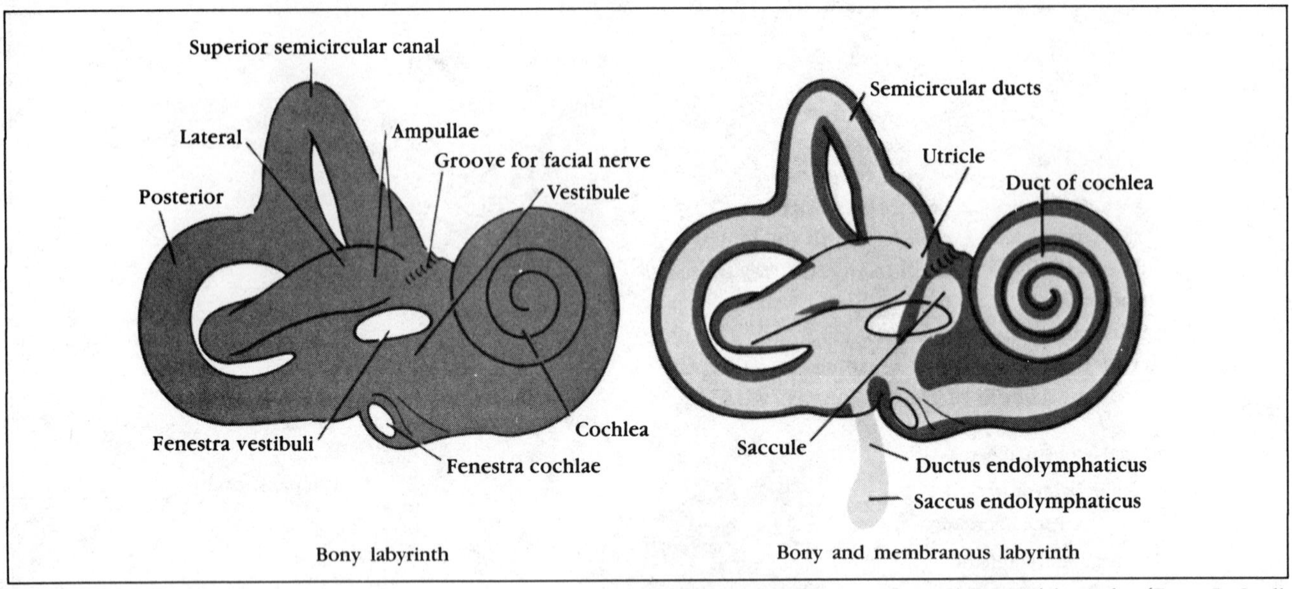

FIGURE 43-11. Bony and membranous labyrinths. (From R. Snell, *Clinical Anatomy for Medical Students* [2nd ed.]. Boston: Little, Brown, 1981.)

The *utricle,* the *saccule,* and the *semicircular canals* function together to maintain equilibrium. These structures are housed in a bony labyrinth that contains a membranous labyrinth composed of the semicircular canals and the two chambers, the utricle and the saccule (Fig. 43-11). Within the utricle and saccule are maculae that provide sensory areas for the detection of the relationship of the head with respect to gravitational pull and other forces. The maculae operate in conditions of acceleration and in static equilibrium. Hair cells within the maculae cause nerve fiber transmission due to the ciliated positions on these cells. Within the semicircular canals a fluid, called *endolymph,* flows and fluid flow in the canal stimulates the sensory nerve fibers that join up with the vestibular nerve. Fluid flow in the opposite direction inhibits these sensory nerve fibers.

The ganglion cells of the vestibular division of the eighth nerve are in the internal auditory meatus, and the dendrites end in the specialized epithelium of the hair cells. The axons pass back to the upper medulla accompanied by the cochlear nerve. On entering the medulla, the fibers pass directly to the cerebellum and to four vestibular nuclei that communicate with the medial longitudinal fasciculus and communicate with the third, fourth, and sixth cranial nerve nuclei and the nuclei of the upper cervical and accessory nerves. This connection results in vestibular influence on movement of the neck, eyes, and head.

A close interrelationship exists between the vestibular nerves and the cerebellum. This relationship accounts for the equilibrium changes that occur with rapid changes in direction. The maculae of the utricle and saccule provide vestibular input to the cerebellum. The influence of the two-way input and output results in coordination of the muscles of the neck and in the coordination required for posture. Interconnection of vestibular nerves to the reticular system may account for the nausea, vomiting, and sweating that results when the vestibular system is stimulated.

Two vestibulospinal tracts arise from the vestibular nuclei. The lateral tract comes from the lateral vestibular nucleus and extends to the sacral level of the cord. The medial tract comes from the medial vestibular nucleus and extends through the cervical level. Impulses descending in these tracts assist in local myotactic reflexes and reinforce the tonus of the extensor muscles of the trunk and limbs, producing extra force to support the body against gravity and to maintain an upright posture.

Communication between the vestibular nuclei and the cerebral nuclei is not established but may exist, since vertigo and dizziness have resulted from cortical stimulation of posterior aspects of the temporal lobe. Disturbances of function of the vestibular system may result in vertigo, nystagmus, and ataxia.

VERTIGO. Vertigo is a disturbance of equilibrium resulting in a sensation of whirling. There are several types of vertigo: (1) acute paroxysmal, (2) chronic, and (3) benign positional.

1. Acute paroxysmal vertigo is exemplified by sudden onset of acute movement, either rotatory and objective, or subjective. If rotatory and objective, external objects seem to be rotating while the person is stationary. If subjective, the person seems to be rotating in relation to the external environment. In addition to rotation, sensations of spinning, falling through space, or being pushed are experienced. Movement of objects or of the self may appear in any plane, horizontally, obliquely, or vertically. Single attacks may occur in acute labyrinthitis.

2. Chronic vertigo is experienced as transient sensations of rotation with sudden head turning. Another type of attack, which may persist for months, is a chronic sense of imbalance.

3. Benign positional vertigo will occur only when the head is in certain postures and will cease when the head is moved out of this position. An attack may occur with the head in a forward or backward position, or when the head is turned to one side. Affected persons learn to avoid the particular posture that causes the attack.

Attacks of vertigo can be disabling since the affected person is often thrown to the ground in reaction to false clues of movement. Nausea, vomiting, and nystagmus commonly accompany acute attacks of vertigo.

NYSTAGMUS. Nystagmus is a disturbance of ocular posture characterized by rhythmic oscillation of the eyes, occurring both in physiologic and pathologic circumstances [1]. Nystagmus can be induced in normal people by irrigation of the external auditory canal with hot or cold water or by rotating a person in a revolving chair. One form of physiologic nystagmus is *opticokinetic nystagmus,* which is induced by having the person look at a repeating pattern passed in a horizontal or vertical direction in front of the eyes.

Pathologically, *vestibular nystagmus* occurs as a response to some disturbance of the synergistic action of the two vestibular organs or their central connections. The nystagmus is always phasic. There is a slow phase in one direction of the eyes and then an opposing quick phase. The direction of nystagmus is designated according to the direction of the fast component, i.e., if the slow phase is to the right and the quick one is to the left, the person is said to exhibit nystagmus to the left. The movement of the eye may be horizontal, vertical, or rotary. The rotary tendency is more prominent whenever there is a lesion involving the labyrinth.

Vestibular nystagmus is associated with vertigo and is increased on turning the head or eyes in the direction of the quick phase. This is seen in dysfunction of the semicircular canals or their peripheral neurons. It is limited in duration because central compensation occurs. If it should persist longer than a few weeks, it is usually because of change in the vestibular pathway [1]. Other causes of pathologic nystagmus are: (1) abnormal retinal impulses, (2) abnormal labyrinthine impulses, (3) lesions of the cervical spinal cord, (4) lesions involving the central paths concerned in ocular posture, (5) weakness of the ocular muscles, and (6) congenital abnormality of unknown etiology.

LABYRINTHINE ATAXIA. *Ataxia* is often striking in vestibular disease. It is characterized by disturbances of equilibrium in standing and walking and does not affect isolated limb movements. It has many features of cerebellar ataxia, e.g., the broad-based gait staggering, leaning over backward or to one side, and deviation from direction of gait. It can usually be differentiated from cerebellar ataxia through association with nystagmus and vertigo. However, causes of ataxias differ, some being caused by degenerative, demyelinating, or inflammatory lesions and others by lesions in the thalamus and subthalamic region near the main cerebellar and sensory pathways. The most common mixed ataxias are (1) the cerebellar and vestibular forms, and (2) the posterior column and cerebellar forms. In multiple sclerosis for example, symptoms of ataxia are mainly of the cerebellar and vestibular forms.

Rapid destruction of one labyrinth causes vertigo, nystagmus, and occasionally some temporary nausea and vomiting. The vestibular nuclei seem to work by comparing signals from both labyrinths. Whenever a labyrinth is destroyed, overcompensation for the input from the other side occurs. Bilateral destruction of both labyrinths does not cause nystagmus or vertigo, but there may be a disturbance of equilibrium for many months.

Assessment of Hearing and Balance

A single effective means of assessing hearing ability is to have the person cover one ear with the hand and whisper a few words softly near the opposite ear, this is repeated for the other ear. If the person is able to perceive these words, the hearing is probably normal. In addition, auditory loss can be determined through the utilization of equipment such as the tuning fork and audiometer. These tools can assist in distinguishing sensorineural hearing loss from conductive loss. A simple test for conductive loss can be demonstrated through the use of a tuning fork. A vibrating tuning fork of 256 Hz is placed on the mastoid process until the individual no longer hears it and is then held in the air next to the external auditory meatus. This is known as the *Rinne's test;* in normal persons, air conduction is more acute and vibrations are heard after bone conduction has ceased. If vibrations are not heard in the air after bone conduction has ceased, the person has conductive deafness. If the vibrating tuning fork is heard at the ear canal after no longer being heard on the mastoid process, the conducting mechanisms through the middle ear are intact and the problem is in the inner ear or its transmissions; the person then has sensorineural loss.

Weber's test is also effective in the identification of hearing loss. A vibrating tuning fork is placed at the vertex of the head; normal perception of the sound is equal in both ears. If conductive loss is present, the sound is louder in the affected ear due to the masking effect of the environmental noise. In the presence of sensorineural damage, sound is heard better in the normal ear.

Audiometry tests the sensitivity of the ear to pure tones at different frequencies through earphones. The audiometer, which is an electronic oscillator, measures hearing objectively and plots it on a graph that represents the percentage of normal hearing based on the average threshold

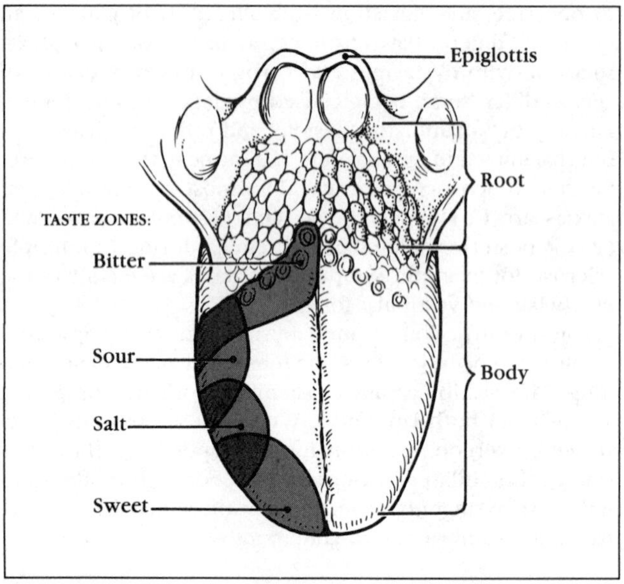

FIGURE 43-12. The dorsal surface of the tongue showing the areas for perception of the sensations of sweet, sour, bitter, and salt.

of normal hearing of a population. Conductive and sensorineural hearing impairments can be distinguished by audiometry.

The vestibular component of the eighth cranial nerve may be assessed if the person's history reveals vertigo with nausea and vomiting. Vestibular function is assessed with the *cold caloric test.* The subject is supine at a 30-degree elevation; after ascertaining no observable defects of the external auditory canal, 5 ml of ice water is introduced into the canal with a soft-tipped catheter. In the normal person a rhythmic jerking of both eyes (nystagmus), vertigo, and nausea are produced. An absent or decreased response indicates impairment of the vestibular system.

Sound Amplification

Sound may be amplified for some individuals through the use of a hearing aid. Some persons with hearing impairments may benefit more from a hearing aid than others. This is best determined by an otologist, although persons with middle ear hearing disturbances generally receive the greatest hearing improvement, while those with inner ear or nerve damage receive the lesser hearing improvement. Hearing aids improve hearing through the mechanical amplification of sound. Thus, the patient's ability to hear per se is not improved.

TASTE

Structure and Function

The sense of taste is a specialized function that is concerned with identification of food. The four primary taste sensations perceived are *sweet, sour, bitter,* and *salt.* The many other taste sensations humans perceive are combinations of the primary sensations along with the olfactory sensation. Specific areas of the tongue are more sensitive to particular sensations (Fig. 43-12).

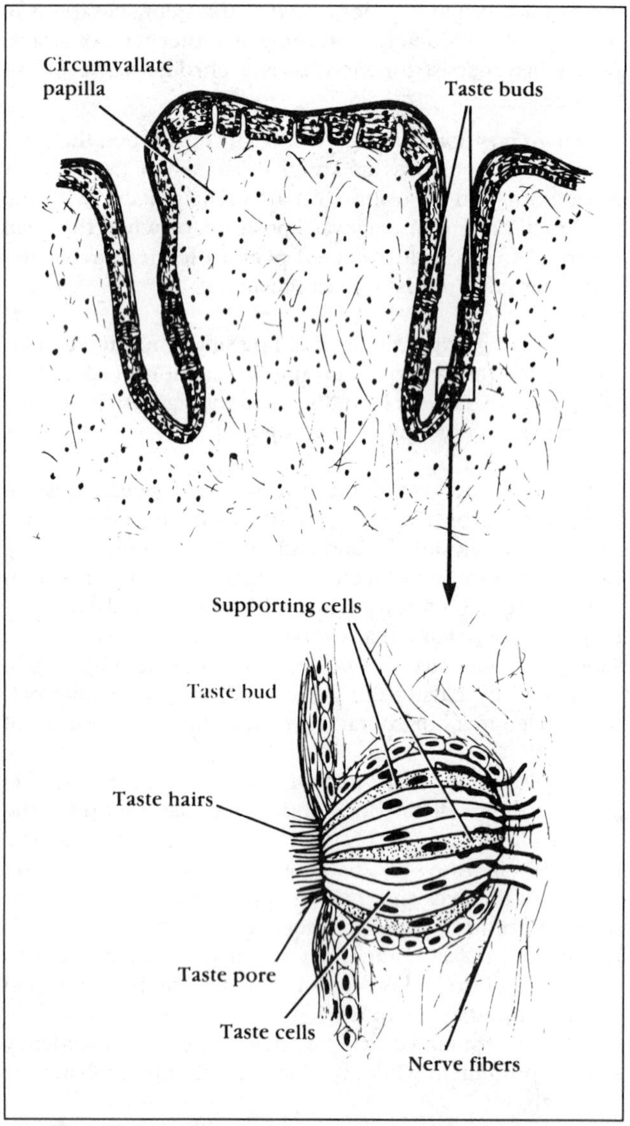

FIGURE 43-13. Microscopic appearance of a taste bud.

Taste buds are the sense organs of taste (Fig. 43-13). These oval structures are located most numerously in the fungiform papillae of the tongue but are also found in the palate, pharynx, and epiglottis. Microvilli project from the buds to the surface and come into contact with the substances dissolved in the fluids of the mouth. This contact is thought to be the basis for the generator potentials. Innervation for the taste bud arrives from its base through small myelinated fibers. Each taste bud is innervated by several nerve fibers and each receives innervation from several taste buds. The life span of a taste bud is approximately 5 days. As they degenerate, new buds are being formed and innervated.

In addition to perception of taste through the taste buds, the sense of smell contributes significantly to the taste perception. Odors of substances taken into the mouth pass to the nasopharynx and stimulate olfactory receptors. Consistency and temperature of ingested substances also contribute to the overall taste perception.

Because taste affects what is consumed, it contributes significantly to the nutritional status and internal environment of the body. However, nutritional needs are not solely dependent on taste. Researchers have shown that people tend to select foods and liquids containing substances in which they may be deficient. This is supported by studies on adrenalectomized animals, which tend to develop a preference for salty substances. Animals that have had the parathyroid gland removed usually show an increased appetite for calcium-containing substances.

Taste Pathways

Innervation from the taste buds to the central nervous system is transmitted through the seventh, ninth, and tenth cranial nerves. The taste buds of the anterior two-thirds of the tongue transmit via the chorda tympani branch of the seventh cranial nerve. The posterior third of the tongue transmits via the ninth cranial nerve, and the remainder of the areas are transmitted by the tenth cranial nerve. All three of these nerves terminate in the medulla oblongata and form the *tractus solitarius.* From this region, second order neurons transmit to the thalamus and then on to the postcentral gyrus of the cerebral cortex, where taste sensation shares projection sites with other somatic sensations.

Taste Disturbances

The sense of taste may be diminished secondarily to other underlying problems, such as dryness of the tongue (hypogeusia), respiratory infections, or aging. It occurs unilaterally in accompaniment with Bell's palsy. Thalamic or parietal lobe lesions may result in impairment or loss of smell on the opposite side of the tongue and parietal lobe seizures may be heralded by an aura of a specific taste. Certain medications may alter the interpretation of taste.

Taste Assessment

In assessing taste, one is examining the function of the eighth, ninth, and tenth cranial nerves. The discrimination of taste in humans is relatively crude, and approximately a 30 percent concentration of a substance is necessary before discrimination is detected. Thresholds of response to substances vary and sensitivity to bitter substances, in particular, is much higher than to other substances. This protective mechanism is significant in that many alkaloid poisonous substances are characteristically bitter.

In the assessment of taste, substances that are sweet, sour, salty, and bitter are assembled. They are individually swabbed on the appropriate area of the tongue and the person is asked to identify the taste sensation. To prevent mixing of the substances applied to the tongue, the individual is asked to rinse the mouth after each sensation has been identified.

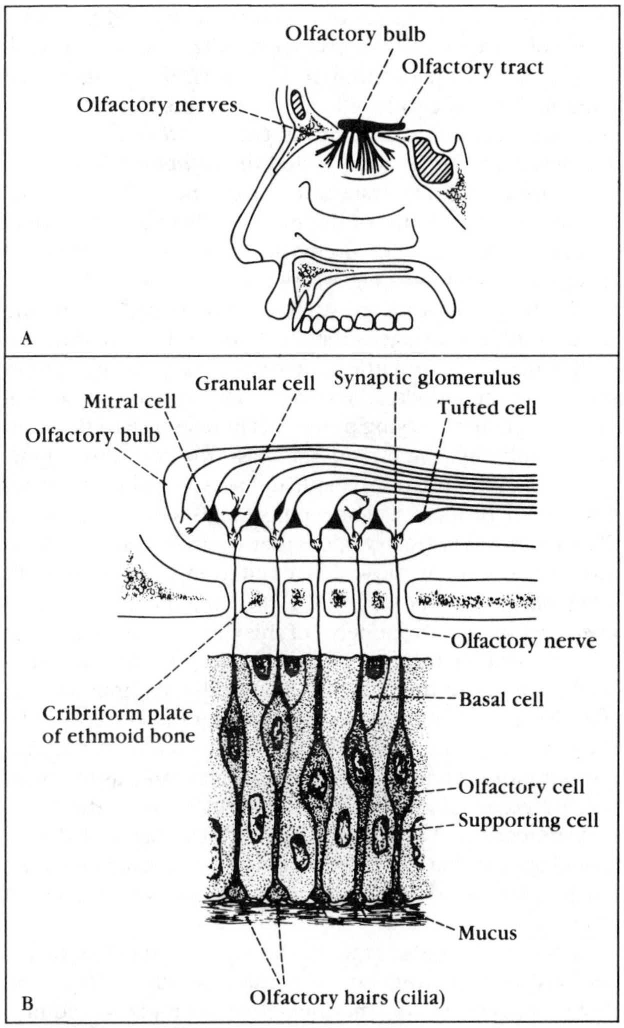

FIGURE 43-14. A. Distribution of olfactory nerves on lateral wall of nose. B. Connections between olfactory cells and neurons of olfactory bulb. (From R. Snell, *Clinical Neuroanatomy for Medical Students*. Boston: Little, Brown, 1980.)

SMELL

Structure and Function

The sense of smell is closely associated physiologically with the sense of taste in humans. Many foodstuffs consumed are perceived partially by taste and partially by smell. Both of these receptors are chemoreceptors that are stimulated by substances in the nose and mouth. Anatomically, they differ in that the apparatus perceiving smell is not relayed to the thalamus or a cortical projection area.

The receptor cells of olfaction are the *bipolar olfactory cells,* which are found in the olfactory mucous membrane. Peripherally, these cells have dendrites that terminate on the surface of the mucus of the nasal cavity and project a group of cilia, or hairlike projections. The axons of the olfactory neurons pass through the *cribriform plate* of the ethmoid bone and enter the olfactory bulb. Here they synapse with second-order neurons, the *mitral cells,* and form a complex plexus of fibers called the *olfactory glomeruli.* Olfactory signals are transmitted from here via the olfactory tract of the axons of the mitral cells and terminate in two principle areas, the prepyriform area and parts of the amygdaloid complex (Fig. 43-14).

Olfactory receptors are stimulated by volatile lipid- and water-soluble substances that are inhaled into the mucosa of the nasal cavity. Little is known about the excitatory process of the individual receptor cells, although researchers have elicited varying potentials in response to different odors. Although the physiologic basis for odor discrimination and differentiation is still unknown, several theories have been proposed. Some physiologists have proposed the existence of primary odors that excite specific cells. An attempt to explain how this excitation of specific cells takes place is proposed by the proponents of the *stereochemical* theory. Proponents of this theory believe that the odor molecules fit into specifically shaped receptor sites on the surface of the olfactory microvilli membrane. Other theorists have attempted to explain odor discrimination by the physical properties of the stimulant such as its molecular vibrations. Electrophysiologic studies have ascertained that different odors stimulate different parts of the olfactory mucosa to varying degrees. On the basis of this, it would appear that olfactory receptors are not specific for a single odor, but rather for a variety of odors to a different degree.

Adaptation is quite rapid in the sense of smell as receptors are readily fatigued by persistent odors. However, newly appearing odors may be detected rapidly. It requires only a small amount of a volatile substance to stimulate the olfactory receptors. Inhalation of irritating substances such as ammonium salts produces pain through stimulation of the trigeminal nerve. In addition, certain respiratory reflexes are initiated by its odors.

Smell Disturbances

Anosmia, the loss of smell, may accompany such disorders as sinusitis, upper respiratory infections, and allergies. Facial injuries involving the cribriform plate and certain tumors involving the olfactory groove may result in the loss of smell. Hysteria may be accompanied by anosmia or *hyperosmia* (increased acuity of smell). Olfactory hallucinations may occur with certain mental illnesses. Specific smells may precede seizures arising from the uncal region.

Smell Assessment

The assessment of the sense of smell can be accomplished simply by requesting the individual to identify common aromatic substances such as coffee, vanilla, or cologne. When doing this, the person is asked to close his or her eyes and occlude the opposite nostril. Although the individual is requested to identify the odor if possible, this ability is less significant than the perception of the odor. Therefore, the individual is asked to identify when he or she initially perceives the odor. The procedure is then repeated for the other nostril and perception is compared.

REFERENCES

1. Clark, R. G. *Essentials of Clinical Neuroanatomy and Neurophysiology* (5th ed.). Philadelphia: Davis, 1975.
2. Guyton, A. *Textbook of Medical Physiology* (6th ed.). Philadelphia: Saunders, 1981.
3. Hubel, D. H., and Wiesel, T. N. Brain mechanisms of vision. *Sci. Am.* 241:150, 1979.
4. Nauta, W. J., and Feirtag, M. The organization of the brain. *Sci. Am.* 241:99, 1979.

CHAPTER 44
ADAPTATIONS AND ALTERATIONS IN HIGHER CORTICAL FUNCTION

LEARNING OBJECTIVES

1. Describe the pathologic changes seen with intracerebral hemorrhages, cerebral thrombosis, and embolism.
2. Locate and discuss cerebral aneurysms and arteriovenous malformations.
3. Relate the clinical manifestations of stroke to the underlying pathologic bases.
4. Define *thrombotic stroke in evolution.*
5. List the etiologic factors of stroke.
6. Explain why rebleeding is a common complication after initial rupture of an intracerebral aneurysm.
7. Discuss the implications of vasospasm with ruptured cerebral aneurysms.
8. Draw or describe the appearance of AVMs.
9. Explain why AVMs rupture and the significance of the location of the bleeding.
10. Define *aphasia.*
11. Differentiate between Wernicke's aphasia and Broca's aphasia.
12. Define the disorders of speech: *anarthria, agraphia, alexia,* and *word-deafness.*
13. Define *apraxia.*
14. Define *agnosia.*
15. Discuss the various types of agnosia.
16. Define *Gerstmann's syndrome.*
17. Discuss the pathophysiology of epilepsy.
18. Differentiate between primary or idiopathic epilepsy and secondary or symptomatic epilepsy.
19. List some of the precipitating factors that may cause seizures.
20. Describe the changes in the electroencephalogram that correlate with three different types of seizures.
21. Discuss laboratory tests used in definitive diagnosis and clinical evaluations of epilepsy.

This chapter concentrates on alterations in cortical and motor activity resulting from stroke (cerebrovascular accident) and epilepsy. Aphasia, apraxia, and agnosia are also included as outcomes of cerebrovascular accidents.

CEREBROVASCULAR ACCIDENTS (CVAs) OR STROKE: PATHOLOGY AND RELATED CLINICAL SIGNS

As is the case with most neuropathology, the site of the lesions is more critical in the production of pathologic signs and symptoms than is the nature or pathology of the lesion. The majority of lesions that affect the motor cortex and its major pathways are vascular in nature and result in either reversible or irreversible anoxic tissue damage. Cerebrovascular accidents are frequently associated with hypertension and atherosclerotic disease. These conditions are closely linked with other risk factors, including hypercholesteremia, cigarette smoking, obesity, and diabetes mellitus. Intracerebral aneurysms are vascular malformations that, on enlargement or rupture, can cause the pathologic signs of stroke. Traumatic injuries, as detailed in Chapter 45, can cause significant alterations in consciousness and many equivalent signs to those of intrinsic CVAs.

The pathology of cerebrovascular accidents may result from ischemia or hemorrhage. Either condition may lead to necrosis of the brain parenchyma. Cerebral infarction refers to cerebral tissue death resulting from ischemia. The resulting infarction is due to a deprivation of blood supply.

Intracerebral Hemorrhages

Cerebral necrosis also may result from intracerebral hemorrhage (bleeding into the brain parenchyma and/or the ventricles of the brain). Intracerebral hemorrhages commonly occur deep within the brain substance, in the region of the basal ganglia. The bleeding may be massive or in multiple foci. The blood in the parenchyma causes extensive neuronal destruction and the central area of hemorrhage is often surrounded by small hemorrhages. The blood is treated like foreign material and eventually is broken down, phagocytosed, and removed from the area. The mechanisms causing intracerebral hemorrhage appear to be many, e.g., a sudden elevation of the blood pressure in the presence of diseased intracranial vessels causing rupture of the vessels. The initial event in an intracerebral hemorrhage may be ischemia produced from an arterial spasm. This may then be followed by rupture of the diseased vessels. The most common cause of subarachnoid hemorrhage (bleeding into the ventricles and subarachnoid space) is the rupture of an intracerebral aneurysm (see pp. 673–674).

Transient Ischemic Attacks

If the tissue ischemia is reversible, the tissue changes are temporary, causing decreased blood supply to an area and focal ischemic clinical signs. These reversible ischemic signs are called transient ischemic attacks (TIAs). The result may be transient episodes of contralateral weakness (hemiparesis), sensory deficits (hemiparesthesias), or visual disturbances [2].

Because intact circulation and a relatively constant flow of blood are required for continuous function of the cerebral cells, syncope (fainting) may result when the general circulation fails suddenly. TIAs are characterized by localized symptoms of cerebral dysfunction, often including syncope.

The symptoms of TIAs seem to result from a cerebral angiospasm or transient impairment of blood flow. The attacks usually last less than 1 hour and are followed by no neurologic impairment. Symptoms may include yawning, headache, vertigo, deafness, diplopia, ataxia, and motor or sensory deficits.

TIAs also may be associated with collateral communications in the intracerebral arterial system that compensate in a short time for the deficits from occlusion of one arterial source.

Diagnosis of TIAs usually requires angiographic evaluation of the site, size, and nature of the pathologic processes in the cerebral arteries. Radiopaque substances are used to outline the cerebral vasculature to locate areas of narrowing or disease.

Ischemic Infarction from Cerebral Thrombosis

Ischemic infarction in the brain is often due to cerebral thrombosis that occurs on an atherosclerotic plaque. Forty-four to seventy-five percent of all CVAs result from thrombosis of a cerebral artery. This type of lesion is often called *atherothrombotic brain infarction (ABI)* [4]. The resulting obstruction to blood flow causes infarction to the area supplied by the artery. The type of infarct produced depends on the amount of hemorrhage that occurs into the area of ischemic necrosis. Infarcts are often divided into red (hemorrhagic) or white (anemic) infarctions. In the first few days, the pale or white infarcts assume a muddy, mottled appearance that is associated with surrounding tissue edema. After about 10 days, liquefaction of the area becomes evident from the release of neuronal lysosomes and other lytic substances into the brain parenchyma [2]. Scar tissue begins to form at the margins of the necrotic area. The necrotic tissue is removed and replaced by cystic scar tissue. Gliosis (proliferation of glial cells) around the area is characteristic and this is followed by polymorphonuclear leukocyte (PMN) exudation leading to removal of the necrotic debris. Therefore, characteristic scar tissue is laid down after the acute inflammation subsides.

Red infarcts also cause tissue destruction. The red blood cells are broken down and removed. The necrotic parenchyma undergoes liquefaction and characteristic scar tissue is formed at the margins of the affected area.

The onset of cerebral thrombosis is usually gradual with periods of progression and periods of improvement. This is apparently due to spread of the thrombus and is called a

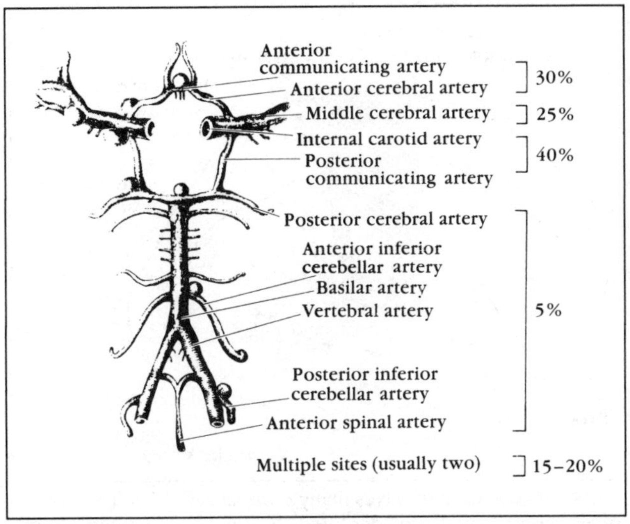

FIGURE 44-1. Common sites of aneurysms. (From J. H. Stein [ed.], *Internal Medicine*. Boston: Little, Brown, 1983.)

thrombotic stroke in evolution. This thrombosis causes the cerebral infarction, which may be associated with a hemorrhage into the brain parenchyma [2]. The symptoms of cerebral thrombosis often begin or are seen in the early morning. These may consist of headache, vertigo, mental confusion, aphasia, and focal neurologic signs, which may present weeks to months before the actual evolved stroke. A full-blown stroke may cause a variety of clinical features. Coma, hemiplegia, and aphasia are common. Aphasia, apraxia, and agnosia are more fully considered in the following section. Flaccidity of the affected side is common in the early period and may be replaced by spasticity.

The recovery from the stroke is variable and depends on the location and the amount of intracerebral damage. Recovery of function in an affected leg usually occurs prior to arm and hand function, which may not return at all.

Cerebral Embolism

Cerebral embolism causes approximately 8 percent of all CVAs [2]. The main source of an embolus is the heart; the embolus frequently lodges in the middle cerebral artery, causing a massive brain infarction. This often results in contralateral hemiplegia, hemianesthesia, and occasionally aphasia, apraxia, and agnosia (see pp. 674–677).

The onset of embolic infarction is always very sudden. With cerebral embolism, there are usually no warning signs. The onset is sudden and the effect is immediate. The clinical picture depends on the artery affected and the amount and location of brain infarction.

Cerebral Aneurysms and Vascular Malformations

Common sources for cerebral bleeding, which also contribute to the etiologic basis of CVAs, include ruptured intracranial aneurysms and vascular malformations. Both of these cerebrovascular problems frequently result in bleeding into the subarachnoid space and are clinically similar.

ANEURYSMS. The etiology of cerebral aneurysms is related to developmental defects and hypertensive atherosclerotic changes. The developmental defects contributing to aneurysm formation involve a weakness in the middle coat (tunica media) of the vessel resulting in an outpouching at the weakened area. These aneurysms are saccular in nature and are referred to as *berry aneurysms*. Berry aneurysms can vary from one to several centimeters in size and generally have a well-defined neck that originates most often near bifurcations in the anterior vessels of the circle of Willis (Fig. 44-1) [3]. Berry aneurysms show the highest incidence of rupture in persons between 30 and 60 years of age and both sexes seem to be affected equally. Of those individuals with developmental cerebral aneurysms, about one-fifth demonstrate multiple aneurysms.

Less common than the developmental aneurysms are those associated with atherosclerotic degenerative changes of the cerebral vasculature. These aneurysms are usually fusiform as a result of weakening of the tunica media from the degenerative atherosclerotic process. The arteries become thin and fibrous, often apparently as a result of long-term hypertension. Although fusiform aneurysms of cerebral arteries may be found in some younger individuals, they generally are found in the over-50-year-old group.

Cerebral aneurysms can remain silent for many years, often going undetected throughout life and being detected only on routine postmortem examination. Cerebral aneurysms become evident when they rupture or compress adjacent nerve tissue, causing focal cerebral disturbances.

The presenting signs and symptoms of subarachnoid bleeding from a ruptured aneurysm may be localized from the pressure exerted on surrounding tissue. Focal localizing signs are related to the region of the brain involved and may include visual defects, cranial nerve paralysis, hemiparesis, and focal seizures. Generalized signs of subarachnoid bleeding include photophobia, fever, malaise, vomiting, abnormal mentation with disorientation, and nuchal rigidity. If conscious, the person complains of a severe headache of a different nature from any experienced previously. Transitory unconsciousness or extended coma may accompany bleeding from ruptured aneurysms. Initial and prolonged coma generally indicates an unfavorable outcome (see also Chap. 45).

The aneurysm decreases in size after rupture and a fibrin clot forms over the site of the rupture. The individual becomes at risk for a rebleed during the first few weeks after the initial bleed. This occurs during the period of clot lysis or breakdown. Rebleeding cerebral aneurysms carry a considerably increased mortality risk.

Diagnosis of ruptured cerebral aneurysms is made by history, clinical examination, lumbar puncture, cerebral angiography, and computer axial tomography (CAT) scanning. The treatment of individuals experiencing ruptured cerebral aneurysms is conservative initially in an effort to stabil-

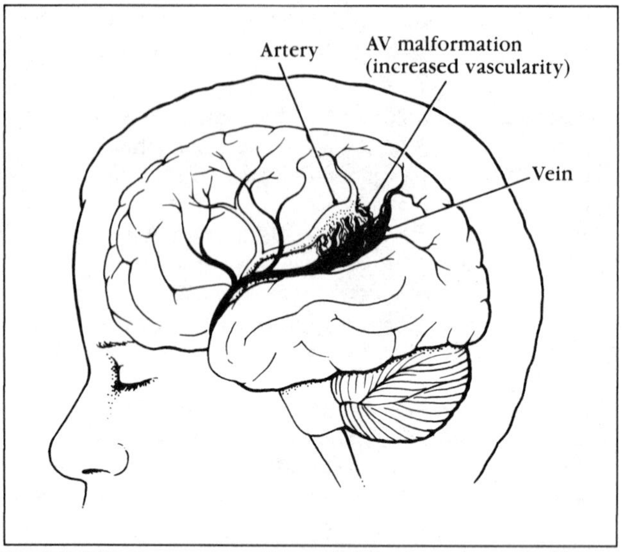

FIGURE 44-2. Appearance of superficial arteriovenous malformation. Vessels appear dilated and tortuous.

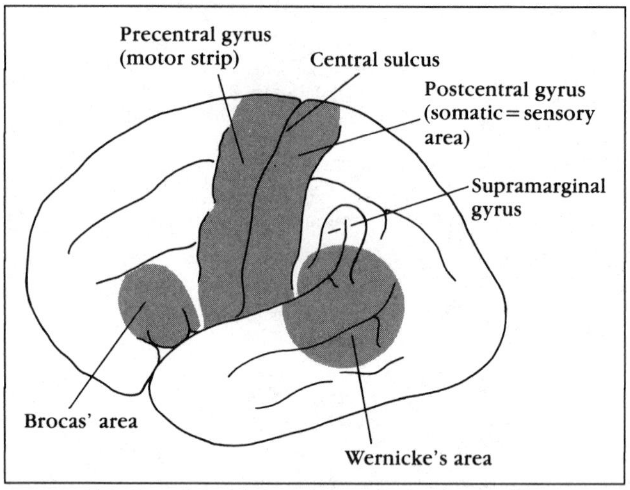

FIGURE 44-3. Speech involves many cortical activities. Two special speech areas have been identified: Wernicke's area and Broca's area. (From D. Dickson and W. Maue-Dickson, *Anatomical and Physiological Bases of Speech*. Boston: Little, Brown, 1982.)

ize the pathologic processes. When the stabilization has been accomplished, surgical intervention is generally utilized to resolve the aneurysm.

An associated problem frequently accompanying ruptured cerebral aneurysms is vasospasm. Because spasm develops within a week or two after the rupture of the aneurysms, it results in the narrowing of the vessel lumen. This may lead to cerebral ischemia and clinically evident neurologic deficits. The precise cause of the vasospasms is unknown, but is thought to be related to certain intrinsic chemicals synthesized in the brain. In most situations, surgery is delayed until the spasms subside. Antispasmotic drugs such as reserpine may be used to control spasms during the time prior to surgery.

ARTERIOVENOUS MALFORMATIONS (AVMs). Vascular malformations that frequently cause a cerebral bleed usually result from a developmental defect in which very few distinguishing characteristics among the cerebral veins, capillaries, and arteries in certain localized regions of the brain are found. The veins frequently appear to connect to the arteries without an intermediate capillary bed. The malformations are referred to as arteriovenous malformations or angiomas (Fig. 44-2). These malformations can be found most commonly on the surface of the cerebral hemispheres although they may appear deeper within the cerebral lobes, the brainstem, or spinal cord. Although AVMs are present from birth, they may not become evident until young adulthood or later. Their presence is evidenced by symptoms of hemorrhage, seizures, headaches, or focal neurologic deficits. A bruit may be audible over the area of the malformation.

The AVM vessels become engorged with very thin walls. The vessels in this state are particularly vulnerable to rupture and bleeding. The bleeding most commonly occurs into the subarachnoid space and, therefore, the presenting symptoms are similar to those observed with ruptured cerebral aneurysms. Additionally, specific findings will reflect the region of the brain that is involved.

Arteriovenous malformations are diagnosed by the clinical findings and by one or more of the following tests: cerebral angiography, lumbar puncture, CAT scan, electroencephalogram (EEG), and radioactive scanning. AVMs are treated with surgical ligation and excision of the feeder vessels into the area, whenever possible. If the location of the AVM does not permit surgical excision, embolization may be utilized to occlude the feeder vessels in an attempt to reduce the blood flow to the AVM.

APHASIA

Language is defined as audible, articulate human speech produced by the action of the tongue and adjacent vocal cords. Speech may be the act of speaking, the result of speaking, the utterance of vocal sounds that convey ideas, or the ability to express thoughts by words. Mechanisms of speech are accomplished through internal symbolization and thought. Language is dependent on retention, recall, visualization, and the integration of symbols. Speech depends on the interpretation of auditory and visual images, which reach the higher human processes during differing states of consciousness and, to some degree, the lesser states of consciousness. Figure 44-3 shows the approximate location of the speech centers in the brain. To speak, one must initially formulate the thought to be expressed, choose appropriate words, and then control the motor activity of the muscles of phonation and articulation. To write, one must involve the motor and sensory impulses of the hand. Simultaneously, an accurate recording of visual and auditory stimuli is necessary before the significance of the words used can be appreciated. Language and speech may become impaired in many ways. Irrespective of the specific cause, the results are generally similar when the brain is damaged.

Aphasia is a defect in speech. Either the ability to comprehend and integrate *receptive language* or the ability to formulate and use *expressive language* or both is impaired. The aphasic individual usually has some impairment of all language modalities. The receptive language modalities are *reading*, which requires visual integration and comprehension of the printed word, and *listening*, which necessitates auditory integration and comprehension of the verbal word. The expressive language modalities are *writing*, which requires visual-motor formulation and use of the printed word, and *speaking*, which requires oral-motor formulation and the use of verbal words.

Aphasia is usually caused by organic disease of the brain. Potentially, the causal lesion in aphasia is located in the left cerebral hemisphere. The left cerebral hemisphere is considered to be dominant in the reception and expression of language. Infrequently, aphasia has occurred in right-sided lesions associated with right-handed individuals. However, the right-handedness has sometimes been forced or induced. In left-handed people, lesions of the left or of the right hemispheres may cause aphasia, but it is more frequent with lesions of the left hemisphere.

When certain portions of the cortex and subcortical associated pathways of the dominant hemisphere are altered by lack of blood supply (loss of oxygen or hemorrhage to the brain tissue), speech patterns become altered, limited, or destroyed, depending on the magnitude of the pathologic process. Vascular disturbances are the most common cause of aphasia. Infarction, caused by thrombotic embolic occlusion of the middle cerebral artery or the left internal carotid artery, is the causal factor in the majority of cases, and is involved with spoken and written language. Infarction, caused by thrombotic or embolic occlusion of the posterior cerebral artery may cause visual disorders. Transitory ischemic attacks and migraine headache may trigger transitory speech disorders. Space occupying lesions, such as intracerebral hemorrhage, intracranial tumors, or infections, also may cause aphasia. Left hemisphere aphasia results from damage to a specific region of the brain, the first and second temporal gyri, the insula, and the posterior part of the third convolution. Visual and auditory impulses reach the cerebral cortex posteriorly, via the occipital lobe and anteroinferiorly, via the temporal lobe. There is extraction of the semantic value of the auditory and visual message and of the symbolic formation of the expressed message in the posterior portion of the temporal convolutions. The anterior part of the region is necessary for the motor realization of the expressed message. There are many cortical areas and association pathways concerned in the integration of the function of speech.

Many combinations of vascular, neoplastic, and traumatic causes and locations of lesions lead to the production of different language patterns. Classifications have been developed to define prominent characteristics, to localize position and size of cerebral lesions, and to assess the language deficit pattern in each category of aphasia. There are several primary types of disorders: (1) Wernicke's aphasia, which causes disturbances of all language activities except for articulation; (2) Broca's aphasia, involving disturbances in spoken and written language with dysarthria (disorder of articulation); and (3) selective disorders of receptive or expressive activities of spoken or written language.

Wernicke's Aphasia

The posterior third of the superior temporal convolution of the dominant hemisphere is called Wernicke's area (see Fig. 44-3). Wernicke's area influences the understanding and interpretation of word symbols. Lesions in other areas, particularly in the posterior half of the dominant hemisphere, the angular gyrus, and the supramarginal gyrus influence speech function, through the involvement of association fibers.

Wernicke's aphasia includes central, receptive, cortical, sensory, auditory, semantic, and conduction aphasia. Affected persons have fluent, spontaneous speech, but comprehension, repetition, and naming are impaired. Expression in spoken language is hindered by difficulty in the choice of words to speak and to write. Repetition, reading aloud, and writing from dictation are deranged. Understanding of spoken language is disturbed. Voices are heard, but the words are without meaning. Speech lacks content and contains much meaningless expression.

Lesions in the Wernicke's area inhibit comprehension in spoken and written language because of its interconnections with the angular gyrus. Lesions of the angular gyrus and posteroinferior part of the parietal lobe may cause acalculia, autopanosia, and disorientation for right and left sides (Table 44-1).

Broca's Aphasia

The lesion in Broca's aphasia is located in the caudal part of the inferior frontal gyrus rostral to the motor area of the tongue, pharynx, or larynx, or involves the pathways carrying impulses from the temporal lobe to this area (see Fig. 44-3). Broca's aphasia includes disorders described as cortical motor aphasia, expressive aphasia, verbal aphasia, and disorders in expression of spoken language. The person may not be able to utter a word or may have extremely limited speech. Simultaneously, he or she will fully comprehend the spoken word and will obey commands. Efforts to speak are frustrated by inability to find appropriate words. Agraphia, a reduction of written language, coexists with that of spoken language and can be more severe in some patients. Agrammatism, when present in spoken language, is present in written language (see Table 44-1).

Selective Disorders of Receptive or Expressive Activities of Spoken and Written Language

The "pure" disorders of receptive and expressive speech may include anarthria, agraphia, alexia, and word-deafness.

TABLE 44-1. Terms used to describe some disorders of higher cortical function

Term	Definition
Acalculia	Inability to solve mathematical problems
Agnosia	Loss of comprehension of auditory, tactile, visual, or other sensations although the sensations and the sensory system are intact
Auditory agnosia	Inability to recognize auditory objects
Tactile agnosia	Inability to identify objects by touch
Visual agnosia	Inability to recognize objects seen
Verbal agnosia	Inability to recognize spoken language
Agrammatism	Inability to arrange words in grammatical sequence or to form a grammatical or intelligent sentence
Anosognosia	Lack of awareness of presence of disease, e.g., paralysis
Apraxia	Inability to carry out a voluntary movement, although the conductive systems are intact
Constructional apraxia	Inability to construct models with matchsticks, cubes, etc., to assemble puzzles, or to draw
Dressing apraxia	Inability to dress or undress
Autotopagnosia	Inability to orient various parts of the body correctly
Dysarthria	Disorder of articulation
Prosopagnosia	Inability to recognize faces and one's own face

In *anarthria*, reading aloud and voluntary speech repetition are disturbed, whereas understanding of spoken and written language and writing remain normal. It usually appears as a sequela of Broca's aphasia.

In *agraphia*, all forms of writing are defective. The lesion may be located in the posterior part of the second frontal gyrus.

In *alexia*, reading of words may be severely impaired but reading of letters is less obstructed than reading words. Language activities may be normal except for the recognition of written symbols. The lesion is located in the lingual and fusiform gyri.

In *word-deafness,* there is impairment in the understanding of spoken language, repetition, and writing from dictation, but all other speech activities are normal. The lesion appears in the superior aspect of the temporal lobe.

APRAXIA

Apraxia is the inability to carry out a voluntary movement, although the conductive systems are intact. There is no paralysis, ataxia, abnormal movement, or sensory loss.

To execute a skilled movement, one must utilize a logical routine. First, the command is received at the primary auditory cortex. This information is then relayed to the auditory association areas for comprehension. The information is relayed by the association fiber systems to the motor association areas in the premotor cortex of the dominant hemisphere. From the dominant premotor cortex, this information is conveyed to the premotor and motor cortexes of the nondominant hemisphere to enable the nondominant hand to perform the learned skilled movement.

Apraxia is caused by damage to the association areas or fibers concerned with voluntary motor activity. Lesions in these areas will cause impairment in accordance with their locations. Lesions of the supramarginal gyrus of the dominant parietal lobe may produce bilateral apraxia (see Fig. 44-3). A lesion of the dominant premotor association areas may produce a bilateral impairment in certain tongue and hand movements. A lesion of the anterior half of the corpus callosum will result in an apraxia of the nondominant hand.

Apraxia of the lips and tongue is fairly common. Apraxia of the limbs may be revealed as dressing apraxia (an inability to dress or undress), and constructional apraxia (an inability to construct models with matchsticks or cubes, or to assemble puzzles, or to draw).

The location of lesions producing the various apraxias is somewhat controversial. All forms of apraxia frequently occur in cases of diffuse brain damage leading to dementia, which suggests that the symptomatic structure of an apraxia may be caused by the mass effect of a lesion rather than its location.

AGNOSIA

Perception occurs when sensory data originating at sensory receptors are forwarded by peripheral and spinal pathways to the primary sensory cortex for analysis and sorting. These data are dispatched to the association areas that contain the memory banks for higher order interpretation, and there the data are translated into codes and symbols of language. This process of recognition of the significance of sensory stimuli is known as *gnosia. Agnosia* is impairment of this faculty of recognition derived from lesions of the visual association areas of the cerebral cortex, even though the primary sensory pathway is intact.

Types of Agnosia

Visual agnosia (inability to recognize objects seen), tactile agnosia (inability to identify objects by touch), and auditory agnosia (inability to recognize auditory objects although auditory sensation is intact) are the three types that may occur. A person with visual agnosia may not recognize a safety pin, but will name it instantaneously if it is placed in his hand. Conversely, one with tactile agnosia will identify visually the safety pin that she was unable to recognize when it was first placed in her hand.

VISUAL AGNOSIA. Visual agnosia is caused by a lesion of the visual association areas. Lesions limited to the visual association areas do not cause blindness. Objects are clearly seen but are not recognized or identified. Visual agnosia is characterized by an inability to recognize any object or shape by sight, although it can be recognized through other modalities, such as touch or smell. Several categories of visual agnosia that have been included in clinical classifications are (1) agnosia for objects, (2) agnosia for colors, and (3) agnosia for physiognomies.

1. *Object agnosia.* Persons suffering from this type of agnosia are not able to recognize objects when they are presented visually.
2. *Color agnosia.* Affected persons are unable to recognize colors, a defect that may be confined to one-half of the visual fields (called *hemiagnosia* for colors).
3. *Agnosia for physiognomies, or prosopagnosia.* The person suffers from an inability to recognize faces, sometimes even his or her own face in the mirror. The affected individual is unable to recognize a familiar face but can identify a person once that person starts to speak.

TACTILE AGNOSIA. Normal tactile recognition is the recognition of an object by feeling without the help of other sensory information. Feeling movements provide impressions until the object is identified. Lesions of the parietal lobe posterior to the somesthetic area produce tactile agnosia.

Tactile agnosia is the inability to identify objects by touch and feeling. It is often called *astereognosis.* There is a loss of some previously acquired factual information from the brain's memory stores. Therefore, there cannot be a comparison of present sensory phenomena with past experience.

AUDITORY AGNOSIA. Auditory agnosia is the inability to recognize auditory objects, although the auditory sensation is intact. The problem of the auditory agnosias is separating them from the sensory aphasias. The first temporal convolution and part of the second temporal convolution of the dominant hemisphere are considered important for auditory recognition.

From the descriptive point of view, auditory agnosia is the inability to recognize familiar concrete sounds, such as animal noises, a sounding bell, or the ticking of a clock (agnosia for nonlinguistic sounds). Other auditory perceptual disorders include verbal agnosia (the inability to recognize spoken language), sensory amusia (the inability to recognize music), and congenital auditory agnosia (primary retardation of speech development, usually associated with mental retardation).

BODY IMAGE

Humans build images of their bodies from sensory impulses from the special senses (skin, muscles, bones, and joints) that provide information of bodily relationships and relationships with the external environment. This concept of body image is stored in the association areas of the parietal lobes.

Lesion involvement of the nondominant parietal lobe, particularly the inferior parietal lobe, may create abnormalities in concepts of bodily image. A lack of awareness of the left side of the body despite intact cortical and primary sensation is exhibited. Lack of awareness of hemiparesis may be noted. An affected person may perceive sensory stimuli applied independently to the two sides of the body, but if sensory stimulus is applied bilaterally simultaneously, one is generally ignored.

Gerstmann's Syndrome

Lesions of the dominant lobes, particularly the supramarginal and angular gyri, may produce one or more of a complex of symptoms known as Gerstmann's syndrome and includes a right-left disorientation (being unable to distinguish right from left). Finger agnosia is exhibited by a failure to recognize one's fingers in the presence of intact sensation and is associated with constructional apraxia. Acalculia and/or dyslexia are common when the lesion involves the angular gyrus.

EPILEPSY

Epilepsy is a symptom, not a disease. An epileptic seizure is a sudden, excessive discharge by neurons of electrical energy in the central nervous system within either a structurally normal or diseased cortex or diencephalon. The discharge may trigger a convulsive movement, interruption of sensation, alteration of consciousness, or some combination of these disturbances. Seizures may originate from diverse factors that are metabolic, toxic, degenerative, genetic, infectious, neoplastic, traumatic, or unknown.

Epilepsy may be linked with increased local excitability, reduced inhibition, or a combination of both factors. Some neurons in identified focal lesions have been identified as hypersensitive and remain in a state of partial depolarization. Increased permeability of their cytoplasmic membranes makes these neurons very susceptible to activation by hyperthermia, hypoglycemia, hyponatremia, hypoxia, repeated sensory stimulation, and even certain phases of sleep. Reduced inhibition may be caused by a lesion of the cortex.

Once the intensity of a seizure discharge has progressed sufficiently, it spreads to adjacent cortical, thalamic, brainstem nuclei, and other brain areas. Excitement feeds back from the thalamus to the primary focus and to other parts of the brain. This process is evidenced by the high-frequency discharge shown on an electroencephalogram. Within the process, a diencephalocortical inhibition intermittently interrupts the discharge and converts the tonic phase to the clonic phase (see p. 680). These discharges become less and less frequent until they cease.

Severe seizures may cause systemic hypoxia with accompanying acidosis from increased lactic acid, which may result in respiratory spasms, airway blockage, and excessive muscular activity. An extremely severe prolonged seizure can cause respiratory arrest or cardiac standstill. Metabolic needs increase markedly during a seizure causing in-

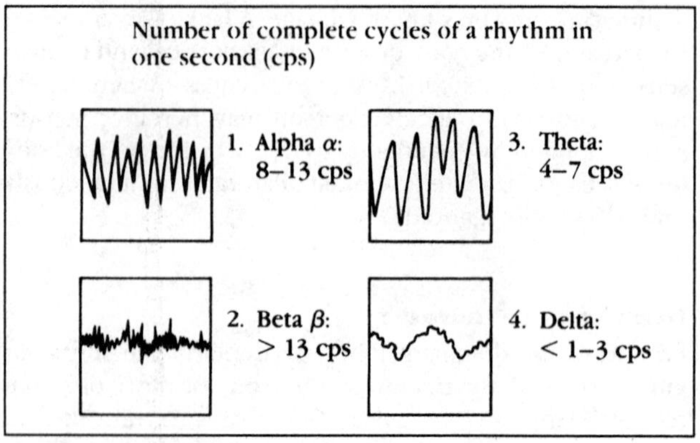

FIGURE 44-4. Frequency of brain waves.

creased cerebral blood flow, glycolysis, and tissue respiration.

Electroencephalography in Epilepsy

Electroencephalogram (EEG) is used routinely in definitive diagnosis and clinical evaluations of epilepsy. The electrical discharges produced by the brain's electrical activity are called *brain waves* and are recorded via electrodes placed on the surface of the scalp. Since the EEG is a surface recording, it reflects the most superficial activity, especially that of the cerebral cortex. An electroencephalogram is recorded while the resting person is awake in a darkened room, or with eyes closed. Movements and external distractions should be minimized. During a recording of the brain's waves, the subject may be asked to hyperventilate. Provocative techniques, photic stimulation, or sleep deprivation may be useful in initiating abnormal electrical activity in some persons.

The normal adult will record a dominant activity in the parietal occipital areas of 8 to 13 cps, identified as "alpha rhythm." In the frontal areas, the dominant activity is of lower amplitude and faster frequency, > 13 cps, and is known as the "beta rhythm." Slower frequency than the "alpha rhythm" is recognized as "slow waves." Those 4 to 7 cps are "theta rhythms," and 1 to 3 cps are "delta rhythms" (Fig. 44-4). Normal variations occur. Age differences are noted on the EEG (Figs. 44-5, 45-6). An infant at 13 months will have dominant awakened activity of 4 to 5 cps; a five-year-old child, 6 to 7 cps, and a 12-year-old, 8 to 9 cps (alpha rhythm) [1].

Two types of abnormalities are described:

1. *Type 1.* Normally, there should be relative symmetry of amplitude and frequency between the two cerebral hemispheres. Abnormality, then, is a difference between the two hemispheres. There may be focal slow waves caused by focal cortical disorders such as an abscess, glioblastoma, meningioma, metastatic tumors, or infarction. Focal spikes indicating an irritable focus and having the quality of sudden excessive neuronal discharge correlate with partial, or symptomatic, seizures.

2. *Type 2.* Abnormalities of this type relate either to the frequency of the dominant awake activity or to the form of the dominant activity. These abnormalities imply pathology of the cerebral cortex in a generalized or diffuse man-

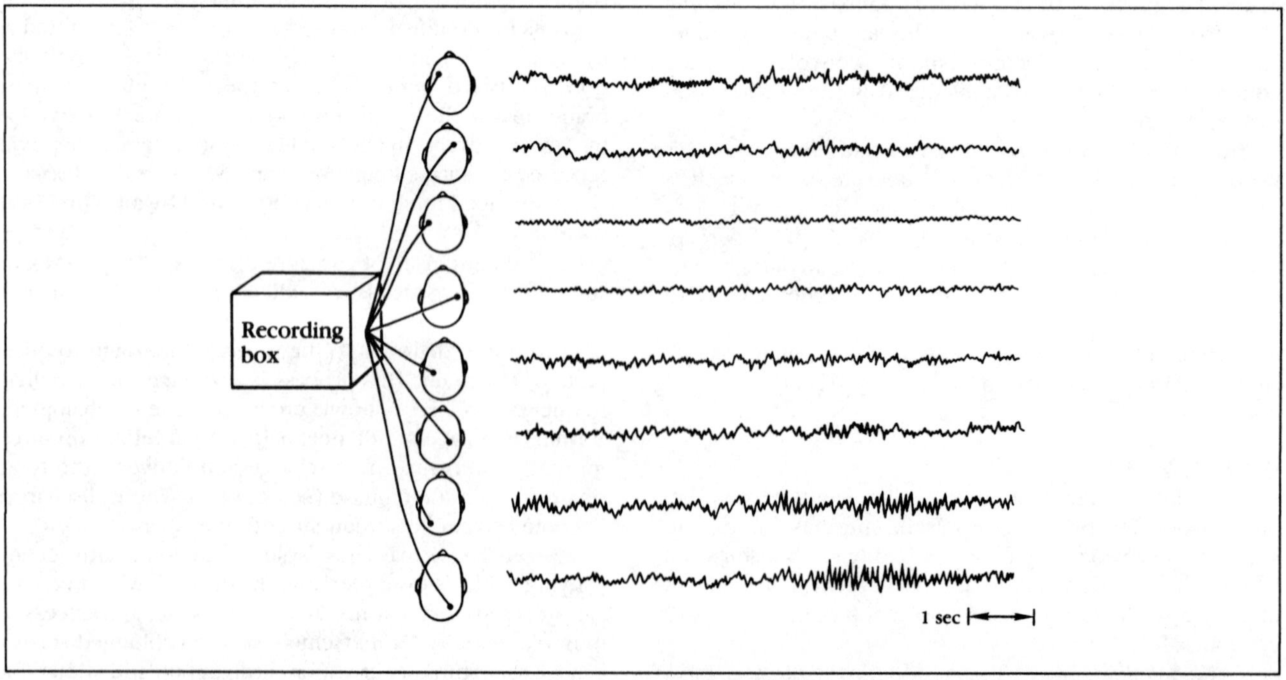

FIGURE 44-5. The normal electroencephalogram in an adult.

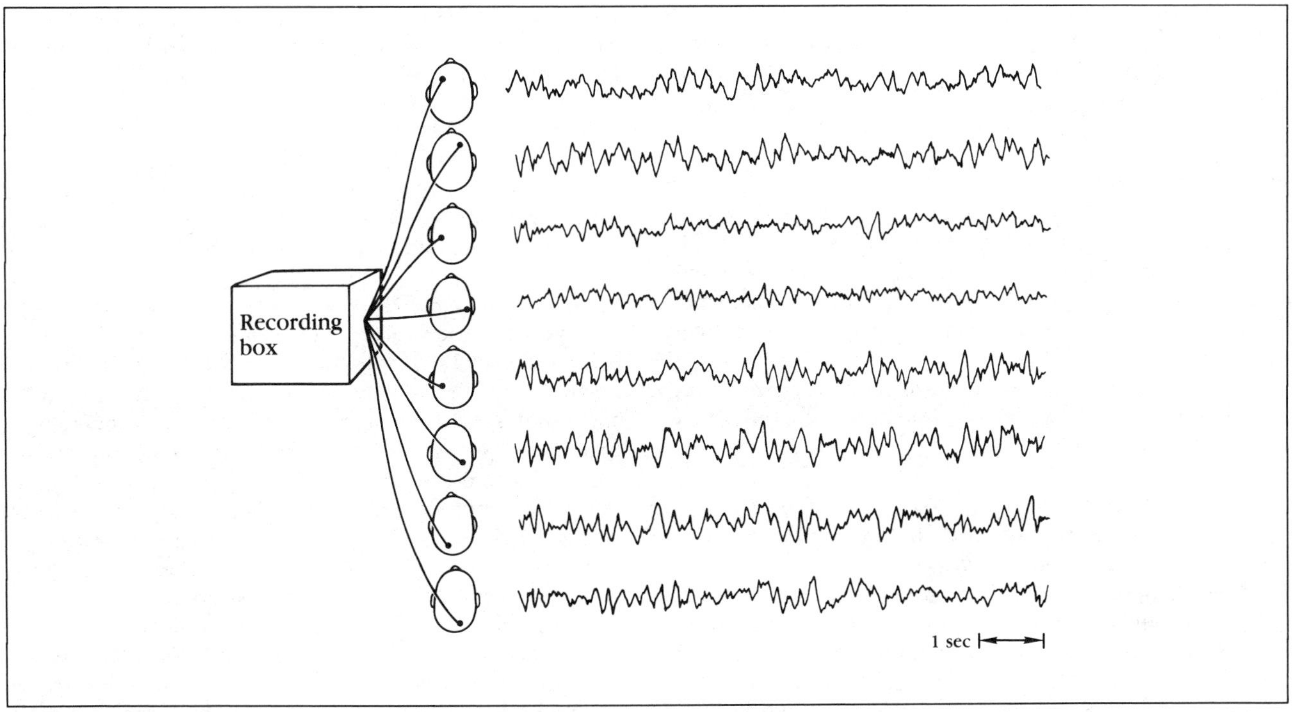

FIGURE 44-6. The normal electroencephalogram in a child.

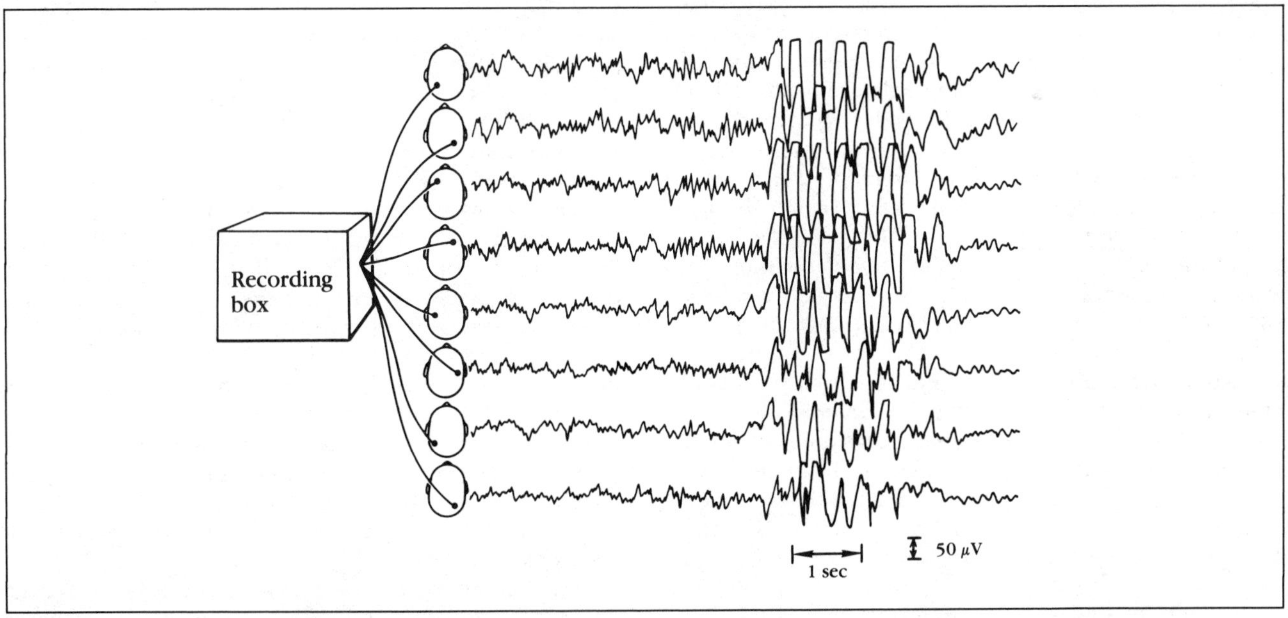

FIGURE 44-7. EEG appearance during a grand mal seizure.

ner. A generalized slow wave may indicate a generalized cortical disorder or a metabolic, or toxic, state. Damage from encephalitis, hypoxia, or hepatic or renal failure, may be deduced from generalized slow-wave activity. Electrical abnormalities are recorded as generalized bursts, 2.5 to 4.0 cps, which can be seen as spikes and slow-wave complexes. This type correlates with petit mal seizures.

Other generalized bursts consisting of polyspike slow-wave complexes correlate with myoclonic seizures. In infantile myoclonic spasms, the electroencephalogram demonstrates continuous high amplitude generalized but often asynchronous spikes and slow waves. This pattern is called ***hypsarrhythmia***. Repetitive fast spikes, 8 to 12 cps, correlate with generalized seizures, specifically the grand mal seizure (Fig. 44-7).

Classification of Seizures

An epileptic seizure is classified as (1) primary or idiopathic, if the origin of the disorder is unknown; or (2) secondary or symptomatic if a definitive etiology is determined.

Primary or Idiopathic Epilepsy

Typical seizure activity may be either generalized or partial. Generalized seizures have bilaterally symmetric epileptigenic foci originating within deep subcortical diencephalic structures, whereas partial seizures usually begin in a cortical focus, but may arise from subcortical structures.

Generalized seizures are the most frequent type. Examples are: absence (petit mal), akinetic, myoclonic, and tonic-clonic (grand mal).

ABSENCE (PETIT MAL). This type of seizure exhibits a characteristic spike-and-wave pattern with 3 cps on the electroencephalogram. The term *absence seizure* is used because the afflicted person, although present physically, is absent concerning higher cortical functions during the seizure. The majority of such persons have normal intelligence and have no significant abnormal physical findings during a neurologic examination. The onset is usually about the age of 5 and attacks are more prevalent in childhood.

The petit mal seizure is characterized by a loss of awareness that may be exhibited by flicking of the eyelids, twitching of facial muscles, or staring into space while general postural tone is preserved. The attack may be precipitated by seeing bright or flashing lights or hearing loud noises and may last from 5 to 30 seconds. Hyperventilation may precede the seizure. Consciousness is abruptly restored after the attack and the interrupted activity is promptly resumed. Memory may be defective only through the seizure. As the affected person reaches adolescence frequency decreases, and the electroencephalogram may eventually show normal discharge. However, these individuals may develop other types of seizures at any time.

MYOCLONIC SEIZURES. Affected individuals have sudden rapid flexion of the limbs and trunk singularly or repeatedly with no loss of consciousness. Loud sounds or bright lights may precipitate myoclonic seizures. These disorders occur with greatest frequency in childhood, but may continue after puberty. Bilateral, synchronous 3-cps discharges on the electroencephalogram are seen during this type of seizure.

Myoclonic spasms occurring in infancy are called "massive spasms," are first noted at 6 to 9 months of age, and continue to age 2 or 3. There is usually associated retardation of psychomotor development and the spasms may be related to other conditions such as phenylketonuria, perinatal brain damage, pyridoxine deficiency, or tuberous sclerosis. Myoclonic spasms may be generalized or multifocal and tend to disappear with growth but other seizure patterns may emerge. A benign form of myoclonus has been described that is associated with sudden myoclonic jerks when falling asleep or when awakening.

AKINETIC SEIZURES. Affected persons experience a sudden loss of consciousness and fall to the ground without contraction or motion. A brief loss of muscle tone is seen but the stance is resumed almost immediately. A history of infantile spasms and mental retardation is often present.

TONIC-CLONIC SEIZURES (GRAND MAL). Electrical disruption with grand mal seizures originates anywhere in the forebrain and usually engulfs the whole forebrain. The epileptic discharge shows nonfocal changes of high amplitude and rapid synchronous bursts on the electroencephalogram (see Fig. 44-7). For several hours preceding the seizure a vague prodomal sensation, epigastric sensation, or muscular twitching may occur. There may be a brief aura lasting for several seconds, which is often described as an olfactory, auditory, or visual sensation. Dizziness or headache also may precede the onset of the seizure.

Following the aura, if present, the individual abruptly loses consciousness, falls to the ground, and suffers generalized tonic contractions followed by clonic contractions of all muscles. Muscle contraction in the tonic phase lasts for a few seconds. The entire body becomes rigid with the arms and legs extended. The jaws become clenched, the head may be retracted, and the eyeballs are rolled backward. Breathing usually ceases during this time. Movements become jerky in the clonic phase as muscle groups contract and relax. The arms and legs contract and relax forcibly. Breathing becomes noisy and stertorous and profuse perspiration is noted. Excessive salivation and loss of bladder or bowel sphincter control may also occur.

Contractions become slower, sometimes irregular, and then stop. The entire seizure may last up to 10 minutes. Spasms of the tongue and jaw may cause biting injuries to the tongue or cheeks. Unconsciousness for the entire seizure is characteristic and may continue up to one-half hour following the seizure. As consciousness is regained, the individual is often briefly confused, fatigued, and drowsy with complaints of muscle soreness. In the early part of the postseizure period, there may be reflex signs characteristic of upper motor neuron disorder (see pp. 688 and 730). Paralysis may follow the attack for a short period of time and is described as postconvulsive *(postictal)* paralysis or *Todd's paralysis.*

Febrile grand mal convulsions are frequently seen under the age of 5 predominantly between 6 months and 3 years of age. Convulsions associated with high fever are generalized and have short duration. Children with febrile seizures have a high familial incidence of this type of seizure and may suffer from nonfebrile convulsions in later life.

Seizures that follow one another without restoration of consciousness are called *status epilepticus,* or seizures without interruption. This disorder is serious, producing exhaustion, hypoxia, acidosis, and other metabolic derangements. Hospitalization and prompt pharmacotherapy are required to prevent irreversible brain damage or death.

Partial Seizures

Partial seizures arise from a focal area. They are characterized by specific repeated patterns of activity and are classified as focal motor, focal sensory, and temporal lobe disorders.

FOCAL MOTOR SEIZURES (JACKSONIAN SEIZURE). This disorder usually originates in the premotor cortex and is responsible for involuntary movements of the contralateral limbs. The discharge from the frontal lobe spreads rapidly into an integrating center, the thalamus, resulting in immediate loss of consciousness. When the seizure starts in one portion of the premotor cortex and spreads gradually to the adjacent region, the clinical manifestations will change accordingly. For example, a focal motor seizure starting in the foot may move up the leg, down the arm and to the face, or the disorder may begin in the hand, spread to the face, and then to the leg. This is called *Jacksonian march*. This type of seizure may last 20 to 30 seconds without loss of consciousness. Conversely, the disorder may spread to the opposite hemisphere attendant with a loss of consciousness. Localizing the lesion may be reflected by where it begins. Despite the greater frequency of focal seizures in young children, the Jacksonian march appears more often in adults and adolescents; focal motor seizures may also occur in certain metabolic derangements.

FOCAL SENSORY SEIZURES. A lesion in the sensory cortex will provoke this type of seizure disorder. A simple, uniform, tactile, auditory or visual experience with complaints of numbness, tingling, "pins-and-needles" sensation, coldness, or a sensation of water running over a portion of the body may be described. If the lesion is in the sensory association area, the experience is more complex and may be visual or auditory. If visual, sensations of light, darkness, or color may be experienced. If auditory, the person may complain of buzzing, roaring in the ears, or hearing voices or words. Consciousness and memory are preserved.

TEMPORAL LOBE PSYCHOMOTOR SEIZURES. Temporal lobe structures, the medial surface of the hemispheres and the limbic system are involved with this disorder. It may be characterized by slow paroxysmal waves in either the anterior or posterior leads of the electroencephalogram. Episodic fluctuations in attitude, attention, behavior, or memory occur. Seizures may begin with an olfactory aura or an unpleasant smell or taste. On other occasions, people may experience hallucinations or perceptual illusions. They may perceive strange objects or people as familiar (déja vu) and familiar objects and people as strange (jamais vu). The person appears to be in a dreamy state and may be unresponsive to vocal stimulation, but mechanically performs a task while the seizure is progressing. Abnormal movements and inappropriate speech may also be associated characteristics.

Later, loss of episodic recall occurs and the behavior is called automatic. Convulsive motor manifestations, when present, include chewing, smacking, licking of the lips, or clapping of the hands. Less frequently, there may be turning of the head and eyes to one side, or tonic spasms of the limbs. Some psychomotor seizures last about a minute, while others may continue for hours.

Secondary or Symptomatic Epilepsy

Secondary seizures are caused by some metabolic or structural underlying disorder. Metabolic disturbances can result fom renal failure, hypoglycemia, hypoxia, hyponatremia, hypernatremia, hypercalcemia, hepatic failure, or withdrawal of drugs.

Meningitis and encephalitis in children lead to strong convulsive tendencies. Following recovery, there may be residual recurrent generalized, focal, or psychomotor seizures.

Many structural lesions are caused by disorders in cerebral blood supply, intracranial tumors, or scarring of the brain. These are described in other areas of Unit 15.

REFERENCES

1. Curtis, B. *An Introduction to the Neuro-Sciences.* Philadelphia: Saunders, 1972.
2. Robbins, S., and Cotran, R. *Pathological Basis of Disease* (2nd ed.). Philadelphia: Saunders, 1979.
3. Stein, J.H. (ed.). *Internal Medicine.* Boston: Little, Brown, 1983.
4. Walter, J.B. *An Introduction to the Principles of Disease* (2nd ed.). Philadelphia: Saunders, 1982.

CHAPTER 45
TRAUMATIC ALTERATIONS IN THE NERVOUS SYSTEM

LEARNING OBJECTIVES

1. Explain the two aspects of consciousness.
2. Discuss the role of the reticular activating system in modulating consciousness.
3. Discuss alterations in the level of consciousness.
4. Explain the etiologic basis of coma.
5. Contrast coma of metabolic origin with coma of structural injury.
6. Discuss the basis of coma from supratentorial and infratentorial lesions.
7. Describe associated functional disturbances commonly found in comatose persons, including altered motor and pupillary responses, respiratory patterns, and eye movements.
8. Differentiate between upper and lower motor neuron lesions.
9. Explain the various types of skull fractures.
10. Differentiate between cerebral concussion and contusion.
11. Discuss type of injury, early and progressive clinical signs and symptoms, and treatment of epidural hematomas, subdural hematomas, subdural hygromas, subarachnoid hemorrhage, and intracerebral hematoma.
12. Differentiate between cytotoxic and vasogenic cerebral edema.
13. Discuss how traumatic injury may occur to each of the cranial nerves and what clinical findings are associated with these injuries.
14. State the normal intracranial pressure.
15. Discuss the etiologic basis of increased intracranial pressure.
16. Describe how intracranial pressure can be measured.
17. Discuss the major types of brain shifts that can occur with increased intracranial pressure.
18. Discuss the medical management of increased intracranial pressure.
19. Discuss the mechanisms of spinal cord injury.
20. Explain the morphologic changes associated with irreversible spinal cord damage.
21. Describe functional alterations in relation to the level of spinal cord injury.
22. Explain the basis for spinal shock and the associated clinical findings throughout its course.
23. Discuss the etiologic basis, physiologic changes, and immediate treatment of autonomic dysreflexia.
24. Describe injuries resulting in intravertebral disk herniation.
25. Identify regions of the vertebral column that are more commonly involved in disk herniation.
26. Discuss diagnosis and treatment of intravertebral herniated disk.
27. Describe the indication for and procedure in the following diagnostic studies in head and spine injuries: x rays, angiography, computerized axial tomography (CAT) scan, echoencephalography, brain scan, pneumoencephalography, ventriculogram, myelography, and electroencephalography.

Trauma to the nervous system can result in major changes in physiologic and psychologic functioning. The alterations in function reflective of the underlying anatomic and physiologic damage to the nervous system are discussed throughout this chapter. Damage secondary to the primary injury of the nervous system, such as cerebral edema and increased intracranial pressure, may be potentially more devastating than the original injury. Many structural and metabolic processes impinging on the brain lead to alterations in consciousness and varying degrees of brain dysfunction. This chapter, therefore, begins with a focus on consciousness and its varying levels that are reflective of specific clinical findings.

CONSCIOUSNESS

The conscious state of human existence involves complex neural phenomena that provide for wakefulness and an awareness of self and environment. Two aspects of consciousness are *content of consciousness* and *arousal* [4]. The former relates to mental activities such as perception of self and memory, and the latter is related to wakefulness. The concept of levels of function within the nervous system is significant in discussing consciousness, as clinically varying levels of consciousness may be observed and these are related to the level of brain function. In essence, as higher levels are no longer functioning due to various disease or traumatic processes, the next lower level can be observed in function. Content of consciousness activities are carried out at the highest level; the cerebral cortex and arousal phenomenon arises from a much lower level at the brainstem structures. The structures necessary for normal consciousness include the central structures of the diencephalon and projections from it, the thalamocortical system, and the reticular activating system of the brainstem. The cerebral cortex is necessary to provide perception to the neural basis of consciousness that evolves from the lower levels of the brain.

The reticular activating system (RAS) plays an important role in modulating wakefulness, arousal, and conscious perception of the environment. It evolves from the deep structures of the brain and brainstem to project onto the cortex. This portion of the RAS is known as the *ascending reticular activating* system. A portion of the reticular activating system bypasses the thalamus on its projectory route, whereas another part terminates in the specific nuclei of the thalamus and from these projects diffusely to the entire cortex. The former is referred to as the *nonspecific* or *diffuse thalamocortical system* and the latter as the *specific thalamocortical system* [2].

Peripheral stimulation is transmitted by the afferent pathways to projection areas on the cerebral cortex via the specific and nonspecific thalamic nuclei for the perception of consciousness. Chapter 42 details the important function of the thalamus in receiving sensory information from various parts of the body and then relaying it onto specific areas of the cortex. This relay involves a three-synapse transmission to its projection site on the cortex and is part of the specific thalamocortical system. Stimulation of the specific thalamic nuclei gives rise to localized primary responses that may not in themselves be sufficient to produce conscious perception.

The nonspecific thalamocortical system, on the other hand, does not project to specific nuclei of the thalamus, but rather transpires the thalamus region in groups of nuclei, including the *midline nuclei*, *intralaminae nuclei*, and *reticular thalamic nucleus*. The nonspecific system conduction involves a multisynaptic path with indistinct boundaries and numerous interconnections with the specific thalamic nuclei, before finally projecting to widely distributed cortical receiving areas.

During sleep and anesthesia, the specific thalamic nuclei transmission remains unchanged whereas the nonspecific system becomes suppressed. In normal wakeful brain functioning there is a continuous activating flow from the nonspecific system that controls the state of consciousness of wakefulness at any given time. This flow is known as the *reticular activating system*. As the activating afferent flow diminishes, sleep states ensue. Major damage to the reticular activating system anywhere rostral to the pons will result in greatly diminished cortical activation, which affects the conscious state.

Investigators have applied electrical stimulation to different areas of the RAS in an attempt to better understand its function. Electrical stimulation of the upper brainstem portion of the RAS has demonstrated immediate waking in the sleeping animal and general activation of the entire central nervous system. In contrast, electrical stimulation of the reticular activating system as it evolves from the thalamic nuclei results in more specific activation of the cortex, which allows for mental activities requiring a more direct focus. During sleep the reticular activating system may be activated by various external and internal stimuli. Some of these prove to be more potent activators than others. Pain is a strong activator of the reticular activating system.

In addition to the stimulation of the reticular activating system from the afferent ascending system, stimulation may also descend from all areas of the cerebral cortex. Particularly strong stimulation arrives from the cortical motor projection areas. It is well known that activity such as walking will ward off sleep, which might otherwise overtake the individual during sitting or reclining.

ALTERATIONS IN CONSCIOUSNESS

The most effective indicator of brain function is the individual's level of consciousness. A wide range of consciousness, from the alert to the comatose state may be observed, and subtle changes that impact diagnosis and management are known to occur within short time spans.

A person with a normal level of consciousness is awake, aware, and interacting appropriately with the environment when not engaged in a period of normal sleep. Therefore, alertness; orientation to time, place, and person; and general responses to the surroundings are evaluated frequently in individuals with cerebral neurologic disturbances. A person whose level of consciousness is deteriorating from normal interactions with the environment may deteriorate slowly or very rapidly to a totally unresponsive state, depending on the underlying neurologic pathology.

A slow deterioration of the level of consciousness will reveal different levels of response that can be observed clinically. The *lethargic* person is somnolent and drowsy and responds sluggishly to verbal and painful stimuli. Heightened stimuli may be necessary to evoke a response and the person may drift back into sleep soon after the stimulation. He or she may be oriented or exhibit occasional disorientation. As brain function deteriorates to lower levels, the lethargy becomes *stupor*. Vigorous and persistent noxious stimuli are utilized to evoke a response as verbal stimuli generally produce little response. The attention span is very short and excessive motor responses may be exhibited.

Further deterioration of brain function is reflected in ensuing *coma*. The first sign is a *light coma* or *semicoma* in which no responses are made to ordinary verbal and tactile stimuli, but motor responses do occur in a reflexive manner to noxious stimuli. *Deepening coma* is observed when reflexive motor responses are no longer elicited in response to vigorous noxious stimulation, and flaccidity of the extremities predominates. Pupillary, pharyngeal, and corneal responses may be minimal or absent. Thermoregulatory mechanisms become erratic and respiratory patterns become irregular.

Coma

The importance of an intact and functioning ascending reticular activating system extending from the midbrain to the hypothalamus, thalamus, and finally to the cerebral cortex has been discussed earlier in this chapter. Disruption of the conscious state is commonly viewed from an etiologic basis of *structural* or *metabolic/toxic* origin.

Persons who are experiencing coma from structural processes have incurred physical damage to the brain, such as contusion, infection, intracerebral bleeding, tumor, edema, or infection. Coma results from structural causes when damage occurs to both cerebral cortices or the brainstem. Brain expansion such as that which occurs in the herniation syndromes may cause secondary damage to the structures necessary for consciousness and result in coma. The distinguishing characteristics of structurally induced coma are focal signs that reflect the area of the brain involved in the structural process. These focal signs are usually initially unilateral processes such as hemiparesis and unilateral pupillary dilation. Without intervention, the focal signs may become bilateral phenomena.

Toxic and metabolically induced coma results from ingestion of certain exogenous nervous system poisons (toxic) or from disease processes producing endogenous materials that interfere with normal brain metabolism.

Additionally, coma may have psychogenic origins. These can be readily distinguished from organic basis by eyelid opening. Active resistance to eyelid opening occurs with

TABLE 45-1. Common etiologic basis for coma

- Structural processes
  - Supratentorial lesions
    - Epidural hematomas
    - Tumors
    - Infections
    - Hemorrhage
    - Subdural hematomas
    - Contusions
    - Edema
  - Infratentorial lesions
    - Hemorrhage
    - Infarction
    - Aneurysms
    - Tumors
    - Contusions
- Endogenous metabolic processes
  - Renal failure (uremia)
  - Diabetic ketoacidosis
  - Electrolyte imbalances
  - Hyperosmolarity
  - Acidosis
  - Hepatic encephalopathy
  - Hypoxia
  - Hypercarbia
  - Hypoglycemia
- Exogenous toxic poisons
  - Sedative drugs
  - Alcohol
- Psychogenic disorders
  - Fainting
  - Hysteria

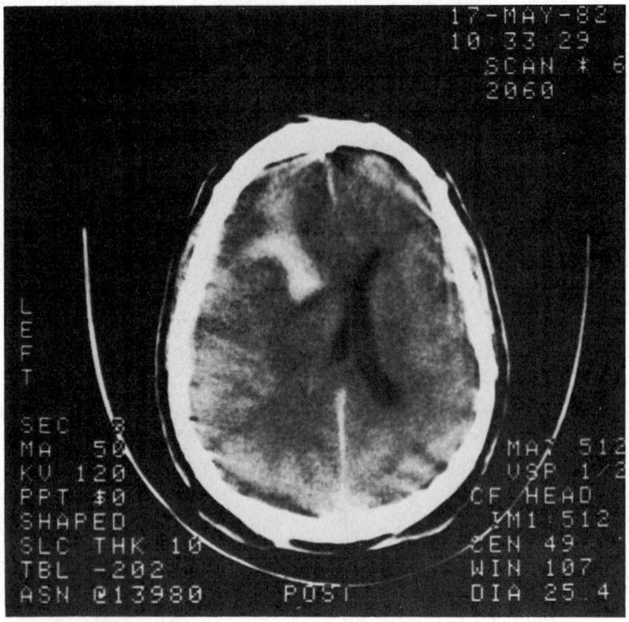

FIGURE 45-1. Intracerebral bleeding in left frontal lobe (light area); compression of left lateral-ventricle with slight compression of midline structures.

psychogenic coma, whereas with true coma, the eyelid is readily opened, falls back into prior position slowly, and remains slightly open. The cold water caloric test is another effective means to distinguish psychogenic coma from organic coma. Nystagmus that occurs during the test indicates that the unresponsiveness is psychogenic [1]. The common causes of coma are summarized in Table 45-1.

CLINICAL FINDINGS IN COMA. Coma has been likened to sleep in the past. Although similarities exist, the two entities are rather distinct. Both lack conscious behavior and electroencephalogram (EEG) recordings tend to show slow rhythms. Nevertheless, the differences are striking. Humans sleeping are arousable and those in profound coma cannot be aroused. Eye movement is lacking in coma resulting from acute neurologic processes, and rapid eye movement (REM) sleep patterns are not present in these victims. As coma becomes chronic, some individuals display periods of restlessness that may be equated with sleep-wakefulness cycles.

SUPRATENTORIALLY INDUCED COMA. Isolated small cerebral hemispheric lesions are not sufficient to cause coma as long as the ascending reticular activating system and its connections to the cortex are intact. However, with progressively larger hemispheric lesions in regions above the tentorium, behavior becomes dulled until the maximum obliteration of the cortex occurs and no content of consciousness is preserved. Supratentorial hemispheric lesions produce coma by enlarging sufficiently to cross midline structures and compress the opposite hemisphere (Fig. 45-1) or by caudal compression of the diencephalon and midbrain. Accompanying dangerous manifestations of hemispheric compressions include herniations of the diencephalon or uncus through the tentorial notch, which results in aggravating vascular obstruction and accentuation of already present ischemia. Likewise, circulation of the cerebral spinal fluid is blocked with transtentorial herniations and the pressure within the cranium rises. Transtentorial herniation is also accompanied by brainstem hemorrhages and ischemia that is thought to be caused by midbrain and pons stretching of the medial branches of the basilar artery.

INFRATENTORIALLY INDUCED COMA. Coma as a result of dysfunction or destruction of areas below the tentorium may evolve from within the brainstem structures and produce destructive effects on the paramedian midbrain-pontine reticular formation. Lesions external to the brainstem may result in compression of this reticular formation. Lesions of the brainstem may involve direct invasive destruction or compression of its blood supply, resulting in brainstem ischemia and eventual necrosis. Brainstem destruction may result from cerebrovascular accidents, neoplasms, nutritional deficiencies, infectious processes, and head trauma.

Lesions external to the brainstem may produce compression by direct pressure on the tegmentum, which directly damages the neural tissue. This may compromise the vascular supply and result in ischemia. Additionally, the mesence-

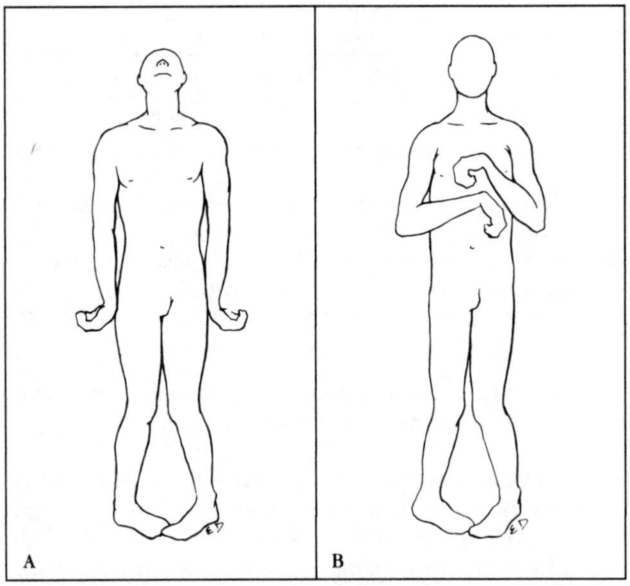

FIGURE 45-2. Abnormal posturing. A. Decerebrate position. B. Decorticate position. (From C. V. Kenner, C. E. Guzzetta, and B. M. Dossey, *Critical Care Nursing*. Boston: Little, Brown, 1981.)

phalic tegmentum may be compressed through an upward herniation of the cerebellum and midbrain through the tentorial notch. This compression results in tissue distortion and vascular obstruction with eventual coma. Expanding lesions of the posterior fossa (cerebellum) are a common cause of upward herniation of structures through the tentorial notch. A downward compression of the brainstem may result from the herniation of the cerebellar tonsils through the foramen magnum. This results in compression and ischemia of the medulla with resultant circulatory and respiratory aberrations.

ASSOCIATED FUNCTIONAL DISTURBANCES WITH COMA. Certain clinical alterations in function may be present in the person with coma that often reflect the level and extent of the underlying brain pathology. These include alterations in consciousness, motor responses, respiratory patterns, pupillary responses, and eye movements.

In evaluating the level of consciousness, the *motor responses* elicited from the individual may be significant in relation to the extent of pathology and depth of coma. Limb movement also offers an excellent opportunity to assess asymmetry of function in the nervous system. However, a consistently justifiable correlation between the level of consciousness and motor responses should not be made, as each of these functions is controlled by separate pathways and stands apart. Nevertheless, lesions at certain levels within the central nervous system result in specific types of motor responses that are readily observable clinically and support the level of pathology. One can systematically assess the individual's level of function.

If no response is elicited from the individual to verbal stimuli, specific stimuli are used to arouse a response. The responses elicited are significant in that they indicate the extent of damage through their appropriateness. Appropriate motor responses to noxious stimuli in the comatose person indicate that the sensory pathways and corticospinal pathways are functioning. An example of an appropriate response to noxious stimulation is an attempt to push the stimulus away. Inappropriate motor responses are stereotyped patterns that indicate the level of damage. *Decorticate* and *decerebrate* motor responses are examples of inappropriate involuntary responses (Fig. 45-2).

The *decorticate* response is observed with the interruption of the corticospinal pathways by internal capsule or cerebral hemispheric lesions and is clinically manifested by a flexion response of the upper extremities and an extension response of the lower extremities. The arms are adducted and in rigid flexion with the hands rotated internally and fingers flexed. The *decerebrate* response is elicited in patients with extensive brainstem damage to the midpontine level as well as large cerebral lesions that compress the lower thalamus and midbrain. Severe metabolic disorders such as hypoglycemia, hepatic coma, and certain drug intoxications may diminish brainstem function and induce a decerebrate response. Characteristic musculoskeletal patterns include extension responses of both upper and lower extremities. Fully expressed, the decerebrate individual exhibits *opisthotonos* (head extended, body arched), posturing with clenched teeth and arms rigidly extended, adducted, and hyperpronated. The legs are stiffly extended and feet plantar flexed. The extent of the decerebrate response correlates with severity of the pathology and is occasionally seen as wavering back and forth between decorticate and decerebrate responses, reflecting physiologic changes. Decerebrate responses of the upper extremities together with flaccidity of the lower extremities indicates more extensive brainstem damage extending even beyond the pons level. In certain persons asymmetry of abnormal responses and normal responses may be observed that are reflective of underlying cerebral pathology. For example, a person may reveal unilateral decorticate response, or may exhibit decorticate response on one side and decerebrate on the other side.

Unilaterally absent motor responses to noxious stimuli indicates interruption in the corticospinal pathways, damage to the reticular activating system at the pontomedullary level, or psychogenic disruption. Hyperreflexia and the presence of the Babinski response support structural lesions of the central nervous system as the origin of the coma. Certain metabolic abnormalities, such as hypoglycemia and uremia, may exhibit the same signs but can be quickly confirmed by laboratory studies.

PARALYSIS. Paralysis, the loss of voluntary movement, is a relatively common occurrence with trauma to the nervous system. Lesions involving the corticobulbar and corticospinal tracts are known as *upper motor neuron lesions* and result in *spastic paralysis* (Fig. 45-3). The lesions involving motor cranial nerves, whose cell bodies are in

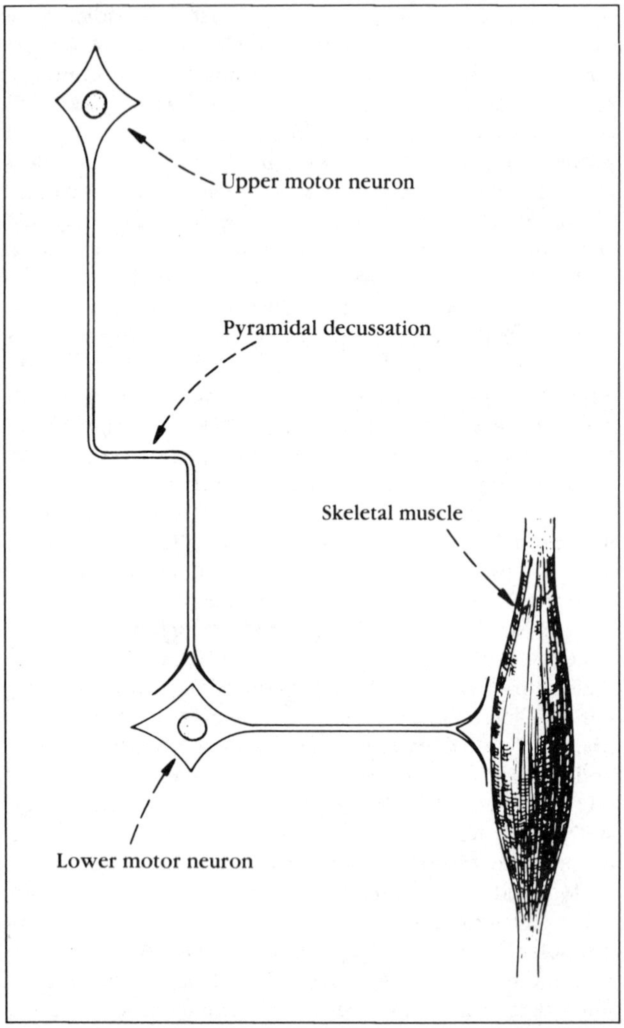

FIGURE 45-3. Traditional concept of motor control. Upper motor neuron lesions produce paralysis, hypertonia, and hyperflexia. Lower motor neuron lesions produce paralysis, hypotonia, areflexia, and muscle wasting. (From M.A. Samuels, *Manual of Neurologic Therapeutics* [2nd ed.]. Boston: Little, Brown, 1982.)

the brainstem nuclei, and spinal nerves, whose cell bodies are in the anterior horn of the spinal cord, are referred to as *lower motor neuron lesions* and result in *flaccid paralysis* (see Fig. 45-3).

The activity of the reflex arc provides the muscle with tone. Interruption of the arc results in atony and a soft, unresponsive muscle associated with lower motor neuron lesions. Voluntary activity and reflex action cannot be elicited when the final common pathway of the lower motor neuron is severed. Deep tendon reflexes are absent in lower motor neuron lesions.

In upper motor neuron lesions the activity of the reflex arc remains intact, although voluntary control movement is lost. The muscle feels hard, is very sensitive to stretch, and is said to be *hypertonic*. Deep tendon reflexes are increased after a period of areflexia immediately following this type of lesion. The characteristics of upper and lower motor neuron lesions are summarized in Table 45-2.

TABLE 45-2. Characteristics of upper motor neuron and lower motor neuron lesions

Upper motor neuron (UMN)	Lower motor neuron (LMN)
Spastic paralysis	Flaccid paralysis
Hyperreflexia (increased deep tendon reflexes)	Hyporeflexia (decreased deep tendon reflexes)
Unilaterally upgoing great toe (Babinski sign)	Absent or normal plantar response
Minimal or no muscle atrophy	Significant muscle atrophy
Fasciculations absent	Fasciculations present

PUPILLARY RESPONSES IN ALTERED STATES OF CONSCIOUSNESS. The close anatomic relationship of fibers controlling pupillary reactions and consciousness provides a valuable guide to the location of the pathologic processes causing coma. Further distinctions of origin of the coma may be assessed in the pupillary responses, as metabolic aberrations leave little effect on the pupils whereas certain structural pathology produces distinct changes.

Pupillary responses are regulated by sympathetic and parasympathetic nervous systems. A balance is normally maintained by the two systems to produce a pupillary aperture appropriate to the prevailing situation. *Mydriasis* (dilation) is produced by the sympathetic nervous system and *miosis* (constriction) by the parasympathetic nervous system. The parasympathetic impulses arrive via the third nerve from the *Edinger-Westphal nuclei* in the midbrain; the sympathetic innervation arrives via a more complex route that originates in the hypothalamus, traverses the brainstem, and travels along with the internal carotid artery into the skull where it reaches the eye through the filaments of the ophthalmic artery and a division of the fifth nerve. Damage to specific areas of the brain produces characteristic pupillary responses that are valuable for diagnostic purposes.

Pupillary size, position, and response to bright light are observed in assessing the neurologic status of the comatose individual. Normal response to bright light in a partially darkened room is a brisk constriction. Other responses may indicate abnormal neurologic processes. Additionally simultaneous pupillary constriction occurs in the opposite pupil (*consensual reflex*). Pupils normally are at midposition and *conjugate* (equally coupled) at rest. The conjugated pupil positioning can be noted by shining a bright light in both eyes simultaneously and observing the light reflection on the same area in each eye. In coma, eyes may exhibit slow random roving movements that may be conjugate or dysconjugate. These movements cannot be mimicked voluntarily, hence, are valuable in differential diagnosis.

Damage to the midbrain results in fixed pupils that are not reactive to light but do fluctuate in size. Pupils that react imply a functioning midbrain, as midbrain lesions generally impinge on both the sympathetic and parasympathetic eye pathways. Lesions affecting the midbrain most commonly result from transtentorial herniation. Other contributing lesions may result from neoplasms and vascular abnormalities affecting the midbrain. Involvement of specific areas of the hypothalamus frequently results in ipsilateral pupillary constriction with ptosis (drooping) and anhidrosis (absence of sweat) of the entire half of the body (*Horner's syndrome*). The combinations of symptoms indicating Horner's syndrome are significant in that they precede progressive neurologic deterioration leading to transtentorial herniation. Pupillary light reflex remains intact with hypothalamic damage.

Pontine lesions interfere with descending sympathetic pathways and thus produce bilateral small pupils. Generally, pupils with pontine involvement react to light, but this may be difficult to discern without a magnifying glass.

Third nerve involvement may be observed in comatose patients when lesions compress the temporal uncus sufficiently to cause herniation and the resultant third nerve compression against the tentorium. Initially a unilateral dilated nonreactive pupil is observed, which may progress to bilateral involvement with expanding cranial pathology.

In assessing pupillary size and reactivity an awareness of certain pharmacologic effects may be useful in determining the origin of coma. Heroin, morphine, and other opiates produce the pontine lesion type of pupils, which are pinpoint and difficult to assess for light reactivity. Ingestion of large amounts of atropine and scopolamine result in dilated, nonreactive pupils, which may give a false impression of a structural lesion. Glutethimide-produced (nonbarbiturate sedative, trade name Doriden) coma results in moderately dilated, nonreactive pupils. Profound anoxia, usually secondary to severely diminished cardiac output, results in dilated, nonreactive pupils.

Metabolically produced coma generally results in pupils that are reactive until the terminal stage and, therefore, provide significant data in differential diagnosis of coma.

EYE MOVEMENTS IN ALTERED STATES OF CONSCIOUSNESS. Vestibuloreflex pathways proximate areas controlling consciousness and, therefore, provide for a useful assessment guide. The *oculocephalic reflex (doll's-head eye reflex)* is assessed by rotating the head from side to side with eyelids kept open. In the positive response eyes deviate conjugatively opposite the head deviation. As the neck is extended, the eyes deviate to a downward gaze, and as it is flexed, the eyes deviate to an upward gaze. The precise physiologic mechanism responsible for this response remains obscure although it is hypothesized that it involves either the vestibular system or the proprioceptive afferents from the neck, or both. Persons with disturbances between the frontopontine pathways exhibit the doll's-head eye reflex while those who are awake with open eyes do not.

Ocular vestibular reflex (cold caloric stimulation) is obtained by introducing up to 50 ml of cold water slowly into the intact patent ear canal. Normal response implies that some intact brainstem function is present and is reflected by an intermittent tonic deviation of the eyes to the side of the irrigated ear.

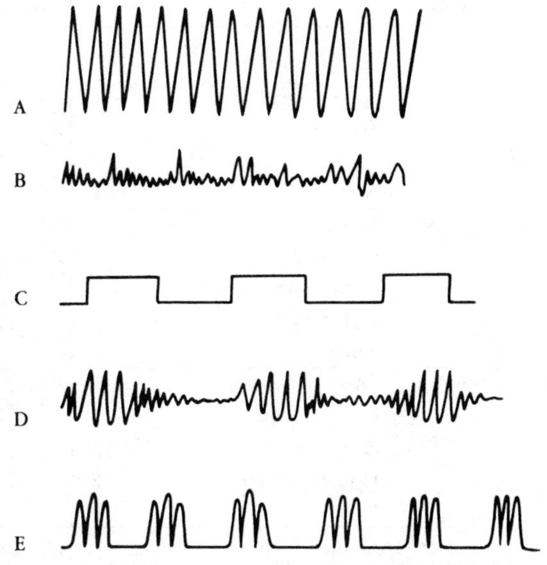

FIGURE 45-4. Respiratory patterns associated with cerebral dysfunction at various levels. A. Central neurogenic hyperventilation (diencephalon). B. Ataxic (medullary). C. Apneustic (pontine). D. Cheyne-Stokes (diencephalon). E. Cluster (high medulla, low pons).

RESPIRATORY PATTERNS IN ALTERED STATES OF CONSCIOUSNESS. Because of the neurologic influences on respiration in various regions of the brain, respiratory patterns observed in persons during coma become useful in its diagnosis (Fig. 45-4). *Central neurogenic hyperventilation* is deep, rapid breathing, which generally indicates dysfunction in the brainstem tegmentum between the midbrain and pons. A respiratory alkalosis is revealed by laboratory findings with a low carbon dioxide tension and high pH values. *Apneustic* breathing consists of a prolonged inspiratory phase followed by an expiratory pause. This respiratory pattern reflects pontine level damage, most generally pontine infarctions secondary to basilar artery occlusions.

Ataxic breathing results from lesions in the reticular activating system of the dorsomedial portion of the medulla and is characteristically a very irregular breathing pattern with irregularly interspersed pauses. The respiratory center tends to be rather hyposensitive and minimal depression, either with mild sedation or sleep, may lead to apnea. Generally, individuals with ataxic respirations who are apneic secondary to depressant drugs or sleep will respond to verbal commands to resume breathing. In severe medullary compression or lesions, ataxic breathing is viewed as a preterminal event.

TABLE 45-3. Glascow coma scale

Coma scale criteria			Time (o'clock)																							
			7	8	9	10	11	N	1	2	3	4	5	6	7	8	9	10	11	M	1	2	3	4	5	6
Eyes open	Spontaneously	4																								
	To speech	3	X	X																						
	To pain	2			X																					
	None	1				X																				
Best verbal response	Oriented	5																								
	Confused	4	X	X																						
	Inappropriate words	3																								
	Incomprehensible sounds	2			X																					
	None	1				X																				
Best motor response	Obey commands	5	X	X																						
	Localize pain	4			X																					
	Flexion to pain	3																								
	Extension to pain	2				X																				
	None	1																								
Glascow coma score (Example findings)			12	12	8	4																				

Cheyne-Stokes respiration is represented by a regular crescendo-decrescendo pattern altering with periods of apnea. It reflects bilateral hemispheric dysfunction with a brainstem that is essentially intact. The hemispheric disturbances resulting in Cheyne-Stokes respiration are generally deep within the brain involving the basal ganglia and internal capsule. This respiratory pattern also accompanies disturbances of metabolic pathogenesis affecting similar cerebral regions, such as occurs with congestive heart failure. Cheyne-Stokes respiration results from an increased sensitivity to carbon dioxide levels, which leads to hyperpnea (increased respiratory rate). As a result, the blood carbon dioxide level falls to below the stimulatory level resulting in a period of apnea. During the apneic period, the carbon dioxide again accumulates to the respiratory threshold level and the cyclic hyperpnea and apnea continue.

Cluster breathing, such as *Biot's* breathing, which is not associated with a regular pattern, may result from damage in the high medulla or low pons region. Lesions in the low brainstem also may lead to frequent yawning and hiccups. The underlying mechanism for this is not clearly understood.

RECORDING OF ASSESSMENTS. Accurate neurologic assessment of the person in a coma is crucial to the correct treatment and best possible outcome. Initial assessment provides a comparative basis for subsequent observations. Changes in neurologic status are particularly important and may reveal serious pathologic processes within the nervous system.

The Glascow coma scale (Table 45-3) is an assessment tool that has received wide acceptance in both the United States and Europe. It provides an objective means for making and recording standardized observations, in relation to eye opening, verbal responses, and motor responses. The best response in each of these categories is checked at regular time intervals and given a numerical value that can range from a low of 3 to 14 for normal persons when totaled in all the categories. It also provides a prognostic guide in that individuals with a Glascow coma scale score of 7 or below generally have a guarded prognosis and those having a score above 7 have a more favorable prognosis.

TRAUMATIC HEAD INJURY

Our highly mechanized society has created an appalling number of traumatic injuries, a great majority of these resulting from the widespread use of the automobile. Many of these injuries involve the head. Mortality resulting from head injury is associated with injury and compression of the brainstem, cerebral contusions and lacerations, large expanding hemispheric lesions, and cerebral edema.

In response to a traumatic force applied to the head, the cranial vault affords protection to the brain by the hair, skin, bone, meninges, and cerebrospinal fluid. These protective encasements absorb energy that is transmitted to the skull when force is applied. However, when the force exceeds absorption capacity it is transmitted to the cranial contents and tissue damage results. The resultant injury frequently correlates with the amount of force applied to the cranial contents. The effects of head trauma may be a direct result of the injury or a secondary tissue response to the injury.

Head injuries lacking obvious external damage with an intact skull are referred to as *closed head injuries*. In contrast, *open head injuries* may reveal penetration of the scalp, skull, meninges, or brain tissue. Closed head injuries frequently result from sudden acceleration-deceleration

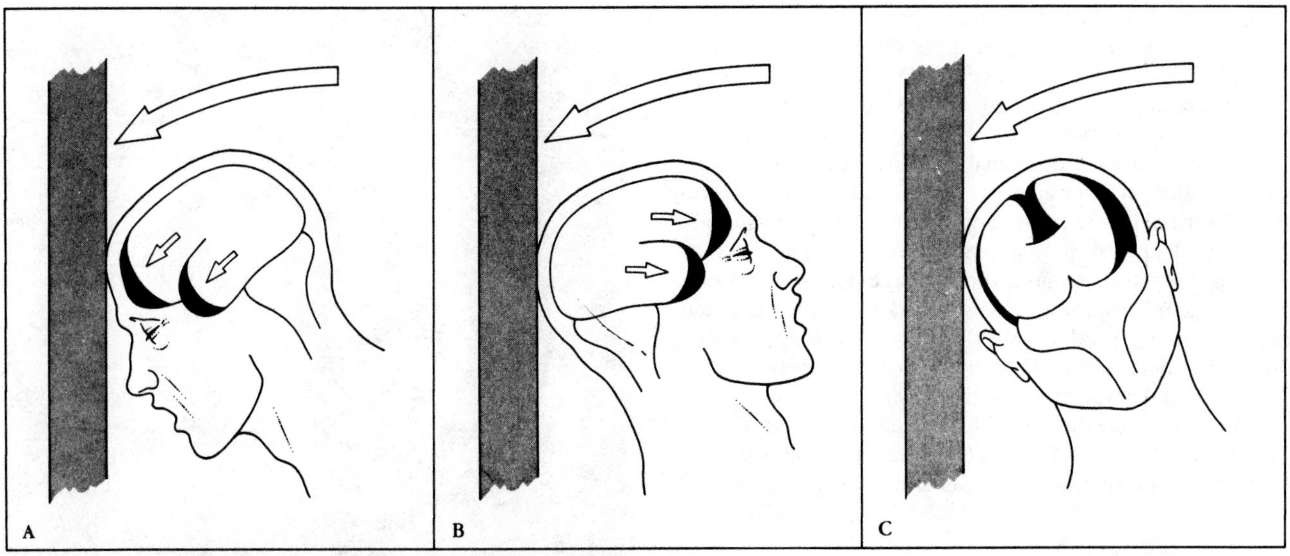

FIGURE 45-5. Cortical contusion with relation to direction of head movement. A. Head moving forward and striking stationary surface—major injury found at tips of frontal and temporal poles. B. Head moving backward and striking stationary surface—major injury found in frontal and temporal lobes (contrecoup). C. Head moving laterally and striking stationary surface—major injury found on side opposite that which strikes surface (contrecoup). Medial surfaces of hemispheres are also injured by impingement on relatively rigid falx. (From S. Budassi and J. Barber, *Emergency Nursing Principles and Practice*. St. Louis: Mosby, 1981.)

accidents (Fig. 45-5). The cranial contents shift to the opposite side of the impact within the rigid skull. This is known as the *contrecoup* injury and may lead to brain tissue contusions and lacerations as the semisolid brain moves over rough projections within the cranial cavity. In addition, rotation of the cerebrum may occur with trauma and result in damage to the upper midbrain as well as areas of the frontal, temporal, and occipital lobes.

Skull Fractures

A blow to the head may result in a variety of skull fractures. Skull fractures may lack significance in themselves unless communication results with the cranial contents or bone fragments are driven into the neural tissue of the brain. Skull fractures may be *linear*, *comminuted*, *compound*, and *depressed*. The most common *linear* fractures are simply line fractures without displacement or communication with cranial contents. *Comminuted* fractures are multiple linear fractures and retain the characteristics of the linear fractures. *Compound* fractures provide communication with the cranial contents and are more serious than linear and comminuted fractures. These may require more extensive observation and treatment. *Depressed* skull fractures result in deformation of the cranial tissue by bone fragments. These fractures decrease the volume of the cranial cavity and may produce uncal herniation. Venous return may be impeded, and secondary hemorrhages in the midbrain and pons may result. Cranial nerves may also be injured by skull fractures.

Concussions

A transient and reversible injury to the brain stem reticular activating system results in a *concussion*. This relatively minor injury in response to mild blows to the head results in brief loss of consciousness due to the temporary physiologic disruption of the reticular activating system. No anatomic injury results and the process is reversible when neuronal function returns. The period of unconsciousness ranges from seconds to as long as a few hours.

Persons suffering concussions are amnesic to the accident and may appear confused for a short period after the accident. The period of amnesia is generally proportional to the severity of the concussion. The longer the period of amnesia the more severe the injury. Generally, neurologic signs normalize rapidly and further deterioration does not result from the concussion after the initial impact.

Contusions

Contusions result in brain tissue destruction at the area of the blow (*coup area*) or at the opposite side of the blow (*contrecoup area*). Cerebral hemispheres, particularly the basal portions, are frequently involved as these areas slide over bony irregularities of the base of the skull. Blows to the back of the head may result in contrecoup injuries to frontal and temporal lobes. A variety of neurologic abnormalities may result from *hemispheric contusions*, even though consciousness may be retained. In contrast, *brainstem contusions* result in loss of consciousness from tissue injury to the brainstem reticular activating system. The period of unconsciousness may range from hours to the individual's lifetime.

Visible bruising occurs with cerebral contusions due to the perivenous hemorrhage that results from the blow to the head. The injured area swells and becomes visibly red and progressively purple due to the venous obstruction and local edema. With large hemorrhages or clusters of small hemorrhages, intracranial pressure increases. EEG recordings directly over an area of contusion reveal progressive abnormalities with the appearance of high amplitude theta and delta waves. Regional hypoxia and acidosis may result in the contused area and produce hyperemia. Cerebral oxygen consumption is reduced by contusions and cerebral lactate production is greatly increased, probably due to the increased regional hypoxia of the contused area and the resultant anaerobic metabolism.

Contusions may be partially reversible, depending on the severity of the blow and the resultant contusions. Lighter blows usually result in faster recovery.

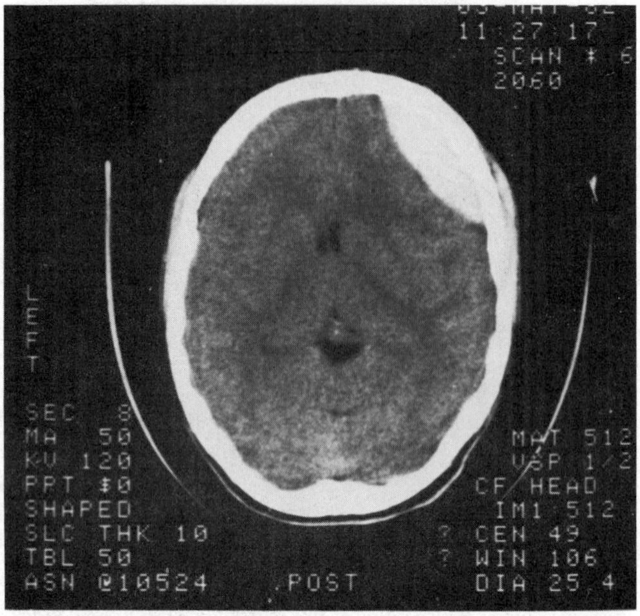

FIGURE 45-6. Epidural hematoma (light area in well-contained round configuration) in right frontal lobe.

Vascular Injuries to the Brain

Potentially catastrophic intracranial processes may result from hemorrhage into the cranial vault from epidural, subdural, subarachnoid, and intracerebral vascular sources. Individuals who have been previously lucid for a period of time following trauma and then begin to deteriorate neurologically are in all probability suffering from cerebrovascular injury and bleeding into the cranial contents. Bleeding into the rigid cranium will result in increased intracranial pressure, which is manifested by its localized or generalized effects on the brain (see pp. 698–701).

EPIDURAL HEMATOMA. A serious sequela to head injuries is the epidural hematoma (Fig. 45-6), a bleeding into the extradural space resulting in compression of the brain toward the opposite side. A common epidural bleed occurs as the result of middle meningeal artery injury in the parietotemporal area. This bleed is frequently accompanied by linear fractures of the skull at the temporal region over the groove of the middle meningeal artery. As the blood volume increases within the cranium, the brain is subjected to increasing pressure and distortion, which generally results in a fatal outcome within 24 hours without surgical intervention.

The individual with an epidural hematoma follows a rather predictable course. After the initial severe blow to the head, a lucid interval of varying length follows, although a brief period of unconsciousness frequently precedes the lucid interval reflecting the concussive effects of head injury. The lucid interval may vary from 10 to 15 minutes to hours and, rarely, days. Progressive loss of consciousness and deterioration in neurologic signs follow as a result of the expanding lesion and extrusion of the temporal lobe through the tentorial opening. *Temporal lobe herniation* compresses the brainstem and presents a rather distinct clinical picture. Deterioration of the level of consciousness results from the compression of the brainstem RAS as the temporal lobe herniates on its upper portion. Contralateral motor deficiencies result due to compression of the corticospinal tracts that pass through the brainstem. Distinct ipsilateral pupillary changes can be observed as the nucleus of the third nerve originates in the brainstem and traverses upward through the tentorial opening. Without intervention, continual bleeding leads to progressive neurologic degeneration as evidenced by bilateral pupillary dilation, bilateral decerebrate responses, and profound coma with irregular respiratory patterns.

Epidural hematomas are identified by the initial clinical picture, CAT scan, x rays, and EEG changes. X rays frequently reveal the linear fracture in the parietotemporal area and the pineal gland displacement by the hematoma. The CAT scan will identify any abnormal masses and structural shifts within the cranium. Electroencephalographic readings may reveal diffuse slowing in the waves over the hematoma, reflecting compression of the underlying structures.

SUBDURAL HEMATOMA. Subdural hematomas (Fig. 45-7) are the most frequently encountered type of meningeal hemorrhage and occur in the *acute*, *subacute*, and *chronic* forms. Bleeding into the subdural space as a result of traumatic injury to vessels may result from either venous or arterial sources, although the venous occurrence is more common. *Acute subdural hematomas* result from severe head injuries and may accompany other manifestations of cerebral trauma such as contusions and lacerations; they may resemble epidural hematomas in the neurologic deficits with rapid deterioration without prompt intervention. Affected persons may be unconscious and rapidly deteriorate, or they may be in a lucid state that deteriorates to

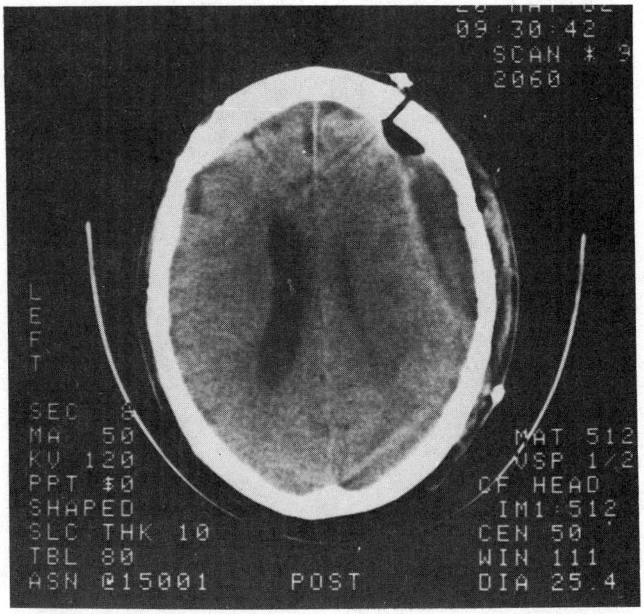

FIGURE 45-7. Subdural hematoma recurring after craniotomy (darker area in right frontoparietal region) showing compression of right ventricle.

drowsiness, stupor, and coma. Signs of brainstem compression may be evidenced by a unilaterally dilated pupil and contralateral hemiparesis. Acute subdural hematomas are identified in the same manner as epidural hematomas. Once diagnosed, the acute subdural hematoma constitutes a surgical emergency and must be treated promptly. The hematoma is generally drained through burr holes. Unfortunately, acute hematomas carry a high mortality, even with surgical intervention.

The *subacute subdural hematomas* carry an improved prognosis because the venous bleeding tends to be slower than in the acute form. The individual is usually in a lucid state after the head injury; this state degenerates to drowsiness, stupor, and coma. The injury may stabilize into a coma for a few days and not exhibit the steady deterioration that accompanies the epidural hematomas. The period of stability is followed by a period of fluctuating neurologic signs that progress to increasing intracranial pressure and eventual fatal outcome without surgical interventions. The presence of subacute subdural hematomas is established by the clinical signs and CAT scanning or x rays.

Chronic subdural hematomas, in contrast, result from very slow bleeding with an insignificant injury. This type of injury is most commonly seen in infants, the elderly, and the apparently demented or alcoholic individual. Because the bleeding slowly accumulates as a clot within the subdural space, a period of hemolysis follows. Cerebrospinal fluid is attracted to the lysed blood through osmosis via the arachnoid membrane. The increasing size of the subdural hematoma impinges further on surrounding capillaries, tearing some of these and initiating further bleeding. This increases the osmotic force even further and contributes to the increase in the overall size of the hematoma. The hematoma may eventually form an encasing membrane around it that may calcify, or it may continue its slow bleed and, lacking proper intervention, may result in transtentorial herniation and a fatal outcome.

Individuals with chronic subdural hematomas may or may not recall injury to the head. They are usually conscious on admission to the hospital and may complain of a generalized dull headache. Some persons with chronic subdural hematomas may be in an obtunded state, confused and disoriented. In the early stages, the individual may exhibit some hemiparesis on the contralateral side. With progressive changes focal seizures, papilledema, homonymous hemianopsia, aphasia, and waxing and waning of the level of consciousness may develop.

Chronic subdural hematomas may be identified by the xanthochromic (yellow appearance) and high protein content of the cerebrospinal fluid. The EEG may show increased slow activity in the theta and delta waves with diminished voltage in the region of the hematoma. CAT scanning, x rays, and arteriography may be helpful in confirming the presence of the hematoma. Subdural hematomas are generally drained through burr holes and may be followed by turning a bone flap to remove any thickened membranes to diminish the possibility of recurrence. The prognosis for chronic subdural hematomas is considerably better when proper intervention has been instituted than for the more acute forms of this hematoma or the epidural hematoma.

SUBDURAL HYGROMA. Subdural hygroma is an excessive collection of fluid under the dura mater, which most commonly results from trauma. Subsequent tearing of the arachnoid allows escape of cerebrospinal fluid into the subdural space. Due to the vascularity of the arachnoid, some vessels are generally damaged, also allowing mixing of cerebrospinal fluid with blood in the subdural space. This CSF blood mixing produces a highly osmotic collection of fluid that continues to pull in fluid; it slowly expands in size.

Confirmation of diagnosis takes place with certainty by burr hole skull opening, although these hygromas may be revealed by CAT scan and other x-ray procedures. Developing signs and symptoms of subdural hygromas following trauma are very similar to those of the chronic subdural hematomas. Relief of symptoms is obtained by draining the fluid if a large collection of fluid-produced neurologic deficits and other pathologic processes are not present.

SUBARACHNOID HEMORRHAGE. Subarachnoid hemorrhage refers to bleeding into the subarachnoid space and may occur spontaneously as a disruption results in the vascular integrity, or as a result of congenital malformations of cerebrovascular beds such as arteriovenous malformations or cerebral aneurysms (Fig. 45-8). However, the most frequent cause of subarachnoid hemorrhage is trauma. Bleeding into the subarachnoid space originates from arterial sources and mixes freely with the circulating cerebrospinal fluid, causing irritation to the contacting central nervous system structures.

Clinical signs identifying subarachnoid hemorrhaging include headache, which is frequently described as severe, violent, or excruciating and seems to occur in the occipital area irrespective of the site of hemorrhage. Some individuals with subarachnoid hemorrhage retain consciousness initially, although about one-half of them experience a delayed onset coma. Conscious individuals complain of visual disturbances such as photophobia or diplopia and deterioration of vision. Fever, malaise, vomiting, and nuchal rigidity may be additional clinical findings. Abnormal mentation with disorientation is not uncommon. The spinal fluid at lumbar puncture is grossly bloody and exhibits increased pressure. Xanthochromia is seen within a few hours of the bleed and persists for about 20 to 30 days. The spinal fluid will also show increased monocytes and protein. Identification of the presence of subarachnoid hemorrhage is made on the basis of clinical signs, cerebrospinal fluid examination, cerebral angiography, and CAT scan analysis. The clinical signs in subarachnoid hemorrhage are generalized and do not focus in the area of involvement; they are, therefore, not significant in localizing the site of hemorrhage.

Subarachnoid hemorrhage may be treated surgically or conservatively depending on the general overall condition of the individual. Those who are obtunded are generally not good surgical risks and are treated conservatively on strict bed rest. Rebleeding is always a possibility and much of the focus of care is directed at its prevention.

INTRACEREBRAL HEMATOMA. Traumatic disruption of cerebral vessels within the cerebral substance may result in varying neurologic deficits depending on the location and amount of bleeding. The shearing forces within the brain substance resulting from brain movement within the skull frequently result in laceration of the vessels and the hemorrhage into the parenchyma. Common sites of intracerebral bleeding occur in the frontal and temporal lobes.

Individuals with intracerebral bleeding may be comatose or may have a lucid period before lapsing into a coma. Motor deficits may be present and decorticate or decerebrate responses may occur. The bleeding site may be identified by CAT scan, such as shown in Figure 45-1, or cerebral arteriography. The cerebrospinal fluid pressure may be elevated and the fluid may appear bloody and xanthochromic.

Intracerebral hematomas may be treated by surgical decompression through burr holes or bone flap removal. Conservative treatment focuses on minimizing cerebral edema and increased intracranial pressure through medications, posturing, and supportive therapy.

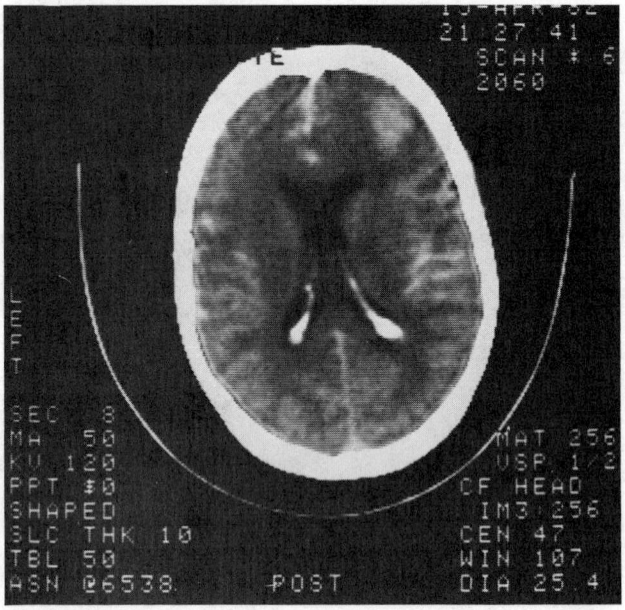

FIGURE 45-8. Subarachnoid bleeding (light diffuse areas throughout brain).

Cerebral Edema

A common and serious sequela to head injury is cerebral edema, wherein the water content in the brain parenchyma becomes excessive. In addition to head injury, cerebral edema may also follow intracranial surgery, brain tumors, hypoxemia, infarctions, and infections. Two distinct types of cerebral edema have been identified: *cytotoxic* and *vasogenic*. *Cytotoxic cerebral edema* reflects cellular dysfunction or injury and occurs secondarily to conditions that produce cerebral hypoxia. The fluid collection is intracellular within most of the cell components of the brain. The sodium pump is not able to remove accumulating intracellular sodium due to ATP deficiency that results from hypoxia. The excess intracellular sodium pulls water into the cell. The *vasogenic* form is a result of damage to or dysfunction in the cerebral blood vessels. Vasogenic edema fluid occurs both intracellularly and intercellularly and has a composition very similar to plasma. This type of cerebral edema reflects an increased permeability of the capillary membranes and widening of the junctions between the cells. The widening of these normally tight junctions allows plasma proteins from the blood to pass into the extracellular spaces. Vasogenic edema occurs commonly with trauma, inflammatory processes, neoplasms, and vascular lesions. *Cytotoxic edema* occurs with certain intoxications, hypoxia, some metabolic disorders, and water overload. It is thought that alteration in the blood-brain barrier occurs in both types of cerebral edema. The mechanism of the alteration in blood-brain barrier is not known but it has been proposed to be associated with loss of cerebral autoregulation. As a result of the malfunction of the blood-brain barrier associated with cerebral edema, the brain becomes more permeable to molecules that normally do not cross this barrier. The significant molecules that escape into the brain parenchyma and contribute to increased brain extracellular osmotic pressure as described earlier especially include the plasma proteins.

As cerebral edema increases within the nonflexible skull clinical signs indicating increased intracranial pressure develop. If the edema progresses, further deterioration of neurologic function due to intracranial shifts or herniations results. The signs indicating increased intracranial pressure, brain shifts, and herniations are discussed on pp. 698–701.

The morphologic changes in the edematous brain as seen at surgery or autopsy are characteristic and striking. The brain appears heavy and boggy. The gyri have lost their normal triangular appearance and the sulci have been obliterated. Sectioning the brain reveals flattened ventricles and an indiscernible subarachnoid space [3].

Management of Head Injuries

After the initial ascertainment of an adequate airway and effective respiratory exchange and the absence of acute shock, a careful history is obtained. If possible, the nature of the accident is obtained and the lapse of time since the accident is noted. This information may assist in localizing the site of injury and give some indication of its degree. Neurologic evaluation of the level of consciousness, pupillary responses, motor activity, and respiratory patterns is obtained for a baseline assessment. In addition to the neurologic signs, a careful examination of the head is made to determine the presence of lacerations, foreign objects, or depressed skull fractures. The ear canals are evaluated for the presence of blood, and otoscopic examination of the tympanic membrane is carried out to assess for a bluish coloration indicating bleeding into the middle ear. The presence of ecchymosis over the mastoid area (*Battle's sign*) is evaluated and may indicate the possibility of a basilar skull fracture. Blood from the ear, if mixed with cerebrospinal fluid (*otorrhea*), will not clot and its drainage leaves a halo effect at the periphery of the drainage on dressings or pillow. Drainage of mixed blood and cerebrospinal fluid from the nose (*rhinorrhea*) has characteristics similar to those of otorrhea.

Individuals with acute head injuries should be treated as if they also sustained a cervical spine injury until it is proven otherwise. Pain, if present, may be associated with the area of neck injury; however, this is not a totally reliable indicator of the presence of spinal cord injury as pain may not be exhibited with all of these injuries and cannot be verified with the unconscious person. Careful palpation of the neck and alignment of the spinous process at the midline of the posterior neck should be done to evaluate for possible cervical cord injury. Immobilization of the neck with sandbags, cervical collars, or head straps to spineboard is undertaken until cervical x rays indicate no abnormalities.

Vital signs reflect the status of the head-injured person and may support the late findings of an increased intracranial pressure or the presence of shock. Elevated temperatures may indicate small brainstem hemorrhages or trauma directly to the thermoregulatory mechanisms of the hypothalamus. Focal seizures may accompany acute head injuries and may be valuable in the localizing of the site of the lesion. Observations of the nature and origin of the onset of the convulsions are invaluable to the overall assessment of the head-injured individual.

ASSESSMENT OF TRAUMATIC DISRUPTION TO CRANIAL NERVES

Persons with head injuries may suffer partial or total loss of function of cranial nerves in the area of the lesion. If the affected individual is conscious, a brief assessment of the function of each of the nerves can be ascertained.

Olfactory Nerve

The first cranial nerve extends from the inferior surface of the frontal lobe and mediates the sense of smell. Disruption of the olfactory nerve may accompany acute head injury, particularly in the presence of basilar skull fractures and fractures of the cribriform plate. The olfactory nerve filaments may be injured in contrecoup injuries following trauma to the occipital or parietotemporal region. Additional disorders responsible for disruption of the sense of smell (*anosmia*) include upper respiratory infections, rhinitis, tumors, meningitis, and subarachnoid hemorrhages.

Assessment of the first cranial nerve can be accomplished simply by requesting the individual to close his or her eyes and identify some common odors such as soap, coffee, or alcohol. Each nostril is tested individually and the patient is asked to occlude one nostril while the other is being tested.

Optic Nerve

The second cranial nerve serves the sensory function of vision. Visual impulses originate in the photoreceptors of the retina and are transmitted via the optic nerve to the optic chiasm and to the various parts of the occipital cortex for recognition and interpretation. Lesions from trauma or intrinsic origins anywhere along these pathways cause specific patterns of visual loss (see Fig. 43-2). Damage to the optic nerve generally results from force to the frontal area of the skull and sudden movements of the brain with the resultant contusion of the optic nerve against the side of the optic foramen. Vision defects may also result from injury to the vessels supplying the optic nerve. Visual loss is maximal directly after injury. If recovery of vision is to occur, it may be anticipated within the first month of injury, as optic nerve atrophy begins about a month after injury. Injury to the occipital lobe may also result in impaired vision; however, pupillary light reflexes in this situation remain intact and prognosis generally is favorable.

Careful clinical evaluation of the visual field can be very significant in determining the site of a lesion. The quadrants of each eye of the cooperative person can be examined individually by superimposing the examiner's eye directly in the visual field of the individual. The examiner closes the eye directly across from the individual's closed eye. The individual is instructed to look directly into the examiner's eye and is asked to signal on first seeing the examiner's finger move into the visual field. This is repeated from each of the four quadrants, the superior and inferior temporal and nasal of each eye. Assuming the examiner's vision to be normal, the individual should see the finger the same time the examiner does. More rudimentary assessments of vision can be done simply by asking the person to count the number of fingers the examiner is holding out. Those who are unresponsive or uncooperative will respond with a blink to a threat motion toward the head if visual fields are at least partially intact.

A frequently encountered visual disturbance is *homonymous hemianopsia* in which corresponding halves of bilateral vision are lost. In addition to trauma, cerebral infarctions, tumors, and abscesses may also cause homonymous hemianopsia. This defect can be recognized by having the individual count all 10 fingers held out by the examiner. Wide turning of the individual's head to visualize all fingers may indicate a homonymous hemianopsia.

Oculomotor, Trochlear, and Abducens Nerves

The third, fourth, and sixth nerves are generally examined together because of their cooperative function in controlling the movements of the eye. In addition, the oculomotor nerve innervates the levator palpebrae superioris muscle, which mediates elevation of the eyelid, and the constrictor muscle of the iris, which alters pupillary aperture in accordance with the degree of illumination. Likewise, convergence and accommodation are mediated by the third nerve. Pupillary responses are more fully discussed on pp. 688–689.

The nuclei of the oculomotor nerve are in the midbrain. The axons traverse ventrally to emerge from the midbrain at the level of the tentorial notch and pass through a portion of the cerebral peduncle. At this level, the nerve is particularly vulnerable to compression from other cerebral structures and its encroachment is reflected by a unilateral pupil change on the ipsilateral side. The nuclei of the trochlear nerve, likewise, are in the midbrain caudal to the oculomotor nucleus, and transmit impulses to the superior oblique muscle. The abducens nuclei are in the lower pons below the fourth ventricle floor and control lateral eye movements by innervating superior, inferior, and medial rectus muscles and the inferior oblique muscle.

Injury to the frontal region of the skull may cause injury to the third, fourth, and sixth nerves. Brainstem trauma may result in difficulties with conjugate movement and paralysis of individual nerves may ensue in some persons. Upward gaze and convergence and lateral eye movements may be interrupted with brainstem lesions. Numerous combinations of third, fourth, and sixth nerve palsies may accompany injuries to the nerves of the superior orbital fissure and may be accompanied by diplopia.

In the assessment of extraocular eye movements, the eyes are observed for conjugate gaze. The eyes are examined in respect to each other and should be aligned parallel in the visual axis when the individual is gazing straight ahead. The extraocular function is evaluated by asking the person to follow the examiner's finger in six cardinal positions.

Trigeminal Nerve

The fifth cranial nerve is a mixed sensory motor nerve and mediates sensations over the entire face and scalp to the vertex, the paranasal sinuses as well as the nasal and oral cavities, and the cornea. The motor component of the fifth nerve innervates the muscles of mastication. The sensory nuclei of the trigeminal nerve are in the gasserian ganglion anterior to the pons and the motor nuclei arise in the midpons region.

The extracranial portions of the fifth nerve are most frequently involved in traumatic injuries. Scalp wounds or compression fractures of the supraorbital area may sever the supraorbital portion of the fifth nerve. This trauma may be identified by the paresthesias, hyperesthesias, and neuralgic pain that lingers in the affected scalp and forehead in some individuals. The infraorbital portion may also be severed in traumatic injury and result in anesthesia of the affected cheek and upper lip.

A frequent cause of disruption of parts of the fifth nerve are tumors arising in the posterior fossa as well as generalized trauma to the cerebellopontine region or local trauma to the face. *Tic douloureux* or *trigeminal neuralgia* occurs primarily in women in their fifth and sixth decades and is manifested by excruciating, unpredictable, paroxysmal pain along part or all of the divisions of the fifth nerve. The cause of this condition remains obscure but it has been known to be exacerbated by infections, emotional upsets, facial movements, and drafts.

Three major divisions of the fifth nerve are the *ophthalmic*, *maxillary*, and *mandibular*. Each of these divisions of the sensory component of the fifth nerve is examined for touch perception and discrimination on both sides of the face. With the individual's eyes closed, the examiner tests areas with a wisp of cotton and a pin, asking the person to identify which area is touched. The *corneal reflex* is assessed by stroking the cornea with a wisp of cotton from the side while the person's eyes are turned to the opposite side to avoid an involuntary blink.

The motor component of the fifth nerve is examined by having the person clench the teeth and open the mouth while the examiner palpates the jaw. Deviation occurs to the affected side in presence of weakness.

FACIAL NERVE. The seventh cranial nerve is a mixed motor and sensory nerve although its primary innervation is motor control of the muscles of facial expression. Its sensory component mediates the sensation of taste perception in the anterior two-thirds of the tongue and innervates the lacrimal and certain salivary glands. The nucleus for the seventh nerve is in the lower pons. Certain cortical innervation of the voluntary movement of the face is transmitted to portions of the seventh nerve nucleus via the corticobulbar tract. Some of these axons cross to the contralateral nuclei and others terminate in the ipsilateral nuclei. High face muscles are innervated by fibers from both contralateral and ipsilateral fibers and the lower muscles are innervated by fibers from the contralateral cortex only. Weakness generated from the effects on the corticobulbar tract are of central origin (upper motor neuron) and cause only contralateral lower face weakness. The ipsilateral facial weakness of an entire side of the face is of peripheral origin (lower motor neuron) from a lesion at the nucleus or the peripheral axon of the seventh nerve.

Dysfunction of the seventh nerve may occur with basilar skull fractures as its location traversing the temporal bone makes it particularly susceptible to injury. Fractures of the petrous portions of the temporal bone may result in injury to the seventh nerve and the resultant facial paralysis. In such situations, the prognosis is generally favorable and function returns with slow recovery that may last for months.

Proximity of the seventh nerve to the middle ear increases the injurious effects of middle ear infections and tumors of the region on the nerve. Central facial paralysis can result from infarctions, lesions, and abscesses of the contralateral cerebral cortex. *Bell's palsy* is an inflammatory response to infections and allergies affecting the seventh nerve within the temporal bone, which results in ipsilateral hemifacial paralysis.

Assessment of the status of the facial nerve includes examination of facial tone and symmetry by requesting the person to wrinkle the forehead, smile, whistle, close the eyes, and show the teeth. The sensory component can be assessed by applying sweet, sour, salty, and bitter substances to the appropriate areas of the anterior tongue and having the person identify what is tasted. The mouth is rinsed between the applied substances.

VESTIBULOCOCHLEAR NERVE. The eighth cranial nerve is composed of the vestibular and cochlear divisions, the former mediating balance and equilibrium and the latter hearing. The nuclei of the acoustic nerve are in the lower pons.

Traumatic head injury may result in loss of hearing due to fractures extending through the middle ear. Severing of the nerve will result in permanent deafness. Hemorrhage into the middle ear will also compromise hearing; however, it does carry a prognosis of some recovery of hearing as the blood clot is absorbed. Edema and contusions of the eighth nerve result in hearing impairments that show recovery with the healing process. Vertigo results from edema or hemorrhage into the labyrinth, which is aggravated by head movement and associated with nausea and vomiting. Although the vertigo may be resolved within 2 or 3 weeks, the person may continue to feel light-headed and reveal signs of ataxia for months after the injury.

Assessment of hearing can be done simply by covering one of the patient's ears and whispering softly near the opposite ear. This is repeated in the other ear. Audibility of whispering is pretty much indicative of normal hearing. Should whispering not be audible to the individual, further testing is indicated. The vestibular component is investigated primarily through a described history of vertigo, unsteadiness of gait, and nausea. Testing is undertaken on the basis of the presence of the above symptoms.

GLOSSOPHARYNGEAL AND VAGUS NERVES. The ninth and tenth nerves are anatomically and structurally similar and, therefore, are examined together. The glossopharyngeal nerve innervates the muscles of the pharynx, posterior one-third of the taste sensation of the tongue, sensations of the tonsils, pharynx, and carotid sinuses, and carotid body. The vagus nerve has widespread innervation of the thoracic and abdominal visceral organs, as well as the larnyx and pharynx. The nuclei of these nerves are in the medulla.

Traumatic injury to the lower brainstem, fractures of the posterior fossa, or vascular injuries at the base of the skull may injure the ninth and tenth nerves, which will be reflected in dysphagia and a diminished or absent gag reflex.

Assessment of the ninth and tenth cranial nerves involves an initial inspection of the soft palate for symmetry. A gag reflex is elicited with a tongue blade contact with the posterior oropharynx. Normally, the palate elevates and the pharyngeal muscles contract. The person is asked to swallow water and the ability to do this without regurgitation is assessed. Speech is noted for signs of abnormal phonation and hoarseness.

ACCESSORY NERVE. The eleventh cranial nerve nuclei are in the anterior gray column of the first few segments of the cervical spinal cord and transmit to innervate the sternocleidomastoid and trapezius muscles to allow lifting or shrugging of shoulders, head rotation, and neck extension. Low brainstem injuries, posterior fossa fractures, and basilar skull fractures may result in injury and paralysis of the eleventh nerve. Additionally, trauma to the neck region may result in impairment of the spinal accessory nerve. Weakness appearing on one side may be suggestive of a stroke, whereas bilateral weakness may support motor neuron diseases or neuromuscular problems.

The functioning of this motor nerve in innervating the sternocleidomastoid is evaluated by having the individual turn the head toward the shoulder while the examiner puts resistance on the movement and assesses the strength of the muscle. This test is repeated on the other side. The functioning of the trapezius is evaluated by having the person raise the shoulders against the resistance applied by the examiner.

HYPOGLOSSAL NERVE. The twelfth cranial nerve is a motor nerve innervating the musculature of the tongue to allow normal articulation and food management in the mouth. Its nucleus is in the floor of the fourth ventricle. The function of the hypoglossal nerve may be jeopardized by trauma to

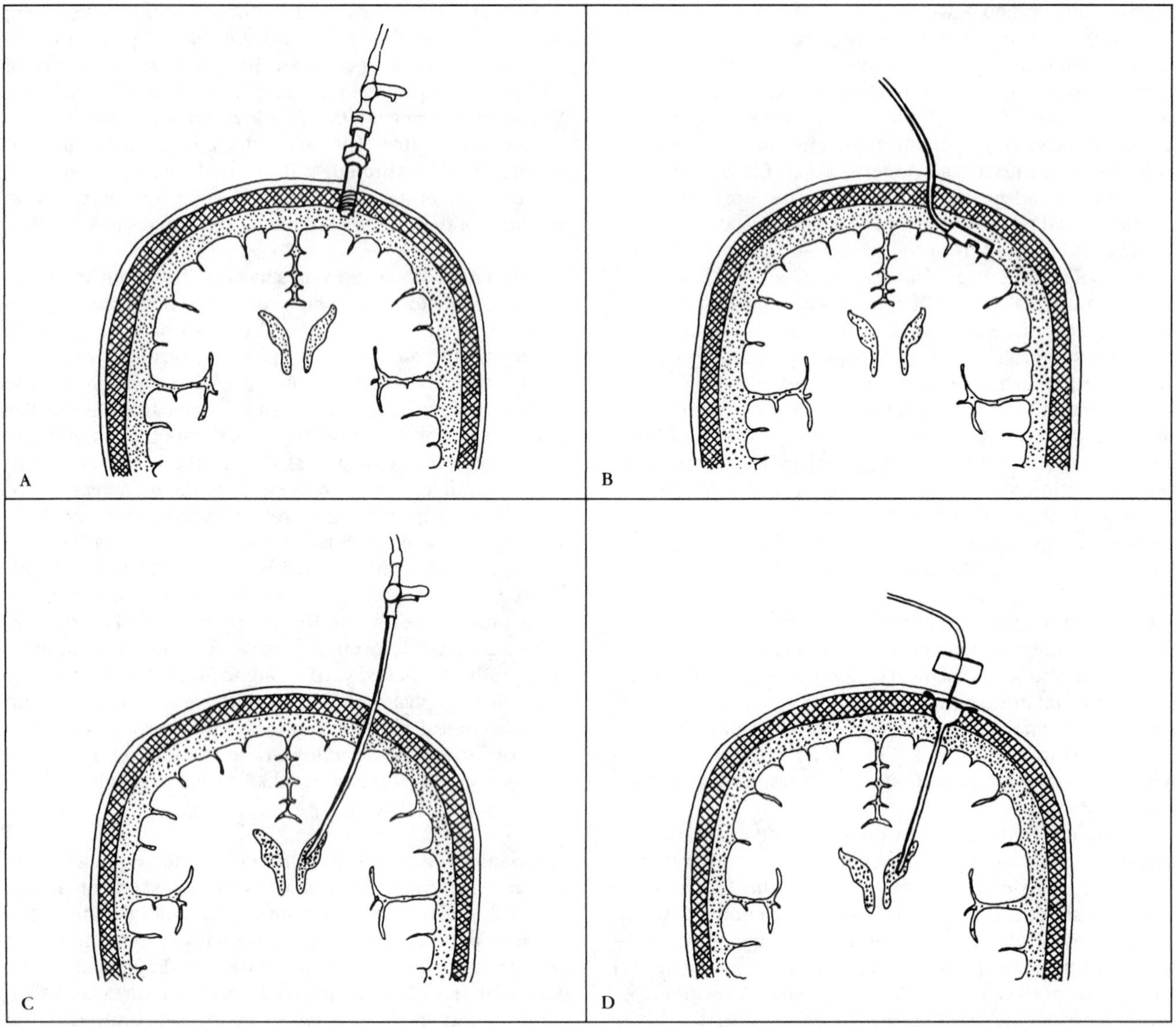

FIGURE 45-9. Devices utilized to measure intracranial pressure. A. Subdural screw. B. Epidural device. C. Intraventricular catheter. D. Intraventricular cannula. (From Massachusetts General Hospital Department of Nursing, *Manual of Nursing Procedures* (2nd ed.). Boston: Little, Brown, 1980.)

the neck as well as to the regions described in the eleventh nerve injuries. Traumatic lesion here may result in unilateral tongue weakness, which is evidenced by deviation of the protruding tongue to the weak side. Bilateral tongue weakness is most commonly associated with disease processes such as amyotrophic lateral sclerosis and poliomyelitis.

The function of the hypoglossal nerve is evaluated by having the individual protrude the tongue and observing for any deviation. The strength of the muscles of the tongue are assessed by the examiner by pushing against the cheek that the person is pressing outward with the tongue. Notation is made of any difficulty with articulation as the examiner and patient are conversing.

INCREASED INTRACRANIAL PRESSURE

Head injuries frequently result in increased intracranial pressure as a result of expanding lesions and accumulation of edema. Without treatment, increased intracranial pressure may compromise neurologic function as well as life itself. Therefore, early diagnosis and treatment are essential to prevent irreversible neurologic damage and death.

In the adult, the cranial vault affords a nonflexible encasement around the brain tissue, extracellular fluid, and cerebrospinal fluid. Although small alterations do occur in the total intracranial volume, the intracranial pressure remains relatively constant. Small increases in volume of one

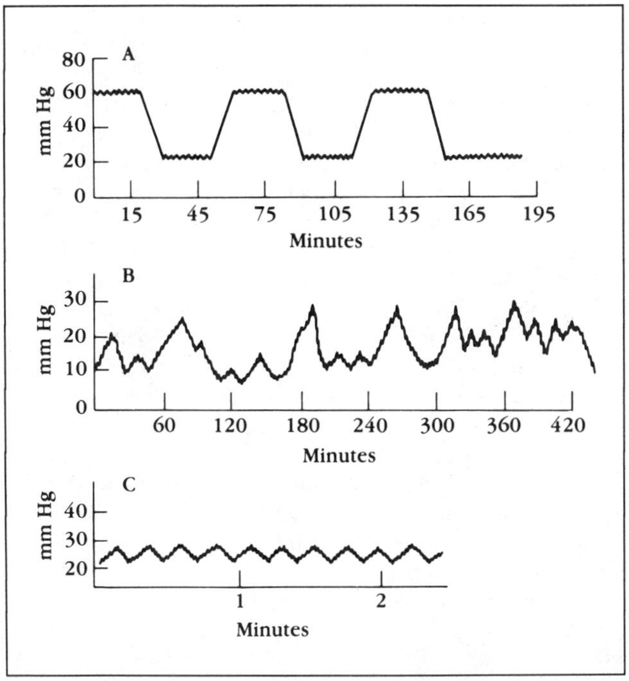

FIGURE 45-10. Generalized shapes of the three types of ICP waves: A, or plateau (top) waves, B (middles) waves, and C (bottom) waves. (From A. Hamilton, *Critical Care Nursing Skills*. New York: Appleton-Century-Crofts, 1981.)

of the cranial components are compensated normally by a decrease in the volume of another. Intracranial cerebrospinal fluid may be shifted to the subarachnoid space of the spine and the vascular bed of the brain may vary according to the existing physiologic conditions. If the small margin of compensation within the cranium is exhausted, the intracranial pressure rises and small increases in volume at this point result in large rises in intracranial pressure. Without intervention, decompensation and death ensue.

Traditional clinical indicators of increased intracranial pressure include: decreased level of consciousness, papilledema, pupillary dilation, peripheral motor changes, decreasing pulse, elevated systolic pressure, decreasing pulse, widening pulse pressure, and respiratory irregularities. The varying presence of these signs indicates the level of brain dysfunction that has occurred as a result of the pathologic process that led to the increased intracranial pressure. Generally, when the classic clinical indicators are present, the individual has reached a state of decompensation and has a poor prognosis for recovery. Treatment is most effective while the brain is in a compensatory state, for once compensatory mechanisms have been used up, the pressure within the cranium rises rapidly. Intracranial pressure monitoring provides a means to detect changes in pressure before clinical signs are evident.

Intracranial pressure is most conveniently monitored through the measurement of the cerebrospinal fluid as pressure is equally transmitted in all directions in fluid. Intracranial pressure changes can be monitored by the use of a subdural screw, an epidural device, or through the lateral ventricles via an intraventricular cannula (Fig. 45-9). Normal intracranial pressures range from 0 to 13 mm Hg or 50 to 200 mm of water. Some fluctuations over the narrow normal range are commonly seen. The pressures measured by these methods are transmitted to a pressure transducer and recording instrument. The mechanical impulses are transmitted to the transducer that converts them into electrical impulses. These appear on an oscilloscope as varying wave patterns (Fig. 45-10). The most significant of these are the plateau waves that are recorded with advanced stages of increased intracranial pressure.

The pressure within the cranium may rise rather abruptly or insidiously. Severely head-injured individuals with rapidly increasing intracranial pressure and intracranial bleeding, frequently have escape of blood into the cerebrospinal fluid, which results in an increased osmotic force, thus increasing cerebrospinal fluid volume. Increased intracranial pressure also occurs with infections, tumors, and hypercapnia. Tissue expansion occurs with inflammatory and neoplastic processes, and the cerebral vasculature increases in size in response to elevated carbon dioxide levels. The expansion of the volume of tissue and cerebrospinal fluid results in compression of cerebral vessels and, in turn, a reflexively higher arterial blood pressure resulting in a lower pulse rate and shifting of cerebral structures. Supratentorial structural displacements result in characteristic clinical changes as previously uninvolved cerebral tissues are being encroached. With progressive expansion, the tissue eventually protrudes through the tentorial notch, which is the single supratentorial opening available.

Intracranial Shifts

Major brain shifts that can occur in response to expanding cerebral pathology are *cingulate herniation*, *transcalvarial herniation*, *central transtentorial herniation*, and *uncal herniation* (Fig. 45-11).

In *cingulate herniation*, lateral displacement of expanding cerebral lesions compresses the cingulate gyrus under the falx cerebri, which results in displacement of the internal cerebral vein. This displacement of the cerebral vasculature, in turn, results in the vessel compression and leads to ischemia, thus further increasing the cerebral contents with the resultant edema. *Transcalvarial herniation* occurs with open head injuries where the brain tissue extrudes through an unstable fractured skull.

Central transtentorial herniation results from lesions of the frontal, parietal, and occipital lobes as they progress to a downward displacement encroaching on the diencephalon and midbrain. Cingulate herniation frequently precedes the central transtentorial herniation. Clinical signs of central transtentorial herniation reflect increasing intracranial pressure and include changes in visual acuity and an increase in the size of the normal blind spot as pressure is exerted on the optic nerve. Papilledema results from optic

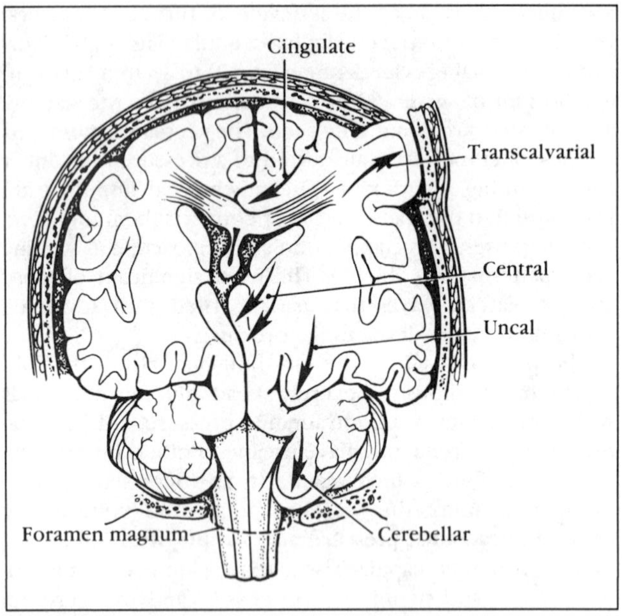

FIGURE 45-11. Major types of intracranial herniations.

nerve compression as interference occurs with venous return from the optic disk. As central expansion progresses caudally, brainstem compression is reflected clinically by a deteriorating level of consciousness. Initially, changes in the level of consciousness may be very subtle. As compression of the corticospinal tract occurs, contralateral weakness or paralysis results and deteriorates to decorticate or decerebrate responses. Early central herniation exhibits pupillary constriction, which leads to moderate dilation without light reflex response as pressure is exerted further to the midbrain region. Wide, fixed dilation is a terminal sign. Respiratory patterns initially may be periodic with yawning and sighing interruptions. This changes to a persistent hyperventilation as central compression continues caudally and, in terminal stages, becomes an ataxic pattern prior to respiratory arrest.

Lesions in the lateral middle fossa or temporal lobe result in *uncal herniation*. Crowding at the tentorial notch results in compression of the third nerve, which results in a unilaterally dilated pupil. This is the classic initial characteristic of uncal herniation. Neurologic deterioration may progress rapidly without successful intervention after the initial pupillary dilation, to nonfunctioning extraocular movement (EOM), hemiplegia, and decerebrate posturing. Terminal stages of uncal herniation resemble central herniation.

Traumatic, rapidly expanding lesions below the tentorium result in rapid loss of consciousness and neurologic

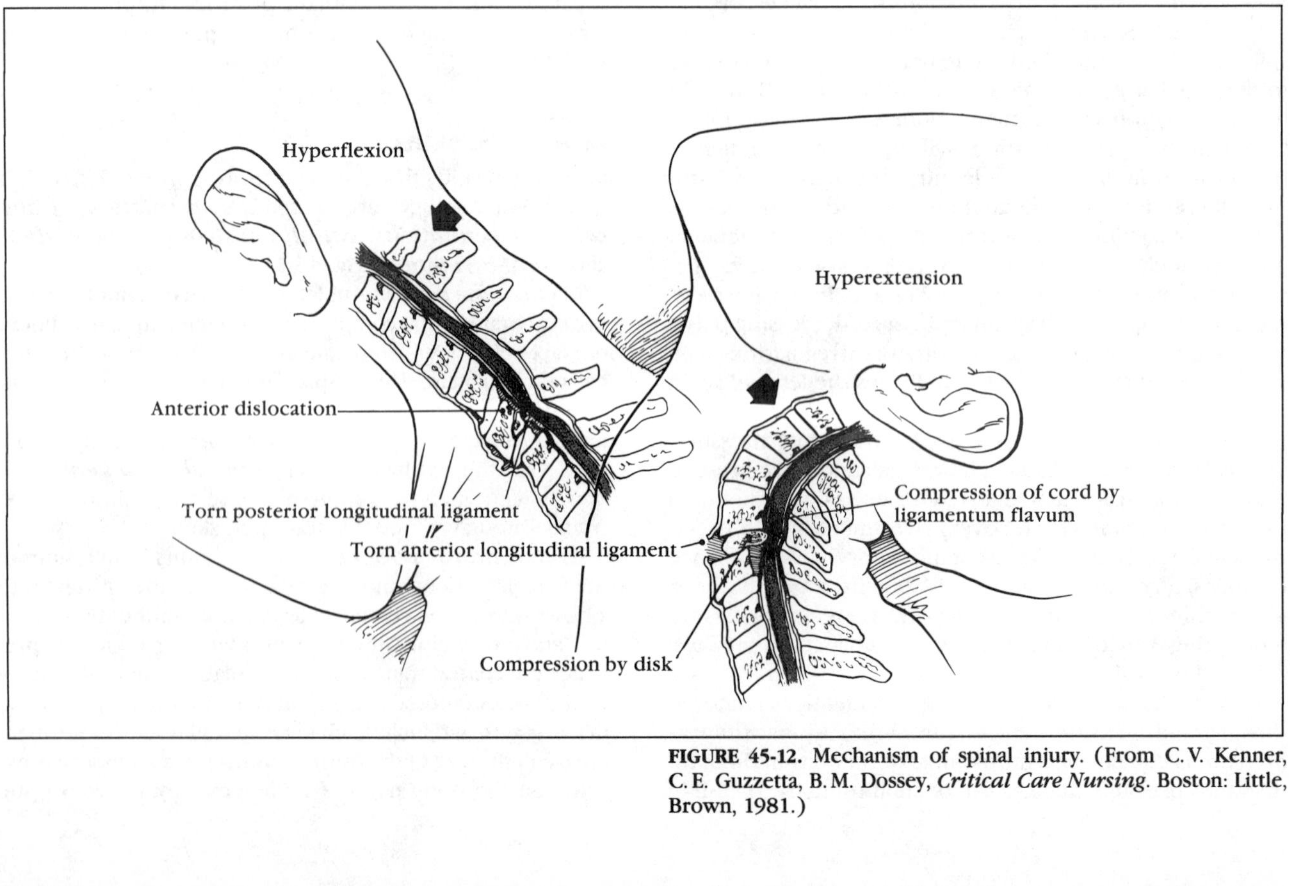

FIGURE 45-12. Mechanism of spinal injury. (From C.V. Kenner, C.E. Guzzetta, B.M. Dossey, *Critical Care Nursing*. Boston: Little, Brown, 1981.)

deficits indicating severe dysfunction. The dysfunction results from the direct effects on the vital centers in the brainstem and the inability of the subtentorial contents to compensate adequately. The cerebellum and midbrain may herniate upward through the tentorial notch. Pontine lesions reflect constricted pupils that may respond minimally to the light reflex. Motor responses vary from flaccidity to flexor to extension responses. Low brainstem breathing patterns such as apneustic and ataxic breathing predominate. Lesions to the medulla result in rapid neurologic deterioration, leading to death as centers controlling respiratory and vasomotor function become dysfunctional.

Management of Increased Intracranial Pressure

Medical management of increased intracranial pressure aims at relieving the pressure to prevent further neurologic deterioration and concomitantly supporting vital functions. Whenever feasible, the underlying cause of increased intracranial pressure is removed. When this cannot be accomplished because of the nature of the lesion, mechanical decompression, hypothermia, osmotic diuresis, corticosteroids, and barbiturates may be utilized. Surgical intervention may be necessary for the removal of intracranial hematomas. Trephines are commonly utilized for exploration of subdural and epidural hematomas, removal of the hematoma, and ligation of the bleeding vessel. Artificial hyperventilation may be utilized to lower the carbon dioxide level of the patient, thus reducing the cerebral blood volume. Mechanical decompression by removal of some cerebrospinal fluid decreases cerebral pressure.

SPINAL CORD INJURY

Injuries to the spinal cord as a result of trauma are increasing every year due to the extensive use of the automobile and increased amount of time people spend in recreation and sports activities. A wide variation is seen in the extent and level of spinal cord injury. A "whiplash" may result in very minor discomfort from the mild flexion-extension type of cord injuries, whereas total quadriplegia from severe fracture dislocations of the cervical vertebral column may result from cord damage. Trauma to the spinal cord can occur at any level although the areas most frequently involved are the cervical spine and lower thoracic spine.

Common mechanisms of spinal cord injury from traumatic impact include the hyperextension or hyperflexion type of injury, frequently accompanied by rotational movement of the cord (Fig. 45-12). The resultant spinal cord damage may be transient or permanent depending on the extent of parenchymal damage. Injuries similar to those that occur to the brain can also occur to the spinal cord including concussion, contusion, hemorrhage, lacerations, and compression. Associated vertebral injuries may lead to spinal cord damage in subluxation, compression fractures, and fracture dislocations of the vertebral column (Fig. 45-13). The extent of cord damage in vertebral injuries is related to the degree of bony encroachment or compression on the cord. Severe injuries result in partial or complete functional transection of the spinal cord.

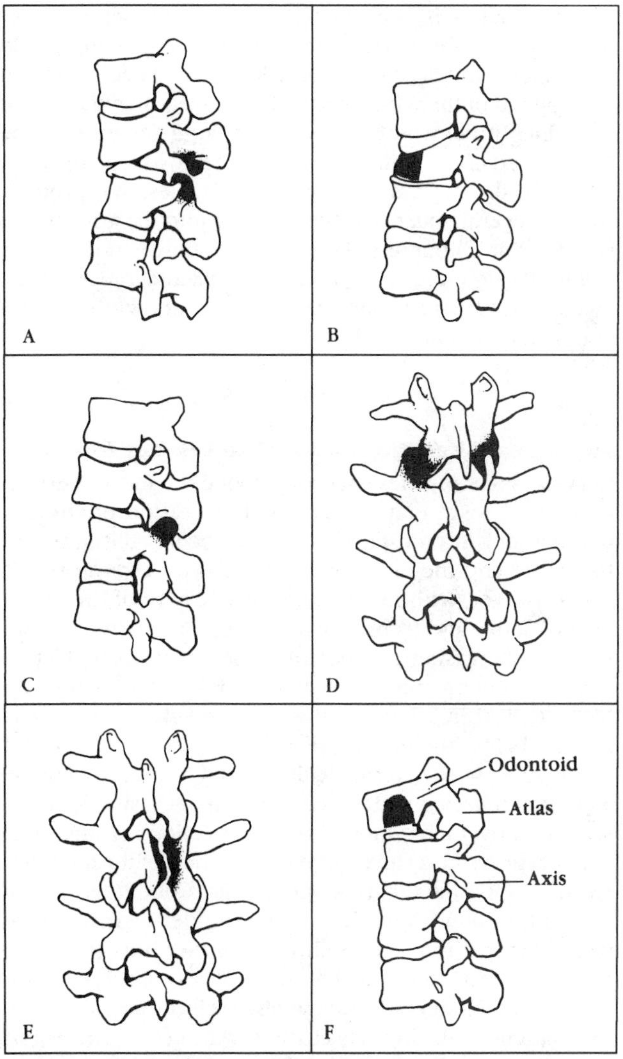

FIGURE 45-13. Common types of vertebral injury. A. Subluxation. B. Compression fracture. C. Bilateral fracture joint dislocation. D. Unilateral facet joint dislocation. E. Posterior arch fracture. F. Odontoid fracture. (From R. Judge, G. E. Zuidema, and F. Fitzgerald, et al. *Clinical Diagnosis: A Physiologic Approach*. Boston: Little, Brown, 1982.)

Morphologic Changes Associated with Irreversible Cord Damage

Experimentally induced spinal cord injury in the laboratory setting on animal subjects has provided insight into the structural changes occurring at varying time periods following the injury. A force strong enough to result in irreversible total paraplegia will cause severe edema and hemorrhage within a few hours, which then leads to massive necrosis and, finally, parenchymal and vessel destruction.

Immediately after cord injury, focal hemorrhages begin in the gray matter and rapidly increase in size until the entire gray matter is hemorrhagic and necrotic. The hemorrhages in the white matter proximal to the gray matter do not coalesce but are associated with massive edema, which envelops all of the white matter. It has been speculated that norepinephrine, which is released in large amounts by the traumatized cord, contributes to the hemorrhagic necrosis caused by direct physical damage [2]. The lesion is progressive for several hours. The hemorrhage into the gray matter is present at 1 hour after injury, fluid in between the axons is found 15 minutes after injury, and disintegration of the myelin sheath and axonal shrinkage occurs within 1 to 4 hours following injury [3].

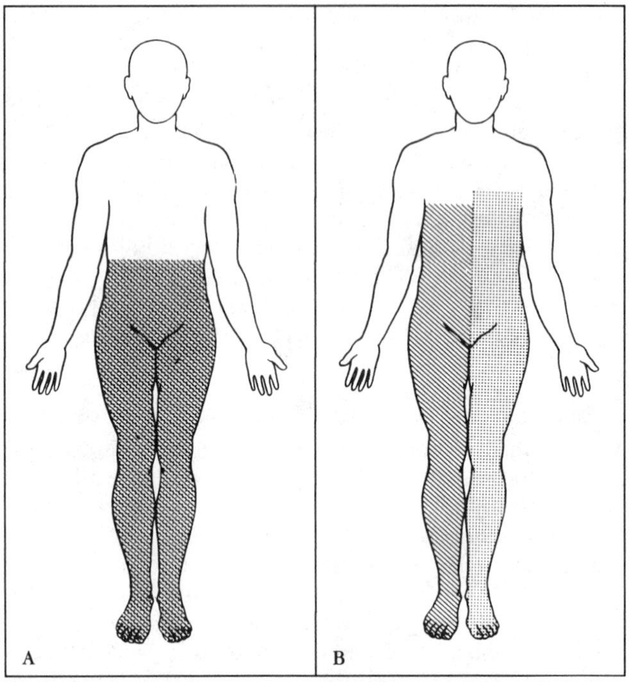

FIGURE 45-14. A. Complete transverse lesion of the spinal cord. B. Brown-Séquard syndrome: lesion on the left side of the spinal cord. (From J. Simpson and K. Magee, *Clinical Evaluation of the Nervous System*. Boston: Little, Brown, 1973.)

Functional Alterations Related to Level of Injury

Cervical spine injuries occurring above the fourth cervical cord (C4) level may be fatal as innervation of the diaphragm and intercostal muscles has been obliterated by the injury and the individual succumbs to respiratory failure. However, with increasing sophistication of the public in knowledge and technique of cardiopulmonary resuscitation, an increasing number of these unfortunate victims arrive at emergency medical facilities. Additionally, the high cervical injuries result in quadriplegia. Patients with injuries below the fifth cervical nerve (C5) level have full innervation of the sternocleidomastoid, trapezius muscles and other muscles, and therefore retain neck, shoulder, and scapula movement. Individuals with lesions at the sixth cervical nerve (C6) level have the function of the shoulder, elbow, and partial function of the wrist. Complete innervation of the rotator muscles of the shoulder is retained and partial innervation is transmitted to the serratus, pectoralis major, and latissimus dorsi muscles. Wrist muscles and the biceps retain innervation allowing for elbow and wrist flexion. Patients with injuries at the seventh (C7) and eighth cranial nerve (C8) level exhibit additional elbow, wrist, and hand function. Innervation is intact to the triceps and common and long finger extensors, enabling elbow extension and flexion, and functional, though weak, finger extension and flexion.

Injuries to the region of the *thoracic* and *lumbar* cord render the victim paraplegic (Fig. 45-14A). Those with high thoracic injury, first thoracic nerve (T1), retain full innervation of upper extremity musculature. Injuries experienced at the sixth thoracic nerve (T6) level allow the person to have an increased respiratory reserve as intercostal innervation is intact. Persons experiencing low thoracic, twelfth thoracic nerve (T12), lesions to the cord have partial innervation to the lower extremities and may, in fact, regain ambulation when supported by long leg braces and assisted by crutches.

Persons who sustain *low lumbar* and *sacral* lesions have full innervation to upper extremities and trunk, hip flexors and extensors, knee extensors, and ankle movement. Therefore, they are able to ambulate with minimal supportive devices.

Functional Alterations Related to Portion of Cord Injured

Central cord lesions can occur at different levels of the spinal cord; the symptoms vary with the extent of hemorrhage and edema as well as with the location. Lesions in the central part of the cord at the cervical level are known as the *central cord syndrome.* Motor weakness occurs with this syndrome in both upper and lower extremities, although the motor weakness is greater in the upper extremities. Loss of pain and temperature sensations occurs above the nipple line and touch perception remains intact.

Brown-Séquard lesions are those that involve only one side of the cord (see Fig. 45-14B). The characteristic symptoms with this syndrome include paralysis and loss of fine touch and two-point discrimination ipsilaterally below the lesion on the same side with contralateral pain and temperature perception loss. *Horner's syndrome* may accompany Brown-Séquard lesions at the cervical level ipsilaterally.

Anterior cord syndrome is reflected by loss of sensitivity to pain and of motor and temperature control below the level of the lesion. Touch, proprioception, and vibratory sense remain intact.

Spinal Cord Transection

Total spinal cord transection results in immediate loss of all voluntary movement from the segments below the transection. The skin and other tissues become permanently anesthetised. Initially, reflex activity is abolished. However, reflex recovery does occur and eventually may become hyperactive.

SPINAL SHOCK. The immediate depression of the cord activity after transection is referred to as *spinal shock* or *posttransectional areflexia*. It results from the interruption of the pathways with the remainder of the central nervous system. The exact mechanisms causing spinal shock and recovery of reflexes are still elusive. It has been speculated that the excitatory effects of alpha and gamma motoneurons on other spinal motoneurons has been lost due to transection of the descending pathways, and that inhibitory spinal internuncial neurons become disinhibited thus resulting in diminished reflexes. Considerable variability of the duration of spinal shock exists in humans. Some reflexes may reappear as early as 2 or 3 days after transection whereas others may not return for 6 weeks. Spinal shock is more pronounced in the segments in the region of the lesion and recovery of reflexes generally occurs last here.

In addition to areflexia in spinal shock, other clinical signs include autonomic deficits, which are reflected in a lowered arterial blood pressure, and poor body temperature control below the area of transection. Because of the depression of the vasoconstrictive action by the sympathetic nervous system, individuals are susceptible to severe postural hypotension. Bowel and bladder reflexes from the sacrum are, likewise, inhibited, and, as a result, the control over these functions is temporarily lost during spinal shock. Flaccid paralysis of skeletal musculature occurs below the transection site.

REFLEX RETURN IN CORD TRANSECTION: FLEXION-EXTENSION REFLEXES. The earliest reflex recovery from spinal shock, about 2 weeks after transection, are flexion reflexes that are evoked by noxious cutaneous stimulation. An example of this withdrawal response is the dorsiflexion of the great toe (Babinski sign) in response to stimulation of the sole of the foot. The presence of complications such as infection and malnutrition may delay the return of the flexion responses. As the flexor reflex recovers, it gradually becomes excited more readily from wider areas of the skin.

As recovery progresses after cord transection, flexor reflexes are interspersed with extensor spasms with ultimate progression to predominantly extensor activity. Individuals with partial cord transections generally exhibit strong extensor spasticity, whereas this seldom occurs with complete transection.

AUTONOMIC REFLEXES. The autonomic spinal reflexes include those controlling reflexive action of the vasomotor reflex activity, reflex diaphoresis, and reflex emptying of the bladder and rectum. Vasomotor reflexes are abolished below the level of transection during spinal shock but with time, tonic autonomic activity returns and wide variances in arterial pressure diminish. Temperature control by the skin is essentially abolished for a time after spinal transection as autonomic innervation for sweating is suppressed. Reflex emptying of the bladder and rectum do occur in individuals with spinal transections after a period of initial atony and increased sphincter tone. Dilation of the bladder with urine eventually overcomes sphincter resistance and overflow incontinence occurs. With progression of time, spontaneous brief contractions of the bladder evolve into larger contractions that are accompanied by bladder sphincter opening and brief micturition. Thus, small amounts of urine are voided with varying amounts of residual urine retained. Sensory stimuli may be utilized to precipitate micturition by tapping on the abdomen, anal stimulation, or stroking the inner aspect of the upper thigh. Downward manual pressure on the lower abdomen over the bladder (Credé's maneuver) is also used to initiate micturition.

Autonomic dysreflexia or *autonomic hyperreflexia* constitutes a cluster of symptoms in which many spinal cord autonomic responses are discharging simultaneously. This syndrome occurs in persons with spinal cord injuries above the seventh thoracic cord (T7) segment. This syndrome can manifest itself any time up to six years postinjury. The symptoms occur in response to a specific noxious stimuli, appear quickly, and may lead to life-threatening situations such as seizures and cerebral hemorrhages. Therefore, emergency measures must be taken rapidly and the precipitation cause must be found and removed.

The symptoms of autonomic dysreflexia are a result of sensory stimuli that produce exaggerated sympathetic discharges, which cause the blood vessels of the skin and splanchnic bed below the level of injury to reflexively vasoconstrict. As a result, the individual will experience a pounding headache, blurred vision, and severe hypertension, which may rise as high as 300 mm Hg. The increased blood pressure distends the carotid sinus and aortic arch baroreceptors that stimulate the vagus nerve to decrease the heart rate in an attempt to lower the blood pressure. Flushing and profuse diaphoresis are present above the level of the injury. Other symptoms that are present include restlessness, nasal congestion, and nausea. Cutes anserina (goose flesh) and pale skin persist below the level of injury. Impulses to the areas below the lesion are blocked so that vasodilation cannot occur. This means that messages for vasodilation below the lesion are interrupted and vasoconstriction continues below the level of the lesion.

Precipitating factors leading to autonomic dysreflexia most commonly include bladder and bowel distention or manipulation. Other triggering stimuli may include decubitus ulcers, spasticity, stimulation of pain receptors, pressure on the penis, and strong uterine contractions. When the symptoms occur, rapid intervention is necessary to lower the blood pressure. The head of the bed is elevated as patients with high cord injuries usually have a lower blood pressure in the sitting position. Next, the source of stimulation must be found and removed. If these measures are not successful in relieving the symptoms, ganglionic blocking agents are given intravenously.

Intervertebral Disk Herniation

Herniation or rupture of the nucleus pulposus of the intervertebral disk is most commonly caused by trauma of varying degrees (Fig. 45-15). Sudden straining of the back in an unusual position and lifting in bent forward position are frequently reported occurrences associated with disk herniation. Herniation of the nucleus pulposus produces pain, sensory loss, and paralysis by pressure on the spinal nerve roots or on the spinal cord. The most commonly affected are the lumbosacral intervertebral disks, which reflect a clinical picture of sciatica. Herniations of the cervical disks occur occasionally and those in the thoracic region are rare.

The clinical findings associated with ruptured or herniated disks are related to the size and location of the extruded material. Single nerve roots may be involved in small lesions; however, several roots may be compressed. Compression of the spinal cord may occur with large lesions and symptoms are reflective of spinal cord tumors.

The vast majority (90%) of the *lumbosacral herniations* occur at the fourth or fifth lumbar interspace. The sciatic symptoms associated with the lumbosacral herniation include pain in the lower back radiating down the posterior surface of one or both legs. In unilateral involvement scoliosis occurs toward the opposite side of sciatic pain and movement of the lumbar spine is limited. Paresthesias in the leg or foot are common. Tenderness is experienced on palpation along the course of the sciatic nerve. Motor weakness occurs in a small percentage of the cases. Hypoesthesia to touch or pinprick is present in about one-half of cases. A decreased or absent ankle reflex is common with herniation of the lumbosacral disc. Coughing, sneezing, or straining may produce radiation of pain along the course of the sciatic nerve.

Herniation of the cervical disks occur most commonly at the level of the fifth through seventh cervical nerves (C5–C7). Displacement of the disk in this region causes stiffness of the neck, shoulder pain radiating down the arm into the hand. Paresthesias may accompany the pain. Weakness and atrophy of the biceps and diminution of the biceps reflex may be present with sixth cervical root involvement. Paresthesias and sensory loss in the index finger, weakness of the triceps muscle, and loss of triceps reflex are indicative of involvement of the seventh cervical root.

DIAGNOSIS AND MANAGEMENT OF HERNIATED DISKS. X-ray findings supportive of a herniated disk show loss of normal curvature of the spine, scoliosis, and narrowing of intervertebral spaces. The most conclusive diagnosis can be demonstrated by myelography, which reveals defects in outline of the subarachnoid space or interruption of the flow of the dye in the presence of herniated disks. An elevated cerebrospinal protein content is an additional supportive finding and complete or partial cerebrospinal fluid block may be present with extrusions in the thoracic or cervical regions.

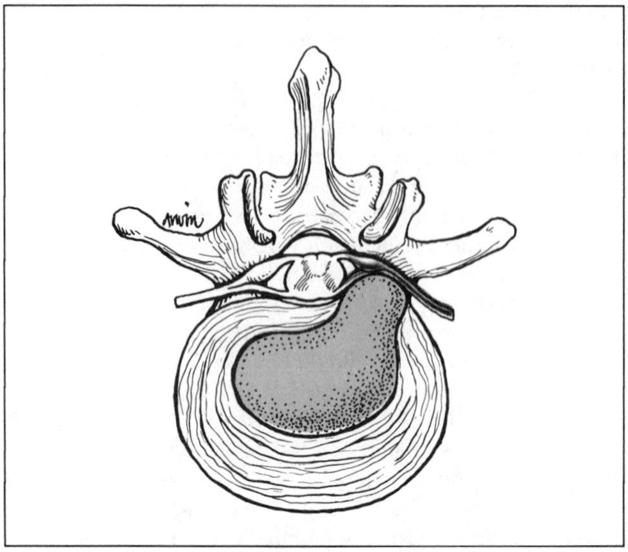

FIGURE 45-15. Herniated disk. (From R. Judge, G. Zuidema, and F. Fitzgerald, *Clinical Diagnosis: A Physiologic Approach*. Boston: Little, Brown, 1982.)

Conservative treatment in the acute stage is focused on bed rest, local heat application, and analgesics. Traction to lower extremities may be utilized initially with lumbosacral disk herniations. Cervical halter traction is indicated for cervical disk involvement. Surgical intervention is indicated if conservative modes of treatment fail and signs of cord compression develop. Simple removal of the disk is commonly performed to relieve the symptoms.

DIAGNOSTIC STUDIES OF NERVOUS SYSTEM ALTERATIONS

A variety of studies may be undertaken to support and expand the impression given from the presenting clinical signs. The diagnostic studies commonly used are described in this section.

Lateral and Posteroanterior (AP) X Rays of Skull and Cervical Spine

X rays are generally done initially as they give certain vital information and can be completed with relative ease. The films will reveal any skull fractures and shifting of the calcified pineal gland, thereby indicating the presence of mass lesions such as subdural hematomas. Fractures, fracture compressions, and subluxations of the cervical spine can be revealed by plain x rays.

Cerebral Angiography

This test provides for localization of substantive subdural hematomas, which show a characteristic vascular area. Vascular lesions such as aneurysms and arteriovenous malformations can be diagnosed effectively by angiography. This invasive procedure involves the injection of a radiopaque dye, such as Iodopyracet, into an arterial blood vessel for the purpose of the visualization of the cerebral circulation. Common injection sites of the contrast media are the internal carotid arteries or the vertebral arteries. Alternate indirect injections may be through the aortic arch or brachial vessels. Occasionally the femoral artery approach is used as some consider this a safer approach.

Computerized Axial Tomography (CAT or CT Scan)

This procedure is a relatively new, very useful, effective, and rapid radiographic modality used for the diagnosis of nervous system lesions. An Electronics and Musical Instrumentation Ltd. (EMI) Scanner uses a narrow moving beam of x ray to scan successive layers of the head. A small computer then processes the accumulated x-ray data by calculating the differences in tissue density in contiguous tissue slices. Pathologic changes can be constructed from the density data in terms of shape, size, and position of structures of the brain. A wide variety of intracranial disorders may be demonstrated by the CAT scan, including traumatic intracranial hematomas, neoplasms, cerebral infarctions, hydrocephalus, intracerebral hemorrhage, and brain abscesses. Certain spinal disorders, such as fractures and cord tumors, can be effectively diagnosed by the CAT scan.

CAT as a neurodiagnostic tool has proved to be more efficient in many situations than conventional radiologic and air studies by virtue of its rapidity, noninvasiveness, and relative reliability in diagnosis.

Echoencephalography

This study is a safe, noninvasive neurologic diagnostic tool that involves the use of an ultrasound generator and receiver that display echo pulsations on an oscilloscope. Permanent recording is done through an attached camera. Echos from deep within the skull "visualize" shifts in midline structures that may be reflective of intracranial trauma, cerebrovascular alterations, or space-occupying lesions. Lateral shifts of the pineal gland are also determined by echoencephalography as well as by plain x ray. The echoencephalogram has been useful as an adjunct to more conventional and accurate neurodiagnostic studies such as the CAT scan and angiography. The limitations in echoencephalography lie in the many chances for error in administering and interpreting the test.

Brain Scan

The *brain scan* is a safe neurodiagnostic technique used primarily for detection of intracranial tumors, abscesses, infarctions, and some subdural hematomas. It is not particularly useful in an acute head injury diagnosis as an intravenous injection of a radioactive substance must be given 1 to 2 hours before scanning. This time span is excessive in many head-injured patients who require rapid diagnosis and rapid treatment. Positive brain scans result when scalp contusions are present. As many acute head injuries are accompanied by scalp contusions, the scan findings may not present an accurate picture of the underlying brain pathology in these situations.

Pneumoencephalography

This procedure is used to diagnose space-occupying lesions and morphologic changes within the ventricular system. It is not feasible for diagnosis in acute head injuries because of the complex invasive nature of the procedure. It is contraindicated in situations where papilledema and increased intracranial pressure is evidenced.

This test involves the replacement of cerebrospinal fluid with air or oxygen by means of a lumbar puncture or, rarely, by cisternal puncture. The air enters the ventricular system primarily through the foramen of Magendie and serial x-ray films are taken to visualize the cerebral structures.

Ventriculography

This test is a variation of the pneumoencephalogram in which CSF replacement with air or oxygen is done directly in the lateral ventricles. This procedure is done in the operating room through skull burr holes and under local anesthesia. The ventriculogram is done for the diagnosis of expanding intracranial lesions.

Myelography

This procedure involves the introduction of a radiopaque substance into the spinal subarachnoid space for the purpose of visualizing spinal canal obstructions. Iophendylate (Pantopaque) is most commonly used and is injected via a lumbar puncture. Prior to the injection of the contrast media, the Queckenstedt's test may be done to determine patency of the spinal canal. This is accomplished by compressing the jugular veins when a lumbar puncture has been made. When the compression is maintained, the cerebrospinal fluid (CSF) pressure is elevated. A unilateral compression results in moderate elevation of CSF pressure, whereas bilateral compression shows an even higher rise. When the compression is terminated, the CSF pressure returns to normal. A failure of the rise and fall of the CSF pressure indicates some obstruction within the spinal canal above the lumbar puncture site.

Myelography is done in the x-ray department on a tilt table so that the patient can be manipulated for spinal canal filling in several positions. With the patient in position and lumbar puncture accomplished, approximately 10 ml of CSF is withdrawn and the radiopaque material is injected slowly. Serial x rays are then taken in various parts of the spinal canal. On completion of the x rays, the contrast media is removed.

Myelography is most commonly used for the diagnosis of intravertebral disk protrusions of herniations. Abnormalities in the x rays indicate incomplete canal filling with contrast media or total obstruction of its flow. In addition to disk abnormalities, tumors and adhesions encroaching on the spinal canal can be demonstrated by myelography.

Electroencephalography (EEG)

A significant tool in assessment of the ongoing spontaneous electrical activity of the cerebral cortex is the electroencephalogram (EEG), which is recorded from the surface of the scalp. Hans Berger, a German psychiatrist, first demonstrated this cerebral activity in the 1930s. Electrodes are placed on the skull and variations in potential are recorded between two cortical electrodes (bipolar record) or between a cortical electrode and an indifferent electrode usually placed on the ear (unipolar record). Simultaneous recordings from numerous portions of the cranium are accomplished by varied systematic electrode placements. The EEG activity reflects the graded potential changes in the cortical neuron dendrites. This cortical activity, in turn, is dependent on stimuli reaching it from deeper brain structures, as has been demonstrated by studies that indicate that the cerebral cortex separated from these structures lacks the normal EEG patterns. Additional support for deep structure effect on the EEG recording is the fact that both cerebral hemispheres generally demonstrate synchronous activity suggesting a pacemaker mechanism in the deeper structures of the brain (see pp. 678–679).

The changes observed in the EEG patterns in response to afferent stimulation are referred to as *desynchronization* of the EEG. This occurs whenever eyes are opened and alpha rhythm is replaced by a high-frequency, low-amplitude activity that exhibits no dominant pattern. Synchronized alpha activity indicates that many dendrite units are firing simultaneously, resulting in a rhythmic discharge. The EEG is affected in frequency and amplitude by the electrode placement, the activity or behavior of the subject, emotional status, biochemical and structural status of the cortex. Oscillations vary from 1 to 50 Hz and scalp voltage amplitude ranges widely according to internal and external environmental conditions.

TYPES OF BRAIN WAVES. The normal EEG depends on the integrity and normal functioning of the cerebral cortex as well as certain structures deep in the brain. Four principal wavebands are commonly recorded in the normal individual's brain function. These include alpha, beta, theta, and delta waves.

The alpha waves make up alpha rhythm that ranges at frequencies of 8 to 13 per second but most commonly occurs at a 9 to 10 per second frequency (Fig. 45-16). *Alpha waves* are recorded symmetrically in most normal adults from the postcentral regions. These are not fully developed until about age 13 and may exhibit greater amplitude on the right side in younger individuals. Alpha waves are

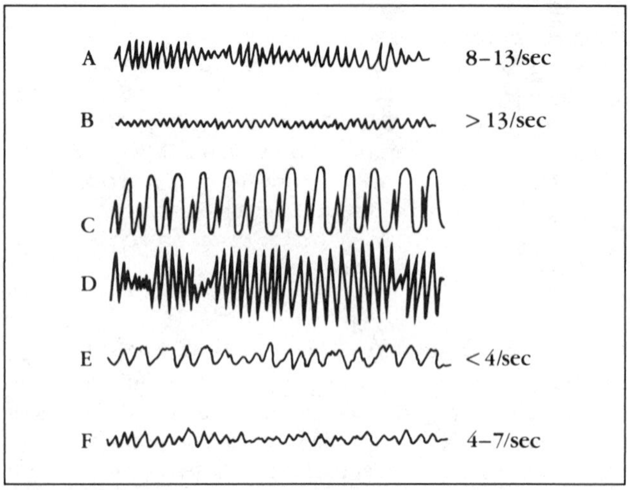

FIGURE 45-16. EEG waves: A. Alpha waves. B. Beta waves. C. Spike and dome waves during petit mal seizure. D. High-frequency spike waves during grand mal seizure. E. Delta waves. F. Theta waves.

present only in the resting person whose eyes are closed. When eyes open the alpha waves disappear and are replaced by an asynchronous rhythm of low voltage. Metabolic aberrations such as anoxia and hypoglycemia slow alpha frequency.

Beta waves are recorded from the precentral portion of the brain and represent activity of the motor cortex (see Fig. 45-16). Their frequency is above 13 cps and the amplitude is generally low. Beta activity may predominate in some people and is seen to replace alpha waves in persons who are tense and anxious. Voluntary movement can block beta wave activity. Closely related to beta waves and recorded from central regions of the brain are *mu waves*. These waves have a relatively high amplitude and a frequency of about one-half of beta waves. Like beta waves, their activity is also blocked by voluntary movement.

Theta waves project a frequency between 4 to 7 cps and an amplitude comparable to that of beta waves (see Fig. 45-16). These are recorded primarily in children and some adults in emotional distress from the parietal and frontotemporal regions of the brain. Visual attention may block theta wave activity.

Delta waves encompass all the electrical rhythms of less than 4 cps (Fig. 45-16). This pattern is observed normally when the individual is in deeper stages of sleep, in young children, and as the dominant rhythm in infants. Presence of delta waves in the awake adult may signify organic brain pathology.

A significant correlation exists between an individual's level of arousal and the dominant frequency of the EEG. Waves appear at 3 or fewer per second in deep sleep states and, as sleep lightens, burst of 10 to 12 waves/second begin to appear at shorter and shorter intervals until the waking state when a continuous more rapid frequency and lower amplitude rhythm dominate. Thus, a direct correlation can be observed in the person's state of arousal and the cortical electrical activity recorded on the EEG.

EEG evaluations are significant in contributing to the diagnostic process of patients with cranial neurologic problems. Characteristic rhythms are observed with the various epileptic seizure attacks (see Fig. 45-16) as well as during the intervals between these attacks. Focal damage to the cortex, either of internal or external origin, is usually reflected by an irregular and abnormal rhythm, which generally is slow and asymmetric with its corresponding hemispheric position.

REFERENCES

1. Finkelstein, S., and Ropper, A. The diagnoses of coma: Its pitfalls and limitations. *Heart Lung* 8:1059, 1979.
2. Guyton, A. *Textbook of Medical Physiology* (5th ed.). Philadelphia: Saunders, 1976. P. 731.
3. Lewis, A. *Mechanisms of Neurologic Disease.* Boston: Little, Brown, 1976.
4. Plum, F., and Posner, J. *The Diagnosis of Stupor and Coma* (3rd ed.). Philadelphia: Davis, 1980. P. 3.

CHAPTER 46
TUMORS AND INFECTIONS OF THE CENTRAL NERVOUS SYSTEM

LEARNING OBJECTIVES

1. Identify the tissue from which central nervous system (CNS) tumors may originate.
2. Describe the classification systems for cranial and spinal tumors.
3. Compare the incidence and malignancy of brain and spinal tumors.
4. Name the brain tumors that occur most often in children and those that occur most often in adults.
5. Describe CNS alterations that lead to focal disturbances and increased intracranial pressure.
6. State what is thought to be the basis for the localized cerebral edema that surrounds brain tumors.
7. Describe CNS alterations that lead to the development of papilledema.
8. State the body's compensatory mechanisms for dealing with increased intracranial pressure.
9. List three types of brain herniations.
10. Describe the clinical manifestations associated with each type of brain herniation.
11. Discuss alterations that occur as a result of the various types of spinal tumors.
12. Identify the classic triad of clinical manifestations that are associated with brain tumors.
13. Describe the basis for the development of the classic triad of clinical manifestations associated with brain tumors.
14. Discuss the clinical manifestations associated with tumors of the frontal lobe, temporal lobe, parietal lobe, occipital lobe, cerebellum, and brainstem.
15. Discuss clinical manifestations associated with the various types of spinal tumors, as well as manifestations associated with the various levels of compression by spinal tumors.
16. List the steps used in diagnosis of CNS tumors.
17. Describe techniques used to diagnose brain and spinal tumors.
18. Compare and contrast characteristics of the various CNS tumors (tissue type, appearance of the tumor, rate of growth, invasive qualities, CNS alterations, and pertinent clinical manifestations).
19. State the two most common primary sites from which metastasis occurs to the brain.
20. State the various routes by which microorganisms reach the CNS.
21. List the ways in which viruses gain access to the body.
22. State the ways in which viruses invade the CNS.
23. Compare and contrast characteristics of the various CNS infections (routes of infection, CNS alterations, pertinent clinical manifestations, and prognosis).

Tumors of the central nervous system and the invasion of this system by infectious organisms are discussed in this chapter. Incidence, alterations within the central nervous system, resultant clinical manifestations, and relevant diagnostic studies are reviewed. However, the topic is vast and the reader is referred to special texts for additional information and study of the subject.

TUMORS OF THE CENTRAL NERVOUS SYSTEM

General Considerations

Tumors of the central nervous system (CNS) include both benign and malignant neoplasms within the brain as well as the spinal cord. These tumors can arise from any of the cells within the CNS. Thus, it is possible to have tumors originating from the glial cells, the neurons, the blood vessels and connective tissue, the meninges, the pituitary gland, and the pineal gland (Fig. 46-1). Metastatic tumors from primary sites throughout the body are also encountered within the CNS.

With the variety and complexity of intracranial tumors, classification of tumors becomes a problem. An adaptation of the Kernahan and Sayre classification is found in Table 46-1. This classification is based on naming the tumor in relation to cells present in the adult nervous system, in vascular tissue, and in developmental defects. A malignancy grading of I to IV is also included, with I being the least malignant.

Classification of intraspinal tumors is done in accordance with the location of the tumor in relation to the dura and spinal cord. Thus, two groups are generally considered: *extradural*, those arising from the extradural space or vertebral bodies, and *intradural*, which includes those arising from the blood vessels, meninges, or nerve roots (extramedullary) and those arising from within the substance of the spinal cord itself (intramedullary) (Table 46-2).

Generally speaking, the location, size, and invasive quality of intracranial and intraspinal neoplasms are responsible for the production of certain neurologic symptoms. The destruction and displacement of tissue, in addition to increased intracranial pressure, causes the onset of specific symptoms. Morbidity and mortality associated with intracranial tumors are high, but advancements in diagnostic techniques, medical therapeutics, and neurosurgical techniques have improved the prognosis. Spinal cord tumors are more easily removed surgically than brain tumors. Thus, if recognized early and removed, prognosis for patients with intraspinal tumors is quite favorable.

Incidence of Central Nervous System Tumors

Primary CNS tumors are not rare. As an intracranial disease, tumor is second in frequency only to stroke.

Although it is difficult to establish an accurate incidence of primary tumors in the general population, Table 46-1

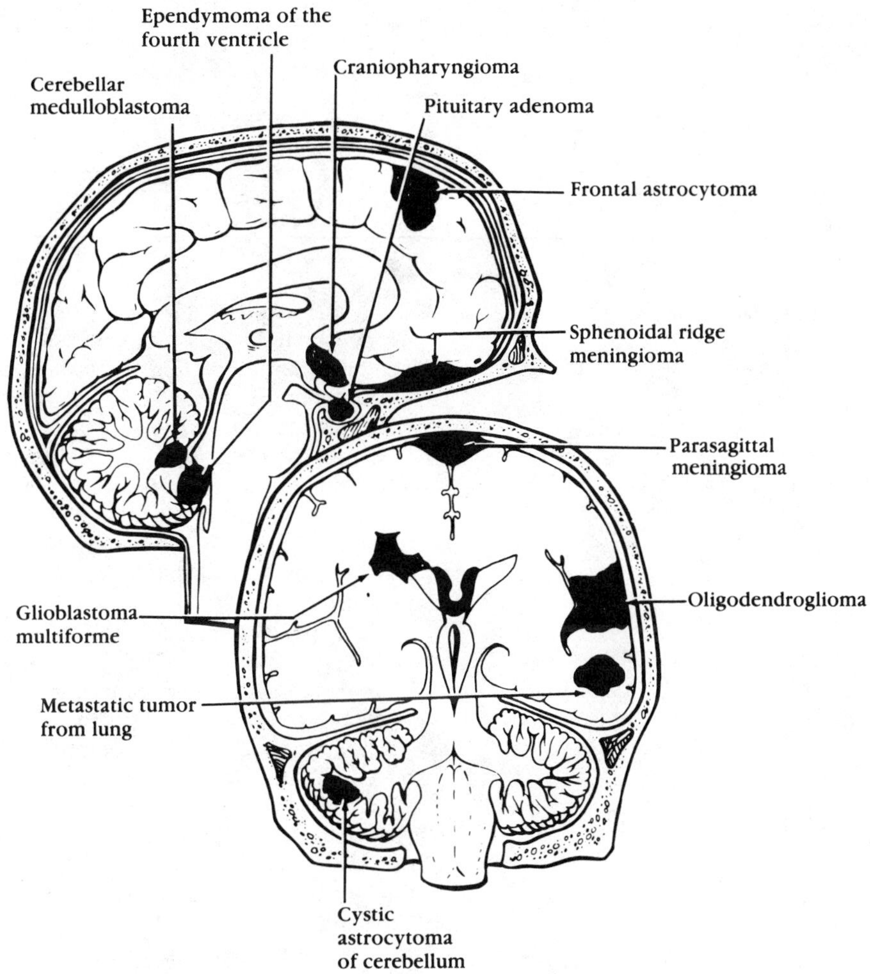

FIGURE 46-1. Common intracranial tumors and the positions in which they frequently occur. Metastatic tumors may localize anywhere. (From M. Snyder and M. Jackle, *Neurologic Nursing: A Critical Care Nursing Focus*. Bowie, Md.: Brady, 1981.)

presents widely accepted percentages of occurrence for the various types of intracranial neoplasms. The brain and its coverings are also involved by neoplasm in 20 percent of all patients who have cancer [1]. Furthermore, according to Russell and Rubinstein, 1.2 percent of all autopsies indicate the presence of tumors of the CNS, dura, or meninges [7].

Although intracranial tumors can occur at any age, there seems to be an increased incidence in young children and again in the fifth and sixth decades of life. Between the ages of 6 and 15 years of age, brain tumors are the second most common malignancy and third most common from birth to 5 years [2]. The more common brain tumors during childhood include: craniopharyngiomas, ependymomas, medulloblastomas, cerebellar and cerebral astrocytomas, brainstem gliomas, optic path gliomas, and pinealomas. In adults, gliomas account for 45 percent of all brain tumors [4]. Furthermore, pituitary adenomas, acoustic neuromas, and meningiomas are more prevalent during adulthood and almost completely absent during childhood.

Intraspinal tumors occur less frequently than those that involve the brain and are rare in children. Of 8784 primary CNS tumors in a Mayo Clinic series of cases, only 15 percent were within the spine [9]. Twenty-five percent of intraspinal tumors are extradural and are generally of a metastatic nature. Seventy-five percent are intradural spinal tumors. Of the intradural tumors, the extramedullary lesions are more frequent than the intramedullary lesions (see Table 46-2). Extramedullary tumors are usually meningiomas or neurofibromas and are more easily removed surgically. Intramedullary tumors consist of the same cellu-

TABLE 46-1. Brain tumors

Tumor	Percent
Tumors of neuroglia cells (gliomas)	40–50
Astrocytoma grade I	5–10
Astrocytoma grade II	2–5
Astrocytoma grade III and IV (glioblastoma multiforme)	20–30
Oligodendroglioma	1–4
Ependymoma grades I–IV	1–3
Tumors of neuronal origin*	
Cerebral neuroblastomas	
Gangliogliomas	
Tumors of primitive or undifferentiated cells	
Medulloblastoma	3–5
Tumors of the meninges	12–20
Meningioma	
Meningeal sarcomas	
Tumors of the pituitary gland	5–15
Tumors of cranial and peripheral nerves and nerve roots	3–10
Neurilemmomas	
Neurofibromas	
Tumors of blood vessels	0.5–1.0
Arteriovenous malformations	
Hemangioblastomas	
Endotheliomas	
Tumors of developmental defects	3–8
Dermoids, teratomas, chordomas, craniopharyngiomas	
Tumors of adenexal structures	0.5–0.8
Pinealomas	
Choroid plexus papillomas	
Metastatic tumors	5–10

*These tumors compose less than 1–3% of the total occurrence of brain tumors.
Source: S. I. Schwartz (ed.), *Principles of Surgery* (2nd ed.). New York: McGraw-Hill, 1974. P. 1646.

lar origins as intracranial tumors and generally infiltrate surrounding tissue. These intramedullary tumors are frequently gliomas (particularly ependymomas), with the astrocytomas, oligodendrogliomas, glioblastomas, hemangioblastomas, and medulloblastomas occurring less frequently.

Alterations Within the Central Nervous System due to Tumors

Brain tumors may be "benign" or "malignant" with regard to histology and morphology of their cellular components. However, it must be remembered that all tumors of the brain are potentially harmful due to their relationship to vital structures. Thus, malignant or harmful effects may be produced by histologically benign lesions.

Brain tumors rarely metastasize to extraneural tissue. However, these neoplasms infiltrate into surrounding nervous tissue, into the meninges, or through the ependymal layer into the ventricles. Once the tumor gains access to the subarachnoid space or ventricular system, and thus the cerebrospinal fluid (CSF) pathways, its spread may occur throughout the entire CNS. This may include the spinal cord and peripheral nerve roots [6].

TABLE 46-2. Intraspinal lesions

Lesion	Occurrence (%)
Extradural	25
Intradural	75
Extramedullary	50
Intramedullary	25

Source: S. L. Robbins, and R. Cotran, *Pathologic Basis of Disease* (2nd ed.). Philadelphia: Saunders, 1979.

Within the confined space of the skull, a growing tumor alters the normally stable volume of the brain, the blood, and the CSF. Thus, as the mass grows, compression of brain tissue as well as alterations in blood and CSF circulation lead to focal disturbances and increased intracranial pressure.

More specifically, tumor growth can produce any of several alterations. Compression of brain tissue and invasion of brain parenchyma cause destruction of neural tissue. Blood circulation may be decreased to such an extent that necrosis of brain tissue occurs. Compression, infiltration of neural tissue, and decreased blood supply may also lead to altered neural excitability with resultant seizure activity. Furthermore, elevation of capillary pressure, due to compression of venules in the area adjacent to the tumor, is thought to be the basis for localized cerebral edema that surrounds the tumor.

As the volume of the intracranial contents is increased, CSF is displaced from the subarachnoid space and ventricles through the foramen magnum to the spinal subarachnoid space. CSF is also displaced through the optic foramen to the perioptic subarachnoid space. With elevations in CSF pressure, particularly in the perioptic subarachnoid space, venous drainage from the optic nerve head and retina is impaired. This is manifested by papilledema or "choked disk." Growth of the mass may also obstruct CSF circulation from the lateral ventricles to the subarachnoid space with resultant hydrocephalus.

Rapid development of any of the previously discussed situations causes a life-threatening increase in intracranial pressure. Compensatory mechanisms exist and include decreased parenchymal cell numbers, decreased intracellular fluid contents, decreased CSF volume, and decreased intracranial blood volume. However, these compensatory mechanisms may take days or months to be effective and are thus not useful with rapidly developing intracranial pressure [8].

Untreated increased intracranial pressure may cause brain herniation. Brain herniations are possible because of the subdivision of the cranial cavity into compartments by the relatively rigid dura. The supratentorial space is divided into right and left halves by the falx cerebri. The cerebellum and occipital lobes are separated by the tentorium. Thus, pressure from a mass causes herniations from one compartment to another compartment to another compartment. Three well-known types of herniations include the *temporal lobe-tentorial herniation*, the cerebellar-foramen magnum herniation, and the subfalcial herniation [1]. Of great importance clinically is the temporal lobe-tentorial herniation in which the medial part of one temporal lobe (usually the uncus) is forced into the tentorial opening. A large amount of pressure is exerted on the midbrain and subthalamic structures. Clinical effects of this herniation are of two types, *central* and *uncal*. The central type is characterized by the following clinical effects: stupor, irregular respirations, small pupils with eventual paralysis of vertical and contralateral gaze, stiffness of neck muscles and decerebrate and decorticate postures with deepening coma. The uncal type is characterized by the following effects: third cranial nerve palsy on the side of the lesion with ptosis, dilated pupils, then paralysis of ocular muscles; decreasing levels of consciousness; respiratory changes with Cheyne-Stokes breathing; hyperpnea; quiet, irregular breathing and finally respiratory arrest; ipsilateral or contralateral hemiplegia with bilateral Babinski signs; the decerebrate posture [1].

The *cerebellar-foramen magnum* herniation is where the inferior, medial parts of the cerebellar hemispheres are displaced downward through the foramen magnum behind the cervical cord. Clinical effects of this herniation include: respiratory disturbances, cardiac irregularity, arching of the neck and back, extension and internal rotation of the limbs, and loss of consciousness [1].

The *subfalcial herniation* is where the medial part of one parietal or frontal lobe is pushed under the falx. Little is known regarding its clinical manifestations [1].

Alterations as a result of intraspinal tumors are largely due to compression of the spinal cord, interference with circulation, and pressure on veins or arteries. Ischemia of cord segments occurs as well as edema below the level of compression. Extradural spinal tumors usually result from extraneural metastases, particularly from the breast or lung, which cause rapid compression of the spinal cord. Hemorrhage due to the metastasis as well as vertebral column collapse add to the compressive effects of extradural tumors.

Extrameduallary tumors are basically of two types, *neurofibromas* and *meningiomas*, and are generally benign. Neurofibromas grow on the nerve root and often form an hourglasslike expansion that extends into the extradural space. Meningiomas grow from the arachnoid membrane. These tumors are commonly found in the posterolateral aspect of the cord. They often result in the Brown-Séquard syndrome, due to the compressive damage to one-half of the spinal cord (see Chap. 45).

As mentioned previously, intramedullary tumors are histologically the same as intracranial tumors. These lesions damage sensory fibers that cross each other in the center of the cord. They also destroy neurons.

Clinical Manifestations of Central Nervous System Tumors

The symptoms produced by intracranial tumors are extremely variable and depend on characteristics of the neoplasm, invasive qualities, location, and rate of growth. However, since these tumors eventually give rise to an increase in intracranial pressure, a classic triad of symptoms usually occurs. These symptoms are headache, vomiting, and papilledema.

Headache is a common symptom of persons with intracranial tumors. The cause is thought to result from displacement and traction of pain-sensitive structures within the skull—cranial nerves, arteries, veins, and venous sinuses. The headache may be dull and is usually temporary. In others, the pain is severe, dull or sharp, and intermittent. It is generally more severe on awakening and tends to improve throughout the day. Typically, it is aggravated by stooping, coughing, or straining to have a bowel movement. In general, the headache has little localizing value with regard to tumor site.

Vomiting is also experienced by many persons with intracranial tumors. It is a result of stimulation of the emetic center in the medulla. Vomiting associated with tumors is not necessarily preceded by nausea and is not related to ingestion of food. It often occurs before breakfast and is frequently projectile in nature.

Papilledema may not be present in the early stages of tumor growth but occurs as intracranial pressure increases. However, in some persons papilledema is not seen even when the intracranial pressure becomes greatly elevated. Hemorrhages may be seen around the optic disk in association with papilledema. Complaints of blurred vision and halos around lights with an enlargement of a blind spot and fleeting moments of dimmed vision (amaurosis fugax) may be elicited.

Other than the classic triad of symptoms, local effects of intracranial tumors occur due to irritation, destruction, or compression of neural tissue in the particular location of the tumor. Generally speaking, supratentorial lesions give rise to paralysis, seizures, memory loss, and visual field defects; infratentorial lesions give rise to cranial nerve dysfunction and ataxia.

Frontal lobe tumors cause disturbed mental status, speech disturbances, hemiparesis, and ataxia. Mental symptoms are manifested by progressive apathy, mild dementia with impairment of memory and intellect, decreased judgment, altered social adaptation, and depression. Aphasia or apraxia may occur when the left or dominant frontal lobe is affected. Pressure on motor areas produces hemiparesis and may result in jacksonian seizures. The unsteady gait as-

TABLE 46-3. Common symptoms of spinal cord tumors

Symptom	Description
Pain in spine, neck, back	Usually gradual onset; may occur suddenly with sudden movement or injury; aggravated by Valsalva maneuver; nocturnal pain predominates due to recumbency (patient may prefer to sleep upright)
Radicular pain	Occurs in the distribution of segmental innervation; aggravated by movement that alters anatomic relationships; causes diagnostic confusion (T8 root involvement may be misinterpreted as ulcer disease)
Medullary referred pain	Shooting or burning over peripheral areas; often bilateral; not influenced by Valsalva maneuver; appears at different sites
Motor disturbances	Motor deficits are caused by lesions of the pyramidal or corticospinal tracts, causing spasticity and increased reflexes and spastic gait; weakness may present as a limp in the guise of muscle stiffness or rigidity
Nonspecific sensory disturbances	Numbness; tingling; coldness

Source: F. McQuat, The insidious spinal cord tumor. *J. Neurosurg. Nurs.* 13:18, 1981.

sociated with frontal lobe tumors may resemble cerebellar ataxia.

Temporal lobe tumors cause sensory aphasia, which begins with difficulty in naming objects. Tinnitus occurs as a result of irritation to the adjacent cortex or temporal auditory receptor. Anterior temporal lobe tumors cause visual field changes that may progress to complete hemianopsia. Psychomotor seizures may occur.

Parietal lobe involvement may include motor-sensory focal seizures, agnosia, hypoesthesia (decreased sensibility to touch), paresthesia, and dyslexia. Visual defects may also occur.

Involvement of the occipital lobe may produce visual field disturbances in the form of homonymous hemianopsia. This may be associated with visual agnosia (loss of comprehension of visual sensation), hallucinations, and convulsive seizures that are preceded by an aura.

Cerebellar tumors produce disturbances in equilibrium and coordination. The specific type of disorder depends on the location and size of the tumor. Disorders of movement may include nystagmus, adiadochokinesis (inability to make rapid alternating movements), asynergia (incoordination of muscle groups), dysmetria (abnormal force of muscular movements), intention tremor, and deviation from a line of movement [5]. Hypotonia may be present. Speech disturbances may be noted with tendency toward staccato or scanning speech. Papilledema is often seen when a cerebellar tumor is present.

Brainstem involvement produces varied effects. There is increasing paralysis of the cranial nerves with paralysis of eye movements, loss of facial sensation, and difficulty swallowing. Lesions of the hypothalamus may produce diabetes insipidus, obesity, disturbances of temperature regulation, and somnolence.

Clinical manifestations associated with spinal cord tumors depend on the type of lesion and the level at which the lesion occurs. A summary of signs and symptoms of spinal cord lesions appears in Table 46-3.

Generally speaking, a soft, slow-growing mass causes gradual compression of the spinal cord with gradually increasing neurologic signs. Malignant and metastatic tumors cause rapid compression of the spinal cord and destruction of the neural tissue.

Extradural tumors usually result from metastasis from primary tumor sites. Local, dull pain is often the first symptom; it is intensified with movements of the spine. Later, due to rapid growth, the spinal cord becomes compressed. Early signs of cord compression include loss of joint position sense, loss of vibration, and spastic weakness below the level in which the lesion occurs. Without surgical removal of the tumor, irreversible damage that may include irreversible paraplegia occurs.

Extramedullary lesions, primarily neurofibromas and meningiomas, are usually benign. There is pain in the back and along the spinal roots. The pain is worse at night and is aggravated by movement or straining. Posteriorly situated tumors produce sensory losses including paresthesia and loss of proprioceptive sense. Sensory loss first occurs below the level of the lesion. Anterior compression of the cord causes severe motor dysfunctions. Lateral cord compression may produce the Brown-Séquard syndrome, in which there is ipsilateral motor weakness and deep sensory loss, as well as contralateral loss of pain and temperature perception below the level of the lesion. Early diagnosis and surgical removal produce good prognosis.

Intramedullary tumors tend to be more histologically benign and have a more benign course than similar intracranial tumors. There is usually a dull, aching pain in the area of the lesion. A dissociated sensory loss occurs in which there is a bilateral sensory loss of pain and temperature that extends through all involved segments; however, there is usually preservation of the senses of touch, motion, position, and vibration. Intramedullary tumors may extend through several spinal cord segments making surgical removal more difficult.

The various levels of compression by spinal cord tumors are as follows: the foramen magnum, the cervical region, the thoracic region, the lumbar-sacral region, and the cauda equina. A summary of signs and symptoms of common root lesions appears in Table 46-4.

TABLE 46-4. Symptoms and signs of common root lesions

Root	Location of pain	Sensory loss	Reflex loss	Weakness and atrophy
C5	Lower neck, tip of shoulder, arm	Deltoid area (inconsistent)	Biceps	Shoulder abductors, biceps
C6	Lower neck, medial scapula, arm, radial side of forearm	Radial side of hand, thumb, index finger	Biceps	Biceps
C7	Lower neck, medial scapula, precordium, arm, forearm	Index finger, middle finger	Triceps	Triceps
C8	Lower neck, medial arm and forearm, ulnar side of hand, fourth and fifth fingers	Ulnar side of hand, fourth and fifth fingers		Intrinsic hand muscles
L4	Low back, anterior and medial thigh	Anterior thigh	Quadriceps	Quadriceps
L5	Low back, lateral thigh, lateral leg, dorsum of foot, great toe	Great toe, medial side of dorsum of foot, lateral leg, and thigh		Toe extensors, ankle dorsiflexors, and evertors
S1	Low back, posterior thigh, posterior leg, lateral side of foot, heel	Lateral foot, heel, posterior leg	Achilles	Ankle dorsiflexion and plantar flexion

Source: J. Simpson and K. Magee, *Clinical Evaluation of the Nervous System*. Boston: Little, Brown, 1970. P. 114.

A tumor in the area of the foramen magnum compresses intracranial contents, nerve roots, and the spinal cord. This causes suboccipital pain. Dermatones C2 and C3 are compressed, which produces weakness of the head and neck. As the tumor extends into the intracranial cavity, increased pressure is produced as well as pressure on the cerebellum and cranial nerve nuclei.

Tumors in the cervical region produce motor and sensory losses in the shoulders, arms, and hands. Bicep, tricep, and brachioradial tendon reflexes may be lost if the lesion occurs in the lower cervical region.

Thoracic lesions may produce pain and tightness across the chest and abdomen. Lower-extremity paresthesia may develop with the loss of abdominal reflexes when the lesion is in the lower thoracic area.

Upper lumbar lesions cause hip flexion weakness, lower leg spasticity, loss of knee jerk reflexes, brisk ankle reflexes, and bilateral Babinski signs. Pain usually occurs in the groin area.

Lower lumbar and upper sacral lesions cause weakness of perineal, calf, and foot muscles. There is often loss of the Achilles reflex.

Lower sacral lesions cause sensation losses in the perianal area. Bladder and bowel control may be impaired.

Lesions in the cauda equina region cause impotence and loss of sphincter control. There is pain in the sacral and perineal areas that often radiates to the legs.

Diagnosis of Central Nervous System Tumors

The following steps are used in diagnosing CNS tumors: (1) A detailed history is elicited and careful neurologic examination is performed. (2) Special radiologic investigations are performed depending on the findings of the neurologic examination. *X rays* of the skull do not visualize the brain itself but reflect changes caused by chronically increased intracranial pressure. These changes include erosion of the sella turcica, calcification of the pineal body or of a lesion, increased density of surrounding bone, or destruction of vertebrae associated with spinal tumors. *Air encephalography* (AEG) performed through a lumbar puncture is useful in outlining tumors that impinge on CSF pathways or displace and distort the ventricles. *Ventriculography* is used to outline the ventricular system through the use of contrast material or air introduced directly into the lateral ventricle. This method is useful especially for persons with increased intracranial pressure in whom a lumbar puncture for the AEG could cause a cerebellar foramen magnum herniation. *Angiography* is useful in detecting displacement of vessels from their normal position due to tumor growth. It also provides information concerning the intrinsic vasculature of the tumor. *Isotopes* are useful because of the breakdown of the blood-brain barrier. This causes an abnormal accumulation of radioactive material that has been introduced by intravenous injection. With isotope scanning, blood supply to the tumor is important and avascular or small tumors may not be detected. More recently, the *computerized axial tomography* (CAT) scan has been the screening procedure of choice because it is noninvasive and nonpainful. CAT scanning involves the use of a computer, which because of various absorptive characteristics of brain tissue, blood, CSF, cyst fluid, and tumors, can process multiple high-speed x rays to produce a pictorial print of transverse sections of the body (see Chap. 45). An *electroencephalogram* (EEG) gives valuable information concerning altered neuron exitability and shows abnormalities in 75 percent of tumor cases [3]. An *echoencephalogram* shows shifts in intracranial contents. A *myelogram* is useful in localizing tumors of the spinal cord. *Lumbar puncture* may be performed to examine the CSF. In the presence of tumors this test usually reveals a normal CSF glucose, an elevated protein level, and sometimes tumor cells. During lumbar puncture a *Queckenstedt jugular compression test* can demonstrate a spinal subarachnoid block. Lumbar puncture is not performed when there is obvious evidence of increased intracranial pressure due to the danger of brain herniation.

Finally, to make a diagnosis, the histologic type of tumor must be determined. This usually requires surgery and tumor tissue examination.

Tumors of the Neuroglia Cells (Gliomas)

Neuroglial tumors or gliomas are classified according to cell type. The glial cells provide support and protection for nerve cells and include astrocytes, oligodendroglia, and ependymal cells. The tumors are named according to the cell type: astrocytomas, oligodendrogliomas, and ependymomas.

ASTROCYTOMAS. Astrocytomas develop from astrocytes. These spider or star-shaped cells infiltrate brain tissue and are frequently associated with various sizes of cysts. Their invasive nature usually makes surgical removal difficult. However, one special cystic type of astrocytoma that grows in the cerebellum has a good prognosis following removal.

Astrocytomas have varying degrees of malignancy. Most are well-differentiated and grow slowly for many years. Gross inspection usually reveals poorly defined gray white infiltrative masses that enlarge and distort underlying CNS tissue. They may be circumscribed occasionally [6]. The initial symptoms are seizures, headaches, and mental disturbances, but these may not develop for several years.

Other astrocytomas are very poorly differentiated, anaplastic astrocytomas that have a rapid rate of growth. On gross inspection, they are larger, more infiltrative lesions resulting in a dismal prognosis with death occurring in months to a few years.

Due to variations in anaplasia, a malignancy grading system of I to IV is used. Differentiated astrocytomas are referred to as grade I or II, anaplastic astrocytomas as grade III, and glioblastoma multiforme as grade IV. Rating systems are highly subjective and clinical usefulness is limited.

GLIOBLASTOMA MULTIFORME. Glioblastoma multiforme is an extremely malignant glioma that frequently arises from undifferentiated astrocytomas. The appearance on gross inspection varies according to the region of the brain in which they arise. Some appear white and firm while others appear yellow and soft [6]. Glioblastomas grow very rapidly, are invasive, and are resistant to various combinations of surgery, radiotherapy, and chemotherapy. Tissue necrosis and brain edema are characteristic with glioblastomas—thus, prognosis is poor. According to Robbins, 90 percent of these patients die within 2 years after diagnosis [6].

OLIGODENDROGLIOMAS. Oligodendrogliomas arise from oligodendroglia, a neuroglia with vinelike processes found sporadically throughout the CNS. Gross examination usually reveals well-defined, gray, globular masses. Masses may contain cystic foci, calcifications, and hemorrhagic areas [6]. These tumors are similar in behavior to astrocytomas in that they generally grow slowly. On occasion, however, rapid growth occurs and these tumors may imitate the glioblastomas. Distinction may be made only on histologic examination. Oligodendrogliomas also have a tendency to form focal calcification.

EPENDYMOMAS. Ependymal cells line the ventricular walls and form the central canal in the spinal cord. Generally, cranial ependymomas appear as fairly well-defined masses that grow by expansion [6]. Ependymomas that arise from ependymal cells lining the walls of the ventricular system fill and obstruct the ventricles and invade adjacent tissue. This can obstruct CSF passage and lead to the development of hydrocephalus.

Ependymomas that arise within the spinal cord represent a large percentage of intraspinal gliomas. Symptoms of spinal ependymomas are related to the spinal level at which they occur. The location of this type of tumor often makes them inaccessible to removal by surgery. Thus, even though these tumors grow slowly the prognosis is poor and death occurs in about 3 years.

Variants of ependymomas include subependymomas and myxopapillary ependymomas. Subependymomas arise from neuroglial tissue beneath the ependymal lining and are comprised of astrocytic and ependymal elements. These small, hard, lobular tumors rarely grow large enough to cause symptoms. Myxopapillary ependymomas are found almost exclusively in the filum terminale. When they are completely removed surgically, prognosis for survival is excellent.

Tumors of Neuronal Origin

Cerebral neuroblastomas arise in precursor cells of neurons. Gross examination reveals well-defined, gray granular masses that may contain areas of necrosis and hemorrhage and cysts [6]. Neuroblastomas are rare and usually occur during the first decade of life. Their rate of growth is rapid and they commonly recur following surgery. *Gangliogliomas* are very rare tumors composed of neuroglial tissue. Gross inspection reveals well-defined masses with granular surfaces. Calcifications and small cysts may be found within the mass. These tumors are usually found in children and young adults, and if the location permits surgical excision the prognosis is good.

Tumors of Primitive or Undifferentiated Cells

Medulloblastomas arise predominantly from primitive cells in the cerebellum. Thus, these tumors have the potential to develop along neuronal or neuroglial lines. Gross inspection generally reveals fairly well-demarcated, gray white masses with indistinct edges [6]. Medulloblastomas occur almost exclusively in children but have been found in adults up to the sixth decade of life. These tumors are highly malignant, grow rapidly, and infiltrate throughout the subarachnoid space with resultant widespread meningeal foci. CSF pathways become blocked and signs of increased intracranial pressure develop. This tumor is associated with increasing ataxia and forceful vomiting. The prognosis is dismal but combinations of surgery, radiotherapy, and chemotherapy can prolong survival.

Tumors of the Meninges

MENINGIOMAS. Meningiomas are primary tumors arising from the meninges. Meningeal constituents that may be involved include arachnoid cells, fibroblasts, or blood vessels. Gross inspection of this tumor tends to reveal tough, gray white, irregular-to-round, lobular masses [6]. Meningiomas are quite vascular and are seen readily with radioisotope scanning. They are usually well circumscribed, encapsulated, and press into surrounding tissue. The tumor may penetrate adjacent bone but widespread infiltration of surrounding nervous tissue is not common. Most of these tumors are benign and grow slowly so that initial symptoms may be overlooked. As the tumor continues to grow, symptoms include seizures, headache, visual impairment, hemiparesis, and aphasia. If the tumor is diagnosed early and if it is located in a position accessible to surgery, complete excision is possible and a good prognosis results.

MENINGEAL SARCOMAS. Spindle-cell sarcomas may arise in the meninges. These are malignant lesions that may metastasize to sites outside the nervous system, particularly to the lungs and lymph nodes.

Tumors of the Pituitary Gland

Pituitary tumors are a special group of nervous system tumors that produce neurologic signs and symptoms when they put pressure on the hypothalamus, optic chiasm, third ventricle, and medial temporal lobe. These tumors arise from the three cell types in the anterior pituitary: basophil cells, which stain blue; eosinophil cells, which stain red; and chromophobe cells, which do not stain. Although pituitary tumors have usually been classified according to cell type, it is more accurate to identify these tumors as functioning (secreting a hormone) or nonfunctioning (nonsecreting). However, the tumor usually contains a predominant cell type. Prognosis depends on the success of treatment, which may include radiation, hypophysectomy, and/or hormone replacement. *Adrenocorticotropic hormone (ACTH) producing pituitary tumors* are primarily composed of basophil cells and are usually so small that adjacent tissue is not compressed. However, they have powerful effects due to hypersecretion of ACTH, which is one of several mechanisms that produce Cushing's syndrome. Symptoms of Cushing's syndrome include weakness, emotional lability, moon face, obesity of the torso, hypertension, salt and water retention, diabetes mellitus, glycosuria, osteoporosis, skin striae over the abdomen, hirsutism, and amenorrhea (see Chap. 32). *Pituitary adenomas inducing gigantism and acromegaly* are primarily composed of eosinophilic cells and are small, rather slow-growing tumors. They cause an increase in the output of growth hormone. If the tumor develops before bone growth is complete gigantism results. Tumor development after bone growth has stopped produces the clinical picture, called acromegaly. These adenomas may grow to such a size that they press on the optic chiasm, causing bitemporal hemianopsia or other visual disturbances. *Nonsecreting pituitary adenomas* are the most common pituitary tumors and are composed primarily of chromophobes. Although the chromophobe cells have no known special function, tumors arising from these cells are rather large and produce symptoms by compression of the pituitary gland, the optic chiasm, the hypothalamus, and adjacent brain tissue. Signs and symptoms that result from this tumor include a sallow appearance, loss of body hair, weakness, amenorrhea, loss of sexual desire, low basal metabolism, hypoglycemia, hypotension, and electrolyte disturbances. As the tumor presses on the optic chiasm, bitemporal hemianopsia is produced and blindness may result (see Chap. 30).

Tumors of the Cranial and Peripheral Nerves and Nerve Roots

Neurilemmomas (schwannomas) and neurofibromas arise from cells that ensheath cranial nerves, peripheral nerves, and nerve roots. The three types of cells within the nerve sheaths include: Schwann cells, perineural cells, and fibroblasts in the epineurium and endoneurium. Although the three cells are similar morphologically, the Schwann cell is generally the primary source of tumors. *Neurilemmomas (schwannomas)* are tumors that arise from the Schwann cells and occur on any of the nerves or nerve roots. The tumors are firm, circumscribed, well-encapsulated, and white to gray in color. Multiple lesions may be found on the same nerve or throughout the body. However, they often involve the acoustic (eighth) nerve, most frequently at the cerebello-pontile angle, or where the acoustic nerve enters the internal auditory meatus. Bilateral involvement of the acoustic nerve occurs in von Recklinghausen's neurofibromatosis. Acoustic nerve neurilemmomas produce the following symptoms due to position and/or functional disruption: impaired hearing, tinnitus, vertigo, loss of caloric vestibular reactivity with horizontal nystagmus, palsies of the fifth and seventh cranial nerves, ataxia, and signs of increased intracranial pressure. Complete surgical removal is usually attempted in order to prevent recurrence of the tumor, but this often produces cranial nerve dysfunctions such as deafness or facial paralysis. *Neurofibromas* arise primarily from Schwann cells and fibroblasts. Gross examination reveals enlargement of the affected nerve or nerve root [6]. Multiple tumors are often present especially when associated with the hereditary disease, von Recklinghausen's neurofibromatosis.

Tumors of the Blood Vessels

Blood vessel tumors include arteriovenous malformations, hemangioblastomas, and endotheliomas. These tumors make up only a very small percentage of brain tumors.

ARTERIOVENOUS MALFORMATIONS (AVM). These malformations, also called *angiomas*, consist of an abnormal collection of blood vessels in which arteries join veins directly rather than through capillaries. The majority of angiomas are in the posterior half of the cerebral hemispheres. The abnormal vessels are present at birth and enlarge with the passage of time. Thus, symptoms may not occur for years although manifestations are often noted between the ages of 10 and 30. As the vessels grow, they may compress the normal brain and weak walls may bleed into the cerebral or subarachnoid spaces. Hemorrhage may be fatal, but in 90 percent of cases bleeding stops and the patient survives [1]. Recurrence of hemorrhage is a constant danger and various modes of treatment have been utilized. Symptoms include seizure, headache, dementia, hemiparesis, and hemiplegia. In some cases there are no clinical symptoms and the AVM is found only on autopsy. *Hemangioblastomas* are neoplasms made up of an aggregation of blood vessels that may also be cystic.

HEMANGIOBLASTOMAS. Hemangioblastomas are found most commonly in the cerebellum but also may occur in the cerebrum. Symptoms include ataxia, dizziness, and signs of increased intracranial pressure. If the cerebellar cyst can be opened and the hemangioblastomatous nodule excised, the prognosis is good. A combination of cerebellar hemangioblastoma in association with cysts of the kidney and pancreas, along with angiomatosis of the retina is known as *Von Hippel-Lindau syndrome*.

ENDOTHELIOMAS. These neoplasms of vascular origin grow around vascular channels. Gross examination reveals a red gray, firm mass that is usually benign. Surgical removal produces a good prognosis [6].

Tumors of Developmental Defects

Developmental tumors arise from cells that have developed abnormally and persist throughout prenatal growth. These include dermoids, teratomas, chordomas, and craniopharyngiomas.

DERMOIDS AND TERATOMAS. *Dermoids and teratomas* may occur anywhere in the CNS but are frequently found in the ventricular system. They may obstruct the third ventricle, the aqueduct of Sylvius, or the fourth ventricle. As a result of embryonic displacement of tissue, these tumors may contain bits of hair, primitive teeth, or other material.

CHORDOMAS. These are rare congenital tumors that are derived from remnants of the primitive notochord. In appearance they are jellylike, gray pink growths and are found near the sella turcica, at the base of the brain, at the cervical or the sacrococcygeal areas. Total surgical removal is impossible due to their highly invasive nature. Symptoms of congenital tumors usually develop within the first 10 years of life and depend on the size and location of the lesion.

CRANIOPHARYNGIOMAS (RATHKE'S POUCH TUMOR). These are tumors derived from "Rathke's pouch," a pouch in the buccopharyngeal embryonic membrane that develops into the anterior lobe of the pituitary. They are most often located posterior to the sella turcica. This tumor is encapsulated and grows as a solid mass or more frequently as a cyst. The cyst often contains thick, brown, oily fluid and often has some degree of calcification. Rupture of the cystic fluid into the subarachnoid space may cause recurrent bouts of a "sterile" meningitis or, in some cases, bacterial meningitis. As the craniopharyngioma grows, pressure is applied to the pituitary gland, the optic chiasm, and sometimes the base of the brain. Symptoms most commonly occur in children and young adults. Surgical removal is possible if the site is accessible.

Tumors of Adenexal Structures

Pineolomas are rare tumors composed of large epithelial cells found in the adult pineal gland. Pineolomas cause symptoms by compressing the aqueduct of Sylvius, causing hydrocephalus and increased intracranial pressure. As the mass destroys the normal pineal gland, melatonin synthesis is reduced, resulting in earlier sexual maturation. Treatment may include a combination of surgery, atrioventricular shunt, and radiotherapy.

Choroid plexus papillomas are rare. Gross inspection reveals well-defined cauliflowerlike papillary masses that often protrude into the fourth ventricle [6]. Although histologically benign, they may cause intraventricular bleeding, hydrocephalus, and increased intracranial pressure. Treatment includes surgery followed by radiotherapy.

Metastatic Tumors

Metastases most commonly occur from primary sites in the breast and lung, but neoplasms of the gastrointestinal tract, genitourinary tract, bone, thyroid gland, and nasal sinuses can also metastasize to the brain and spinal cord. Signs and symptoms are as varied as the location, size, and number of lesions present. Intracranial metastases most often appear in individuals who already have symptoms of far-advanced cancers but occasionally produce the initial symptoms. Even with combinations of surgery, radiotherapy, and chemotherapy, prognosis is poor.

INFECTIONS OF THE CENTRAL NERVOUS SYSTEM

General Considerations

Central nervous system tissue is not immune to viral, bacterial, or other infections. The infection usually arises initially in another region of the body. Organisms can gain access to the CNS in several ways: (1) by spread from adjacent structures—the nasal sinuses, the skull, the middle ear; (2) by entrance through penetrating wounds; and (3) through the bloodstream. Once infectious organisms enter the CNS they can spread rapidly by way of the CSF, leading to widespread devastating results.

Diagnosis of any CNS infections depends on evidence of the infective organism along with changes in pressure, glucose, and protein levels of the CSF. The CNS alterations and clinical manifestations vary according to the type of infection present. The general categories presented in this chapter include viral infections, myelitis, pyogenic infections, tuberculous infections, neurosyphilis, fungal infections, protozoal infections, metazoal infections, rickettsial infections, disorders due to bacterial exotoxins, and postinfectious/postvaccinal diseases.

Viral Infections

A virus may gain access to the body orally, through the respiratory system, by animal or mosquito bites, or across the placenta to the fetus. Once inside the body, viruses make their way to the CNS via the cerebral capillaries and the choroid plexus, through peripheral nerves, and possibly by penetrating olfactory mucosa [1].

Within the CNS, viruses apparently affect specific, susceptible cells. The pathologic effects then are considerably different. Viral damage to the CNS may be due to direct viral invasion of cells with subsequent lysis (acute encephalitis), to selective lysis with resulting demyelination (progressive multifocal leukoencephalopathy), to immune responses to viral antigens (acute disseminated encephalomyelitis) and, in some cases, to cellular destruction without apparent inflammatory or immune response. Viruses may also remain latent in cells for months or years until circumstances trigger acute infections (see Chap. 7).

Encephalitis (Viral)

Encephalitis is an infection of the brain in which a wide range of symptoms are manifested. These symptoms include headache, high fever, confusion, convulsions, and restlessness, which progresses to stupor and coma. There may also be focal CNS impairment such as hemiparesis, asymmetry of Babinski signs and tendon reflexes, involuntary movements, ataxia, and difficulty in speaking or understanding. Brainstem involvement may be manifested by facial weakness or ocular palsies. CSF analysis usually reveals increased numbers of lymphocytes, normal to slightly increased pressure, slightly increased protein, normal glucose, and normal chloride. A comatose state may persist for days, weeks, or months following the acute infection. Residual effects may include behavior and personality changes, mental deterioration, parkinsonism, paralysis, or persistant seizures. The specific signs and symptoms that predominate depend on the type of virus producing the encephalitis. A wide variety of viruses cause encephalitis. The more common ones are reviewed in this chapter.

ARTHROPOD-BORNE (ARBO) VIRUS ENCEPHALITIS. This large group of viruses commonly causes encephalitis. The various viruses seem to occur in certain geographic locations and during certain seasons. Except for tick-borne arboviruses, all of these viruses have vertebrate hosts with mosquito vectors. The principal site of infection is the brain. Clinical manifestations among the different arboviruses are similar; however, they may vary with age. A more abrupt onset of fever and convulsions is common in children.

Eastern equine encephalitis is an infrequent cause of encephalitis but is the most serious of the arboviruses because it causes extensive destruction of the cerebral cortex. When there is clinical evidence (1 in 19 cases) of encephalitis due to this virus, there is an associated high mortality of close to 80 percent [6]. Those who survive often have residual effects that include blindness, deafness, mental retardation, emotional disorders, and hemiplegia. The greatest change in CSF is evidence of large numbers of polymorphonuclear leukocytes.

Western equine encephalitis may involve the upper spinal cord as well as the brain. Mortality is lower than with eastern equine encephalitis, generally in the range of 8 to 19 percent [6].

St. Louis encephalitis involves the cerebral cortex and spinal cord. In addition there is a more prominent meningeal reaction. Although any age group may develop this infection, the symptoms are usually more severe in adults. Depending on the various epidemics, the mortality ranges from 2 to 20 percent [6].

California encephalitis and *tick-borne encephalitis* both produce meningoencephalitis. *Tick-borne encephalitis* can also produce polioencephalomyelitis, which produces paralysis of the upper extremities and may cause a 30 percent mortality in epidemics [6].

HERPES SIMPLEX. Herpes simplex may produce illness in any age group, especially children and young adults. Most frequently the disease is associated with type 1 herpes simplex virus, which is also the common cause of oral mucosal lesions. Type 2 herpes simplex virus causes genital infection and, when present in the mother, produces acute encephalitis in the neonate. Neonatal herpes simplex encephalitis is usually acquired following passage through an infected birth canal [1]. CNS alterations are more common in the medial and inferior portions of the temporal lobes and orbital gyri of the frontal lobes. The lesions include hemorrhagic necrosis and perivascular infiltrates. CSF reveals an increased protein, an increased number of lymphocytes, and the presence of red cells due to the hemorrhagic nature of the lesions. Serologic tests and brain biopsy are used to confirm a diagnosis of herpes simplex encephalitis. Clinical manifestations include headache, fever, convulsions, confusion, stupor, and coma in addition to focal disturbances related to lesions in specific portions of the temporal and frontal lobes. Mortality is estimated to be almost 70 percent, but treatment with the antimetabolite adenine arabinoside A has reduced the mortality to 28 percent [10].

SUBACUTE SCLEROSING PANENCEPHALITIS (SSPE). This illness is usually found in children and is related to infection by the measles virus. Granular regions, areas of focal destruction, and proliferation of neuroglial cells are found in the CNS. CSF reveals increased protein, increased gamma globulin fraction, and high levels of measles antibody. There is also evidence of measles antigen in neurons and glial cells. Bursts of high-voltage and sharp waves are found on EEG examination. The illness occurs in stages: (1) Initially, personality changes occur. (2) Intellectual deterioration, seizures, and visual disturbances follow. (3) Rigidity, progressive unresponsiveness, and signs of autonomic dysfunction cause death within a few months or years.

POSTENCEPHALITIC PARKINSONISM (VON ECONOMO'S DISEASE). This disease is also referred to as encephalitis lethargica or sleeping sickness. It is thought to have occurred in association with a viral pandemic during World War I. Although the virus was never identified, the signs, symptoms, and pathologic alterations were indicative of a viral infection. CNS alterations include meningeal infiltrates and perivascular cuffing with lymphocytes, neuronal destruction, and proliferation of neuroglial tissue. Manifestations of the illness are headache, irritability, fatigue, dizziness, and confusional psychosis. Although 20 percent of the victims died, the survivors retained some neurologic dysfunction [1]. After months, or even years, many survivors developed symptoms that were clinically similar to parkinsonism (see Chap. 47). Since the 1930s, few cases, if any, have been identified.

RABIES. Clinical cases of rabies in humans are rare but once a clinical case of rabies is established, it is almost always fatal. This dreaded viral disease can affect anyone who has sustained a bite through the skin by a rabid animal (usually dogs, cats, bats, foxes, racoons, or skunks) with an incubation period that varies from 14 days to 3 months. Survival of inoculated victims depends on specific postexposure prophylaxis.

The virus makes its way to the CNS via the peripheral nerves. Alterations within the CNS include brain edema, neuron degeneration, and vascular congestion. Inflammatory reactions seem to be greatest in the basal nuclei, midbrain, and medulla. The spinal cord, sympathetic ganglia, the dorsal root ganglia may also be involved. Negri bodies, which are oval shaped, eosinophilic, cytoplasmic inclusions are a characteristic histologic feature of rabies.

Clinical manifestations of rabies occur in stages beginning with generalized malaise, fever, and headache. The general symptoms, along with numbness in the area of the wound, are diagnostic of the illness in its early stage. Within 24 to 72 hours following the general symptoms, there is an excitement phase marked by extreme fear, violent spasms of the larynx when swallowing that lead to hydrophobia, and dysphagia, which leads to salivating with "frothing from the mouth." Facial numbness, dysarthria, seizures, and a confusional psychosis accompany this phase. Finally, there are alternating periods of stupor and mania, flaccid paralysis, coma, and respiratory failure. Death usually occurs within 2 to 7 days following the onset of neurologic symptoms.

PROGRESSIVE MULTIFOCAL LEUKOENCEPHALOPATHY (PML). PML most often occurs in middle-aged persons who have either a chronic debilitating disease such as rheumatoid arthritis or a neoplastic disease, or in those who are receiving immunosuppressive therapy. Opportunistic viruses cause CNS alterations including widespread demyelinization of white matter, particularly of the cerebral hemispheres, brainstem, cerebellum, and rarely, the spinal cord. The CSF usually remains normal. Diagnosis of lesions may be facilitated by computerized axial tomography [1]. Symptoms of this viral disease include hemiparesis, visual field defects, aphasia, ataxia, dysarthria, confusion, and eventually coma. Death occurs within 3 to 6 months following the onset of symptoms.

VIRAL SPONGIFORM ENCEPHALOPATHY ("SLOW VIRUS"). This is a group of unconventional viruses that have incubation periods lasting from months to years, do not produce an inflammatory reaction in tissue, and do not cause an immune reaction in the host. "Slow" viruses are linked with two conditions occurring in humans, subacute spongiform encephalopathy and kuru, and in similar conditions occurring in animals (scrapie in sheep and transmissible encephalopathy in mink).

SUBACUTE SPONGIFORM ENCEPHALOPATHY (CREUTZFELDT-JAKOB DISEASE, TRANSMISSIBLE VIRAL DEMENTIA). This disease, which usually occurs in late middle age, produces CNS alterations mainly in the cerebral and cerebellar cortex, and occasionally the basal ganglia. Alterations include neural degeneration, gliosis, and a spongelike condition in affected areas. Although serologic studies and CSF are normal, there is usually an associated, distinctive EEG pattern of diffuse nonspecific slowing, which changes to sharp waves or spikes on an increasingly flat background [1].

The early clinical manifestations include personality changes, memory loss, visual abnormalities (distortions of shape, decreased visual acuity), and delirium. These symptoms are followed rapidly by dementia, myoclonic contractions, dysarthria, and ataxia, which eventually give way to stupor and coma, although myoclonic contractions continue. Death usually occurs within 1 to 2 years following the onset of symptoms.

KURU. Kuru, the first "slow" viral infection documented in humans, is found in the Fore natives of Papua-New Guinea. The disease is associated with cannibalism in this tribe. Although the CNS alterations are similar to those associated with subacute spongiform encephalopathy, the spongelike conditions are more prominent in the corpus striatum and cerebellum [6]. Clinical manifestations include progressive cerebellar ataxia, shivering tremors, abnormal extraocular movement, incontinence, progression to complete immobility, and dementia in the terminal stage. Following the onset of symptoms death usually occurs within 3 to 6 months.

Aseptic Meningitis Complex (Benign Viral Meningitis)

These are general names for disorders in which there is evidence of meningeal irritation, although pyogenic organisms, parasites, or fungi are not found in CSF. Thus, a virus is expected to be the causative agent. The following viruses have been found in over one-third of the patients with aseptic meningitis complex: mumps, Coxsackie virus, lymphocytic choriomeningitis virus, and ECHO virus. Most individuals recover from these viral illnesses.

Viruses Acquired Congenitally

Viruses are capable of crossing the placenta to reach the fetus, especially during the first trimester of pregnancy. These viruses often produce devastating effects on the fetus. Although it is possible for many types of viruses to infect the fetus, the most common ones include *rubella* and *cytomegaloviruses* (CMV).

Congenital *rubella* often occurs during the first 10 weeks of gestation. The virus invades the fetus's brain and contributes to the establishment of severe mental retardation, seizures, and motor defects. Other manifestations may include low birth weight, abnormally small eyeballs, pigmentary retinal degeneration, glaucoma, cloudy cornea, cataracts, neurocochlear deafness, enlarged liver and spleen, jaundice and patent ductus arteriosus or intraventricular septal defects [1]. These severe effects are preventable by ensuring that women receive the rubella vaccine prior to becoming pregnant.

Cytomegaloviruses (CMV) usually infect the fetus early during the first trimester of pregnancy and may produce cerebral malformation. Later, although the brain is normally formed, CMV may produce inflammatory necrosis in various parts of the brain. Nervous system effects of this infection may include mental defects, convulsions, microcephaly, and often hydrocephalus. Other manifestations include enlarged liver and spleen, jaundice, melena, hematemesis, and petechiae [1]. Whether a fetus has been infected by CMV cannot be determined until birth (and in some cases several years following birth) since the infection is not apparent in pregnant women.

Myelitis (Inflammation of the Spinal Cord)

POLIOMYELITIS. Since the advent of the Salk vaccine in 1955 and the oral Sabin vaccine in 1958, cases of paralytic poliomyelitis are uncommon. The synonym for poliomyelitis is "infantile paralysis"; however, the disease occurs in all age groups. The disease is known to occur throughout the world and a peak incidence occurs during the summer months.

The human intestinal tract is the main viral reservoir for the ribonucleic acid (RNA) virus, which infects through the fecal-oral route. Incubation lasts from 1 to 3 weeks. The virus then penetrates intestinal walls, invades the bloodstream, and is carried throughout the body.

CNS alterations include destruction of nerve cells, as well as cellular infiltration, edema, and severe inflammatory processes, which produce tissue necrosis and hemorrhages. Although the entire CNS may be involved, the predominant site of alterations is the anterior horn of the spinal cord. Examination of CSF usually shows no evidence of the virus during the clinical disease but protein levels are elevated, glucose is normal, and increased lymphocytes are present.

The majority of people infected with the virus experience no symptoms, or only a vague illness because of the failure of the virus to invade the CNS. However, even following CNS invasion, clinical effects range from a mild, nonparalytic form of the disease to a severe, paralytic form. This variation in symptoms is related to the severity of the inflammatory response and to the degree to which nerve cells are injured.

Nonparalytic poliomyelitis produces general symptoms of fever, headache, listlessness, anorexia, nausea, vomiting, sore throat, and aching muscles. At this point, the disease may be resolved. However, with increasing irritability, restlessness, muscle tenderness and spasms, neck and back pain, neck stiffness in addition to Kernig's and Brudzinski signs, the paralytic form of the disease is often imminent.

Paralytic poliomyelitis is often divided into three types: *spinal*, *bulbar*, and *encephalitic*. This division is primarily useful as a descriptive mechanism, since there is often a combination of these types during the course of the disease. Spinal involvement may include muscle weakness with fasciculations, diminished reflexes in association with progressive abdominal and limb muscle weakness, eventual paralysis (the level varying among different age groups), and muscle atrophy. Bulbar involvement causes impairment in the ability to swallow, disturbances of respiration and vasomotor control, and progressively slowing respirations. Cyanosis and hypertension may occur, followed by hypotension and circulatory collapse. The mortality is as high as 75 percent when there is accompanying paralysis of phrenic and intercostal muscles [1]. Involvement of the high brainstem and hypothalamus produces encephalitic symptoms that include restlessness and anxiety initially, progressing to stupor and coma [1].

HERPES ZOSTER ("SHINGLES"). Herpes zoster infection occurs more commonly in adulthood, particularly with advancing age, and in persons with an underlying systemic disease. The development of this illness is not completely understood. It is thought that herpes zoster infection represents a reactivation of varicella virus infection that persists in the nerve ganglia following a primary infection with chickenpox. Individuals who have herpes zoster infection usually have a past history of chickenpox. Nervous system alterations include congested, edematous, and hemorrhagic dorsal root ganglion. There is also disintegration of ganglion cells. Painful, vesicular skin eruptions, which harbor varicella zoster virus, are associated with involvement of the corresponding dorsal root ganglion or *gasserian* ganglion. The most frequently involved dermatomes are T5 and T10; however, any dermatome may be involved. In some cases there is accompanying sensory loss and motor palsies. Although most individuals recover, the process is often slow and painful. The pain may persist for months or even years, causing much despair for the person.

Pyogenic Infections

The brain or its coverings can be infected by pyogenic (pus-forming) microorganisms. Bacteria enter the CNS by spread from adjacent cranial structures, through the bloodstream; in a few unfortunate cases the infection is iatrogenic (for example, from a lumbar puncture or contaminated scapel). Once within the CNS, the results of pyogenic microorganisms may be disastrous.

BACTERIAL MENINGITIS (LEPTOMENINGITIS). The leptomeninges and subarachnoid space are primary targets for invasion by pyogenic microorganisms. Once an infection enters any part of the subarachnoid space, it spreads quickly throughout CSF pathways. Thus, an inflammatory reaction is set up in the pia and arachnoid and in the ventricles. Any microorganisms entering the body may cause meningitis. However, some bacteria are more prominent and seem to be more prevalent in certain age groups. According to Robbins, *pneumococcus* organisms are commonly cultured in very young patients and adults over 40 years of age, *E. coli* in the neonatal period, *H. influenzae* in infants and young children, and *N. meningitidis* in adolescents and young adults [6]. Spinal fluid cultures usually reveal the causative agent.

Alterations within the CNS include swelling and congestion of the brain and spinal cord, as well as exudate within the subarachnoid space. In severe cases, inflammatory cells can produce occlusions of vessels that penetrate the brain with subsequent areas of necrosis. The CSF reveals elevated protein levels, decreased glucose, decreased chloride, elevated pressure (above 180 mm water), and the presence of thousands of leukocytes.

Clinical manifestations of acute pyogenic meningitis are fever, headache, pain with eye movement, photophobia, neck and back stiffness, positive Kernig's sign, generalized convulsions, drowsiness, and confusion. Stupor, followed by coma and death may occur without prompt and adequate treatment.

Residual effects are also a danger due to destruction of the meningeal framework. Potential residual effects include optic arachnoiditis, meningomyelitis, and chronic meningoencephalitis with hydrocephalus. Again, with prompt diagnosis and antibiotic therapy, these residual effects are less common.

BRAIN ABSCESS. Approximately one-half of all brain abscesses are secondary to infection in the nasal cavity, middle ear, and mastoid cells. The remaining cases are due to primary focus of infection elsewhere in the body, particularly the lungs or pleura, heart, and distal bones (Fig. 46-2). Streptococci are often the causative organisms.

An abscess is formed when an inflamed area, caused by an invading organism, liquifies and begins to accumulate white blood cells. A fibrous capsule is formed in an effort to contain the pus. As the brain expands, nerve tissue is compressed and destroyed. Chronic inflammation and edema surround the abscess. The CSF reveals an increased protein level and an increased white cell count. If the abscess ruptures into the subarachnoid space or ventricles, organisms can be cultured from CSF. Other diagnostic techniques that may be used are skull x rays, CAT scanning, EEG, arteriography, and ventriculography.

The most frequent initial clinical manifestation is headache, with other symptoms being similar to those produced by growing masses within the brain. Notably, the increased intracranial pressure and focal complaints related to the location of the abscess are important. In addition, a brain abscess can rupture and lead to other complications such as sinus thrombosis, ventriculitis, or meningitis. Mortality from brain abscesses has been greatly reduced due to successful combinations of antibiotic therapy and surgery.

SUBDURAL EMPYEMA. Empyema refers to pus in a body cavity; thus, subdural empyema is a suppurative process in the subdural space. These usually occur between the dura's inner surface and the outer surface of the arachnoid. The most common causative organisms are *Staphylococcus aureus* and the streptococci. Infective organisms usually speed to the subdural space by spread from thrombophlebitis or by erosion through bone or dura from the frontal sinuses, ethmoid sinuses, middle ear, or mastoid cells.

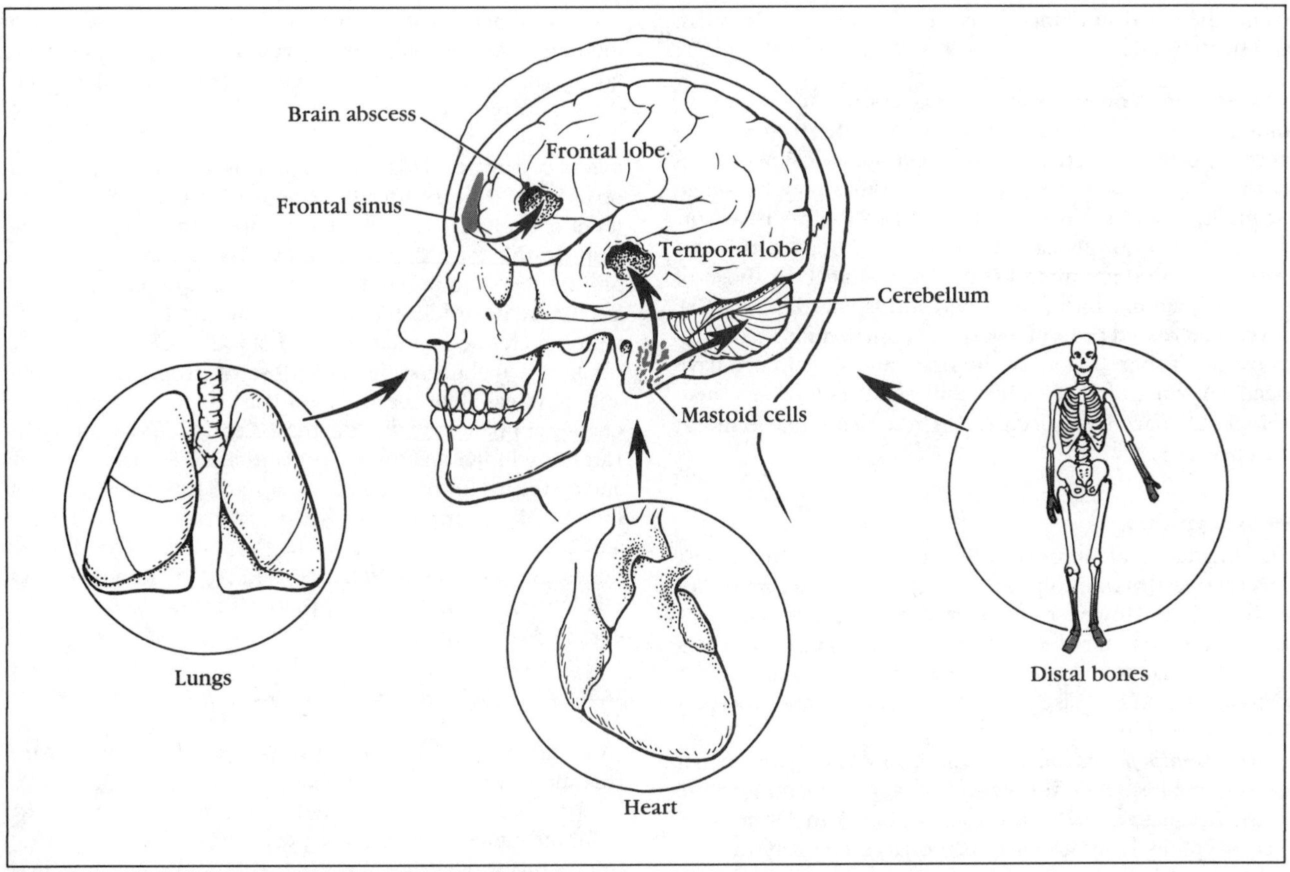

FIGURE 46-2. Origins and locations of cerebral abscesses.

Exudate is found on the undersurface of the dura. As the empyema grows, pressure is applied to the underlying cerebral hemisphere. Thrombophlebitis of cerebral veins that are near the subdural empyema can lead to ischemic necrosis of the cortex. CSF reveals elevated pressure, increased protein, normal glucose, and an increased number of lymphocytes.

Many affected persons have a history of chronic mastoiditis or sinusitis. Clinical manifestations that indicate that the infection has spread to the subdural space include fever, general malaise, a localized headache that becomes generalized, associated vomiting, and neck stiffness. As the empyema enlarges, focal neurologic signs, lethargy, and coma develop. Prognosis depends on the success of surgery and antibiotic therapy, as well as the extent to which neurologic deficits have occurred.

Tuberculous Infections

Tuberculous meningitis and tuberculomas of the brain and spinal cord are usually secondary to a tuberculous focus in another part of the body. Thus, as better public health measures and modern antituberculous therapy help control the incidence of tuberculosis, the incidence of tuberculous meningitis and tuberculomas of the brain and cord are also decreased.

TUBERCULOUS MENINGITIS. Tuberculous meningitis is caused by *Mycobacterium tuberculosis*. This condition has a slower onset and more chronic course than pyogenic meningitis. The base of the brain and the spinal cord become compressed by shaggy, necrotic, fibrinous yellow exudate. There may also be large areas of caseation and tiny tubercles around the blood vessels [6]. CSF reveals increased pressure, elevated protein, decreased glucose (but not as low as values observed in pyogenic meningitis), and the presence of polymorphonuclear leukocytes and lymphocytes. With careful technique in obtaining a specimen, tubercle bacilli may be recovered from CSF.

Clinical manifestations depend on the chronicity of the disease and the extent of pathologic processes. However, in general, adults have headache, fever, lethargy, confusion, neck stiffness, and positive Kernig's and Brudzinski signs. Young children more frequently undergo vomiting, irritability, and seizures.

Due to the slow onset of this illness, neurologic damage may be present before treatment is sought. Then, even though the patient survives, there may be lasting effects, such as recurrent seizures, retarded intellectual development, mental disturbances, visual disturbances, deafness, and hemiparesis.

TUBERCULOMAS OF BRAIN AND SPINAL CORD. Tuberculomas, though rare in the United States, constitute from 5 to 30 percent of all intracranial space-occupying lesions in underdeveloped countries [1]. Tuberculomas may be single or multiple and contain a core of caseation necrosis surrounded by a fibrous capsule. Within the brain and spinal cord they produce neurologic effects similar to those of other expanding intracranial and intraspinal lesions. CSF reveals increased protein levels and a small number of lymphocytes. Tuberculomas of the brain and spinal cord have been known to calcify while still small before any neurologic changes have occurred. These are often found at autopsy.

Neurosyphilis

The incidence of neurosyphilis has decreased in the last several decades due to prompt diagnosis and treatment of early syphilis. However, the overall incidence of syphilis is increasing, particularly in younger people. Thus, since it is estimated that only 30 percent of all cases are reported, the potential for an increase in the development of neurosyphilis is very real [6].

Treponema pallidum is a spiral, motile organism that causes syphilis. Once this organism is introduced into the body, it usually invades the CNS within 3 to 18 months. Neurosyphilis is progressive in the large majority of individuals and includes several forms: asymptomatic neurosyphilis, meningovascular syphilis, general paresis, and tabes dorsalis (see Chaps. 49, 51).

Meningitis is the initial event in all forms of neurosyphilis but the severity of symptoms varies among the different forms. CSF is the most accurate, sensitive indicator that an active neurosyphilitic infection is present. Changes in CSF include positive serologic tests—the Venereal Disease Research Laboratory (VDRL) slide test, the Kolmer test, the fluorescent treponemal antibody absorption (FTA/ABS) test, and the treponema immobilization (TPI) test; increased protein; presence of increased lymphocytes, plasma cells, and mononuclear cells; and an abnormal colloidal gold curve.

ASYMPTOMATIC NEUROSYPHILIS. As the name asymptomatic neurosyphilis implies, there are usually no physical signs or symptoms of the meningitis. This form of the disease is recognized by changes in CSF, which, if treated, prevent further development of the disease.

MENINGOVASCULAR SYPHILIS. This form of neurosyphilis commonly develops 6 to 7 years after the original infection. CNS alterations include infiltration of meninges and blood vessels with plasma cells and lymphocytes, inflammation of arteries, and fibrosis, which leads to occlusion of vessels. The vascular lesions are referred to as Heubner's arteritis. Miliary gummas may also be seen in the meninges.

Clinical manifestations are similar to those of a low-grade meningitis as well as a cerebrovascular accident and mental derangement. Unless treated, neurologic deficits continue to progress.

GENERAL PARESIS. This form of neurosyphilis usually develops 15 to 20 years after the original infection. Early treatment of syphilis has decreased the incidence of general paresis. In this form of neurosyphilis, the parenchyma of the brain is involved due to the presence of spirochetes. There is a diffuse destruction of cortical neurons. Plasma cells and lymphocytes accumulate around blood vessels.

Clinical manifestations are those of progressive mental and physical deterioration. Initially, slight memory loss, changes in behavior, and decreased ability to reason occur. Later, the individual develops elaborate delusional systems and disregard for moral and social standards. Physically, the individual experiences dysarthria, tremor of the tongue and hand, muscular hypotonia, hyperactive tendon reflexes, Babinski signs, seizures, and Argyll Robertson pupils. Without treatment the prognosis is poor and death occurs in 3 to 4 years.

TABES DORSALIS. Tabes dorsalis, like general paresis, occurs 15 to 20 years after the onset of infection. This form of neurosyphilis is also uncommon now due to improved, early treatment with penicillin.

CNS alterations include degeneration of the posterior columns, fibrosis around the posterior roots, and destruction of proprioceptive fibers in the radicular nerves. These changes produce various symptoms with the most common being lightening pains (sudden sharp pains lasting only a portion of a second), ataxia due to sensory defects, and urinary incontinence. Visceral symptoms include vomiting and bouts of sharp epigastric pain that extends around the body. Other clinical manifestations may include Argyll Robertson pupils, Charcot joints due to repeated injury to insensitive joints, absence of a vibration sense and deep tendon reflexes, as well as a Romberg sign. Although treatment with penicillin can arrest the disease process, residual effects such as urinary incontinence, lightening pains, visceral crises, and Charcot joints may persist indefinitely.

Fungal Infections

Fungi infect the CNS less commonly than bacteria and viruses. Their effects can be similar to bacterial infection but more difficult to treat. Fungal infections may produce brain abscesses, meningitis, meningoencephalitis, and thrombophlebitis of vessels within the CNS. As with other infections, fungal infections of the CNS are usually secondary to a primary source of infection elsewhere in the body. In addition fungal infections may be a complication of another disease process or related to immunosuppressant drugs.

Fungi usually spread to the CNS by way of the bloodstream. Once within the CNS, fungi cause an inflammatory reaction and a purulent exudate involves the meninges. In some cases, an invasion of vessel walls results in vasculitis and thrombosis with subsequent nervous tissue infarction. The process develops slowly over a period of days or weeks. Clinical manifestations are similar to those of tuberculous meningitis. In addition, hydrocephalus is a frequent related complication. CSF reveals elevated pressure, increased protein, decreased glucose levels, moderate pleocytosis (increased number of lymphocytes), and often the isolation of the infective organism.

Many types of fungi may invade the CNS; the most common infections are cryptococcosis, coccidioidomycosis, and mucormycosis.

CRYPTOCOCCOSIS (TORULOSIS). Common soil fungi, the cryptococci, are the most frequent cause of fungal infection of the CNS. This condition, which usually arises secondary to a pulmonary infection, produces cysts and granulomas in the cortex and occasionally in the deep white matter and basal ganglia. These cysts contain large numbers of organisms. *Cryptococcus neoformans* is recovered from spinal fluid. Mortality, even in the absence of preexisting diseases (lymphomas and Hodgkin's disease), is close to 40 percent [1].

COCCIDIOIDOMYCOSIS. *Coccidioides immitis* produces a relatively mild, flulike illness involving the respiratory organs. Commonly occurring in the southwestern United States, coccidioidomycosis may become a chronic, diffuse, granulomatous disease that spreads throughout the body. The meninges and CSF become involved with resultant pathologic and clinical manifestations similar to those of tuberculous meningitis. When the meninges become involved, treatment is difficult. Amphotericin B is the only effective drug and even with this treatment the disease is often fatal.

MUCORMYCOSIS. Mucormycosis is a rare opportunistic infection occurring in very debilitated patients. One of the primary sites of invasion is the nasal sinuses. From the nasal sinuses the organism may spread along invaded vessels to periorbital tissue and the cranial vault. Nervous tissue infarctions occur as a result of vascular occlusion. The cerebral form of mucormycosis is rapidly fatal.

Protozoal Infections

MALARIA. *Plasmodium vivax* produces the most common form of malaria. This organism does not actually invade brain tissue but the parasitized red blood cells block microcirculation, thus leading to tissue hypoxia and ischemic necrosis. The vessel blockage within the brain leads to glial necrosis, which causes drowsiness, confusion, and seizures. Quinine is used for treatment and is helpful unless the cerebral symptoms are far advanced.

Plasmodium falciparum produces a form of malaria that has more severe symptoms. The parasite fills capillaries, and Dürck's nodes (small foci of necrosis surrounded by glia) are found in brain tissue. CSF reveals elevated pressure and contains white blood cells. Clinical manifestations include focal neurologic signs, headache, seizures, aphasia, cerebellar ataxia, hemiplegia, hemianopsia and, eventually, coma. Cerebral malaria due to *P. falciparum* is usually rapidly fatal.

TOXOPLASMOSIS. *Toxoplasma gondii* produces an infection that is either acquired or congenital. The organism is transmitted by eating raw beef or by contact with cat feces.

Acquired toxoplasmosis that produces clinical effects are rare. However, in clinical cases the white and gray matter contains necrotic lesions that harbor *T. gondii.* Symptoms are similar to meningoencephalitis.

Congenital toxoplasmosis causes much destruction of the neonatal brain. Signs of infection are fever, rash, seizures, and enlarged liver and spleen, which may be present at birth. However, in many cases, clinical manifestations of the illness are not present for days, weeks, or months. These clinical effects include hydrocephalus, retardation, cerebral calcification, and chorioretinitis.

AMEBIASIS. Infection with amebae may occur after swimming in lakes or ponds. The causative organisms are usually of the *Naegleria* genus and there is a prevalence of cases in the southeastern United States.

CNS alterations include abscesses in the cortex and purulent exudate involving the meninges. CSF findings are similar to those of bacterial meningitis. The disease is rapidly progressive with nausea, vomiting, fever, neck stiffness, focal neurologic signs, seizures, and eventually coma. This illness is usually fatal within a week of onset due to the resistance of *Naegleria* to treatment.

TRYPANOSOMIASIS. Several strains of *Trypanosoma brucei* produce African "sleeping sickness," which is transmitted by the tsetse fly. Two epidemiologic patterns are described: Gambian (Middle and West African) and Rhodesian (East African). The Rhodesian type is more severe with intercurrent infections and myocarditis dominating the clinical picture. Within 2 years following infection with the Gambian form, trypanosomes produce meningoencephalitis, with thickening of the meninges and cerebral edema. Symptoms range from somnolence to convulsions and coma. The mortality depends on the effectiveness of treatment and the degree of CNS involvement.

Trypanosoma cruzi produces Chagas' disease in Central and South America, rarely in North America. The organism is transmitted by biting bugs commonly called "assassin bugs." Chagas' disease is either acute or chronic. The acute form of the disease is more prevalent in children and produces fever, enlarged liver and spleen, myocardial involvement with congestive failure, and eventually involvement of the lungs, meninges, and brain. Months or years after an acute attack of Chagas' disease, the chronic form of the disease may develop with subsequent meningoencephalitis.

TRICHINOSIS. *Trichinella spiralis* enters the body when raw or insufficiently cooked pork is eaten. Within two to three days early symptoms of the disease are apparent and are mainly due to the invasion of muscle by larvae, producing muscle weakness and tenderness. Three to six weeks following ingestion, larvae invade the nervous system. Lymphocytic and mononuclear infiltration of the meninges, as well as focal gliosis, occurs. Symptoms of CNS involvement include headache, confusion, neck stiffness, seizures, and occasionally coma. Though trichinosis is usually not fatal, seizures and neurologic deficits may continue indefinitely.

Metazoal Infections

CYSTICERCOSIS. Ingestion of encysted eggs of pork tapeworm, *Taenia solium*, produce cysticercosis. This disease is most common in South American countries. The larvae spread throughout the body and develop cysts in any body tissue. Cystic nodules within the brain produce symptoms similar to those of brain tumors. Jacksonian epilepsy is a common manifestation. Prognosis depends on the extent of neurologic damage.

ECHINOCCOSIS (HYDATID DISEASE). This disease is caused by the ingestion of larvae of the canine tapeworm, *Echinococcus granulosus*. The larvae invade the liver, lungs, bones and, less frequently, the brain. The larvae become encysted and are at first microscopic. However, within 5 or more years the cysts may grow to massive sizes of 25 cm or more [6]. Thus, within the brain symptoms similar to those associated with brain tumors are produced. The amount of local destruction throughout the body determines the prognosis.

Rickettsial Infections

Rickettsial infections are relatively rare in the United States. These infections are caused by microorganisms that are obligate intracellular parasites with multiplication occurring only within living cells of susceptible hosts. Their cycle involves an animal reservoir and an insect vector (ticks, fleas, lice, mites, and humans). Epidemic typhus involves only a cycle with lice and humans.

Major rickettsial diseases include epidemic (primary) typhus, louse-borne murine (endemic) typhus, flea-borne, scrub typhus or tsutsugamushi fever, mite-borne; Rocky Mountain spotted fever, tick-borne; and Q fever, tick- and airborne. Within the CNS rickettsial diseases can produce lesions in the gray and white matter. Focal gliosis along with mononuclear leukocytes produce characteristic "typhus nodules."

All the rickettsial diseases, except Q fever, have similar pathologic and clinical effects. A 3- to 15-day incubation period is followed by the abrupt onset of fever, chills, headache, and weakness followed by a generalized macular rash. During the second week after the onset of fever, the CNS becomes involved producing apathy, dullness, intermittent episodes of delirium, then eventually stupor, and coma. Occasionally, in untreated cases there are focal neurologic manifestations and optic neuritis. CSF may be completely normal. Q fever is not accompanied by a rash and produces symptoms similar to those of a low-grade meningitis.

Mortality due to typhus is greatest during epidemics. Antibiotic therapy has reduced fatality rates to less than 10 percent, for typhus, and 3 to 10 percent for Rocky Mountain spotted fever. Fatalities are rarely associated with scrub typhus and Q fever [6].

Disorders Due to Bacterial Exotoxins

Bacterial exotoxins can have powerful effects on the CNS. The major diseases produced by these toxins are tetanus, diphtheria, and botulism.

TETANUS. *Clostridium tetani* produces tetanus following the contamination of penetrating wounds or the umbilical cord of the newborn with spores. The bacilli produce two exotoxins: a tetanolysin and a tetanospasmin. Neurotoxic effects are produced by tetanospasmin. Most of the toxin enters the peripheral ending of the motor neuron from the bloodstream, travels up the fibers to the spinal cord, and crosses the synaptic cleft to the inhibitory neuron, where it prevents the release of glycine. Glycine is a neuromuscular transmitter secreted mainly in the synapses of the spinal cord, and it acts as an inhibitor. The action of tetanospasmin is through an affinity for the sympathetic nervous system, the medullary centers, the anterior horn cells of the spinal cord, and the motor end plates in skeletal muscle. It produces uninhibited motor responses leading to the typical muscle spasm.

The incubation period varies from several days to several months. Usually, symptoms occur within 2 weeks following wound contamination. The initial manifestation is usually difficulty opening the jaw (trismus); thus, the synonym "lockjaw." There is generalized muscle stiffness with eventual muscle spasms (tetanic seizures or convulsions). These convulsions are very painful and can occur spontaneously or in response to the slightest stimuli. Facial spasms produce a characteristic sardonic smile (risus sardonicus). Contractions of back muscles produce a forward arching of the back (opisthotonous). Spasms of glottal, laryngeal, and respiratory muscles cause difficulty in breathing and frequently lead to death due to asphyxia. In established clinical cases of tetanus, the overall mortality is 50 percent [1]. However, the disease is prevented with active immunization with tetanus toxoid. Also, prompt administration of antitoxin may prevent the development of clinical manifestations.

DIPHTHERIA. *Corynebacterium diphtheriae* produces an acute infection, diphtheria. Although open wounds in any part of the body can provide entry for this organism, the usual portal of entry is the oral cavity. The incubation period is 1 to 7 days. During this time the organism becomes established and proliferates at the site of implantation, usually the throat and trachea. The bacteria produce exotoxin that is absorbed by the blood and carried to the CNS and heart. Local neurologic manifestations occur within 5 to 12 days and include vomiting, dysphagia, and nasal voice due to palatal paralysis. Blurred vision and loss of accommodation occurs in the second or third week due to ciliary paralysis. Between the fifth and sixth weeks, weakness and paralysis of the extremities may occur. Most neurologic disturbances disappear slowly and individuals usually improve completely, if respiratory obstruction or cardiac failure does not supervene. The disease is prevented with immunization, or prompt administration of antitoxin may prevent clinical manifestations.

BOTULISM. *Clostridium botulinum* can contaminate and produce exotoxins in food such as fruits, vegetables, and meats that are kept for long periods of time without refrigeration. When ingested, the toxin resists gastric digestion, is absorbed by the blood and then travels to the nervous system. The botulinus toxin acts only on the presynaptic endings of neuromuscular junctions and autonomic ganglia. It prevents the release of acetylcholine but does not cross the blood-brain barrier, thus having little effect on the CNS. Symptoms occur within 2 to 36 hours following ingestion of the contaminated food. Neural symptoms may or may not be preceded by nausea and vomiting. The individual may develop cranial nerve palsies, blurred vision, diplopia, ptosis, strabismus, hoarseness, dysarthria, dysphagia, vertigo, deafness, constipation, and progressive muscle weakness. Tendon reflexes may be absent. Sensation remains intact and the person is conscious throughout the illness. Even with prompt administration of antitoxin, death occurs in more than one-half of cases due to paralysis of respiratory muscles.

Postinfectious/Postvaccinal Diseases

Acute disseminated (postinfectious) encephalomyelitis, acute inflammatory polyradiculoneuropathy (Guillain-Barré syndrome), and Reye's syndrome often occur during or shortly after viral infection or rarely after vaccinations for smallpox, rabies, or typhoid. These conditions often require an individual susceptibility to the virus or viral effects.

ACUTE DISSEMINATED (POSTINFECTIOUS) ENCEPHALOMYELITIS. Postinfectious encephalomyelitis develops 2 to 4 days following a rash and is thought to be an autoimmune response to myelin, which is triggered by a virus [6]. Demyelination occurs in the region of the brainstem and spinal cord. In addition the meninges are infiltrated by inflammatory cells. Clinical manifestations include headaches, stiffness of the neck, lethargy, and eventually coma. One-third to one-half of patients die in the acute phase of the illness. Neurologic residual effects are severe in patients who survive.

GUILLAIN-BARRÉ SYNDROME. Guillain-Barré syndrome is thought to be the result of an autoimmune reaction triggered by a virus in the peripheral nerves. Nervous system alterations include inflammatory infiltrate around vessels throughout the cranial and spinal nerves, demyelination, and axon destruction. CSF reveals an elevated protein level and pleocytosis. Clinical manifestations include proximal to distal weakness or paralysis of extremities, hypotonia, areflexia, pain, and paresthesias. Weakness that progresses to total motor paralysis of respiratory muscles can result in death. Autonomic dysfunction may occur with resultant hypertension, orthostatic hypotension, sinus tachycardia, and loss of sweating. Individuals who survive the acute phase of the disease usually recover completely; however, in some cases there are residual motor or reflex deficits in the lower extremities (see p. 735).

REYE'S SYNDROME. Reye's syndrome seems to occur following viral infections such as chickenpox or a respiratory virus, although the relationship between the virus and pathologic changes is not understood. It is characterized by the onset of acute encephalopathy 10 days to 2 weeks postviral infection. Cerebral edema is produced, as well as fatty changes in the liver and renal tubules. The disease is also characterized by hypoglycemia and increased serum ammonia levels. Clinical manifestations include persistent vomiting, delirium, seizures, stupor, and eventual coma. This disease carries a 60 percent mortality, which appears to be improving due to earlier diagnosis and supportive treatment.

REFERENCES

1. Adams, R., and Victor, M. *Principles of Neurology* (2nd ed.). New York: McGraw-Hill, 1981.
2. Hausman, K. Brain tumors in children. *J. Neurosurg. Nurs.* 10:8, 1978.
3. McDonald, J., et al. *Central Nervous System Tumors in Clinical Oncology for Medical Students and Physicians: A Multidisciplinary Approach* (5th ed.). New York: American Cancer Society, 1978.
4. Nelson, G. Current approaches in the treatment of malignant gliomas of the brain. *J. Neurosurg. Nurs.* 6:109, 1974.
5. Price, S. A., and Wilson, L. M. *Pathophysiology: Clinical Concepts of Disease Processes* (2nd ed.). New York: McGraw-Hill, 1982.
6. Robbins, S., and Cotran, R. *Pathological Basis of Disease* (2nd ed.). Philadelphia: Saunders, 1979.
7. Russel, D., and Rubinstein, L. *Pathology of Tumors of the Nervous System* (4th ed.). Baltimore: Williams & Wilkins, 1977.
8. Schwartz, S. I. (ed.). *Principles of Surgery* (3rd ed.). New York: McGraw-Hill, 1979.
9. Sloof, J., Kernohan, J., and Mallarty, C. *Primary Intramedullary Tumors of the Spinal Cord and Fillum Terminale.* Philadelphia: Saunders, 1964.
10. Whitley, R. et al. Adenine arabinoside therapy of biopsy-proved herpes-simplex encephalitis: National Institute of Allergy and Infectious Diseases Collaborative Antiviral Study. *N. Engl. J. Med.* 297:289, 1977.

CHAPTER 47
DEGENERATIVE AND OTHER ALTERATIONS IN THE NERVOUS SYSTEM

LEARNING OBJECTIVES

1. Contrast the terms *disability* and *handicap*.
2. Differentiate between primary and secondary disabilities.
3. Identify examples of developmental, congenital, and degenerative alterations in the nervous system.
4. Explain why the site of a neurologic alteration has a greater impact on the production of clinical signs than does the nature of the lesion.
5. Identify examples of congenital and developmental alterations in the motor areas of the brain and cord.
6. Identify examples of developmental and degenerative alterations in the upper voluntary motor areas of the nervous system leading to progressive weakness, tremor, and/or spastic paralysis.
7. Contrast upper and lower motor neuron paralysis.
8. Describe alterations in the lower voluntary motor areas of the nervous system leading to transient or permanent sensory or motor changes, and/or flaccid paralysis.
9. Describe the structural basis for signs and symptoms of bulbar palsy.
10. Explain the physiologic basis for medical treatment of muscle weakness and fatigue related to inadequate transmission of impulses across the myoneural junction.
11. Describe pathologic changes in the extrapyramidal motor system resulting in the loss of normal automatic or spontaneous body movements.
12. Describe pathologic changes in the extrapyramidal system resulting in the generation or facilitation of abnormal movements.
13. Identify examples of structural alterations affecting higher cerebral functions such as memory and judgment.
14. Define prognostic terms such as *recovery*, *stabilization*, *progression*, *recurrence*, *remission*, and *exacerbation*.

PROGRESSIVE NEUROLOGIC DISABILITIES

Primary Disabilities

A *primary disability* is the direct result of a pathologic process resulting in a structural and functional alteration. Primary disabilities may be due to congenital disorders, genetic disorders, injuries or disease, and, unlike cardiovascular or skeletal disorders, are usually referred to in terms of the functional, rather than structural, alteration. For example, terms such as *spastic quadriplegia* or *right homonymous hemianopsia* are more frequently used than such phrases as *demyelination of the.... tracts* or *anoxia of the .... branch of the.... nerve* for problem definition.

A reason for referring to primary neurologic alterations in functional terms is that often the nature of the lesion is very hard to identify early in the course of the disease. Also, the description of the dysfunction helps to pinpoint the site of the lesion, even if it does not give much evidence as to the nature of it. The location of changes in the nervous system dictate the expression of signs and symptoms no matter whether the lesions that interrupt the generation of transmission of nerve impulses are developmental, infectious, degenerative, vascular, neoplastic, or traumatic. Therefore, a lesion that interrupts the pyramidal tracts in the brain or cord tends to produce spastic paralysis, whether it is due to neuronal anoxia or to an inborn metabolic defect in the nerve cells. Similarly, an imbalance between the neurotransmitters in the basal ganglia will result in abnormalities of movement whether it is due to degeneration of dopamine-projecting neurons following carbon monoxide poisoning, or to the dopamine-blocking or binding effects of phenothiazine drugs.

The degenerative and other neurologic disorders selected as examples in the following pages share common signs and symptoms because they cause structural or chemical alterations in common locations in the brain. Because their causes vary greatly, their treatment and prognoses are quite different, even when initial symptoms seem identical.

Secondary Disabilities

Secondary disabilities are often associated with primary neurologic disorders in that they are problems caused by restrictions or conditions imposed due to presence or treatment of a primary disability. These secondary problems may arise from forced inactivity, such as a muscle contracture that occurs in a paralyzed limb. Secondary disabilities also may arise from injurious activity; for example, when a paralyzed extremity is not supported properly its weight may cause subluxation of the associated joint. Most of the secondary disabilities associated with primary neurologic disease are progressive and may be threatening to function and even to life, even if the primary disorder is resolved. Secondary disabilities are usually as preventable as they are crippling.

Organic disease of the nervous system tends to be long-term and is not always characterized by recovery. If a person does recover from a neurologic disease, such as neurosyphilis, full function may not be regained, even though the causative agent has been eliminated. Residual primary damage or secondary disabilities may linger or be permanent. Even if a cure is complete, or when a disorder such as Guillain-Barré syndrome is self-limiting, it usually takes a long time for full function to return.

Disability Versus Handicap

Since the term *disability* simply means deficit or impairment, health care providers usually prefer it over the older term, *handicap*, which carries the connotation of disadvantage. Whether the alteration is as common as senile atherosclerotic dementia or as rare as amyotrophic lateral sclerosis, individuals, families, and health care providers all find it difficult to sustain motivation and to marshal resources when the prognosis for function and for life itself is poor.

PARALYZING DEVELOPMENTAL OR CONGENITAL DISORDERS

Developmental disorders occur when neurologic structures fail to develop to full size, fail to develop mature function, or when they develop abnormally. Usually the causes of developmental defects are not known. Congenital diseases are those present at birth; the classification includes clinically apparent genetic disease and that which occurs during fetal life as a result of infection, anoxia, malnutrition, or some other traumatic or toxic factor.

Both developmental and congenital disorders may be characterized by progressive signs or they may show signs that stabilize with or without treatment. If the alterations are in the voluntary motor areas in the cerebral cortex or the pyramidal tracts of the brain or cord (the upper motor neuron), *spastic paralysis* (characterized by sporadic involuntary muscle jerks or spasms) usually results. Spastic paralysis with normal or hyperactive reflexes below the level of the lesion indicates that the reflex arc is intact even if it is no longer influenced by the moderating control of the higher cerebral centers. Muscles remaining under the influence of the reflex arc alone tend to develop muscle contractures causing them to permanently shorten and decrease in size because of the sustained hypertonicity with eventual permanent fibrotic changes. If alterations occur in the peripheral nervous system or in any part of the system where the reflex arc is interrupted, the result is usually hypoactive or absent reflexes with a *flaccid or limp paralysis*. Lower motor neuron damage leaves muscles devoid of innervation and without tone. Typically they atrophy and are permanently replaced with connective tissue and fat.

Spina Bifida

Spina bifida is a developmental disorder of the vertebral canal. During embryogenesis, the bony arch of the canal fails to close completely. If this is the only defect, it is called

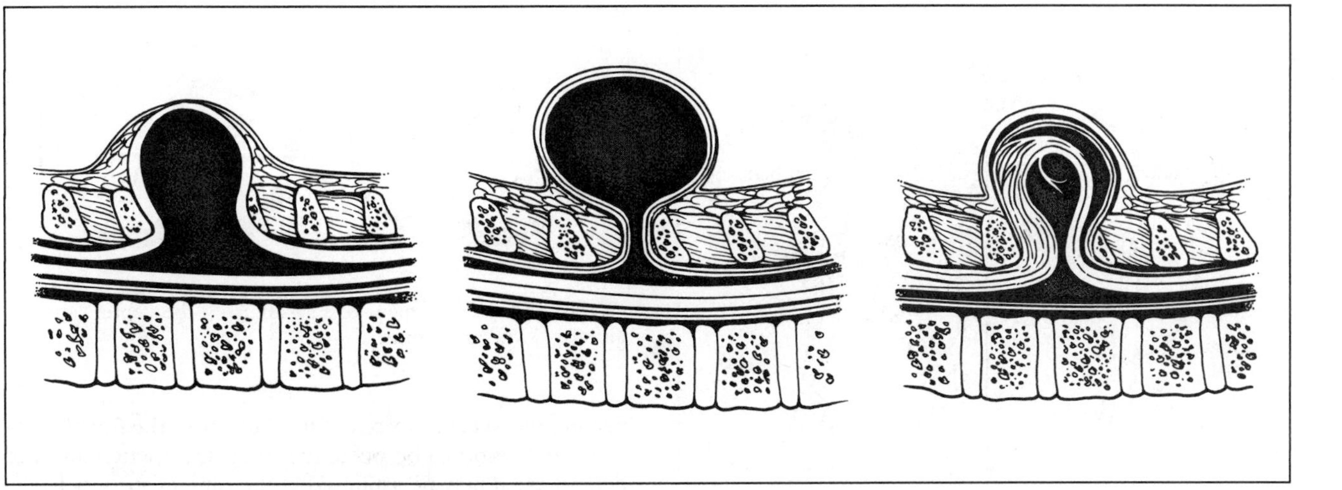

FIGURE 47-1. Appearance of types of spina bifida: syringomyelocele, meningocele, and meningomyelocele.

spina bifida occulta because there are no signs of neurologic deficit to advertise its presence. The bony defect is only identifiable by x ray or palpation. The cause of this developmental defect is unknown, although various theories link it with prenatal infection, prenatal drug usage, or heredity [10].

Unfortunately, spina bifida is often associated with a defect in the closure of the neural tube (Fig. 47-1). Such defects can range from a closed but dilated central cord canal (*syringomyelocele*) to a sac protruding through the bony defect containing meninges (*meningocele*) and/or elements of the spinal cord (*meningomyelocele*). These sacs may leak cerebrospinal fluid if the skin covering is incomplete. Additional defects such as abnormal neural tissue or a fistula also may be associated with this type of spina bifida. Occasionally, in the occipital area, brain elements may protrude through a defect in the skull; this impairment is referred to as an *encephalocele*.

Spina bifida occulta may occur with no clinical signs or symptoms. However, it is possible for late signs such as persistent or intermittent eneuresis, (the most common symptom) late walking, or even chronic cold feet to be traced to a previously undetected intradural lesion.

Several forms of spina bifida can be diagnosed in utero by amniocentesis, or at birth by the presence of the sac protruding through the defect in the vertebral arch. If the sac is a meningocele, it is possible for the individual to show no signs of neurologic deficit, although hydrocephalus may occur after surgical repair. The meningomyelocele is accompanied by signs of neurologic damage, the extent of which is dependent on the size and level of the lesion and the presence of dysplastic neural tissue. If the defect occurs in the lumbosacral area, flaccid paralysis of the lower limbs and absence of sensation below the level of the lesion are usual. Sphincter control is also affected in both bowel and bladder. These neurologic deficits occur because the defect and abnormal tissue often involve all or most of the lumbosacral spinal cord along with the nerve roots entering and exiting in the lumbosacral area. Alterations in blood supply due to pressure, trauma, or infection may also contribute to the interruption of the reflex arcs in the area. If the tip end of the conus terminalis is intact, some external bowel sphincter control due to an intact reflex arc may be present [10].

Prognosis for life and function are excellent with spina bifida occulta and after surgical repair of a meningocele, especially in the absence of hydrocephalus. Approximately 50 percent of children who survive surgical treatment for meningomyelocele will reach adulthood and some may learn to walk with braces and crutches. The primary disabilities of meningomyelocele may be resolved, but complications result from secondary disabilities, especially immobility.

Syringomyelia

The cause of syringomyelia remains unknown. It may be a developmental disorder. Unlike spina bifida, syringomyelia is characterized by the onset of progressive motor symptoms in the adult. Weakness and spastic paralysis as well as alterations in sensory function all may progress steadily or intermittently throughout the remainder of life.

Syringomyelia seems to be a developmental disorder involving the outlets in the fourth ventricle of the brain. It is present throughout embryogenesis but does not become symptomatic until the normally microscopic central canal of the spinal cord balloons and forms fluid-filled cavities in the nervous tissue of the cord itself (Fig. 47-2). A pathologic cavity caused by retained cerebrospinal fluid, called a *syrinx*, results, thus the name syringomyelia.

As with most developmental defects, the cause of syringomyelia is unknown, but the disorder may occur in association with other developmental defects such as spina bifida or hydrocephalus. Usually signs and symptoms of syrinx formation occur sometime after the age of 30, although they may begin at any age. The nature of the clinical signs depends on the level and size of the cavities, and which

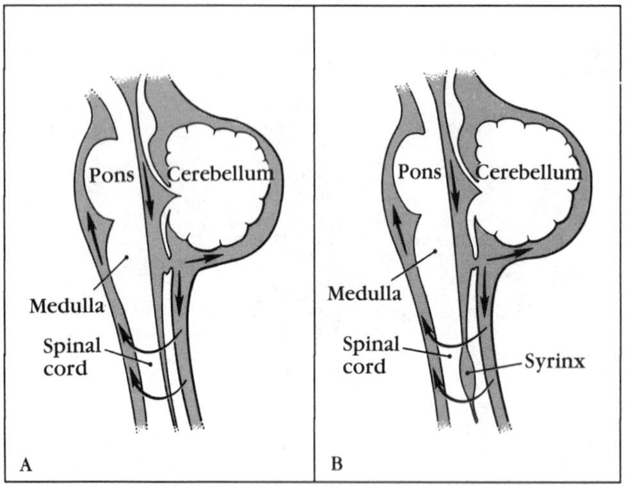

FIGURE 47-2. Syringomyelia. A. Normal circulation. B. Presence of syrinx in spinal column.

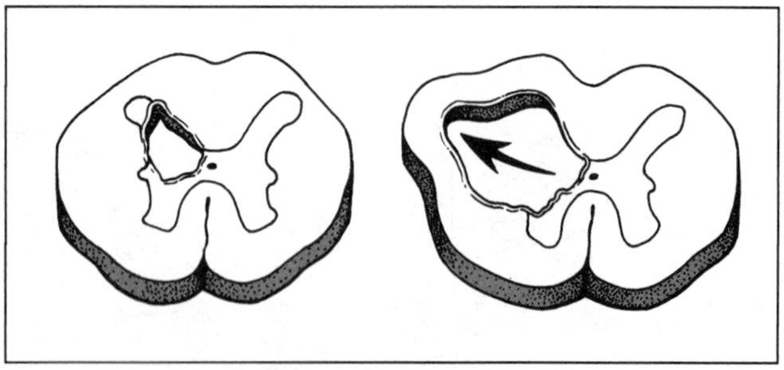

FIGURE 47-3. Development of a syrinx from the center outward into the dorsal gray horns.

structures are affected. Typically, the syrinx develops from the center of the cord outward in the direction of the dorsal gray horns (see Fig. 47-3). Since pain and temperature fibers cross immediately in the cord, and are relayed by the cells in the dorsal gray horns of the cord, the loss of these sensations with analgesia and thermoanesthesia are early signs of the onset of syringomyelia. If the syrinx spreads anteriorly toward the anterior horn cells, signs of lower motor neuron damage with small muscle atrophy occur. Signs and symptoms develop asymmetrically at first, but cord compression may become so severe that a complete paraplegia results.

The lower cervical and upper thoracic areas of the cord most frequently develop syrinx-related alterations. If the brainstem is affected initially or by extension, it is termed *syringobulbia*. Characteristic symptoms of medullary involvement result from cranial nerve damage and include weakness of facial and palatal muscles, laryngeal palsy, wasting of the tongue, loss of pain and temperature sensation, or onset of trigeminal pain. Occasionally dizziness may occur. Severe medullary involvement may be lethal.

In syringomyelia, the cerebrospinal fluid remains normal unless its circulation becomes obstructed. The cord enlarges in the areas of syrinx formation, and signs and symptoms may be suggestive of spinal cord tumor, multiple sclerosis, or amyotrophic lateral sclerosis. Later, manifestations of poorly healed, painless injuries with trophic skin lesions confirm the diagnosis of syringomyelia.

Clinical manifestations may be stationary for years, or slow progression may lead to death from brainstem involvement or from secondary problems such as extensive decubiti, renal infection, or pneumonia. Symptomatic treatment is aimed at preventing lethal and crippling secondary disabilities. If attempted early in the disease, surgical decompression of the medulla and fourth ventricle by removal of the posterior rim of the foramen magnum has yielded promising results in arresting and occasionally reversing the sensory losses. If the outlets in the fourth ventricle are found to be occluded, they are opened and the central canal may be aspirated at the time of surgery [3].

Hydrocephalus

The term *hydrocephalus* simply means an increased quantity of cerebrospinal fluid (CSF) within the ventricles of the cerebrum. If the cerebrospinal fluid pressure is normal or only sporadically increased with gradual cortical atrophy, the symptoms tend to begin slowly and relate to memory and judgment deficits, speech disorders, alterations in gait, some spasticity, and the signs of a simple dementia. If the pressure is elevated due to excess formation, faulty circulation, or inadequate resorption of CSF, the symptoms tend to be more abrupt in onset and more severe.

The most common cause of hydrocephalus is obstruction to the flow of cerebrospinal fluid (Fig. 47-4). In the fetus or neonate, the obstruction may result from cerebellar dysplasia, tumor, or developmental abnormalities of the cerebellar tonsils, the medulla, the cerebral aqueduct, or the fourth ventricle. In the older person, the obstruction may be due to trauma, infection, or tumor. If the obstruction is within the ventricles, the disorder is classified as *noncommunicating*, or *obstructive, hydrocephalus*. If CSF can gain access to the subarachnoid space and is then not absorbed by the arachnoid villi, it is classified as a *communicating hydrocephalus*. This type of hydrocephalus may be associated with postmeningitic or posthemorrhagic states. Excess formation of cerebrospinal fluid is rare and may be caused by choroid plexus tumors. Noncommunicating types of hydrocephalus due to faulty circulation or obstruction cause enlargement of the ventricular system. This eventually leads to signs of increased intracranial pressure and increased head size in adults and to bulging fontanels in infants. The treatment of choice is the removal of the obstruction. Prognosis depends on the cause and the severity of the obstruction and on the timing and effectiveness of the treatment.

Clinical manifestations of hydrocephalus depend on the age and rapidity of onset, as well as on the nature and success of the treatment. A newborn infant who exhibits a grossly enlarged head, widely separated cranial sutures,

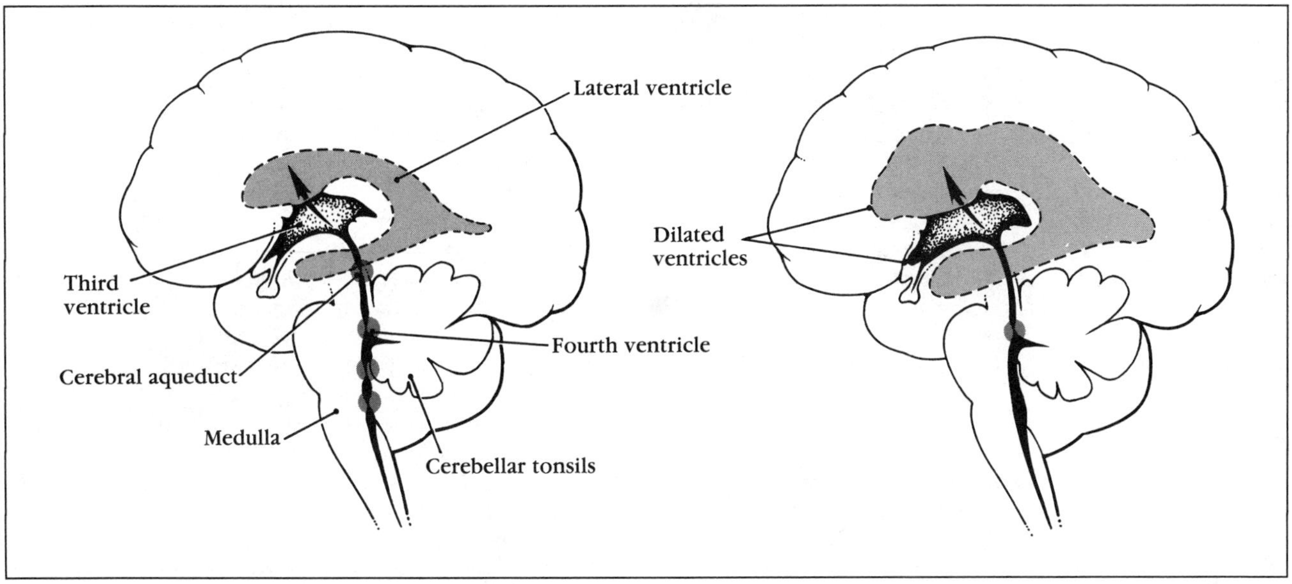

FIGURE 47-4. Schematic representation of areas of possible obstruction to spinal fluid and resulting ventricular enlargement.

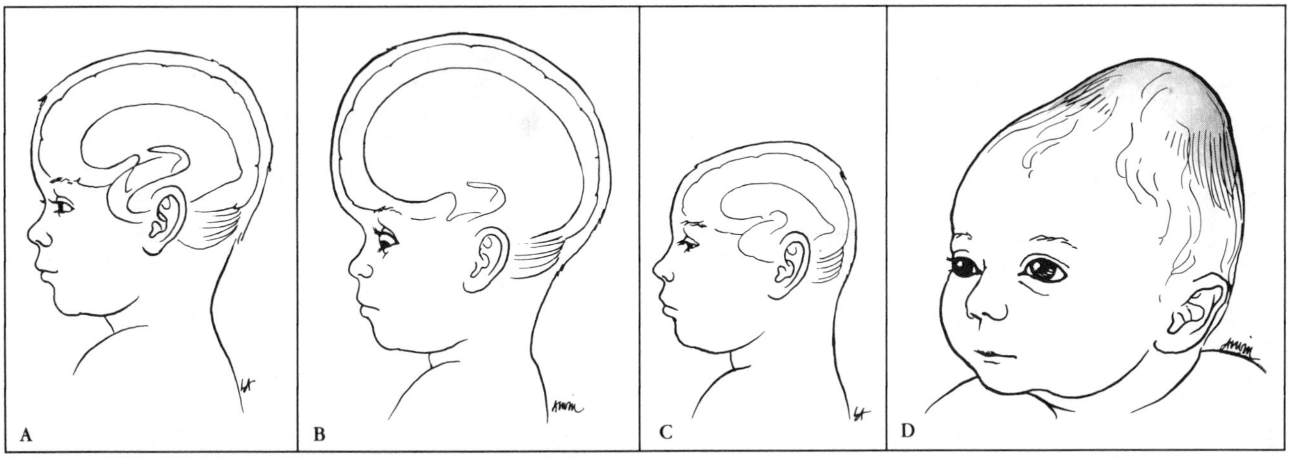

FIGURE 47-5. Some cephalic shapes. A. Normal. B. Hydrocephalus. C. Microcephalus. D. Molding. (From R. Judge, G. Zuidema, and F. Fitzgerald, *Clinical Diagnosis: A Physiologic Approach*. Boston: Little, Brown, 1982.)

and protruding eyes usually has irreversible signs of prolonged pressure, such as blindness from optic atrophy, paralysis, and mental retardation. In other infants, rapidly increasing head circumference, feeding problems, irritability, delayed motor skills, high-pitched cry, or turned down (setting sun) eyes are signs of developing hydrocephalus (Fig. 47-5). Because cerebral expansion is permitted by the open sutures and fontanelles of infancy, classic signs of increasing intracranial pressure such as headache, vomiting, or altered vital signs are usually minimal or absent. When the onset is in older children or adults whose cranial sutures have closed, headache and vomiting are often early signs and develop with much less trapping of CSF and greater CSF pressure increases.

Diagnosis is achieved by clinical observation of a head circumference increase in infants and by demonstration of dilated ventricles. Computerized axial tomography (CAT) scan often can demonstrate the ventricular dilatation and the cause. In the absence of available CAT scanning, a combination of skull x rays, angiography, and/or air studies can identify the existence of hydrocephalus.

Cranial Malformations

Arrested brain growth is the cause of the cranial malformation called *microcephaly*, or small head. The premature suture closure frequently associated with microcephaly results from the arrested brain growth and is not a cause of it.

This developmental defect in brain growth may be caused by first trimester irradiation, by German measles or other infections, or by heredity. There is no treatment for the severe mental retardation of microcephaly, which is often accompanied by cerebral palsy and/or seizure activity.

Craniosynostosis is early closure and ossification of one or more of the sutures in the skull, which occurs before brain growth is arrested. Early recognition and immediate surgery to create artificial sutures are necessary to decompress the brain and to limit the extent of neurologic damage caused by increasing intracranial pressure. If treatment is absent or delayed, this pressure can cause exophthalmos, optic atrophy, seizures, and mental retardation.

Cerebral Palsy (CP)

The term *cerebral palsy* is used to include a wide variety of nonprogressive brain disorders occurring during intrauterine life, during delivery, or during early infancy. Cerebral palsy by definition is a syndrome of motor disabilities, although it may be accompanied by mental retardation and/or seizure disorders. Causes are multiple and include cerebral developmental disorders such as microcephaly, intracranial hemorrhage, cerebral anoxia, or poisoning by toxins such as excessive bilirubin in the blood (kernicterus).

Clinical manifestations of cerebral palsy depend on the areas of the brain that sustain damage. Three main groups of CP have been described according to the dominant presenting signs. The *paralytic cerebral palsies* are the result of damage to the cortical motor cells and the pyramidal tracts in the brain. Typically, these are manifested as spastic paraplegias, quadriplegias, or hemiplegias. The *dyskinetic cerebral palsies* are caused by damage to the extrapyramidal system and are characterized by abnormal movements of athetoid, choreiform, or dystonic nature. The *ataxic cerebral palsies* indicate cerebellar damage and typically involve problems of incoordination and gait disturbances. Mixed CP presentations may combine any of the above.

Symptoms are present and nonprogressive from birth or early infancy, and diagnosis is usually made early in the preschool years. Treatment is aimed at preventing crippling secondary disabilities and providing special education to maximize useful function.

DISORDERS CHARACTERIZED BY PROGRESSIVE WEAKNESS OR PARALYSIS

Progressively paralyzing neurologic disorders affect the pyramidal system of the brain or cord, or the final common pathway between the cord and the muscle. They may result from dietary deficiencies, autoimmune disorders, genetic defects, infectious diseases, or they may be idiopathic. If the reflex arc remains intact, the usual sign is a spastic paresis or paralysis with normal or hyperactive reflexes. If the lower motor neuron or final common path is interrupted, the result is flaccid paralysis with diminished or absent reflexes. If the damage is spread throughout the motor system, as in amytrophic lateral sclerosis, spasticity will be present until the final common pathway is interrupted, when characteristic flaccidity and atrophic wasting of muscles will predominate. Prognosis and treatment depend on the nature of the disease and the availability and use of treatment.

Myasthenia Gravis (MG)

This chronic disease, seen in young adults and progressing with remissions and exacerbations, is characterized by abnormal muscle fatigability. The fatigue results in a typical drooping of eyelids (ptosis) and jaw, nasal voice, slurred speech, and weakness of the proximal extremities; all symptoms worsen during the day, but improve with rest or with the use of anticholinesterase drugs such as neostigmine. Eventually, muscle fibers may degenerate and weakness, especially of the muscles of the head, neck, trunk, and limbs, may become irreversible. Hyperplasia of the thymus is frequently associated and approximately 12 percent of afflicted persons have a thymoma. Reflexes may remain normal or reflect fatigue, decreasing with each repeated test. There appears to be no sensory alteration.

A number of primary muscle disorders cause clinically similar fatigue in the muscles, but myasthenia gravis is the only disorder that responds to anticholinesterase drugs. Myasthenia gravis involves progressive failure of the neuromuscular junctions to conduct an impulse. It is now believed to be an autoimmune disease with cellular and humoral factors playing a part [11]. As a result of the autoimmune reaction, the acetylcholine receptor sites in the voluntary muscles apparently sustain damage and cause the muscles to become less responsive to nerve impulses. As a result, the neurotransmitter, acetylcholine, is less effective in producing the desired depolarization in the affected muscles and muscle contractions become less effective with each rapidly succeeding nerve impulse.

The observed relationship between myasthenia gravis and disorders of the thyroid such as thyroiditis or thyrotoxicosis is believed to be due to a common disturbance of the immune system, expressed in different ways. Even today, the exact nature of these disturbances is not fully understood, nor is their relationship clear. Many experts postulate that genetic characteristics may constitute risk factors for autoimmune disorders such as myasthenia gravis, thyroiditis, or even diabetes mellitus [2].

During the early active stage of myasthenia gravis, while the characteristic remissions and exacerbations are occurring and before muscle atrophy sets in, some individuals may respond well to the surgical removal of the thymus. It is believed by many that an early thymectomy may decrease the level of autoimmune activity before much permanent damage is sustained by the acetylcholine receptor sites in the voluntary muscles. Plasmapheresis is another method of treatment aimed at removing antiacetylcholine receptor antibodies from the blood to decrease the autoimmune activity [2]. Steroids are usually given to suppress the production of antibodies. Anticholinesterase drugs are administered to prevent the breakdown of the acetylcholine at the myoneural junction. Too much anticholinesterase drug activity may produce a skeletal muscle weakness that resembles the myasthenic defect. This phenomenon is called cholinergic crisis or depolarization block [1]. It is hard to differentiate clinically between a cholinergic crisis and a myasthenic crisis, or disease exacerbation. Most individuals in a crisis state are treated for cholinergic crisis, withdrawn from the anticholinesterase drugs, and maintained on assisted respiration until the type of crisis can be identified.

The course of myasthenia gravis is variable. Some persons do not develop other symptoms than the initial ocular muscle fatigue and weakness. Others, who exhibit more generalized symptoms, respond well to the standard treatment for years. A small percentage of afflicted persons suffer the acute, fulminating disease accompanied by muscle atrophy and have poor response to all treatment. Death from myasthenia gravis usually occurs within the first 5 to 10 years of onset, when the disease is most acute. Lethal crises are not usually seen late in the disease and the damage sustained tends to remain constant or to be compensated for by other muscles. Death occurring after many years of MG is usually due to the secondary problem of immobility, resulting in pneumonia.

Subacute Combined Degeneration of the Cord

Vitamin B_{12} deficiency, usually occurring as a part of pernicious anemia, (see Chap. 14) can produce a degeneration of the white matter in the lateral and posterior spinal cord, as well as peripheral polyneuropathy and slight cerebral atrophy. Neurologic manifestations begin gradually and usually are accompanied by the classic megaloblastic anemia. Unusual sensations such as tingling, numbness, or pain are often the first symptoms of neurologic degeneration. These paresthesias are followed by motor signs of weakness and incoordination. The paresthesias and motor signs both tend to begin in the lower limbs and move to the upper limbs and trunk as the disease spreads up the posterior and lateral cord. With progressive and untreated degeneration of the cord, sensory ataxia and either spastic paralysis with hyperactive reflexes or flaccid paralysis with absent reflexes may occur in all four limbs, being the most severe in the lower limbs. If the degeneration is confined to the posterior columns, incoordination is predominant. If the degeneration is more lateral, weakness and paralysis are most characteristic. The nature of the paralysis is influenced by the presence or absence of peripheral neuropathy and the status of the reflex arc. In addition to these motor signs, individuals may suffer optic atrophy and/or nystagmus if the second or third cranial nerve is affected. The other cranial nerves are rarely affected. The cerebral atrophy may result in impaired memory, confusion, paranoid behavior, irritability or depression.

Eventually, the damaged peripheral nerves can regenerate, with improvement in sensory symptoms, coordination, and reflexes, but spasticity and signs of cerebral atrophy are unlikely to disappear, since central nervous system damage is not reversible.

Clinically similar disorders such as neurosyphilis or multiple sclerosis must be ruled out by gastric acid evaluation, blood tests for megaloblastic anemia, and bone marrow evaluation for red cell formation abnormalities. Serum B_{12} evaluation may be done or tests may be made of vitamin B_{12} absorption, using radioactive vitamin B_{12}.

Guillain-Barré Syndrome (Acute Idiopathic Polyneuritis)

This acute, frequently postinfectious polyneuritis may be due to an allergic response or some type of hypersensitivity reaction. The initial symptoms usually follow a febrile illness, vaccination, injury, or surgery by a few days or weeks. Guillain-Barré syndrome has no predilection for any age group, sex, or race and when an infectious etiology can be demonstrated, it is usually viral.

The anterior gray matter of the cord and more vascular dorsal nerve roots are usually affected first with segmental peripheral and spinal nerve root demyelination. Phagocytic cells have been shown to break through the basement membrane of the Schwann cell and cause the demyelinization [7]. As a result, both sensory and motor dysfunction occur. Flaccid paralysis may occur suddenly, affecting all four limbs simultaneously or spreading upward from the lower limbs (ascending paralysis). It may involve the muscles of the neck, the trunk, and cause respiratory paralysis. Occasionally some vague sensory changes occur prior to the paralysis that include nausea, or pain in the back, limbs or head. However, the paralytic symptoms are usually the chief problem. Variant autonomic dysfunction may occur and may include orthostatic hypotension, tachycardia, and other manifestations. Reflexes are usually diminished or lost, but occasionally remain normal even with severe muscular weakness. Paresthesias in the affected limbs are common and include numbness, tingling, and pain. When the onset of flaccid paralysis is sudden and symmetric, and when it is accompanied by sensory changes, diagnosis of Guillain-Barré syndrome can be made by clinical observation and history alone. Muscular atrophy is not common but may be seen when axon loss is severe. Cerebrospinal fluid (CSF) protein becomes markedly elevated after the first few days of illness.

When death occurs, it is usually due to respiratory arrest or pneumonia. For survivors of respiratory problems, the prognosis for life and for eventual recovery of function is good. Eighty-five percent make a complete recovery in 4 to 6 months but others may have severe residual disabilities. Treatment with steroids, adrenocorticotropic hormone (ACTH), or other immunosuppressant drugs may or may not be beneficial in altering the course of the disease.

Multiple Sclerosis (MS)

MS is a relatively common inflammatory, demyelinating disease of the central nervous system that results in diverse manifestations of neurologic alteration. The cause or causes of MS are unknown, but it probably is an autoimmune disorder influenced by a genetic susceptibility. While no single virus has been incriminated in the causation of the disease, elevated antibody titers to measles virus have been demonstrated [7]. This suggests the possibility that a latent viral infection precipitates the disease. Dietary deficiencies and acute viral infections have also been studied as etiologic agents. Stress and trauma seem to play a role in precipitating the onset of the disease or in precipitating an exacerbation of the symptoms. MS is more common in colder climates and its onset generally occurs between the ages of 20 and 40 years.

The disease usually begins rather suddenly with the occurrence of a set of focal symptoms of visual disturbance or of motor dysfunction in one or two limbs. The causative lesion or plaque is found predominantly in the white matter of the central nervous system with loss of the myelin sheaths that normally act as insulation around nerve fibers. Loss of myelin slows, blocks, or distorts nerve impulse transmission. During the course of the disease, some of the myelinated fibers may regenerate and associated symptoms disappear. Eventually gliosis occurs in the lesions and scar tissue replaces the myelin and may replace the axis cylinders themselves. From this gliosis comes the term *sclerosis*, meaning induration or scarring. Initial symptoms may be transient and are frequently followed by complete, or nearly complete recovery as the myelin is replaced. Periods of remission are common. Later alterations become permanent with remissions and exacerbations limited to new symptoms superimposed on a baseline of disability. This permanence in symptoms is due to eventual disruption and destruction of the nerve cells themselves, even though this is initially a disease of the myelin sheaths rather than the cells. If the lesions are predominantly in the pyramidal tracts of the cerebrum and/or spinal cord, the symptoms will be motor in nature. If they affect the lateral spinothalamic or posterior tracts of the cord, sensory changes will be noted. Weakness or spastic paralysis of the limbs and sphincters with hyperactive reflexes are common. Sexual dysfunctions, with impotence in males and alterations in vaginal sensations in females, are common and disturbing aspects of sensorimotor changes. Paresthesias such as pain, numbness, or tingling may be noted in the limbs and/or the face. Emotional changes may range from emotional lability to sustained euphoria or severe depression.

Brainstem lesions often contribute to emotional lability and also produce symptoms of cranial nerve injury. The optic, oculomotor, trochlear, and abducens nerves and the vestibular branch of the auditory nerve are especially common sites of damage. Visual signs and symptoms range from nystagmus to diplopia to visual dimness to patchy or complete blindness. Occasionally pupillary abnormalities may be noted. Dizziness may be mild, or it may be severe and associated with nausea and vomiting. Speech may be difficult due to spastic weakness of facial and speech muscles. Dysphagia makes eating difficult with an increased danger of aspiration. Cerebellar lesions also affect speech, producing a slurred, uncoordinated type of articulation. Other signs such as intention tremor of the hands, head tremor, and/or staggering gait are indicative of cerebellar lesions.

Although early clinical manifestations may be limited to effects of alteration in the cerebellar area, the brainstem, or the cerebrum, late multiple sclerosis usually affects all parts of the central nervous system. The classic triad of Charcot described in 1868, which occurs late in the disease, includes nystagmus, intention tremor, and speech disorders. Spastic paraplegia, incontinence, and extreme emotional lability are also typical of the late stages of MS.

MS is diagnosed by evaluating the clinical picture, observing the pattern of remission and exacerbation of symptoms, and ruling out other diseases such as subacute combined degeneration of the cord. Studies of antibodies in the blood or cerebrospinal fluid often show gamma globulin abnormalities in the established MS case. Other changes in the CSF are inconsistent and nonspecific.

The prognosis varies from a progression to death in less than 6 months or a benign course for over 20 years without shortening or altering productive life. However, even when the MS victim survives to old age, the last years are often spent as a spastic paraplegic, with visual disorders, incontinence, dysarthria, and lack of emotional control. Death is often due to secondary disorders such as pneumonia or septic decubiti.

Treatments for MS range from special high-vitamin, low-fat diets, to steroids, to core-cooling of the body and have failed to consistently influence the course of the disease.

Amyotrophic Lateral Sclerosis (ALS)

ALS or progressive muscle atrophy is another primary neurologic disease that affects motor function and results in alterations of gait and paralysis. It is a noninflammatory disease of the upper and lower motor neurons, with demyelination secondary to axon degeneration. Unlike MS, which classically is characterized by remissions and exacerbations, ALS usually steadily progresses to death within 2 to 6 years [7]. Premature aging of nerve cells due to some environmental or genetic factor, nutritional deficiencies, heavy metal poisoning, metabolic defects, or even a smoldering virus have all been identified as possible causes or contributors to ALS.

Loss of the motor cells in the cerebral cortex can result in signs of upper motor neuron damage, with weakness or spastic paralysis and hyperactive reflexes. This is especially likely to occur in the lower limbs. Damage to cranial nerves in the medulla produces signs of ***bulbar palsy***, either of the spastic or flaccid type. Bulbar palsy refers to weakness or paralysis of the muscles supplied by the medulla. Commonly upper and lower motor neuron damage are mixed in ALS, and where reflexes are interrupted, muscle atrophy secondary to denervation and loss of muscle tone occurs. In these areas, diminished reflexes or flaccid paralysis occur. Muscle atrophy is often seen in the upper limbs and tongue.

Degeneration may occur anywhere within the pyramidal

system, the anterior motor cells of the spinal cord, and/or the ventral nerve roots. It does not characteristically affect peripheral nerves. The muscle fasciculations or twitching frequently seen in the upper limbs and/or tongue are believed to be due to accumulating excessive neurotransmitter at the myoneural junction, rather than being caused by abnormal spontaneous discharges of degenerating nerve cells [5].

The onset of ALS usually occurs after the age of 50 with a 2:1 incidence of men over women. One common early sign may be muscle fasciculations of the tongue when there is brainstem involvement. Fasciculations may also be seen in the hands or upper limbs and are small local muscle contractions that occur when a muscle is tapped or moved passively [5]. Whenever the brainstem is affected, slurred speech and weakness of the palate and facial muscles may occur. Reflexes may be normal, hyperactive, or diminished depending on whether it is mixed with lower motor neuron damage. If lower motor neuron damage is present, muscle wasting will occur in the tongue or other muscles. Eventually swallowing is affected and speech may become unintelligible.

Weakness and clumsiness are first noted in the distal portions of the upper limbs and wasting of the muscles of the hand is characteristic. Sexual dysfunctions, such as impotence, are an early sign, but bowel and bladder sphincters are not usually affected until late in the disease. Characteristically there is no sensory alteration in ALS. Paralysis of the trunk and respiratory muscles occurs late in the course of the disease if bulbar palsy does not cause death first. Death is often due to pneumonia or respiratory failure.

Diagnosis of ALS is based on characteristic clinical signs such as upper limb weakness, wasting of hand muscles, and muscle fasciculations. Disorders such as syringomyelia, cord tumors, and neurosyphilis usually have pain and sensory changes associated but must be ruled out diagnostically. The absence of muscle atrophy and lack of muscular response to edrophonium hydrochloride rules out a diagnosis of myasthenia gravis. Biopsy of muscle and electromyograms show denervation atrophy in ALS.

Prognosis is worst when the brainstem is affected first. Life expectancy is best when the degeneration remains confined to the lower motor neurons of the middle and lower spinal cord for a long time. However, it is rare for individuals to survive longer than 10 years after onset, and death can occur within a year. Treatment is symptomatic with no beneficial effects from antiinflammatory and immunosuppressive drugs.

DISORDERS CHARACTERIZED BY ABNORMAL MOVEMENTS

Abnormal movements often indicate alterations in the extrapyramidal motor system. This system is not clearly understood so that the relationship of the pathology and structural alterations with the clinical manifestations is not clear. Abnormal movements often result from alterations and reflect a disturbance in the balance between the excitatory and inhibitory neurotransmitters in the basal ganglia. The neurotransmitters involved apparently are dopamine, acetylcholine, and gamma aminobutyric acid (GABA). The basal ganglia most often affected are the four that make up the corpus striatum: the caudate, putamen, globus pallidus, and the claustrum. In some disorders, such as early parkinsonism, conscious effort can suppress these movements temporarily, but typically they return when the person relaxes or is distracted.

The abnormal movements that result are of different types but may be painful or incapacitating. Types of abnormal movement range from the fine, rhythmic quivering of tremor to the violent, irregular jerking or twisting movements of *ballismus*. *Dyskinesias* or alterations in voluntary muscle movement, and *dystonias*, or alterations in muscle tone (such as rigidity), are both classified as abnormalities of movement. *Fixed or intermittent muscle spasms*, such as are characteristic of torticollis, may be included unless they are due to muscle rather than nerve damage. *Choreas* are irregular muscle twitchings that may become so severe that they contribute to death from exhaustion. *Athetosis*, or athetoid movements, are slow, repeated, purposeless muscle movements that may affect only the digits or the entire body.

There are many causes of extrapyramidal dysfunction. Cerebral anoxia and/or trauma in utero or during delivery may produce an athetoid cerebral palsy or a spastic cerebral palsy or both. The characteristic tremors of parkinsonism may be produced by therapy with the major tranquilizers of the phenothiazine family or by carbon monoxide poisoning. The exhausting muscle twitchings of chorea may be due to a genetic defect or to an infectious disease. As with all neurologic disorders, abnormal movements give more clues about which structures are damaged than about what has damaged them. Therefore, a very complete physical exam and a thorough family history may be more important than laboratory results in identifying the source of the problem.

Parkinsonism (Paralysis Agitans)

When the levels of dopamine in the corpus striatum are decreased, a primary neurologic disorder called parkinsonism or a parkinsonian syndrome may result. *Parkinson's disease* refers to parkinsonism of unknown etiology that occurs between the ages of 50 and 80.

Dopamine is one of the more than 40 chemicals known or thought to be chemical transmitters in the brain. This monamine transmitter appears to be concentrated in areas such as the substantia nigra with dopamine-containing neurons projecting to other areas such as the corpus striatum. In the corpus striatum, dopamine seems to play an important part in the control of complex movements [6].

Various lesions and cellular alterations noted in the corpus striatum itself (especially the caudate, the putamen, and the globus pallidus) and the substantia nigra are commonly present in parkinsonism, but their significance in

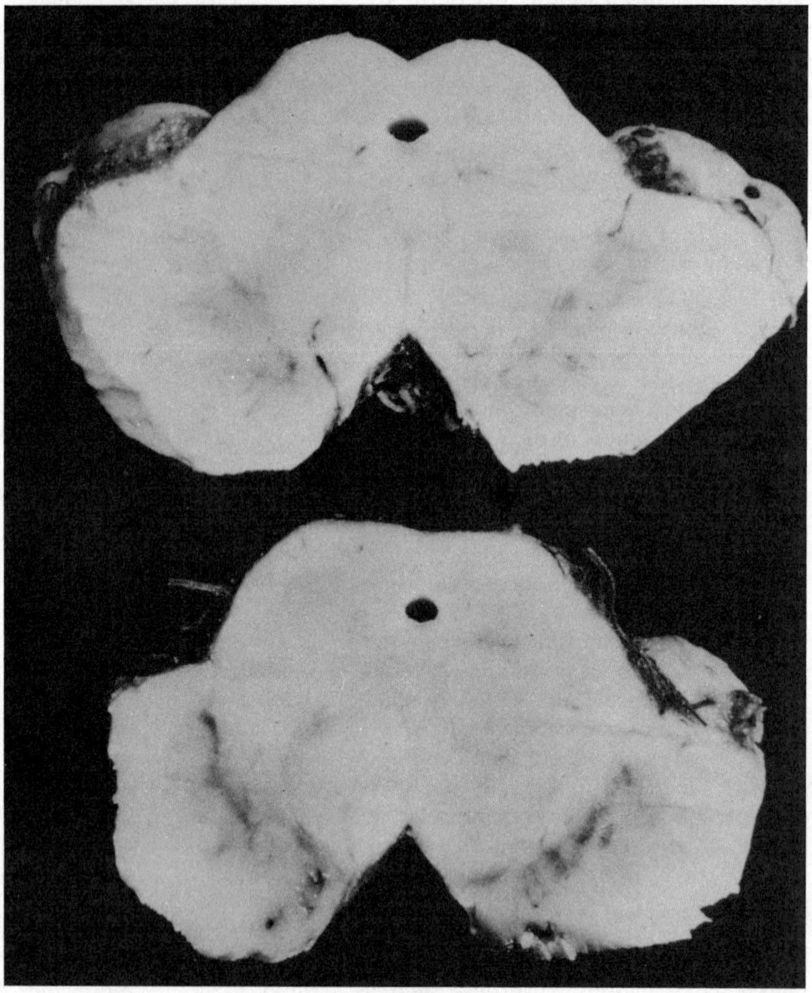

FIGURE 47-6. Brainstem in parkinsonism. There is decreased pigmentation in the substantia nigra as compared to normal (*below*). (From F. Miller, *Peery and Miller's Pathology* [3rd ed.]. Boston: Little, Brown, 1978.)

terms of cause and effect is not known (Fig. 47-6). If the dopamine fibers projecting to the corpus striatum degenerate, permanent or progressive muscle rigidity and/or the tremors of parkinsonism result. If the dopamine in the corpus striatum is blocked or bound temporarily by a drug such as chlorpromazine, the typically reversible rigidity and/or tremors of the parkinsonian syndrome occur.

Usually parkinsonism is characterized by a masklike facial expression and infrequent blinking, due to diminished automatic movements. Speech is quiet and monotonous. Mental ability is usually unaffected. Spontaneous, automatic movements, such as swinging the arms when walking, also diminish and cease. The body posture becomes stooped with apparent flexion of the limbs. The characteristic gait progresses with small, shuffling steps that pick up speed as the person travels. The afflicted person suffers increasing muscle rigidity in both extensor and flexor muscles that may be jerky or spastic in nature. Rather than losing voluntary function, the person finds it increasingly difficult to initiate a voluntary act and the actions tend to be slow and clumsy. The tremor of parkinsonism commonly occurs in the hands, ankles, head, and/or mouth during periods of rest. It can be suppressed with conscious effort for brief periods and usually disappears with sleep. If fingers and thumb are both involved, the tremor may be described as a "pill-rolling" tremor. Intention tremor, which refers to a tremor occurring during the performance of a precise movement, can also occur. Both resting and intention tremor become worse under emotional stress although extreme provocation may result in the quick, efficient performance of complex motor functions. Other symptoms such as heat intolerance and excessive salivation, are due to autonomic system dysfunction.

If the symptoms of parkinsonism are due to dopamine-binding or blocking by drugs such as chlorpromazine, the symptoms usually disappear when the drug is withdrawn or decreased. If the symptoms are due to a discrete episode of cerebral anoxia or trauma, such as carbon monoxide poisoning or head injury, they may stabilize. However, most cases of parkinsonism are characterized by progressive disability until death occurs from secondary problems such as pneumonia in 10 or more years after the onset of the disease. Diagnosis is based on evaluation of signs and symptoms and by ruling out other diseases with muscle rigidity or tremor, such as multiple sclerosis or neurosyphilis.

Levodopa (L-dopa) is the treatment of choice for most parkinsonism patients who are experiencing progressive disability. It crosses the blood-brain barrier and is converted to dopamine in the central nervous system. It may be administered with other drugs to reduce its toxic effects on the rest of the body [1].

Drug-Induced Dyskinesias and Dystonias

The major tranquilizers have many effects on the extrapyramidal nervous system. Besides the drug-induced parkinsonian syndrome, which usually occurs early in therapy, there may be a number of other effects, some of which are reversible and some permanent. Dyskinesias are embarrassing, rhythmic, involuntary movements such as chewing or smacking. Dystonias are spasms that jerk the face, head, or limbs in a painful and/or frightening way. Both can occur alone or in association with more typically parkinsonian symptoms soon after major tranquilizer therapy is begun. Usually they respond well to anticholinergic therapy and are probably caused by a relative increase in cholinergic activity in the presence of a sudden reduction in the level of dopamine in the basal ganglia. The anticholinergic therapy seems to temporarily restore the balance [8]. *Akathisia* or a feeling of restlessness in the muscles is more difficult to treat and may require dose reduction or a change in drugs [4].

Dyskinesias and dystonias also may occur during levodopa therapy. They usually disappear as the levodopa is decreased. Unfortunately, these symptoms may appear before the tremor of parkinsonism is under control, which means that if the dose of levodopa is increased enough to control the tremor, the dyskinesias or dystonias may become intolerable. If the levodopa dosage is decreased to eliminate the dystonias, the tremor may become much worse.

When dyskinesias occur late in a tranquilizer-therapy regimen, or appear after the drug has been discontinued (tardive dyskinesias), they may be evidence of permanent, irreversible change in the extrapyramidal nervous system. This change may be in the dopamine receptors themselves. These tardive dyskinesias do not respond well to anticholinergic therapy, as do early dyskinesias, although they also seem to be due to a disturbed balance in the brain between acetylcholine and dopamine [8].

Torticollis

Torticollis, or wry neck, is an intermittent or sustained dystonic contraction of the cervical muscles on one side of the neck, due to hysteria, drug therapy, or organic neurologic disease. It may occur as one of the painful dystonias seen in early phenothiazine therapy or, rarely, it may accompany primary parkinsonism. When it occurs in association with primary or secondary parkinsonism, it may be due to a relative increase in cholinergic activity in the brain associated with a striatal dopamine deficiency [8].

The angle of head rotation depends on which muscles are affected; the affected muscles often hypertrophy in response to the constant or frequent powerful muscle contractions. The spasm may occur suddenly and painfully which is characteristic of the drug-induced dystonias and also of hysteria. The contraction also can occur very slowly. Primary muscle fibrosis following trauma or abnormalities of the cervical spine must be ruled out as the cause of this disorder. If major tranquilizers are being used, reduction in dose and/or anticholinergic therapy may prove useful. Psychotherapy and/or relaxation therapy may be helpful for hysterical torticollis. Unfortunately, if the cause of the torticollis is a lesion in the corpus striatum, the prognosis for cure is poor [11].

Huntington's Chorea

Huntington's chorea is a familial disorder that is characterized by a progressive degeneration of the cerebral cortex as well as of the basal ganglia. In addition to the dramatic choreiform movements for which it is named, there is progressive deterioration of higher intellectual functions such as memory and judgment, to the point of severe dementia and death. This disease is transmitted as an autosomal dominant trait.

In Huntington's chorea the neurotransmitter GABA (gamma aminobutyric acid) is seen to be markedly reduced in the degenerating areas of the brain. Acetylcholine also seems to be reduced, resulting in an imbalance between the three transmitters, GABA, acetylcholine, and dopamine. When dopamine predominates, chorea results [9]. When chorea is the major motor symptom, degenerative lesions are especially common in the caudate. In those occasional cases in which rigidity and tremor predominate, lesions seem to be more likely in the putamen. However, in many cases of Huntington's chorea, lesions are common throughout the corpus striatum, and in the thalamus as well [11]. As is usual with extrapyramidal disorders, the full significance of these lesions is not fully understood.

GABA is believed to be an inhibitory transmitter and the neurons that degenerate in the corpus striatum are inhibitory neurons [6]. As a result, increasingly violent choreiform movements begin to occur in the face, neck, and arms during middle age and may be the first signs of neurologic disease. In addition to the chorea or less commonly, widespread muscle rigidity and tremors, a dementia occurs that is characterized by impulsiveness, loss of judgment and memory, irritability or apathy, delusions or hallucinations, and suicidal tendencies. The dementia seems to result from atrophy of the cerebral cortex especially over the frontal lobes [11].

When a family history of Huntington's chorea exists, diagnosis is made by this history and confirming physical examination of symptoms. With a negative family history, diseases such as neurosyphilis must be ruled out. Usually this disease progresses to death from pneumonia or heart failure in 10 to 20 years. No treatment is known to have any effect on the progression of the disease.

DISORDERS CHARACTERIZED BY MEMORY AND JUDGMENT DEFICITS

Dementia is a term used to refer to an organically caused syndrome of impaired intellectual functions. There is widespread deterioration in the cerebral cortex, especially in the frontal lobes. Characteristically, decreasing quality of judgment, loss of abstract thinking and reasoning, and diminished memory are accompanied by emotional changes ranging from apathy to lability, by decreasing personal cleanliness, by increasing impulsiveness, and by confusion and disorientation.

There are many causes of dementia, but in most cases it is a rare or late accompaniment to characteristic symptoms of the individual problem. The examples presented here have been selected because dementia is the prime symptom and demonstrates similarity between vascular, infectious, and other types of lesions. No cure for dementia exists but the pathologic process may be arrested with subsequent therapy for residual problems.

Senile Dementia

Cerebral atherosclerosis may contribute to the development of transient ischemic attacks or cerebrovascular accidents of a focal nature. Cerebral atherosclerosis can also produce the symptoms of dementia secondary to diffuse small cerebral infarctions and widespread cerebral anoxia. The term *senile dementia* may be used for the results of diffuse cerebral atherosclerosis; generally it refers to a condition of decreasing intellectual capability with increasing disorientation and emotional lability beginning in the aged individual. Most frequently, the disorder seems to be due to a decreasing blood supply and cerebral anoxia resulting in cortical degeneration. Sensory deprivation and overmedication in the institutionalized elderly person may also be contributing factors to the progression of senile dementia.

Alzheimer's Disease (Presenile Dementia)

This progressive cerebral degeneration begins to be symptomatic during the middle years, usually after the age of 40, being most common between 50 and 65 years of age. Cortical degeneration is most marked in the frontal lobes, but atrophy occurs in all areas of the cortex. The disease does not appear to be genetically linked and its cause remains unknown. A number of lesions may be noted in the cortex and basal ganglia. Enzyme and other chemical changes have also been noted but their significance is not known [11].

Pathologically, degeneration of neurofibrils especially in the frontal, parietal, and occipital cortices is seen. The brain changes are visible first as microscopic plaques, which consist of a core surrounded by fibrous tissue, and later as striking atrophy of the cerebral cortex.

Early symptoms include loss of memory, carelessness about personal appearance and speech disturbances that progress to complete disorientation, severe deterioration in speech, incontinence, and stereotyped, repetitive movements. Progression to severe dementia is relentless and occurs over a period of 5 to 10 years. Death from secondary causes such as septic decubiti or pneumonia may occur. Diagnosis of Alzheimer's disease is usually made after other conditions that can cause dementia have been ruled out. No treatment seems to have a significant effect on the course of the disease.

Neurosyphilis

It is believed that the causative spirochete, *Treponema pallidum*, reaches the nervous system during the second stage of a syphilitic infection, although neurologic symptoms may not occur for months or years. During this period, the cerebrospinal fluid will give a positive VDRL. If neurologic symptoms appear within a few years of the initial infection, they tend to be focal in nature and respond well to antibiotic therapy. However, when the onset of neurologic symptoms is delayed for a longer period of years, the earliest symptoms reveal widespread pathology and do not respond as well to therapy.

In the second stage of syphilis, the symptoms of neurosyphilis are transient and vague including headache and intermittent pains in the trunk and limbs. Rarely, acute meningitis or encephalitis occur and may result in seizures and/or coma [11]. A few years after this early stage, inflammation of arterial walls and meningitis often occur, occasionally manifesting a communicating hydrocephalus. Symptoms of the vascular pathology and meningitis include seizures, headache, anxiety, and signs of cranial nerve damage such as palsies, neuralgia, dizziness, or deafness [11].

Blood tests for syphilis are usually positive in secondary and early tertiary neurosyphilis. The cerebrospinal fluid is positive and generally the serum protein and mononuclear cell count are elevated. These tests, used to confirm the diagnosis of neurosyphilis and to monitor the response to antibiotic therapy indicate success when cell count falls, the protein, content decreases, and eventually changes occur in the VDRL.

General paresis occurs approximately 20 years after the initial infection and the spirochetes seem to invade the brain parenchyma and cord tissue, rather than staying in the meninges and blood vessels. As a result, lesions are spread diffusely over the cerebral cortex, the basal ganglia, and sometimes the cerebellar cortex. Early symptoms include impaired memory and concentration. Later, characteristic personal carelessness, impulsiveness, incontinence, and signs of both receptive and expressive aphasia develop. Seizures are common as are irregular and miotic pupils. The pupillary reaction to light is diminished or absent even though the pupils may accommodate to distance changes; this condition is called an *Argyll Robertson pupil*, which evidences midbrain damage. This pupil is especially suggestive of neurosyphilis, although similar pupil changes may be seen in other disorders, such as alcoholic polyneuropathy. Because of damage to the cortical motor cells and pyramidal tracts, voluntary motor function decreases and reflexes become hyperactive unless the cord is invaded, in which case reflexes may diminish or disappear. The untreated end result of general paresis is usually a bedridden, incontinent, confused, hallucinating person who is susceptible to all the secondary problems of immobility. Penicillin or erythromycin are curative drugs for syphilis, and no tolerance to the drugs appears to be developed by the organism.

REFERENCES

1. Albanese, J. A. *Nurses' Drug Reference*. New York: McGraw-Hill, 1982. Pp. 379–381.
2. Anchi, T. Plasmapheresis as a treatment for myasthenia gravis. *J. Neurosurg. Nurs.* 13:23, 1981.
3. Haerer, A., and Currier, R. D. *Neurology Notes* (5th ed.). University of Mississippi Medical School, 1974. P. 95.
4. Harris, E. Extrapyramidal side effects of antipsychotic medication. *Am. J. Nurs.* 81:1324, 1981.
5. Hartley, F. D. A nurse's view: Amyotrophic lateral sclerosis. *J. Neurosurg. Nurs.* 13:89, 1981.
6. Iverson, L. The chemistry of the brain. *Sci. Am.* 9:141, 1979.
7. Robbins, S., and Cotran, R. *Pathologic Basis of Disease* (2nd ed.). Philadelphia: Saunders, 1979.
8. Rosal-Greif, V. Drug-induced dyskinesias. *Am. J. Nurs.* 82:66, 1982.
9. Stripe, J., et al. Huntington's disease. *Am. J. Nurs.* 79:1428, 1979.
10. Vigliarolo, D. Managing bowel incontinence in children with meningomyelocele. *Am. J. Nurs.* 80:105, 1980.
11. Walton, J. N. *Brain's Diseases of the Nervous System* (8th ed.). New York: Oxford University Press, 1977. Pp. 456, 457–466, 580–581, 610, 619–620, 1023, 1184.

BIBLIOGRAPHY

Bartol, G. J. Psychological needs of spinal cord injured person. *J. Neurosurg. Nurs.* 10:171, 1981.

Boltshauser, E., et al. Permanent flaccid paraplegia in children with thoracic spinal cord injury. *Paraplegia* 19:227, 1981.

Bracken, M. B., et al. Psychological response to acute spinal cord injury: An epidemiological study. *Paraplegia* 19:271, 1981.

Brock, M., and Dietz, M. (eds.). *Intracranial Pressure: Experimental and Clinical Aspects*. New York: Springer-Verlag, 1972.

Butterworth, J. F., et al. Flaccidity after head injury: Diagnosis, management and outcome. *Neurosurgery* 9:242, 1981.

Chusid, J. *Correlative Neuroanatomy and Functional Neurology* (17th ed.). Los Altos, Calif.: Lange, 1979.

Conway, B. *Pediatric Neurologic Nursing*. St. Louis: Mosby, 1977.

Davis, J., and Mason, C. *Neurological Critical Care*. New York: Van Norstrand Reinhold, 1979.

de la Torre, J. C. Spinal cord injury: Review of basic and applied research. *Spine* 6:315, 1981.

Dye, O. A., et al. Long-term neuropsychological deficits after traumatic head injury with comatosis. *J. Clin. Psychol.* 37:472, 1981.

Easton, K. C. Emergencies in the home: Head, neck and back injuries. *Br. Med. J.* 282:2099, 1981.

Epstein, B. *The Spine: A Radiological Text and Atlas*. Philadelphia: Lea & Febiger, 1976.

Feiring, E. (ed.). *Brock's Injuries of the Brain and Spinal Cord and Their Coverings* (5th ed.). New York: Springer, 1974.

Findelstein, S., and Ropper, A. The diagnoses of coma: Its pitfalls and limitations. *Heart Lung* 8:1063, 1979.

Fischer, R. P., et al. Postconcussive hospital observation of alert patients in primary trauma center. *J. Trauma* 21:920, 1981.

Foo, D., et al. Post traumatic acute anterior spinal cord syndrome. *Paraplegia* 19:201, 1981.

Ginnity, S. W. Assessment of cervical cord trauma by the nurse practitioner. *J. Neurosurg. Nurs.* 10:193, 1981.

Gudeman, S. K., et al. Computed tomography in the evaluation of incidence and significance of post traumatic hydrocephalus. *Radiology* 141:397, 1981.

Gurdjian, E. S. *Impact Head Injury*. Springfield, Ill.: Thomas, 1975.

Guttmann, L. *Spinal Cord Injuries: Comprehensive Management and Research* (2nd ed.). Oxford, England: Blackwell, 1976.

Guyton, A. *Textbook of Medical Physiology* (6th ed.). Philadelphia: Saunders, 1981.

Hardy, A., and Rossier, A. *Spinal Cord Injuries*. Acton, Mass.: Publishing Sciences Group, 1975.

Howell, T., et al. Depression in spinal cord injured patients. *Paraplegia* 19:204, 1981.

Hudak, C., Lohr, T., and Gallo, B. *Critical Care Nursing* (3rd ed.). Philadelphia: Lippincott, 1982.

King, L. R., et al. Pituitary hormone response to head injury. *Neurosurgery* 9:229, 1981.

Kunkel, J., and Wiley, J. Acute head injury: What to do when... and why. *Nurs. 79* 9:22, 1979.

Lazure, L. Defusing the dangers of autonomic dysreflexia. *Nurs. 80* 10:52, 1980.

Levin, H. S., et al. Ventricular enlargement after closed head injury. *Arch. Neurol.* 38:623, 1981.

Lewis, A. *Mechanisms of Neurological Disease*. Boston: Little, Brown, 1976.

Lindgren, S., et al. Acute head injuries: Cooperative efforts in clinical assessment. *J. Neurosurg.* 25:32, 1981.

Merritt, H. H. *A Textbook of Neurology* (6th ed.). Philadelphia: Lea & Febiger, 1979.

Pierce, D., and Nickel, V. (eds.). *The Total Care of Spinal Cord Injuries*. Boston: Little, Brown, 1977.

Plum, F., and Posner, J. *The Diagnosis of Stupor and Coma* (3rd ed.). Philadelphia: Davis, 1980.

Powner, D. (ed.). Coma: Cessation of therapy and decision making process. The University of Pittsburgh School of Medicine Symposium. *Heart Lung* 8:1057, 1979.

Outcome of non-traumatic coma (Editorial). *Br. Med. J.* 4:428, 6283:3, 1981.

Rimel, R. W. A prospective study of patients with central nervous system trauma. *J. Neurosurg. Nurs.* 13:132, 1981.

Rimel, R. W., et al. Disability caused by minor head injury. *Neurosurgery* 9:221, 1981.

Robbins, S., and Contran, R. *Pathological Basis of Disease* (2nd ed.). Philadelphia: Saunders, 1979.

Rockswold, G. L. Evaluation and resuscitation in head trauma. *Minn. Med.* 64:81, 1981.

Rossier, A. *Rehabilitation of the Spinal Cord Injury Patient*. Summit, N.J.: Ciba-Geigy Corp., 1975.
Schochet, S., and McCormick, W. *Essentials of Neuropathology*. New York: Appleton-Century-Crofts, 1979.
Sipkins, J. H., et al. Severe head trauma and acute renal failure. *Nephron* 28:36041, 1981.
Spencer, P. S., and Schaumberg, H. H. *Experimental and Clinical Neurotoxicology*. Baltimore: Williams & Wilkins, 1980.
Stone, J. L., et al. Traumatic subdural hygroma. *Neurosurgery* 8:542, 1981.
Swann, I. J., et al. Head injuries at an inner city accident and emergency department. *Injury* 12:274, 1981.
Taylor, J. Increased intracranial pressure. *Nurs. 83* 13:44, 1983.
Taylor, J., and Ballenger, S. *Neurological Dysfunction and Nursing Interventions*. New York: McGraw-Hill, 1980.
Vick, N. *Grinker's Neurology* (7th ed.). Springfield: Thomas, 1976.
Wehrmaker, S., and Wintermute, J. *Case Studies in Neurological Nursing*. Boston: Little, Brown, 1978.
Weiner, H., and Levitt, L. *Neurology for the House Officer* (2nd ed.). Baltimore: Williams & Wilkins, 1978.
Yashon, D. *Spinal Injury*. New York: Appleton-Century-Crofts, 1978.
Young, M. S. A bedside guide to understanding the signs of intracranial pressure. *Nurs. 81* 11:59, 1981.
Zuidema, G., Rutherford, R., and Ballenger, W. *The Management of Trauma* (3rd ed.). Philadelphia: Saunders, 1979.

UNIT 16
REPRODUCTION

Sharron Schlosser
NORMAL AND ALTERED MALE AND FEMALE FUNCTION

Shirley Freeburn
Joan Hurlock
ENDOCRINE MECHANISMS OF REPRODUCTION
DISORDERS OF REPRODUCTION

Ann Edgil
GENETIC DISORDERS

Unit 16 emphasizes the male and female reproductive physiology and the common pathologic problems associated with them. Chapter 48 provides an overview of the anatomy and physiology of the male reproductive system. Chapter 49 presents alterations in the prostate, penis, scrotum, testis, and epididymis. Chapter 50 discusses normal female anatomy and physiology along with laboratory and diagnostic aids in the examination of the female system. Chapter 51 details some of the common alterations in female function including menstrual problems, infections, and benign and malignant conditions. Chapter 52 presents a concise overview of genetics and includes principle of inheritance, patterns of transmission of genetic traits, and chromosomal disorders. This chapter is intended to provide a basic reference for the student to utilize in identifying genetic abnormalities.

The reader is encouraged to utilize the learning objectives as study guides and to supplement material presented here with some of the suggested reading at the end of the unit.

CHAPTER 48
NORMAL MALE FUNCTION

LEARNING OBJECTIVES

1. Describe the development and function of the male sexual organs.
2. List three functions of the male reproductive system.
3. Discuss the process of spermatogenesis.
4. List and discuss the factors involved in determining male fertility.
5. List and discuss the stages of the male sexual act.
6. Identify the functions of testosterone.
7. Describe the production and degradation of testosterone.
8. Discuss the influence of the hypothalamus and anterior pituitary on the production of testosterone and spermatogenesis.
9. Briefly describe three diagnostic tests used to determine male reproductive alterations.

Reproductive function is an integral facet of the human body. Survival of the species is dependent on proper functioning of the reproductive system. This chapter provides an overview of normal male reproductive physiology and function.

PHYSIOLOGIC ANATOMY

The male reproductive organs include both essential and accessory organs. The essential organs are the testes, which are responsible for production of the sperm, while accessory organs include the epididymis, vas deferens, seminal vesicles, ejaculatory ducts, prostate gland, and urethra. The supporting structures of the scrotum, penis, and spermatic cords are also considered to be accessory organs. Figure 48-1 shows the male genitourinary anatomy.

Testes

The testes are two ovoid glands suspended in the scrotum by attachment to both scrotal tissue and spermatic cords. The testes consists of many lobules, each of which contains the *seminiferous tubules* and *interstitial cells of Leydig*. Spermatogenesis occurs in the seminiferous tubules, while the interstitial cells are responsible for secretion of testosterone, the male hormone (see p. 748).

Epididymis

The epididymis is a very tortuous genital duct that serves as a passageway for the sperm. It is located on top of the testes and is divided into three parts: (1) a head, which is connected to the testes, (2) a body, and (3) a tail, which is continuous with the vas deferens (Fig. 48-2). Sperm are

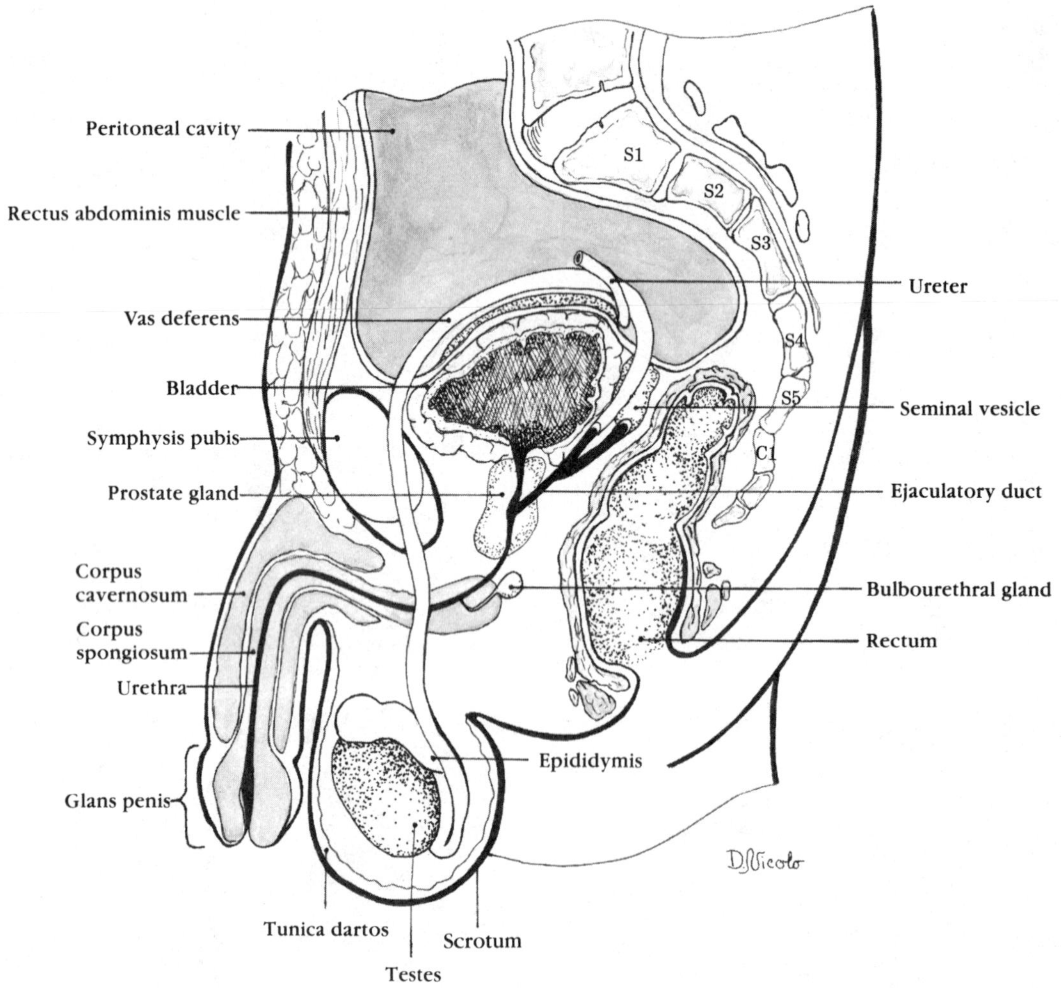

FIGURE 48-1. Side view of male genitourinary anatomy. (From M. A. Miller and P. Brooten, ***The Childbearing Family: A Nursing Perspective*** [2nd ed.]. Boston: Little, Brown, 1983.)

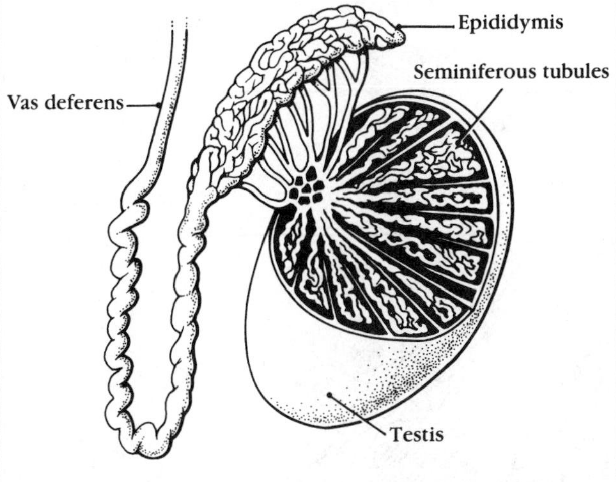

FIGURE 48-2. The vas deferens in relationship to the tubules of the testis and epididymis.

stored in the epididymis from 18 hours up to 10 days. During this storage, the sperm mature, develop the power of motility, and become capable of fertilization.

Vas Deferens

The vas deferens is an uncoiled tube or duct serving as an extension of the tail of the epididymis. This duct ascends from the scrotum into the abdomen where it passes over the bladder. On the posterior of the bladder the duct enlarges into the ampulla of the vas deferens and joins with the duct from the seminal vesicle to form the ejaculatory duct (Fig. 48-2).

The vas deferens also serves as a storage site for the majority of the sperm. During the storage period, sperm metabolism continues and large amounts of carbon dioxide are formed and secreted into the surrounding fluid. The resulting acidic pH inhibits activity of the sperm during storage. However, on release to the exterior, the sperm again exhibit the power of motility [1].

Seminal Vesicles

The seminal vesicles are two pouches that are lined with secretory epithelium and are located directly behind the urinary bladder (Fig. 48-3). They produce a viscous alkaline fluid that contributes about 30 percent of the seminal fluid volume. This thick fluid is rich in fructose, an energy source for sperm metabolism. Fluid from the seminal vesicles also contains citric acid, five amino acids, and prostaglandins.

Ejaculatory Ducts

The ejaculatory ducts are two short tubes that descend through the prostate gland and terminate in the urethra. As

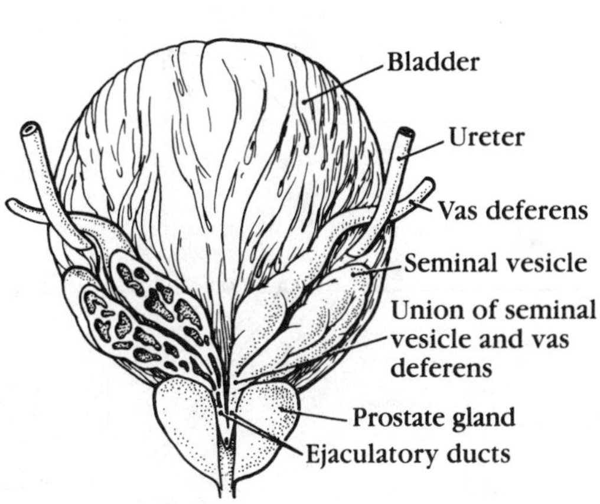

FIGURE 48-3. The seminal vesicles, union with the vas deferens, and entrance into the prostate gland.

previously mentioned, they are formed by union of the vas deferens and seminal vesicle ducts.

Prostate Gland

The prostate is a chestnut-sized gland located just below the bladder. It surrounds the ejaculatory duct and about an inch of the urethra and functions primarily to secrete a thin, milky, alkaline fluid that comprises about 60 percent of the seminal fluid volume. This fluid is discharged into the urethra during emission and helps to neutralize the acidic fluid of the male urethra and female vagina.

Urethra

The urethra serves as the terminal portion of the seminal fluid passageway. It is about 18 to 20 cm in length and passes through the prostate gland and the penis, terminating at the external urethral orifice. Located along the urethra are the glands of Littré, which supply mucus. The urethra also receives alkaline fluid from the bulbourethral glands.

Bulbourethral Glands

The bulbourethral glands are two pea-sized glands located just below the prostate gland. The alkaline secretions from these glands constitute less than 5 percent of the seminal fluid volume.

Penis

The penis is covered by a loose layer of skin and contains three compartments of erectile tissue, two corpora cavernosa and the corpus spongiosum (see Fig. 48-1). Corpora cavernosa are larger and parallel to each other. The corpus spongiosum is smaller, lower than the corpora cavernosa, and contains the urethra. Distally, the corpus spongiosum

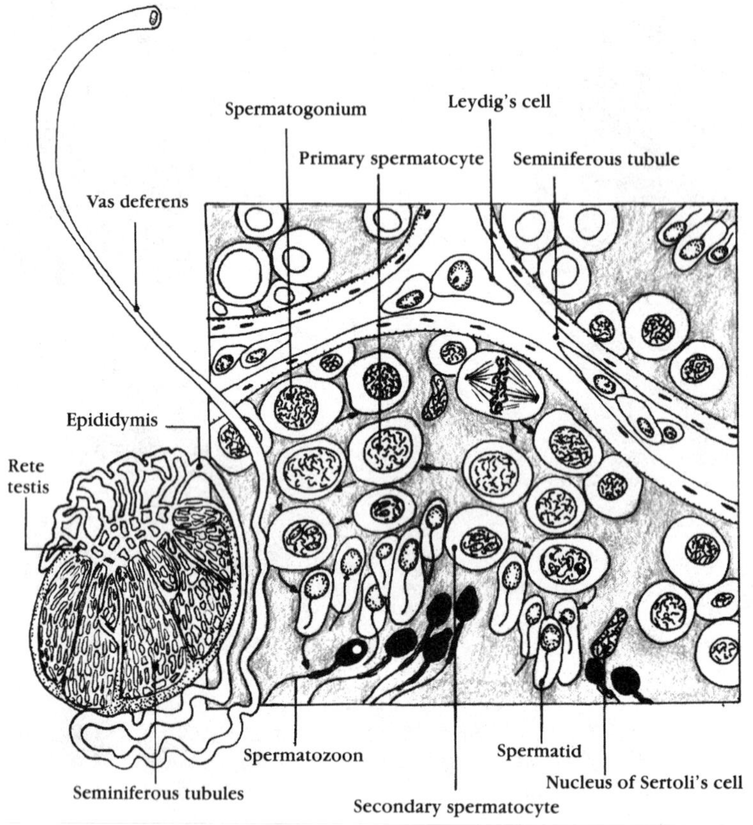

FIGURE 48-4. Male ductal system and developing reproductive cells. The detail on the right shows spermatogenesis and the seminiferous tubule. (From M. A. Miller and P. Brooten, ***The Childbearing Family: A Nursing Perspective*** [2nd ed.]. Boston: Little, Brown, 1983.)

expands to form the glans penis. In the uncircumcised male, a fold of loose skin covers the glans. The erectile tissue is spongelike and contains large venous sinuses, interspersed with arteries and veins. Sexual stimulation results in dilation of the arteries and arterioles and distention of the cavernous spaces with blood. Filling of the erectile tissue then results in erection of the penis. The penis serves two functions: (1) It contains the urethra, which acts as a passageway for urine. (2) It also serves as the organ of copulation for the male.

MALE REPRODUCTIVE FUNCTIONS

The male reproductive system serves the following primary functions: (1) spermatogenesis, (2) performance of the male sexual act, and (3) hormonal regulation of male sexual function.

Spermatogenesis

The seminiferous tubules of the newborn male's testes contain primitive sex cells called *spermatogonia*. They are located in two to three layers in the outer border of the tubular epithelium (Fig. 48-4). At approximately the age of 13, spermatogenesis begins in all the seminiferous tubules. This development occurs as a result of stimulation by the adenohypophyseal (anterior pituitary) gonadotropic hormones. A lengthier discussion of this influence is found on pp. 752–753.

During spermatogenesis, a series of meiotic divisions occurs. The primary spermatocyte divides into two secondary spermatocytes, which subsequently divide and produce four spermatids (Fig. 48-5). During this process each cell retains one of each pair of 23 chromosomes. Of the 23 chromosomes, one is the sex chromosome.

In the process of spermatid production, each cell loses most of its cytoplasm and elongates into a sperm, which consists of a head, neck, body, and tail (Fig. 48-6). The head is formed when nuclear material rearranges and the cell membrane contracts around it. This part of the sperm is responsible for fertilization of the ovum while the tail portion of the sperm is responsible for its rapid motility.

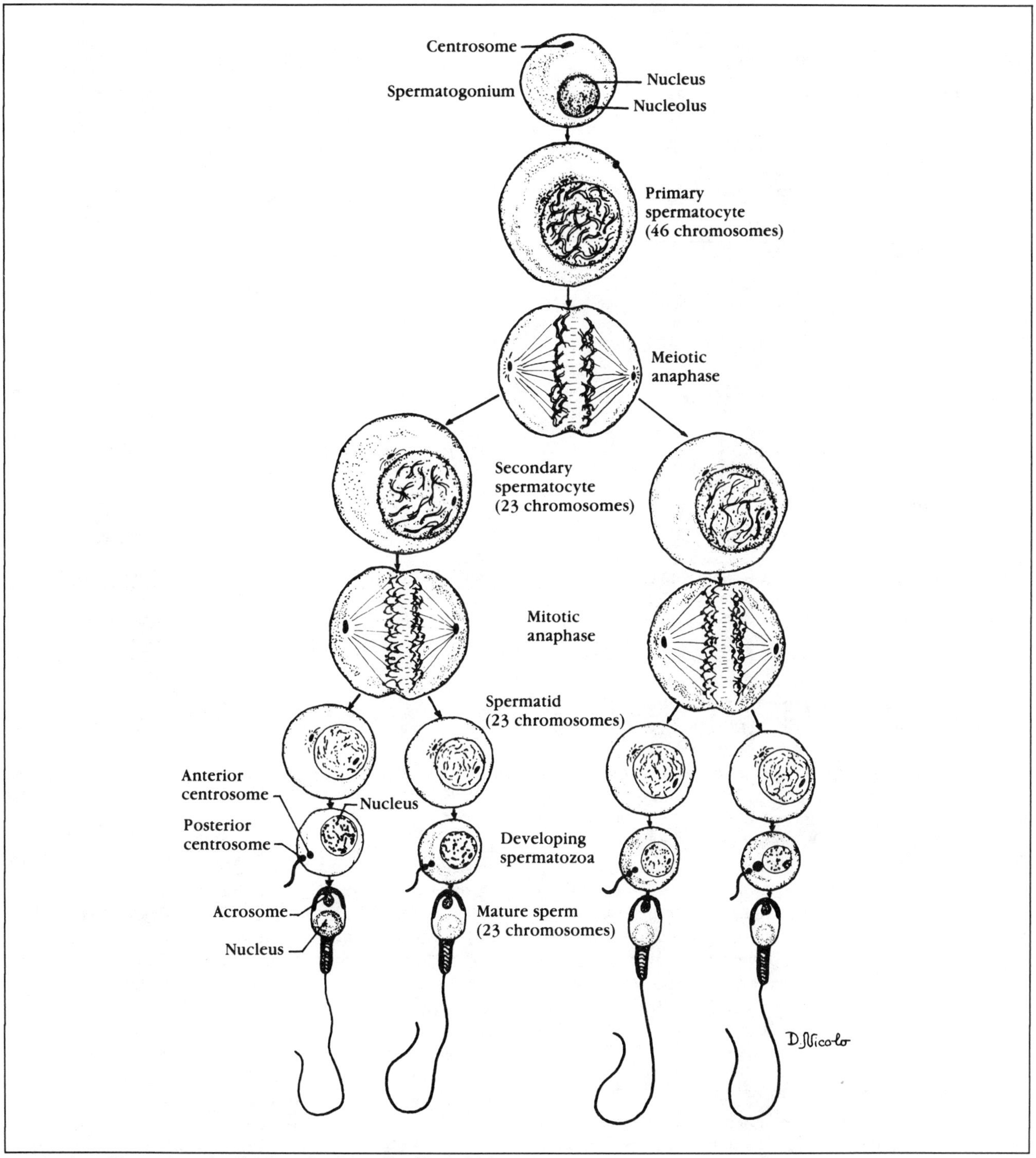

FIGURE 48-5. Maturation of male reproductive cells. (From M. A. Miller and P. Brooten, *The Childbearing Family: A Nursing Perspective* [2nd ed.]. Boston: Little, Brown, 1983.)

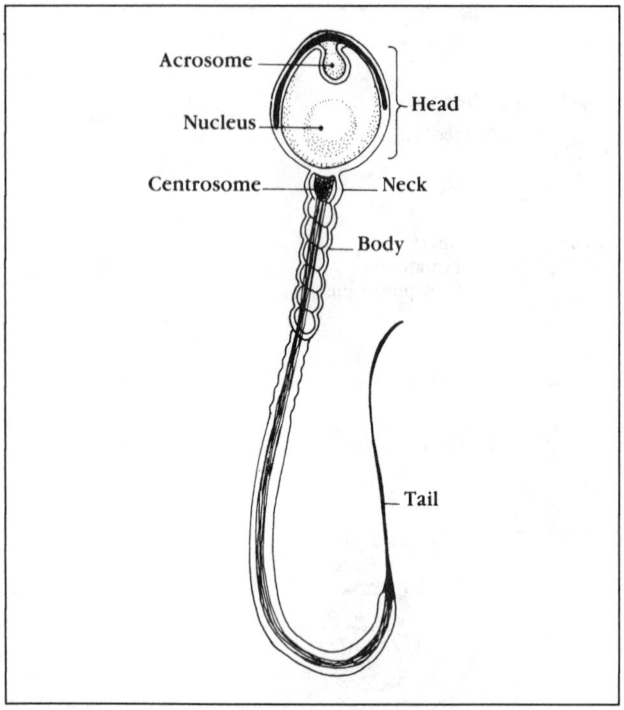

FIGURE 48-6. The mature sperm, consisting of a head, neck, body, and tail. (From M. A. Miller and P. Brooten, *The Childbearing Family: A Nursing Perspective* [2nd ed.]. Boston: Little, Brown, 1983.)

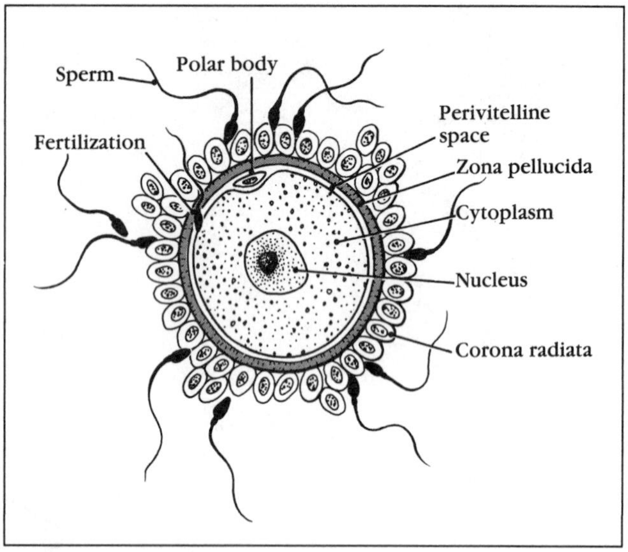

FIGURE 48-7. Fertilization of an ovum.

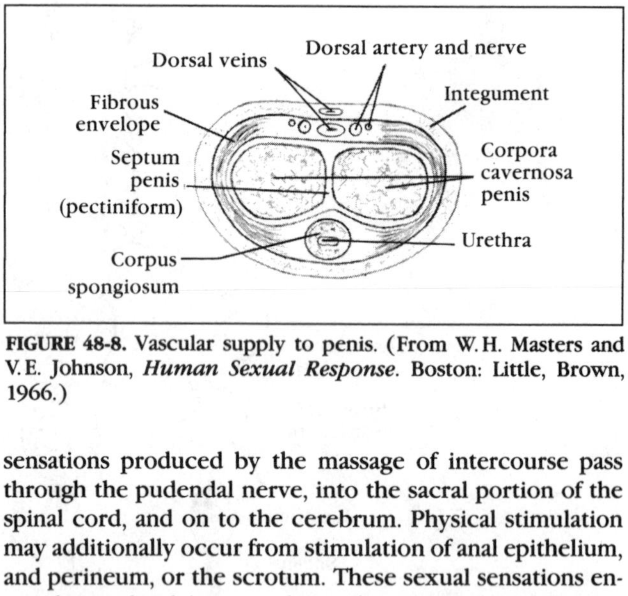

FIGURE 48-8. Vascular supply to penis. (From W. H. Masters and V. E. Johnson, *Human Sexual Response*. Boston: Little, Brown, 1966.)

Fertility

Actual male fertility is dependent on the following: (1) the quantity of semen ejaculated, (2) the number of sperm per milliliter, and (3) the motility and morphology of the sperm. The seminal fluid volume ejaculated with each coitus averages 400 million sperm in a fluid volume of approximately 3 ml. When the number of sperm in each milliliter drops below 20 to 50 million, ***infertility*** (defined as the inability to conceive after 12 months of adequate exposure in unprotected intercourse) and/or ***sterility*** (absolute inability to conceive) frequently result. The acrosome on the head of the sperm produces the enzymes ***hyaluronidase*** and several proteinases. It is believed that these enzymes are necessary to remove the outer cell layers of the ovum. However, only one sperm is responsible for the actual fertilization of the ovum (Fig. 48-7).

The Male Sexual Act

In the field of sexual behavior, humans differ from all other living creatures. In animals, for example, sex drive and behavior are instinctual and dependent on hormones. With humans, the initiation of the sexual act may begin through physical or psychic stimulation. Thoughts and dreams of sexual intercourse may produce erection and ejaculation in the male.

The most important source for stimulation of the male sexual act is physical stimulation of the glans penis. Sexual sensations produced by the massage of intercourse pass through the pudendal nerve, into the sacral portion of the spinal cord, and on to the cerebrum. Physical stimulation may additionally occur from stimulation of anal epithelium, and perineum, or the scrotum. These sexual sensations enter the pudendal nerve from the perineal and scrotal nerves and then enter the sacral portion of the spinal cord to be transmitted to the cerebrum.

The first effect of sexual stimulation is erection of the penis. Normally, the penis is flaccid due to constriction of the arterioles supplying the vascular spaces of the penis (Fig. 48-8). Sexual stimulation results in a stimulation of parasympathetic nerves and inhibition of sympathetic nerves to the arterioles. As a result, the penile arterioles dilate while the veins constrict. Blood is forced into the vascular spaces and erectile tissue. The blood flow, under pressure, produces a ballooning effect of the erectile tissue resulting in a hard and elongated penis. This stage terminates the first part of the sexual act, which is termed *erection*.

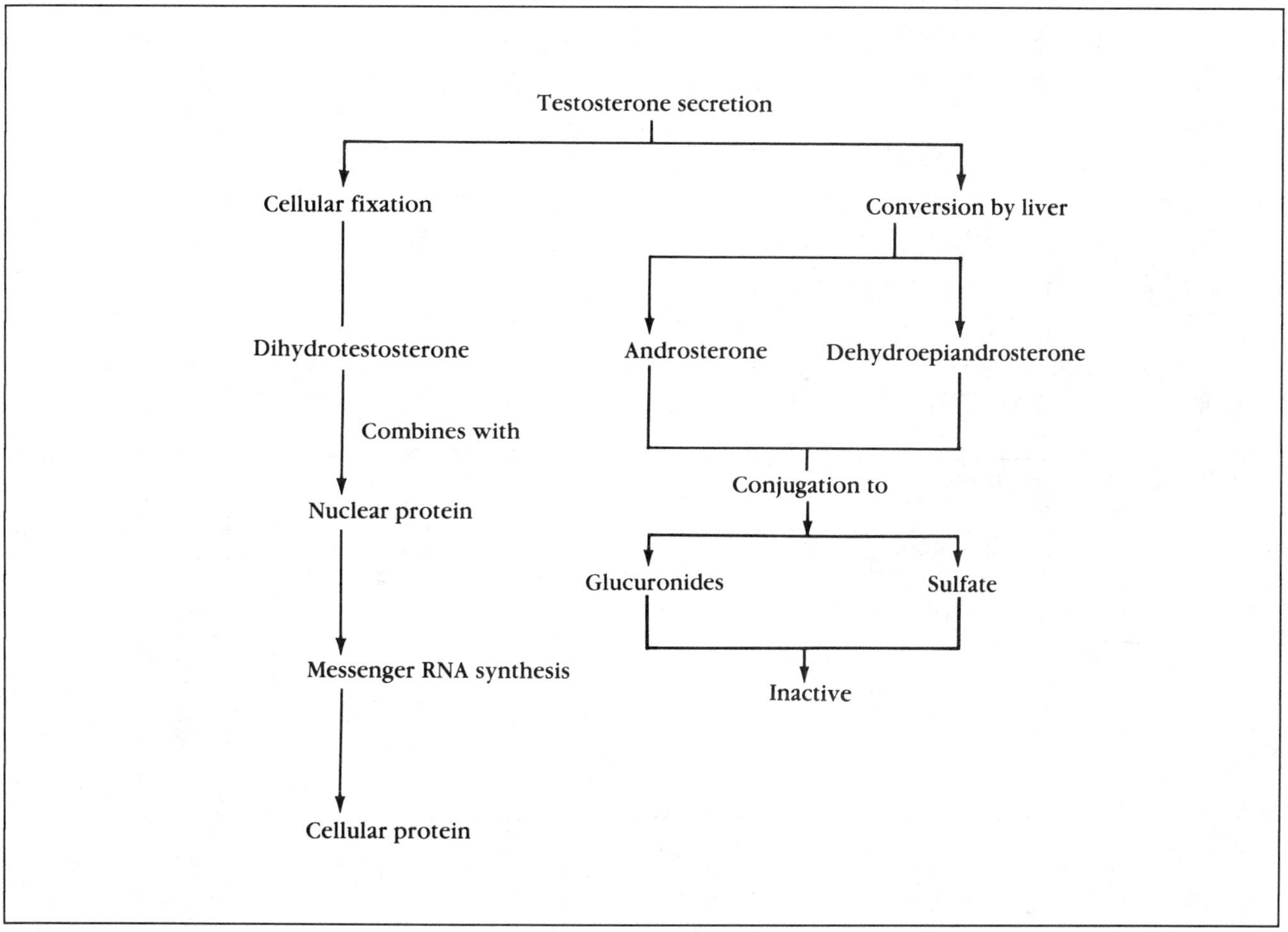

FIGURE 48-9. Fate of testosterone after secretion by testes. Part of the hormone becomes fixed in tissues to perform intracellular functions and part is degraded by the liver.

During this first stage of the male sexual act, lubricating fluid is discharged from the bulbourethral glands and the glands of Littré, a result of parasympathetic stimulation.

The second stage of the male sexual act involves two processes: *emission* and *ejaculation*. Emission is initiated when sympathetic impulses are emitted by reflex centers in the spinal cord, which pass to the smooth muscle of the genital ducts, producing contractions and forcing the sperm and seminal fluid into the internal urethra. Filling of the internal urethra then initiates impulses that result in contractions of the skeletal muscle at the base of the penis. During these contractions, the sphincter at the base of the bladder constricts, preventing the expulsion of urine, as seminal fluid and sperm are expelled through the external urethral orifice. This activity is termed ejaculation and culminates the male sexual act.

Hormonal Regulation of Male Sexual Functions

Testosterone is the active male hormone secreted by the testes. It is produced by the *interstitial cells of Leydig*, which are located between the seminiferous tubules. The testosterone released by these cells circulates in the bloodstream only 15 to 30 minutes before it is fixed in tissues to perform intracellular functions or is degraded by the liver. Once testosterone enters the cells it is converted to *dihydrotestosterone* to perform its functions. Dihydrotestosterone combines with a nuclear protein, promotes messenger ribonucleic acid (RNA) synthesis, which then enhances cellular protein production. Testosterone not fixed in tissues is converted in the liver into androsterone and dehydroepiandrosterone. These forms are conjugated into glucuronides or sulfates and are excreted in bile or urine as 17-ketosteroids (Fig. 48-9). The inactivation process for testosterone accounts for the ineffectiveness of oral administration of this hormone. Testosterone serves the following functions: (1) controls development of male secondary sex characteristics, (2) regulates metabolism, (3) affects fluid and electrolyte balance, and (4) inhibits anterior pituitary secretion of gonadotropins. These functions are further described in this section.

Testosterone is responsible primarily for the distinguishing male characteristics. As early as the second month of embryonic life, chorionic gonadotropin from the placenta

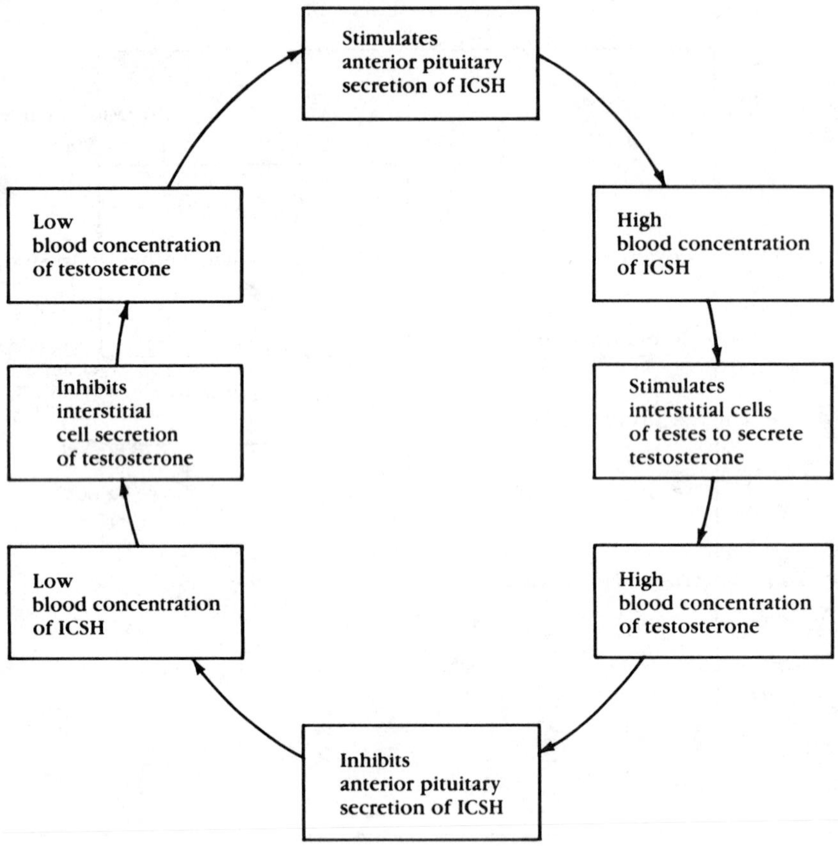

FIGURE 48-10. Illustration of negative feedback mechanism for the secretion of ICSH and interstitial cell secretion of testosterone. (From C. Anthony, *Textbook of Anatomy and Physiology*. St. Louis: Mosby, 1979.)

stimulates production of small amounts of testosterone, which is believed to be responsible for the development of the penis, scrotum, prostate gland, seminal vesicles, and genital ducts in the fetus. During childhood, virtually no testosterone is produced until puberty at which time a rapid increase in secretion is noted. Following puberty and continuing until maturity at approximately the age of 20, testosterone produces an enlargement of the penis, scrotum, and testes.

Testosterone stimulates protein anabolism, which is directly responsible for virilization of the male. The secondary sexual characteristics—muscular development and strength; hair growth on the face, axilla, and chest; bone growth; and deepening of the voice—are manifestations of this process. In affecting bone growth, testosterone is also responsible for early uniting of the epiphyses and shafts of long bones, which stops the growth process. The basal metabolic rate (BMR) increases under the influence of this hormone.

Testosterone secondarily increases sodium, potassium, calcium, and water retention. The hormone levels can affect the fluid balance through influencing ion retention by the kidneys. It is a method to retain substances necessary to effect the anabolic process.

High levels of testosterone inhibit secretion of gonadatropins by the anterior pituitary.

Gonadotropic Hormonal Control of Male Sexual Functions

In the male, the anterior pituitary is responsible for secretion of the following sexual hormones: (1) follicle-stimulating hormone (FSH) and (2) interstitial cell-stimulating hormone (ICSH). The latter hormone may also be referred to as the luteinizing hormone (LH).

ICSH stimulates the Leydig cells to produce testosterone. A rise in the blood level of testosterone provides a negative feedback to the anterior pituitary, thus reducing the levels of FSH and ICSH. A drop in ICSH level inhibits se-

TABLE 48-1. Normal hormone levels

Hormone	Age	Blood	Urine
Testosterone			
Male	Adult	0.3–1.0 gm/dl (average = 0.7)	47–156 gm/24 hours (average = 70)
	Adolescent	0.10 gm/dl	
Female	All ages	0–0.1 gm/dl (average = 0.04)	0–15 gm/24 hours (average = 6)
17-Ketosteroids			
Male and female	All ages	25–125 gm/dl	
Male	10 years		1–4 mg/24 hours
	20–30 years		6–26 mg/24 hours
	50 years		5–18 mg/24 hours
	70 years		2–10 mg/24 hours
Female	10 years		1–4 mg/24 hours
	20–30 years		4–14 mg/24 hours
	50 years		3–9 mg/24 hours
	70 years		1–7 mg/24 hours
Chorionic gonadotropin			
Male			0

cretion of testosterone. As testosterone levels drop, the anterior pituitary is again triggered to secrete ICSH (Fig. 48-10). Chorionic gonadotropin, in the fetus, has properties like those of ICSH. Thus, it stimulates the interstitial cells in the testes, the production of testosterone, and the development of the penis, scrotum, prostate gland, seminal vesicles, and genital ducts in the fetus.

FSH is the hormone responsible for the conversion of the spermatogonia into sperm. Without FSH spermatogenesis will not occur, but without testosterone the sperm will not mature. The secretion of FSH and ICSH is controlled not only by testosterone but also by the follicle-stimulating hormone releasing factor (FSHRF) and the luteinizing hormone releasing factor (LHRF). These releasing factors are secreted by the hypothalamus and conducted through the blood flow channels, called the hypothalamo-hypophyseal portal system, between the hypothalamus and the pituitary glands. Stress and emotions affect the secretions by the hypothalamus and usually decrease the releasing factor secretion.

PHYSICAL, LABORATORY, AND DIAGNOSTIC TESTS

In study of the male reproductive system, both physical examination and laboratory studies are important. Physical examination allows for the detection of redness, swelling, discharge, or abnormal masses, while laboratory evaluation centers on testicular function. Primary laboratory studies include measurement of testosterone secretion and examination of seminal fluid.

Physical Examination

The physical examination includes inspection and palpation of the external genitalia and a rectal examination. After visualization of the external genitalia, the examiner palpates the scrotal contents for any abnormal masses. A rectal exam concludes the examination and is performed to detect the size and texture of the prostate or the presence and location of any masses. Prostatic massage may also be performed in order to obtain a sample of prostatic secretions.

Testosterone Measurement

Testosterone, a 19-carbon hormone responsible for development of male sexual characteristics, degrades into androsterone and dehydroepiandrosterone, which can be measured as 17-ketosteroids. Approximately one-third of 17-ketosteroid excretion in the male can be attributed to testosterone and its products.

Testosterone levels, measured directly, are particularly helpful in assessment of hypogonadism, impotence, cryptorchidism, and pituitary gonadotropin functions in the male. Male hypogonadism and Kleinfelter's syndrome in men can be associated with a decreased testosterone level.

In women, testosterone measurement may assist in the diagnosis of ovarian and adrenal tumors. Adrenal neoplasms, benign and malignant ovarian tumors, adrenogenital syndrome in women, and Stein-Leventhal syndrome with virilization are frequently associated with an increased testosterone level. Table 48-1 depicts normal laboratory values for testosterone production; these values may vary slightly.

High levels of 17-ketosteroids may be found in testicular tumors or adrenal cortical hyperplasia. Prior to puberty spermatogenesis rarely occurs as a result of testosterone production.

Semen Examination

Semen evaluation is of particular importance in assisting infertile couples. A specimen examination of the seminal fluid, an important diagnostic test, is best collected through masturbation, which provides a complete specimen of ejaculate. This method also protects sperm mor-

TABLE 48-2. Semen examination

Sperm count	50–60 million/ml
Volume	3–6 ml
Morphology	60% of sperm motile; 50% of normal morphology
Liquefaction	Complete in 15–20 minutes

phology and motility, which may be affected by rubber condoms.

Semen examination includes a sperm examination along with the quantity of fluid. Semen viscosity is studied and morphology, and motility of the sperm are examined. Wide variations have been found in the normal sperm count. Most authorities consider greater than 50 to 60 million sperm/ml to be normal. However, pregnancies have been documented with lower levels. The normal volume of ejaculate is 3 to 5 ml. Infertility has been associated with both lower and higher volumes.

The morphology and motility of sperm may also be factors in infertility even when the count is normal. High percentages of inactive or abnormally formed sperm are associated with infertility [2]. Viscosity of seminal fluid may vary. Initially thick, the seminal fluid must liquify to encourage normal motility of the sperm. This liquefaction is usually complete in 15 to 20 minutes. Normal semen test findings are summarized in Table 48-2.

Testicular Biopsy

Testicular biopsy may be indicated if the semen examination reveals no sperm or if a tumor is suspected. Biopsy may reveal abnormalities of the epididymis or vas deferens that may block the emission of normal sperm. It also aids in the diagnosis of testicular atrophy.

REFERENCES

1. Guyton, A. *Textbook of Medical Physiology* (6th ed.). Philadelphia: Saunders, 1981.
2. Yen, S. S. C., and Jaffe, R. B. *Reproductive Endocrinology: Physiology, Pathophysiology and Clinical Management.* Philadelphia: Saunders, 1978.

CHAPTER 49
ALTERATIONS IN MALE FUNCTION

LEARNING OBJECTIVES

1. Differentiate between prostatitis, benign prostatic hyperplasia, and carcinoma of the prostate.
2. Discuss the staging of prostatic carcinoma.
3. Define *phimosis*, *hypospadias*, *epispadias*, *balanitis*, *hydrocele*, *varicocele*, *torsion of testis*, and *cryptorchidism*.
4. Discuss sexually transmitted diseases (STDs) including causative organism, clinical manifestations, and diagnosis.
5. Describe the four types of testicular germ-cell tumors.
6. List and describe the three major stages of testicular tumors.

Alterations in male function may be very disturbing to a man since they represent a threat to how he feels about himself and his ability to reproduce. Alterations can occur in any reproductive organ at virtually any age. This chapter includes some of the congenital anomalies, infections, malignancies, and venereal diseases, which are discussed in relation to the various reproductive organs affected.

PROSTATE

Alterations in prostate function generally occur in adult life and include (1) degeneration, (2) prostatitis, (3) benign prostatic hyperplasia, and (4) carcinoma of the prostate.

Degeneration

The prostate gland maintains its normal adult size until approximately the age of 40 to 50 years. At this point, in some men it begins to decrease in size. This atrophy is associated with a decrease in testosterone level and usually produces no symptoms.

Prostatitis

Prostatitis is infection of the prostate gland that may result from (1) ascending infection of the urethra; (2) descending infection from the bladder or kidneys; (3) hematogenous spread from teeth, skin, gastrointestinal, or respiratory systems; or (4) lymphogenous spread from rectal bacteria. It also occurs in three different forms: (1) acute bacterial, (2) chronic bacterial, or (3) chronic abacterial (also called prostatosis).

Manifestations of acute bacterial prostatitis include chills and fever, dysuria, urinary frequency and urgency, as well as hematuria. It may also be associated with suprapubic, perineal, or scrotal pain and purulent urethral discharge. On rectal examination the prostate is enlarged and tender. The seminal vesicles may also be palpated since infection of these organs frequently accompanies prostatitis. Pus cells and bacteria are present in the urinalysis with specific organisms such as the gonococcus and staphylococcus organisms being identified. Appropriate antibiotics, analgesics, and sitz baths—if instituted early—usually lead to good results. Chronic infection may follow if the infection is not adequately treated.

Chronic bacterial prostatitis may represent a continuation of acute prostatitis that did not completely respond to antibiotics. Clinical manifestations may include low-grade fever, dull perineal pain, nocturia, and dysuria. However, chronic bacterial prostatitis may also be asymptomatic. In chronic bacterial prostatitis, the infection is more resistant to antibiotic therapy. Prostate massage may be implemented to help drain the bacteria.

Abacterial chronic prostatitis is the third and most common form of prostatitis [4]. Symptoms are usually mild and include low back pain, urinary frequency and urgency with rectal, urethral, or perineal discomfort. Physical examination reveals a nontender prostate with normal urinalysis and prostate fluid. Abacterial chronic prostatitis may be related to excessive alcohol or caffeine intake.

Benign Prostatic Hyperplasia

Benign prostatic hyperplasia (BPH) is a common condition, the incidence of which gradually increases in men over 50 years of age and occurs in about 80 percent of men over the age of 80 years [6]. Hyperplasia occurs in the periurethral glands, producing adenomas that appear as large, fairly discrete nodules, located in the median and lateral lobes.

Enlarging nodules compress the prostatic portion of the urethra producing symptoms of urinary obstruction. The man may experience difficulty in starting the urinary stream, which is smaller than normal and less forceful. He may also experience frequency and nocturia. The median lobe enlarges and pushes upward on the bladder. Bladder muscles thicken and diverticula may develop, which results in incomplete emptying of the bladder and urinary stasis. Compression of the urethrovesical junction leads to reflux. Hydroureter and/or hydronephrosis may also occur and eventually may cause renal insufficiency.

The cause of BPH is unknown but it is not always progressive. It may be associated with an increase in estrogen from the adrenal gland as the testosterone levels decline with age.

Diagnosis is based on history and physical exam, x-ray examinations, laboratory studies, and instrumentation examination. Prior to any diagnostic studies or examinations, a complete history of any specific signs or symptoms is obtained. The rectal exam is especially useful in determining the size and condition of the gland. Both an intravenous pyelogram (IVP) and voiding cystourethrogram help to determine the condition of the kidneys and degree of bladder emptying. Specific laboratory studies include routine urinalysis, culture and sensitivity, and renal function studies, i.e., blood urea nitrogen (BUN) and creatinine. Instrumentation studies include catheterization for residual urine and cystoscopy. Cystoscopy allows the examiner to visualize the urethra and bladder. Bladder tone and diverticula may be noted and the size of the prostate estimated. The usual treatment is surgical removal of enlarged tissues. More conservative treatment may include prostatic massage, hot sitz baths, chemotherapy, catheterization, and urethral dilation.

Cancer of the Prostate

Cancer of the prostate is among the leading cancers found in men. It ranks third in cause of death from cancer in all men with only lung and colorectal cancers having a higher incidence [4]. In men over age 75, it is the leading cause of death. It is primarily seen in men over 50 years of age, but when it is seen in younger men it usually is an aggressive tumor.

Adenocarcinoma is the usual form of prostatic cancer. It

occurs most frequently in the posterior lobe; hard fixed nodules can be palpated on rectal exam. In the early stages, prostatic cancer produces no symptoms. For this reason metastasis is common with the most frequent sites being bone, lung, lymph nodes, and liver. Early symptoms are those of urethral obstruction, and at this time it is usually associated with metastasis.

The most accepted classification of prostatic adenocarcinoma divides the disease into four stages. Stage A represents a small localized lesion. It is clinically unsuspected and not detectable on rectal exam. This stage is most frequently found at autopsy or during surgery for BPH. Stage B represents a localized lesion palpable on rectal exam. In both stages, the acid-phosphatase levels are usually normal but there may be some elevation in stage B. Stage C involves an extracapsular extension of the lesion. It is palpable on rectal exam and may involve the seminal vesicles and pelvic nodes. The acid phosphatase level may be elevated. In stage D distant metastasis to various organs has occurred. Bone metastasis results in an elevation of alkaline phosphatase.

Probably the most beneficial of all diagnostic tools is the rectal exam. This exam should be included in annual examinations of all men over 40 years. Since most tumors arise in the posterior lobe palpation is usually easy. Additional diagnostic studies include (1) acid phosphatase, (2) alkaline phosphatase, (3) biopsy of any detectable lesion of posterior lobe, and (4) bone scans or x rays of spine and pelvis if scans are unavailable. Cystoscopy and lymphangiography also aid in diagnosing the extent of the disease.

Treatment is dependent on the stage of the disease, the patient's age, and symptoms. It generally consists of (1) radiation therapy; (2) radical prostatectomy, transurethral resection, or orchiectomy; (3) chemotherapy; or (4) hormone therapy. According to the 1982 edition of *Cancer Facts & Figures*, there has been an improvement from 50 to 63 percent in 5-year survival rates in prostatic cancer [1].

PENIS

Phimosis

Phimosis is a condition in which the orifice of the prepuce is too small for retraction over the glans penis. Frequently it is congenital but it may also follow infection or injury. It predisposes the man to secondary infection and scarring since secretions and smegma accumulate in the area. Forcible retraction of the foreskin may lead to constriction, swelling, and pain of the glans penis. Circumcision is the treatment of choice.

Hypospadias

At about 7 to 8 weeks gestation, the embryo develops a genital tubercle and two genital swellings. In the male infant the genital tubercle develops into the penis. The two swellings develop into two folds (urethral and scrotal), which descend and fuse. This fusion closes the urethra in the penis and forms the scrotum. Failure of these folds to fuse on the ventral side results in the congenital anomaly hypospadias. The urethral orifice is located on the underneath side of the penis. The condition is also associated with undescended testicles and chordee, or curvature of penis. If the anomaly is so severe that the infant's sex is questionable, chromosomal studies are initiated. Surgical repair is aimed at straightening the penis and formation of a urethra terminating as centrally as possible.

Epispadias

Epispadias results from fusion failure on the dorsal side of the penis. The urethral opening is located on this surface rather than centrally. Epispadias occurs less frequently than hypospadias and is often associated with exstrophy of the bladder. Surgical repair is aimed at establishment of a normally functioning urethra and penis.

Balanitis

Balanitis is an inflammation of the glans penis. It is seen most frequently in uncircumcised males with poor hygiene. It may result from venereal disease. Clinical manifestations include redness, swelling, pain, and purulent drainage. Infection may cause adhesions and scarring. Cultures and sensitivity are done to diagnose the organism in order to offer appropriate antibiotics. Circumcision may be indicated in uncircumcised males.

Sexually Transmitted Disease

Sexually transmitted disease (STD) is a relatively new term used to refer to those diseases that can be transmitted through sexual intercourse or intimate contact. For many years these conditions were referred to as venereal disease and included primarily gonorrhea and syphilis. STD, however, is more inclusive and also refers to herpes genitalis, chancroid, granuloma inguinale, and lymphogranuloma. The last three occur infrequently and will be discussed only briefly.

GONORRHEA. Gonorrhea is the most common of all the sexually transmitted diseases. It is now occurring in epidemic proportions in the United States, affecting 2 million Americans each year [4].

The causative organism in gonorrhea is *Neisseria gonorrhoeae*, which appears as a gram-negative diplococcus. Within 2 to 10 days of exposure, urethritis occurs with the person noting a purulent discharge from the urethral meatus. The discharge is clear at first but soon becomes white or even green. It may be accompanied by itching, burning, and pain of the meatus, especially during voiding. In 10 to 20 percent of males with gonorrhea there may be no symptoms. In the absence of prompt treatment, infection is likely to spread to involve the prostate, seminal vesicles, and epididymis. With chronic or prolonged infection, abscesses, tissue destruction, and scarring may result. Urethral strictures may lead to hydronephrosis while epididymitis may cause sterility. Other complications that may occur from gonococcal bacteremia include suppurative arthritis, acute bacterial endocarditis, and suppurative meningitis.

Diagnosis is confirmed by smear or culture of urethral discharge. Treatment with penicillin is instituted immediately and is usually curative. In persons sensitive to penicillin or with gonococcal strains resistant to penicillin, other antibiotics such as tetracycline may be utilized. Cultures should be repeated following treatment to ensure the eradication of the gonococcus organism. Single infection with the gonococcus organism does not confer immunity.

SYPHILIS. Syphilis is less common than gonorrhea but more serious. Serologic screening has been shown to be successful in detecting syphilis, resulting in a dramatic decline of the disease in the 1950s [6]. It is estimated that 70 percent of cases remain unreported. In 1977, 10.4 cases per 100,000 population were reported [3].

The causative organism in syphilis is the spirochete *Treponema pallidum*. It can be transmitted through sexual contact, by personal contact, or by an infected mother to her unborn fetus. If the disease is untreated three stages may occur: (1) primary, (2) secondary, and (3) tertiary.

Primary syphilis develops following an incubation period of 10 days to 3 months. The first symptom is the development of an ulcer, referred to as a chancre, usually on the penis. The chancre appears as a painless ulcer with raised hardened edges. Usually the chancre heals spontaneously and serology tests are normal. Diagnosis at this time is based on identification of the spirochete from the ulceration. Another symptom of primary syphilis is painless swelling of lymph glands near the ulceration.

Secondary syphilis begins with the development of a generalized, usually maculopapular, rash. Other lesions may be follicular, pustular, or scaling. Large elevated plaques, termed *condylomata lata*, develop on the genitalia. Spirochetes are present in all lesions, especially the condylomata lata. Generalized lymphadenopathy also occurs. Approximately 4 to 12 weeks after the beginning of the second stage, all symptoms disappear and the patient enters a latent period. Serology tests at this time are positive. Following the latent period the patient may experience a spontaneous cure, remain latent permanently, or enter the third stage, or tertiary syphilis. When the spontaneous cure develops all of the serologic tests return to normal.

Tertiary syphilis develops in about one-third of those having untreated syphilis. It can affect any body part but especially the heart and central nervous system. Chronic inflammation of bones and joints may also occur. Gummas, large necrotic areas, may develop in the liver, bones, and testes. Gummatous lesions in the central nervous system are rare but meningovascular syphilis more commonly causes infiltration of the meninges and blood vessels by lymphocytes and plasma cells [6]. Neurosyphilis refers to the loss of cortical neurons due to large numbers of spirochetes throughout the brain parenchyma. The effect of neurosyphilis is dementia and behavioral changes that progress to psychotic behavior and ataxic paresthesias. Finally, loss of position, deep pain, and temperature sensation occur. The average interval from infection to symptomatic neurosyphilis is 20 to 30 years.

Early diagnosis depends on identification of the spirochete from the lesions. After approximately 4 weeks blood serology tests such as the Kahn, Wasserman, and VDRL are reliable. Examination findings and biopsies also aid in the diagnosis. Treatment is with antibiotics, preferably penicillin.

Infection with *Treponema pallidum* confers immunity on the infected person. Both syphilitic reagin and treponemal immobilizing serum antibodies are produced after 1 to 4 months. Treponemal immobilizing antibodies are specific and probably account for the active immunity. Syphilitic reagin is the basis for both the complement fixation and flocculation diagnostic tests.

HERPES GENITALIS. Genital herpes is the second most common sexually transmitted disease. It is caused by herpes virus hominis (HVH) type 2, one of the herpes simplex viruses. Type 1 refers to the common cold sore or fever blister, found primarily above the waist. HVH type 2 produces single or multiple vesicles that rupture spontaneously after 24 to 72 hours. Painful reddened ulcers develop that eventually scab and heal. Genital herpes is highly contagious when the vesicles rupture. Lesions of 0.5 to 1.5 cm in size are found on the glans penis, prepuce, buttocks, and inner thighs. Accompanying symptoms include dysuria, pain, fever, edema, and bilateral inguinal lymphadenopathy. Since no cure has been identified, recurrent infections may occur but these are generally milder than the primary infection. Transmission to pregnant women and to the fetus or newborn infant can result in disseminated fetal infection and fetal death.

CHANCROID. Chancroid is an acute disease process that produces a soft chancre, a shallow, ragged ulcer on the penis. This condition is prevalent worldwide, especially in Southeast Asia, Africa, and South America. It is caused by the gram-negative bacillus, *Hemophilus ducreyi*. Regional lymph nodes may become swollen and tender. Suppuration from lymph nodes and the necrotic chancre occur. Culture or biopsy aid in diagnosis and sulfisoxazole (Gantrisin) and good hygiene allow healing in 2 to 4 weeks.

GRANULOMA INGUINALE. Granuloma inguinale is a chronic disease process caused by the gram-negative bacillus, *Donovania granulomatis*. It begins as a papule and progresses to a spreading necrotic ulcer with extensive scarring. It has a low degree of infectivity and progressively involves the skin and lymphatics of the groin and inguinal areas. Smears and biopsy aid in differentiation from other

STDs. Antibiotic treatment with tetracycline will result in complete healing.

LYMPHOGRANULOMA. This condition is caused by the *Chlamydia trachomatis* organism. It is characterized by a small vesicle, usually on the penis, which progresses to ulceration, lymphatic involvement, and obstruction. A skin test with Frei antigen is utilized to confirm the diagnosis.

Carcinoma of the Penis

Carcinoma of the penis is an extremely rare condition that progresses slowly. The prepuce and glans are primarily affected and onset is often associated with chronic infection. Early circumcision seems to prevent development of the squamous cell carcinoma, which first appears as a gray crusted papule. The papule gradually enlarges and produces necrotic ulceration in the center. Early diagnosis may result in a cure by local excision and circumcision, if necessary. Larger lesions involving the shaft of the penis and/or the inguinal nodes may require penile resection or amputation.

SCROTUM, TESTIS, EPIDIDYMIS

Hydrocele

A hydrocele is an accumulation of clear or straw-colored fluid within the sac enclosing the testis and epididymis, the tunica vaginalis. It is the most common cause of scrotal enlargement [6]. Frequently it develops without a known cause but also occurs following epididymitis, orchitis, injury, or neoplasm. In the newborn, it results from late closure of the processus vaginalis. The condition may be asymptomatic or the affected person may complain of pain or tension in the scrotal sac. Treatment may include aspiration or incision if the hydrocele is large or uncomfortable, or if palpation of testes is impossible. The condition must be differentiated from a testicular mass, which is usually demonstrated by a translucent rather than an opaque mass on transillumination studies.

Varicocele

Varicocele refers to the abnormal dilation of the venous plexus of the testis. Onset is usually between 15 and 25 years of age and usually affects the left side. Occurrence on the right side is strongly suggestive of a tumor obstructing a vein above the scrotum. Palpation reveals dilated and tortuous veins often described as "a bag of worms." Clinically, the primary concern relates to the production of subfertility. Both motility and numbers of sperm are decreased because of the increased warmth created by vascular engorgement. The condition is usually asymptomatic, but symptoms may include complaints of a dragging sensation or a dull pain in the scrotum. Surgical ligation of the internal spermatic vein is reserved for more severe conditions or to increase sperm count.

Torsion of the Testis

Torsion of the testis is an infrequent cause of enlargement. It results from rotation of the testis within the tunica vaginalis, which cuts off the blood supply to the testis. It occurs primarily during adolescence and usually follows physical exercise. With twisting of the spermatic cord and testis venous obstruction occurs, resulting in vascular engorgement and sometimes extravasation of blood into the scrotal sac.

The first symptom is usually sudden onset of severe pain in the testicular area. This pain is unrelieved by rest or support and may radiate into the groin. Other manifestations include scrotal edema, testicular tenderness, and perhaps nausea and vomiting. If the torsion cannot be reduced surgery must be performed immediately to preserve fertility.

Cryptorchidism

Cryptorchidism is the term given to incomplete or maldescent of the testis. The testis may remain in the abdomen or may be arrested in the inguinal canal or at the puboscrotal junction. It may be unilateral or bilateral and when unilateral is somewhat more common on the right [6].

The cause of cryptorchidism is unknown. However, it has been associated with a shortened spermatic cord, testosterone deficiencies, narrowed inguinal canal, or adhesions of the pathway. Correction of the condition is necessary if sterility is to be avoided because after puberty a progressive atrophy of the testis occurs. Spermatogenesis decreases and the cells may be replaced by collagenous fibrous tissue. Because there is a direct relationship between cryptorchidism and testicular cancer, surgical placement in the scrotum is recommended.

Testicular Tumors

Testicular tumors are the most common cause of testicular enlargement. They occur primarily in males between 15 and 30 years of age, are predominantly malignant, often metastasize before diagnosis, and 95 percent arise from germ cells [6]. The benign tumors usually arise from the interstitial cells of Leydig or Sertoli cells.

Dixon and Moore have identified four types of testicular germ cell tumors: (1) seminoma, (2) embryonal carcinoma, (3) teratoma and teratocarcinoma, and (4) choriocarcinoma [2]. Seminomas are the most common of these and appear as gray white fleshy masses. Most seminomas remain localized until late in the course when metastasis occurs to regional and aortic lymph nodes. Because of their sensitivity to radiation, seminomas are best treated with radiation.

Embryonal carcinomas are highly malignant tumors that exhibit a wide variety of cell types. These tumors may be seen in both adults and children. Small, gray white nodules are formed, which do not usually invade the entire testis. Metastasis to the lymph nodes, liver, lungs, and bones is frequent. Elevated serum levels of alphafetoprotein (AFP) and/or chorionic gonadotropin (CG) helps to differentiate this type of tumor from other testicular tumors [6].

Teratoma and teratocarcinoma are tumors with various cellular types. Testicular enlargement and invasiveness are less than in the seminomas but greater than in embryonal carcinomas. Metastases generally follow the lymphatic system but may involve many other structures.

Choriocarcinomas are small gray tumors that may not be palpable. Early, distant metastasis usually causes death within a year of diagnosis. Characteristically they produce both cytotrophoblastic and syncytiotrophoblastic cells identical to those formed in the placenta. These cells are responsible for secretion of chorionic gonadotropins which, when found in men, aids in the diagnosis of choriocarcinoma.

Four stages of testicular progression have also been identified. Stage 1 is subdivided into Stage 1A, which includes tumors confined to one testis without evidence of metastasis, and stage 1B, in which the iliac or paraaortic nodes are involved. Stage 2 requires clinical or x-ray evidence of metastasis to lymph nodes below the diaphragm. Stage 3 includes lymph nodes above the diaphragm or metastasis to other body organs such as lungs and liver [5].

Palpation provides the most important diagnostic aid and most testicular tumors can be identified relatively early in the course of the disease. Once a mass has been identified, a biopsy is necessary to determine if it is malignant. In addition to chemotherapy and radiation, orchiectomy may be performed.

Orchitis

Orchitis refers to an inflammation of the testes. It most commonly occurs as a complication of mumps, since the mumps virus is excreted through the urine. Orchitis may also be acquired as an ascending infection of the genital tract. Treatment includes bed rest, scrotal support, warm compresses, and antibiotics, if indicated. Clinical manifestations include pain, swelling, chills, and fever. It may be bilateral or unilateral and may result in sterility or impotence.

Epididymitis

Epididymitis occurs when disease-producing organisms in the urine, urethra, prostate, or seminal vesicles spread to the epididymis. Acute epididymitis may result from a sexually transmitted organism, such as *Neisseria gonorrhoeae*. It also occurs as a complication of prostatectomy. Symptoms include pain, chills, fever, and malaise with scrotal swelling so great that it interferes with ambulation and produces congestion of the testis. Necrosis and fibrosis may occlude the genital ducts and result in sterility. Treatment includes bed rest, scrotal elevation, sitz baths, hot or cold applications, and antibiotics appropriate for the organism.

REFERENCES

1. American Cancer Society. *Cancer Facts & Figures*. New York: American Cancer Society, 1982.
2. Dixon, F.J., and Moore, R.A. Testicular tumors: Clinicopathological study. *Cancer* 6:427, 1953.
3. Holmes, K. Syphilis. In K.J. Isselbacher, et al. (eds.), *Harrison's Principles of Internal Medicine* (9th ed.). New York: McGraw-Hill, 1980.
4. Luckman, J., and Sorensen, K.C. *Medical-Surgical Nursing: A Psychophysiologic Approach* (2nd ed.). Philadelphia: Saunders, 1980. P. 1845.
5. Maier, J.G., et al. An evaluation of lymphadenectomy in the treatment of malignant testicular germ cell neoplasms. *J. Urol.* 101:356, 1969.
6. Robbins, S., and Cotran, R. *Pathologic Basis of Disease* (2nd ed.). Philadelphia: Saunders, 1979.

CHAPTER 50
NORMAL FEMALE FUNCTION

LEARNING OBJECTIVES

1. Describe the development and function of the female sexual organs.
2. List the functions of estrogen, progesterone, prolactin, and prostaglandins.
3. Describe the hypothalamic and pituitary influence on the menstrual cycle.
4. List and discuss the three phases of the menstrual cycle.
5. Describe the phases involved in the female sexual act.
6. Discuss the process of oogenesis.
7. Describe the process of fertilization and implantation.
8. Define *menopause* and discuss the physiologic basis for the associated symptoms.
9. Define the various diagnostic tests utilized in diagnosis of female reproductive alterations.
10. Recall normal values for laboratory tests utilized in diagnosis of female reproductive alterations.

Reproduction is a universal and natural process necessary for continuation of the human species. Yet this physiologic occurrence has often been surrounded by fantasy, myth, and superstition. Cultural attitudes and assumptions have helped perpetuate these misconceptions. It is the intent of this chapter to provide a realistic overview of the anatomy and physiology fundamental to an understanding of alterations in female reproductive function.

PHYSIOLOGIC ANATOMY

The female reproductive organs include both essential and accessory organs. The essential organs are the ovaries, which are responsible for the production of the ovum. The accessory organs include the following: (1) the fallopian tubes, uterus, and vagina, which serve as ducts (Fig. 50-1); (2) Bartholin's, Skene's, and the mammary glands; and (3) the external genitalia (Fig. 50-2).

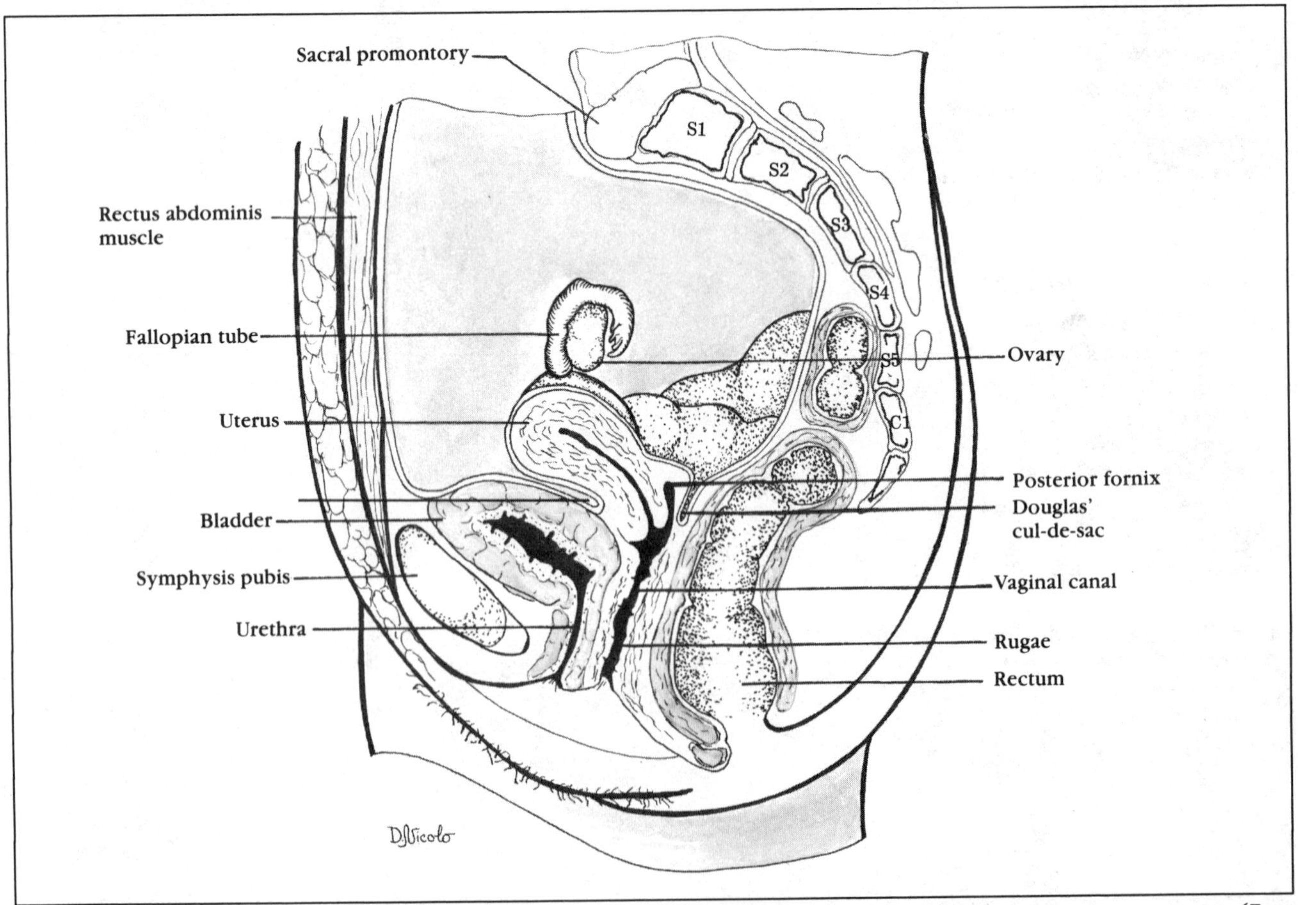

FIGURE 50-1. Side view of female genitourinary anatomy. (From M.A. Miller and D.A. Brooten, ***The Childbearing Family: A Nursing Perspective*** [2nd ed.]. Boston: Little, Brown, 1983.)

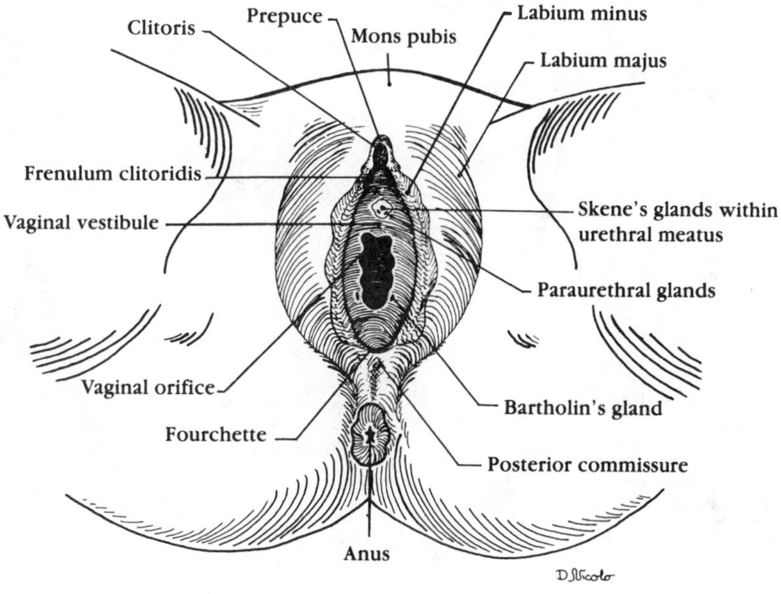

FIGURE 50-2. External female genitalia. (From M.A. Miller and D.A. Brooten, *The Childbearing Family: A Nursing Perspective* [2nd ed.]. Boston: Little, Brown, 1983.)

Ovaries

These essential reproductive organs of the female are two nodular glands located on either side of the uterus. Each ovary is attached by (1) the mesovarian ligament, (2) the ovarian ligament, and (3) the suspensory ligament (Fig. 50-3). The mesovarian ligament attaches the ovary to the back of the broad ligament, while the ovarian ligament attaches the ovary to the uterus. The suspensory ligament is an extension of the broad ligament beyond the fallopian tubes. The ovaries perform the vital functions of ovulation and hormone secretion, functions discussed in more depth later in this chapter.

The ovary is covered with germinal epithelium and consists of three portions: (1) cortex, (2) medulla, and (3) hilum (Fig. 50-4). The outer portion is the cortex, which is composed of fine areolar stroma, blood vessels, and follicles containing ova at various stages of development. The medulla is the central portion and is composed of stroma or connective tissue, smooth muscle, blood and lymph vessels, and nerves. The innermost portion is the hilum, which is composed of nerves, blood vessels, connective tissue, and the hilar cells, which secrete steroid hormones.

Uterus

The uterus is a pear-shaped organ consisting of three parts: (1) the fundus, located above the entrance of the tubes; (2) the body, located below the entrance of the tubes; and (3) the cervix, which is the lowest and narrowest portion (Fig. 50-5). It functions in the processes of menstruation, pregnancy, and labor.

The uterine walls are composed of three layers: (1) the endometrium, (2) the myometrium, and (3) the peritoneum, also known as the perimetrium. The endometrium is the mucous membrane lining of the body of the uterus. It consists of three layers of tissue: (1) the stratum compactum, (2) the stratum spongiosum, and (3) the stratum basale. The ***stratum compactum*** is the surface layer and consists of partially ciliated simple columnar epithelium. The ***stratum spongiosum*** is the spongy middle layer of loose connective tissue. Both the stratum compactum and stratum spongiosum slough during menstruation and following delivery. The ***stratum basale*** is the dense inner layer that attaches to the myometrium.

The myometrium is the thick middle layer consisting of three layers of smooth muscle fibers supported by connective tissue. This layer blends into the endometrium and provides great strength for the uterus. The myometrial layer is thickest in the fundus, which allows for more force during the contractions of labor, aiding in the delivery process.

The third layer of the uterine wall is the peritoneum. It consists of a serous membrane covering almost all of the uterus. On the anterior surface, the peritoneum is reflected onto the bladder below the internal os of the cervix.

The uterus is supported mainly by the levator ani muscles and eight ligaments, which include two broad ligaments, two uterosacral ligaments, a posterior, an anterior, and two round ligaments. The round ligaments are fibromuscular cords that extend from the upper outer portion of the uterus through the inguinal canals and terminate in

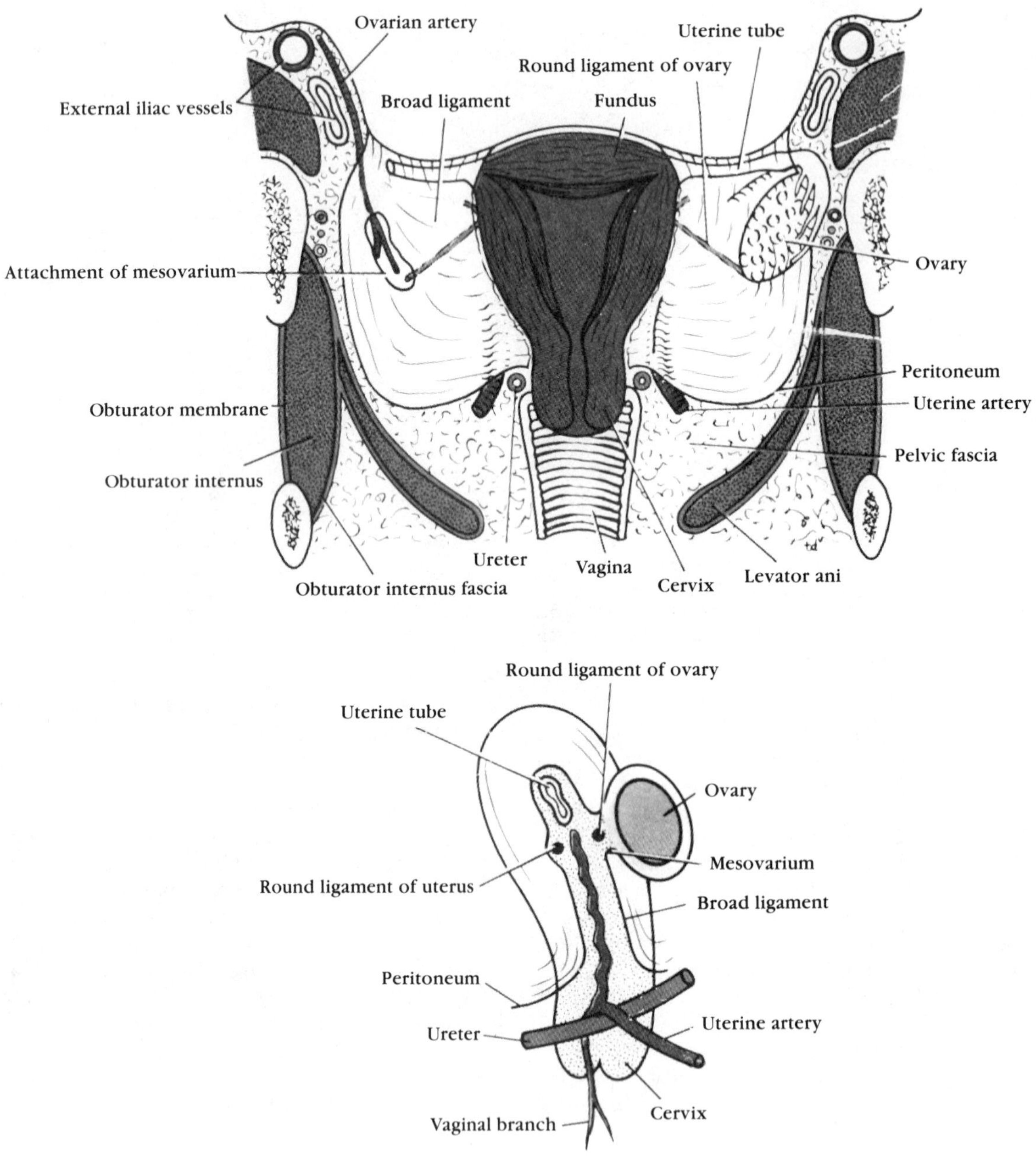

FIGURE 50-3. Coronal section of pelvis, showing uterus, broad ligaments, and right ovary on posterior view. The left ovary and part of the left uterine tube have been removed. Below, uterus on lateral view. Note structures that lie within broad ligament. (From R. S. Snell, *Clinical Anatomy for Medical Students* [2nd ed.]. Boston: Little, Brown, 1981.)

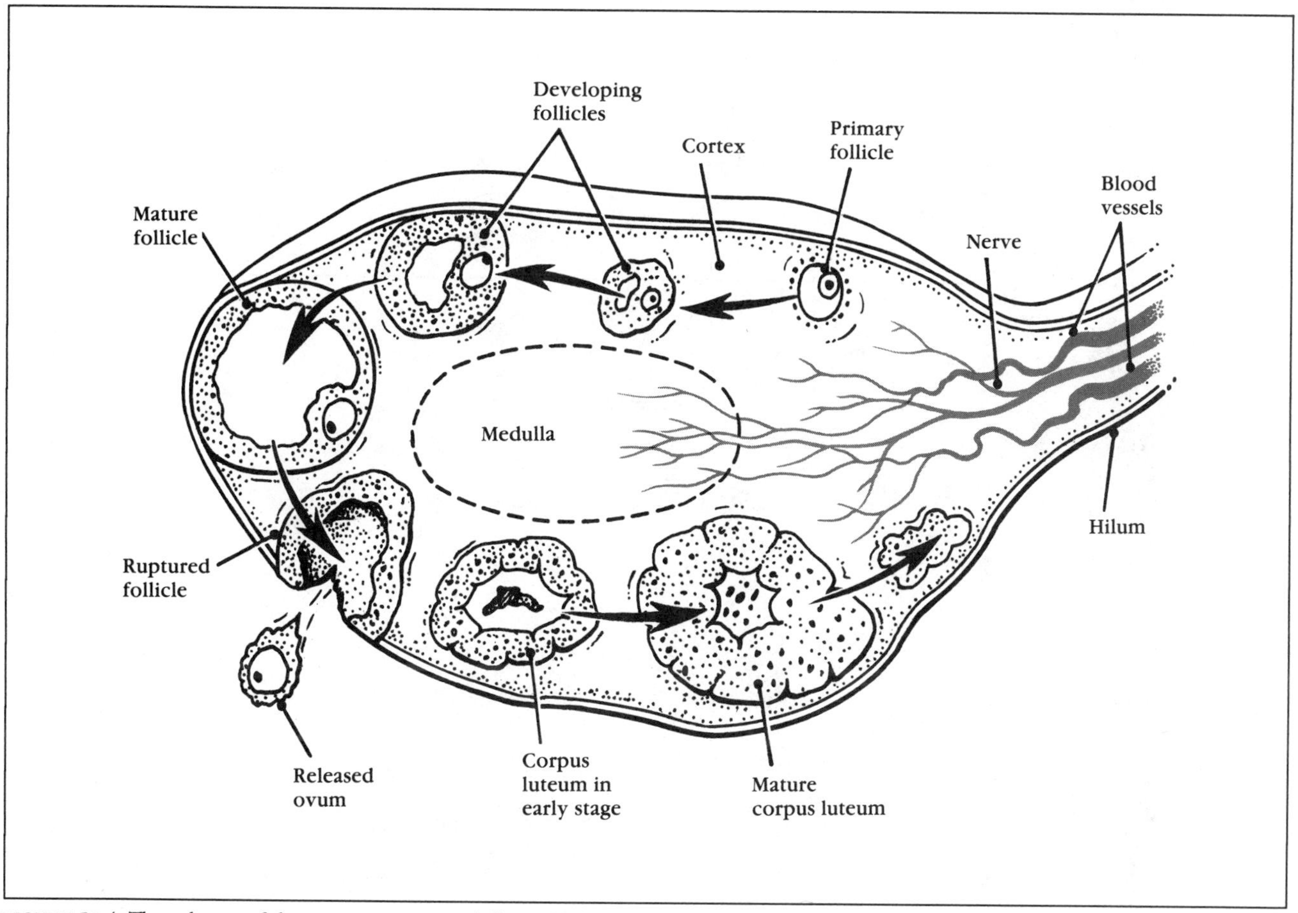

FIGURE 50-4. Three layers of the ovary: cortex, medulla, and hilum.

the labia majora. The outer ligaments are extensions of the peritoneum (Fig. 50-6).

Two of these ligaments are of particular importance because of the pouches they form. The posterior ligament forms the rectouterine pouch (or cul-de-sac of Douglas) as it extends from the posterior surface of the uterus to the rectum (see Fig. 50-1). This is the lowest point of the pelvic cavity.

The anterior ligament forms the uterovesical pouch as it extends from the anterior uterus to the posterior bladder. However, this pouch is not as deep as the rectouterine pouch.

Fallopian Tubes

The fallopian tubes are slender muscular tubes about 10 cm in length. They are attached at the upper outer angles of the uterus. These structures serve as the passageway through which the ova travel to the uterus, as well as the normal site for conception.

The fallopian tubes consist of four sections: (1) the interstitial section, (2) the isthmus, (3) the ampulla, and (4) the infundibulum (Fig. 50-7). The interstitial section is very short, very narrow, and lies within the muscular wall of the uterus. The isthmus is the straight part with a thick muscular wall and narrow lumen. It is adjacent to the uterus and is the usual site for tubal ligations. The ampulla is the dilated lateral section, which is thin-walled with a highly folded lining. The wide distal opening near the ovary is the infundibulum, or fimbriated end. Through muscular action the fimbriae wave back and forth to create a current that moves the ova toward the infundibulum.

Vagina

The vagina is a musculomembranous canal located between the rectum and urethra. It extends upward from the vulva to the midpoint of the cervix. It functions as the passageway both for the menstrual flow and the fetus during delivery.

The vagina consists mainly of smooth muscle and mucous membrane continuous with the uterus. The mucous membrane is arranged in small transverse folds called rugae. The vagina contains no glands, but the epithelial cells of the mucosa undergo changes in response to estrogen. Without the influence of estrogen the epithelium is thin and consists almost entirely of basal cells. The mucosal

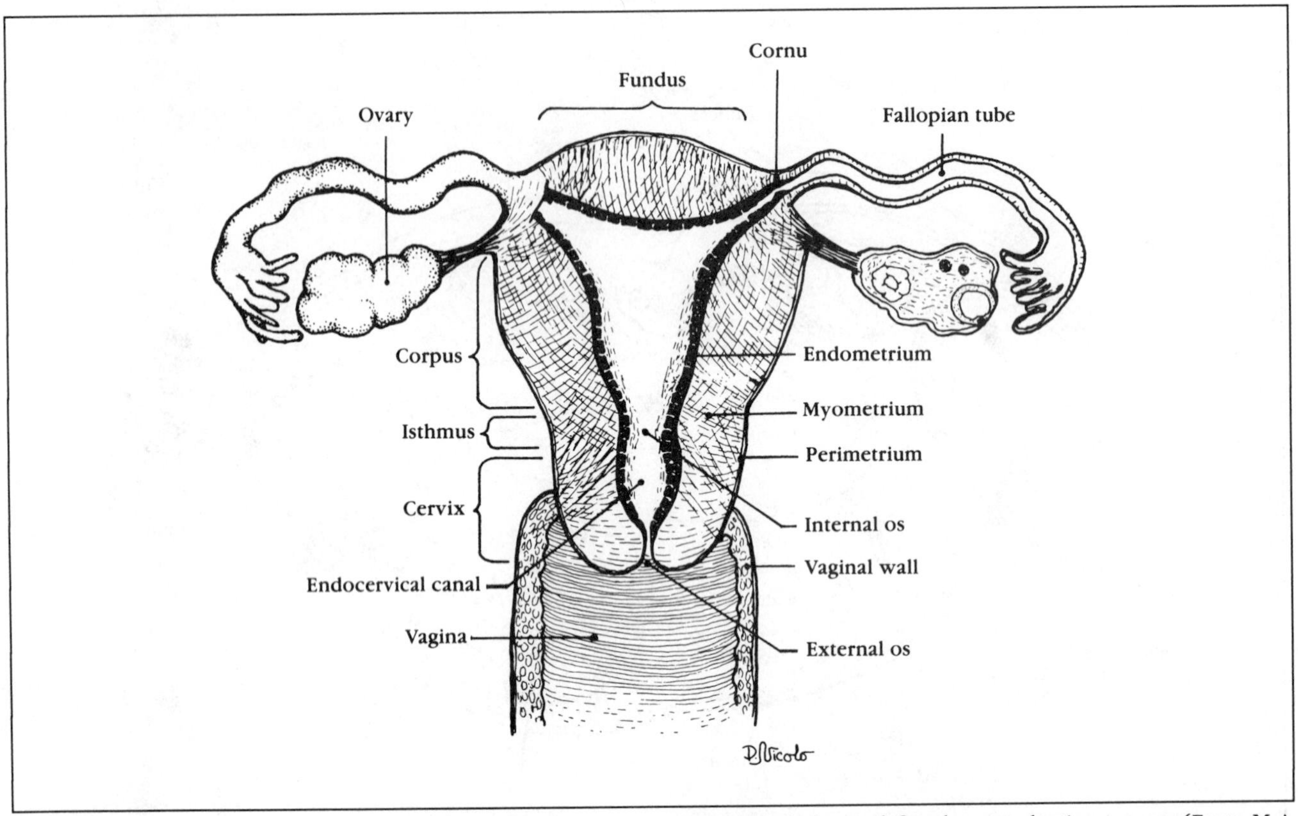

FIGURE 50-5. Internal female reproductive organs. (From M.A. Miller and D.A. Brooten, *The Childbearing Family: A Nursing Perspective* [2nd ed.]. Boston: Little, Brown, 1983.)

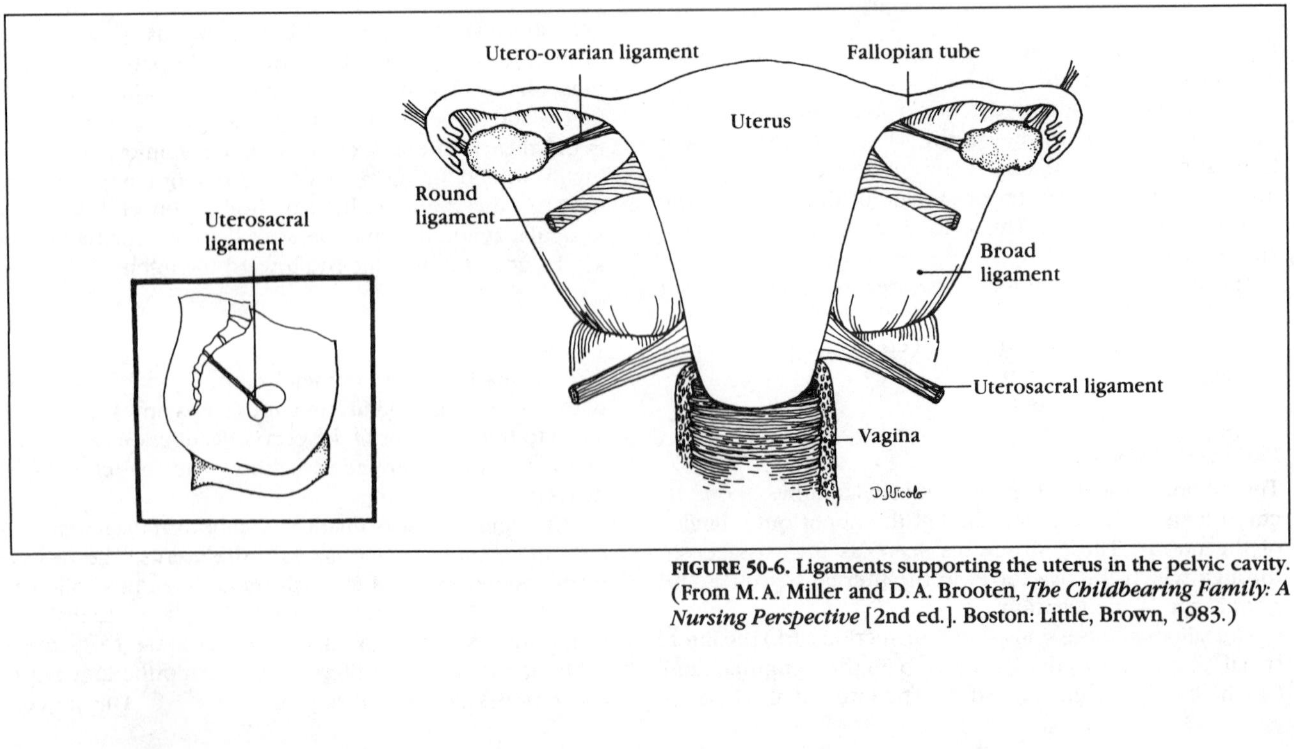

FIGURE 50-6. Ligaments supporting the uterus in the pelvic cavity. (From M.A. Miller and D.A. Brooten, *The Childbearing Family: A Nursing Perspective* [2nd ed.]. Boston: Little, Brown, 1983.)

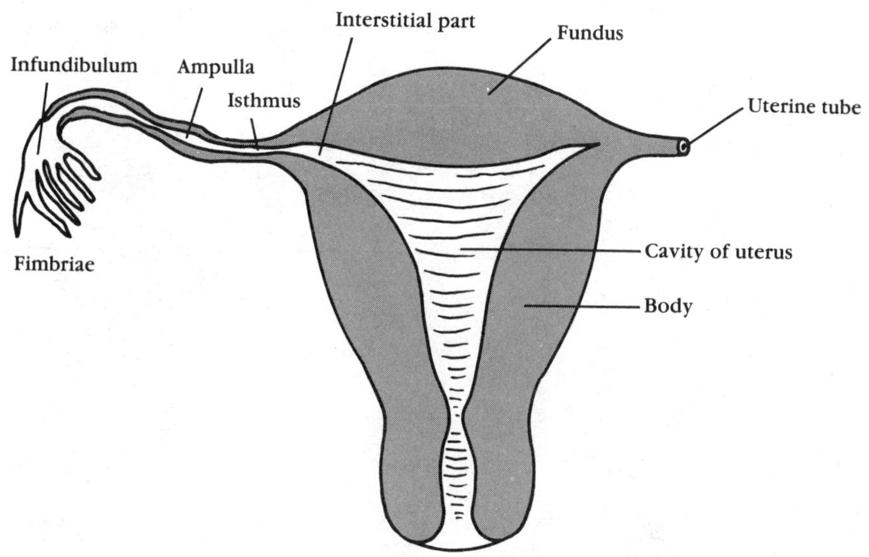

FIGURE 50-7. Different parts of uterine tube and uterus. (From R. S. Snell, *Clinical Anatomy for Medical Students* [2nd ed.]. Boston: Little, Brown, 1981.)

cells also contain a considerable amount of glycogen. These characteristics provide the basis for such diagnostic tests as the Pap test, Schiller test, and vaginal smears.

Bartholin's Glands

The Bartholin's (or greater vestibular) glands are two bean-shaped mucus-secreting glands located on each side of the vaginal orifice (see Fig. 50-2). Secretion is increased during sexual excitement and moistens the inner surfaces of the labia in preparation for intercourse. The duct may become obstructed or infected, particularly by the gonococcus organism, and Bartholin's cyst or abscess may be formed.

Skene's Glands

Skene's glands are tiny mucus-secreting glands located just posterior to the external urethral meatus (see Fig. 50-2). The mucus from the Skene's glands, along with mucus from glands in the urethra, functions to keep the urethral opening moist and lubricated. The Skene's glands are also susceptible to infection by the gonococcus organism, which is difficult to eradicate from this location.

Mammary Glands

The mammary glands, or breasts, are two skin glands located over the pectoral muscles and attached by a layer of connective tissue. They consist of (1) a nipple and surrounding areola, (2) lobes, (3) ducts, and (4) fibrous and fatty tissue (Fig. 50-8).

The nipple, a cylindrical projection near the center of the breast, is located approximately in the fourth intercostal space. It is surrounded by a pigmented, circular area and is perforated by ductal openings. Stimulation of the nipple results in engorgement and muscle contraction, which produces nipple erection.

The mature female breast is made up of 15 to 20 lobes arranged around the nipple. Each lobe is further composed of a number of lobules. Inside each lobule are the alveoli which contain both myoepithelial and acini cells. The acini cells serve as secretory cells in lactation, while the myoepithelial cells contract to force milk into the ducts.

Each lobule is drained by intralobular ducts that empty into the lactiferous duct. The lactiferous ducts dilate into a reservoir, called the lactiferous sinus, just before it opens in the nipple. Lobes and ducts are separated by fibrous tissue while fatty tissue contributes to breast size.

Lymph drainage of the breast is very important, especially in breast cancer. Generally lymph vessels follow the lactiferous ducts and eventually drain into the central axillary nodes (Fig. 50-9). This creates drainage of the superficial and areolar as well as glandular parts of the breast.

During puberty, breast development is controlled by estrogen and progesterone production. Estrogen is responsible for growth of the gland and ducts while progesterone stimulates development of the secreting cells. The function of the breast is secretion of milk to nourish the newborn infant.

External Genitalia

The external genitalia, commonly called the vulva, consists of: (1) the mons pubis, (2) the labia majora, (3) the labia minora, (4) the clitoris, (5) the urinary meatus, (6) the

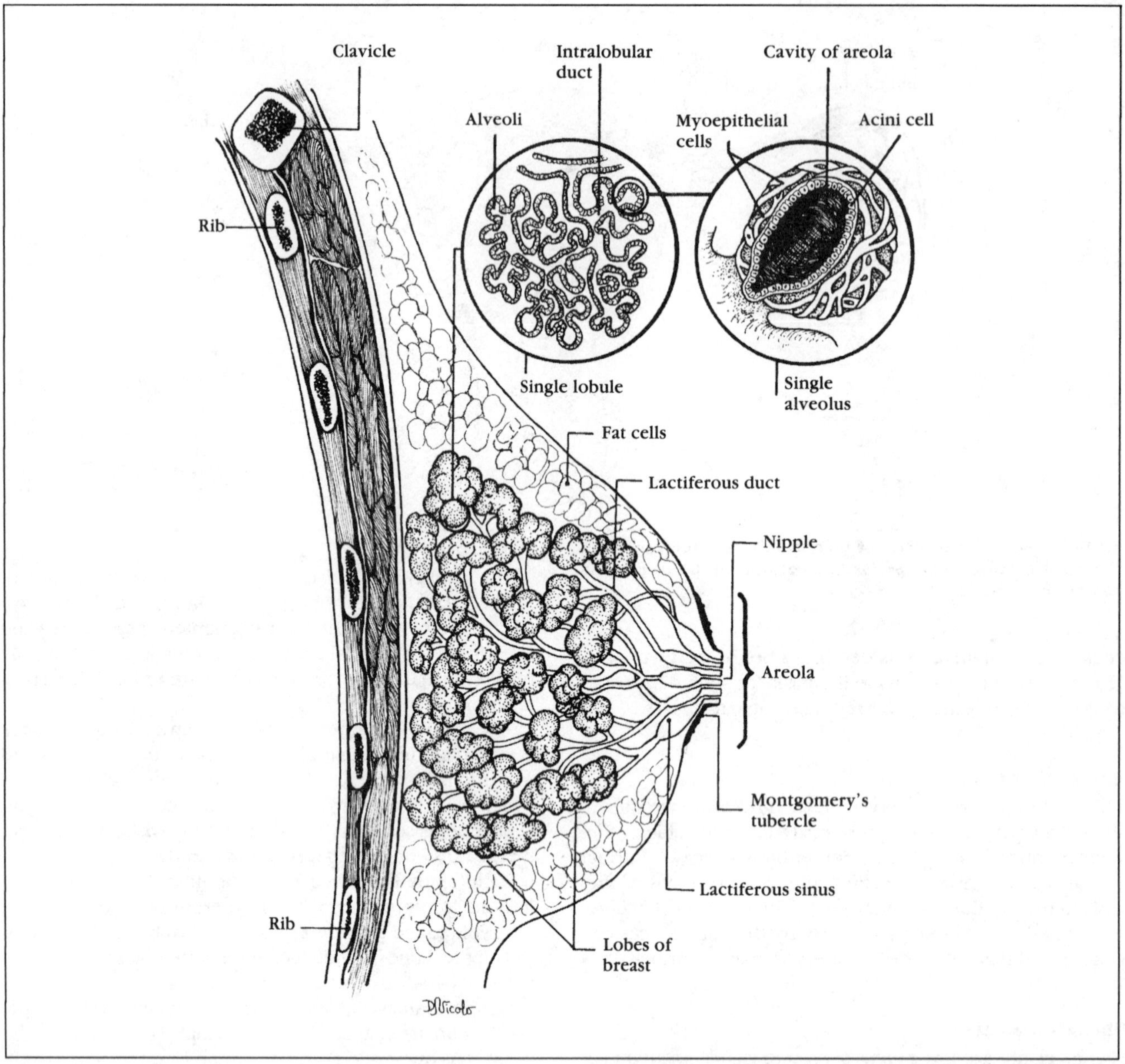

FIGURE 50-8. Breast and ductal system. (From M.A. Miller and D.A. Brooten, *The Childbearing Family: A Nursing Perspective* [2nd ed.]. Boston: Little, Brown, 1983.)

vaginal orifice and (7) the vestibule (see Fig. 50-2). Bartholin's glands are sometimes considered parts of the vulva.

FEMALE REPRODUCTIVE FUNCTIONS

Female reproductive functions, which begin with puberty and end with menopause, fall into two phases: (1) preparation of the body for conception and gestation, and (2) the period of gestation. The specific functions include the reproductive cycle, the production of female hormones, the female sexual act, and gestation.

The female reproductive cycle involves many periodic changes throughout the life span or from menarche to menopause. Successful reproductive function is dependent on changes that occur in the ovaries, endometrium, myometrium, breasts, vagina, and endocrine glands, and on changes in body temperature regulation. Even the woman's emotions are affected by these changes. Various organs respond differently to the changes but all can be related to the menstrual cycle.

Hypothalamic Influence

Cyclic changes in the reproductive cycle begin with hormonal changes initiated by the hypothalamus, which is considered to be a part of both the nervous and hormone systems. Both physical and emotional stressors can affect

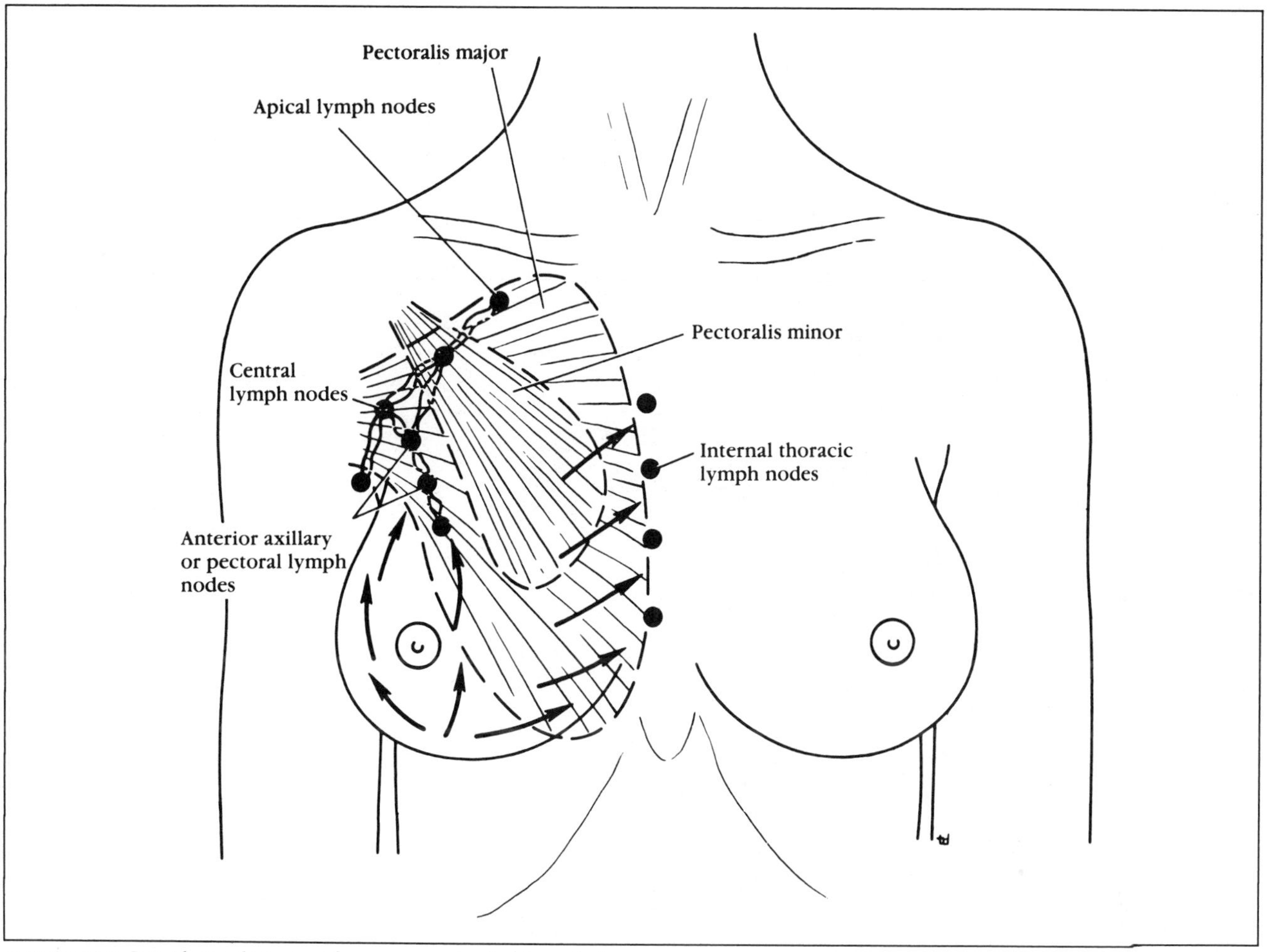

FIGURE 50-9. Lymphatic drainage of mammary gland. (From R.S. Snell, *Clinical Anatomy for Medical Students* [2nd ed.]. Boston: Little, Brown, 1981.)

menstrual regularity through the nervous control of the hypothalamus. Depending on the messages it receives, the hypothalamus then secretes hormones called *releasing* or *inhibiting factors*, which act directly on the pituitary gland. Neurosecretory substances that are secreted by the hypothalamus and transported through the hypothalamo-hypophyseal portal system to the anterior pituitary include: (1) follicle-stimulating hormone releasing factor, (2) luteinizing hormone releasing factor, and (3) luteotropic hormone inhibiting factor. These factors act on the anterior pituitary to control the secretion of this gland. *Oxytocin*, secreted by the posterior pituitary but formed in the hypothalamus, functions to increase uterine contractions during labor and to move milk from breast glands to nipples during suckling of the infant.

Pituitary Influence

The anterior pituitary secretes two hormones that directly influence reproductive function. These are follicle-stimulating hormone (FSH) and luteinizing hormone (LH). Both FSH and LH act directly on the ovary to control ovulation along with estrogen and progesterone production. The release of FSH and LH is also regulated by feedback effects of estrogen and progesterone on the hypothalamus. In addition, the anterior pituitary secretes *prolactin*, also called luteotropin hormone or LTH. Prolactin acts on the breasts to control lactation following delivery. The release of prolactin is prevented by the prolactin-inhibiting factor which is controlled by high levels of estrogen and/or progesterone. Suckling and low estrogen levels stimulate prolactin production.

The Menstrual Cycle

The menstrual cycle involves cyclic changes that are repeated approximately every 28 days. This process may vary some in individual women but has three phases: (1) the menstrual phase, (2) the proliferative phase, and (3) the secretory phase. The proliferative and secretory phases are separated by the process of ovulation.

THE MENSTRUAL PHASE. The menstrual phase begins with the onset of the menses and lasts approximately 5 days with an average blood loss of 30 to 150 ml, the amount of

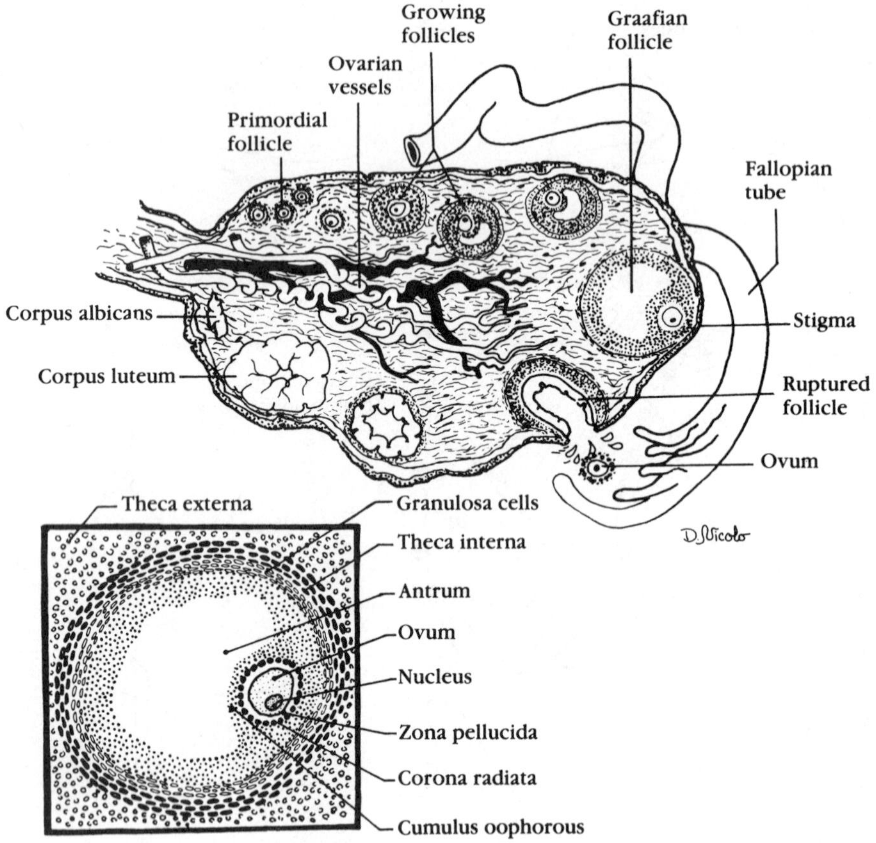

FIGURE 50-10. The ovary, showing maturation and release of ovum. Inset (in box) shows a developing graafian follicle. (From M.A. Miller and D.A. Brooten, ***The Childbearing Family: A Nursing Perspective*** [2nd ed.]. Boston: Little, Brown, 1983.)

which varies widely with individual women. During the menstrual phase the blood levels of both estrogen and progesterone are low. This phase also involves a degeneration and sloughing of the stratum compactum and most of the stratum spongiosum.

THE PROLIFERATIVE PHASE. The proliferative phase follows the menstrual phase and is accompanied by changes in the ovary, endometrium, and myometrium. The cyclic changes result from changes in gonadotropin and estrogen levels.

Low levels of estrogen in the menstrual phase signal the production of FSH by the anterior pituitary. In the ovary FSH production then stimulates the primary follicles. At this time a number of follicles begin the maturation process. Soon only one, the graafian follicle, begins to dominate while the others recede. This follicle gradually moves to the surface of the ovary (Fig. 50-10). The follicle contains the ovum and is surrounded by a layer of granulosa cells, which are further surrounded by specialized cells called the theca interna and theca externa. Estrogen is secreted by the theca interna while the granulosa cells supply nutrition for the ova. As the follicle increases in size, fluid begins to collect inside, pushing the ovum to one side. It is surrounded on the outside by granulosa cells, called the cumulus oophorus. A clear membrane also develops and surrounds the ovum. This inner surrounding is termed the zona pellucida. Outside the zona pellucida and inside the cumulus oophorus is a single layer of cells called the zona radiata. While these changes are occurring within the follicle, the anterior pituitary also begins a gradual secretion of LH, which stimulates increased estrogen production by the follicles. High levels of estrogen then signal the hypothalamus, which stops the production of the FSH releasing factor. Production of LH continues, resulting in a surge of LH about 12 hours prior to ovulation. This surge of LH then triggers ovulation within 1 to 24 hours. The mature ovum is then extruded from the ovary with both the zona pellucida and corona radiata surrounding it.

During this same period of time, changes are also occurring with the endometrium and myometrium. These

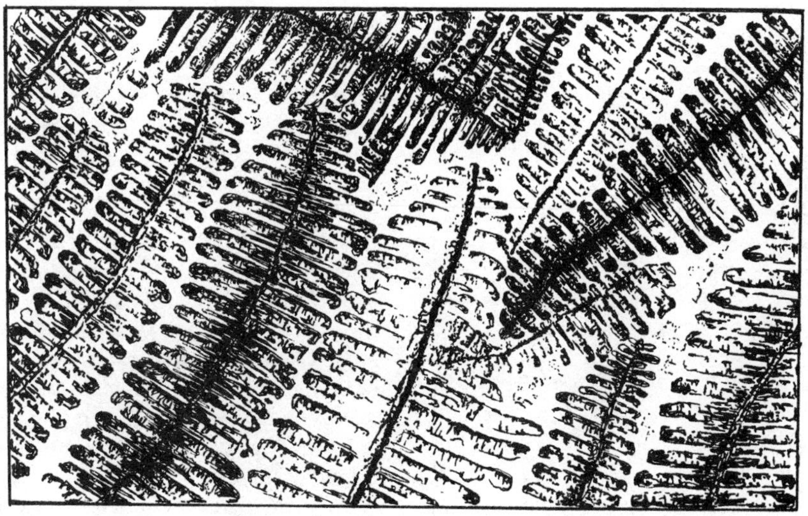

FIGURE 50-11. Diagram of fern pattern seen on microscopic examination of cervical mucus at midcycle in normal menstruating women. (From M.A. Miller and D.A. Brooten, *The Childbearing Family: A Nursing Perspective* [2nd ed.]. Boston: Little, Brown, 1983.)

changes are controlled primarily by blood levels of estrogen. The endometrium thickens as the endometrial cells and arterioles grow longer and more coiled. There is also an increase in water content of the endometrium and contractions of the myometrium.

OVULATION. Ovulation serves to divide the proliferative and secretory phases of the menstrual cycle and usually occurs 14 days before the onset of the next menstrual cycle. In a number of women it is accompanied by low abdominal pain, termed *mittelschmerz*. The escape of fluid or blood from the follicle is believed to produce peritoneal irritation that causes the abdominal pain.

Ovulation is also accompanied by changes in cervical mucus. Cervical mucus increases in amount as it becomes clear and thin. Under the influence of high estrogen levels it forms a ferning pattern when allowed to dry on a slide (Fig. 50-11).

OOGENESIS. Unlike the continuous production of sperm in the male, the process of oogenesis involves the cyclic production of a single ovum. Immediately prior to ovulation the primary oocyte undergoes its first meiotic division, resulting in a secondary oocyte containing 23 chromosomes and most of the cytoplasm. A second body is formed and is referred to as a first polar body. This first polar body receives 23 chromosomes but little cytoplasm. In the event of fertilization the secondary oocyte undergoes a mitotic division. Both cells again contain 23 chromosomes but only one receives the majority of cytoplasm. It is this cell that is termed the *mature ovum*. The second cell is known as a second polar body. Figure 50-12 illustrates the maturation of one mature ovum.

SECRETORY PHASE. The secretory phase begins with ovulation and is characterized by (1) formation of the corpus luteum in the ovary, (2) production of progesterone and estrogen, (3) secretory changes in the endometrium, and (4) decreased contractions in the myometrium. In the ovary, follicle walls now collapse with some hemorrhage into the cavity, forming a corpus hemorrhagia. Under the influence of LH the granulosa cells hypertrophy, take on a yellow color, and become known as luteal cells. This golden body, the corpus luteum, continues to function for about 7 to 8 days. Its primary function is the secretion of progesterone and some estrogen. In the absence of fertilization, luteal cells begin to degenerate, causing a decrease in estrogen and progesterone levels. Eventually the corpus luteum is converted into the corpus albicans, which moves to the center of the ovary and finally disappears.

The production of progesterone by the corpus luteum leads to secretory changes in the endometrium that create a favorable environment for pregnancy. Increase in the endometrium at this time is believed to be due to swelling from increased water content rather than cellular proliferation. The endometrium becomes more vascular with coiled spiral arteries located close to the surface. The changes produce a thick, succulent environment, rich in glycogen and ideal for implantation of the fertilized ovum.

Progesterone is also associated with a decrease in myometrial contractions. In addition, women may notice

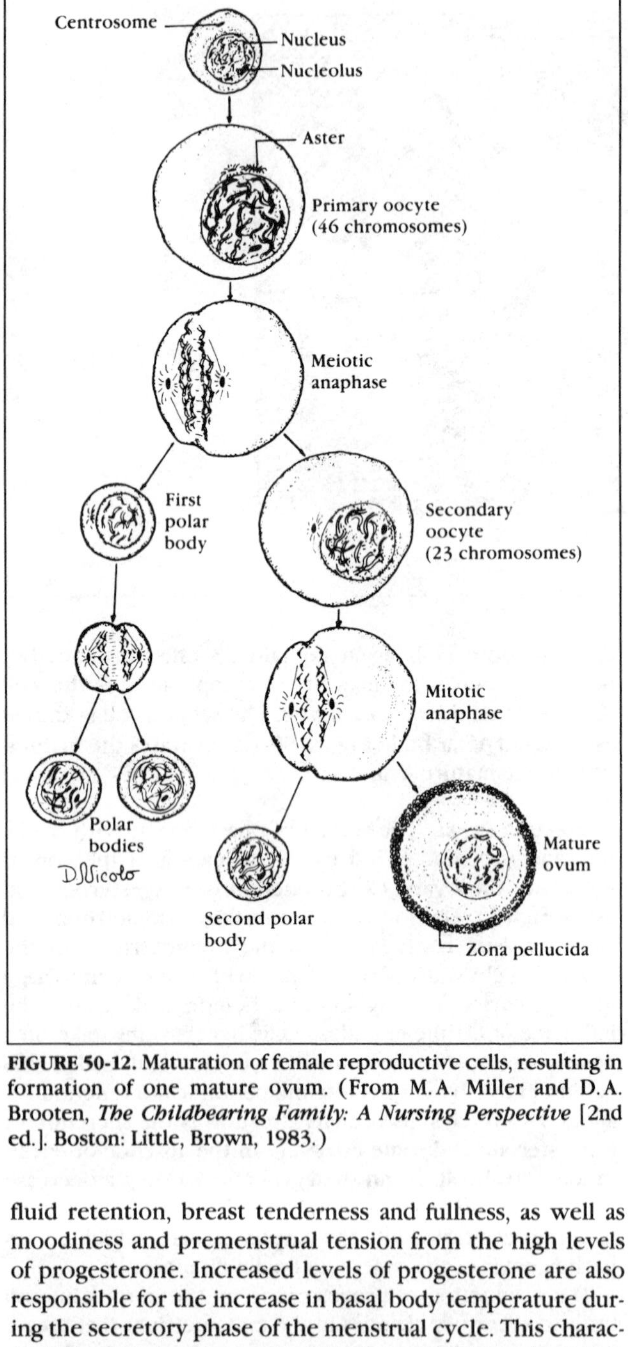

FIGURE 50-12. Maturation of female reproductive cells, resulting in formation of one mature ovum. (From M.A. Miller and D.A. Brooten, *The Childbearing Family: A Nursing Perspective* [2nd ed.]. Boston: Little, Brown, 1983.)

fluid retention, breast tenderness and fullness, as well as moodiness and premenstrual tension from the high levels of progesterone. Increased levels of progesterone are also responsible for the increase in basal body temperature during the secretory phase of the menstrual cycle. This characteristic of progesterone provides the basis for basal temperature studies in fertility problems.

In the absence of fertilization and implantation, progesterone secretion falls, which is a signal for the beginning of a new cycle. Degenerated endometrium sloughs, the hypothalamus begins its secretion of releasing factors, and the cycle begins again.

Production of Female Hormones

Estrogen and progesterone are the two primary female hormones. Other hormones include androgen, prolactin, and prostaglandins.

ESTROGEN. Estrogen is a general term for a class of hormones predominantly found in the female. It is a steroid hormone secreted primarily by the ovary and by the placenta during pregnancy with a small amount being secreted by the adrenal cortices. There are a number of natural estrogens but only three are potent enough to cause physiologic effects: (1) estradiol, (2) estrone, and (3) estriol. The major estrogen, estradiol, is the most potent (12 times that of estrone) but the ovary secretes about 4 times more estrone. Both estradiol and estrone can be identified in venous blood from the ovary, while estriol is oxidized mainly in the liver from estradiol and estrone.

Following secretion by the ovary, estradiol and estrone either enter cells to perform their functions or are oxidized principally in the liver to estriol. The liver is also responsible for the inactivation of estrogens through conjugation with sulfuric acid and glyconuric acid. The glyconurides and sulfates are then excreted in the bile. Estrogens found in extracellular fluids are primarily in the form of estroprotein, another process accomplished in the liver. This inactivation process accounts for the ineffectiveness of the natural estrogens when administered orally. Conditions causing a depression of liver function may also be associated with increased estrogen levels because of the absence of the inactivation process.

In the clinical setting two other forms of estrogen may be used: (1) synthetic estrogens and (2) conjugated estrogens. The synthetic estrogens are of particular importance because of their potency when administered orally.

Estrogen affects the cellular proliferation and development of the female secondary sexual characteristics as well as the previously described effect on the menstrual cycle.

Throughout childhood very small quantities of estrogen are produced but, at puberty, the levels become greatly increased. As a result of estrogen influence, the sexual organs, including the breasts, ovaries, fallopian tubes, uterus, and vagina, increase in size while the external genitalia enlarge [3]. Vaginal epithelium thickens and differentiates into layers that increase the resistance of the vagina to injury and infection. The epithelium also increases its glycogen levels, which are acted on by Doderlein's bacilli to create an acidic pH. Estrogens also influence the contour of the female body by effecting the fat deposits in the vulva and mons pubis, the growth of the pelvis, and the distribution of axillary and pubic hair.

The onset of puberty is associated with a very rapid growth rate in the female. However, estrogens produce an early uniting of the epiphyses and shafts of the long bones, causing female growth to cease earlier than male growth. Estrogens also affect calcium and phosphate retention, which is important in menopause when the estrogen levels are greatly reduced.

Estrogens exert an influence on the skin and capillary walls. Under the influence of estrogen, the skin becomes soft, smooth, and thicker than that of a child. It is also more vascular. For this reason women may bleed more when cut or note increased skin warmth. In addition the capillary walls become stronger. When estrogen levels are low there is a greater tendency toward bruising.

PROGESTERONE. Progesterone is often considered the hormone of pregnancy because of its effect on the endometrium and myometrium (see pp. 771–772). It is produced almost exclusively by the corpus luteum in the nonpregnant female and by the placenta during pregnancy. Chemically, natural progesterone is very similar to estrogen. Its potency is less than estrogen and it is secreted in larger amounts. It is degraded shortly after secretion to pregnanediol and is excreted in this form in the urine.

In addition to its uterine effects, progesterone also affects the breast. While estrogen is responsible for breast growth, progesterone is responsible for maturation of lobules and alveoli so that they may become secretory when stimulated by prolactin.

ANDROGENS. Female androgens are secreted in very small amounts by the adrenal gland and ovaries [3]. However, in disruptions of female function the amount of secretions can become significant and result in masculine hair distribution, acne, and deepening of the voice.

PROLACTIN. Prolactin is a protein hormone secreted by the anterior pituitary. Suckling in breast feeding and low estrogen levels stimulate its release. High estrogen and progesterone levels trigger the release of prolactin inhibiting factor from the hypothalamus, thus preventing its secretion. Prolactin stimulates production of milk by the acini cells in the alveoli. Pituitary gland tumors can cause milk production, even in the absence of pregnancy.

PROSTAGLANDINS. Prostaglandins are a group of potent lipids. Controversy exists as to whether they are truly hormones [6, 7]. Regardless of classification they are gaining importance in the study of reproductive physiology.

Prostaglandins have been grouped into three areas: prostaglandin A, E, and F (PGA, PGE, and PGF). Each group exerts different actions on various systems of the body. Prostaglandins are synthesized from phospholipids in various body tissues. Phospholipase A, an enzyme, is responsible for liberation of essential fatty acids from the phospholipids. The essential fatty acids are then converted to PGE or PGF by prostaglandin synthetase. PGA is the result of additional metabolism of PGE (Fig. 50-13).

Prostaglandins are degraded primarily in the lungs soon after entering the circulation. For this reason, the actions of prostaglandins seem to be primarily local.

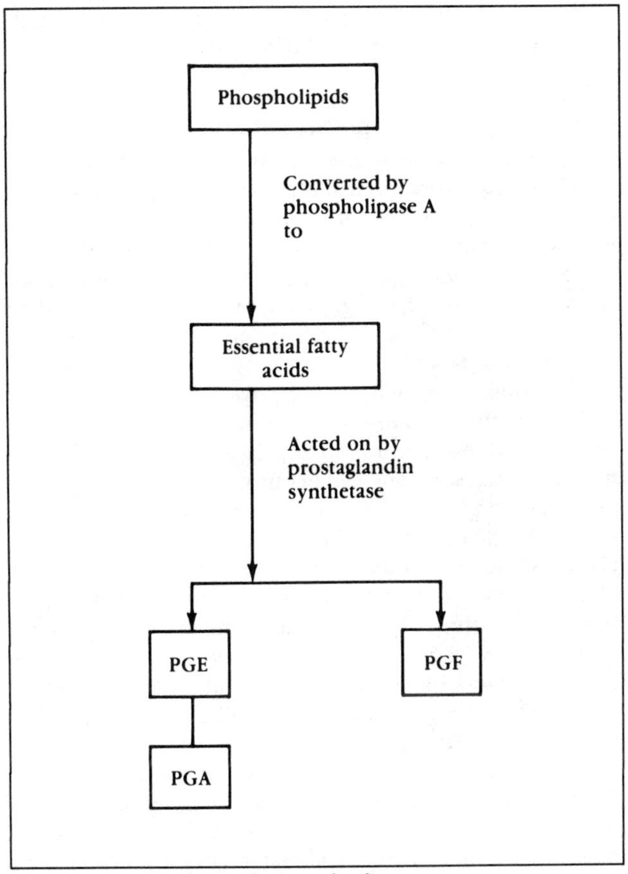

FIGURE 50-13. Synthesis of prostaglandins.

TABLE 50-1. Levels of prostaglandins in different phases of the menstrual cycle

Prostaglandin	Proliferative phase	Midluteal phase	Menses
PGE_2	13–26 ng/100 ng tissue	13–26 ng/100 ng tissue	52 ng/100 ng tissue
$PGF_{2\alpha}$	10–25 ng/100 ng	67 ng/100 ng tissue	67 ng/100 ng maintained

Sources: H. J. Clithroe and V. R. Pickles, The separation of the smooth muscle stimulants in menstrual fluid. *J. Physiol. (Lond.)* 156:225, 1961; and J. Downie, N. L. Poyser, and M. Wunderlick, Levels of prostaglandins in the human endometrium during the normal menstrual cycle. *J. Physiol. (Lond.)* 236:456, 1974.

Although there are many different prostaglandins, only PGE_2 and PGF_2 primarily affect reproduction. Both PGE_2 and $PGF_{2\alpha}$ have been identified in endometrial tissue where both exert a stimulating effect on the uterus. Studies have confirmed that levels of prostaglandins vary with the menstrual cycle (Table 50-1). Elevated levels of PGE_2 and $PGF_{2\alpha}$ have now been identified as a possible factor in primary dysmenorrhea. Currently, PGE_2 is being used to induce uterine contractions for intrauterine fetal death, missed abortion, and hydatidiform mole.

Female Response In the Sexual Act

The female response in the sexual act is a normal physiologic process. Every woman is a diverse individual who has different levels of response. However, the physiologic events of sexual response tend to occur in an orderly sequence. This sequence of events and responses is summarized in the four phases of sexual response identified by Masters and Johnson: (1) excitation, (2) plateau, (3) orgasm, and (4) resolution.

Excitation begins with either physical or psychic stimulation. The first response to this sexual stimulation is vaginal lubrication. This lubrication is a result of vasodilatation and congestion and can occur within 10 to 30 seconds of stimulation. Transudation of fluid, not secretion, account for this lubrication since the vagina contains no secretory glands. Other characteristics of the excitement phase include (1) engorgement and enlargement of the labia, clitoris, and uterus, (2) enlargement and ballooning of the vagina, (3) elevation of the uterus and cervix, as well as nipple erection. Blood pressure and pulse increase and the "sex flush" may appear as a measleslike rash on epigastrium, chest, and throat.

The plateau phase is reached as sexual arousal is increased. Characteristics of this phase include retraction of the clitoris against the symphysis, narrowing of the vaginal opening, increased length and diameter of the vagina, deep red coloring of the labia minora, and complete elevation of the uterus. Breast size may also increase in the plateau phase and the sex flush may spread over the shoulders, inner surface of arms and, perhaps, abdomen, back, and thighs. Respiratory rate also increases late in the plateau phase.

During orgasm, vasocongestion reaches its maximum and stimulates the reflex stretch mechanism. As a result, rhythmic contractions occur in the uterus, outer one-third of the vagina, and perhaps the rectal sphincter. Rhythmic contractions may also be noted in the arms, legs, abdomen, and buttocks.

During resolution, the final phase of sexual response, the body returns to its preexcitement phase. Within 10 to 15 seconds the clitoris returns to normal and normal color returns to the labia minora. Ten to fifteen minutes are required for the vagina to return to normal and the cervical os remains open for about 30 minutes. Unlike the man, who experiences a refractory period during resolution when he is incapable of sexual stimulation, some women are capable of multiple orgasms without dropping below the plateau phase. Resolution then follows the last orgasm.

Gestation

Gestation, which begins with fertilization of the ovum and continues throughout the development of the fetus, represents a normal physiologic function of the body. This normal process is the basis of many complete and comprehensive texts. Therefore, the discussion will be limited to gestation from conception through placental formation to provide the basis for a discussion of the alterations in normal pregnancy, which are covered in Chapter 51.

Conception generally occurs in the outer one-third of the fallopian tube and mitotic divisions begin immediately. Cellular division continues and after approximately 3 to 4 days the cell mass is referred to as a *morula*. At this point it enters the uterus where it remains free but moves toward the site of implantation. The morula consists of both an inner and an outer cell mass. The inner cell mass will develop into the embryoblast and finally the embryo, while the outer cell mass forms the trophoblast and finally the placenta. As cellular division continues, the embryoblast becomes located at one pole while the trophoblast forms the outer wall (Fig. 50-14). The zygote is now referred to as a blastocyst.

After about 7 days, the trophoblasts are in direct contact with the endometrium and the process of implantation begins. The trophoblast consists of two layers: (1) cytotrophoblast or inner layer, and (2) syncytiotrophoblast or outer layer. This outer layer of syncytial cells has the ability to erode the endometrial tissue (now referred to as decidua) and produce maternal lakes of blood. Cytotrophoblastic cells begin to send out fingerlike projections producing chorionic villi. Fetal capillaries also form in the chorionic villi so that maternal-fetal exchange can occur. As pregnancy continues villi beneath the embryo continue to grow while those on the other side degenerate and form the chorion. This process continues until implantation and placental formation are complete.

Menopause

Menopause, the cessation of menstruation, marks the final phase of the female reproductive function. The transition or gradual change in ovarian function is termed *climacteric*. The average age of menopause in the United States is 50, but may occur before the age of 45 or after 50. Menopause is complete when the woman has experienced no menstrual periods for a period of 1 year.

In some women, menopause occurs abruptly with complete cessation of menstruation after normal periods. In other women, there is a gradual cessation characterized by decreased amounts of bleeding with monthly cycles, periods of amenorrhea, and finally complete cessation of normal periods. Menopause is accompanied by decreased estrogen levels and reversal in estrogen forms. The production of all estrogens by the ovary decreases. The primary estrogen seen in menopause is estrone, which is derived from androstenedione and fat conversion.

Menopause is frequently associated with other physiologic changes and symptoms. These include (1) hot flashes, (2) changes in reproductive organs, (3) cardiovascular dis-

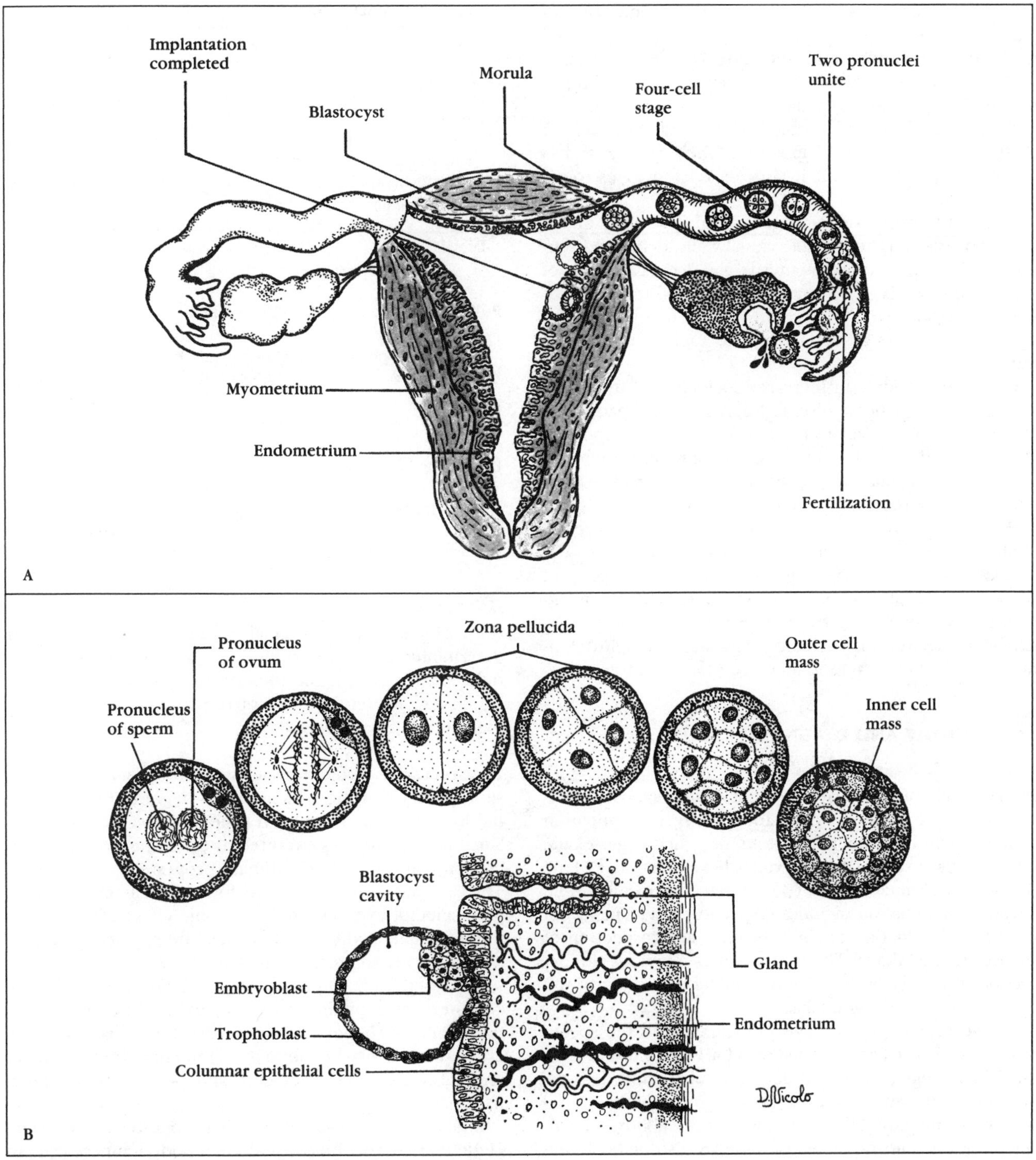

FIGURE 50-14. Implantation of the blastocyst. A. Serial representation of ovum from ovulation to implantation. B. Blastocyst beginning implantation (zona pellucida has been lost). (From M.A. Miller and D.A. Brooten, *The Childbearing Family: A Nursing Perspective* [2nd ed.]. Boston: Little, Brown, 1983.)

ease, (4) osteoporosis, and (5) nervousness and psychologic problems.

The most common, most universal symptom associated with menopause is hot flashes. It begins as a feeling of warmth in the chest and progresses upward over the neck and face. It may be accompanied by flushing of the skin in these areas and profuse diaphoresis. The exact cause has not been determined but it appears related to estrogen withdrawal.

Changes in reproductive organs include atrophy of the labia, dryness and thinning of vaginal walls, decreased support of bladder, rectum, and uterus, and decrease in size of uterus and cervix. The changes are all associated with lower estrogen levels and account for such complaints as dyspareunia, stress incontinence, and vaginal itching and burning.

Evidence supports an increased incidence of hypertension, stroke, and heart disease following menopause [4]. Decreased estrogen levels are also linked to osteoporosis and increased bone fragility. Estrogen administration has been shown to halt the process in young women having had premature removal of the ovaries.

Psychologic symptoms associated with menopause include nervousness, depression, headache, insomnia, decreased sex drive, memory loss, vertigo, and a feeling of worthlessness and hopelessness. There has been no identified connection between these symptoms and estrogen levels. Therefore, the basic personality and cultural influences are of more importance in determining treatment.

LABORATORY AND DIAGNOSTIC AIDS

Gynecologic Examination

Probably one of the most important of all diagnostic tools available is the physical examination. Physical examination of the female reproductive system, or gynecologic exam, involves three steps: (1) the external examination, (2) the speculum examination, and (3) the bimanual examination. External examination includes inspection and palpation of the breasts, palpation of the abdomen, and inspection of the external genitalia. These procedures allow for the detection of masses, redness, and swelling or lesions of the breasts and external genitalia.

The second step of the gynecologic exam is the speculum exam. This examination allows for visualization of the cervix and vaginal wall and detection of redness, lesions, swelling, or unusual discharge. Specimens for other laboratory tests—including Pap smear, wet smear, gonorrhea cultures, vaginal smears, or biopsies—may also be collected at this time.

The final step of the gynecologic exam is the bimanual examination. This examination allows for palpation of the uterus, ovaries, and fallopian tubes. Conclusion of the bimanual exam involves either a rectal or rectovaginal exam. At this point the examiner is able to palpate such pelvic structures as the posterior surface of the uterus, the uterosacral ligaments, and the cul-de-sac of Douglas.

TABLE 50-2. Normal hormone levels

Hormone	Blood	Urine
Pregnanediol		
Male		<1.5 mg/24 hours
Female		
Proliferative phase		0.5–1.5 mg/24 hours
Luteal phase		2–7 mg/24 hours
Postmenopausal		0.2–1.0 mg/24 hours
Estrogens (total)		
Male		4–25 μg/24 hours
Female		4–60 μg/24 hours with increase in pregnancy
Prolactin	<20 ng/ml	
Progesterone		
Proliferative phase	<1.0 ng/ml	
Luteal phase	<2.0 ng/ml	
FSH		6–50 mouse uterine units/24 hours
Luteinizing hormone		
Proliferative phase	<70 mIU/ml	
Luteal phase	>70 mIU/ml	
Estriol		10–20 mg/24 hours

Hormone Levels

Both bioassay and chemical methods are available for determining ovarian hormone levels. However, these are time-consuming, difficult to perform or to standardize, and expensive. Therefore, most of the studies to detect hormone levels are indirect.

PROGESTERONE. Progesterone is a steroid that is degraded shortly after secretion. Most of this degradation occurs in the liver with the major end product being pregnanediol. Since pregnanediol is excreted in the urine, its rate of excretion can be used to estimate progesterone formation. This estimate must be done by chemical means since pregnanediol exerts no progesteronic effects. Standardization of results is difficult, but the generally accepted normal values are summarized in Table 50-2.

Increased levels of progesterone may be associated with (1) luteal cysts of the ovary, (2) arrhenoblastoma of the ovary, and (3) hyperadrenocorticism (see Chap. 32). Decreased levels may be found in (1) amenorrhea, (2) threatened abortion, (3) fetal death, and (4) toxemia of pregnancy.

Indirect methods of determining progesterone levels include endometrial biopsy and basal body temperature. An endometrial biopsy is useful in determining the stage of the menstrual cycle and therefore infers the level of hormone production. In studying basal body temperature charts, a substantial rise of 1°F implies that ovulation has taken place and that progesterone secretion is adequate.

ESTROGEN. One very useful laboratory test in the study of estrogen levels is a 24-hour urinary estriol excretion. Since

TABLE 50-3. Classifications of Pap smear findings

Class	Original	CIN system	Category	Other descriptive terms
I	Absence of atypical or abnormal cells	Normal	Benign	Negative
II	Atypical cytologic picture, but no evidence of malignancy	Inflammatory	Benign	Atypical
III	Cytologic picture suggestive of, but not conclusive for, malignancy	Mild CIN	Mild CIN	Mild dysplasia
IV	Cytologic picture strongly suggestive for malignancy	Severe CIN	Severe CIN	Carcinoma in situ
V	Cytologic picture conclusive for malignancy	Cancer	Malignant	Invasive cancer

estriol is produced by the placenta it represents both fetal and placental activity. A significant drop (40% less than the mean of three previous values) may indicate that the fetus is in jeopardy, since urinary estriol excretion increases as pregnancy progresses. Incomplete 24-hour urine specimens as well as pyelonephritis have been known to affect the results. Normal findings are 10 to 20 mg/24 hours.

Changes in cervical mucus and epithelial cells of the vagina are good indicators of estrogen production. Cervical mucus undergoes very definite changes in response to estrogen and progesterone production. Spinnbarkheit and ferning are two characteristics of cervical mucus that can easily be studied. Spinnbarkheit refers to the elasticity of cervical mucus. This allows the examiner to draw it out into a long thin thread of 15 to 20 cm at the time of ovulation. During minimal estrogen production threads only reach 1 to 2 cm.

Ferning refers to the pattern created when cervical mucus, under the influence of estrogen, dries (see Figure 50-11). Ferning results when sodium chloride in the mucus crystallizes. Estrogen secretion increases the sodium chloride content of cervical mucus while progesterone decreases it. Therefore, the level of estrogen without progesterone determines the presence of a ferning pattern. This pattern is fullest and most complete at the time of ovulation.

Vaginal smears are also useful in determining estrogen levels since the vaginal cells also undergo cyclic changes. Estrogen thickens the vaginal epithelium. Glucose excretion also corresponds to estrogen secretion. Both are highest at the time of ovulation.

Smears

PAP SMEAR. A specimen for Pap smear is best collected from the cervical canal and the squamocolumnar junction near the external os during the speculum examination. Dry cotton swabs are used to collect cervical canal secretions while a small wooden spatula is used for the squamocolumnar specimen. The specimen is then transferred to a glass slide where it is fixed for staining and microscopic examination. The primary purpose of a Pap smear is screening for abnormal cervical cells and indication for more extensive testing. It may also help in detecting cancer of the endometrium and vagina.

Classification of Pap smear results varies widely from institution to institution. The original Papanicolaou classification identified five classes of smears ranging from class I, which was normal, to class V, definitely malignant. A more recent classification uses three major classifications: (1) benign, (2) precancerous, and (3) malignant. The precancerous classification includes the cervical intraepithelial neoplasia (CIN) also referred to as dysplasia. Other clinicians use a verbal description to indicate their findings. A summary of the various classifications is found in Table 50-3.

WET SMEAR. Wet smears are especially beneficial in diagnosing the cause of vaginitis. In this procedure a specimen of vaginal discharge is placed on a slide, mixed with a drop of saline solution or potassium hydroxide, and examined under the microscope for *Candida*, *Trichomonas*, or other bacteria. However, it is not conclusive for gonorrhea.

Biopsy

ENDOMETRIAL BIOPSY. An endometrial biopsy involves insertion of a curet through the cervix. It is placed against the uterine wall and slowly withdrawn. It is best to repeat the procedure on different walls of the uterus in order to obtain a more complete specimen.

Endometrial biopsy is especially useful in evaluation of dysfunctional bleeding. It may be helpful in diagnosis of endometrial cancer. However, there is increased risk that scattered growths may be missed. Another use for endometrial biopsy is in infertility studies. This is best performed just prior to onset of menses or day 22 of the menstrual cycle. However, it can interfere with pregnancy if conception has occurred.

CERVICAL BIOPSY. A punch biopsy instrument is used in the physician's office to obtain samples of cervical tissue. This can aid in more precise diagnosis of questionable lesions. It is also helpful in removal of small polyps.

CONE BIOPSY. Cone biopsy, also referred to as conization, is a hospital procedure. It involves the removal of a cone-shaped specimen of cervical tissue, removal of any visible lesions, as well as removal of tissue specimens of the squamocolumnar junction and cervical canal. It may be used as follow-up to Pap smear or punch biopsy.

OPEN BREAST BIOPSY. Breast biopsy involves surgical intervention for removal of a lump. A frozen section can be done for immediate classification, while more extensive pathologic studies will require more time.

NEEDLE BIOPSY. In needle biopsy of a breast lesion, the physician inserts a needle into the lesion and aspirates its contents. This procedure may be performed in the office but must be followed up as necessary.

VULVAR BIOPSY. Punch biopsy forceps can be utilized to obtain adequate tissue. Frequently the gross appearance is normal and staining procedures must be utilized to identify the affected area.

Radiography

HYSTEROSALPINGOGRAM. Hysterosalpingogram is an x-ray examination of the uterus and fallopian tubes. A small cannula is inserted through the cervix. A radiopaque dye is then injected into the uterus and fallopian tubes. Filling of the uterus and tubes can be observed on the fluoroscopy screen. Spot films may also be made. Hysterosalpingogram is especially useful in noting the size and shape of the uterus and tubes as well as tubal obstruction.

MAMMOGRAPHY. Mammography is an x-ray examination of the breasts. It is useful in the detection of early lesions that cannot be palpated and the exact location of deep tumors. It may be useful in predicting malignancy. As with any x-ray procedure radiation exposure occurs and the procedure is not recommended for routine screening except in women over the age of 35 who have a high risk of developing a malignancy.

Other Procedures

COLPOSCOPY. The colposcope is a binocular diagnostic instrument that allows magnified (10–20 x) viewing of the cervix and vaginal walls. It is mounted on a tripod and maintains no contact with the patient during the exam. Colposcopy is useful in follow-up on abnormal Pap smears, to identify abnormal areas for biopsy, and to examine lesions on the vulva. Colposcopy is also recommended in follow-up of women whose mothers took DES (diethylstilbestrol) during pregnancy; it may also be employed for the woman with dyspareunia and bleeding with intercourse. Each procedure involves the following five observations: (1) vascular pattern, (2) color tone, (3) intercapillary distance, (4) borderline against normal tissue, and (5) surface pattern [5].

LAPAROSCOPY AND CULDOSCOPY. Both laparoscopy and culdoscopy are surgical procedures that allow the physician to visualize the pelvic area through a lighted tube. The procedures are performed to note the condition and position of the various organs, or whether scarring, presence of endometrial tissue, or infection exist. A tubal ligation may also be performed through the laparoscope.

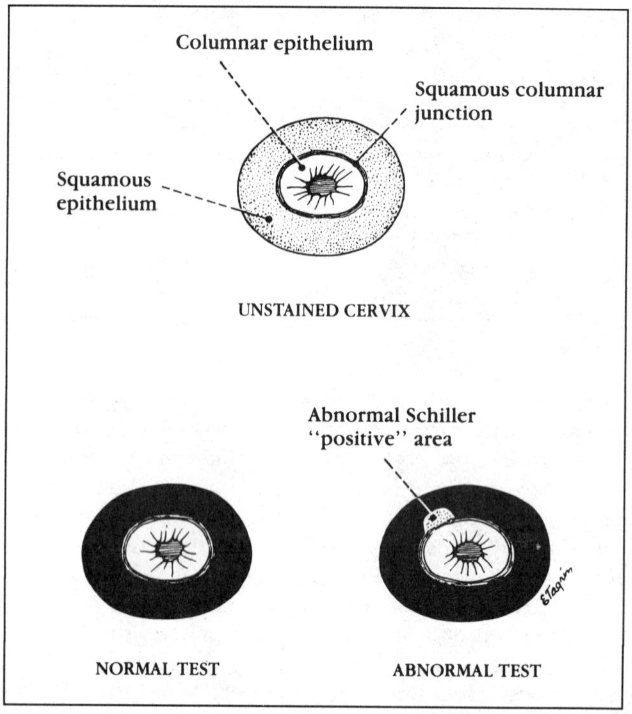

FIGURE 50-15. Schiller's test. (From T.H. Green, Jr., and R.C. Knapp, Gynecology. In G.L. Nardi and G.D. Zuidema [eds.], *Surgery: A Concise Guide to Clinical Practice* [4th ed.]. Boston: Little, Brown, 1982.)

ULTRASOUND. Ultrasound, also referred to as sonography, is a noninvasive technique particularly useful in providing pictures of the soft tissue structure of the body. Little preparation is necessary except that the individual must have a full bladder. The distended bladder, with 200 to 400 ml of urine, is used as a reference point and to displace the pelvic organs for better visualization. Overdistention can distort the findings.

An ultrasound transducer serves both as a transmitter and receiver. It converts an electrical signal into ultrasound energy, which is transmitted into the body and then reflected from tissues of different densities. These reflections of ultrasound energy are then received by the transducer and converted again to electrical energy for recording. The procedure is virtually painless and requires from 5 minutes up to 30 minutes or more for completion.

Ultrasound has become a valuable diagnostic tool in both obstetrics and gynecology. In obstetrics, ultrasound is especially useful to confirm pregnancy, to establish or confirm dates or placental location, to rule out large or small size for gestational age, fetal position, and hydrops. Gynecologists now utilize ultrasound to assist in the diagnosis of uterine malformations, hydatidiform mole, malignancies, ovarian masses, pelvic inflammatory disease, tubal malformations, and pelvic abscess or hematoma.

SCHILLER TEST. The Schiller test is a very simple procedure that involves painting the cervix with Schiller's solution or similar iodine solution. A normal cervix, which contains glycogen, appears mahógany brown from absorption of the iodine. However, abnormal areas, containing no glycogen, remain a light brown. The primary usefulness of the Schiller test is in locating the exact area for biopsy (Fig. 50-15).

CULTURES. Cultures are most helpful in the diagnosis of the specific organism responsible for an infection. A specimen is collected from the infection site with a sterile cotton swab and placed immediately in an appropriate medium. The specimen is then sent to the lab where it is incubated and checked for growth and sensitivity. If gonorrhea is suspected, special precautions should be undertaken to ensure an anaerobic environment. Special media may also be used to reduce growth of other bacteria.

THERMOGRAPHY. Thermography is the photographic display of infrared rays from skin temperature over the breast. An elevation of skin temperature is seen in breast cancer because of increased blood flow in the area. This procedure does not always detect early cancers and false positives are quite common.

RUBIN'S TEST. Rubin's test involves the injection of carbon dioxide through a cannula and into the uterus. If one or both fallopian tubes are open referred shoulder pain will be felt. The value of this test is to determine the patency of at least one tube.

HUHNER'S TEST. Huhner's test is an examination of cervical mucus. Ideally it is performed during ovulation and within several hours of intercourse. Cervical mucus is collected with an eyedropper or cotton swab and examined under a microscope. It is a simple procedure used in screening infertility cases since the examiner can note the characteristics of the cervical mucus as well as the numbers and activity of sperm present.

REFERENCES

1. Clithroe, H. J., and Pickles, V. R. The separation of the smooth muscle stimulants in menstrual fluid. *J. Physiol.* (Lond.) 156:225, 1961.
2. Downie, J., Poyser, N. L., and Wunderlick, M. Levels of prostaglandins in the human endometrium during the normal menstrual cycle. *J. Physiol.* (Lond.) 236:456, 1974.
3. Kolodny, R. C., et al. *Textbook of Human Sexuality for Nurses.* Boston: Little, Brown, 1979.
4. Luckman, J., and Sorenson, K. C. *Medical-Surgical Nursing: A Psychophysiologic Approach* (2nd ed.). Philadelphia: Saunders, 1980.
5. Parsons, L., and Sommers, S. C. *Gynecology* (2nd ed.). Philadelphia: Saunders, 1978. P. 1010.
6. Selkurt, E. E. (ed.). *Basic Physiology for the Health Sciences* (2nd ed.). Boston: Little, Brown, 1982. P. 512.
7. Stewart, F. H., et al. *My Body, My Health: The Concerned Woman's Guide to Gynecology.* New York: Wiley, 1979. P. 16.

CHAPTER 51
ALTERATIONS IN FEMALE FUNCTION

LEARNING OBJECTIVES

1. Define *endometriosis*.
2. List the clinical manifestations of endometriosis and the pathologic basis.
3. Distinguish between primary and secondary dysmenorrhea.
4. Discuss the role of prostaglandins in dysmenorrhea.
5. Define *dysfunctional uterine bleeding*.
6. Distinguish between primary and secondary amenorrhea.
7. Compare and contrast the forms of vaginitis regarding causative organism, clinical manifestations, and diagnostic studies.
8. Distinguish between cervical erosion and eversion.
9. Define *toxic shock syndrome* and list the clinical manifestations.
10. Discuss sexually transmitted disease (STD) including causative organism, clinical manifestations, diagnosis, and treatment.
11. Compare and contrast uterine fibroids and cancer.
12. Distinguish between functional ovarian cysts, benign neoplastic tumors of the ovary, and ovarian cancer.
13. Compare and contrast the three types of trophoblastic disease.
14. Discuss the sequential process of cellular proliferation of cervical cancer.
15. Describe the effects of diethylstilbestrol administration on mothers and offspring.
16. Describe the staging systems of cancer of the ovary, breast, cervix, and endometrium.
17. List the three influences on breast cancer currently under study.

For many women alterations in female function represent a threat to body image and self-concept. Feelings of femininity may be altered. Alterations may occur in all reproductive organs and with no consideration of age. Alterations considered in this chapter include menstrual problems; infectious conditions; and benign, premalignant, and malignant conditions.

MENSTRUAL PROBLEMS

Endometriosis

Endometriosis refers to the abnormal location of endometrial tissue. Two types of endometriosis, internal and external, are described. *Internal endometriosis*, or adenomyosis, refers to the location of aberrant endometrial tissue within the myometrium. *External endometriosis* refers to the location of endometrial tissue outside the uterus. Sites for external endometriosis include (1) the outer surface or perimetrium of the uterus, (2) fallopian tubes, (3) ovaries (most common site), (4) bladder and rectal surfaces, (5) uterine ligaments, (6) cul-de-sac, (7) rectovaginal septum, (8) appendix, and (9) bowel. On occasion aberrant tissue may also be found in laparotomy scars, vulva, vagina, and umbilicus (Fig. 51-1). In this chapter the term *adenomyosis* is used to refer to internal endometriosis and *endometriosis* refers to external endometriosis.

Endometriosis is characterized by functional aberrant endometrium that responds to hormonal stimulation as normal uterine endometrium does. This tissue grows and thickens under cyclic hormonal influence in the same manner as normal endometrium. As estrogen and progesterone are withdrawn this tissue reacts with bleeding. Early lesions appear as tiny red blue spots surrounded by puckered scar tissue. Larger masses may form when the smaller lesions coalesce. These are usually located on the serosal layer of the involved organs. In the ovary, lesions may take the form of *endometriomas*, cystic lesions lined with functioning endometrium. Bleeding within the cysts results in a thick, chocolate-colored fluid, thus the term *chocolate cysts* (Fig. 51-2). Adhesions result when bleeding occurs into the peritoneal cavity and lead to fixation of involved pelvic structures.

The exact cause of endometriosis is unknown but there are two primary theories that are accepted: (1) retrograde menstruation, and (2) metaplasia. The *retrograde menstruation* theory, known as Samson's theory, states that during menstruation, endometrial tissue is regurgitated through the fallopian tube into the pelvic cavity where it implants.

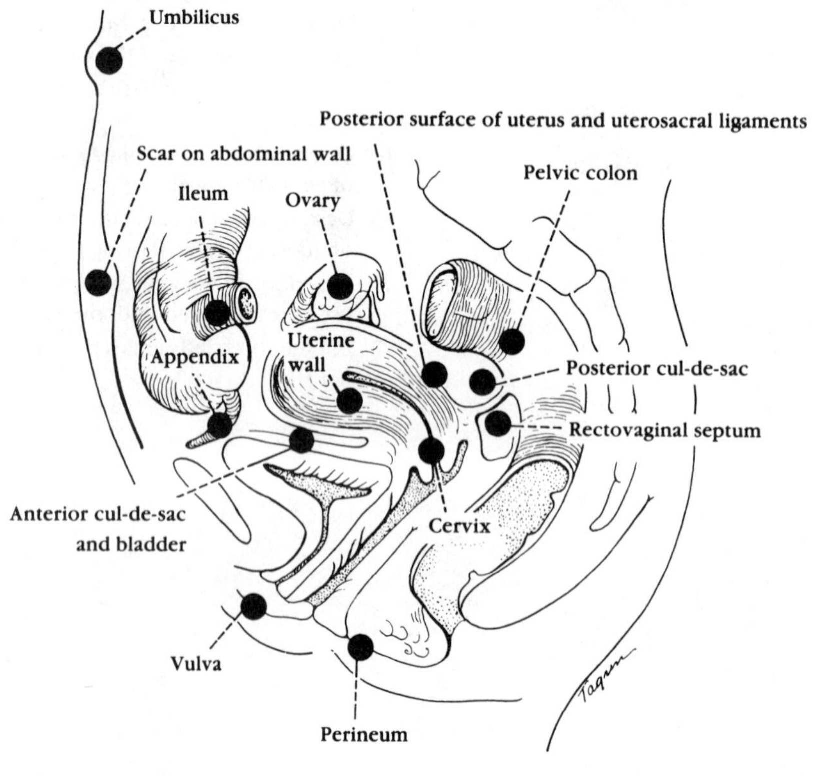

FIGURE 51-1. Sites of occurrence of endometriosis. (From T. H. Green, Jr., *Gynecology: Essentials of Clinical Practice* [3rd ed.]. Boston: Little, Brown, 1977.)

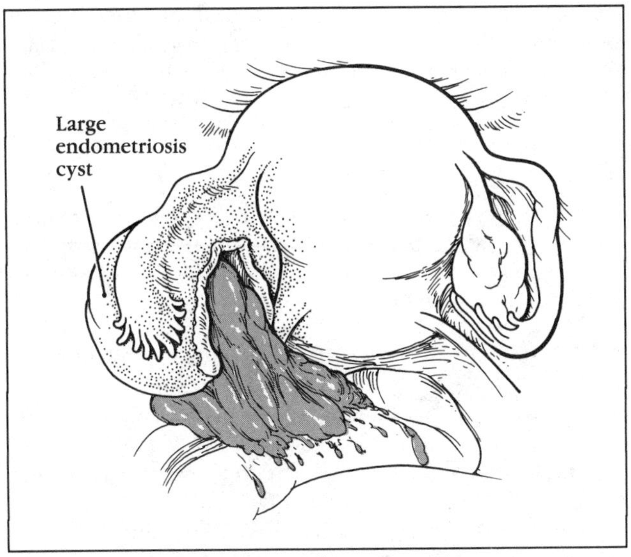

FIGURE 51-2. Endometriomas with cyst formation.

The *metaplasia theory* suggests that the undifferentiated coelomic epithelia of the embryo remain dormant until menarche. This tissue then begins to respond to estrogen and progesterone in a similar way as other endometrial tissue.

Clinical manifestations are dependent on the location of lesions. The most common symptom is low abdominal and/or pelvic pain associated with the menstrual period, such as backache and cramps beginning just prior to or with the onset of menses. The pain increases throughout menstruation and subsides afterward. It is commonly described as a dull, bearing-down type of pain. The cause of the pain is irritation from hemorrhage of the aberrant tissue or distention. Occasionally a chocolate cyst may rupture with signs of acute abdomen. Sterility and/or infertility may result from extensive scarring of the ovaries and tubes. Dyspareunia reflects uterine involvement, dysuria reflects bladder involvement, and pain on defecation occurs with rectal involvement.

No specific laboratory test is available for diagnosis of endometriosis. Physical examination may reveal small nodular masses on pelvic organs that enlarge during menstruation and are rarely movable (Fig. 51-3). Laparoscopy or exploratory surgery are the most beneficial since they allow visualization of the lesion.

The treatment of choice depends on the woman's symptoms, age, and childbearing desires. In early endometriosis, treatment consists of analgesia and regular follow-up care. With severe symptoms, surgery is indicated. Surgery in women desiring children is usually aimed at removal of as much endometrial tissue as possible with preservation of uterus and ovaries. Hormone therapy that prevents ovulation or produces pseudopregnancy may also help in the younger woman.

In adenomyosis, endometrial tissue has invaded the myometrium. The invasion may be diffuse or localized and

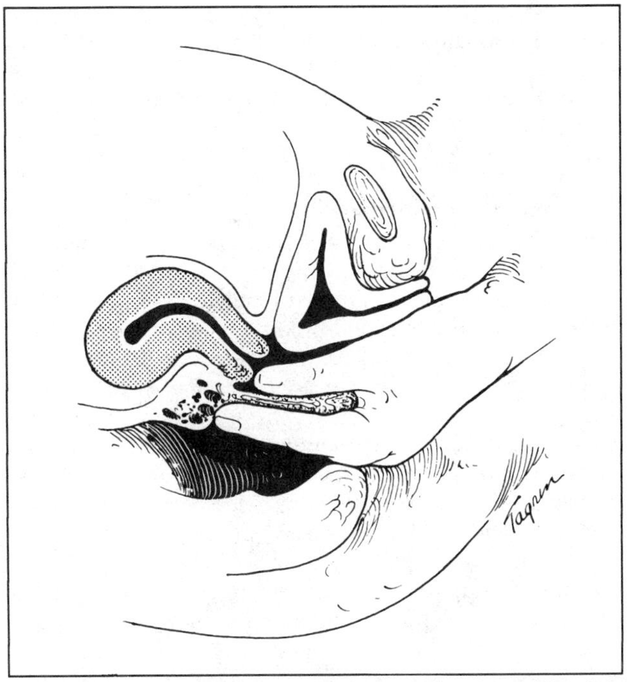

FIGURE 51-3. Rectal examination in the typical patient with pelvic endometriosis. The tender nodularity of the uterosacral ligaments and cul-de-sac and the fixed retroversion of the uterus are almost diagnostic of the disease. (From T. H. Green, Jr., *Gynecology: Essentials of Clinical Practice* [3rd ed.]. Boston: Little, Brown, 1977.)

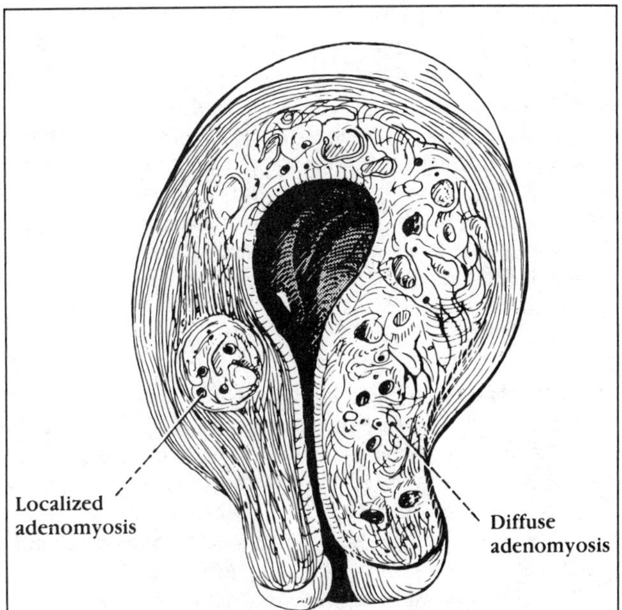

FIGURE 51-4. Adenomyosis of the uterus. Diffuse involvement of the uterine wall (right) and the localized form, the so-called adenomyoma (left). (From T. H. Green, Jr., *Gynecology: Essentials of Clinical Practice* [3rd ed.]. Boston: Little, Brown, 1977.)

results in an enlarged uterus (Fig. 51-4). This buried endometrium is usually nonfunctional. Symptoms include menorrhagia, dyspareunia, dysmenorrhea, and generalized pelvic discomfort. The usual treatment is hysterectomy, which is indicated by symptoms.

Premenstrual Syndrome

Premenstrual syndrome is a term used to collectively cover the discomforts noted, prior to the onset of monthly menses. The symptoms vary with individuals but most frequently include headache, breast tenderness, abdominal heaviness and bloating, edema, weight gain, backache, nervous irritability, mood changes, crying spells, depression, insomnia, and anxiety. These symptoms become worse 7 to 10 days prior to menses and subside when the menstrual flow is well established. The exact cause of premenstrual discomfort is unknown. However, it is believed to be associated with estrogen and progesterone levels.

Treatment is symptomatic and varies with individuals. The most frequently employed treatments include diuretics, dietary restriction of sodium, tranquilizers, and sedatives.

Dysmenorrhea

Dysmenorrhea may occur as a single entity or as part of the premenstrual syndrome. Dysmenorrhea means painful menstruation and is commonly referred to as cramps. There are two types of dysmenorrhea: (1) primary and (2) secondary. *Secondary dysmenorrhea* is caused by organic pelvic disease and is discussed in the appropriate section. *Primary dysmenorrhea* is the term used to refer to painful menses unrelated to an obvious physical cause. It usually begins with the establishment of ovulatory cycles. Spasmodic primary dysmenorrhea is usually characterized by sharp cramping sensations the first day or two of menses. This type may improve in monthly cycles reestablished following pregnancy. Congestive primary dysmenorrhea frequently occurs in association with premenstrual syndrome. It is characterized by a dull aching pain prior to onset of menses.

The cause of primary dysmenorrhea remains unknown. However, one theory attributes the cause to the secretion of prostaglandins, especially PGE_2, which have a stimulating effect on the uterine muscle. Nausea, vomiting, and diarrhea associated with dysmenorrhea have also been attributed to prostaglandins [6]. Other factors considered among possible causes of primary dysmenorrhea include acute anteflexion of the uterus, estrogen-progesterone imbalance, and hypersensitivity of the individual to pain.

The more common treatments include (1) hormones, (2) analgesics, (3) prostaglandin synthetase, (4) optimum health maintenance, and (5) psychotherapy. Hormone therapy is aimed at preventing ovulation since anovulatory cycles are rarely painful. Antiprostaglandins include aspirin, indomethacin, rosyn, and ibuprofen (Motrin). These drugs may be administered prior to the onset of menses to inhibit prostaglandin synthesis. The drugs may not only inhibit prostaglandin synthesis but also block its action. Mild analgesics may also be administered.

Abnormal Uterine Bleeding

Abnormal uterine bleeding is usually a symptom of some underlying disease process rather than a disease entity itself. A number of descriptive terms are used to describe abnormal uterine bleeding:

Metrorrhagia or intermenstrual bleeding—bleeding between periods
Menorrhagia or hypermenorrhea—excessive menstrual flow
Polymenorrhea — abnormally frequent menstrual bleeding
Oligomenorrhea—abnormally infrequent menses
Hypomenorrhea—deficient menstrual flow
Amenorrhea—absence of menstrual flow
Perimenopausal bleeding—irregular bleeding prior to menopause
Postmenopausal bleeding—bleeding occurring 1 year or more after menopause

The multiple causes of abnormal uterine bleeding can be grouped into four major categories: (1) complications of pregnancy, (2) organic lesions, (3) constitutional diseases, and (4) true dysfunctional uterine bleeding. Complications of pregnancy include abortion, trophoblastic disease, and ectopic pregnancy. Organic lesions include conditions associated with pelvic diseases such as infection, tumors, and polyps. Constitutional diseases include conditions such as hypertension, blood dyscrasias, and hormonal dysfunction. No pelvic disease is found but symptoms are reflected through abnormal uterine bleeding. The last category, dysfunctional uterine bleeding, represents abnormal bleeding associated with endocrine dysfunction. This category is explored further in the next section and the other categories are discussed in other portions of this chapter as they are related to specific conditions.

DYSFUNCTIONAL UTERINE BLEEDING. The term *dysfunctional uterine bleeding* is frequently used interchangeably with anovulatory bleeding. It refers to abnormal bleeding that is the result of endocrine dysfunction. It is associated with an absence of ovulation. Therefore, no corpus luteum is formed, no progesterone produced, and no secretory changes occur in the endometrium. The endometrium becomes hyperplastic. As estrogen levels decrease from degenerating follicles, withdrawal bleeding occurs. Occasionally dysfunctional uterine bleeding results from inadequate production of progesterone following ovulation.

Psychogenic uterine bleeding may be included in dysfunctional uterine bleeding when both organic and constitutional causes have been ruled out. The influence of emotional stimulation on the hypothalamus and the resultant influence on the gonadotropic hormones were discussed in Chapter 50. Emotions may also directly affect the uterine blood vessels and produce bleeding.

Diagnosis is made following a complete and thorough menstrual history. Physical examination reveals pelvic lesions and aids in the diagnosis of constitutional diseases. Additional laboratory studies include thyroid function, complete blood count (CBC), and platelet count to rule out blood dyscrasias. Studies to determine the presence of ovulation include estrogen and progesterone studies, endometrial biopsy, and spinnbarkheit and ferning studies of cervical mucus. During the climacteric, both cytologic studies and biopsy are important to rule out cancer.

AMENORRHEA. Amenorrhea is not a disease entity. It may indicate a very serious condition or be completely normal, as in pregnancy. Amenorrhea may be either primary or secondary. *Primary amenorrhea* refers to a failure to begin menstrual cycles. *Secondary amenorrhea* occurs following a variable period of normal function. Causes of amenorrhea may be physiologic, anatomic, genetic, endocrinologic, constitutional, or psychogenic. Physiologic causes include pregnancy, lactation, menopause, and adolescence. Anatomic factors include congenital anomalies, hysterectomy, and endometrial destruction. Genetic factors include Turner's syndrome and hermaphroditism. Dysfunction of the hypothalamus, pituitary, ovary, thyroid, or adrenal glands may also produce amenorrhea. Malnutrition, obesity, drug addiction, diabetes, and anemia are all constitutional problems that can prevent menstrual periods. Psychogenic factors include psychosis and anorexia nervosa.

Specific diagnostic tools, in addition to the history and physical exam, include thyroid function studies, serum prolactin level, buccal smear, skull x rays, progesterone challenge test, and hormone values.

REPRODUCTIVE TRACT INFECTIONS

Trichomonas Vaginitis

Trichomoniasis is a vaginal infection caused by the single-celled protozoan, *Trichomonas vaginalis* (Fig. 51-5A). The organism may remain dormant for extended periods of time and prefers a basic vaginal pH. It has been identified in the male urethra and prostate, so it serves as a frequent source of reinfection for the female. The incidence of *Trichomonas* infection is higher in women with multiple sexual partners due to its venereal nature.

Trichomonas produces an intense itching and burning of the vulva and vagina. It is accompanied by a moderate to profuse discharge that is thin, frothy, greenish-yellow to greenish-white in color with a foul odor. Examination of the cervix may reveal small deep red spots referred to as "strawberry spots." Microscopic examination of a wet smear reveals the one-cell protozoan with four flagellae. Cultures are rarely done to confirm the diagnosis.

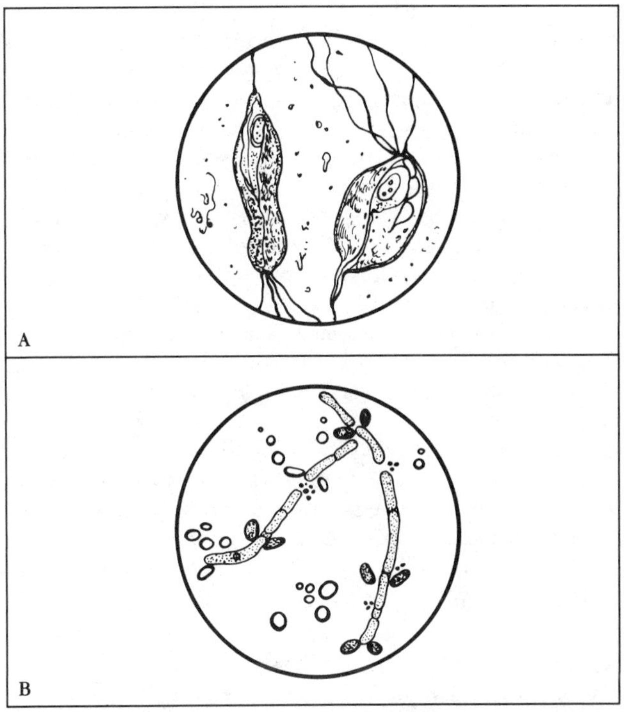

FIGURE 51-5. Fresh vaginal smear preparations. A. Microscopic appearance of *Trichomonas vaginalis* organisms. B. Microscopic picture in candidal vaginitis. (From T. H. Green, Jr., *Gynecology: Essentials of Clinical Practice* [3rd ed.]. Boston: Little, Brown, 1977.)

The treatment of choice is a trichomonacidal drug, Flagyl (metronidazole). It is effective in eradicating the organism in 90 percent of cases. However, it may be accompanied by severe side effects and should be used only after confirmed diagnosis of *Trichomonas*. Side effects of the drug include leukopenia, nausea, diarrhea, headache, and alcohol intolerance. The drug has been found to produce cancer in mice and birth defects in guinea pigs and mice. Therefore, its use is avoided in pregnant women or those suspected of being pregnant. Alternative treatment includes AVC cream or suppositories, Aci-Jel, Tricofuron suppositories or powders, and Floraquin.

Candidiasis

Candidiasis is a vaginal infection produced by the fungus *Candida albicans* (Fig. 51-5B). It is also referred to as moniliasis, thrush, and yeast infection. The fungal organism normally is found on the skin and in the digestive tract and may be found in the vagina of some asymptomatic women. Symptoms occur when there is an overgrowth of the organism, which occurs most frequently during pregnancy, following antibiotic therapy, in diabetics and women on oral contraceptives. Infants may become infected at delivery and develop thrush. During pregnancy and in women on oral contraceptives the levels of estrogen are high, resulting in high glycogen levels, which are favorable for fungal growth. It is believed that systemic antibiotics also suppress the normal bacterial flora found in the vagina and in diabetics the vaginal environment is "sweeter," both of which create a favorable environment for fungal growth. The yeast infection produces a heavy, white cottage cheese–like discharge that is odorless. Complaints of severe itching, dysuria, dyspareunia, and perineal burning are common. The vulva appears erythematous and inflamed. Speculum exam may reveal white plaques on the vaginal wall. Diagnosis is confirmed by wet smear examination with potassium hydroxide.

Antifungal preparations such as mycostatin (Nystatin), Monistat, and Gyne-Lotrimin are the treatments of choice. These medications are used as topical drugs and inserted into the vagina where they exert a local action on the organism. Absorption is poor from the skin and mucous membrane in the vagina. Gentian violet swabs and suppositories may also be used but they produce staining and sometimes allergic reactions. Lactinex tablets or eating yogurt may be helpful in restoring the normal bacterial flora following antibiotic therapy.

Hemophilus Vaginalis Vaginitis

Hemophilus vaginalis, also referred to as *Gardenerella* has now been identified as the causative organism in vaginitis previously referred to as nonspecific vaginitis. It is a gram-negative bacillus of the type *Corynebacterium vaginalis*. It is spread through sexual contact and elimination of the infection requires treatment of both sexual partners.

The most outstanding symptom is a heavy gray discharge with the presence of only mild irritations. Diagnosis is made by identification of cells dotted with small short bacilli. Cultures may be done for additional confirmation. Ampicillin or tetracycline may be administered orally for systemic effect. Milder cases may be treated with sulfonamide creams or suppositories such as Sultrin, Gynben, Furacin, or Gantrisin. Flagyl may also be used.

Atrophic Vaginitis

Atrophic vaginitis refers to inflammation of the atrophied epithelium in postmenopausal women. It produces an irritating vaginal discharge with pruritis and swelling with secondary dyspareunia and dysuria. Red "strawberry spots" may be found on the vaginal wall. Bleeding may occur from trauma to the thin epithelium but malignancy must be ruled out. Estrogen therapy is utilized to convert the epithelium to the more normal thick, stratified squamous layer.

Cervicitis

Cervicitis refers to inflammation of the cervix, which may be acute or chronic. Acute cervicitis usually occurs with other acute reproductive tract infections. Causative organisms include *Staphylococcus, Streptococcus, E. coli,* and *Gonococcus* organisms. Speculum examination reveals an edematous congested cervix with purulent discharge. Symptoms may include dyspareunia, backache, dull pain in lower abdomen, and urinary frequency and urgency. Pain may be noted on palpation. Cultures and smears are done to allow identification of the causative organism and appropriate antibiotic therapy is then instituted.

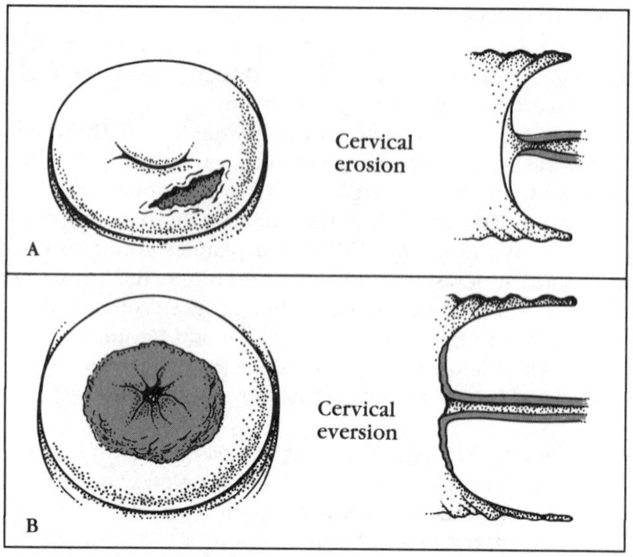

FIGURE 51-6. A. Cervical erosion. B. Cervical eversion.

Many women exhibit some form of chronic cervicitis. It may follow acute infections, childbirth trauma, or abortion. The cervical canal is primarily affected but there are no characteristic findings of the cervix. The only symptom may be a mucopurulent vaginal discharge or occasionally there may be paracervical or low back pain. Abnormal bleeding is rare and often indicates cervical cancer. Physical examination may reveal cervical erosions, cervical eversions, or Nabothian cysts. *Cervical erosion* refers to an area of the surface of the cervix in which the surface epithelia are partially or totally absent. It appears red and raw. Columnar cells are more likely to exhibit this characteristic than squamous cells since they are not as curable. *Cervical eversion* refers to a portion of the cervix in which columnar epithelium of the cervical canal extend outward (Fig. 51-6). The characteristic squamocolumnar junction is then located along the outer edge of the lesion. Eversion occurs more frequently in women taking oral contraceptives, young, never-pregnant women, and in the daughters of women who took diethylstilbestrol during pregnancy. There is an increase in mucoid secretions. In an attempt to repair the eversion, the squamous cells begin to grow inward. As this invasion progresses, the mucus-secreting glands are obliterated. Their secretions are then trapped beneath the epithelium, producing *Nabothian cysts*. These cysts are filled with normal mucus, are not infected, and produce no symptoms.

The primary concern in diagnosing cervicitis is screening for cervical cancer since the lesions are not easily differentiated by the naked eye. In addition to cultures, the

TABLE 51-1. Toxic Shock Syndrome case definition

Fever (temperature ≥38.9°C [102°F])
Rash (diffuse macular erythroderma)
Desquamation, 1–2 weeks after onset of illness, particularly of palms and soles
Hypotension (systolic blood pressure ≤90 mm Hg for adults or <fifth percentile by age for children <16 years old, or orthostatic syncope)
Involvement of three or more of the following organ systems:
GI (vomiting or diarrhea at onset of illness)
Muscular (severe myalgia or creatine phosphokinase level ≥2 × ULN)
Mucous membrane (vaginal, oropharyngeal, or conjunctival hyperemia)
Renal (BUN or Cr ≥2 × ULN or ≥5 white blood cells/high-power field—in the absence of a urinary tract infection)
Hepatic (total bilirubin, SGOT, or SGPT ≥2 × ULN)
Hematologic (platelets ≤100,000/μl)
Central nervous system (disorientation or alterations in consciousness without focal neurologic signs when fever and hypotension are absent)
Negative results on the following tests, if obtained:
Blood, throat, or cerebrospinal fluid cultures
Serologic tests for Rocky Mountain spotted fever, leptospirosis, or measles

ULN = upper limits of normal.
Source: Centers for Disease Control, *Morbidity and Mortality Weekly Report*. 29:442, 1980.

Pap smear, colposcopy, and biopsy are the most important screening aids.

Silver nitrate, douches, and antibiotics are relatively ineffective methods of treatment because of the depth of the lesion. Small areas may be treated with thermal cautery or cryosurgery. Entire areas are treated in depth; healing and reepithelialization then take place. The sloughing cervical tissue produces an annoying discharge that may be treated with antibiotic creams for 7 to 10 days. Complete healing may take 6 to 8 weeks.

Toxic Shock Syndrome

Toxic shock syndrome (TSS) is a relatively new entity first recognized and reported in 1978 [8]. At that time it was thought to be related to *Staphylococcus aureus*. Since then it has gained notoriety as a condition occurring most often in menstruating women who use tampons. The causative agent is believed to be a toxin produced by *Staphylococcus aureus*.

The link with tampons is most interesting since the unused tampons of women developing TSS contained no *S. aureus* [2]. There are theories to support the tampon link. One theory states that bacteria are nourished by carboxymethyl cellulose, which is found in tampons [1]. The other indicates that conditions for bacterial growth are improved through use of superabsorbent tampons [3].

Clinical manifestations of TSS include (1) elevated temperature, sudden in onset, (2) vomiting and diarrhea, and (3) an erythematous macular rash, which is found especially on palms of hands and soles of feet. The sunburnlike rash progresses to peeling of palms of hands and soles of feet about 10 days later. Renal dysfunction may develop with decreased urinary output. Hypotension and shock may develop. Laboratory studies usually reveal an elevated blood urea nitrogen (BUN), serum creatinine, bilirubin, and creatine phosphokinase. Additional complications associated with TSS include disseminated intravascular coagulation, shock lung, and acidosis. Table 51-1 summarizes all criteria for diagnosis.

Treatment varies depending on extent of symptoms. However, it may include (1) antibiotics (pencillinase-resistant penicillin) or cephalosporins, (2) intravenous colloid to prevent fluid loss from blood vessels, (3) ventilation therapy, (4) heparin, (5) blood transfusion, and (6) correction of acid-base imbalance.

Pelvic Inflammatory Disease

Pelvic inflammatory disease (PID) is a general term used to refer to any infection of the upper reproductive tract (above the cervix). More precise terms such as endometritis, endoparametritis, salpingitis, oophoritis, and pelvic peritonitis should be used to indicate specific areas of involvement. Common causes of PID include *Gonococcus*, *Staphylococcus*, *Streptococcus*, and *Chlamydia trachomatis* organisms. It often occurs following delivery or abortion or in women using intrauterine devices (IUD) as a means of contraception.

Symptoms include the sudden onset of severe pelvic pain, chills and fever, nausea, vomiting, and a heavy, purulent vaginal discharge with foul odor. Vaginal bleeding may also be present.

One of the most important diagnostic tools in PID is a complete and thorough history. Specific information of most importance is history of previous reproductive tract infection, delivery, abortion, pelvic surgery, onset of pain, date of last menses, sexual history, and contraceptive means. Specific diagnostic tests include cultures of any discharge, CBC, and possibly ultrasound studies if pelvic abscess is suspected.

Medical regimen depends on the cause, acuteness, and extent of the infection. Hospitalization with bed rest and appropriate intravenous antibiotics may be indicated. Analgesics may be ordered for pain. Removal of an IUD is indicated when one is present. Surgical drainage is usually recommended for an abscess. The importance of follow-up care cannot be overemphasized. Untreated or inadequately treated PID may result in infertility and/or sterility.

Gonorrhea

Gonorrhea is the most frequent of all the sexually transmitted diseases (STD). It is caused by the gram-negative diplococcus, *Neisseria gonorrhoeae*. This organism thrives in the warm, moist environment of mucous membranes. It may spread rapidly during menstruation because of the favorable environment produced by the blood. It does not survive well outside the body and exhibits increasing resistance to penicillin. It is almost exclusively a sexually transmitted disease but it can be contracted by the infant during delivery or by persons who have skin breaks that contact the discharge. Occasionally, it may be found in the throat, eyes, or rectum. Gonorrheal infection does not produce lasting immunity.

Women who contract gonorrhea are frequently asymptomatic. When symptoms are present, they may include green or yellow vaginal discharge, dysuria, urinary frequency, pruritis, and red swollen vulva. Rectal discharge may be noted with rectal infection. Both Skene's glands and Bartholin's glands may be involved.

Conclusive diagnosis must be made on the basis of cultures since there are no serology tests for diagnosis. Culture media usually contain antibiotics to inhibit other bacterial growth and should be placed in an atmosphere of increased carbon dioxide. Bacterial growth should be apparent within 24 to 48 hours if gonorrheal organisms are present.

The treatment of choice continues to be penicillin. Sexual partners should be treated concurrently and intercourse should be avoided until repeat cultures indicate a cure.

Genital Herpes

Genital herpes is a highly contagious venereal condition caused by the herpes simplex type 2 virus. Following an attack with the virus, the sores heal and disappear. The virus then remains dormant in the nerve cells and sores appear whenever the virus is triggered to multiply. Factors known to trigger outbreak of symptoms include colds, fever, severe sunburn, menstruation, gastrointestional upset, and stress.

The first attack of genital herpes is usually the worst and is characterized by small, extremely painful blisters. Prior to the appearance of blisters, the individual may notice a tingling or burning sensation possibly followed by intense itching. Secondary infection may occur when the blisters rupture. The initial infection may be accompanied by fever, swelling, and enlarged, painful lymph nodes. Fever and enlarged lymph nodes are less likely to occur with subsequent attacks.

There is no known cure at this time for herpes. A number of agents have been used with varying success. These include iodine solutions, chloroform, immunotherapy, BCG vaccine, nitrous oxide, ether, and photoinactivation with a light-sensitive dye and fluorescent light. A new drug, acyclovir (Zovirax) has recently been released by the FDA [4]. Alone it is inactive. When in contact with the virus it is converted to an active form by an enzyme, thymidine kinase, produced by the virus. It hastens healing, decreases transmissibility, but has no effect on recurrence.

Infection with herpes can be painful and annoying to the woman; however, it can represent a life-threatening situation to an unborn baby. It can produce abortion or premature delivery. Delivery of the baby through an infected vagina increases the chance that the infection will be passed to the baby. Herpes infection in a newborn can produce brain damage or death. Therefore, a cesarean birth is advisable.

Another primary concern for women with herpes virus is the increased risk of cervical cancer. It is now suspected that herpes may be a factor in the development of cervical cancer [6].

Syphilis

Syphilis, another of the sexually transmitted diseases, is caused by the spirochete, *Treponema pallidium*. Due to its size it is visible only with dark-field microscopy. It is sensitive to both drying and temperature and normally enters the skin through moist mucous membranes. However, it has also been known to enter the skin through breaks in the skin.

The course of untreated syphilis is divided into three stages: *primary syphilis*, *secondary syphilis*, and *tertiary syphilis* (see Chap. 46). Within 24 hours after the spirochete has entered the body, it spreads throughout. Within 3 weeks the first symptom, a chancre, appears at the site of entry. The chancre is usually a painless, hardened lesion that may resemble a pimple. It frequently goes undetected at this stage. Infection is highly contagious at this time and the chancre usually disappears within 2 to 6 weeks with or without treatment. At this point blood remains contagious.

The second stage, termed secondary syphilis, appears at variable times, up to 6 months later. It is characterized by fever, headaches, loss of appetite, sore mouth, loss of hair, and a nonitching body rash. The rash is noted especially on palms of hands and soles of feet. In the genital area *condylomata lata* (wartlike, flattened areas) may form, which are moist, broad-based, and swarming with spirochetes. Syphilis in this stage remains highly contagious and spirochetes may even cross the placenta to an unborn baby. Untreated, the characteristics of secondary syphilis will also disappear.

After a period of several years the condition progresses to tertiary syphilis and eventually is no longer contagious. About two-thirds of infected persons remain symptom-free; however, serology tests will remain positive and the spirochetes can affect an unborn baby if the woman becomes pregnant. For the other one-third of patients, the disease progresses and develops into late clinical syphilis. Gummas (benign nodular skin lesions) may develop. The spirochetes may attack the brain, liver, heart, or spinal cord and cause blindness, aneurysms, paralysis, insanity, and senility.

In the early stages diagnosis is made only by dark-field microscopy. After the antigen-antibody reaction has occurred, serology tests such as the VDRL, FTA-ABS (Fluorescent Treponemal Antibody-Absorption), TPI (*Treponema Pallidum* immobilization), TPHA (*Treponema Pallidum* hemoagglutinin assay), and RPR (rapid plasma reagin) can be utilized. The VDRL is the most widely used because of cost and simplicity. However, both false-positive and false-negatives are more likely to occur with this test. The next most favorable is the PTA-ABS test. Both the TPHA and RPR are used for screening large populations.

The treatment of choice for syphilis is penicillin. It must be given in doses appropriate to the stage of syphilis. In persons with known drug sensitivity to penicillin, the choice is tetracycline. Because of its teratogenic affect on unborn babies, tetracycline should not be administered to pregnant women. In these cases the treatment of choice becomes erythromycin. Treatment should be initiated at any point of diagnosis during pregnancy to prevent further damage to the baby.

BENIGN CONDITIONS OF THE FEMALE REPRODUCTIVE TRACT

Uterine Fibroids

Uterine fibroids, also referred to as *leiomyomas*, *myomas*, or *fibromyomas*, are second only to pregnancy as the most common cause of uterine enlargement. Twenty to fifty percent of women between the ages of 30 and 50 have some evidence of these growths. They are more commonly found in black women [7]. Actually, fibroids are masses of muscle and connective tissue that are stimulated by estrogen. Diagnosis is most often made on the basis of physical examination. However, ultrasound, x rays, and dilatation and curettage may aid in diagnosis differentiation.

The tumors occur singly or in groups. Size varies from the size of peas to that of an apple or cantaloupe. They are firm, smooth, and spherical in shape. Sectioning of a fibroid tumor reveals a pinkish-white, whorled, and lined muscle bundle.

Position in the uterine wall determines the type or classification of the tumors (Fig. 51-7). Intramural or interstitial tumors are found in central portions of the uterine wall. These are the most common. Submucosal tumors are located between the endometrium and uterine lining. Projection into the uterine cavity with subsequent distortion and enlargement of the endometrium may cause excessive menstrual bleeding and habitual abortion. Subserous tumors lie beneath the serous lining of the uterus and project outward into the abdominal cavity. Subserous tumors may also extend outward on a stalk, which is *pedunculated*.

Many fibroids are asymptomatic. However, as they enlarge the patient may experience excessive or prolonged bleeding during regular monthly cycles, urinary frequency, constipation, abdominal fullness, low abdominal pain, dysmenorrhea, and infertility. Abnormal bleeding usually occurs with submucous tumors because of the increased amount of endometrium to build and slough. Enlargement of tumors can produce pressure on the bladder, urethra, rectum, or nerves. Infertility or habitual abortion occur most frequently with submucous tumors because of distortion of the endometrium and uterine cavity. Enlarging fibroids have also been known to interfere with delivery of a full-term baby.

The course of treatment is determined by age, parity, symptoms, and condition of the individual. No treatment at all is needed for asymptomatic persons. Women approaching menopause are usually observed at regular intervals, since a withdrawal of estrogen results in a stationary or decreasing size of the fibroids. Hysterectomy may be indicated for the woman desiring no additional children or with bleeding problems.

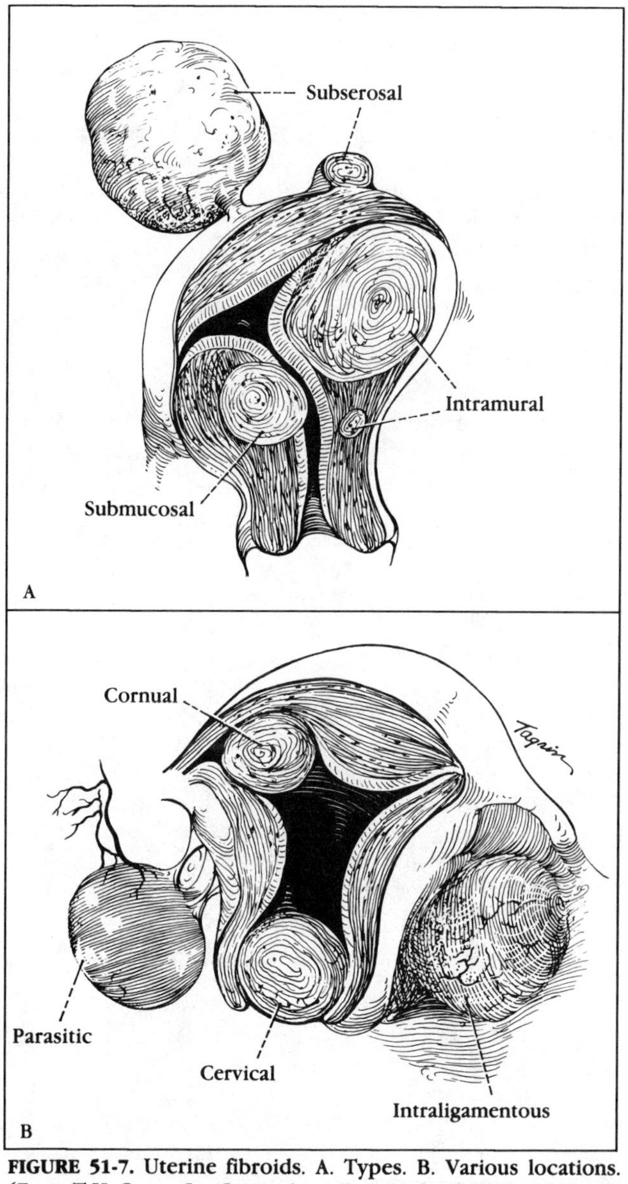

FIGURE 51-7. Uterine fibroids. A. Types. B. Various locations. (From T. H. Green, Jr., *Gynecology: Essentials of Clinical Practice* [3rd ed.]. Boston: Little, Brown, 1977.)

Functional Ovarian Cysts

Functional ovarian cysts are the result of normal ovarian function and account for more than 50 percent of ovarian enlargements. A functional follicular cyst results when a maturing follicle fails to rupture an ovum. Instead it continues to enlarge and produce estrogen. A corpus luteum cyst occurs when the corpus luteum fails to degenerate normally. It continues to grow and produce progesterone.

Ordinarily functional ovarian cysts produce no symptoms. They may be noted on periodic examination and usually are seen to disappear following the next menstrual cycle. Occasionally, when a functional cyst ruptures it tears an ovarian vessel. Intraperitoneal bleeding occurs and the extent of symptoms is related to the amount of hemorrhage. With excessive bleeding, abdominal pain may be severe in onset requiring hospitalization and surgery.

Benign Neoplastic Tumors of the Ovary

Occurring less often than functional cysts, benign neoplasms are more important. They may grow to be quite large and secrete hormones. Classification is by cellular origin: (1) germ cell, (2) germinal epithelium, (3) gonadal stroma, and (4) nonspecialized stroma. Three of the most common benign neoplasms are: (1) benign cystic teratomas or dermoid cysts, (2) benign serous cystadenomas, and (3) mucinous cystadenomas.

Dermoid cysts represent about 15 to 20 percent of all ovarian neoplasms and arise from germ cells. They are found most frequently in women 18 to 35 years of age. The tumor is gray, smooth, and contains tissue from all three germ layers, commonly skin, hair, and sebaceous glands.

Benign serous cystadenomas arise from germinal epithelium and with mucinous cystadenomas account for about 50 percent of benign ovarian neoplasms. Those most frequently affected are women between 40 and 50 years of age. Occurrence may be unilateral or bilateral. Tumors are pearly gray in color, lobulated, and filled with a clear, yellow fluid that becomes brown if there is bleeding in the cyst. *Psamma bodies*, which are small, calcified granules, may be found in the cell wall. Papillary serous cystadenomas may develop into malignancies.

Mucinous cystadenomas also arise from germinal epithelium and are usually unilateral. They are usually larger than serous cystadenomas, contain no psamma bodies, and contain a thick, straw-colored fluid.

Most ovarian tumors are asymptomatic and are noted on routine pelvic examination. Once they are enlarged enough to produce pressure, the woman may complain of pain on defecation, dyspareunia, heaviness, and sterility. Increased enlargement may result in abdominal distention, dyspnea, and anorexia. Menstrual irregularities, masculinization, and feminization may occur if hormones are produced. Complications include rupture, hemorrhage, possible infection, and torsion of pedicle cyst. The treatment of choice is surgical removal of the tumor since it will increase in size and may undergo malignant changes.

Benign Breast Alterations

The two most common benign breast alterations are: (1) fibrocystic disease, and (2) fibroadenoma. Fibrocystic disease is the most common of all female breast lesions affecting approximately 1 in 20 women. Characteristically the lesion becomes nodular from fibrous thickening. It may be tender, especially prior to menstruation, and exhibit cystic formation. Complaints of dull, heavy pain and a sense of fullness that increases prior to menstruation are characteristic. Aspiration may be utilized to aid in diagnosis. The exact cause is unknown but it is thought to result from abnormal or exaggerated response of the breast tissue to cyclic hormonal stimulation. It is a benign breast neoplasm consisting of proliferative ductal epithelium and fibrous stroma.

The second most common benign breast tumor is fibroadenoma. Physical examination reveals a well-outlined, solid, firm lump that moves freely. It occurs most often in younger women 15 to 40 years of age being the most common breast lesion in the adolescent female. The cause of this condition is unknown but estrogen stimulation is suspected since it occurs primarily in younger women and rarely after menopause. Treatment is surgical removal of the lump. Recurrence is common.

PREMALIGNANT AND MALIGNANT CONDITIONS

Trophoblastic Disease

The term *trophoblastic disease* is used to refer to three complications of uterine pregnancy: (1) hydatidiform mole, (2) chorioadenoma destruens, and (3) choriocarcinoma. Hydatidiform mole is usually benign with malignant potential, while choriocarcinoma is a highly aggressive malignancy.

HYDATIDIFORM MOLE. Hydatidiform mole represents a malformation of the placenta. It is characterized by absence of embryo development, conversion of the chorionic villi into marked vesicles with a clear, thick, sticky fluid, and production of human chorionic gonadotropin (HCG).

Clinical manifestations include (1) intermittent bleeding, (2) excessive increase in uterine size, (3) no evidence of fetal development, (4) spontaneous abortion, and (5) markedly elevated HCG levels. The patient may experience intermittent bleeding following amenorrhea. The passage of dark brown vaginal discharge may be accompanied by passage of watery discharge containing the characteristic vesicles. Even by the sixteenth to twentieth weeks, no fetal heart tones are noted, no fetal movement felt, and ultrasound reveals no fetal skeleton. HCG levels may be as much as 10 times higher than those associated with normal pregnancy [6]. Hyperemesis gravidarum, bilateral ovarian cysts, and toxemia of pregnancy prior to the twenty-fourth week have also been noted with hydatidiform mole.

Diagnostic tools include dilatation and curettage (D and C), histologic studies, HCG levels, and sonography. Histologic studies can be done on tissue passed spontaneously or from dilatation and curettage. Curettage scrapings usu-

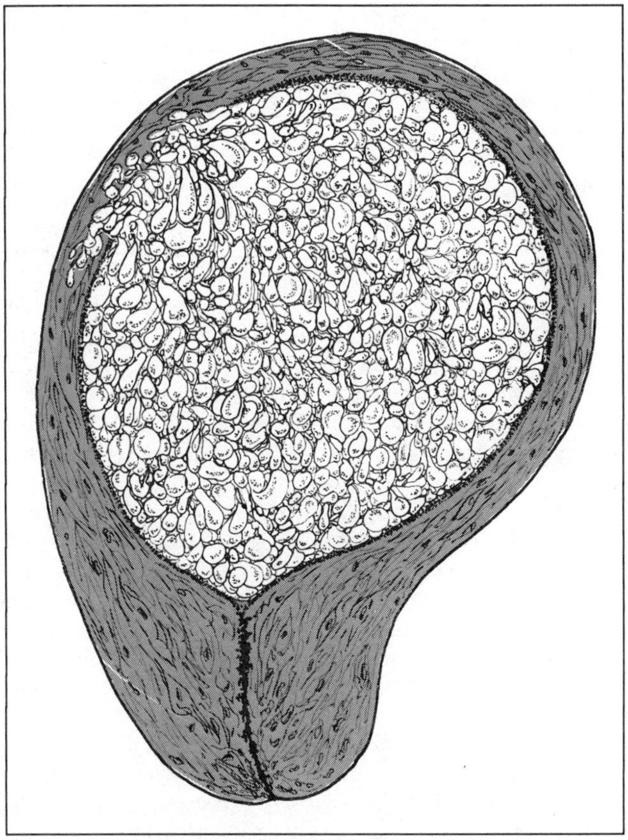

FIGURE 51-8. Hydatidiform mole. (From M.A. Miller and D. Brooten, *The Childbearing Family: A Nursing Perspective* [2nd ed.]. Boston: Little, Brown, 1983.)

ally include both superficial and deep tissue to determine any invasiveness. Sonography reveals a characteristic pattern of hydatidiform mole, which helps in differentiation (Fig. 51-8).

Treatment of choice is evacuation of the uterus as soon as possible after diagnosis. Possible means for evacuation of uterine contents include: (1) dilatation and curettage, (2) suction curettage, and (3) hysterectomy. Following this HCG levels are initially checked every week, gradually moving to every other week, and finally monthly for a 1-year period. Ordinarily, HCG levels return to normal within a week or so. If HCG levels are still elevated at 4 weeks, approximately 50 percent of the affected persons will develop choriocarcinoma unless chemotherapy is instituted. Occasionally, chemotherapy may be instituted as a prophylactic measure. Chemotherapeutic agents include the folic acid antagonists methotrexate and actinomycin D.

CHORIOADENOMA DESTRUENS. Chorioadenoma destruens is the term given to an invasive hydatidiform mole. It is characterized by the presence of chorionic villi deep within the myometrium. Penetration of the uterine wall with rupture and hemorrhage are possible.

Curettage may not be successful in removal of the lesion because of the depth of invasion. Chemotherapy with methotrexate or actinomycin D is usually initiated since response of the lesion is good. HCG levels are done regularly until normal levels are attained. Thereafter, they are done at monthly intervals for 1 year.

CHORIOCARCINOMA. Choriocarcinoma is a malignant tumor of the trophoblast occurring most frequently in the uterus. It is characterized by sheets of immature cells (cytotrophoblasts and syncytiotrophoblasts) that invade the uterine wall producing necrosis and hemorrhage. Chorionic villi are not present. Occasionally, choriocarcinoma may be found in the ovaries.

The only symptom noticed may be irregular bleeding or continual bleeding after a delivery or abortion. Frequently, the first symptoms noted are related to metastasis. Since the most common site of metastasis is the lung, hemoptysis may be the first complaint. Other metastatic sites include the vagina, brain, liver, and kidney. HCG levels remain markedly elevated.

Prior to the use of chemotherapeutic agents, the prognosis for a woman with choriocarcinoma was extremely grim, with death within 1 to 2 years. The *1982 Cancer Facts & Figures* lists choriocarcinoma among 14 cancers that today are being cured primarily because of chemotherapy [1]. Among the chemotherapeutic agents utilized are methotrexate, actinomycin D, chlorambucil, and vincristine. The response of lung metastasis is also very good while lesions in the brain and liver respond poorly. Prognosis continues to be directly related to amount of metastasis, duration of disease, and HCG titer.

Endometrial Carcinoma

Cancer of the endometrium may be increasing in incidence and is the third most frequent cancer in women [5]. It affects primarily postmenopausal women, with peak occurrence around 55 years of age.

Experimental evidence has been found to link endometrial cancer with ingestion of exogenous estrogens. Endogenous estrogen production unbalanced by progesterone may contribute to its incidence in early menopause. Additional factors that seem to increase the risk of endometrial cancer include obesity, diabetes, hypertension, and family history of uterine cancer. It is also more prevalent among white women in higher socioeconomic levels [7].

In many cases malignant changes are preceded by abnormal cell maturation. Adenomatous hyperplasia has been known to occur both spontaneously and as a result of estrogen drugs. If untreated, the process progresses to an in situ lesion in which the cells are larger and more disoriented. Nuclei may be found in varying locations with varying size and staining characteristics. About 85 percent of endometrial malignancy is adenocarcinoma. Cells may be well-differentiated as in in situ lesions or so undifferentiated that no glandular pattern is seen. The lesion represents a slow-growing tumor with late metastasis. Metastasis occurs first to the cervix and myometrium with later involvement of the vagina, pelvis, and lungs.

Staging or extension of lesion from the site of origin and grading of cellular differentiation of endometrial cancer is possible only after removal of the uterus and subsequent pathologic studies. Therefore, it is of little value in determining initial therapy. The grades of endometrial cancer are I through III with grade I representing well-differentiated cells and grade III undifferentiated. The Federation Internationale de Gynecologie et Obstetrique (FIGO) has adopted a staging system of five major stages:

- Stage 0: Carcinoma in situ
- Stage I: Tumor confined to the corpus uteri
- Stage II: Tumor involves both the corpus and cervix
- Stage III: Tumor extends outside the uterus, but not outside the true pelvis
- Stage IV: Tumor involves bladder, rectum, or extends outside the true pelvis

The first sign of endometrial cancer is abnormal uterine bleeding. It may range from light irregular bleeding with intermenstrual spotting to heavy prolonged periods when it occurs prior to menopause. Following menopause any bleeding should be suspicious. Another early sign may be marked leukorrhea. Both reflect erosion and ulceration of the endometrium. Later signs may include cramping, pelvic discomfort, lower abdominal or bladder pressure, bleeding after intercourse, or swollen lymph nodes.

The most important diagnostic tool is probably dilatation and curettage since it allows more comprehensive study. Routine Pap smears have limited usefulness unless metastasis has occurred. Both endometrial biopsy and washing may reveal abnormal endometrial tissue.

Stage 0 endometrial cancer is considered curable with hysterectomy. Stage I and II disease is treated with radiation and surgery. Chemotherapy is quite ineffective. Progesterone therapy may be utilized, especially in recurrent disease.

Cervical Cancer

The incidence of cancer in the cervix continues to decline from its position as second most frequent female cancer. It occurs more frequently in the 30- to 50-year-old woman. It has been found to occur most frequently in women (1) who began intercourse prior to the age of 20, (2) of low socioeconomic status, (3) who are black, (4) who receive DES during pregnancy, (5) who have had many sexual partners, and (6) who are multiparous. There also seems to be an emerging link with the sexually transmitted diseases, especially genital herpes infection. Chronic cervicitis and unrepaired cervical lacerations seem to predispose to malignancy [5].

Cancer of the cervix is most frequently of the squamous cell type and represents a sequential process of cellular proliferation. It usually begins in the transformation zone of the squamocolumnar junction as a basal cell hyperplasia. As the hyperplasia extends toward the surface it becomes known as dysplasia and refers to the disorderly cellular arrangement in the upper layers of the epithelium. The nuclei of these cells are enlarged and stain darkly. Some cells may even be multinucleated. The number of atypical cells determines the classification: (1) mild dysplasia, (2) moderate dysplasia, or (3) severe dysplasia. Spontaneous regression has been known to occur at this point.

The next stage in the sequential process is carcinoma in situ. This stage represents an involvement of the entire epithelial cell layer and is referred to as "intraepithelial neoplasm." The term *cervical intraepithelial neoplasia* (CIN) is currently being used to refer to all dysplasia and carcinoma in situ since the potential for progression and metastasis exists.

There are three forms of invasive cervical cancer: (1) fungating, (2) ulcerative, and (3) infiltrative. The fungating tumor is a nodular thickening of the epithelium, which may project above the mucosa. The ulcerative lesion represents a sloughing necrosis of the central portion of the tumor. Infiltrative invasion represents a downward growth into the stroma. As metastasis continues there is spread to the bladder, rectum, lymph nodes, and eventually the lungs, bones, and liver may be involved. The slow process of metastasis is believed to take as long as 10 years following the diagnosis of carcinoma in situ. However, in more rapidly growing lesions, invasion can occur in 3 to 4 years.

Since early cervical cancer is asymptomatic, early diagnosis and staging of the lesion is essential. Routine Pap smears have probably done more than any other diagnostic tool to detect early cervical cancer. Early CIN can also be detected by Pap smears. Colposcopy, cervical biopsy, and conization can be utilized to confirm the diagnosis.

Following is the FIGO recommendation for staging of cervical cancer:

- Stage 0: Carcinoma in situ
- Stage I: Carcinoma limited to the cervix
- Stage II: Carcinoma extends beyond the cervix and involves the upper two-thirds of the vagina
- Stage III: Carcinoma involves the lower one-third of the vagina and has become fixed to the pelvic wall
- Stage IV: Carcinoma involves the rectum, bladder, or extends beyond the true pelvis

Laser surgery, electrocautery, and cryosurgery are procedures aimed at removal of the lesion in early stage cancer. Total hysterectomy, radical hysterectomy, radiation therapy, or pelvic exenteration may be indicated as the extent of malignancy increases.

DES Exposure

The first synthetic estrogen was released in the early 1940s. It was used to prevent miscarriage, lactation following delivery, and as hormone therapy for dysfunctional uterine bleeding during postmenopause. In the late 1960s it became linked with adenocarcinoma of the vagina, vaginal adenosis, squamous cell carcinoma of the cervix and vagina, cervical dysplasia, as well as congenital abnormalities of both male and female offspring and impaired sperm production.

Cancer of the vagina is a very rare condition, most frequently seen in women over the age of 50. It usually is the squamous cell type, but adenocarcinoma has been identified in a number of adolescent girls whose mothers received DES during pregnancy.

Vaginal adenosis is a benign condition in which the transformation zone of the squamocolumnar junction extends over the vaginal portion of the cervix and may involve the vaginal walls. This condition is extremely common in DES daughters and may predispose them to adenocarcinoma. Question also arises as to the progression of adenosis to squamous cell cancer of the cervix and/or vagina.

Lowered fertility rates have been identified in both male and female offspring of DES mothers. Irregular or infrequent menstrual periods are seen in females. Low sperm counts, abnormally shaped sperm, and decreased ejaculate volume have been noted in males. Congenital anomalies in males include undescended as well as underdeveloped testicles, testicular cysts, and abnormal meatal openings.

The most important factor in treatment of DES problems is identification of those exposed and follow-up care every 6 to 12 months. Children of women known or suspected of DES exposure should have regular exams beginning at puberty. Routine exams should include Pap smears and colposcopy exam. Precancerous cell changes can be found early and appropriate therapy initiated.

Ovarian Cancer

Ovarian cancer is the most lethal of all pelvic cancer in women; it is the fourth most frequent cause of cancer death in women in the United States [1]. The reason for this is the advanced stage of the disease when diagnosis is made. It occurs most frequently in women around 50 years of age.

There is no diagnostic tool for early detection of ovarian cancer. If detected early it is by chance and on routine periodic exams. Any ovarian enlargement in the postmenopausal women and any ovary larger than 5 cm in diameter regardless of age should be suspected.

Ovarian cancer is difficult to diagnose from gross inspection until it invades the ovarian wall or seeds tumor cells in the peritoneal cavity. The epithelial form is usually cystic in nature, while the appearance is a solid form when it involves the stoma and connective tissue [5].

Initial treatment in any woman with ovarian cancer is surgical. Total hysterectomy with bilateral salpingo-oophorectomy and omentectomy is recommended. Supplementary therapy when indicated includes radiation and chemotherapy. Chemotherapeutic agents include the alkylating drugs such as Myleran, Leukeran, Cytoxan, and Alkeran.

Grading and staging systems are also utilized in ovarian cancer. Ovarian tumors are graded I through IV from well-differentiated to undifferentiated. One accepted staging classification follows:

- Stage I: Tumor limited to one or both ovaries
- Stage II: Tumor involves one or both ovaries with pelvic extension
- Stage III: Tumor growth with widespread intraperitoneal metastasis
- Stage IV: Tumor growth involves metastasis outside the peritoneal cavity

Breast Cancer

The most frequent site of cancer in the woman is in the breast. Breast cancer is also the leading cause of death from cancer in women. The cause of breast cancer is not known but three theories have been associated with it: (1) viral influence, (2) hormonal influence, and (3) genetic influence. It has been discovered that mouse mammary tumor virus (MMTV) can be transmitted through a mother's milk and produce cancer in suckling mice. The enzyme reverse transcriptase, found in oncogenic virus particles, has also been identified in human milk samples with viruslike particles. The hormonal influence receives some support from the risk factors associated with breast cancer: (1) early menarche and/or late menopause, (2) no children or children born after age 30, and (3) history of fibrocystic disease. All of these patients are exposed to long periods of ovarian function with high estrogen levels. Having a history

TABLE 51-2. Staging and TNM classification for breast malignancy

Stage 1	T_1	(tumor 2 cm or less)
	N_0	(no palpable axillary nodes)
	M_0	(no evident metastasis)
Stage 2	T_0	(no palpable tumor)
	T_1	(tumor 2 cm or less)
	T_2	(tumor less than 5 cm)
	N_1	(palpable axillary nodes with histologic evidence of breast malignancy)
	M_0	(no evidence of metastasis)
Stage 3	T_3	(tumor more than 5 cm; may be fixed to muscle or fascia)
	N_1 or N_2	(fixed nodes)
	M_0	(no evidence of metastasis)
Stage 4	T_4	(tumor any size with fixation to chest wall or skin; presence of edema, including peau d'orange; ulceration; skin nodules; inflammatory carcinoma)
	N_3	(supraclavicular or intraclavicular nodes or arm edema)
	M_1	(distant metastasis present or suspected)

Source: W. J. Phipps, B. C. Long, and N. F. Woods, *Medical Surgical Nursing* (2nd ed.). St. Louis: Mosby, 1983.

of breast cancer increases one's risk factor and also supports the theory of genetic influence.

Breast cancer is usually discovered by the woman. She notes a single lump, which is painless, nontender, and movable. It most frequently is found in the upper outer quadrant. The tumor may arise in either the ducts or lobules and may be either infiltrating or noninfiltrating. As the condition progresses the tumor becomes adherent to the pectoral muscles and fixed. Dimpling and retraction of the skin may develop. *Peau d'orange* skin may be noted with dimpling that resembles the skin of an orange in the area of tumor involvement. Metastatic sites include lymph nodes, lungs, bones, adrenals, brain, ovaries, and liver.

In addition to breast self-examination, mammography, thermography, and ultrasound may be utilized for diagnosis. Mammography is a major diagnostic tool, since it allows detection of breast masses before they are palpable. Breast biopsy allows confirmation of diagnosis.

The treatment for breast cancer is highly individualized. Surgical procedures ranging from lumpectomy to radical mastectomy may be employed depending on the individual situation. Supplementary therapy includes radiation, endocrine therapy, and chemotherapy. A grading system for breast cancer is important in comparing the effectiveness of various treatments. Table 51-2 provides a summary of the widespread grading system.

REFERENCES

1. American Cancer Society. *Cancer Facts & Figures*. New York: American Cancer Society, 1982. P. 5.
2. Centers for Disease Control. Follow-up on Toxic-Shock syndrome. *Morbidity and Mortality Weekly Report* 29:441, 1980.
3. Gold, M. Toxic shock. *Science* 80:8, 1980.
4. Nurses' Drug Alert. Acyclovir for genital and other herpesvirus infections. *Am. J. Nurs.* 82:1124, 1982.
5. Parsons, L., and Sommers, S. C. *Gynecology* (2nd ed.). Philadelphia: Saunders, 1978.
6. Robbins, S. L., and Cotran, R. *Pathologic Basis of Disease* (2nd ed.). Philadelphia: Saunders, 1979.
7. Stewart, F. N., et al. *My Body, My Health: The Concerned Woman's Guide to Gynecology*. New York: Wiley, 1979. P. 356.
8. Todd, J. Toxic-shock syndrome associated with phage-group I *Staphylococci. Lancet* 2:1116, 1978.

CHAPTER 52
GENETIC DISORDERS

LEARNING OBJECTIVES

1. List the three broad types of genetic disorders.
2. Briefly discuss the chromosome set (karyotype) of human species.
3. Differentiate between the terms *homozygous* and *heterozygous*.
4. Define *allele, genotype,* and *phenotype*.
5. Draw a Punnett square to compute the progeny of specific genotypes.
6. Briefly describe autosomal dominant inheritance patterns.
7. Briefly describe autosomal recessive inheritance patterns.
8. Briefly describe X-linked dominant inheritance patterns.
9. Briefly describe X-linked recessive inheritance patterns.
10. Explain the three types of chromosomal aberrations.
11. Compare the inheritance pattern of multifactorial disorders with the inheritance pattern of single-gene disorders and chromosomal disorders.
12. Identify at least one disease or disorder that is determined by each type of inheritance pattern.

Genes control the functions of the cell by determining what substances are synthesized within the cell. The genes also control the transmission of characteristics from parents to children. This chapter describes the principles of heredity, the classification of genetic disorders, and the fundamental role of the gene in inheritance patterns. The effect of alterations in the genes and chromosomes has resulted in a vast array of genetic diseases, and apparently all diseases are a product of or are affected by the genotype [6].

Gregor Mendel, an Austrian monk, is credited with discovering the basic principles of heredity. Mendel's laws were derived from his experiments with garden peas in which he crossed varieties with distinct characteristics and followed the *progeny* (offspring) of the crosses for at least two generations. Nearly 40 years later, in 1900, three workers (de Vries in Holland, Correns in Germany, and Tscheronak in Austria) rediscovered Mendel's findings. The field of genetics has since developed from the reports of the rediscovery of his laws.

PRINCIPLES OF INHERITANCE

As reported by Mendel, the principles of inheritance describe gene activity during gametic formation and fertilization. Referred to as Mendel's laws, these principles are essential to the study of heritable disorders. The principle of segregation describes the separation of *alleles* during gamete formation and their recombination during fertilization. The principle of dominance explains the expression of a trait that is manifested in a person when the gene is present on only one chromosome. The principle of independent assortment describes the random distribution of alleles in gamete formation.

CLASSIFICATION OF GENETIC DISORDERS

Generally genetic disorders are classified into three broad types: (1) single-gene disorders, (2) chromosome disorders, and (3) multifactorial disorders. Analysis of the genetics of any disorder first requires its categorization into one of these types. Table 52-1 shows examples of a wide variety of conditions that can be caused by genetic abnormalities.

Single-gene disorders are those disorders that are known to be due to a single mutant gene. The mutation may be present on both chromosomes of a pair or on only one chromosome of a pair. In the latter case the matching gene on the partner chromosome is a normal gene. Single-gene disorders are easily recognized as hereditary as they usually exhibit obvious and characteristic *pedigree* patterns, a characteristic distribution pattern of a specific trait in a family. Although the upper limits of frequency of these disorders is about 1 in 2000, most such disorders are rare [9].

Chromosome disorders are those disorders in which the defect is due to an excess or deficiency of the chromosome or segments of the chromosome. Unlike single-gene disorders caused by a mutant gene, chromosomal disorders can exhibit normal genes on the extra chromosome. One such example is Down's syndrome which results from an extra chromosome 21. Chromosome disorders affect about seven babies per thousand births and account for about one-half of all spontaneous first-trimester abortions [3].

TABLE 52-1. Common examples of genetic disorders

Disorder	Classification	Genetics
Huntington's chorea	Single-gene disorder	Autosomal dominant
Cystic fibrosis	Single-gene disorder	Autosomal recessive
Hypophosphatemia (vitamin D–resistant rickets)	Single-gene disorder	X-linked dominant
Hemophilia	Single-gene disorder	X-linked recessive
Down's syndrome	Chromosome disorder	Trisomy 21
Turner's syndrome	Chromosome disorder	45, X
Cleft lip/palate	Multifactorial	?

Multifactorial disorders as with chromosome disorders are not due to a single-gene mutation but instead result from a combination of small variations in genes that, when combined with environmental factors, produce serious defects. Although they do not show the distinct pedigree patterns of single-gene disorders, multifactorial disorders tend to cluster in families. It is estimated that as many as 10 percent of the population is affected by these disorders [7].

PATTERNS OF TRANSMISSION OF SINGLE-GENE TRAITS

The gene concept or gene theory explains how hereditary material is transferred and maintains its identity from one generation to another. All the information required to direct the formation and the function of any organism, including humans, is contained by threadlike structures of protein in cells called chromosomes.

The *karyotype* (characteristic chromosome constitution) of each species defines the species chromosome number and morphology. In humans the cell most commonly used for study of chromosomes is the small lymphocyte of peripheral blood. After the lymphocytes are grown in a nutrient medium, colchicine is added to stop cell division in metaphase. Application of a hypotonic solution causes the cells to swell, separating the chromosomes from each other. They are placed on a glass slide and stained. Following this process the chromosomes are photographed, cut out, and arranged into seven groups according to the length of the chromosome and the position of the centromere. A normal male karyotype is shown in Figure 52-1. Normal human somatic cells contain 23 pairs

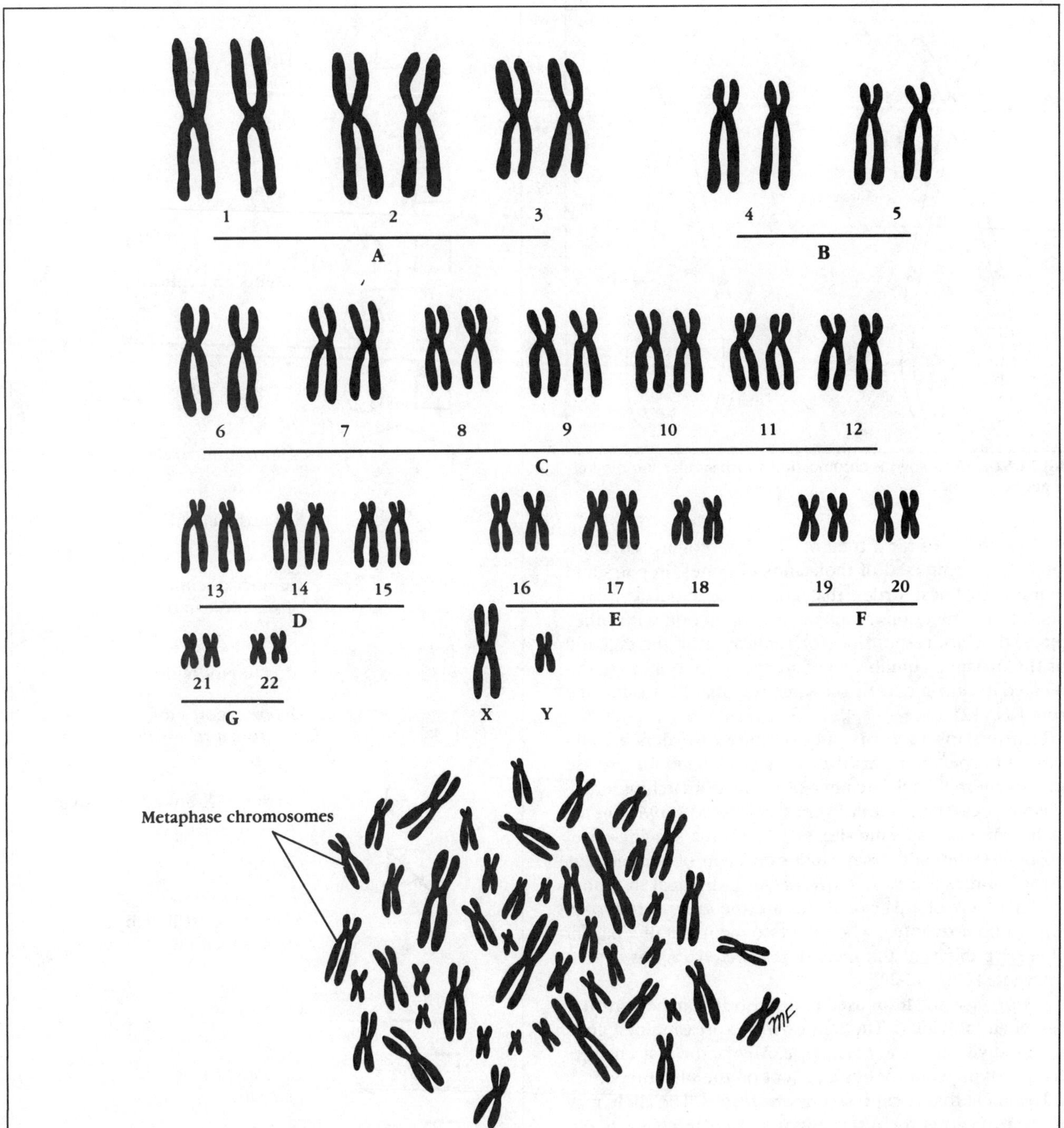

FIGURE 52-1. Structure of chromosomes in a human male karyotype. Note the seven groups of chromosomes that are grouped according to size and shape. (From R. S. Snell, *Clinical Histology for Medical Students*. Boston: Little, Brown, 1984.)

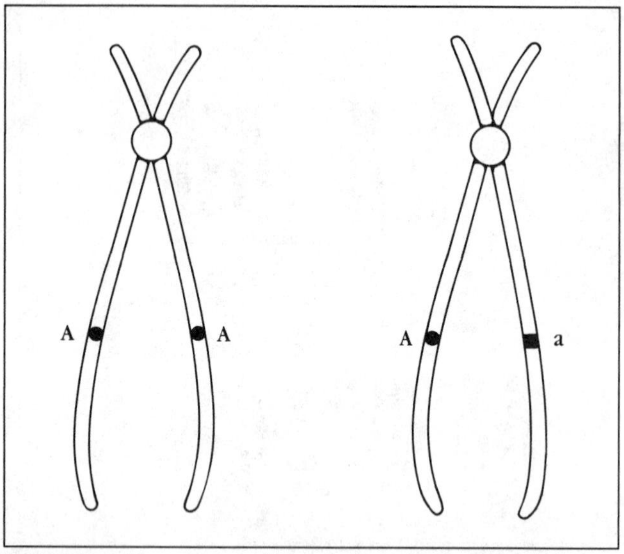

FIGURE 52-2. Homologous chromosomes with similar and dissimilar genes.

of chromosomes for a total of 46. Homologous chromosomes are composed of thousands of genes, in pairs and arranged in linear order, that control or regulate a specific cellular function. Alone or in conjunction with other genes, they are responsible for replication of the cell and for the dynamic equilibrium of an organism. Genes are duplicated in almost exactly the same way that RNA is formed from DNA [2].

Transmission patterns in hereditary disorders are described in specific terms that must be defined for precise understanding. Each member of a pair of matching chromosomes carrying similar genes is labeled *homologous*. Each gene has a specific site, or *locus*, on a specific chromosome. Genes at the same locus on a pair of homologous chromosomes are called *alleles*. An individual in whom two members of a pair of alleles are the same is *homozygous* (a homozygote); when the two members of a pair of alleles are different the individual is *heterozygous* (a heterozygote) (Fig. 52-2).

Genotype is the term used to describe the gene constitution of an individual. The trait or the expression of a gene in an individual is the *phenotype*. Any factor that changes the genotype will produce an effect on the phenotype.

The allele that is expressed is *dominant*. The allele may be homozygous or heterozygous. An allele that is expressed only when it is homozygous is *recessive*. Although the terms dominant gene and recessive gene are commonly used, it is the trait (phenotype) rather than the gene itself that is dominant or recessive. In genetic disorders, a *dominant disorder* is one in which the person who carries the gene (either heterozygous or homozygous) is clinically affected. To be clinically affected by a recessive disorder the individual must be homozygous for the gene. When only one gene is present (X-linked disorders) a recessive disorder will be expressed.

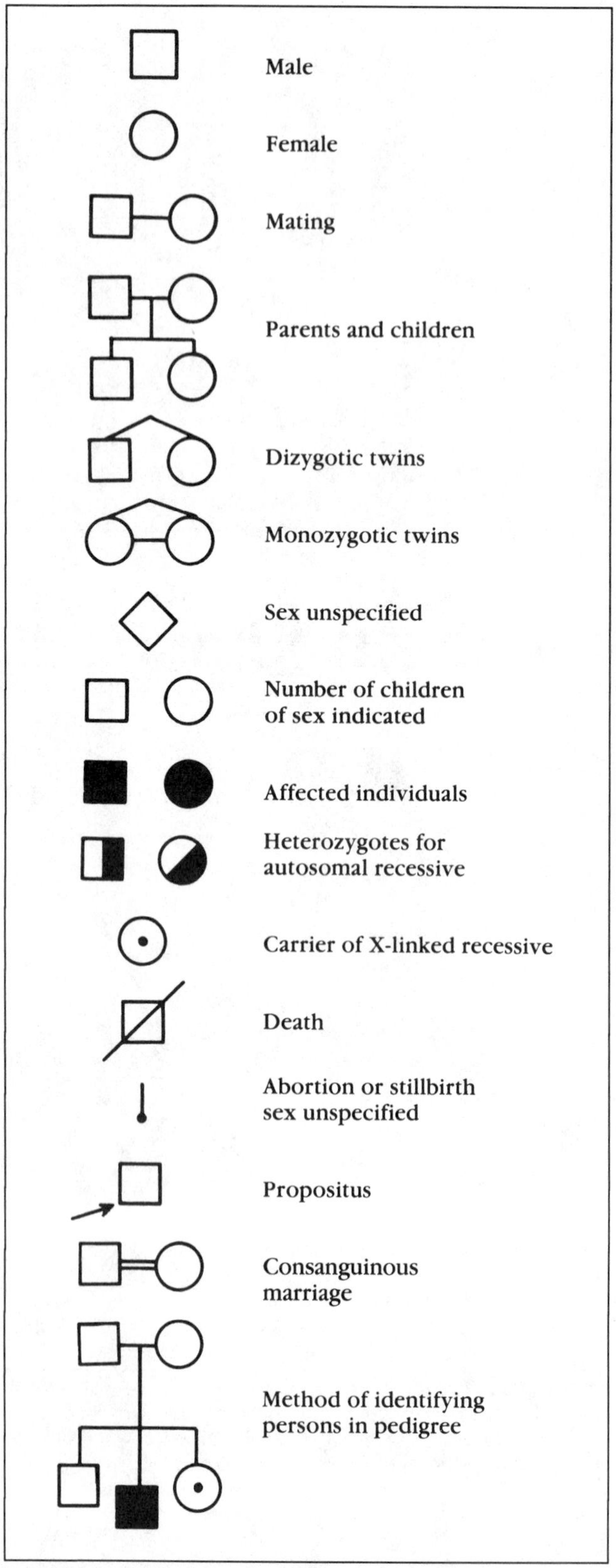

FIGURE 52-3. Symbols used in pedigree charts.

Single-gene phenotypes occur in fixed proportion. The pedigree patterns of such traits are dependent on whether the gene is located on an autosomal chromosome or on the sex (X) chromosome and whether it is dominant or recessive. These factors allow four basic patterns of inheritance for single-gene traits. These patterns are (1) autosomal dominant, (2) autosomal recessive, (3) X-linked dominant, and (4) X-linked recessive.

These patterns of single-gene inheritance can be exhibited in a *pedigree chart*, which is a schematic method for classifying data. Some symbols used in constructing a pedigree chart are shown in Fig. 52-3. Gene symbols are always expressed in italics. Usually a capital letter is used to signify a dominant gene and the lower case of the same letter is used to signify the corresponding recessive allele. In this method a genotype may be shown as *TT* or *Tt*.

An example of a phenotype determined by a single pair of autosomal alleles is the ability to taste phenylthiourea (PTC). The bitter taste of the drug is detected by persons with the dominant gene but cannot be detected by persons homozygous for the recessive allele. Therefore, the genotype *TT* (homozygous dominant) and *Tt* (heterozygous dominant) would be able to taste the drug and be classified as phenotypes, taster. The genotype *tt* (homozygous recessive) would not be able to taste the drug and would be classified as phenotype, nontaster.

Figure 52-4 illustrates the use of a Punnett square to compute the progeny of a heterozygous (*Tt*) male and female. Mendel's laws of dominance, segregation, and independent assortment are utilized for this computation. As shown in each offspring there is a 25 percent risk of being a dominant homozygote (*TT*) and a 50 percent risk of being a heterozygote (*Tt*). Both of these genotypes produce the phenotype taster. There is a 25 percent risk of being a recessive homozygote (*tt*) and the phenotype nontaster.

Figure 52-5 illustrates all possible mating types involving a single pair of autosomal alleles. Using the same trait of PTC taster, for an example, there are three possible genotypes for each male and female and there are six mating types. The mating type *Tt x tt* is the usual pattern of inheritance for an autosomal dominant trait and the mating type *Tt x Tt* is the usual pattern of inheritance for an autosomal recessive trait.

Sperm \ Ova	*T*	*t*
T	*TT*	*Tt*
t	*Tt*	*tt*

FIGURE 52-4. Progeny of *Tt* and *Tt* mating.

Genotypes	*TT*	*Tt*	*tt*
TT	*TT/TT*	*TT/Tt*	*Tt/Tt*
Tt	*TT/Tt*	*TT/Tt/tt*	*Tt/tt*
tt	*Tt/Tt*	*Tt/tt*	*tt/tt*

FIGURE 52-5. Mating types and expected progeny for a pair of autosomal alleles T and t.

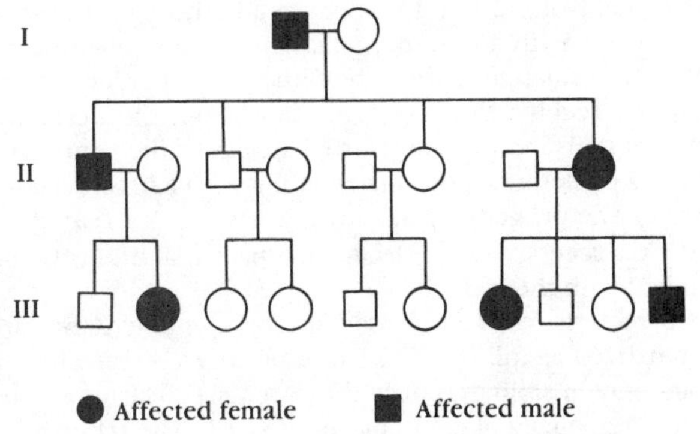

FIGURE 52-6. Stereotype pedigree of autosomal dominant inheritance.

Autosomal Dominant Inheritance

In autosomal dominant inheritance the abnormal allele is dominant and the normal allele is recessive. The phenotype is the same for both homozygous and heterozygous genotype persons having the particular allele. Although there are five patterns of inheritance involving autosomal dominant genes, as previously stated, the pattern of heterozygous (*Tt*) and homozygous (*tt*) is the most common. The stereotype pedigree of this pattern is shown in Figure 52-6. When either parent is heterozygous for the autosomal dominant allele (in this case the father) and the other parent is homozygous for the normal allele, each child has a 50 percent risk of receiving the dominant allele and thus being affected. Each child will receive a normal allele from the normal parent. Although one-half of the children may receive the dominant allele, the chances are independent in each zygote formation (principle of independent assortment), and the ratio of affected children may be different than 1 : 1. Since the allele is autosomal and not X-linked, either sex may be affected. All affected children will have an affected parent unless the disorder results from a fresh mutation.

Characteristics of an autosomal dominant inheritance are summarized as follows: (1) Affected persons have an affected parent. (2) Affected persons mating with normal persons have affected and unaffected offspring in equal proportion. (3) Unaffected children born to affected parents will have unaffected children. (4) Males and females are equally affected. (5) Traits can be identified on a pedigree chart except in instances of fresh mutations (most of these mutations in humans occur without known reason). Irradiation, from x rays, atomic energy, radium, or from the atmosphere, is known to cause mutations in genes [4].

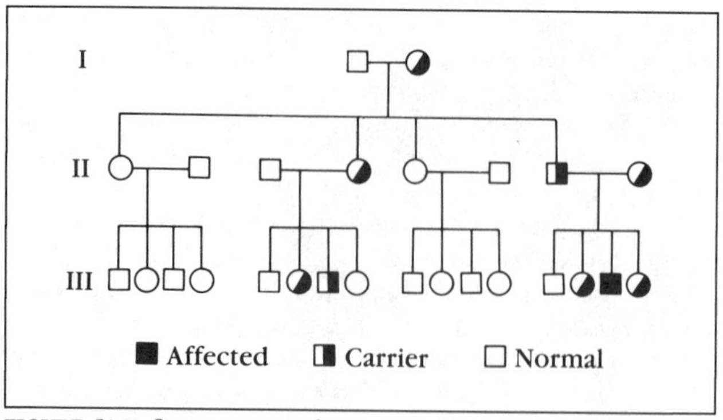

FIGURE 52-7. Stereotype pedigree of autosomal recessive inheritance.

Autosomal Recessive Inheritance

In autosomal recessive disorders the abnormal allele is recessive. In order for the trait to be expressed in a person he/she must be homozygous for the abnormal allele. As the dominant or normal allele masks the trait, most persons who are heterozygous for an autosomal recessive allele go undetected. Only when two heterozygous individuals mate (the most common pattern in autosomal recessive inheritance) and the offspring receives the recessive allele from each parent is the trait expressed. *Consanguinous* marriages (of persons who are blood relatives) may increase this probability.

When a heterozygous person mates with a homozygous normal person each offspring receives a normal allele from the normal parent and cannot express the trait. Figure 52-7 illustrates a stereotype pedigree of autosomal recessive inheritance. Note in line I that when a homozygous normal male mates with a heterozygous female each offspring receives a normal gene from the father. Fifty percent of the offspring receive the recessive allele from the heterozygous mother and are, therefore, carriers of the gene. Line III shows a heterozygous male mating with a heterozygous female. The progeny of this mating have a 1 : 4 risk of receiving a recessive allele from each parent and thus being affected with the trait.

Characteristics of an autosomal recessive inheritance are summarized as follows: (1) The trait characteristically appears only in siblings, not in the parents. (2) Males and females are equally likely to be affected. (3) The recurrence risk is one in four for every birth. (4) Both parents are heterozygous or carriers of the recessive allele. (5) The parents of the affected child may be consanguinous.

X-Linked Inheritance

Of the 23 pairs of chromosomes that determine the karyotype of the human, 22 pairs are autosomes and one pair is the sex chromosomes. Unlike the 44 autosomes that can be arranged in 22 homologous pairs, the two sex chromosomes are of unequal size. The X chromosome is a large submetacentric chromosome while the Y chromosome is a small acrocentric chromosome. Designations are based on the position of the centromere of the chromosome. Note in Figure 52-1 the large chromosomes in groups 1 to 3 (*A*) have approximately median centromeres (metacentric chromosomes). Chromosomes in groups 4 and 5 (*B*) have submedian centromeres (submetacentric chromosomes). The two sex chromosomes in the female are XX and in the male are XY. In fertilization of the ovum if the sperm contributes an X chromosome the product will be a female (XX), and if the sperm contributes a Y chromosome the product will be a male (XY).

Transmission of genes on the sex chromosomes follows the same principles of heredity as on the autosomes. The difference in the patterns of inheritance results from morphologic and gene complement differences in the sex chromosomes. The X chromosome carries many genes that are not matched on the Y chromosome. To date, no known medically significant genes located on the Y chromosome have been identified. It seems that its major importance is sex determination. Therefore, for practical purposes the genes located on the X chromosomes are the genes involved in sex-linked inheritance; thus, they will be discussed as X-linked inheritance.

Females (XX) can be homozygous for genes located on the X chromosome, whereas males (XY) have only one X chromosome. Genes located on the male's one X chromosome (hemizygous) have no counterparts on the Y chromosome. Because the Y chromosome is smaller than the X chromosome and is not homologous to it, traits determined by X-linked genes are expressed in the male. Simply stated, the genes on the X chromosome of the male are expressed because they are not matched by corresponding genes on the Y chromosome. These genes on the X chromosome cannot be transmitted from father to son as fathers contribute a Y chromosome to sons, but are transmitted to all daughters through the one X chromosome. However, recessive mutant genes on the X chromosome of a female may not be expressed because they are matched by normal genes in the other X chromosome. A gene that is X-linked may be indicated as X_H to represent a dominant gene and X_h to represent its recessive allele.

X-LINKED DOMINANT INHERITANCE. Genetic disorders caused by X-linked dominant genes are rare. The main characteris-

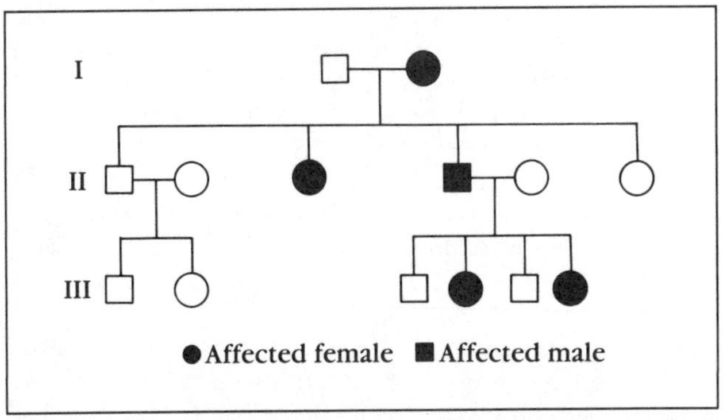

FIGURE 52-8. Stereotype pedigree of X-linked dominant inheritance.

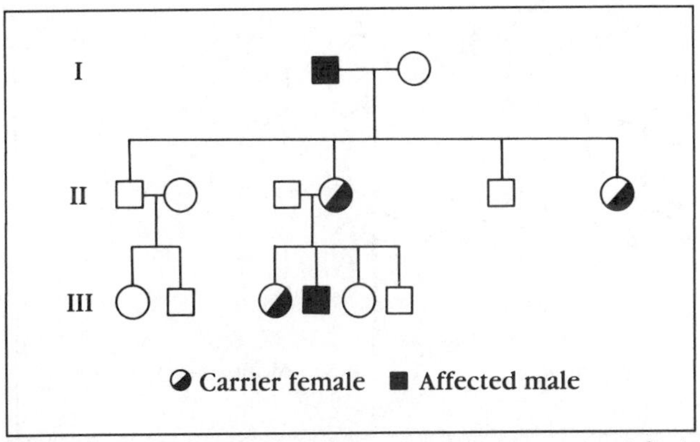

FIGURE 52-9. Stereotype pedigree of X-linked recessive inheritance.

tic of this inheritance pattern is that an affected male transmits the gene to all his daughters and to none of his sons. The affected female may transmit the gene to offspring of either sex (Fig. 52-8).

Characteristics of X-linked dominant inheritance are summarized as follows: (1) Affected males have normal sons and affected daughters. (2) Affected females (heterozygous) have a 50 percent risk of transmitting the abnormal gene to each daughter or son. (3) The disorder tends to be more severe in males (hemizygous) than in females (heterozygous).

X-LINKED RECESSIVE INHERITANCE. Several genetic disorders associated with a recessive gene on the X chromosome have been identified. Again, the inheritance pattern of these disorders results from the morphologic difference in the X and Y chromosome. Remember that the Y chromosome is structurally different from the X chromosome and is not homologous in regard to gene complement. The recessive gene located on the one X chromosome of the male is not repressed by a dominant allele on the Y chromosome and is thus expressed. The recessive gene is expressed in the female only if she is homozygous ($X_b X_b$). Therefore, X-linked recessive disorders are practically restricted to males and are rarely seen in females. Only the mating between an affected male and a carrier female can result in an affected female.

Males affected with an X-linked recessive disorder as with an X-linked dominant disorder cannot transmit the gene to sons, but will transmit it to all daughters. An unaffected female who is heterozygous for the recessive gene will transmit it to 50 percent of her sons and daughters. Figure 52-9 gives a stereotype pedigree of X-linked recessive inheritance.

Characteristics of X-linked recessive inheritance are summarized as follows: (1) Males are predominantly affected. (2) Affected males cannot transmit the gene to sons but transmits the gene to all daughters. (3) Female carriers have a 50 percent risk of affected sons and a 50 percent risk of carrier daughters.

CHROMOSOMAL DISORDERS

Chromosomal aberrations (deviations from normal) may be either numerical or structural and may affect either autosomes or sex chromosomes. Rarely are both simultaneously affected. Chromosome aberrations where there are two or more cell lines with different chromosome numbers are called *mosaics*. In these situations one or more of the cell lines are abnormal.

Numerical Aberrations

Deviations or abnormalities in chromosome number are classified in terms of loss or gain of chromosome sets. As discussed earlier, the normal chromosome number in humans is 2N = 46 and N = 23. To compare abnormalities with the normal karyotype several terms must be defined.

Somatic cells with two sets of chromosomes are said to be *diploid* (double) or 2N; whereas gametes with a single set of 23 chromosomes are *haploid* (single) or N. An exact multiple of the haploid number is *euploid*. Euploid numbers may be 3N (*triploid*) or 4N (*tetraploid*). Chromosome numbers that are exact multiples of N but greater than 2N are said to be *polyploid*. *Aneuploid* is a chromosome complement that is abnormal in number but is not an exact multiple of N. Aneuploid may be *trisomic* (2N + 1 chromosome) or monosomic (2N − 1 chromosome). Any chromosome number that deviates from the characteristic N and 2N is *heteroploid*.

Disjunction is the normal separation and migration of chromosomes during cell division. Failure of the process or nondisjunction in a meiotic division, resulting in one daughter cell receiving both homologous chromosomes and the other receiving neither, is the primary cause of aneuploidy. If this deviation in normal process occurs during the first meiotic division, one-half of the gametes will contain 22 chromosomes and one-half will contain 24. Any gamete produced in this manner contains an abnormal chromosome and, if joined with a normal gamete, will produce either a monosomic (2N − 1) or trisomic (2N + 1)

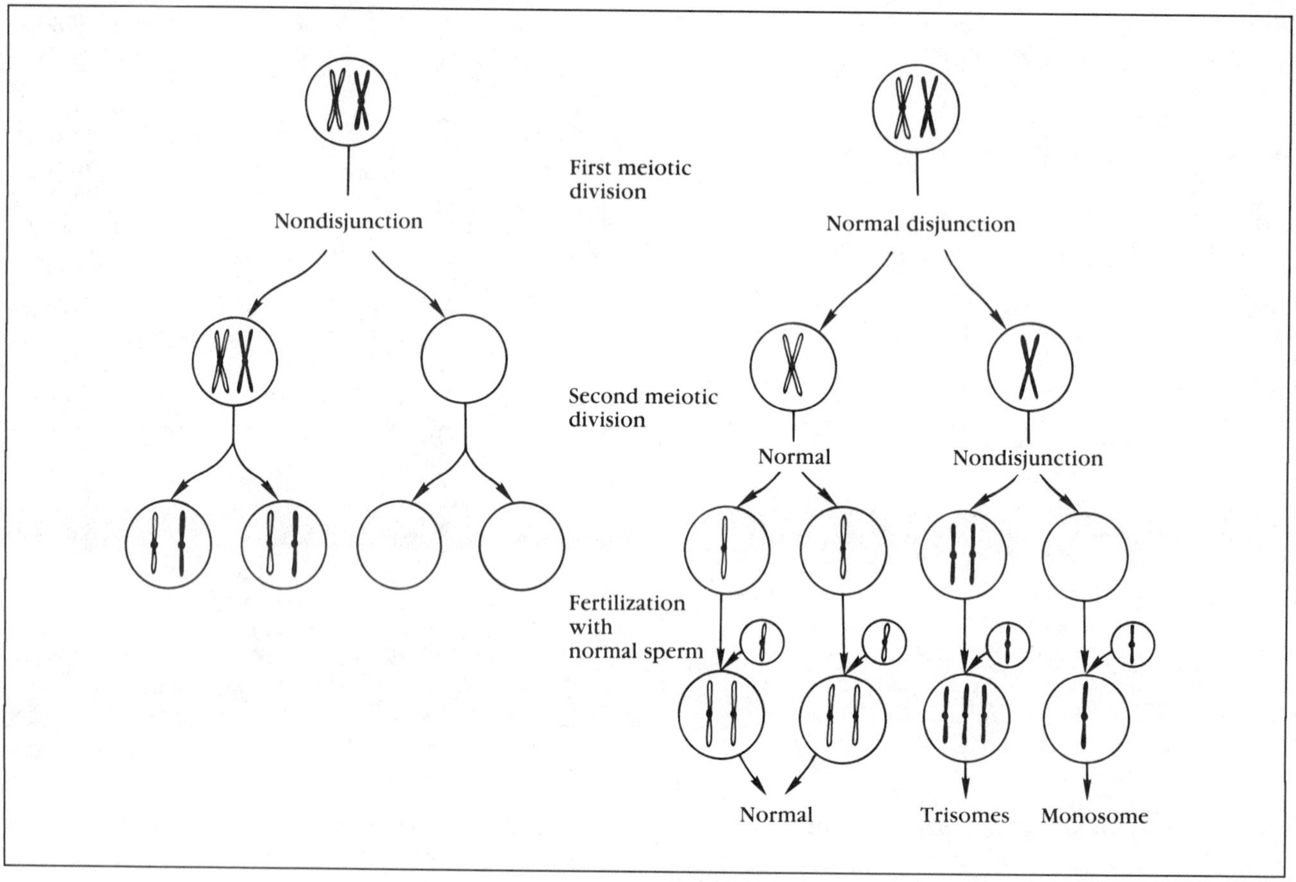

FIGURE 52-10. Process of nondisjunction at the first and second meiotic division of the ovum and fertilization with normal sperm.

cell. Normal disjunction and nondisjunction at the first and second meiotic division of the ovum are illustrated in part I and part II of Figure 52-10. Part III shows the union of normal sperm with gametes with varying chromosome complement. A common example of a disorder that results from an abnormality of chromosome number is trisomy 21 or Down's syndrome. This disorder can result when nondisjunction of chromosome 21 occurs at meiosis producing one gamete with an extra chromosome 21 (N + 1 = 24) and one gamete with no chromosome 21 (N − 1 = 22). Union of the 24 chromosome gamete with a normal sperm produces a 47 chromosome zygote, trisomy 21.

Structural Aberrations

Deviations in normal structure of chromosomes result from breakage and reassembly of the chromosome material in an abnormal arrangement. These changes in chromosome structure may be either stable (persist through future division) or unstable (fail to undergo cell division).

Stable types of structural abnormalities include:

1. Deletion, or loss of a portion of a chromosome. The missing segment may involve a terminal portion of the chromosome resulting from a single break or an interstitial section resulting from two breaks.
2. Duplication, presence of an extra piece of chromosome. A deleted segment of one chromosome becomes attached to another chromosome. The chromosome that lost the segment becomes a deletion.
3. Inversion—the linear arrangement of genes on a chromosome is broken and the order of the genes complement is reversed in the process of reattachment.
4. Translocation, transfer of part of one chromosome to a nonhomologous chromosome. In this process both chromosomes break and rejoin in an abnormal arrangement.
5. Formation of isochromosomes, division of the two arms of a chromosome rather than the two chromatids. This process results in metacentric chromosomes (the centromere is central).

Mosaics

Nondisjunction occurring in cell division other than gametogenesis results in two or more cell lines with different chromosome numbers. Persons with at least two cell lines with different karyotypes are labeled *mosaics*. Although several different mosaics have been described, most of the cases of different cell lines involve sex chromosome constitution.

Sex Chromosome Aberrations

In comparison to other hereditary disorders, sex chromosome aberrations are fairly common. Of the types found in males, the incidence is about 1 in 400 births, and of the types found in females about 1 in 650 births [8].

Most sex chromosome abnormalities are due to numerical aberration resulting from nondisjunction during meiosis. The disorders are described by the total number of chromosomes present. A normal male is 46 XY and a normal female is 46 XX. Any variation from these normals would constitute a disorder. The most common genotype with female phenotype is 45 X (Turner's syndrome) and with male phenotype is 47 XXY (Klinefelter's syndrome).

MULTIFACTORIAL INHERITANCE

Multifactorial inheritance includes the disorders in which a genetic susceptibility combined with the appropriate environmental agents interacts to produce a phenotype that is classified as disease.

Although the term *polygenic* is sometimes used to describe multifactorial disorders, it more accurately describes disorders determined by a large number of genes, each with a small effect, acting additively [1]. To date, there is no method of determining the exact effects of environmental factors on the contribution and/or the additive effects of genes in determining a trait in an individual [8]. For this reason multifactorial inheritance is more difficult to analyze than other types of inheritance. These traits tend to cluster in families but their genetic patterns are not clearly predictable as with single-gene traits and chromosome disorders.

A characteristic of multifactorial inheritance is a unimodal distribution of a trait in the population. Some normal characteristics are also distributed unimodally and have family patterns that are characteristic of multifactorial inheritance [8]. Two common traits are stature and intelligence. The correlation between relatives with such traits is proportional to their genes in common (inherited from a common ancestral source). The more distant the relationship, the fewer their genes in common [5].

The threshold model of multifactorial inheritance helps explain many of the features of the family distributions of many disorders. It is based on collecting information on the frequency of the malformation in the general population and in different categories of relatives. Through this method of analysis the empiric risk of the disorder can be estimated. Knowledge of the nature of the genetic and environmental factors in the pathogenesis of the disorder is not considered.

REFERENCES

1. Fraser, F.C. The multifactorial/threshold concept: Uses and misuses. *Teratology* 14:276, 1976.
2. Guyton, A.C. *Textbook of Medical Physiology* (6th ed.). Philadelphia: Saunders, 1981.
3. Hook, E.B., and Porter, I.H. *Population Cytogenetics: Studies in Humans*. New York: Academic, 1977.
4. McKusick, V.A. *Mendelian Inheritance in Man* (5th ed.). Baltimore: The Johns Hopkins Press, 1975.
5. Porter, I.H. *Heredity and Disease*. New York: McGraw-Hill, 1968.
6. Robbins, S., and Cotran, R. *Pathologic Basis of Disease* (2nd ed.). Philadelphia: Saunders, 1979.
7. Stern, C. *Principles of Human Genetics* (3rd ed.). San Francisco: Freeman, 1973.
8. Thompson, J.S. *Genetics in Medicine*. Philadelphia: Saunders, 1980.
9. Whaley, L.F. *Understanding Inherited Disorders*. St. Louis: Mosby, 1974.

BIBLIOGRAPHY

American Cancer Society. *Cancer Facts & Figures*. New York: American Cancer Society, 1982.

Anthony, C.P., and Thibodeau, G.A. *Textbook of Anatomy and Physiology* (10th ed.). St. Louis: Mosby, 1978.

Athey, P.A., and Hadlock, E.P. *Ultrasound in Obstetrics and Gynecology*. St. Louis: Mosby, 1981.

Auclair, C.A. Consequences of prenatal exposure to diethylstilbestrol. *J. Obstet. Gynecol. Neonat. Nurs.* 8:35, 1979.

Bettoli, E.J. Herpes: Facts and fallacies. *Am. J. Nurs.* 82:924, 1982.

Burke, S.R. *Human Anatomy and Physiology for the Health Sciences*. New York: Wiley, 1980.

Campbell, C.E., and Herten, R.J. VD to STD: Redefining venereal disease. *Am. J. Nurs.* 81:1629, 1981.

Clark, A.L., Affonso, D.D., and Harris, T.R. *Childbearing: A Nursing Perspective* (2nd ed.). Philadelphia: Davis, 1979.

Clithroe, H.J., and Pickles, V.R. The separation of the smooth muscle stimulants in menstrual fluid. *J. Physiol.* 156:225, 1961.

Conklin, M., et al. Should health teaching include self-examination of the testes? *Am. J. Nurs.* 78:2073, 1978.

Dixon, F.J., and Moore, R.A. Testicular tumors: Clinicopathological study. *Cancer* 6:427, 1953.

Downie, J., Poyser, N.L., and Wunderlich, M. Levels of prostaglandins in the human endometrium during the normal menstrual cycle. *J. Physiol.* 236:465, 1974.

Dwyer, J.M. *Human Reproduction: The Female System and the Neonate*. Philadelphia: Davis, 1976.

Edwards, M.S. Venereal herpes: A nursing overview. *J. Obstet. Gynecol. Neonat. Nurs.* 7:7, 1978.

Fischbach, F.T. *A Manual of Laboratory Diagnostic Tests*. Philadelphia: Lippincott, 1980.

Gorringe, R., Lee, M.M., and Voda, A. The mammography controversy: A case for breast self-examination. *J. Obstet. Gynecol. Neonat. Nurs.* 7:7, 1978.

Green, T.H., Jr., *Gynecology: Essentials of Clinical Practice* (3rd ed.). Boston: Little, Brown, 1977.

Guyton, A.C. *Textbook of Medical Physiology* (6th ed.). Philadelphia: Saunders, 1981.

Himmell, K. Genital herpes: The need for counseling. *J. Obstet. Gynecol. Neonat. Nurs.* 10:446, 1981.

Hoeft, R.T., and Jones, A.G. Treating metastasis with estramustine phosphate. *Am. J. Nurs.* 82:829, 1982.

Jones, A.G., and Hoeft, R.T. Cancer of the prostate. *Am. J. Nurs.* 82:826, 1982.

Kelly, T. *Clinical Genetics and Genetic Counseling*. Chicago: Year Book, 1980.

Kolodny, R.C., et al. *Textbook of Human Sexuality for Nurses*. Boston: Little, Brown, 1979.

Lilienfeld, A.M., Levin, M.L., and Kessler, I.I. *Cancer in the United States*. Cambridge, Mass.: Harvard University Press, 1972.

Luckmann, J., and Sorensen, K. C. *Medical-Surgical Nursing: A Psychophysiologic Approach* (2nd ed.). Philadelphia: Saunders, 1980.

Maier, J. G. An evaluation of lymphadenectomy in the treatment of malignant testicular germ cell neoplasms. *J. Urol.* 101:356, 1969.

Markett, C. L., and Urspring, H. *Developmental Genetics*. Englewood Cliffs, N.J.: Prentice-Hall, 1971.

Martin, L. L. *Health Care of Women*. Philadelphia: Lippincott, 1978.

Masters, W. H., and Johnson, V. E. *Human Sexual Response*. Boston: Little, Brown, 1966.

McKusick, V. A. *Human Genetics* (2nd ed.). Englewood Cliffs, N.J.: Prentice-Hall, 1969.

McKusick, V. A. *Mendelian Inheritance in Man: Catalogs of Autosomal Dominant, Autosomal Recessive, and X-Linked Phenotypes* (5th ed.). Baltimore: The Johns Hopkins Press, 1978.

Miller, M. A., and Brooten, D. A. *The Childbearing Family: A Nursing Perspective* (2nd ed.). Boston: Little, Brown, 1983.

Moody, P. A. *Genetics of Man* (2nd ed.). New York: Norton, 1975.

Morton, N. E. *Outline of Genetic Epidemiology*. New York: Karger, 1982.

Neil, E., and Keele, C. A. *Samson Wright's Applied Physiology* (12th ed.). New York: Oxford University Press, 1971.

Nora, J., and Fraser, F. *Medical Genetics: Principles and Practice* (2nd ed.). Philadelphia: Lea & Febiger, 1981.

Novitski, E. *Human Genetics*. New York: Macmillan, 1977.

Nurses' Drug Alert. Acyclovir for genital and other herpes virus infections. *Am. J. Nurs.* 82:1124, 1982.

Ohno, S. *Sex Chromosomes and Sex-Linked Genes*. New York: Springer-Verlag, 1967.

Pansky, B. *Dynamic Anatomy and Physiology*. New York: Macmillan, 1975.

Pardue, S. F. Hydatidiform mole: A pathological pregnancy. *Am. J. Nurs.* 77:836, 1977.

Parsons, L., and Sommers, S. C. *Gynecology* (2nd ed.). Philadelphia: Saunders, 1978.

Robbins, S. L., and Cotran, R. *Pathologic Basis of Disease* (2nd ed.). Philadelphia: Saunders, 1979.

Roberts, W. *The Reproductive System: Disease, Diagnosis, Treatment*. Bowie, Md.: Brady, 1973.

Romney, S. L., et al. *Gynecology and Obstetrics: The Health Care of Women*. New York: McGraw-Hill, 1975.

Schottelius, B. A., and Schottelius, D. D. *Textbook of Physiology*. St. Louis: Mosby, 1978.

Schuster, C. S., and Ashburn, S. S. *The Process of Human Development: A Holistic Approach*. Boston: Little, Brown, 1980.

Selkurt, E. E. (ed.). *Basic Physiology for the Health Sciences* (2nd ed.). Boston: Little, Brown, 1982.

Simpson, J. L. *Disorders of Sexual Differentiation: Etiology and Clinical Delineation*. New York: Academic, 1977.

Sloane, E. *Biology of Women*. New York: Wiley, 1980.

Smith, D. W. *Recognizable Patterns of Human Malformation* (2nd ed.). Philadelphia: Saunders, 1976.

Srivastava, P. K. *Basic Genetics for Health Professionals*. Littleton, Mass.: PSG, 1979.

Stewart, F. H., et al. *My Body, My Health: The Concerned Woman's Guide to Gynecology*. New York: Wiley, 1979.

Sutton, H. E. *An Introduction to Human Genetics* (2nd ed.). New York: Holt, Rinehart & Winston, 1975.

Thompson, H. E., and Bernstine, R. L. *Diagnostic Ultrasound in Clinical Obstetrics and Gynecology*. New York: Wiley, 1978.

Tobiason, S. J. Benign prostatic hypertrophy. *Am. J. Nurs.* 79:286, 1979.

Wallach, J. *Interpretation of Diagnostic Tests: A Handbook Synopsis of Laboratory Medicine* (3rd ed.). Boston: Little, Brown, 1978.

Watson, J. E. *Medical-Surgical Nursing and Related Physiology* (2nd ed.). Philadelphia: Saunders, 1979.

Whaley, L. F., and Wong, D. L. *Nursing Care of Infants and Children*. St. Louis: Mosby, 1979.

Widmann, F. K. *Clinical Interpretation of Laboratory Tests* (8th ed.). Philadelphia: Davis, 1979.

Willson, J. R., and Carrington, E. R. *Obstetrics and Gynecology* (6th ed.). St. Louis: Mosby, 1979.

Wroblewski, S. S. Toxic shock syndrome. *Am. J. Nurs.* 81:82, 1981.

Yen, S. S. C., and Jaffe, R. B. *Reproductive Endocrinology: Physiology, Pathophysiology and Clinical Management*. Philadelphia: Saunders, 1978.

Yunis, J. J. *Molecular Structure of Human Chromosomes*. New York: Academic, 1977.

Ziegel, E. E., and Cranley, M. S. *Obstetric Nursing* (7th ed.). New York: Macmillan, 1978.

UNIT 17
AGING

Metta Fay Street
ALTERATIONS THAT RESULT FROM AGING

Virginia Earles
AGING

Aging is not a disease process but is the result of yearly wear and tear on the systems of the body. It is associated with an increase in and perhaps inevitable association with disease, the development of which is highly individualized. Factors predisposing people to disease include such things as heredity, culture, race, and nutritional status. Chapter 53 presents some of the biologic theories of aging and a summary of biologic effects of aging on the body systems. The timetable of aging changes varies with individuals, but as age progresses the general changes are almost inevitably seen.

The discussion in this chapter organizes pathologic processes seen in the aged person. Each of these changes is discussed in greater depth in other units in the text. The reader is encouraged when studying the objectives to also refer to the other areas of the textbook that refer to the pathologic process under study.

CHAPTER 53
AGING

LEARNING OBJECTIVES

1. Discuss important research on the aging process, especially that done by Hayflick and Moorhead, and Verzar and associates.
2. Describe the biologic cellular theories: the free radical, the crosslink, the immunologic, and the genetic aging theories.
3. List the general effects of aging.
4. Describe the causes and effects of nervous system alterations.
5. Relate anatomic alterations in the cardiovascular system to the physiologic changes that result.
6. Describe how the arterial changes cause an alteration in blood flow and pressure.
7. Specifically, discuss causes and effects of hypertension in the elderly.
8. Describe the physiologic result of respiratory changes due to aging.
9. Explain why elderly persons are at risk for the development of respiratory failure following stressful situations.
10. Compare renal function at age 20 with that at age 65.
11. List common organisms that can cause cystitis in elderly men and women.
12. Describe the effects of lack of estrogen in postmenopausal women.
13. Describe the effects of hormone changes in elderly men.
14. Briefly discuss the multiple factors that cause digestive disturbances in the elderly.
15. Characterize the alterations in body movement that occur as a consequence of aging.
16. Explain the factors involved in increased risk of bone fractures.
17. List the joint changes that are commonly seen, at what age they begin, and when they become symptomatic.
18. Describe the characteristic changes in skin, nails, and hair.
19. Explain how sensory alterations affect adjustment in the aging process.
20. Discuss the factors causing alterations in drug metabolism.
21. List at least two cancers that are more common in the aged than in the younger population.

Research into the causes of aging has been going on for centuries, yet no researcher has been able to specifically identify any single causative factor. More questions are being asked and research has intensified as people live to an older age. What is aging? Why do we age and what can be done to prolong life? It is very difficult to define what aging is or to establish the facts about aging. One might think defining aging should be simple; yet there seems to be much confusion about it. Much of the confusion arises from the difficulty of distinguishing between normal aging and changes secondary to disease. Health and longevity are affected by a number of factors, such as heredity, culture, race, and nutrition. As we learn more about age-related changes in the body's ability to respond to stress, we will be able to refine strategies for the care of the aged.

From the time of conception life is a continuous process of change. The process of change is highly individualized and the rate and degree of aging varies widely. The inevitability of aging and death has been a source of mystery and concern over the ages. Science and medicine have focused on preventing and curing illness in the earlier stages of life, which has resulted in an increased life expectancy in the United States. Worldwide, however, longevity for human beings has not increased. The variability of life span for humans seems to be a function of genetic and environmental factors. Total life span seems to be limited to 90 to 105 years regardless of mitigating circumstances. This limitation supports the belief that aging is an innate process.

Medicine has long focused on diagnosis and cure-directed treatment. These objectives may prove difficult to attain in older persons. In the elderly, more often than not, multiple problems are present simultaneously. Degenerative changes and certain diseases worsen with age and can be superimposed one on the other. Important warning signs are frequently misinterpreted by an older person because of concomitant symptoms prior to illnesses. Two of these age-related changes are altered temperature response and pain perception. In the older person, elevation in temperature may not occur or may occur late in the presence of an acute infection. Pain, usually a motivation to seek medical assistance, may not be viewed in that context by the elderly. Many older persons look on pain as a burden of old age and not as an important indicator of problems.

Elderly persons are more prone to infections than are younger persons for several reasons. Alterations in the circulatory system result in a decreased blood supply, and insufficiencies in immune factors combine to increase the chance of infection. The production of antibodies that fight disease is depressed partially because their production is somewhat dependent on nutritional supply. Many elderly persons, particularly those living alone, do not have a nutritious diet and therefore do not have optimal nutritional reserves for antibody production. Also important in the lowered resistance of the elderly to infection are the degenerative changes occurring in the immune system with advancing years [23]. The elderly are susceptible to greater numbers of infectious diseases than younger persons and have a higher mortality as a result.

BIOLOGIC THEORIES OF AGING

Until the nineteenth century, most of the interest in the aging process focused on ways to prevent it. The ancient Egyptians tried to find the fountain of youth. Hippocrates (c.460–377 B.C.) perceived aging as stemming from a decrease in body heat, a natural, irreversible, and unavoidable phenomenon. Galen (c.130–201 A.D.) had a similar theory postulating that the increased coldness and dryness of aging resulted from changes in body humor.

Leonardo Da Vinci (1452–1519) stimulated later development of theories of biologic aging through his descriptions and drawings. He studied anatomy with passion throughout his life. He investigated all aspects of anatomy with scientific intention and his sketches were drawn to illustrate purely scientific matter. While in Florence, Italy, he lived in a hospital where he dissected more than 30 bodies of men and women of all ages. His illustrations were accompanied by descriptions done with minute detail [6]. From Da Vinci's time through the nineteenth century many theories on the aging process have developed.

One of the main problems encountered in researching theories is the fact that so much of the research is approached with the biases unique to the multiple disciplines, rather than an unbiased, interdisciplinary approach. Disciplines such as biology, sociology, and psychology have all arrived at different explanations for the changes that occur with the aging process. Some theories have been thoroughly researched and verified, whereas other theories do not enjoy the support of clinical testing or the acceptance of the medical community.

Despite multiple postulates, no one theory has gained general acceptance. The theories do, however, generate questions and spur further investigation. The major theories of the aging process establish a frame of reference for understanding various changes that occur with aging. Birren [2] states that humans age in three ways: biologically, psychologically, and sociologically. In the older adult, these three aspects of development are not as closely intermeshed as they are in the younger adult and in the formative years of life.

To better understand differences between theories of aging and certain processes that take place within the aging organism, it is necessary to examine some of the commonly occurring aging processes. These processes frequently form the basis for various theories of aging. Of importance to the aging research is the work of Hayflick and Moorhead [18] regarding the number of times cells replicate themselves. Their findings, which have since been confirmed by other researchers, have shown that the number of times normal diploid human fibroblasts can replicate themselves in vitro is limited. Hayflick reports that "the sum of population doublings undergone by normal fetal human fibroblasts both before and after preservation is always equal to 50 ±10" [18]. Cells isolated from older persons show progressively fewer doublings before finally stopping. The cultured human fibroblast has become a widely used object of research into the causes of aging as a result of Hayflick's studies.

Other researchers have found that the homeostatic mechanisms that govern immunity and cell replication decrease as a person grows older. It has been shown that as a person ages, both the cell division process and ribonucleic acid (RNA) synthesis of protein slow down. There is also an increasing heterogenicity of cells in terms of size, shape, and mitotic capabilities.

Also common in metabolism of the older person is the phenomenon of increasing collagen cross-linking, a process discovered in the early 1950s by Fritz Verzar and other researchers in Switzerland. Cross-linkages are stable molecules that prevent division of deoxyribonucleic acid (DNA) strands in the normal cell reproductive cycle. Cross-linkage molecules accumulate and affect proteins in elastin and collagen resulting in cell deaths. The cell deaths result in a decreased elasticity of blood vessels and skin [12].

This section describes the following biologic cellular theories: The free radical theory, the cross-link theory, the immunologic theory, and the genetic aging theory [9]. No one theory answers all the questions but each provides a clue to the aging process and certain interrelationships that do appear to exist.

The Free Radical Theory

Free radicals are parts of molecules that have broken off or molecules that have had an electron stripped from their structure. These broken pieces damage or alter the original structure or function of other molecules by attaching themselves to them. According to Krohn, oxygen is highly reactive, and oxidation of protein, fat, carbohydrate, and other elements in the body results in the formation of these free radicals [20]. Free radical end products and compounds are not useful, and some cause cellular disruption. In the aging process, free radical compounds appear to increase faster than the body cells can repair the damage. Some scientists consider the cell membrane as the key to survival and believe that the greatest damage could be perpetrated by free radicals at this level [9].

When DNA is irradiated, for example, it responds with free radical formation and establishes aberrant cellular development that affects aging. Vitamin E and coenzyme Q are thought to protect the mitochondria from the hazards of the free radical activity. Vitamin E may function as an antioxidant and binding agent in the antioxidation process, which leads to support for the use of antioxidants such as vitamin E in an attempt to delay cellular aging [27].

Free radical activity is also introduced into the body by such environmental factors as smog, by-products of the plastics industry, gasoline, and atmospheric ozone. The human body appears to be bombarded from both external and internal sources of free radicals. If this theory is as fundamental to aging as proponents believe, careful monitoring of the environment and proper food selection should lead to healthier aging.

The Immunologic Theory

The theory currently receiving the most attention, particularly in relation to its potential for therapy or prevention of aging, is the theory based on changing immunologic function. The immunologic theory asserts that aging is an autoimmune process. The body's immune system fails to recognize its own cells as the cells change with age. Autoimmune responses damage or destroy cells, leading to cell death [12]. Tissue damage and increased susceptibility to infection may be caused by the presence of autoantibodies and decreased numbers of immunocompetent cells (see Chap. 9). Whether the diminished capacity for immune responses is a cause of aging is not known, but it certainly is the source for many of the disease problems of the aged. These include an increased incidence of autoimmune disease, cancer, and infection of all types.

The immune system has multiple components that are altered in different ways during aging. Aging affects all parts of this system, but especially the T cells. A decline in T cell–dependent immune function begins at sexual maturity with the onset of involution of the thymus gland. This factor is associated with an increased incidence of diseases such as cancer and autoimmune diseases. The macrophages that play a major role in protecting the body against infection, do not seem to diminish in number as the body ages. The B cell number stays elevated but responsiveness to stimulation by antigens decreases markedly, probably because of dependence on T cell stimulation.

The involution of the thymus gland appears to be the key to the aging of the immune system. Whether it is caused by the changing hypothalmic regulation or factors intrinsic to the cells of the gland itself remains unknown.

The Cross-Link Theory

"The cross-link theory, sometimes called the collagen theory, suggests that strong chemical reactions create strong bonds between molecular structures that are normally separate. Cross-link agents are so numerous and varied in the diet and in the environment that they are impossible to avoid" [9]. Connective tissue changes are an indicator that cross-linkage has occurred. Collagen, which makes up a large part of the proteins of the body, is responsible for maintaining strength, support, and structural form. As a result of the chemical action of cross-linkage, aging collagens become more insoluble, chemically stable, and rigid, resulting in inhibition of cell permeability. Passage of nutrients, metabolites, antibodies, and gases through the blood vessel walls is inhibited. The linings of the lungs and gastrointestinal tract are also affected.

Elastin, another of the fibrillar proteins found in connective tissue, is very prone to cross-linkage. It differs from collagen on the basis of its chemical composition and physical properties. Both elastin and collagen respond to cross-linkage in the same manner. Aging elastin becomes frayed, fragmented, and brittle, leading to multiple changes in connective tissue throughout the body. A good example of this is skin changes with loss of skin turgor along with dryness, loss of elasticity and tone. Cross-linkage can also affect cell division because its molecules can prevent division of the strands of the DNA. If only one strand is affected, no damage results. However, if the cross-link molecule attaches itself to both sides of the DNA, the cell will die because division is prevented. The cell deaths have a profound effect on the elasticity of blood vessels and skin. As a result of the changes in collagen and elastin, cross-linkage is thought to be a primary cause of aging.

The Genetic Aging Theory

The genetic aging theory is based on the belief that the life span is programmed before birth into the genes in the DNA molecule. This means that a person fortunate enough to have long-lived parents or grandparents will have a life expectancy longer than it would have been with short-lived parents. Gender also makes a difference in predicting longevity, since built-in genetic material seems to favor the female. In all countries of the world women live longer than men by approximately 6 years. Race is also a factor in predicting longevity. Whites of both sexes have a longer life expectancy than blacks [30].

BIOLOGIC EFFECTS OF AGING ON BODY SYSTEMS

Many physical and chemical changes that occur as a person ages have been identified through research even though the exact causes of aging cannot be isolated. Some of the changes are harmful in that they interfere with the healthy function of cells and tissues. Other changes have not been found to be harmful. Research will continue into the aging process and the identification of causes of harmful effects of aging will lead to findings that can delay or decrease these effects.

In aging there is a gradual diminution in the functional capacity of the organ systems. It must be realized, however, that the aging process is extremely variable among different individuals. Chronologic age, therefore, is a poor index of physiologic age or of performance. Advancing years are not necessarily equated with illness. A 90-year-old person may feel young and be able to care for all his or her needs even though activities may be somewhat slowed. However, if one problem is identified, others must be looked for because multiple diseases are characteristic of the health problems of the elderly [24].

General Effects of Aging

In the older adult, as in younger persons, the various parts of the body form an integrated whole and the function of the entire organism depends on the function of each system. Characteristic changes in the anatomy and physiology of the various body systems occur even though there is a general slowing of cell division. The older adult's body reacts more slowly to stressors in the internal and/or external environment. Adaptation can occur, however, in a suitable environment.

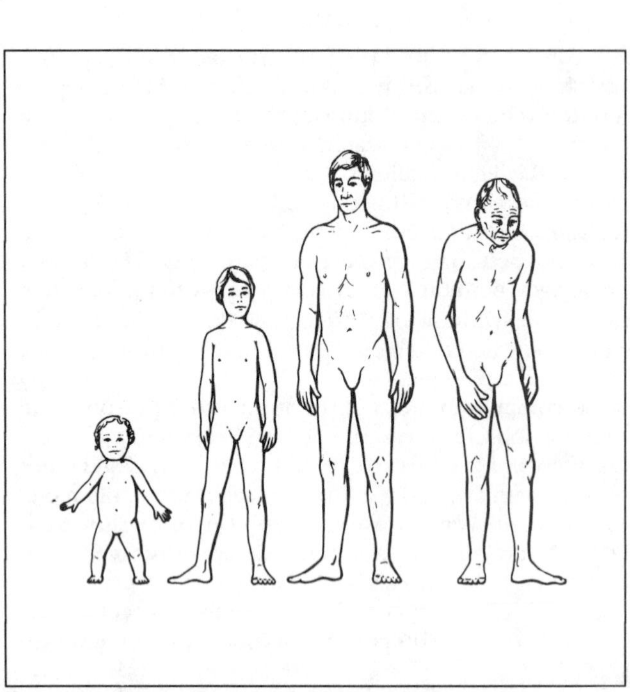

FIGURE 53-1. Changes in proportion throughout the life span.

The aging person characteristically presents an altered appearance. Stature is lost, body proportions are changed, skin is dry and wrinkled, hair is thinning and grey, and there is a change in body movement characterized by slowness, stiffness, and diminished coordination and balance. The intervertebral discs become thin as do the vertebrae themselves, leading to the reduction in height. The thoracic curve of the vertebral column increases, resulting in a kyphosis. The cervical curve increases to compensate, causing a tilting of the head. The height loss, therefore is in the trunk. The length of the long bones is unchanged. The effect then is a short-trunked, long-limbed relationship, which is just the opposite of that of the child (Fig. 53-1). The kyphosis of the thoracic vertebrae plus other changes in lung elasticity result in an increased anterioposterior diameter of the chest.

The total body composition is altered. Reduction of lean tissue occurs, with an increase of fat laid down within mesenteric or perinephritic areas rather than in subcutaneous fat. Decreased subcutaneous fat leads to increased skin folding. Total body potassium, water, and intracellular fluid decrease. The bone mineral mass is reduced with increased bone porosity. The total effect of these losses is a reduced density of the body.

Weight changes are characteristic. In men, the average maximum weight is 172 pounds at ages 35 to 54. This falls to 166 pounds at ages 55 to 64. In women, the average maximum weight is 152 pounds at 55 to 65, 146 pounds at ages 65 to 74, and 138 pounds at ages 75 to 89. Women's weight declines less proportionately than men's [26].

Visible changes in movement are primarily a function of the altered nervous system with diminished muscle strength and joint mobility contributing only minimally to this change. Movement is an extremely complex activity requiring integration of many portions of the nervous system. Intact sensory information going to the brain must be coupled with integration of cortical, basal ganglionic, and cerebellar function. The extrapyramidal system is subject to early changes in function due to diminished presence of neurotransmitters. Vascular supply to all portions of the brain is critical to coordinated function for movement. Locomotion then becomes increasingly precarious with aging and alterations in movement characterize the appearance of the elderly.

Fasting blood sugar, blood volume, serum pH, red blood cell count, and osmotic pressure are unchanged with aging in the absence of disease. The ability to respond to severe stresses is altered, however. For example, normal pH may be well maintained under normal circumstances but should ventilatory failure or metabolic acidosis occur, the elderly person will take much longer to restore normal pH. Responses to events such as infection may be diminished or slowed. An elderly person may have an infectious illness with subnormal or normal temperature and a normal heart rate.

A general reduction in the accuracy of sensory input in the elderly is characteristic. Changes in the accommodation of the lens result in a decreased acuity of vision. *Presbyopia*, impairment of vision due to increasing age, usually occurs early in the fifth decade of life and serves as a signal that the aging process has begun. Auditory acuity begins to fade with the initial loss of high-frequency tones. *Presbycusis*, a progressive, bilaterally symmetrical perceptive hearing loss, starts at about the fourth decade, but the effects are usually not noticeable to the person at the outset.

Nervous System

The general integrative effects of aging are strongly affected by alteration in the central nervous system. Because of its dependency on oxygen, the central nervous system responds to change in the circulatory system, such as arteriosclerosis, which can lead to decreased oxygen supply. A decreased oxygen supply to the brain leads to changes in mental acuity, sensory interpretation, movement, and a generally reduced capacity to cope with multiple environmental events. The onset of such changes is extremely variable from one individual to another.

The transmission strength of signals from the brain to the body parts decreases due to the fact that the number of neurons decrease with age. The signals become slightly blurred and the threshold for arousal of an organ system may be altered. It is known that overstimulation in the older individual can lead to anxiety and tension. The increased recovery time within the autonomic system causes an organ to take longer to return to base level activity after stimulation.

The muscular weakness frequently seen in the aged is due mostly to disuse atrophy or may be due to pharmacologic side effects and decreased hormone secretion. Nerve impulses decrease their rate of conduction by about 10 percent, which may lead to ischemia, the general lowering of basal metabolism, and temperature changes in nerve fibers [4].

The reasons for change in function of the central nervous system are not specifically known. The cardiovascular changes in blood vessels, such as atherosclerosis and arteriosclerosis, which tend to increase with age, may lead to a degree of hypoxia. Hypoxia may, in turn, cause disequilibrium in the central nervous system. The primary changes may be due to degenerative changes in the neuronal system or may result primarily from circulatory failure [12].

There are also physical changes in the brain. The brain loses an average of 100 gm in weight between 25 and 70 years of age. Diminished number of neurons result, with the loss being greater in some areas than others. Up to 45 percent loss has been noted in some cortical areas, while 25 percent loss may be seen in the cerebellum. Little loss in the brainstem structure occurs. Atrophy of the convolutions of the brain is common with widening of the sulci and gyri, especially in the frontal lobe. Dilatation of the ventricles also commonly occurs. Despite these anatomic changes there is little loss of the total amount of DNA, nucleic acid, or protein. The intracellular accumulation of lipofuscin pigment has been extensively studied. A major accumulation of this pigment is in storage vacuoles and is quantitatively correlated with age. The amount per cell varies, but there can be enough to fill the cytoplasm and force the nucleus into an abnormal position. Despite the obvious and apparently significant nature of this material and the interest that it has engendered, it is not known if the presence of lipofuscin has any actual effect on cell function [4].

Due to the physiologic and metabolic changes in the brain and the reduced oxygen consumption, less intracellular energy is produced; glucose utilization is diminished and cerebral blood flow is reduced. The EEG of the older adult remains within the normal limits of other age groups except that it is about one cycle slower.

Substantial metabolic changes within the synaptic complexes are related to neurotransmitter production. Changes in neurotransmitter effects are known to be related to many brain functions related to neuroendocrine events such as sleep, temperature control, and especially mood. Depression is associated with reduced levels of norepinephrine in the brain, a common situation in elderly persons. Despite the changes enumerated previously, intellectual function in the aging adult seems to be sustained.

The effects of general changes in the brain are associated with the common characteristics of the elderly. These include decreasing motor strength, lack of dexterity and agility, difficulties in association, retrieval, and recall, diminished memory and cognitive ability and change in affect, and often depression. The behavior resulting from these changes causes concern to the person and significant others.

Cardiovascular System

Under normal circumstances the aging heart adapts and allows the person to maintain an average level of activity. Anatomic and physiologic changes cause a falling stroke volume and cardiac output. The heart begins to have difficulty adapting to the workload, especially when unusual demands are made on it. Also if the workload is increased by such problems as hypertension, valvular disease, or myocardial infarction, alteration in cardiac adaptation can result.

ANATOMIC CHANGES. Anatomic changes in the heart lead to diminished contractility and filling capacity. Loss of muscle fiber in the heart with localized hypertrophy of individualized fibers is due to an increased amount of collagenous material that surrounds every fiber. Thickening of the semilunar and atrioventricular valves causes increased resistance to blood flow. The end result is a heart encased in a more rigid collagen matrix, which leads to the diminished contraction and decreased filling capacity of the heart chambers.

PHYSIOLOGIC CHANGES. The numerous physiologic changes that occur in the heart include alterations in the conduction system, loss of contractile efficiency and decreased levels of circulating catecholamines. Harris states that after age 60, peripheral vascular resistance increases 1 percent per year [17]. The change in peripheral resistance coupled with the anatomic and physiologic changes previously described produces numerous changes in the capacity of cardiac performance. The cardiac index (*cardiac output*) falls by 0.79 percent per year with stroke volume decreasing at the rate of 0.7 percent per year. Heart work (stroke volume × mean systolic blood pressure) decreases at the rate of 0.5 percent per year [19]. The heart rate increase that occurs in response to stress is less effective and the range of optimal heart rate narrows. A mild tachycardia or bradycardia may lead to a significant deficit in blood flow in vital organs.

All these factors combined result in a heart that no longer has the capacity to meet all the demands that it met in earlier years. Excessive fluid load, excessive work load (as in shock or hemorrhage), or insult to the heart muscle, such as ischemia or infarction, are met by a heart muscle unable to compensate. Inadequate output relative to demands occurs leading to many circulatory problems, such as cardiogenic shock and congestive heart failure. Even in situations of mild stress, all organs are less well perfused and therefore function inadequately.

CONDUCTION SYSTEM. The changes in the conduction system of the heart of the elderly are due to anatomic changes in the conduction system per se and to ischemia due to interrupted blood supply through the coronary arteries. Disturbances of the autonomic nervous system and the local chemical (ionic) environment of the pacemaker cells may initiate arrhythmias. The conduction impulses may be blocked at some point or parts of the system may become irritable and susceptible to irregular discharge. Digitalis administration is a common cause of arrhythmias in the elderly that can be potentiated by low serum potassium. A real danger exists when potassium-depleting diuretics are used in association with digitalis. Cardiac arrhythmias contribute to poor cardiac output and may result in cardiac arrest.

ARTERIAL CHANGES. Blood vessels are markedly affected by degenerative changes in aging, particularly the arteries. Basic to the problems of all arteries is the progressive stiffness due to the cross-linkage effect on elastin and smooth muscle with an increase in the amount of collagen present. This generalized problem in the arteries leads to increased peripheral resistance. The major arteries demonstrate these changes as follows [19]:

1. The tunica intima becomes thickened and less smooth as arteriosclerotic streaks are accumulated.
2. In the tunica media, muscle fibers are replaced with collagen or connective tissue and calcium material.
3. The ability to expand or stretch decreases due to the changes of the intimal layers.
4. Higher blood pressures become common in the older adult, resulting from the decreased interior diameter of the artery and the diminished stretchability.
5. The aorta and its branches tend to dilate and become tortuous.

In addition, there is the development of *atherosclerosis*. Fatty streaks in the intima have been found to be present in the first year of life. These may or may not be related to the subsequent development of atherosclerotic changes. As a person ages, atheromatous plaques increase, resulting in raised areas with a central core of degenerative lipid on the tunica intima. These atheromatous plaques are most numerous in the major arteries, particularly the aorta, iliac, coronary, and carotid arteries. They also occur frequently in the renal and femoral arteries. Pathologically they cause two problems: (1) thrombosis and occlusion in the lumen of the artery, and (2) destruction of the tunica media due to interrupted nutrition leading to aneurysm. Aneurysms occur most typically in the abdominal or thoracic aorta.

Arterial changes are widespread and result in diminished circulation to all organs and tissues. Of particular consequence is the reduced circulation to the brain and to the kidneys. Renal plasma flow, without evidence of disease, drops 53 percent between ages 20 to 90 years. The circulation drops 23 percent from 20 to 80 years of age.

VENULAR CHANGES. The thin-walled veins have valves formed from the internal layer that assist the blood to flow toward the heart, but prevent a reversal of the flow. Veins are capable of constricting and enlarging, of storing large quantities of blood and making this blood available when it is required by the circulation, and can actually propel blood forward [16].

Since muscle contraction in the legs provides for upward propelling force for venous return, every time the legs are moved or the muscles are tensed a certain amount of blood is propelled toward the heart. Varicose veins occur when the valves of the venous system are destroyed. The inactivity of the older adult, constricting clothing, and crossing legs at the knees can result in ruptured valves. Varicose veins are quite common in older adults. The venous stasis that occurs with varicose veins further complicates the circulatory problems.

A major vascular problem of aging is that of venous thrombosis and pulmonary emboli. One study speculates that 10 to 25 percent of all persons reaching 65 will have had venous thrombosis of some type [32]. Immobilization from increased sitting time and bed rest increases the risk of thrombosis.

HYPERTENSION. The prevalence of hypertension increases substantially with age, even though hypertension is not an essential aspect of aging. There is a gradual increase in systolic pressure with age, due to decreased aortic elasticity. The increase in diastolic pressure is less marked and results from an increased resistance in the peripheral blood vessels. The diastolic pressure tends to level off in later life. Cardiac output and blood volume are also factors in the regulation of blood pressure. Blood pressure is elevated through increased resistance to blood flow due to arteriolar constriction. Blood pressure lowers when arteriolar relaxation reduces resistance to blood flow.

Benign essential hypertension is the most common type in persons over 70, with more than 90 percent of all cases being placed in this category [10]. Elevated pressure usually develops slowly with little untoward effect in benign essential hypertension. Malignant hypertension is found in individuals who exhibit an accelerated course and a diastolic pressure of 110 mg Hg and a systolic pressure of 200 mm Hg [13]. This type of hypertension is rarely found in persons over 70 years of age. Clients with either type of elevated pressures may develop cardiovascular, renal, or cerebral problems due to secondary organ damage. Complications due to hypertension account for over 50 percent of the deaths in the United States.

Hypertension contributes considerably to diseases of the cardiovascular system. It is associated with increased incidence of coronary artery disease and myocardial infarction, and with hemorrhagic problems and infarcts in the brain. It is also associated with major hemorrhage from cerebral arteries and resultant strokes.

The incidence of cerebrovascular disease increases with age. There are two major sources of serious damage to the brain via the vascular system. One is infarction of areas of the brain due to occlusion of cerebral arterial vessels. The other is hemorrhage. The infarction is by far the more common. The hemorrhage has a more serious prognosis. Events that may precipitate a cerebrovascular accident are [22]:

1. Marked or sudden reduction in blood pressure
2. Decrease in cardiac output
3. Diminution of circulating blood volume
4. Anemia
5. Increase in blood viscosity

Transient cerebral ischemic attacks may occur prior to major strokes. These attacks are due to arterial occlusion or hypotension. The occlusive phenomena occur most frequently with the carotid artery. In this case, the signs are hemiparesis, hemianopsia, aphasia, and loss of vision in one eye. The vertebral artery is more often involved with hypotensive states causing a falling forward on the knees without loss of consciousness, vertigo, vomiting, dysarthria, visual blurring, or diplopia [5].

The baroreceptors in the aorta and carotid arteries become less sensitive to pressure changes with age. This results in a slow response to postural changes and sudden changes in position may cause dizziness or syncope. Pressure on the carotid sinus may cause serious slowing of the heart rate and may be elicited by twisting and turning of the head.

Respiratory System

Alterations in the respiratory system in the aged impose many limitations that are not always obvious when the person is at rest, but appear on exertion or stress. Under usual circumstances older persons are capable of maintaining usual daily activities but various changes make them more susceptible to pulmonary infections. Among aged individuals, influenza and pneumonia are the fourth leading causes of death with bronchitis, emphysema, and asthma ranking eighth [11].

ANATOMIC CHANGES. Loss of elasticity affects the older person's pulmonary compliance and results from increased cross-linkage in collagen and elastin fibers around the alveolar sacs. Pressure builds up within the alveolar sacs during inspiration, some of which tends to be retained during expiration, and finally results in an increased residual air volume. In addition, there is a decrease in the quantity of air that can be taken in during normal breathing. This is also affected by the fact that older persons take shallower and more frequent breaths than younger persons [28].

Changes in the costal cartilage result in a diminution of chest wall compliance, which is further complicated by skeletal deformities of the thorax and postural changes such as stooped shoulders. In the older adult the changes in the muscular system lead to a decline in the strength of muscles that assist respiration. Degeneration of the intervertebral disks of the thoracic spine results in an increased anterioposterior diameter of the chest and a chest wall that is less compliant during respiration.

The end result of the loss of elasticity, the muscle weakness, and the changes in the structure of the chest is difficulty in expiration of air. The pulmonary function studies are altered as a result of this reduced capacity to empty the lungs. The total lung capacity is changed little, but the vital capacity is gradually and progressively reduced. The forced expiratory volumes and maximum breathing capacity are both reduced, while the residual volume and the functional residual capacity of the lungs are increased. The residual volume increases 40 percent between 20 and 70 years. The maximum breathing capacity is diminished by 50 percent by age 60. Actual air flow is reduced 20 to 30 percent.

FUNCTIONAL CHANGES. The partial pressure of arterial oxygen gradually falls with aging. With the structural and mechanical changes described above, the bases of the lungs are ventilated less and less. The part of the lung being well perfused is the part of the lung not being ventilated. Blood must be shunted to the ventilated upper portions of the lung. The redistribution of blood is usually insufficient to compensate and the arterial partial pressure of oxygen falls. The problem becomes worse when the elderly person lies down, and nocturnal hypoxemia may be a major cause of confusion. The partial pressure of arterial oxygen declines with age, averaging 77 mm Hg in the seventh decade [7]. The partial pressure of carbon dioxide, however, remains the same unless there is disease superimposed on the diminished ventilation; this is probably due to the higher rate of diffusion of carbon dioxide.

The main functional respiratory problems in the elderly person without pulmonary disease are reduced ventilation of all alveoli, especially at the bases of the lungs, and reduced oxygen partial pressure in the arterial blood. This deficit may not impair function under baseline conditions with minimal physical exertion. The changes in capacity to increase the work of breathing due to structural changes in the chest wall, and the structural changes that reduce the maximum breathing capacity, however, put the elderly person at risk. The need to increase oxygen intake rapidly or to blow off carbon dioxide rapidly due to acidemia may cause decompensation and rapid respiratory failure in an elderly person with no respiratory disease per se. Sudden increases in physical activity, or sudden psychologic stress may overwhelm a respiratory system that handles moderate stress well.

In addition to the changes described above, which are normal alterations with aging, most persons in modern Western society have lung changes due to chronic environmental pollution. The inhalants such as smoke, various industrial end products, and the end products of combustion of petrochemicals have a profound effect on respiratory function. They cause decreased ciliary action, increased mucus production, and deposition of foreign materials in the functional alveoli and in intercellular spaces. These pollutants have two main effects: (1) increase of the obstructive component in lung function, or (2) decrease of the compliance of the lung tissue through deposits of foreign material increasing its stiffness. The latter situation is common among miners and industrial workers who constantly inhale coal dust, asbestos, and the like. The predominant clinical problem is the presence of an increased obstructive component. Smoking, being around smokers, bronchial constriction due to exposure to a wide variety of irritants, and chronic bronchitis with large increases in mucus production all cause increased obstruction in the airways contributing to trapping of air in the alveoli, structural changes (emphysema), and markedly diminished ventilation. In addition, the unevenness of the changes results in perfusion difficulties in that some pulmonary arterial blood receives oxygen and some does not. The interaction of the aging effects and environmental effects on lung function cannot be separated. Aging is continuous and environmental effects on the lungs are long-term and continuous. One has to assume that all elderly persons have some degree of diminished ventilation along with alterations in ventilation and perfusion.

An elderly person with little previous problem, may develop respiratory failure rather rapidly following stress, such as surgery, excessive exercise, a sudden rise in environmental pollution (as in smog crises), or infection such as pneumonia. The assumption must be made that all elderly people are at risk for respiratory failure. Respiratory failure is evidenced by a diminishing PaO_2 and a rising $PaCO_2$ associated with a drop in the arterial pH. Potential causes of respiratory failure are surgery, the use of depressant drugs, lung infections, bed rest, pulmonary edema due to circulatory problems, and pulmonary embolism. Pulmonary embolism is frequently seen in elderly patients who are immobilized due to bone fractures or other conditions requiring bed rest. Any acute situation such as trauma, burns, or myocardial infarction in the elderly may be complicated by respiratory failure. The potential of unrecognized pulmonary changes, particularly those due to environmental effects, is present in all patients over 40. Pulmonary function tests on middle-aged or elderly persons facing elective surgery are necessary to be prepared to prevent respiratory failure during the postoperative period (see also Chap. 25).

Genitourinary System

Genitourinary problems in older adults are common problems that many of the aged are reluctant to discuss. They frequently postpone seeking treatment because of embarrassment. The problems are bothersome and frequently thought of as another sign of growing old. Renal problems are potentially life-threatening and become more so because of delay in detection and treatment.

ANATOMIC CHANGES IN THE KIDNEYS. The urinary tract undergoes many changes with age. The kidneys are affected by involutional processes related to time. Also, there is a normal age-related change in renal vascular anatomy and function, independent of disease. The nephrons begin to degenerate and disappear by the seventh month in utero. The normal young adult has approximately 800,000–1,000,000 nephrons in each kidney. These gradually degenerate and are reduced by one-third to one-half by the seventh de-

TABLE 54-1.

	At birth	Young adult	Over 65 Years	Percentage loss
Kidney mass	50 gm	270 gm	185 gm	31
Kidney volume	20 ml	250 ml	200 ml	20
Filtering surface area	.02 sq m	1.6 sq m	0.9 sq m	43

cade. The changes in kidney size, volume, and filtering surface over the life span are shown in Table 54-1 [15].

Renal vascular changes begin before birth and increase with age. Each kidney has approximately one million nephrons at birth. The nephrons increase in size, but not in number until maturity. There is some loss of nephrons in the normal physiologic aging changes in the urinary tract. The loss of nephrons accelerates as one ages, so that by the age of 85 the number decreases by 30 to 40 percent. In addition to the loss of nephrons, there is some degeneration of the remaining nephrons. The degeneration starts as a sclerosis or scarring of the glomeruli, followed by atrophy of the afferent arterioles. The glomeruli, deep in the cortex of the kidney, retain one capillary which enlarges and acts as a shunt between the afferent and efferent arterioles. The compensation that does occur results from enlargement of the remaining nephrons. Despite the enlargement of the nephrons there is a decrease of about 30 percent in the net weight of the kidney.

FUNCTIONAL CHANGES IN THE KIDNEYS. It is to be expected, due to the loss of nephrons, or functional units of the kidneys, that there will be a decline in function. The kidneys do not concentrate the urine as well because of the loss of nephrons. However, under normal circumstances, the kidneys are capable of maintaining the acid balance. The renal filtration rate decreases about 6 percent per decade as the general circulation decreases. As general arteriosclerosis occurs throughout the body, the arterioles in the kidneys are also affected. The result is that some of the blood is diverted to other parts of the body and is not filtered through the glomerular filtration system [12].

The kidneys of an older adult can respond to emergencies almost as well as those of a young person, even though the changes described are present. Even minor stress can cause disruption in kidney function and the aged kidney has difficulty in restabilizing.

DISEASES AND PROBLEMS WITH AGING KIDNEYS. Renal function in the elderly may be compromised by one or more of the following problems [29]:

1. Inadequate fluid intake
2. Fluid loss due to vomiting or diarrhea
3. Shock due to hemorrhage
4. Acute or chronic cardiac failure
5. Septicemia due to gram-negative bacteria
6. Injudicious use of diuretics

These situations may result in renal ischemia and acute renal shutdown if not promptly corrected. The minimum urinary output should be 400 ml daily. Any output of 20 ml per hour or less may herald acute renal failure. Acute renal failure (ARF) is a frequent problem in the elderly and carries a mortality in persons 70 years and over of 80 percent. The dangers of ARF include: (1) fluid overloading leading to congestive heart failure and pulmonary edema, and (2) a rising serum potassium, which may cause cardiac arrest.

Diseases of the kidneys, regardless of the cause, create long-term problems. Due to the various pathologic events associated with the disease, the aged have a combined effect from the ravages of disease coupled with the normal changes. The most frequent chronic kidney disease seen in the elderly is pyelonephritis. The physiologic problems associated with chronic kidney disease are hypertension, sodium and water retention, marked sodium or water loss, retention of potassium, and loss of serum protein. The greatest problem in chronic renal disease is the inability of the kidneys to handle changing concentrations of hydrogen ion. The responses to increased hydrogen ion concentration are slowed and diminished, leading to metabolic acidosis.

A number of antibiotics often used in infections of the elderly are nephrotoxic; they include tetracycline, cephaloridine, and gentamycin. Occasionally, penicillin will have this effect. It is not uncommon for an elderly patient who develops an infection and is treated by one of these antibiotics to have septic shock and renal shutdown. It is difficult to ascertain under such circumstances whether the renal failure is caused by the antibiotic or the shock associated with the infection. Parsons suggests that the indiscriminate use of antibiotics produces more renal failure than the sepsis for which they are prescribed [25].

BLADDER CHANGES AND PROBLEMS. Two of the most common and bothersome problems the elderly encounter are nocturnal frequency of micturition and urinary incontinence. Changes that contribute to these problems are: loss of muscle tone resulting in relaxation of the perineal muscles in the female; prostatic hypertrophy in the male; bladder diverticuli; sphincter relaxation; and altered bladder reflexes. Frequently there is a reduced bladder capacity and often residual urine. Incomplete emptying of the bladder predisposes the elderly person to infection. *Escherichia coli* is the most frequent cause of bladder infection in women, while *Proteus* is the most common in men. Bladder infections can result from poor hygienic practices or from anything that impedes urinary flow — such as neoplasms, strictures or a clogged indwelling catheter. Urine may become alkaline in the presence of an infection, leading to the formation of small inorganic salt calculi. Hematuria, gross and/or microscopic, may be found with urinary tract infections (see Chap. 27).

GYNECOLOGIC CHANGES IN THE AGED WOMAN. In the elderly woman objective findings are directly related to the effects of estrogen deprivation. A general atrophy occurs in the reproductive system causing a reduction in the size of the uterus and the cervix; the vaginal walls become thinner; changes take place in mucous secretions and vaginal tissues become more friable and susceptible to irritation and infection. Due to the diminished vaginal secretions, the vagina has a loss of normal flora that create an acid environment to protect the canal. Atrophic changes result in a vulva that is pallid, has a loss of subcutaneous fat, and is accompanied by a flattening and folding of the labia. Other findings include a thinning and change in hair patterns, plus a thinning and sagging of the breasts. Breast tissue changes result from the replacement of atrophying glandular tissue with fat.

SEXUAL CHANGES IN THE AGED MAN. Physiologic changes in the elderly man are also due to lowered hormone production. The reduction of hormone production in the male is much more gradual than in the female. Cellular changes in the testes occur but no significant change in the weight is noted. Fat content increases in testicular cells, accompanied by a decrease in the number of cells. The number of sperm ejaculated decrease by up to 50 percent by age 90. Sperm change in size and shape and lose their fertilization ability [2]. Androgen production begins to decline at age 30 and continues to decline until the age of 90 [12].

Most elderly men have some benign prostatic hypertrophy, which is considered to be a normal aging change. The changes in the prostate results in a prostate that is more fibrous and has irregular thickening. The incidence of prostatic cancer increases with age (see Chaps. 28 and 49).

Gastrointestinal System

NORMAL ANATOMIC CHANGES. Problems with the gastrointestinal system are the source of many complaints voiced by older persons. The problems range from simple dyspepsia to carcinomatous conditions. Gastrointestinal cancer occurs with increasing frequency after middle age. The aged population has a high incidence of gastrointestinal problems such as peptic ulcers, biliary tract disease, and intestinal obstructions.

Contributing to the high incidence of these problems are many normal aging processes. The grinding surface of the molars have worn down and many aged persons have lost most or all of their teeth. With the loss of chewing ability most elderly persons eat soft food, thereby developing gum and digestive problems. Altered taste sensation, due to a decline in taste buds on the tongue, fosters a poor appetite and this can result in malnutrition.

ESOPHAGEAL CHANGES AND PROBLEMS. Changes in esophageal motility begin to occur with aging. Degenerative changes in smooth muscle that lines the lower two-thirds of the esophagus result in a delay in esophageal emptying, dilatation of the esophagus, and an increase in nonpropulsive contractions [4]. Obstructive phenomena can occur as a result of tumors, rings, or strictures.

The risk of hiatal hernia in persons over 50 years of age may be as high as 40 to 60 percent. Small hiatal hernias are so common that they are frequently considered a normal finding in x-ray studies [28]. Difficulty in swallowing is one of the primary symptoms. Hiatal hernias can mimic pulmonary distress and angina; therefore x-ray studies should be done to verify diagnosis.

STOMACH CHANGES AND PROBLEMS. The stomach mucosa becomes thinner and less hydrochloric acid and enzymes are produced. A common finding in the elderly is pernicious anemia because vitamin B_{12} is dependent on the intrinsic factor in gastric secretions. Cell changes in the stomach lining results in atrophic gastritis in 50 percent of the people by age 70 [12]. The prevalence of peptic ulcers increases with persons over 60 but associated epigastric pain is not as acute in older persons as it is in affected younger persons.

COLON CHANGES AND PROBLEMS. The elderly person is particularly at risk for constipation because of decreased physical exercise, decreased food and water intake, and low-residue dietary patterns. Diverticulosis is considered a disease of aging. The majority of diverticuli occur in the sigmoid colon and are asymptomatic. A high percent of cancer in aged persons occurs in the colon. Constipation is one of the most frequent complaints of the elderly. In a large percentage of the elderly constipation is due to cultural eating patterns, decreased exercise, decreased gastric mobility due to vascular changes, low fluid intake, and the ingestion of drugs such as antihypertensives and sedatives. The problem of constipation in the elderly is compounded by the abuse of purgatives, laxatives, and enemas.

Musculoskeletal System

One of the most visible changes characteristic of the aging person is that of a change in the pattern of movement. Successful characterization of an aging person by an actor nearly always includes alterations in body movement. Changes of posture, increased muscular rigidity, slowness of movement, and lack of coordination and stability are characteristic. Changes in neuromuscular function result from the combined effect of changes in the muscles, the peripheral motor neurons, the myoneural synapses, and the central nervous system. Diet, heredity, and hormonal balances also have an influence.

CHARACTERISTIC CHANGES IN ANATOMIC STRUCTURE AND FUNCTION. There is a general wasting of skeletal muscles due to loss of muscle fibers. Muscle strength, endurance, and agility are affected by the decrease in muscle mass. All muscle activity in the elderly is affected by the degree of oxygen supply and its alterations, which are due to circulatory and respiratory function. The peripheral motor neurons also have some decrease in protein synthesis with thickening at the myoneural junction and decrease in acetylcholine.

The general decrease in movement, coupled with muscle stiffness and slowness particularly in initiating movement in the aging person, is attributable primarily to changes in the extrapyramidal system. A resting tremor may also be present. These changes are considered normal. If the extrapyramidal function becomes severely impaired, Parkinson's syndrome, chorea, or dystonia of various types may appear.

With age, in addition to the wasting of skeletal muscles, a loss of bone minerals causes the bones to become more brittle. Some joints stiffen and lose motion, while other joints become more mobile because of stretching of the ligaments. A reduction in height results from hip and knee flexion, kyphosis of the dorsal spine, and shortening of the vertebral column.

DEGENERATIVE ARTHRITIS. Discomfort, disability, or deformity frequently accompanies musculoskeletal changes. Arthritis and degenerative changes in the tendons are often the causes for pain in the shoulders, elbows, hands, hips, knees, feet, and spine. Older persons suffering from arthritis express subjective complaints of fatigue, weakness, weight loss, and numbness of the hands and feet. Degenerative arthritis is a noninflammatory disorder of movable joints. It is characterized by bone hypertrophy, deterioration, and abrasion of articular cartilage. This type of osteoarthritis occurs more often in women than in men [18].

RHEUMATOID ARTHRITIS. Rheumatoid arthritis is a chronic systemic inflammatory disease of connective tissue that is commonly seen in the aged but occurs at all ages. This disease occurs 2 to 3 times more often in women than in men, and in persons with a family history of rheumatoid arthritis. The joints in rheumatoid arthritis are reddened, stiff, swollen, warm to the touch, and extremely painful. Bursae and subcutaneous nodules over prominences may be present. Deforming flexion contractures may also be present. The person will detail symptoms that include fatigue, weakness, malaise, weight loss, fever, and anemia [22]. Theories have been advanced to explain the cause of rheumatoid arthritis, although the exact cause is not known. One theory is that microorganisms such as streptococci, staphylococci, and diphtheroids are the causative agents. Another theory states that the presence of autoantibodies supports the autoimmune nature of rheumatoid arthritis [13] (see also Chaps. 11 and 37).

FRACTURES AND RISK OF FALLING. Cerebral vascular disease is another cause of disability and difficulty in locomotion of the elderly. Arteriosclerosis of the carotid arteries and the vertebral arteries resulting in ischemia may cause transient paralysis or transient light-headedness, poor balance, and falling episodes. When such events occur, the person becomes anxious and tense about moving, and thereby coordination is reduced even further. Older persons who fear falling tend to take fewer and fewer risks; the result is increased immobility. The person who has had a stroke tends to have a hemiparesis or hemiplegia. Those who recover from such episodes tend to have some motor disability that creates difficulty in walking, postural changes both in sitting and standing, residual spasticity and footdrop. These factors put the person at risk for future falling.

Injury from falling is a very real problem for the elderly. Fractures of the hip and wrist are frequent. Head injury is a frequent outcome of falling and the subsequent hospitalization and surgery also carry high risk for the elderly.

The bone becomes increasingly vulnerable to injury through mechanical stress. Two main processes occur as a natural course of events in aging, osteoporosis and osteoarthritis. As in all the other systems, it is difficult to know where natural aging ends and disease begins. However, the nature of the changes and the fact that they occur in most all persons who live long enough lend credence to the belief that they are normal aging states.

OSTEOPOROSIS. Osteoporosis is basically caused by an imbalance between bone formation and bone absorption. In osteoporosis, bone absorption increases. This affects primarily trabecular bone, but also the cortices of long bones. The "outer surfaces of long bones continue to grow slowly (normally) throughout life, but in osteoporosis, the inner surfaces are resorbed at a slightly faster rate. The end result in the long bone is a bone slightly longer in external diameter but with thinner walls and with markedly diminished trabecular bone in its ends. Vetebral bodies, which have a larger percent of trabecular bone, are more severely affected by this process [1]." In osteoporosis, there is evidence of decreased calcium absorption from the gastrointestinal tract. Also, there is some relationship with gonad deficiency since osteoporosis is greatly increased in postmenopausal women. Immobilization and lack of weight bearing on the skeletal system causes osteoporosis at any age. Also excess levels of cortisone, either exogenous or endogenous, will cause the condition. Regardless of the underlying pathologic process, the osteoporosis occurs to a degree in all elderly persons, but is much more marked in women.

The primary problem related to osteoporosis is the tendency for bone fracture, most frequently of the vertebrae and the femur. In elderly persons, it has been found through studies by Brockehurst and his associates, that 34 percent of the time the fractured femur was due to an accident [3]. Twenty-five percent of the time the fracture was due to a "drop attack." The "drop attack" is a sudden fall due to postural instability resulting from changes in the hind brain and cerebellum. The person suddenly falls to the ground without warning or with a momentary vertigo. In examining all the causes of falls, for the 384 persons studied by Brockehurst, the most frequent cause of falling was tripping. The second most frequent was loss of balance, and the third most frequent was "drop attack." Forty-three percent of the total sample had neurologic diseases.

Kyphosis or curvature of the spine, in older persons, frequently occurs as a result of osteoporosis of the vertebrae. Vertebral atrophy also occurs. Due to the progressive degeneration, the number of cells diminish, the water content decreases, the tissues lose turgor and become friable. The combined changes in the vertebrae and disks result in a curvature of the spine. The resultant kyphosis causes problems such as decreased respiratory capacity of the chest wall, and increased problems due to impingement on various spinal nerves from the narrowed disks and vertebral changes. These problems are most often related to the lumbar and cervical spine. Compression fractures of the spine are also common.

JOINT CHANGES. Joint problems with the elderly include (1) erosion of the cartilagenous surface of the joints, (2) degenerative changes of the soft tissue in the joint, and (3) calcification and ossification of the ligaments, especially those around the vertebrae. The name given to the degenerative processes of the joint is *osteoarthritis*. Once again, it is difficult to determine how much of this process is normal aging because it is present in all persons to some degree. It begins at age 20, and by age 50 radiologic changes are present. Five percent have symptoms by age 50, and by age 60, 15 percent of men and 25 percent of women have symptoms.

The cartilage of the joint loses elasticity, becomes dull and opaque, and then softens and frays, denuding the underlying bone. The underlying bone develops a proliferation of fibroblasts and new bone formation takes place. At the joint margins, extensive proliferation produces bony outgrowths, or spur formation. When spurs project into the joint they can cause considerable pain and limitation of motion. Pieces of cartilage and bone may break off to form loose bodies in the joint that require surgical removal.

Changes in joints are probably due to the results of long-term trauma. When overgrowth of the bone margins occurs on the fingers, most often in women, it may only be unsightly. "When it occurs about the hip, the femoral head may become trapped, painful and immobile. This is the most common cause for hip replacement [12]." The cartilagenous disks that exist between the vertebrae undergo the same pathologic changes that take place in the other joints. The degenerative changes are contributed to by the predisposing factors of aging, extensive involvement in physical activities leading to injury, excessive use of the joint, and obesity. These pathologic changes are accompanied by pain and limitation of motion.

Skin and Dermal Appendages

CHANGES IN THE SKIN, NAILS, AND HAIR. Next to musculoskeletal changes, changes in the integument are the most obvious and disturbing changes for the aging person. Due to the loss of elasticity, wrinkles, lines, and drooping eyelids occur. Exposed areas such as the hands develop age spots, or excessive skin pigmentation. The skin becomes dry, thin, fragile, and more prone to injury. Nails become dry and brittle. Toenails become susceptible to fungus infection and appear thickened. There is a lifting of the nail plate. The rate of change is very individual and is dependent on such factors as nutrition, genetics, emotions, and environment.

A number of skin problems occur due to the changes in the skin. The loss of water, which is the basis for many problems in the elderly, results from atrophy of all skin layers, with diminished vascularity and decreased elasticity. The lack of water in skin tissues leads to pruritis and decubitus ulcers, which are real problems for the aged. Lesions on the skin, such as tumors, warts, or keratoses may arise with no pain. On the other hand, lesions such as herpes zoster may be very painful.

Sebaceous and sweat glands become less active and contribute to the dry skin. The older person frequently has overgrowths of epidermal tissue which are cosmetic problems, but rarely need surgical excision. *Senile telangiectasia*, small scarlet growths scattered over the skin increase in number after middle age. *Hyperkeratotic warts*, raised brown or black epidermal overgrowths, are also found in increased numbers as a person ages. The latter two types of lesions, along with several less frequently occurring lesions, have no clinical significance and do not require removal unless irritated by clothing or jewelry [10].

Another inevitable change resulting from aging is the loss of pigment or greying of the hair. The onset and degree of greying varies greatly. There is also a generalized thinning of the hair, contributed to by a decrease in the density of hair follicles. In older females, the hair appears finer and more sparse, with loss of axillary and pubic hair. Often an increase in facial hair is noted due to decreased estrogen production after menopause. The older male will frequently have hair growth in ears and nares and the eyebrows grow more bushy. The older male is more susceptible to alopecia than women, with genetics playing a part in the degree and rapidity of balding.

Sensory System

Few persons escape sensory deficits as they age. The elderly become more vulnerable to injury, more isolated from society, and less able to care for their personal needs as these deficits occur. Sensory deficits occur in the areas of sight, hearing, taste, smell, and touch, interfering with the ability to communicate, to exchange experiences, and to express feelings.

VISUAL CHANGES. As a person ages, changes take place in both the structural and functional aspects of the eyes. Eyelids become thinner and wrinkled, and skin folds result from loss of orbital fat, leading to proptosis. Inversion or eversion of the lids is a common occurrence and the conjunctiva is thinner and more fragile. *Arcus senilis*, a bluish-grey ring may occur close to the corneal limbus and is visible against the darker pigments of the eye. Arcus senilis is a harmless change and does not affect visual acuity. Light brown patches may occur in the iris, changing its appearance but not the iris' ability to regulate pupil size. The lens of the eye may develop age changes which may cause visual problems. The lens becomes less elastic. This loss of elasticity is termed presbyopia (see Chap. 43).

Cataracts may develop as a result of loss of soluble proteins and the lens loses its transparency. The cloudy, hazy lens results in visual loss. Reduced transmission of light causes distant objects to become hazy and the individual's presbyopic reading glasses will no longer be necessary. Surgical excision may become necessary if the cataract becomes too dense.

Glaucoma is another major eye problem that affects the aged. Glaucoma accounts for about 10 percent of all blindness in the United States. Intraocular pressure rises rapidly in acute glaucoma and slowly in chronic glaucoma. Peripheral vision and night vision are both affected. The decline in peripheral vision may occur slowly and interferes with driving ability. Medications and surgery are now available to treat glaucoma. Early treatment is essential because the blindness resulting from glaucoma is irreversible.

HEARING CHANGES. The aging person may develop changes in the functional ability of the ears as well as external changes in appearance. According to a National Public Health Service survey in 1964, at least 30 percent of the population over age 65 (which represents about 24 million people) suffer from a significant hearing loss.

The external ear undergoes very little change other than some slight elongation of the ear lobes. The amount of cerumen decreases but contains a greater amount of keratin which becomes easily impacted and difficult to remove. Impacted cerumen can block sound waves and cause a temporary hearing loss until the cerumen is removed.

Sclerosis or atrophy of the tympanic membrane affects the middle ear in a reduction of sound waves reaching the inner ear. Loss of cells at the base of the cochlea causes inner ear and retrocochlear loss of efficiency. The loss of the ability to hear high-frequency sounds occurs first, and this is followed by the loss of ability to hear lower frequencies. The term used to describe the progressive hearing loss in the aging is *presbycusis*.

Exposure to excessive noise, recurrent otitis media in younger years, trauma to the ear, and certain drugs are contributing factors to hearing loss in the aging. Persons living or working in highly industrialized areas experience more hearing loss than those in nonindustrial areas.

OTHER SENSORY CHANGES. The aging process does not have as dramatic an effect on the senses of taste, smell, and touch as it does on vision and hearing, but these sensations are also reduced. There is an obvious decrease in ability to taste sweet and salty flavors, due to a decrease in the number of taste buds. Diet becomes an important factor because the aging person tends to eat more sweets and salt food more heavily. The sweets lead to obesity and increased dental problems and the salt may aggravate a hypertensive problem when one exists. Olfactory function may diminish, resulting in inability to smell, which also interferes with appeal to the appetite. The inability to smell can present a hazard in the case of fire or smoke.

A decrease in tactile sensation may be noted by the older person having difficulty in discriminating temperature changes. Older persons tend to get burned more frequently because of this change in touch. Minor injuries occur as a result of occasional unawareness of pain or pressure.

DRUGS AND THE ELDERLY

Many studies have shown that elderly women outnumber elderly men 2:1. They take up more of the physician's time, receive more drugs than do men, and have more adverse drug reactions. Elderly women, as a rule, are more apt to live alone and are more likely to make errors in taking their medications. Frequently the elderly do not purchase all prescriptions ordered by their physicians because of low incomes [2].

The elderly use one-third of all prescribed drugs in this country. Most take multiple drugs and also use over-the-counter drugs frequently [14]. Lamy states "all drugs can pose certain heightened risks to elderly patients and all can decrease a patient's mental, physical, and functional status" [21]. A person's nutritional status may be impaired by long-term use of certain drugs. The elderly person is the least able to tolerate injudicious use of drugs because many physiologic changes make them respond to medication in more variable ways than young adults. The physiologic changes of aging result in a system that is less able to distribute, metabolize, and excrete drugs. The liver, kidneys, and heart are the systems most involved with drug excretion and metabolism. Since these systems may have lost some of their efficiency, drugs may accumulate, leading to toxic effects. The cumulative effects of trauma, prior illnesses, accidents, and disabilities further reduce the aging person's ability to handle drugs.

One of the factors that contributes to the physiologic metabolism of drugs is that absorption of drugs from the gastrointestinal tract is greatly reduced, which may be due to reduced circulation to the gastrointestinal tract. A second factor involved is that of distribution. The total body composition has changed with a higher percentage of fat tissue and less lean tissue and water. Drugs that are selectively used in different tissues will be affected. Also the body size has decreased. This means that the concentration of the drug in the body will be higher for standard dosages.

There is a decrease of 20 percent in plasma binding by albumin in the elderly. Drugs that are normally plasma-focused are therefore increased in concentration in the tissues. A third major change in handling of drugs in the elderly is metabolism of the drug by the liver. The actual rate of metabolism by the liver is diminished by poor circulation to the liver and by a reduction in the available hepatic enzymes with age. Any disease of the liver will aggravate this considerably. Some of the most common drugs metabolized by the liver that will have increased half-life in the elderly are the antidepressants diazepam (Valium) and chlordiazepoxide (Librium). The fourth major problem in the use of drugs for the elderly is the reduced excretion due to diminished renal function. Renal function is markedly reduced as people age and the ability to excrete drugs is also markedly reduced. Drug action in the elderly is also altered by changes in tissue responses. There may be an increased threshold to the drug's actions. Also there may be a decrease in the number of receptive sites for the drug coupled with a decrease in the necessary enzymes.

Listed high among drugs that can be dangerous to the elderly are antibiotics such as tetracyclines and gentamycin. Antibiotics are excreted by the kidneys and reduced kidney function can lead to toxic accumulation of the drugs. Mental disturbances, gastrointestinal side effects, and rashes are toxic effects that can occur [31]. When diuretics, which cause potassium loss, are given in combination with digoxin the danger of arrhythmias is greatly increased. The effect of the digitalis on the conduction system is greatly enhanced by low serum potassium. Many of the antihypertensives have diverse side effects, but they all possess the ability to cause hypotension. Orthostatic hypotension can lead to falls and fractures. Elderly persons should be warned of this possibility, and when on antihypertensives they should be cautioned not to rise too rapidly from a supine or sitting position.

The elderly person does not display the toxic effects of digoxin, such as gastrointestinal and ocular symptoms, usually found in younger adults. This makes digoxin one of the drugs that places the older client in grave risk. Digoxin blood levels are not always a good guide to toxicity because the elderly client reacts in a different fashion. Electrocardiogram changes and confusion appear more readily in the elderly and should be anticipated with digoxin.

Many elderly persons develop nutritional problems from long-term use of medications such as laxatives. Mineral oil can interfere with absorption of nutrients and vitamins in the intestinal tract and its use should be discouraged.

AGING AND CANCER

Cancer is a serious problem, regardless of a person's age. In childhood, cancer is the second leading cause of death. The cancers of childhood are often due to inherited problems and immediate environmental problems. This incidence of cancer and aging advance together until the age of 80 [11]. Even though the prevalence of cancer is higher in the aged, certain types of cancer are diagnosed less frequently; these include cervical cancer and sarcoma. Neoplasia is detailed in Unit 6. Specific malignancies are discussed in the related units.

There is a marked relationship between decreased efficiency of the immune system and increased vulnerability to carcinoma. Persons treated with immunosuppressants for purposes of organ transplantation have shown an increased incidence of cancer. It may be that the immune system is active throughout life, destroying aberrant, potentially tumor-inducing cell changes, and it is only with reduced capacity for such activity that aberrant cells are allowed to grow [8].

Several factors are associated with cancer; however the exact etiology of cancer has not been discovered. It is known that constant irritation from smoking a pipe can cause oral cancers, chewing tobacco can result in cancer of the mouth, and smoking cigarettes can lead to carcinoma of the lung. Environmental factors such as air pollution, food additives, asbestos, and certain chemicals have been found to be carcinogenic. According to the National Research Council, current evidence indicates that most common cancers are influenced by diet, although there are no precise estimates of diet's impact on cancer. Support exists for a viral cause of certain malignancies (see Chap. 13).

Chemical carcinogens produce different effects at different periods of life span. Chemical carcinogenesis occurs more readily in the aged. The assumption is that there is either an accumulated effect on the DNA of the cell or an accumulated risk for a cell to become malignant. Breast cancer, however, is a serious problem in aged women, not only due to the malignancy, but also because of damage to the self-image.

The majority of persons having carcinoma of the colon are in the older age group. Cancer of the colon is usually a very slow-growing tumor and remains localized for a long period of time. Early surgical removal is beneficial.

Cancer of the prostate affects 54,000 men yearly; 90 percent of these are over the age of 50 when the tumor is diagnosed. Cancer of the prostate is known to metastasize to the pelvis, vertebrae, and other bony sites as well as to the brain.

Cancer of the lung is increasing in incidence. A great deal of evidence has been found to link carcinoma of the lung to a history of smoking. Formerly a high percentage of lung cancer occurred in men, but lung cancer in women is increasing due to the increase in the number of women who smoke.

Acute leukemia, lymphosarcoma, and myeloma are malignancies with a high incidence in the aged population. Hodgkin's disease tends to run a rapid course in the aged. Malignancies can occur in any part of the body of the aged as they can in younger aged population.

REFERENCES

1. Barzel, U. Common Metabolic Disorders of the Skeleton in Aging. In W. Reichel (ed.), *Clinical Aspects of Aging*. Baltimore: Williams & Wilkins, 1978.
2. Birren, J. E., and Schaie, K. W. (ed.). *Handbook of the Psychology of Aging*. New York: Van Nostrand Reinhold, 1977.
3. Brockehurst, J. C., et al. Fracture of the femur in old age: A two-centre study of associated clinical factors and the cause of the fall. *Age and Aging* 7:7, 1978.
4. Carnevali, D. L., and Patrick, M. *Nursing Management for the Elderly*. Philadelphia: Lippincott, 1979.

5. Carter, A. The Neurologic Aspects of Aging. In I. Rossman (ed.), *Clinical Geriatrics*. Philadelphia: Lippincott, 1971.
6. Clark, K. *Leonardi Da Vinci*. London, England: Cambridge University Press, 1939.
7. Dhar, S., Shastri, S., and Robalgi, L. Aging and the respiratory system. *Med. Clin. North Am.* 60:1121, 1976.
8. Donovan, M. I., and Pierce, S. G. *Cancer Care Nursing*. New York: Appleton-Century-Crofts, 1976. Pp. 218–233.
9. Ebersole, P., and Hess, P. *Toward Healthy Aging*. New York: Van Nostrand Reinhold, 1977.
10. Engleman, K., and Brunwald, E. Elevation of Arterial Pressure. In K. J. Isselbacher, et al. (eds.). *Harrison's Principles of Internal Medicine* (9th ed.). New York: McGraw-Hill, 1980.
11. Epiopoulos, C. *Gerontological Nursing*. Hagerstown, Md.: Harper & Row, 1979.
12. Forbes, E. J., and Fitzsimons, V. M. *The Older Person: A Process for Wellness*. St. Louis: Mosby, 1981.
13. Futrell, M., et al. *Primary Health Care of the Older Adult*. Duxbury, Mass.: Duxbury Press, 1980. Pp. 301–305.
14. Goldberg, P. B. How risky is self-care with OTC medicines? *Geriatric Nurs.* 1:279, 1980.
15. Goldman, R. Aging of the Excretory System. In C. Finch and L. Hayflick (eds.), *Handbook of the Biology of Aging*. New York: Van Nostrand Reinhold, 1977.
16. Guyton, A. C. *Textbook of Medical Physiology* (6th ed.). Philadelphia: Saunders, 1981.
17. Harris, R. Cardiac Problems: Treating the Geriatric Patient. In E. W. Busse (ed.), *Theory and Therapeutics of Aging*. New York: Medcom, 1973.
18. Hayflick, L. Current theories of biological aging. *Fed. Proc.* 34:9, 1975.
19. Kohn, R. Heart and Cardiovascular System. In C. Finch and L. Hayflick (eds.), *Handbook of the Biology of Aging*. New York: Van Nostrand Reinhold, 1977.
20. Krohn, P. L. *Topics in the Biology of Aging*. New York: Wiley, 1965.
21. Lamy, P. P. Drugs and the elderly: A new look. *Fam. Comm. Health* 5:34, 1982.
22. Locke, S., and Galaburda, A. Cerebrovascular Disorders in Later Life. In W. Reichel (ed.), *Clinical Aspects of Aging*. Baltimore: Williams & Wilkins, 1978.
23. Makinodan, T. Immunology of aging. *J. Am. Geriatr. Soc.* 24:249, 1976.
24. Malasanos, L., et al. *Health Assessment*. St. Louis: Mosby, 1977.
25. Parsons, V. What decreasing renal function means to aging patients. *Geriatrics* 32:93, 1977.
26. Rossman, I. Anatomic and Body Composition Changes with Aging. In C. Finch and L. Hayflick (eds.), *Handbook of the Biology of Aging*. New York: Van Nostrand Reinhold, 1977.
27. Sacher, G. A. Life Table Modification and Life Prolongation. In C. E. Finch and L. Hayflick (eds.), *Handbook of the Biology of Aging*. New York: Van Nostrand Reinhold, 1977.
28. Schrock, M. M. *Holistic Assessment of the Healthy Aged*. New York: Wiley, 1980.
29. Shapiro, W., Parish, J., and Kohn, A. Medical Renal Diseases in the Aged. In W. Reichel (ed.), *Clinical Aspects of Aging*. Baltimore: Williams & Wilkins, 1978.
30. Shock, N. W. Age changes in some physiologic processes. *Geriatrics* 12:40, 1957.
31. Winsberg, F. Roentgenographic Aspects of Aging. In I. Rossman (ed.), *Clinical Geriatrics*. Philadelphia: Lippincott, 1971. Pp. 267–281.
32. Wright, I. Venous Thrombosis and Pulmonary Embolism. In W. Reichel (ed.), *Clinical Aspects of Aging*. Baltimore: Williams & Wilkins, 1978.

INDEX

INDEX